Handbook of Sensory Physiology

Volume VII/4

Visual Psychophysics

By

M. Alpern · E. Aulhorn · H. B. Barlow · E. Baumgardt
H. R. Blackwell · D. S. Blough · M. A. Bouman · R. M. Boynton
B. H. Crawford · J. M. Enoch · A. Fiorentini · P. Grützner
H. Harms · E. G. Heinemann · L. M. Hurvich · W. Jaeger
D. Jameson · D. H. Kelly · D. H. Krantz · Y. LeGrand
L. Matin · J. D. Moreland · J. Nachmias · L. A. Riggs
K. H. Ruddock · P. L. Walraven · N. Weisstein · G. Westheimer
B. R. Wooten · W. D. Wright · D. Yager

Edited by

Dorothea Jameson and Leo M. Hurvich

With 297 Figures

Springer-Verlag Berlin · Heidelberg · New York 1972

ISBN 978-3-642-88660-7 ISBN 978-3-642-88658-4 (eBook)
DOI 10.1007/ 978-3-642-88658-4

Softcover reprint of the hardcover 1st edition 1972

Preface

This volume on Visual Psychophysics documents the current status of research aimed toward understanding the intricacies of the visual mechanism and its laws of operation in intact human perceivers. As can be seen from the list of contributors, the problems of vision engage the interest and experimental ingenuity of investigators from a variety of disciplines. Thus we find authors affiliated with departments of biology, medical and physiological physics, ophthalmology, physics, physiology and anatomy, psychology, laboratories of neurophysiology, medical clinics, schools of optometry, visual and other types of research institutes.

A continuing interplay between psychophysical studies and physiological work is everywhere evident. As more information about the physiological basis of vision accumulates, and new studies and analyses of receptor photochemistry and the neurophysiology of retina and brain appear, psychophysical studies of the intact organism become more sharply focused, sometimes more complex, and often more specialized. Technological advances have increased the variety and precision of the stimulus controls, and advances in measurement techniques have reopened old problems and stimulated the investigation of new ones.

In some cases, new concepts are being drawn in to help further our understanding of the laws by which the visual mechanism operates; in other cases, ideas enunciated long ago have been reevaluated, developed more fully, and reified in terms of converging evidence from both psychophysical experiments and unit recordings from visual cells.

The organization of the volume is self-evident. It starts with simple light perception and issues of absolute threshold. Phenomena related to spatial stimulus patterns are then considered, and they are followed by discussions of visual responses to temporal as well as spatial stimulus variations. Problems of the moving eye and perceived visual direction are then analyzed. Wavelength is then considered as a major stimulus variable, and a number of chapters are devoted to color vision and color deficiencies. The final three chapters treat problems of measurement theory, the relation between electrical and psychophysical measures in intact humans, and animal psychophysics.

It is our hope that this volume will inform graduate students as well as other visual scientists about the current status of the issues that are engaging the attention of the psychophysicist today, and that it will provide both the background and the challenge to those who may want to contribute their own expertise to the continuing research.

We are indebted to the following publishers and organizations for permission to redraw and use figures from their publications: Academic Press, Inc., American Association for the Advancement of Science, Bergmann Publishers, Dr. W. Junk Publisher, Henry Kimpton, Musterschmidt Verlag, Physical Society of London, Rockefeller University Press, Springer-Verlag, Charles C. Thomas Publisher, John Wiley and Sons, Inc.

We should like also to thank the following journals: Acta Ophthalmologica, Acta Physiologica Scandinavica, American Journal of Ophthalmology, Anales Sociedad Española de Física y Química, Archives of Ophthalmology, Atti Fondazione Giorgio Ronchi, British Journal of Ophthalmology, British Medical Bulletin, Comptes Rendus Académie des Sciences, Documenta Ophthalmologica, Electroencephalography and Clinical Neurophysiology, Gerontologia, Graefe's Archiv für Ophthalmologie, Investigative Ophthalmology, Japanese Psychological Research, Journal of Experimental Psychology, Journal of General Physiology, Journal of Neurophysiology, Journal of Physiology, Journal of the Optical Society of America, Klinische Monatsblätter für Augenheilkunde, Kybernetik, Nature, Ophthalmologica, Optica Acta, Perception and Psychophysics, Proceedings of the Royal Society of London, Psychological Review, Psychonomic Science, Transactions of the Ophthalmological Society of the United Kingdom, Vision Research, and Zeitschrift für Vergleichende Physiologie.

Philadelphia, February 1972

DOROTHEA JAMESON
LEO M. HURVICH

Contents

List of Contributors

ALPERN, Mathew, Department of Ophthalmology, Vision Research Laboratories, University Medical Center, University of Michigan, Ann Arbor, Michigan 48104, USA

AULHORN, Elfriede, Universitäts-Augenklinik, D-7400 Tübingen, Germany

BARLOW, Horace B., Department of Physiology-Anatomy, University of California, Berkeley, California 94720, USA

BAUMGARDT, E. †, F-75 Paris, France

BLACKWELL, H. Richard, Institute for Research in Vision, Ohio State University Research Center, Columbus, Ohio 43212, USA

BLOUGH, Donald S., Department of Psychology, Brown University, Providence, Rhode Island 02912, USA

BOUMAN, Maarten A., Department of Medical and Physiological Physics, University of Utrecht, Utrecht, The Netherlands

BOYNTON, Robert M., Center for Visual Science, University of Rochester, Rochester, New York 14627, USA

CRAWFORD, Brian H., Applied Optics Section, Department of Physics, Imperial College of Science and Technology, London, SW7 2BZ, Great Britain

ENOCH, Jay M., Department of Ophthalmology, Washington University, School of Medicine, St. Louis, Missouri 63110, USA

FIORENTINI, Adriana, Laboratorio di Neurofisiologia del C.N.R., I-56100 Pisa, Italy

GRÜTZNER, Peter, Universitäts-Augenklinik, D-7800 Freiburg, Germany

HARMS, Heinrich, Universitäts-Augenklinik, D-7400 Tübingen, Germany

HEINEMANN, Eric G., Department of Psychology, Brooklyn College of the City University of New York, Brooklyn, New York 11210, USA

HURVICH, Leo M., Department of Psychology, University of Pennsylvania, Philadelphia, Pennsylvania 19104, USA

JAEGER, Wolfgang, Universitäts-Augenklinik, D-6900 Heidelberg, Germany

JAMESON, Dorothea, Department of Psychology, University of Pennsylvania, Philadelphia, Pennsylvania 19104, USA

KELLY, Donald H., Stanford Research Institute, Menlo Park, California 94025, USA

KRANTZ, David H., Department of Psychology, University of Michigan, Ann Arbor, Michigan 48104, USA

LeGrand, Yves, Muséum National d'Histoire Naturelle, F-75 Paris 5e, France

Matin, Leonard, Department of Psychology, Columbia University, New York, New York 10027, USA

Moreland, J. D., School of Optometry, University of Waterloo, Waterloo, Ontario, Canada

Nachmias, Jacob, Department of Psychology, University of Pennsylvania, Philadelphia, Pennsylvania 19104, USA

Riggs, Lorrin A., Department of Psychology, Brown University, Providence, Rhode Island 02912, USA

Ruddock, K. H., Applied Optics Section, Department of Physics, Imperial College, London, SW7 2BZ, Great Britain

Walraven, Pieter L., Institute for Perception TNO, Soesterberg, The Netherlands

Weisstein, Naomi, Department of Psychology, Loyola University, Chicago, Illinois 60626, USA

Westheimer, Gerald, Department of Physiology-Anatomy, University of California, Berkeley, California 94720, USA

Wooten, Billy R., Biological Laboratories, Harvard University, Cambridge, Massachusetts 02138, USA

Wright, William D., Applied Optics Section, Department of Physics, Imperial College, London, SW7 2BZ, Great Britain

Yager, Dean, Department of Psychology, Brown University, Providence, Rhode Island 02912, USA

Chapter 1

Dark and Light Adaptation: Psychophysics

By

HORACE B. BARLOW, Berkeley, California (USA)

With 12 Figures

Contents

I. Introduction

In the most general sense, dark and light adaptation simply mean getting accustomed to lesser or greater levels of environmental illumination. The importance and efficiency of the mechanisms involved are not obvious subjectively because they function so well. Changes of average luminance by factors of 10, 100, or 1000 occur frequently and pass largely unnoticed; it is only when luminance changes by a much larger factor that we are seriously inconvenienced, either by the temporary blindness resulting from the slowness of regeneration of rhodopsin, or by the unpleasant glare resulting from our inability to reduce our pupil area to the same extent as the domestic cat. Psychophysical measurements show that, though we may not be vividly aware of them, great changes of visual performance nonetheless occur, and the main purpose of this chapter is to describe them.

Diverse mechanisms enable the eye to function well over a great range of light intensities. Pupil responses, the dual (photopic and scotopic) receptor system, and pigment migration are known to play some part, and have been understood up to a certain level for many decades. The limited objective in this review will be to mention them, to refer to relevant sources, and to point out the overall role they may play in adaptation. It is the retina itself that is the main site of adaptation, and one of the results of psychophysical studies is to show precisely what is accomplished by the complex neural interactions that take place there. First the meaning of the word "adaptation" must be discussed because it is used ambiguously; when the ambient illumination is changed, visual performance changes, and the eye is said to adapt to the new luminance, but the change is not instantaneous and may take many minutes to complete. Sometimes the word is used to refer exclusively to the temporal changes of threshold, especially the slow decline during dark adaptation; alternatively it may be used to refer to the changes in performance when the eye is in equilibrium at various levels. In this chapter we distinguish between steady state adaptation and temporal adaptation. In the former, the eye is given time to reach an equilibrium at a particular adapting level and variations of visual performance are described as a function of that level; the increment threshold relationship typifies this type of study. (See Blackwell, chapter 4 this volume.) In temporal adaptation the eye is not in equilibrium, and performance is studied as a function of the time that has elapsed since the adapting level was changed. The classical dark adaptation curve that shows well separated cone and rod portions is the best known result of this type of investigation. Two sections are devoted to these two classes of investigation, and the final section deals with experiments that have shown an unexpectedly close relation between them.

Abnormalities of dark adaptation have recently been studied (Carr, Ripps, Siegel, and Weale, 1966a, b; Carr and Ripps, 1967) but will not be discussed further here. This is also a suitable point to mention previous reviews of dark adaptation. The earlier ones were concerned largely with the rivalry between photochemical and neural explanations of psychophysical facts; Hecht (1937), Lythgoe (1940) and Craik and Vernon (1941) exemplify these. Most of their theories can now be discarded, though Craik's views (1938) are possibly seminal. More recent theoretical review articles are those of Pirenne (1962), Rushton (1965a) and Dowling (1967). Rushton is strongly concerned with the quantitative aspects of the problem, and in their latest paper Alpern, Rushton, and Torii (1970) may have achieved a satisfactory formulation. Dowling is primarily concerned with placing the physiology in the appropriate anatomical structures, and in this field also striking advances are being made (Werblin and Dowling, 1969). We are coming tantalizingly close to being able to give an account of dark and light adaptation that will fulfill the aims of all these authors, but this article has a more modest objective. Psychophysical studies show what changes occur in dark and light adaptation, and our aim is to describe these changes as concisely as possible. Many of the facts fit well the theoretical views I have myself put forward previously (Barlow, 1964a, 1964b), but there are also discrepant facts which will be mentioned in due course.

II. Accessory Mechanisms of Adaptation

Pupillary Changes

The constriction of the pupil in response to light is one of the best known reflexes. Since the human pupil area in bright light is about 1/10 its area in darkness, its variation obviously cannot reduce the total range of retinal luminances by more than 1 log unit. Its amplitude of response is greater for some temporal frequency components than it is to steady light (STARK, 1968), but this cannot increase the range of its effectiveness, and it can at best be regarded as an inefficient homeostatic device if all it accomplishes is a reduction of input range from 10^{11} to 10^{10}. In looking for possible additional significance of the pupil reactions several possibilities should be born in mind. In non-human species the range of light control may be very much greater; indeed there is some indication that the cat can oppose the edges of its slit pupil and exclude all light. Second, a special advantage of constriction may be to protect the pigments from bleaching; the pupil can dilate much more quickly than pigment can regenerate, and it is therefore an excellent mechanism for rapid adaptation. Third, one should bear in mind that seemingly trivial advantages may become extremely significant in a competitive situation; thus an animal whose pupil can dilate a little more may acquire a distinct competitive edge at dusk, and this could make the difference between starvation and plenty. Finally one should recall that pupil constriction brings improved optical resolution (WESTHEIMER, 1965a; CAMPBELL and GUBISCH, 1966); since resolution may be limited either by too little light, or by poor optical image quality, there is clearly an optimum pupil diameter for each illumination, and it makes more sense to regard the pupil response as image-quality-optimising rather than as a homeostatic reflex that grossly fails to stabilize image luminance (CAMPBELL and GREGORY, 1960).

Rods and Cones: Duplicity Theory

MAX SCHULTZE'S (1866) histological studies of the retina of many species of vertebrates led him to the conclusion that there were two families of photoreceptor cells. The most consistent differences were the shapes of the pigment-containing outer segments (long and rod-like in rods, short and conical in cones) and the presence of a highly refractile body in the inner segment of cones. There were many other differences, but these were frequently no greater than inter-species differences, or the differences found between receptors of the same family located in different portions of the same retina. Even the most reliable distinguishing characteristic fails occasionally; for instance the outer segments of the rods of Newts are conical, whereas the outer segments of the foveal cones of man are long and almost cylindrical. In these two cases the family is determined by contrast with the short, sharply tapered cones of the Newt, or by observing that the long, slightly tapered foveal cones of man have many of the other characteristics of typical conical cones in the neighbouring retina. The electron microscope (COHEN, 1968) has shown other differences, notably in the connection between extracellular space and outer segment saccules which exists in cones but not rods. Whether this will be a more constant characteristic of the two families remains to be determined.

SCHULTZE noticed that cones were relatively commoner in diurnally active species than in nocturnal ones. PARINAUD (1898) related this to night blindness in humans, and VON KRIES (1896) to the shift of the peak spectral sensitivity in nocturnal vision. Thus the idea of a double retina — the duplicity theory — came about, and in 1937 HECHT reviewed the very impressive body of evidence showing that almost all quantitative measures of visual performance could be split into two segments, a low luminance level portion attributable to rods and called "scotopic", and a high luminance level portion attributable to cones and called "photopic". HECHT'S theoretical interpretations of the nature of the photoreceptor processes are now quite unacceptable, but they only occupy a small portion at the end of his review; the main part of it should be referred to for more detailed information on the separation of scotopic and photopic visual functions. In general it can be said that scotopic vision is mediated by rhodopsin in rods, has low spatial resolution (see WESTHEIMER, chapter 7, this volume), low temporal resolution (see KELLY, chapter 11), gives no sense of color (see LEGRAND, chapter 15), has a high lower limit to the Weber fraction ($\Delta I/I$) and is best a few degrees away from the fovea. By contrast, photopic vision is mediated by three types of cones containing different photochemical pigments, has high spatial and temporal resolution, mediates color vision, has a low limiting value to $\Delta I/I$, and is best in the fovea and immediately surrounding area.

STILES and CRAWFORD (1933) discovered another difference: for photopic vision, light entering the periphery of the pupil is less effective than light entering the centre, and this is attributable to the cones being more sensitive to light entering along their axes rather than obliquely. (See CRAWFORD, chapter 18, this volume.) This directional sensitivity is not detectable in scotopic vision mediated by rods (STILES, 1939). Naturally it is tempting to relate the difference to the refractile body in the inner segment of cones tending to focus axial light on to the photosensitive pigment. This speculation receives considerable support from observations of parallel light passing through isolated retinas and observed from the outer side; the ends of all types of receptors are more brightly illuminated than the interspaces, but if the observing microscope is appropriately focused, the light passing through cones can be seen to be concentrated in bright spots (TANSLEY and JOHNSON, 1956). The ability of the receptors to concentrate light is confirmed by estimates (RUSHTON, 1956) of the photosensitivity of rhodopsin in situ, which is greater than expected from the in vitro measures even after allowance is made for the orientation of the pigment molecules in the outer segments. In the case of the cones, the apparent photosensitivity is even higher (RUSHTON, 1963); this is a paradoxical finding in view of their lower visual sensitivity, but it fits the greater directional sensitivity of cones, and seems to demonstrate clearly the role of SCHULTZE'S refractile body in the inner segment.

Why are rods more sensitive than cones? The greater length of their outer segments must be a factor, since it presumably increases the total optical density of pigment. However, it is worth looking more closely at how much more sensitive the rods actually are. Consider the minimum *quantity* threshold; this is the threshold measured at the optimal wavelength for each system using a small, brief, test light, for which the threshold quantity of light is minimum. Using this measure, it is surprising to find that the human fovea, which contains no rods, is only a few times less sensitive than the 15° periphery, where rod sensitivity is maximum. However, the situation is very different if one considers the minimum *intensity* threshold; this is the threshold measured with a large area, long lasting, test stimulus, which allows the maximum degree of spatial and temporal summation. Using light of 527 mm, for which scotopic and photopic relative visibilities are equal, the cones require 10^4 times the intensity required for rods. Thus the great advantage of scotopic vision appears to lie in greater spatial and temporal summation, which presumably results from properties of the neural connections between receptors and ganglion cells. There will be more to be said, however, after the concept of "dark light" has been explained, for the lower dark light of rods is a more basic difference between scotopic and photopic systems. This characteristic of each system immediately indicates that rods operate at levels of ambient illumination below the range where cones operate.

A word should be said here about the "blue sensitive" cones. These differ from other cones, and resemble rods, in three respects: they have poor optimum spatial (BRINDLEY, 1954) and temporal (BRINDLEY, DUCROZ, and RUSHTON, 1966) resolution, a higher value of their lower limit for $\Delta I/I$ (STILES, 1954), to which GREEN (1969) attributes their low temporal resolution, and they may be absent from the very center of the fovea. (WALD, 1968; see JAMESON, chapter 14, this volume.) If these properties are attributable to the nervous pathway, it seems possible that "blue" cones either have the same type of pathway as the rods, or use the rod pathway in the light adapted state, when rods are saturated. Some interaction of this sort might lie behind the curious discovery (HOUGH and RUDDOCK, 1969) that the Purkinje shift occurs abnormally in tritanopic individuals who presumably lack "blue" cones.

Pigment and Receptor Migration

These adaptive mechanisms are found in non-mammalian vertebrates, especially ganoids, amphibians, and birds. They serve to shield the rods in dim light without shielding cones in bright light, both mechanisms cooperating to achieve this result: in dark adaptation the rods are fully exposed to light falling on the retina, whereas in the light pigment migrates alongside them and even in front of them, thus shielding them from light. The cones, when they migrate, do so to keep ahead (vitreal) of the advancing pigment, thus maintaining their exposure to light in light adaptation. WALLS (1942) gives a good qualitative description of these changes, but quantitative information is lacking.

III. Steady State Retinal Adaptation

Desensitization

It is a familiar fact that self-luminous objects appear dimmer when the ambient illumination is raised: a blazing fire seems to be extinguished by direct sunlight, and bright stars vanish with the dawn. The same basic phenomenon shows up in other ways. For instance, the adjectives black, white, or grey refer to the reflectance of an object, not its luminance. Presumably this confers a selective advantage because reflectance is the more constant attribute of an object and hence a more reliable aid to identification, but the physiology behind it is the fact that the eye responds primarily to contrast, not the absolute level of illumination. In the laboratory, the capacity to detect contrast is studied as the difference threshold, Weber's law, or incremental sensitivity: here we refer to the reduction in the ability to detect increments of luminance at higher adaptation levels as "steady state desensitization". This is to distinguish it from temporal adapting effects, and to emphasize that it is the desensitizing effect of the adapting light that is of interest.

Many different experimental situations have been used to investigate this, but the conditions chosen by STILES and his colleagues, and their method of plotting the results on double logarithmic coordinates, have many advantages. (See ENOCH, chapter 21.) The adapting field is large, and the subject looks at it, or a closely similar luminance, for some minutes before the threshold-determining test exposures are made. This test stimulus is smaller than the adapting field, and exposed as a fairly brief flash so that the test area can be compared both simultaneously and successively with the adapting field. The characteristics of the test stimulus make an important difference to the result (see Fig. 3), and we shall return to this.

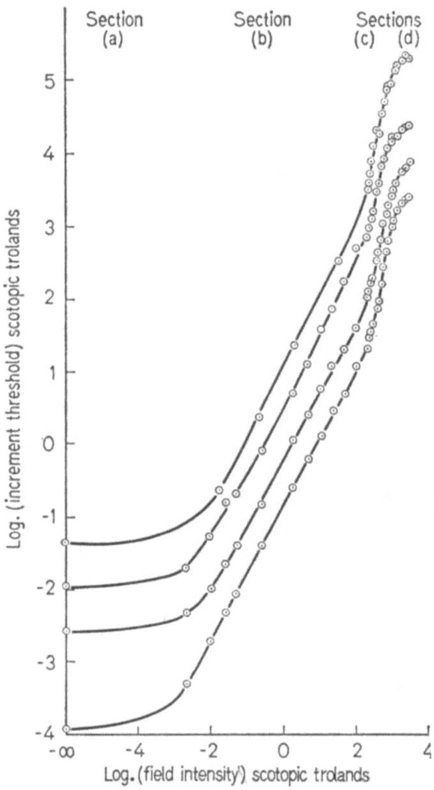

Fig. 1. Desensitization by adapting light. The test stimulus was 9° diameter exposed for 0.2 sec, and centered 9° from the fovea in a 20° adapting field. The mean results for each of four subjects show that the rod increment threshold is increased by increasing adapting field intensity. The lowest curve is correctly placed; the others are displaced upwards by 0.5, 1.0, and 1.5 log units (AGUILAR and STILES, 1954)

In Fig. 1 the log of the incremental threshold luminance is plotted against log of the adapting field luminance. Curves similar to it have been obtained under an enormous variety of conditions intended to isolate single visual mechanisms. In this example AGUILAR and STILES (1954) were able to follow the incremental sensitivity of the rods over the whole of their functional range. They used a 9° diameter test stimulus exposed for 0.2 sec, centered 9° from the fovea, and superimposed on a 20° adapting field. The rods would be expected to determine threshold at low adapting luminances, but when the increment threshold had been raised 2 or 3 log units, cones would normally take over (see Fig. 2). To avoid this AGUILAR and STILES used a blue-green light for the test stimulus in order to favor the rods, and for the desensitizing adapting field, they used red light that favored cones, thereby desensitizing them more and preventing their threshold from dropping below that of the rods. They also made the light from the test field enter the periphery of the pupil, where the directional effect reduces its effectiveness on cones but not rods, and they tested for the intrusion of cones by comparing the effectiveness of light entering the centre and the periphery of the pupil.

The main features of Fig. 1 are the central straight portion (Section b) with a slope nearly equal to 1 on these log-log coordinates. This is terminated at the low end by a horizontal plateau (Section a) and at the upper end by a steeply rising portion (Section c), with transition zones between. At still higher luminances, cones enter and a new plateau can be seen (Section d). Clearly the curves can be characterized by the vertical position of the straight portion and by the background levels where it starts and finishes. Over the linear portion, Weber's law is a good approximation: $\Delta I = KI$, and the position of the line defines the value of the Weber constant, $K = \Delta I/I$. In this case it averaged 0.21; lower values would have been obtained with a longer stimulus duration, and much lower values are obtainable for cones.

The transition from the horizontal plateau is best defined by the background level at which the extrapolated linear portion intersects the plateau value. If we assume an internal source of excitation ("dark light") which acts like real light and adds to it, then this intercept determines its value, I_0. The horizontal plateau and linear portion are in fact well described by $\Delta I = K(I + I_0)$. The dark light is an extremely important characteristic of the rod system because its low value compared to the cones is what enables the rods to operate at low luminance levels. Fig. 2 (STILES, 1954) shows the results obtained under conditions where the test stimulus did not favour the rods and the adapting field did not favour desensitization of cones. The curve breaks into two; the upper one belongs to the cones and it is characterized by a value of I_0 many log units above that of the lower, rod segment. Because of this, the rods are more sensitive at low adapting levels in spite of the combination of adapting and test wavelengths that is much more favourable to cones. Our discussion of the mechanism of bleaching recovery adaptation will show again that it is precisely this low dark-light of the rods that is affected. It is elevated by bleached pigment, and its subsequent decline as pigment is resynthesized underlies the familiar dark adaptation curve of Fig. 7.

The steepening of the curve at high adapting luminances is called "saturation". FUORTES, GUNKEL, and RUSHTON (1961) showed that it occurred at the same scotopic luminance regardless of the wavelength of the adapting field, and therefore it is not a result of interference by cones. Fig. 1 shows that the saturation effect begins at about 100 scotopic trolands; this would cause about 200 quantal absorptions per rod each second, and would correspond to about 6 cd/m² with a natural pupil in daylight. The cause of saturation is not known for certain but it receives a natural explanation in terms of the maximum possible hyperpolarization of S-potentials

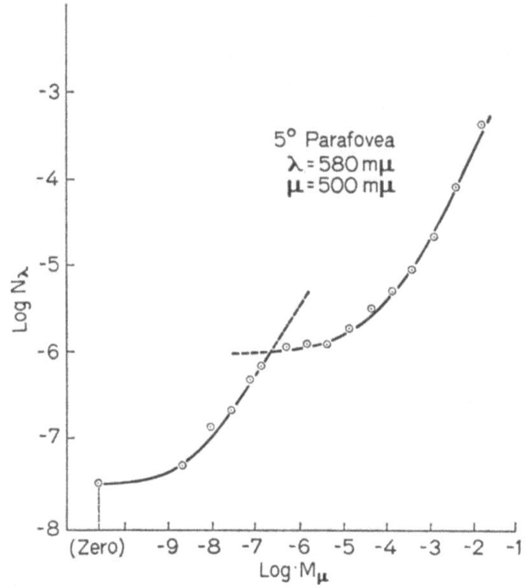

Fig. 2. At low background levels (M_μ) the increment threshold (N_λ) is determined by the rods, but at background levels higher than $\log M_\mu = \bar{7}.3$ the cones become more sensitive to incremental stimuli of this wave length (580 nm). For each curve the value of the background at the intersection of horizontal and sloping asymptotes defines I_0, the "dark light" of each system, and it is clearly the low dark light of rods that gives them the advantage at low background luminances. N_λ and M_μ are expressed in erg. sec^{-1} deg^{-2}, and the test stimulus was 1° diam. and 0.06 sec duration (Stiles, 1959)

(Alpern, Fulton, Rushton, and Torii, 1969), or of receptors (Werblin and Dowling, 1969). Penn and Hagins (1969) show that the effect of illumination is to reduce the resting current produced by unilluminated rods, and this appears to be done by increasing the resistance of the outer segments (Toyoda, Nasaki, and Tomita, 1969). Clearly this process could never reduce the current below zero, which explains the upper limit to the hyperpolarization of the receptors under light.

Saturation has not been observed in cones. Brindley (1959) showed that the difference threshold is constant over an extremely wide range of luminances. At the higher levels, discrimination is performed on the after images rather than the original flash presentations. and it rises steeply at high luminances. However, in this case, unlike the rods, the steep rise occurs only when the luminance is great enough to bleach a large proportion of the cone pigment.

The linear portion in Fig. 1 has a slope very near 1, but this is exceptional, and results from the use of a large area test stimulus (9° diam.) and relatively long exposure (200 msec). If either of these is reduced, the slope is decreased, and for small areas and brief exposures it is close to 1/2 for adapting luminances covering a range of several log units (BARLOW, 1957; BOUMAN, 1961). This parallels the square-root-law behaviour of an ideal detector limited only by quantum fluctuations: $\Delta I = K\sqrt{I}$ (ROSE, 1942; DEVRIES, 1943, and see BAUMGARDT, chapter 2, this volume.) It appears that the square-root-law and Weber's law are limits; with most types of stimulus the slope (on log-log coordinates) is intermediate between 1/2 and 1. There is also a tendency for the slope to become steeper at higher luminances. The square-root-law does, however, hold for cones if small enough, brief enough, stimuli are used, as shown in Fig. 3 (BARLOW, 1958b). This figures shows that the value of the dark light of cones is unaffected by the parameters of the test stimulus, and this is also true for rods, as is shown in Fig. 10.

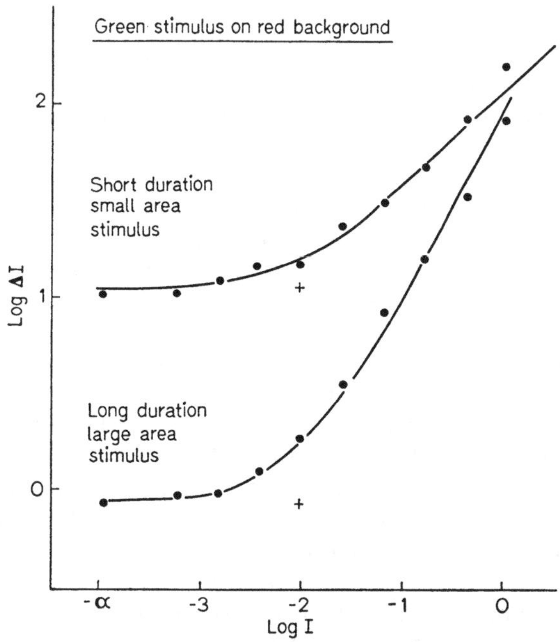

Fig. 3. Dependence of the slope of the increment threshold relation upon the area and duration of the test stimulus in the green (π_4) colour system. Foveal fixation. Lower curve, stimulus 55 min diameter, 1 second duration: upper curve, 5.2 min diameter, 7 msec duration. The separation of the curves has been reduced by 1 log unit (BARLOW, 1958b). + indicates the intersection of sloping and horizontal asymptotes, and is at nearly the same background for each curve, showing that estimates of I_0 for one system are not affected by stimulus area and duration

Spatial and Temporal Summation and Resolution

When increment threshold is determined as a function of the area or duration of the test stimulus another aspect of the desensitizing effect of adapting light becomes evident. At all adapting luminances increasing the area or prolonging the duration of the test stimulus lowers the incremental threshold luminance; however, at low backgrounds the reduction of threshold is greater and continues out to larger areas and longer times. Thus the maximum area and duration of complete summation are greater at low backgrounds than at high (BARLOW, 1958a), and the extent of the additional decrease of threshold for large, long, stimuli can be judged by noting the increased separation of the curves of Figs. 3 and 10 at low backgrounds. Clearly changes of performance of this sort cannot result solely from photochemical bleaching or alterations of receptors, and must involve changes in the neural mechanisms.

The loss of summating ability at higher backgrounds is accompanied by improved resolution; it is as if the retina changed to resemble a finer grained film being operated at a faster frame repetition frequency at higher luminances. This change is partly accomplished by switching from rods to cones, but within each system there is also an improvement of resolution with adaptation level. Evidence for these changes was originally obtained by classical measures of acuity and flicker fusion frequency as a function of luminance, and such experiments are summarized by HECHT (1937), and more recently by PIRENNE (1962). In these experiments the limit to resolution, whether spatial or temporal, was determined by decreasing the size of a test object such as a grating, or increasing the flicker rate, until the stimulus appeared spatially or temporally uniform; this value was then determined for different luminances. More complete information can be obtained at each adaptation level by holding the mean luminance constant and varying the percentage modulation at each frequency in turn until the non-uniformity can just be detected. In this way one not only observes the highest frequency passed (the cut-off), but also how lower frequencies are attenuated. Instead of using square-wave modulation with time and distance, it is convenient to use sinusoidal variation of luminance, since the response to any arbitrary wave form can be predicted from the response to sine waves if the system is linear. (See WESTHEIMER, chapter 7, and KELLY, chapter 11, this volume.) The resulting sets of curves, an example of which in the spatial domain is shown in Fig. 4 (DAITCH and GREEN, 1969), are called "modulation (or contrast) transfer functions" (m.t.f.). They show that the improved resolution at high luminances is not achieved by a bodily shift of the whole curve; instead a peak develops at medium frequencies and the transmission of higher frequencies is improved relative to the low frequencies. If one considers the transition from unpeaked to peaked functions that occurs as the mean luminance is raised, one sees that the frequencies at the peak and higher are favored relative to lower frequencies and spared some of the desensitizing effects that result from raising mean luminance.

It is clear that these results on resolution are very closely related to those observed by varying the area and duration of the test stimulus in incremental sensitivity curves. The low spatial frequencies approximate Weber's law, but sensitivity for the high frequencies rises less steeply, and the peaks of the m.t.f. functions approach the square-root law found with small, brief, stimuli. This is shown in Fig. 5, where the 0.5 cycle/degree and 2.5 cycle/degree results of DAITCH and GREEN have been replotted to show their similarity to increment threshold curves (Fig. 3 and 10).

Similar changes occur in the temporal domain (KELLY, 1969), and these adjustments of spatial and temporal properties allow the retina to extract more

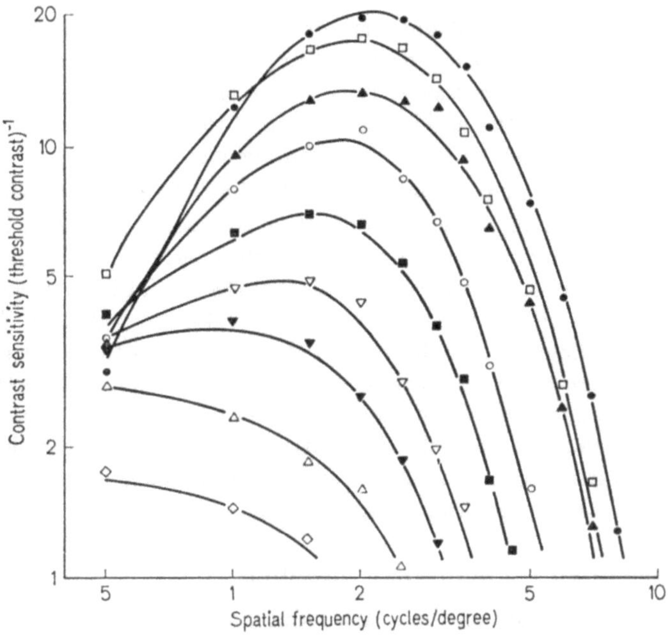

Fig. 4. Contrast sensitivity of the peripheral retina at varying luminances and spatial frequencies. Target 8° × 3° centered 12° from fovea. Contrast is $(I_{max} - I_{min}) \div (I_{max} + I_{min})$. Mean luminances from lowest curve upwards, in log trolands: —2.5, —2.0, —1.5, —1.0, —0.5, 0.0, 0.5, 1.0, 1.5. For the higher spatial frequencies contrast sensitivity is greatly improved by raising the luminance, but for the lowest frequency it is only slightly improved. (Daitch and Green, 1969)

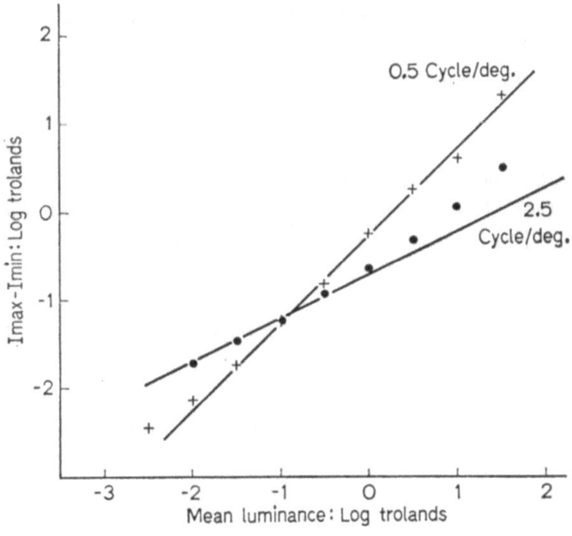

Fig. 5. Results of Fig. 4 (Daitch and Green, 1969) replotted to show their relation to increment threshold curves. Log $(I_{max} - I_{min})$ in trolands is plotted against log (mean luminance) for 0.5 and 2.5 cycles/degree. The line through the low frequency points has a slope of 1 (Weber's Law), whereas the line approximating the high frequency points has a slope of 1/2 (the square-root law)

information about high spatial and temporal frequencies at high image luminances. At low luminances, this information would have very low signal/noise ratio because quantum fluctuations are relatively large; when the image becomes less noisy the retina changes its properties and is able to extract the new information. Thus these adaptive changes are seen to be truly advantageous.

Though more difficult it is also possible to show that intensity discrimination at a particular level is improved by adaptation to that level (CRAIK, 1938). This is shown most clearly by comparing quantum efficiencies since this is an absolute measure of efficiency and comparisons maintain their validity even when test conditions vary (ROSE, 1948; CLARK JONES, 1959; BARLOW, 1962a). At moderate adapting levels, efficiency is highest when the luminances to be discriminated do not differ greatly from the adaptation level, and for such luminances the efficiency is lowered by changing the adaptation level in either direction (BARLOW, 1962b). This brings out the fact that the desensitization and rise of threshold that accompany adaptation to a particular average luminance does not necessarily represent a decrease of performance at all tasks.

Spatial Spread of Steady State Desensitization

Light falling uniformly on the retina reduces the sensitivity to added light. Is this desensitization a purely local effect, or does light falling on one region desensitize neighboring regions? This is a difficult question to answer satisfactorily in human vision because of the impossibility of maintaining absolutely steady fixation and the limitations of methods of stabilizing the retinal image (BARLOW, 1963). In spite of this difficulty CRAWFORD and WESTHEIMER have done psychophysical experiments with careful voluntary fixation, and their results reveal a new phenomenon. They show that light falling close to a particular test area desensitizes that area as expected, but they also show that light falling further away has the opposite, sensitizing, effect.

CRAWFORD (1940) used a test area (1/2 deg. diam.) that is larger than the desensitizing zone in the fovea and almost as large as the desensitizing zone in scotopic vision in the periphery. However, his experiments were the first to reveal the sensitizing effect. The desensitizing effect was maximum when the adapting field diameter was slightly greater than the test area. When it was further enlarged, the threshold for the test stimulus fell to a lower value, so that light falling one or two degrees away from the test area actually had a sensitizing effect for the detection of light falling within the test area. WESTHEIMER (1965b, 1967) has refined the experimental conditions and shown that it occurs in both scotopic and photopic vision.

Figure 6 shows that the sensitizing effect of the annular zone only occurs when some desensitization by adapting light falling in the centre has occurred. In this respect it resembles lateral inhibition of ganglion cell responses (BARLOW, FITZHUGH, and KUFFLER, 1957) and interaction of horizontal cells and bipolars (WERBLIN and DOWLING, 1969); thus sensitization by the annulus is almost certainly inhibition of steady-state desensitization and is probably brought about by horizontal cells.

WESTHEIMER (1970) showed that rods act independently of cones, and McKEE and WESTHEIMER (1970) showed that when cones are involved the action spectrum for the sensitizing effect depends upon which of STILES' π systems is mediating detection of the incremental test stimulus; if it was the "red" (π_5) system, then the action spectrum for desensitization resembled π_5, and similarly for the "green" system, π_4. These results have important implications with regard to the organization of receptors, horizontal cells, and bipolar cells in human colour vision.

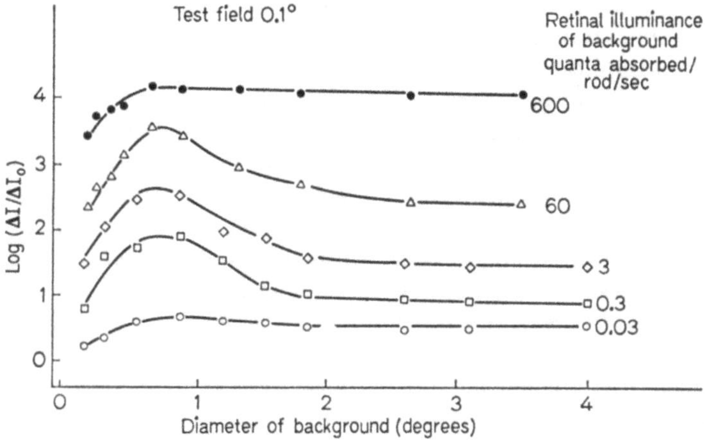

Fig. 6. Increment threshold of the peripheral retina measured in the centre of an adapting field of variable diameter at five different luminances. At the middle three luminances, the background elevates the threshold maximally when it is nearly 3/4 deg. in diameter; addition of further annuli of adapting light to create larger adapting fields has the effect of lowering thresholds. These annuli diminish the desensitizing effect of adapting light on and close to the test spot. Note that this does not occur at the lowest luminance, where thresholds are only about 3 × the absolute threshold and the adapting light has caused little desensitization. At the highest it also fails to occur, but at this luminance level cones determine the threshold, whereas rods are responsible at the lower levels (WESTHEIMER, 1965b)

IV. Temporal Retinal Adaptation

Initial Stages

We have seen how the incremental threshold is changed by changing the background upon which the test flash is superimposed, and how this influence spreads spatially; now we look at the speed of these changes. One can divide the effects into two parts: first there are rapid changes which take place within a few seconds of the change in luminance; second there are persistent after-effects of strong light adaptation from which the eye takes many minutes to recover. The latter have been shown to be closely related to the bleaching and resynthesis of photo-sensitive pigments, and these are considered in the next section. Here we consider the rapid changes that occur for both upward and downward changes of adapting luminance.

CRAWFORD (1947) outlined the major features; if the adapting light is of 1/2 second duration, the threshold rises rapidly to a peak at onset, then declines within a few tenths of a second to a nearly level plateau, shows a tendency to rise transiently again at offset, and then declines rather more slowly to the dark value. A curious feature that has attracted considerable attention is the fact that the threshold rise at onset (and again at offset) occurs when the test flash is delivered before the change of background luminance, that is, before the physical event that causes the threshold rise; this is less surprising if one recalls the long reaction time of a visual response, and backward masking phenomena such as metacontrast. (See Boynton, chapter 9, and Weisstein, chapter 10, this volume.)

Baker (1963) has reviewed these rapid temporal changes of adaptive state and has suggested that central as well as peripheral neural factors must be responsible. Clearly the rapid attainment of near-equilibrium values of the increment threshold has important implications for the mechanisms of steady state desensitization: for instance, bleaching of pigment to an equilibrium level is very much slower, and therefore is not responsible. Amacrine cell depolarization (Werblin and Dowling, 1969) has about the right time course to account for the transient elevations of threshold if amacrines antagonize the bipolar's input to the ganglion cell. It will be a difficult task to give a complete theory of this type of phenomenon because turning on or off an adapting field itself causes an intense sensation. In its presence, it is difficult to assess whether or not further change has occurred and subjectively one is very much aware of this difficulty near the onset and offset of an adapting field. Perhaps one should be surprised at how quickly the eye recovers from changes of the average input level that might cause disastrous overloads in a sensitive electronic system.

Bleaching Recovery Adaptation

The eye takes many minutes to recover from exposure to photopic levels of illumination, and "Dark Adaptation" is often associated exclusively with experiments like that shown in Fig. 7 (Hecht, Haig and Chase, 1937). After exposure

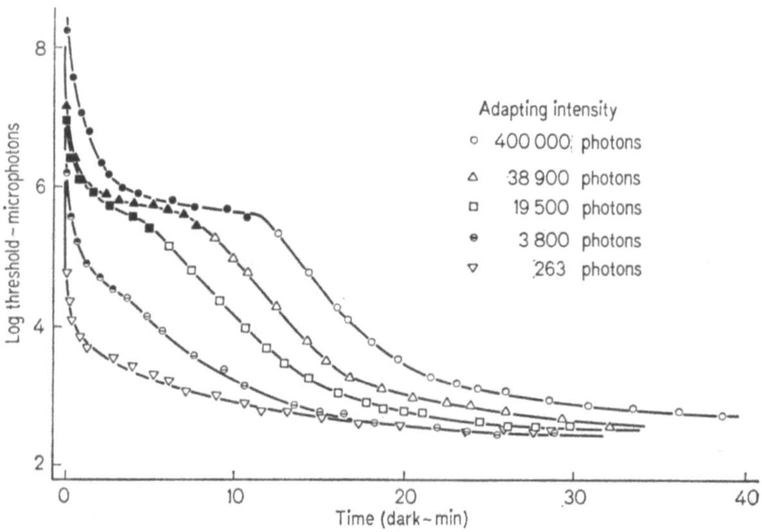

Fig. 7. The course of dark adaptation following different degrees of light adaptation. Threshold was the luminance of the violet test light that enabled an opaque black cross to be seen. The filled-in symbols indicate that a violet colour was apparent at threshold, whereas the empty symbols indicate that it was colourless. Photons = trolands (Hecht, Haig, and Chase, 1937)

to the adapting light, the subject was in darkness except for the weak test stimulus; in this case threshold was taken as the luminance of a 0.2 sec flash that just enabled the subject to see a large dark cross. After the strongest light adaptation, threshold fell to 1/100,000th of its initial value during a period of about 30 minutes. This occurred in two stages. The initial decline is due to increasing sensitivity of cones while the delayed drop to a lower value is mediated by the rods, which have a higher threshold than cones in the earlier stage. This is established by the presence of a colour sensation at threshold in the early part, by spectral sensitivity curves obtained on the first plateau and after complete dark adaptation, and by much other evidence. These changes occur in the retina, for dark adaptation can be followed using the electroretinogram or single unit discharges, where central structures certainly play no part. The outstanding question is the cause of the slow decline of threshold of rods and cones.

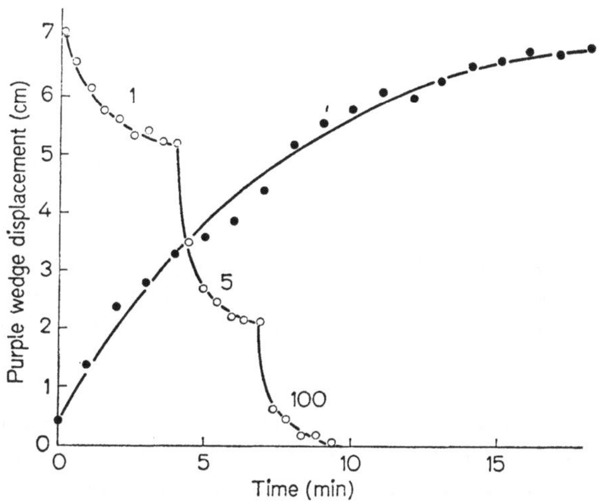

Fig. 8. Bleaching and resynthesis of rhodopsin in the human eye (CAMPBELL and RUSHTON, 1955). Empty circles: effect of bleaching the dark-adapted retina with lights of intensities 20,000, 100,000, and 2,000,000 trolands. Filled circles: time course of regeneration in the dark; this curve should be compared with the right-most curve of Fig. 7 showing the recovery of threshold following a comparable bleach

At an early stage it was thought that this was associated with the regeneration of photopigments, but even in 1929 HECHT doubted if sensitivity itself was linearly related to the pigment concentration, as the simple photochemical hypothesis suggested. It became clear that this was not the case when rhodopsin was measured in the intact human eye (RUSHTON, CAMPBELL, HAGINS, and BRINDLEY, 1955; CAMPBELL and RUSHTON, 1955). Fig. 8 shows CAMPBELL and RUSHTON'S measurements of rhodopsin bleaching and resynthesis. The rising curve shows how rhodopsin was regenerated after a nearly complete bleach, and it should be compared with the rightmost curve of Fig. 7; clearly rhodopsin resynthesis is not far from complete by the time the rod threshold drops below the cone plateau.

The relation between sensitivity and pigment concentration is logarithmic; this first became clear for human cones (Rushton, 1957, 1963, 1965a) and was later established for human rods by using a rod monochromat (Rushton, 1961a, b). Meanwhile Dowling (1960) found the relation in rat rods by measuring the threshold for eliciting the b-wave of the electroretinogram following exposure to a

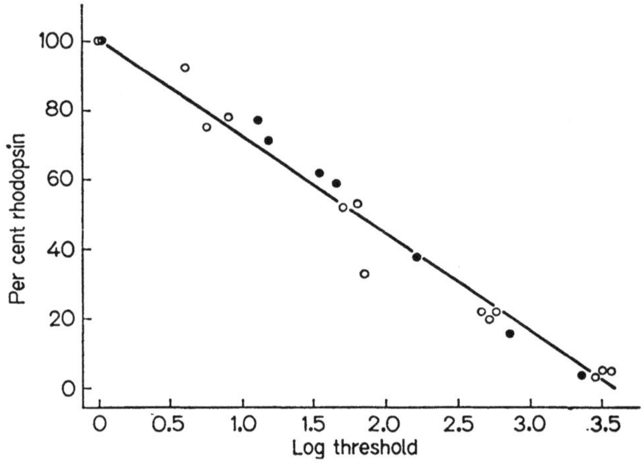

Fig. 9. The relation between rhodopsin content of the retina and the visual threshold in animals dark adapted after exposure to bright light (empty circles), and in animals night-blind due to Vitamin A deficiency (filled circles). In both instances the same relationship is observed: the log threshold rises linearly with fall in rhodopsin concentration (Dowling, 1960)

bleaching light, and comparing this with rhodopsin concentrations measured in the eyes of rats killed and frozen at the same time after a bleach. His results are shown in Fig. 9; the log of the threshold varies with rhodopsin concentration so that

$$\frac{\theta}{\theta_0} = e^{\alpha r} \quad (1)$$

where θ/θ_0 is the factor by which threshold has been elevated, r is the proportion of rhodopsin bleached, and α is a constant.

Although it is log of threshold that is proportional to photopigment bleached in rat rods, human rods, and cones, there are interesting differences between the value of the constant α (Eq. (1)) in these three cases: for human cones the value is about 4, for rat rods 8, and for human rods 40. The high value of α for human rods means that the threshold is raised by a very large factor for small bleaches. When 10% is bleached, it is already elevated nearly 100 ×, and this explains why the rod threshold did not drop below the cone plateau until 12 minutes after bleaching in the top curve of Fig. 7 for it took that long for 90% of the rhodopsin to be regenerated, as shown in Fig. 8.

The relationship of Eq. (1) is not at all what one would expect if the regeneration of photopigment lowered threshold simply by causing a larger proportion of incident light to be absorbed, and the exponential relation is urgently in need of theoretical explanation. In attempting this, some additional points should be born in mind. First is DOWLING'S important discovery that the relation between threshold and proportion of rhodopsin present is the same when rhodopsin is reduced by dietary deficiency as it is when reduced by bleaching. Second, we may note that Eq. (1) can hardly be true for very large bleaches, for it implies a finite threshold when all rhodopsin has been bleached. Third. Eq. (1) will be modified when we come to consider equivalent background lights and the dark light of bleaching: this development leads us to look for a reason why bleached rhodopsin makes the receptors become "noisy" and transmit signals as if they were constantly being stimulated by light: bleaching recovery adaptation becomes a special case of steady state desensitization.

The typical biphasic dark adaptation curve illustrated in Fig. 7 is obtained only after preadaption sufficiently intense to bleach a large proportion of the rhodopsin in the retinal rods. RUSHTON (1961 a) gives the following equation for calculating the proportion of rhodopsin bleached by short preadaptations:

$$\mathrm{Log}_{10}(1 - r) = -It/(2 \times 10^7)$$

where r is the fraction bleached, I is the retinal illumination in scotopic trolands, and t is the duration of exposure to the preadapting light. The duration must be considerably shorter than 240 seconds, the half time of regeneration (RUSHTON, 1961 a) for the equation to hold; in the work of HECHT *et al.* (1937) illustrated in Fig. 7 the duration of exposure was 120 seconds which would allow some regeneration. However their luminances are presumably photopic, and if these opposing sources of error are assumed to cancel each other one calculates bleaches of 99.6 %, 41.8 %, 23.3 %, 5.2 %, and 0.35 % for the five curves shown.

If dark adaptation depends on the amount of rhodopsin bleached, we naturally ask the question "How does the duration of preadaptation affect subsequent dark-adaptation ?" The simple answer would be that it is independent of preadaptation duration, and depends solely on the amount of rhodopsin bleached. From HAIG'S (1941) results this appears to be approximately true. He varied preadaptation intensities and durations, and found that the rod portion of dark adaptation occurred earlier following shorter or weaker preadaptations. He also found that, at a given level above the final threshold, the curve fell more steeply for the weaker preadaptations. However, these differences seemed to depend solely upon the product of intensity and duration; provided duration was less than 4 minutes, it had no independent effect, as expected if the quantity of rhodopsin bleached is the determining factor. Even at longer durations when this reciprocity law broke down, the time course of dark adaptation was the same if the delay before the rod portion of the curve was reached was the same.

CRAWFORD (1946) confirmed the validity of the reciprocity for some conditions, but pointed out that it only held for the rod portion of dark adaptation. He also found some exceptions when longer durations of preadaptation at lower luminances produced slower dark adaptation, even though they must have resulted in lower amounts of bleached rhodopsin. However, it has more recently become doubtful whether a constant bleach always results when intensity and duration are reciprocally related. HAGINS (1955) showed objectively that this was not true for very brief flashes, and BRINDLEY'S (1959) experiments show that the reciprocity relation also breaks down for large bleaches of cone pigments. DOWLING and HUB-

Bard (1963) found that resynthesis of rhodopsin was delayed after bleaches by brief flashes. Rushton and Baker (1963) also found abnormal dark adaptation in cones following bleaching by brief flashes, and Rushton (1964) showed that these effects might be caused by molecules that have received multiple quantum hits instead of the single one that is usually sufficient. Further Rushton and Henry (1968) showed that depletion of 11-cis retinaldehyde may slow down resynthesis after prolonged bleaching, and Rushton (1968) showed that, under carefully selected conditions, cones can "steal" 11-cis retinaldehyde, slowing down its utilization by rods in regeneration of rhodopsin. These apparent exceptions to reciprocity can probably be interpreted as complex consequences of the fact that threshold is determined by the proportion of rhodopsin (or cone pigment) in the bleached state; that is, they confirm that the concentration of opsin in rods and cones determines threshold during dark adaptation. Donner and Reuter (1965) suggest that rate of regeneration rather than concentration is important, but Weinstein, Hobson, and Dowling (1967) show that rate is not the important factor, and this is confirmed by Rushton, Fulton, and Baker (1969).

Dowling (1963) distinguished between a rapid "neural" phase of dark adaptation and a slow phase determined by the concentration of rhodopsin. Donner and Reuter (1967) suggested that the rapid phase is related to metarhodopsin concentration, but Frank and Dowling's (1968) experiments did not support this.

It is worth emphasizing that the typical biphasic curves of Fig. 7 are only obtained under extreme conditions. The highest preadapting intensity, which took 2 minutes to bleach almost all the rhodopsin, was about 10^9 times the lowest luminance required to see the cross in a 0.2 sec exposure, and nearly 10^{10} times the lowest detectable luminance for large areas exposed for several seconds (4.4×10^{-5} scotopic trolands; Pirenne, 1962). Even the lowest preadapting exposure lasted 2 minutes at a luminance about 10^7 times the minimum detectable, and recovery from this was almost complete in only 10 minutes. It is clear from these considerations that the biphasic curve that one considers typical for the course of dark adaptation is really only an extreme case. The special interest of these curves lies in their connection with photochemical bleaching, though the functional relation between threshold and bleaching remains unexplained. It is also worth commenting that the slowness of recovery after exposure to intense lights must be disadvantageous to the owner of the eye, and this contrasts sharply with the previously described changes in performance with varying illumination that can be seen to be adaptive in the true sense of that word.

V. Equivalent Background and Bleaching Recovery

The Crawford Transform

For many years all discussions of dark adaptation were dominated by the argument as to whether bleaching and resynthesis of rhodopsin caused the sensitivity changes, or whether these represented neural changes resulting from intense stimulation. As a result of the developments to be described in this section we now understand that both factors are involved, and know something about their relationship. It is interesting to observe that this development, like many other observations by STILES and CRAWFORD referred to in the previous sections, stemmed from the practical investigations of glare and the temporary loss of sensitivity caused by bright lights that were carried out at the National Physical Laboratory during the 20's and 30's. A bright glare source reduces sensitivity to other sources seen in its neighborhood. This is caused, at least to a large extent, by the light physically scattered in the optic media causing a veiling light in the retinal region responsible for signalling the presence of the neighbouring source. The veiling light, of course, raises threshold by what we have called "steady state desensitization". When STILES and CRAWFORD (1932) measured threshold-elevating effects, they found that these depended not only upon the luminance and location of the glare source, but also upon the parameters of the test stimulus. However, the amount of steady state desensitization produced by a uniform adapting field was affected by the parameters of the test stimulus in exactly the same way; thus the effectiveness of the glare source could be expressed uniquely in terms of an "equivalent veiling luminance" without bothering with the parameters of the test stimulus, which were irrelevant for those purposes.

This was a natural development when dealing with the threshold elevation caused by concurrent exposure to a glare source, but having found its usefulness in those circumstances STILES and CRAWFORD naturally turned to the concept of "Equivalent background brightness" when they found that the threshold elevation *following* exposure to a preadapting light was also dependent upon the parameters of the test stimulus. Under these circumstances the concept had lost its physical basis, but it still made it possible to express the after-effects of light exposure by a single time dependent quantity that was independent of the characteristics of the test stimulus. It has subsequently turned out that pupil diameter and the subjective appearance of the after-image are also correctly predicted by I_E, the equivalent background brightness.

The notion was discussed by STILES and CRAWFORD (1932), and the first evidence of its usefulness provided by CRAWFORD (1937, 1947). BLAKEMORE and RUSHTON (1965a, b) tested its validity over a greatly extended range for scotopic vision. By using a rod monochromat, they were able to cover 7 log units of threshold variation following preadaptations that bleached 50% of the rhodopsin. Fig. 10 shows the dark adaptation curves obtained with a 1 second exposure of a small (5 minute) and large (6 degree) test area. Clearly the threshold drop during dark adaptation is very different in the two cases. After dark adaptation was complete, they measured the two increment threshold curves on the right, and these show that there is a similar difference in the desensitization produced by a uniform adapting field. Equivalent Background Brightness is defined as the background that elevates the increment threshold to the value of the threshold with zero background at a certain time during dark adaptation; when this is plotted as a function of time a single curve results, as shown in Fig. 11. BLAKEMORE and RUSHTON also extended the concept to cover resolution of two gratings with dark and light bars subtending 7 or 11 minutes. The dark adaptation curves for resolution had different shapes and extents, but again this was mirrored in the increment threshold curves for resolution, so that Equivalent Background Brightness for these test conditions and detection of a 10 minute disc all follow the same time course. In another extension (BLAKEMORE and RUSHTON, 1965b) they tested for the additivity of

"Equivalent Background Light" and real light, finding that no departure from linear summation could be detected.

In a different series of experiments, DUCROZ and RUSHTON (1966) investigated the Equivalent Background Brightness of cones that had been bleached. Their

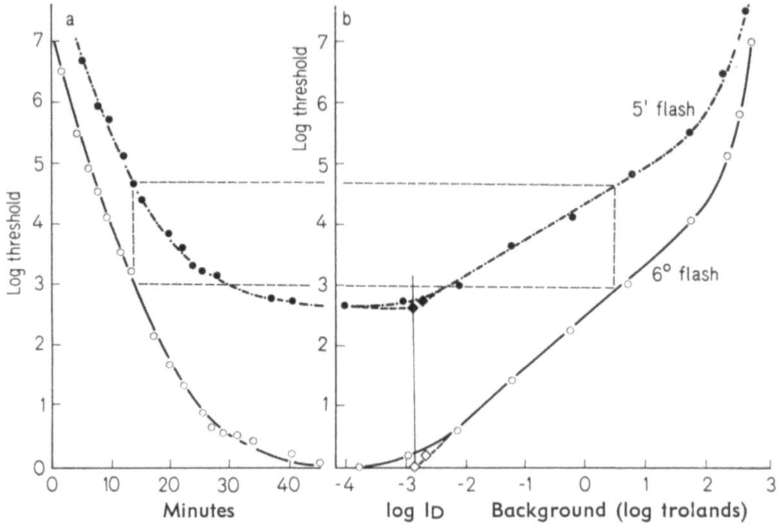

Fig. 10. The Crawford transform in a rod monochromat. a) left half, dark adaptation curve, log threshold plotted against time in the dark following intense preadaptation. b) right half, increment threshold curve, log threshold plotted against log background field. Threshold flash subtending 6°, empty circles; subtending 5′, filled circles. Dark adaptation differs for the two test stimuli,but the same difference is observed when a background light causes desensitization (BLAKEMORE and RUSHTON, 1965a)

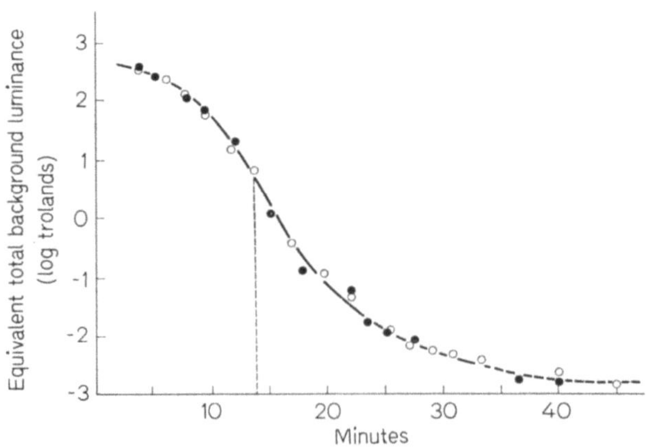

Fig. 11. Replot of Fig. 10 to show log equivalent background luminance as a function of time in the dark. A horizontal line drawn across Fig. 10 at any level of log threshold cuts the left curve at a "time in the dark" and the right curve at a "background luminance." These two quantitites are plotted against each other in this figure, empty circles for 6° test flash, filled circles for 5′. The equivalent background light is invariant for size of test stimulus (BLAKEMORE and RUSHTON, 1965a)

results show that STILES' π_1 ("blue"), π_4 ("green") and π_5 ("red") systems each generates its own dark light under bleaching, and that these operate nearly independently of each other after bleaching, as they do in the increment threshold situation.

At this point we should revise Eq. (1), p. 16, and derive the quantitative relation between Equivalent Background Light, I_E and pigment bleached. In the conditions used by BLAKEMORE and RUSHTON, Weber's Law is nearly true, so $\theta(I)/\theta_0 = (I + I_0)/I_0$. $\theta(I)$ is the increment threshold on a background of intensity I, θ_0 is the absolute threshold, and I_0 is the dark light (p. 7). According to the Equivalent Background Light formulation, we postulate a light $I_E(t)$ at time t in dark adaptation that raises threshold to a value $\theta(t)$ exactly as a real light would. So

$$\frac{\theta(t)}{\theta_0} = \frac{\theta(I_E)}{\theta_0} = \frac{I_E + I_0}{I_0}.$$

Now from DOWLING and RUSHTON's empirical results

$$\frac{\theta}{\theta_0} = \exp(\alpha r),$$

and it follows that

$$I_E = I_0 \exp(\alpha r) - I_0. \tag{2}$$

Notice that this only holds for values of I_E below rod saturation (100 scotopic trolands). If it held for large values of r, $\log(I_E + I_0)$ would decline exponentially throughout dark adaptation, but Fig. 11 shows that this is not the case. Threshold, on the other hand, does decline exponentially even when the amount bleached is large.

The view naturally adopted at this point would be that receptors containing a proportion r of bleached pigment signal messages indistinguishable from those caused by illumination at the intensity I_E when the receptors contain very nearly their full complement of pigment. This interpretation of dark adaptation in terms of the receptors becoming "noisy" (BARLOW, 1964a) fits everything that has so far been described with regard to threshold changes, and it has received striking support from two further observations.

The pupil diameter constricts when entering light is raised, and ALPERN and CAMPBELL (1962) showed that it also constricted when I_E was raised by bleaching rhodopsin. Furthermore this constriction depends upon impulses coming up from the eye: BORNSCHEIN (1958) showed that pressure blinding arrested the flow of impulses up the optic nerve, and pressure blinding after the bleach causes dilation of the pupil, followed by reconstriction upon release of pressure. Thus it seems that the dark light of bleaching not only desensitizes like real light, it also causes pupillary constriction like real light.

It may seem surprising that one is not vividly aware of these impulses that are causing pupillary constriction, and the Stiles-Crawford Equivalent Background light would have been taken seriously at an earlier time if there had been an intense subjective counterpart. It is true that there is the positive after-image, and CRAIK and VERNON (1941) tried to find its role in dark adaptation, but they concluded that it was too weak and transient to play much part. However, at that time the importance of image movement in maintaining the vividness of subjective images was not fully appreciated. When after-images are compared with stabilized retinal images, they are seen to be exactly as persistent and bright as the equivalent background light (Barlow and Sparrock, 1964). In Fig. 12 a circular after-image was matched to a surrounding annulus seen in stabilized vision, and at the same time sensitivity to a light superimposed on the after-image was measured. This matching

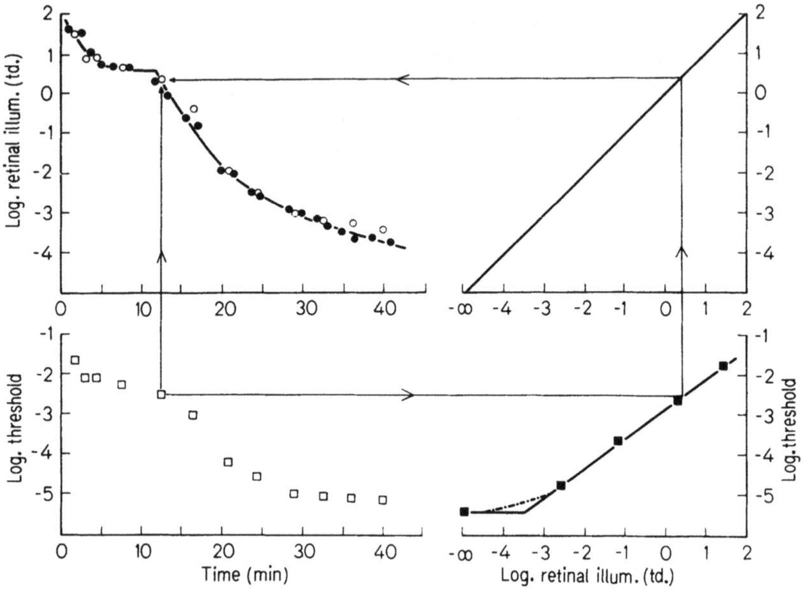

Fig. 12. Comparison of equivalent background luminance and equivalent luminance of the positive after-image. The after-image of an intense flash was surrounded by an annular screen viewed as a stabilized retinal image. The luminance of the annulus was adjusted to match the after-image, and the values at various times in the dark are plotted as filled circles, top left. The lower half of the figure shows (left) the threshold measured over the after-image as a function of time in the dark, and the increment threshold in the same area (right). These enable the equivalent background luminance to be obtained, and these values are plotted as open circles at top left. The positive after image has the luminance required to account for the equivalent background light (Barlow and Sparrock, 1964)

brightness declined as the threshold declined, and after it levelled off the increment threshold in the area of the after-image was measured. The equivalent background brightness determined by the Crawford transform at a particular moment in dark adaptation was found to be equal to the brightness that matched the after image at that moment.

Mechanism of Bleaching Recovery Adaptation

So far everything has fitted the view that the dark-light of bleaching is exactly the same in its effects on the retina as real light. Summarizing, it correctly predicts: (a) That changing test stimulus area will have the same effect on threshold during dark adaptation following bleaching, as when measured against adapting fields of varying luminance (Crawford, 1937, 1947; Blakemore and Rushton, 1965a, b).

(b) That the pupil will be constricted following bleaching, as it is during exposure to an adapting field (ALPERN and CAMPBELL, 1962). (c) The brightness of an after-image determined by matching it to a real field in stabilized conditions is the same as the dark light of bleaching determined from dark adaptation curves and increment threshold curves (BARLOW and SPARROCK, 1964). There are, however, objections, some of which might be surmountable but others are not easily disregarded. The difficulties arise in three instances: comparisons between the effects of non-uniform spatial distributions of real light and dark light; comparisons between their effects on temporal aspects of retinal performance; and comparisons between their effects on S-potentials.

RUSHTON (1965b) measured the dark-adaptation curve after bleaching the retina with an array of small dots separated from each other by 30 minutes of arc. Confirming earlier results (RUSHTON and WESTHEIMER, 1962), he found that the threshold elevating effect was proportional to the average amount bleached; since $I_E = \exp$ (large constant $\times$ amount of rhodopsin bleached), this gives a very different result from averaging I_E. However, when one tests the threshold elevating effect of a similar array of real luminous dots, the desensitizing effect is approximately proportional to the average luminance. This latter part of the experiment was done without stabilizing the dot-array, and somewhat different results are obtained if one measures threshold with small rather than large test stimuli. Furthermore the contrast in real light images of this sort probably does not exceed 10 : 1 or 20 : 1, whereas the dark light contrast is enormous because of the amplifying effect of the $\exp(\alpha r)$ relation. Nonetheless, one suspects that there may be a difference between the spatial spread of the desensitizing influences of real light and of dark light.

This suspicion is strengthened by WESTHEIMER'S (1968) experiments. He found that his sensitization effect (see p. 12) could not be produced by darklight: dark adaptation curves for a test flash on a 1° bleached spot were indistinguishable from those on a 3° bleached spot. Furthermore he could get no evidence of sensitizing interactions between spots and annuli composed of real and dark light. Unfortunately these experiments were performed without stabilization, and it is not altogether fair to compare the effect of the extremely stable after-image with those of the shifting real image. It is true that TELLER, ANDREWS, and BARLOW (1966) obtained evidence for the sensitizing effect of the real light annulus in stabilized image experiments, but the stabilization had only been held for a fraction of a minute in these tests, compared to many minutes for after-images.

Differences between the effects of real and dark light have been established with greater certainty for temporal processes in the retina. CONE (1964) found that the amplitude of the ERG was very similarly affected by adapting backgrounds of real light, and by the dark light of partial bleaching. The latency, however, was not affected equally, and MAFFEI and POPPELE (1968) found that the frequency spectrum of the ERG differed even when the amplitude had been equally reduced. ERNST'S (1968) psychophysical experiments probably reflect the same difference.

Finally there appear to be differences between the intracellular potentials. NAKA and RUSHTON (1968) reported that S-potentials are sustained in response to real light, but not in response to dark light, and STEINBERG (1969) confirms this in the cat.

Thus the present evidence indicates that the receptors can influence later stages in two different ways. Apparently real light a) gives the visual image which one sees, b) constricts the pupil, c) causes steady state desensitization, d) causes relative sensitization for high spatial frequencies, e) speeds up the process to emphasize high temporal frequencies, and f) causes sustained S-potentials. Dark light, on the other hand, behaves like real light with respect to a) to d), but does not speed up the process and does not cause sustained S-potentials.

The nature of the equivalent background light is one of the most puzzling aspects of the problem of light and dark adaptation, and the difficulties of reconciling different results suggests that some of them may actually be erroneous. However, the evidence from intracellular recording is not complete, and one can still hope for a resolution of the difficulties from this source.

VI. Resumé

Within the last twenty years profound advances have been made in understanding visual adaptation. Many of the psychophysical facts were known before then, as were the elementary facts about bleaching and regeneration of photolabile visual pigments, but now we know that log (threshold elevation) is directly proportional to the amount of pigment bleached. The idea of equivalent background light is nearly thirty years old, but now we have much better evidence for the validity of the concept and appreciate its relationship with positive after-images. The question of the origin of the equivalent background, and its exact relationship with activity evoked by real light, is a major unsolved problem, but acceptance of the concept abolishes the rivalry between photochemical and neural factors as explanations for adaptive changes.

Exposure to an adapting field, or to the equivalent background light of bleached pigment, causes desensitization and changes of summation and resolution. These are the changes that allow the eye to function effectively over an enormous dynamic range, and enable it to extract more information from high intensity images that are less perturbed by quantum fluctuations. These are also the changes, summarized in a few words, that require explanations at a cellular level. The picture of dark adaptation that emerges from psychophysical experiments thus provides an essential link between our knowledge that man's versatile vision suits him for an ecological niche extending through night and day, and the mechanisms being discovered by cellular neurophysiologists.

Acknowledgement. Preparation of this chapter was aided by grant EY 00276 from the National Eye Institute, U. S. Public Health Service.

References

Aguilar, M., Stiles, W. S.: Saturation of the rod mechanism at high levels of stimulation. Optica Acta **1**, 59—65 (1954).

Alpern, M., Campbell, F. W.: The behaviour of the pupil during dark-adaptation. J. Physiol. (Lond.) **165**, 5P—6P (1962).

— Fulton, A., Rushton, W. A. H., Torii, S.: Effect of adaptation on the retinal nerve code. Nature (Lond.) **224**, 712—713 (1969).

— Rushton, W. A. H., Torii, S.: The attenuation of rod signals by backgrounds. J. Physiol. (Lond.) **206**, 209—228 (1970).

Baker, H. D.: Initial stages of dark and light adaptation. J. opt. Soc. Amer. **53**, 98—103 (1963).

Barlow, H. B.: Increment thresholds at low intensities considered as signal noise discriminations. J. Physiol. (Lond.) **136**, 469—488 (1957).

— Temporal and spatial summation in human vision at different background intensities. J. Physiol. (Lond.) **141**, 337—350 (1958a).

— Intrinsic noise of cones. In: Visual Problems of Colour, Vol. 2, pp. 617—630. London: H. M. Stationery Office 1958b.

— A method of determining the overall quantum efficiency of visual discriminations. J. Physiol. (Lond.) **160**, 155—168 (1962a).

— Measurements of the quantum efficiency of discrimination in human scotopic vision. J. Physiol. (Lond.) **160**, 169—188 (1962b).

— Slippage of contact lenses and other artifacts in relation to fading and regeneration of supposedly stable retinal images. Quart. J. exp. Psychol. **15**, 36—51 (1963).

— Dark adaptation: a new hypothesis. Vision Res. **4**, 47—58 (1964a).

— The physical limits of visual discrimination. In: Photophysiology, Vol. 2, pp. 163—202. Giese, A. C. (Ed.) New York: Academic Press 1964b.

— Fitzhugh, R., Kuffler, S. W.: Change of organization in the receptive fields of the cat's retina during dark adaptation. J. Physiol. (Lond.) **137**, 338—354 (1957).

— Sparrock, J. M. B.: The role of after-images in dark adaptation. Science **144**, 1309—1314 (1964).

Blakemore, C. B., Rushton, W. A. H.: Dark adaptation and increment threshold in a rod monochromat. J. Physiol. (Lond.) **181**, 612—628 (1965a).

— — The rod increment threshold during dark adaptation in normal and rod monochromat. J. Physiol. (Lond.) **181**, 629—640 (1965b).

Bornschein, H.: Spontan- und Belichtungsaktivität in Einzelfasern des N. Opticus der Katze. I. Der Einfluß kurzdauernder retinaler Ischämie. Z. Biol. **110**, 210—222 (1958).

Bouman, M. A.: History and present status of quantum theory in vision. In: Sensory Communication, Ch. 21, pp. 377—401. Rosenblith, W. (Ed.) Boston: M.I.T. Press 1961.

Brindley, G. S.: The summation areas of human colour-receptive mechanisms at increment threshold. J. Physiol. (Lond.) **124**, 400—408 (1954).

— The discrimination of after-images. J. Physiol. (Lond.) **147**, 194—203 (1959).

— Du Croz, J. J., Rushton, W. A. H.: The flicker fusion frequency of the blue-sensitive mechanism of colour vision. J. Physiol. (Lond.) **183**, 497—500 (1966).

Campbell, F. W., Gregory, A. H.: Effect of pupil size on acuity. Nature (Lond.) **187**, 1121—1123 (1960).

— Gubisch, R. W.: Optical quality of the human eye. J. Physiol. (Lond.) **186**, 558—578 (1966).

— Rushton, W. A. H.: Measurement of the scotopic pigment in the living human eye. J. Physiol. (Lond.) **130**, 131—147 (1955).

Carr, R. E., Ripps, H.: Rhodopsin kinetics and rod adaptation in Oguchi's disease. Invest. Ophthal. **6**, 426—436 (1967).

— — Siegel, I. M., Weale, R. A.: Rhodopsin and the electrical activity of the retina in congenital night blindness. Invest. Ophthal. **5**, 497—507 (1966a).

— — — — Visual functions in congenital night-blindness. Invest. Ophthal. **5**, 508—514 (1966b).

Clark Jones, R.: Quantum efficiency of human vision. J. opt. Soc. Amer. **49**, 645—653 (1959).

Cohen, A. I.: New evidence supporting the linkage to extracellular space of the outer segment saccules of frog cones but not rods. J. cell Biol. **37**, 424—444 (1968).

Cone, R. A.: The rat electroretinogram I: contrasting effects of adaptation on the amplitude and latency of the b-wave. J. gen. Physiol. **47**, 1089—1105 (1964).

Craik, K. J. W.: The effect of adaptation on differential brightness discrimination. J. Physiol. (Lond.) **92**, 406—421 (1938).

— Vernon, M. D.: The nature of dark adaptation. Brit. J. Psychol. **32**, 64—81 (1941).

Crawford, B. H.: The change of visual sensitivity with time. Proc. roy. Soc. (Lond.) B **123**, 69—89 (1937).
— The effect of field size and pattern on the change of visual sensitivity with time. Proc. roy. Soc. (Lond.) B **129**, 94—106 (1940).
— Photochemical laws and visual phenomena. Proc. roy. Soc. (Lond.) B **133**, 63—75 (1946).
— Visual adaptation in relation to brief conditioning stimuli. Proc. roy. Soc. (Lond.) B **134**, 283—302 (1947).
Daitch, J. M., Green, D. G.: Contrast sensitivity of the human peripheral retina. Vision Res. **9**, 947—952 (1969).
De Vries, Hl.: The quantum character of light and its bearing upon the threshold of vision, the differential sensitivity and acuity of the eye. Physica **10**, 553—564 (1943).
Donner, K. O., Reuter, T.: The dark adaptation of single units in the frog's retina and its relation to the regeneration of rhodopsin. Vision Res. **5**, 615—632 (1965).
— — Dark adaptation processes in the rhodopsin rods of the frog's retina. Vision Res. **7**, 17—62 (1967).
Dowling, J. E.: Chemistry of visual adaptation in the rat. Nature (Lond.) **188**, 114—118 (1960).
— Neural and photochemical mechanisms of visual adaptation in the rat. J. gen. Physiol. **46**, 1287—1301 (1963).
— The site of visual adaptation. Science **155**, 273—279 (1967).
— Hubbard, R.: Effects of brilliant flashes on light and dark adaptation. Nature (Lond.) **199**, 972—975 (1963).
DuCroz, J. J., Rushton, W. A. H.: The separation of cone mechanisms in dark adaptation. J. Physiol. (Lond.) **183**, 481—496 (1966).
Ernst, W.: The dependence of critical flicker frequency and the rod threshold on the state of adaptation of the eye. Vision Res. 8, 889—900 (1968).
Frank, R. N., Dowling, J. E.: Rhodopsin photoproducts: Effects on electroretinogram sensitivity in isolated perfused rat retina. Science **161**, 487—489 (1968).
Fuortes, M. G. F., Gunkel, R. D., Rushton, W. A. H.: Increment thresholds in a subject deficient in cone vision. J. Physiol. (Lond.) **156**, 179—192 (1961).
Green, D. G.: Sinusoidal flicker characteristics of the colour sensitive mechanisms of the eye. Vision Res. **9**, 591—601 (1969).
Hagins, W. A.: The quantum efficiency of bleaching of rhodopsin in situ. J. Physiol. (Lond.) **129**, 22P—23P (1955).
Haig, C.: The course of rod dark adaptation as influenced by the intensity and duration of pre-adaptation to light. J. gen. Physiol. **24**, 735—751 (1941).
Hecht, S.: The nature of the sensitivity of animals to light. J. opt. Soc. Amer. **18**, 264—286 (1929).
— Rods, cones, and the chemical basis of vision. Physiol. Rev. **17**, 239—290 (1937).
— Haig, C., Chase, A. M.: The influence of light-adaptation on subsequent dark adaptation of the eye. J. gen. Physiol. **20**, 831—850 (1937).
Hough, E. A., Ruddock, K. H.: The Purkinje Shift. Vision Res. **9**, 313—315 (1969).
Kelly, D. H.: Diffusion model of linear flicker repsonses. J. opt. Soc. Amer. **59**, 1665—1670 (1969).
Lythgoe, R. J.: The mechanism of dark adaptation. Brit. J. Ophthal. **24**, 21—43 (1940).
Maffei, L., Poppele, R. E.: Transient and steady state electroretinal responses. Vision Res. 8, 229—246 (1968).
Mckee, S. P., Westheimer, G.: Specificity of cone mechanisms in lateral interaction. J. Physiol. (Lond.) **206**, 117—128 (1970).
Naka, K. I., Rushton, W. A. H.: S-potential and dark-adaptation in fish. J. Physiol. (Lond.) **194**, 259—269 (1968).
Parinaud, H.: La Vision. Paris: Octave Doin 1898.
Penn, R. D., Hagins, W. A.: Signal transmission along retinal rods and the origin of the electroretinographic a-wave. Nature (Lond.) **223**, 201—205 (1969).

PIRENNE, M. H.: Visual functions in man. In: The Eye, Vol. 2, Ch. 1—11, pp. 3—218. DAVSON, H. (Ed.) New York-London: Academic Press 1962.

ROSE, A.: The relative sensitivities of television pick-up tubes, photographic film, and the human eye. Proc. Inst. Rad. Eng. **30**, 293—300 (1942).

— The sensitivity performance of the human eye on an absolute scale. J. opt. Soc. Amer. **38**, 196—208 (1948).

RUSHTON, W. A. H.: The difference spectrum and the photosensitivity of rhodopsin in the living human eye. J. Physiol. (Lond.) **134**, 11—29 (1956).

— Physical measurement of cone pigments in the living human eye. Nature (Lond.) **179**, 571—573 (1957).

— Dark-adaptation and the regeneration of rhodopsin. J. Physiol. (Lond.) **156**, 166—178 (1961a).

— Rhodopsin measurement and dark-adaptation in a subject deficient in cone vision. J. Physiol. (Lond.) **156**, 193—205 (1961b).

— Cone pigment kinetics in the protanope. J. Physiol. (Lond.) **168**, 374—388 (1963).

— Flash photolysis in human cones. Photochem. and Photobiol. **3**, 561—577 (1964).

— Cone pigment kinetics in the deuteranope. J. Physiol. (Lond.) **176**, 38—45 (1965a).

— Bleached rhodopsin and visual adaptation. J. Physiol. (Lond.) **181**, 645—655 (1965b).

— The Ferrier Lecture, 1962. Visual Adaptation. Proc. roy. Soc. (Lond.) B **162**, 20—46 (1965c).

— Rod/cone rivalry in pigment regeneration. J. Physiol. (Lond.) **198**, 219—236 (1968).

— BAKER, H. D.: Effect of a very bright flash on cone vision and cone pigments in man. Nature (Lond.) **200**, 421—423 (1963).

— CAMPBELL, F. W., HAGINS, W. A., BRINDLEY, G. S.: The bleaching and regeneration of rhodopsin in the living eye of the albino rabbit and of man. Optica Acta **1**, 183—190 (1955).

— FULTON, A. B., BAKER, H. D.: Dark adaptation and the rate of pigment regeneration. Vision Res. **9**, 1473—1480 (1969).

— HENRY, G. H.: Bleaching and regeneration of cone pigments in man. Vision Res. **8**, 617—632 (1968).

— WESTHEIMER, G.: The effect upon the rod threshold of bleaching neighbouring rods. J. Physiol. (Lond.) **164**, 318—329 (1962).

SCHULTZE, M.: Zur Anatomie und Physiologie der Retina. Arch. mikr. Anat. **2**, 175—286 (1866).

STARK, L.: Neurological Control Systems. New York: Plenum Press 1968.

STEINBERG, R. H.: The rod after-effect in S-potentials from the cat retina. Vision Res. **9**, 1345—1356 (1969).

STILES, W. A.: Color vision: The approach through increment-threshold sensitivity. Proc. nat. Acad. Sci. (Wash.) **45**, 100—114 (1954).

STILES, W. S.: The directional sensitivity of the retina and the spectral sensitivities of the rods and cones. Proc. roy. Soc. (Lond.) B **127**, 64—105 (1939).

— CRAWFORD, B. H.: Equivalent adaptation levels in localized retinal areas. In: Report of a Joint Discussion on Vision, pp. 194—211. Physical Society of London: Cambridge: University Press 1932.

— — The luminous efficiency of rays entering the eye pupil at different points. Proc. roy. Soc. (Lond.) B **112**, 428—450 (1933).

TANSLEY, K., JOHNSON, B. K.: The cones of the grass snake's eye. Nature (Lond.) **178**, 1285—1286 (1956).

TELLER, D. Y., ANDREWS, D. P., BARLOW, H. B.: Local adaptation in stabilized vision. Vision Res. **6**, 701—705 (1966).

TOYODA, J. I., NOSAKI, H., TOMITA, T.: Light induced resistance changes in single photoreceptors of Necturus and Gekko. Vision Res. **9**, 453—463 (1969).

VON KRIES, J.: Über die Funktion der Netzhautstäbchen. Z. Psychol. Physiol. Sinnesorg. **9**, 81—123 (1896).

WALD, G.: Blue-blindness in the normal fovea. J. opt. Soc. Amer. **57**, 1289—1301 (1967).

WALLS, G. L.: The Vertebrate Eye and its Adaptive Radiation. Cranbrook Institute of Science, Bloomfield Hills, Michigan 1942. (Republished, Hafner, N. Y. 1963).

WEINSTEIN, G. W., HOBSON, R. R., DOWLING, J. E.: Light and dark adaptation in the isolated rat retina. Nature (Lond.) **215**, 134—138 (1967).

Werblin, F. W., Dowling, J. E.: Organization of the retina of the mud puppy, *Necturus maculosus*. II. Intracellular recording. J. Neurophysiol. **32**, 339—355 (1969).
Westheimer, G.: Visual acuity. Ann. Rev. Psychol. **16**, 359—380 (1965a).
— Spatial interaction in the human retina during scotopic vision. J. Physiol. (Lond.) **181**, 881—894 (1965b).
— Spatial interaction in human cone vision. J. Physiol. (Lond.) **190**, 139—154 (1967).
— Bleached rhodopsin and retinal interaction. J. Physiol. (Lond.) **195**, 97—106 (1968).
— Rod-cone independence for sensitizing interaction in the human retina. J. Physiol. (Lond.) **206**, 109—116 (1970).

Chapter 2

Threshold Quantal Problems

By

E. Baumgardt*, Paris (France)

With 7 Figures

Contents

I. From Physical Stimulus to Light Sensation

There is no light, but we may see light. Light is a sensation and thus has no physical existence. Between the energy flux of electromagnetic radiation of a given bandwidth, called the stimulus, and the light sensation, there are physical, chemical, physiological and psychological events.

The first physical event is the absorption of radiant energy by the visual receptors of the retina. This absorption takes place by finite steps called quanta, each of which carries the energy

$$h\nu$$

where h is Planck's constant, and ν the frequency of the radiation. Since

$$\nu = \frac{c}{\lambda}$$

* This chapter was completed in February, 1969, shortly before Dr. Baumgardt's death.

where c is the velocity of the radiant energy in the medium in question and λ its wavelength, the energy of a quantum may be specified as

$$E_q = \frac{1}{\lambda} \times hc .$$

For normal levels of illumination (daylight), light sensations are evoked in man for $400 \leqq \lambda \leqq 750$ nm (one nm $= 10^{-9}$ m) but there are no real spectral limits for vision. Infra-red sensations have been reported for wavelengths up to 1100 nm (GRIFFIN *et al.*, 1947), and ultra-violet ones appreciably below 400 nm, if high luminance levels are used (DE GROOT, 1934).

Planck's constant h is equal to 6.625×10^{-27} erg sec, and $c = 3 \times 10^{10}$ cm sec^{-1} in air. If λ varies between 400 and 750 nm, E_q varies between 2.5×10^{-12} and 4.7×10^{-12} erg. These are very small amounts of energy that correspond to a few electron volts.

The absorption of quanta by the visual pigment of receptor cells leads to at least one chemical event that is indispensable for triggering a light sensation. In retinas that contain rhodopsin, when a quantum is absorbed a molecule of the latter shifts to prelumirhodopsin, i.e., from the cis-form to the trans-form (HUBBARD and KROPF, 1958).

This first chemical event is followed by many others, but as yet there is no proof that the latter are indispensable for vision. CONE (1967) showed that within less than half a microsecond after absorption, the first electrophysiological event can be observed in the retina. This is the first cornea-positive part of the early receptor potential (ERP) which can be recorded after very strong stimulation (see BROWN and MURAKAMI, 1964).

Since the fundamental work of HECHT *et al.*, (1942) we have known that a single quantum absorbed by a human rod triggers an intraretinal response and that a small number of such responses may provoke a light sensation in man. This has been confirmed by several other authors (VAN DER VELDEN, 1944; PEYROU and PIATIER, 1946; BAUMGARDT, 1949). The absorption of a quantum of any wavelength must give rise to the same sequence of events in a given rod receptor, for the spectral efficiency curve of scotopic vision, after correction for light losses in the ocular media, coincides with the absorption curve of rhodopsin. However, it is probable that a low amount of energy is delivered by the absorbing pigment molecule, as has been suggested by STILES (1948). CROUZY (1963) showed that the sensitivity of the human visual organ effectively reaches the limits imposed by spontaneous stimulus fluctuation. He emphasizes that what has to be considered is not the number of quantum absorptions, but the action potentials generated in the retina. He believes these two quantities to be proportional on the average, but it is clear that the factor of proportionality varies with light adaptation.

YEANDLE (1958) has shown that "quantum-bumps" may be observed in the Limulus eye, and further work by ADOLPH (1964), by DOWLING (1968) and by BORSELLINO and FUORTES (1968) has confirmed his observation. SCHOLES (1965) finds also that in locust, at low illumination levels, the discharge frequency is proportional to the luminance and that Bloch's law (see below) holds.

RICCÒ (1877) showed that there is spatial summation in the human eye, i.e., that by enlarging the stimulated retinal area one may reduce the absolute threshold for vision. If one quantum were sufficient to trigger a threshold sensation, the mean threshold would not vary with changes in stimulated area. Thus it is self-evident that in order to trigger a sensation, the absorption of more than one quantum is needed.

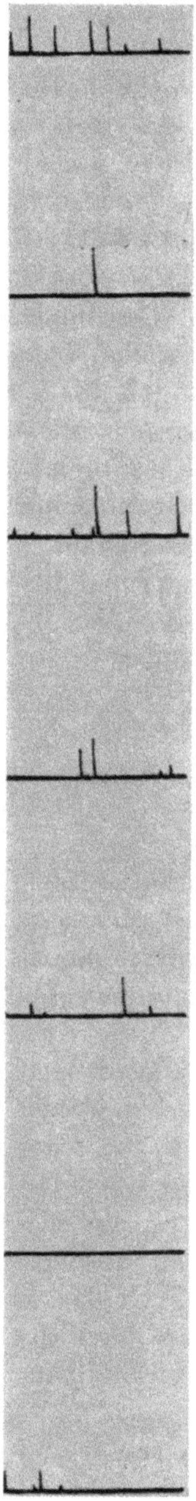

Galifret and Piéron (1950) showed by psychophysical measures, analyzed in connection with histological and electrophysiological results obtained by other scientists, that the absorption of one quantum is unable to trigger a light sensation.

Denton and Pirenne (1954) observed day-to-day variability of the order of 0.20 log unit. A normal observer will thus have a threshold which may vary roughly between one and two-and-a-half times its minimum value when measures are made over a long period of time. This has been confirmed by Zegers (1959).

II. The Variability of Weak Stimuli and the Probability that they will Trigger a Sensation

It has long been known that weak stimuli sometimes give rise to a sensation, but sometimes do not. This observation is true for any type of sensation and it has been studied extensively in vision.

Since any source of visible radiant energy emits a considerable number of quanta in any small solid angle per unit of time, absolute threshold stimuli cannot be obtained by the use of ordinary sources without filters or corresponding devices for attenuation. Since quantum emission is considered to be a random event in space and time, the threshold stimulus should possess the same characteristics. In a given space element, a randomly

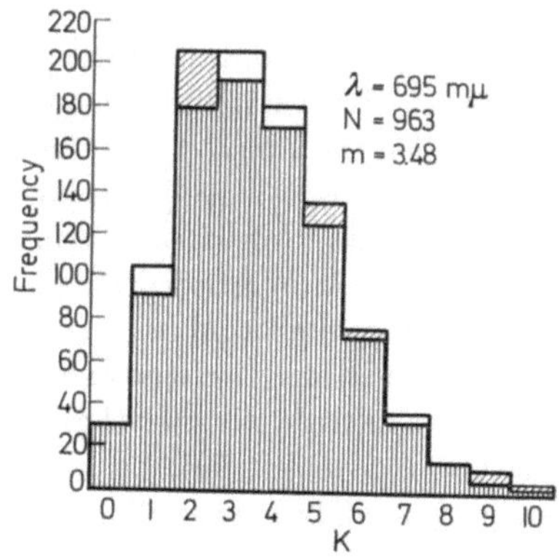

Fig. 1. Left: Sample recording on cathode ray oscilloscope. Each spike corresponds to one quantum absorption by the cathode of the photomultiplier. Mean absorption by 8 ms flash: $m = 3.48$. Luminous emission constant (±0.9%). Right: Statistics of 963 spikes recorded, compatible with Poisson's law. The quantities in excess of the expectation are hatched, the opposite ones are empty (after Baumgardt, 1957)

fluctuating energy in time should be observable. If this were true, the absolute threshold could not be a constant energy value but must be a variable one. Thus the mean threshold value should sometimes trigger a light sensation, sometimes not. This is what we observe in fact, and the question arises whether this fact is due to the quantum fluctuation or not.

This is a fundamental question which will be treated in the last section of this chapter. In the present section we will show that a positive answer to this question is possible, by proving that the theoretical quantum fluctuation really exists.

After GARLICK and WRIGHT (1952) had reported some qualitative results, BAUMGARDT (1957) obtained this proof with a 20-stage photomultiplier followed by a cathode ray oscilloscope and a photographic device. At the temperature of solid CO_2, this multiplier emits 12 thermionic electrons per second at its cathode, corresponding to a mean of one-tenth during the 8 milliseconds of each trial. Thus for about four mean quanta absorptions per trial, the probability of "false" quantum spikes was about 2.5%. Fig. 1 shows a sample of photographs and a graph of the statistical distribution of quantum absorption[1]. Between 0 and 10 absorptions per trial were observed; the frequency distribution is compatible with the Poisson distribution that applies here, because the observed event, a quantum absorption, has a very low probability as compared with the probability of the emission of a quantum during the duration of a single trial.

III. Absolute Visual Thresholds

A. General Considerations

A threshold is defined by a convention. Usually, the convention is 50% probability of perception of a difference in luminance, quality (color), size, etc., and this includes absolute thresholds where comparison is made between absence or presence of a luminous sensation *at the expected time and in the expected region of the monocular or binocular field.*

When the number of quanta contained in a stimulus is not as small as it is at absolute threshold, its relative variability decreases. For $n \geqq 25$, there is practically no difference between the Poisson and the normal distribution. In the latter case, the relative variability is inversely proportional to the square root of the number N of random events considered. Thus, the influence of the physical random distribution of quantum absorptions is particularly large at absolute threshold and at very low background luminances. A straightforward calculation shows that the observed increment or contrast thresholds at levels far above the absolute threshold are considerably higher than those necessarily caused by quantum absorption fluctuations (ROSE, 1948).

For this reason, in this chapter we will consider only absolute thresholds and increment thresholds at very low levels of background luminance.

There is an unlimited number of different absolute threshold values in night vision in a given species, e.g., man. Indeed, retinal position, retinal area, form,

[1] There are two numerical errors in the 1957 original: λ_{425} should read λ_{445}, and $N = 263$ should read $N = 963$.

duration and wavelength of a stimulus are parameters for any combination of which there is an absolute threshold, i.e., a threshold in dark adaptation.

The measurement of absolute thresholds and of increment thresholds at very low luminances involves particularly severe working conditions. Normally, 45 minutes of dark adaptation suffices, but if the observer enters the experimental room where his threshold is to be measured having come from outside, and especially from a high luminance environment such as the seashore in summer or a sun-flooded snow landscape, hours of dark adaptation may be necessary. Coffee, tea, alcohol, or smoking are also likely to change the threshold (WEINSTEIN and ARNULF, 1946).

There are different methods for determining thresholds but not all of them are equally useful for absolute threshold measures. Thus, the flicker-fusion method does not work and scaling methods are easier to handle at higher levels. "Yes-no" methods imply the use of personal criteria, and the false alarm ratio poses a problem that is not easy to resolve. (See NACHMIAS, chapter 3, this volume).

A constant-stimulus method with randomized stimulus presentation is considered to be the best "yes-no" method. But "blanks" are always required in order to assess the observer's reliability.

A temporal forced-choice method consists in comparing sensory impressions for several time intervals demarcated by auditory signals and in selecting that one interval which seems to have contained the test flash. BLACKWELL (1953) has described a four-interval forced-choice method in which personal criteria do not (or nearly not) interfere with the final result. (See also BLACKWELL, chapter 4, this volume).

The author believes such methods to be more suitable than others for absolute threshold or near threshold measures.

B. The Minimal Threshold in Scotopic Vision

The issue at hand is the measurement of the lower limit of the absolute threshold. Now, threshold may be expressed as an energy or as a luminance. The latter definition is of considerable practical interest and it has been treated extensively by PIRENNE *et al.* (1957). For 22 young subjects who observed for 15 seconds using both eyes and the natural pupil, the mean threshold for a continuing stimulus of white light of 2400° K color temperature subtending a visual angle of 47 degrees in diameter was found to be 0.75×10^{-6} cd/m². The variability from observer to observer is not negligible. The lowest threshold measured was 0.4×10^{-6} cd/m², the highest 2×10^{-6} cd/m². The reader will find an extensive bibliography in DAVSON (1962) which appears to the author as adequate now as it was about eight years ago. The lowest energy necessary to elicit a visual sensation is of the order of 80 quanta of 507 nm radiation at the level of the cornea. Values down to 25 quanta have also been measured, but during the last 25 years only by BOUMAN and his associates (e.g., BOUMAN and VAN DER VELDEN, 1947). These values seem unlikely, as emphasized by BARLOW (1956). Most of the mean values measured for individual observers or for groups of observers fall between 50 and 100 quanta (EYSTER, 1907; BARNES and CZERNY, 1932; HECHT *et al.*, 1942; PEYROU and PIATIER, 1946; BAUMGARDT, 1959; MARRIOTT *et al.*, 1959).

Values less than about 50 quanta under the most favorable conditions – brief flashes and small visual angle, about 9° to 20° outside the fovea – are likely to be related to defective experimental conditions for the following reason. LUDVIGH and MCCARTHY (1938) and SAÏD and WEALE (1959) measured the transparency of the ocular media for radiation of different wavelengths. For 507 nm, and in peripheral vision, one may safely assume that about 50% of the radiant energy arriving at the cornea reaches the retina, where about 70% of this energy enters the rods, the remaining 30% entering cones or interstices between receptors. *In situ* measures by RUSHTON (1956) show that the optical density of the rod pigment in man, rhodopsin, is approximately 0.15 for $\lambda = 500$ nm. It thus appears that about 10% of the energy that enters the eye can be absorbed by the rods.

If frequency of seeing is plotted as a function of the logarithm of the energy of a stimulus flash, an S-shaped curve results. This curve is compared to Poisson sums, $F_n(x)$, of different slopes, where each of the latter corresponds to a parameter n: 1, 2, . . . :

$$F_n(x) = \sum_{r=n}^{\infty} \frac{e^{-x} x^r}{r!}$$

where x is the number of acting, i.e., absorbed, quanta, since at the absolute threshold, quantum efficiency is 1, as WILLIAMS (1965) has particularly emphasized.

The steepness of these curves described by a parameter n' is an estimate of n, the lowest number of quanta absorbed in order to yield a threshold response, as HECHT *et al.* had postulated. PIRENNE and MARRIOTT (1959) proved that n' is a *lower limit* of n. Any variability of the observer's sensitivity and any disturbing factor linked to the measuring procedure necessarily flattens the response curve and thus yields n' smaller than n. (See Fig. 2.)

No frequency-of-seeing (or psychometric) curve that fits a Poisson sum of parameter $n' < 3$ is known, except for the one published by VAN DER VELDEN (1944) who found n' between 2 and 3 and not less than 2.5. Even this extremely low value of n' would imply an absolute threshold of at least 25 quanta at 507 nm

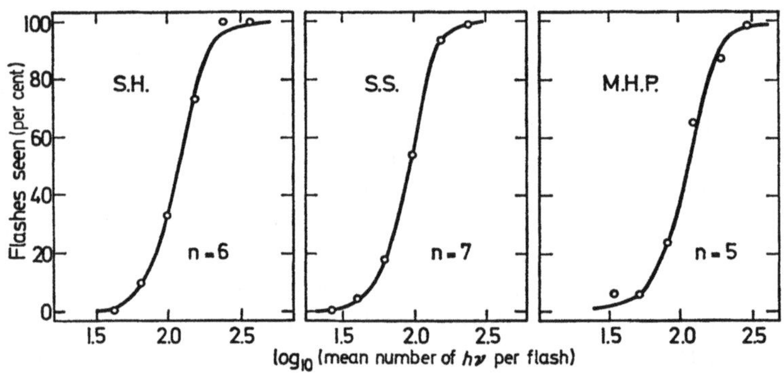

Fig. 2. Relation between the average energy content of a flash of 510 nm radiation, in number of quanta, measured at the cornea, and the frequency with which it was seen by three observers. Test field 10′ of arc in diameter, retinal position 20° peripherally, flash duration 10^{-3} sec. The curves are the Poisson sums for n-values of 5, 6 and 7. (from HECHT *et al.*, 1942)

at the corneal level. Thus, abnormally low energy values of absolute threshold as well as particularly flat response curves may be due to abnormal variability of the observer's sensitivity, and/or to the absence of the necessary precautions for assessing the observer's reliability. The latter may be measured by the frequency of "false positives" or "false alarms", which requires the use of a significant proportion of blanks. It is of interest to note that HECHT *et al.*, and BAUMGARDT (1959, 1960) used very reliable observers whose false positive rate was zero or less than 1%. The steepness of their response curves implies $5 \leqq n' \leqq 8$, which corresponds to not less than 50 to 80 quanta at the corneal level. This fits very well the physical energy measures of these authors, and is confirmed by several authors before 1939 and by all since then, except for BOUMAN and his collaborators. *We are thus led to the conclusion that in these experiments the uncertainty of seeing is predominantly due to fluctuations in the actual numbers of quanta absorbed by the retinal rods*[2].

C. The Minimal Threshold in Foveal Vision

Since the end of the 19th century, astronomers and physicists have been interested in measuring the lowest energy threshold of vision, but few measures have been made of the foveal absolute threshold under experimental conditions that really guarantee a possibility of reaching such a threshold. We will discuss these conditions in the next section; it is sufficient to state here that foveal thresholds should be measured with small test stimuli of short duration. This has been done by BOSWELL (1908), who found a mean threshold corresponding to 625 quanta of 555 nm at the corneal level. BOUMAN and VAN DER VELDEN (1947) determined thresholds that ranged from 467 to 790 quanta of 555 nm radiation, MILLER (1959) measured 2420 quanta, and MARRIOTT (1963) obtained values that ranged from 490 to 872 quanta of 555 nm radiation with a mean of 602 quanta. The mean threshold seems to be of the order of 600 quanta of 555 nm if we do not include MILLER'S result, which is clearly outside the range of all others so far obtained.

In order to compare cone and rod sensitivities, one may choose the wavelength where the curves V_λ and V'_λ cross. (See LE GRAND, chapter 15, this volume). This is at about 528 nm. Here, the cone threshold should be about 1.25 times the threshold for 555 nm light, which means about 750 quanta at 528 nm. BAUMGARDT and SMITH (1967) found that for 4 observers, the ratio of foveal cone threshold to rod threshold ranges between 7.0 and 12.9, with a mean of 10.9, when $\lambda = 528$ nm. If 750 is divided by 10.9 it yields a rod threshold of about 57 quanta at 528 nm, which is compatible with the known results. Thus, rod vision is approximately

[2] HALLETT (1963) has thoroughly analyzed the spatial summation work in vision. He states that for a given test object, variation between observers is sufficiently striking to justify dividing them in two groups, A and B, according to whether summation is large or small at a given excentricity. He presents limited evidence for the co-existence of two sizes of receptive fields, and also discussess the role of technique.

The difficulty seems to be located in the latter. BOUMAN and his collaborators, for example, belong to group B (which is the minority group) until 1950, but in 1952, BOUMAN and BLOKHUIS show very clearly A-values. This is an additional reason why we should not take into consideration too low energy levels of the absolute threshold for brief small test flashes that strike the most sensitive region of the retina.

10 times more sensitive than cone vision, if small test stimuli of the order of 1 square minute of arc are used at 528 nm. (See Fig. 3.)

It is equally interesting to compare the threshold number of quanta necessary for cone and for rod vision when both are measured for the most sensitive conditions, i.e., with 555 nm light for foveal cones and 507 nm light for rods. Since the mean of the cone threshold is about 600 quanta, that for rod vision is about 80, the rod/cone efficiency for small retinal areas is of the order of 7.5.

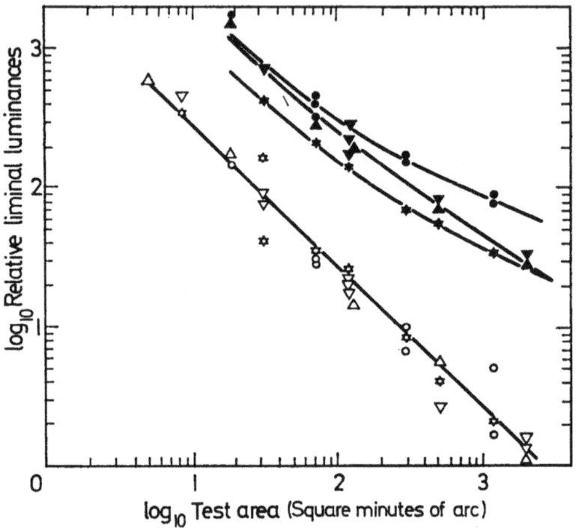

Fig. 3. Filled symbols represent liminal luminances in foveal vision, empty symbols the same in peripheral vision; $\lambda = 528$ nm, four observers (after BAUMGARDT and SMITH, 1967)

Since the optical density of the foveal receptor pigments is of the order of 0.10 (see RUSHTON, 1959), a light sensation in foveal vision arises by the absorption of about 38 quanta at 555 nm, when we take into account the mean threshold of 600 quanta at the corneal level and all the absorption and reflection losses between the cornea and the cones.

MARRIOTT (1963) rejects the hypothesis of BOUMAN and VAN DER VELDEN (1948) and BOUMAN and WALRAVEN (1957) that the absorption of two quanta within any small area of the fovea is the necessary and sufficient condition for detection of a brief foveal stimulus. By examining foveal frequency-of-seeing curves, MARRIOTT demonstrates that if there are independent units in the central fovea such that the excitation of any one suffices for vision, at least five quanta must be absorbed within an independent unit to excite it. He also notes that the frequency-of-seeing curves of BOUMAN and WALRAVEN (1957) actually exclude the 2- and 3-quanta theory proposed by these authors. MARRIOTT (1963) used 9 observers, whose parameters n' (deduced from the slopes of the psychometric response curves) range from 13 to 67. As we know, $n' \leq n$, thus these values seem not to be incompatible with the evaluation of the absolute foveal threshold for very small and brief stimuli by physical methods. It is clear that for foveal absolute threshold we are not led to conclude firmly that uncertainty of seeing is predominantly due to fluctuations in the numbers of quanta absorbed, as we had concluded for peripheral vision.

In all observations reported here, in Section III, C, "yes-no" methods were employed, except for the experiments reported by BAUMGARDT and SMITH who used a forced-choice method. Ordinarily, a constant-stimulus method with randomized stimulus sequence and intermingled blanks is used.

IV. The Laws of Spatial and Temporal Summation at and near Absolute Threshold

A. Riccò's Law of Total Spatial Summation

In foveal as well as in peripheral vision, experiments have shown that the absolute threshold energy does not vary when the angle subtended by the test flash does not exceed a certain limit which depends on several factors. These are retinal location, wavelength and duration of the test flash. Total spatial summation is called Riccò's law. In the following, we assume an exposure time t of the flash which is sufficiently short to avoid possible interference between temporal and spatial laws.

In foveal vision, Riccò's law holds up to about 7 minutes of arc in dark adaptation, with a natural pupil, 30 millisecond exposure time, and long-wave stimulation (BAUMGARDT, 1949). Use of an artificial pupil reduces the range over which Riccò's law is valid. For long-wave light, Riccò's law did not hold between 2 minutes and 7 minutes of arc if artificial pupils of 1 millimeter and of 4 millimeters were used. In the very small range between 1.12 minutes and 1.79 minutes of arc, Riccò's law holds for "green" stimuli. It has not been tested for "red" stimuli in this range. HILLMANN (1958) measured foveal thresholds with white light. She finds departures from Riccò's law which vary among her 4 observers. One of them shows total summation for test fields up to 8 minutes in diameter, the others show somewhat less summation. This interpretation of HILLMANN's figures differs from her own in that she seems to conclude that even between 1.2 minutes and 5.0 minutes test-field diameter Riccò's law does not apply. Some authors, e.g., BOUMAN and VAN DEN BRINK (1952), have defined spatial summation as the largest spatial separation between two stimuli of very small diameter such that the sum of the threshold energies of the two stimuli is equal to the threshold energy when the two stimuli are superimposed on the same retinal area. This definition results in smaller spatial limits for the validity of Riccò's law than does the one where only one stimulus is delivered and the variable is its angular diameter or its largest angular dimension. Systematic research to explain this difference on a quantum basis has not yet been undertaken. It seems probable that the mean distance between two quantum absorptions must be less than a limiting value which depends on physiological factors related to the nervous network behind the photoreceptors.

In peripheral vision at 8 to 20 degrees outside the fovea, Riccò's law seems to hold up to about 1 degree of test field diameter (BAUMGARDT, 1949; GRAHAM and MARGARIA, 1935; HALLET *et al.*, 1962; WEALE, 1958; WEINSTEIN and ARNULF, 1946).

The WEINSTEIN and ARNULF paper merits particular attention for it contains a comprehensive study of spatial summation in the central fovea as well as at 1°, 7°, 12°, 18°, 20°, and 35° outside the fovea. The circulation of this paper has been very limited, and where it is cited in treatises on physiological optics, one generally finds only a brief summary that far from exhausts the rich material of the original.

Among the 7 observers in this study there were only 3 (A, B and H) who fixated correctly, B observing separately with both of her eyes. The mean values obtained for 4 eyes, for test field diameters from 1.33 minutes of arc up to 8.10°, show that spatial summation increases steadily from the foveal center to the 35° peripheral position, where it attains a diameter of the order of 2°. These results are consistent with those of the authors cited above, but they are more complete and representative.

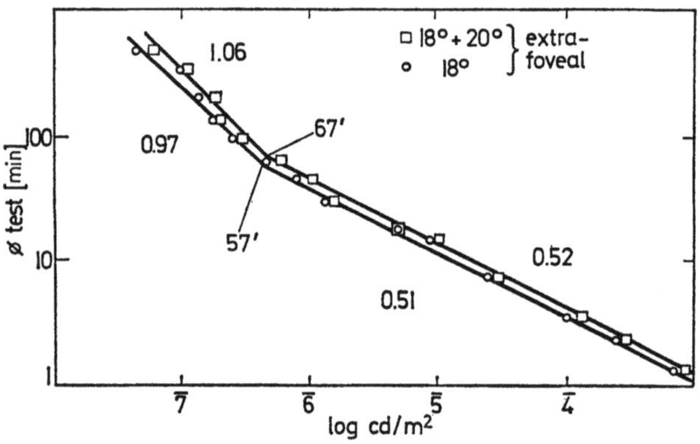

Fig. 4. Liminal test diameter as a function of test luminance. White stimuli at 18° and 20° peripherally, steady stimulation (3 eyes: 18°; 2 eyes: 20°). For small test diameters, Riccò's law applies; between about 1° and 3°, Piper's square-root law fits the measured points. Plotted from numerical results in WEINSTEIN and ARNULF (1946)

Fig. 4 shows the mean results for 3 eyes for the 18° retinal position, and the main results for the same 3 eyes together with those for 2 additional eyes at 20° peripherally. Spatial summation appears to be complete up to about 62 minutes of arc in test field diameter. The corresponding values for 7°, 12°, and 35° are respectively: 32′, 45′, 1°58′. At 12°, there were only 2 observers (3 eyes), but we have added the results for observer H at the 10° peripheral position. There is not enough space to show all the graphical data. It suffices here to emphasize that the *mean* of the slopes of all regression lines calculated by computer for test field diameters greater than, respectively, 32′, 45′, 62′, 1°58′ (for the four different eyes) fits Piper's law very precisely. This means that the absorption of about 8 quanta within a retinal area that contains roughly 10,000 rods (see ØSTERBERG, 1935), may trigger a threshold sensation. Let us call A_0 (square degrees or deg²) the limiting area such that for retinal areas less than or equal to A_0, Riccò's law holds.

B. Bloch's Law of Complete Temporal Summation

Bloch (1885) showed that the threshold is constant if the stimulus duration is less than a certain limit τ. This law is sometimes erroneously called the Bunsen-Roscoe law, which applies to photochemical reactions. At threshold, the range within which Bloch's law holds may depend on retinal location, wavelength and the angle subtended by the stimulus.

In foveal vision, Herrick (1956) reports that $\tau = 99$ milliseconds (ms) for scotopic supra-threshold levels. Johnson and Bartlett (1956) show that in the human ERG, for criterion *b*-wave amplitude at low luminances, $I \times t =$ a constant, where I is the liminal energy, if $t \leqq 100$ ms. For zero background luminance and a test field of 5.9 degrees subtense, Barlow (1958b) found total summation up to 100 ms. Clark and Blackwell (1959) (see also Blackwell, 1963) report results indicating that $\tau = 87$ ms at threshold, and Thomas (1965), in a study of Mach-bands, shows that τ is approximately 80 ms even for supra-threshold conditions. Thus τ appears to be of the order of 100 ms in foveal vision at threshold.

In peripheral vision at 12° from the fovea, for a white test stimulus of 1.2 degrees diameter, Bloch's law holds for durations as low as 4×10^{-6} seconds (Baumgardt, 1949). A device described by Baumgardt and Segal (1946) was used for this research. Brindley (1952) showed Bloch's law to hold down to 4×10^{-7} seconds. The upper limit for Bloch's law is 100 ms according to Baumgardt and Hillmann (1961) who showed that this law holds for "red" and "blue-green" light at 20 degrees from the fovea for circular test fields that varied between 3.43 minutes and 8 degrees in diameter. Barlow (1958b) gets the same result up to 27.6 deg² of test area, at 6°30′ from the fixation point.

We may thus adopt a time limit of $\tau = 100$ ms so that for stimulus durations $t \leqq \tau$ total energy summation occurs, i.e., for these durations the absolute threshold energy is the lowest possible, for foveal as well as peripheral vision, at least up to 20 degrees away from the fovea.

C. Piper's Law of Partial Spatial Summation

Piper's (1903) law describes a relation of partial summation, i.e., the square-root law of summation. Let E_A be the threshold energy, A the stimulated retinal area, then Piper's law states that

$$E_A = E_0 \times A^{-0.5},$$

where E_0 corresponds to $A \leqq A_0$.

The generality of this law is no longer assumed, for it certainly does not necessarily hold if the retinal structures are non-homogeneous throughout the stimulated area, as pointed out by Hallett (1963). But even under these conditions it *may* hold, as shown by Baumgardt (1959). Fig. 5 demonstrates a typical case of Piper's law. No power other than -0.5 can describe the results.

It is clear that Piper's law does not immediately take over from Riccò's law when A increases and becomes larger than A_0, as shown by Hillmann (1958). When $\log E_A$ is plotted as a function of $\log A$, the slope of the resulting curve is -1 for the Riccò part and -0.5 for the Piper part. Between these two regions, an intermediate segment of the function has slopes between these two values. Finally, when A becomes very large, E_A = a constant, which corresponds to the absolute threshold determinations by PIRENNE *et al.* (1957), for test stimuli of 47 degrees in diameter. Since Piper's law cannot hold within very large areas unless they are

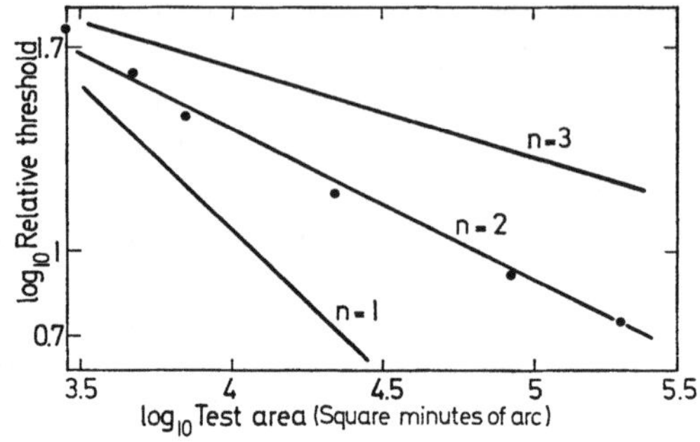

Fig. 5A

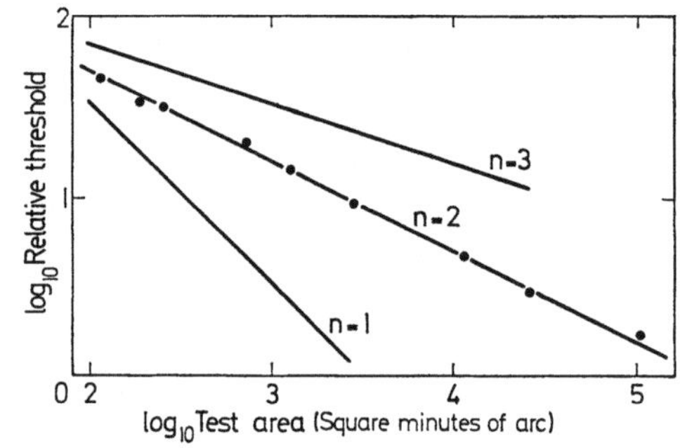

Fig. 5B

Fig. 5. A: Piper's square-root law applies for 479 nm stimulation for test diameters from 1° up to 8°; B: The same law applies for 670 nm stimulation from 12.3′ of arc up to 6°. Both experiments: 15° peripherally (after BAUMGARDT, 1960)

centered on the fovea – in this case this law may, but does not necessarily, hold – one cannot assume any single uniform law for test stimuli of diameters greater than 8°, even if their centers are sufficiently far from the fovea (BAUMGARDT and HILLMANN, 1961). It is highly probably that the same result would be obtained if the stimulus were projected at a 14-degree instead of a 20-degree peripheral retinal position, since the retinal structure does not change very much between 10 and 24 degrees peripherically.

D. The Inverse-Square Law of Partial Temporal Summation

This law is the temporal counterpart of Piper's law. It was proposed by VAN DER VELDEN (1944) and shown by him to apply. For reasons which are probably only partially the same as for Piper's law, it holds only up to limited values of the independent variable t, and for higher values the relation shifts to E_t = a constant.

Of particular difficulty here are involuntary eye-movements and blinks, as well as multiple stimulus detections. Thus it is not clear what value should be taken for t such that for higher values of t, E_t = a constant. It certainly is equal to or greater than 1 second, as shown by BAUMGARDT and HILLMANN, and by KECK (1937) who used 2 flashes of 20 ms duration each, and presumably used foveal vision, notwithstanding the absence of a fixation device. KECK finds partial summation at threshold up to 3 seconds. BAUMGARDT and HILLMANN obtained measures only up to 1 second, and found square- or cube-root laws between 100 ms and 1 second. For long exposure times, where summation is only partial, BLONDEL and REY (1911) propose an empirical relation called Blondel and Rey's law:

$$E \times t = E_\infty (t + t_0),$$

where E_∞ is the threshold for indefinitely long exposures, and t_0 is a time constant. Studies by PIÉRON (1920a, b) have shown that the results are better described by the relation

$$E \times t^n = \text{a constant},$$

where n is different in the fovea ($n = 2/3$) from its values in extra-foveal parts of the retina. No dependence on wavelength is observed.

E. Summation Laws for Large and Long-Lasting Stimuli

Little work that is very precise has been done concerning these issues. The early measures of GRAHAM and MARGARIA (1935) are at variance with the values of BAUMGARDT and HILLMANN, who tried to explain why the former investigators (whose "neutral" filters were probably spectrally selective) had found Bloch's law to hold only for very small values of t, when A was increased. GRAHAM and MARGARIA's measures are at variance with BARLOW's figures (1958b) as well. BAUMGARDT and HILLMANN's results are shown in Fig. 6.

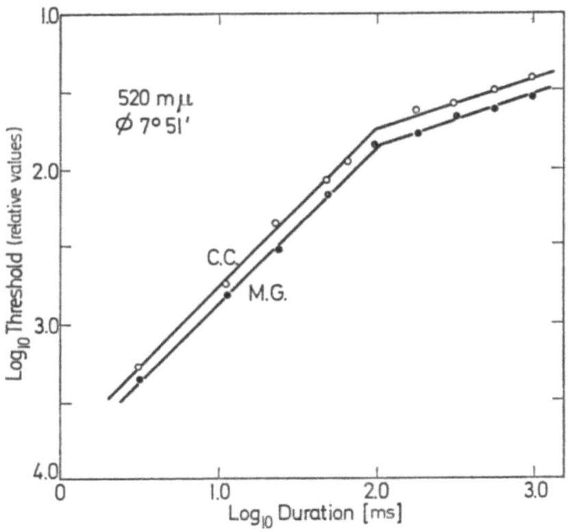

Fig. 6. The intensity-time relation at 20° peripherally; $\lambda = 520$ nm. It clearly appears that for both observers, Bloch's law holds precisely up to 100 ms, even for a test size of 7° 51′, i.e., 48.6 square degrees (from BAUMGARDT and HILLMANN, 1961)

Since the mid-1950's, there has been a tendency to show that, even at absolute threshold, A_0 and τ are not independent constants, i.e., that they are not really constants. One of the best known studies of this issue is that of Barlow cited

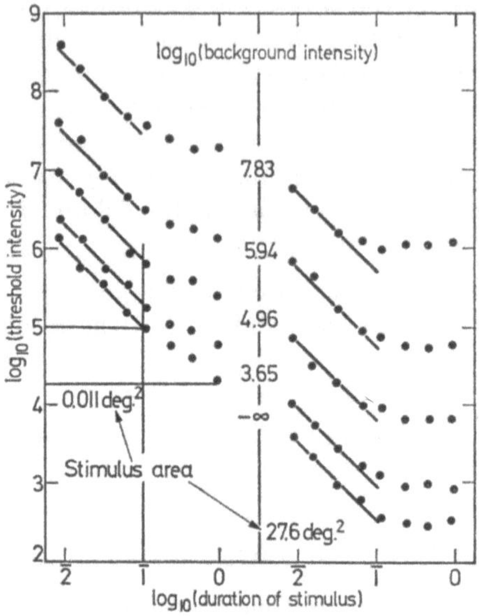

Fig. 7A

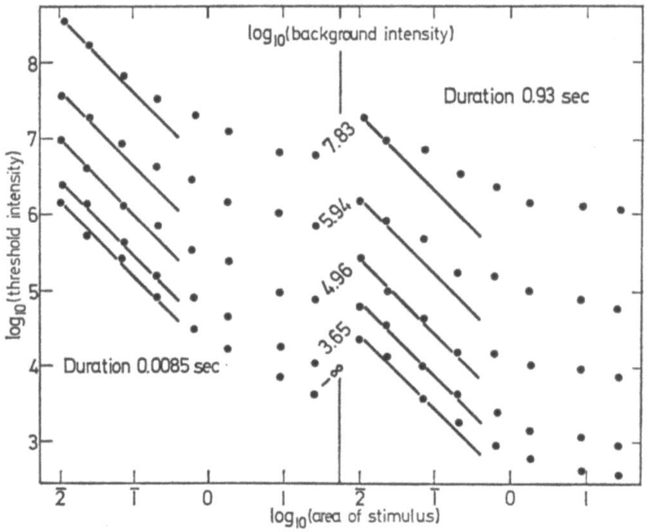

Fig. 7B

Fig. 7. A: Temporal summation at incremental and absolute threshold for a circular field centered 6° 30′ from the fixation point. Duration in seconds. The straight lines have gradient —1. Note that in dark-adaptation the greatest duration at which complete summation occurs is not significantly different for the 0.011 deg² field and the 27.6 deg² field. B: Spatial summation at incremental and absolute threshold for a circular field centered 6° 30′ from the fixation point. Areas in degrees. The straight lines have gradient − 1. For short flashes, Riccò's law holds up to a value between 0.2 deg² and 0.6 deg² (after Barlow, 1958b)

above. He showed that for supra-threshold levels, A_0 and τ tend toward lower values, and that with a 27.6 deg² field, there is no temporal summation for $t > 0.1$ second. His figures do not show any significant difference at zero background luminance between τ for a 0.011 deg² field and τ for a 27.6 deg² field. His graphs show a trend but no more. See Fig. 7. This becomes particularly clear when we examine his plot of log threshold luminance for a 100 ms flash of 0.011 deg² on a zero background field. This value reads about 5.0, and for a flash of 1-second duration the value is about 4.27, which makes a difference of 0.73 log unit. This difference is too high by at least 0.25, probably even 0.30, (Baumgardt and Hillmann, 1961; also unpublished results obtained by Baumgardt and Ferlampin).

In the next and final section, we will discuss the fundamental question of whether the absolute threshold is determined by quantum fluctuation, or if it is due, more or less, to intrinsic noise. If the latter point of view is adopted, the absolute threshold is equivalent to an increment threshold on a zero background field, i.e., there would be no "real" absolute threshold. On the contrary, if one considers the absolute threshold as determined by the mean number of nervous events related to quantum absorptions at the lowest possible sensation level, there is a "real" absolute threshold.

In Section V, we will mention or discuss some of the most important contributions to this particularly interesting and difficult problem. Indeed vision is only one of the many senses, and it is highly probable that real absolute thresholds either exist or do not exist for all of them. Thus our problem is in fact a fundamental one.

V. Are Absolute Thresholds Increment Thresholds?

A. Theories Based on the Assumption that Absolute Thresholds are Limited by Intrinsic Noise

Fechner (1860) suggested that detection of a stimulus might be limited by the intrinsic noise of the visual system. In fact, in complete dark adaptation, the visual field does not appear black, but all observers report visual sensations which are variously referred to as „Eigengrau", „Eigenlicht", „Augenschwarz", "cloudy appearance", etc. We know that "black" can be perceived only by contrast, and that it is due to a phenomenon of neural inhibition.

Noise has been studied intensively by engineers since the Second World War, particularly in order to improve electronic devices such as photocells, photomultipliers, etc. This type of technical research is probably at the origin of numerous currently popular theories of detection. Here we can simply mention some of them, e.g., Blackwell (1963), Blakemore and Rushton (1965), de Vries (1943), Green and Swets (1966), Pirenne (1944), Rose (1948), Swets (1961), Swets *et al.* (1961), and Tanner and Swets (1954). (See also chapters 3 and 4 by Nachmias and Blackwell.) We will discuss here the representative work of Barlow 1956, 1957, 1958a, b), of Denton and Pirenne (1954), of Treisman (1964, 1966), of Treisman and Watts (1966), and in the second part of this section we will comment on them.

Hecht (1945) suggested that the effect of a single light quantum might be confused with a spontaneous excitation occurring in a single rod, but that a critical number of such spontaneous events in a given retinal area and at a given time would be quite improbable. He thus appears as the precursor of modern noise theories. Denton and Pirenne took a second step in this direction. They calculated an *upper limit* of spontaneously activated rhodopsin molecules *in situ* which they thought likely to be at the origin of intrinsic noise, and the value they found was 44 molecules per 0.1 second per deg^2.

In their calculation, Denton and Pirenne make the assumption that a signal is perceived if its value is at least 3 times the standard deviation of the noise. This value is reasonable, for it results in not more than 3% false positives. This is a false-alarm rate which 5 of the 7 very reliable observers of Hecht *et al.*, and of Baumgardt (1960) did not reach and which was slightly exceeded by 2 of them.

Thus, Denton and Pirenne adapted a signal-to-noise theory to vision, but they concluded that the effective noise in the retina may be of negligible importance even at absolute threshold. If we want to calculate a *probable* noise level rather than an upper limit, the proportion of 500 nm radiation incident on the retina that is absorbed by the rods should be put at 0.21 instead of 0.10. This accords with the results of Rushton (1956) who measured the rod density of man *in situ* and found a value of 0.15 at about 500 nm, and it also takes into account the fact that 70% of the retinal area is covered with rods between about 10 and 25 degrees outside the fovea (at 7 degrees this proportion is slightly smaller). Moreover, the threshold energy content of the conditions assumed by Denton and Pirenne – retinal area stimulated 1 deg^2, stimulus duration 0.1 second – is certainly less than 100 quanta, most probably near 80 rather than near 200 quanta. When these values are substituted for those of Denton and Pirenne, the *probable noise* per functional unit of 1 deg^2, during the exposure of 0.1 second, would be about 18 quanta rather than 44. The threshold would be $3 \times \sqrt{18} = 12.75$ mean quantum absorptions which is, however, about 60% too high. Only the use of a lower signal/noise level at threshold (1.87 instead of 3) could make the noise hypothesis fit with experiment, but this would necessarily reduce the observer's reliability and introduce a false-positive rate of 6.2%, which is unacceptable.

Barlow (1956) suggests that noise in the optic pathway limits its sensitivity, and he subjects this idea to an experimental test. He formulates his noise hypothesis quantitatively and attempts to show that it can account for his experimental results. He calculates the "maximum allowable noise", which is expressed as a number x of random, independent events that are confusable with the absorption of a quantum of radiation.

Barlow's fundamental assumption is that the absolute threshold is, in fact, a threshold of discrimination or an increment threshold. (See Barlow, chapter 1, this volume, for the application of this view to adaptation.) The background field is not external, but an internal "black" light, possibly caused by thermal decomposition of rhodopsin molecules contained in the rods. He thus follows very closely Denton and Pirenne, but he does not agree with their hypothesis that the noise to be accounted for might be the "smaller" noise of a functional neural sub-unit, even linked to a larger one, if the stimulus field is projected onto this sub-unit only. BARLOW (1957) very clearly assumes that the noise that limits threshold is due to the largest independent neural unit present, even if the test stimulus "covers" only a part of it.

BARLOW'S (1956) experiment consists in measuring the absolute threshold under conditions similar to those used by HECHT *et al.*, i.e., dark adaptation, peripheral vision 20 degrees nasal to the fixation point, stimulus duration 2.4 ms, diameter 7.5′ of arc, light beam 2.1 mm diameter entering the center of the natural pupil, narrow-band radiation centered at 495 nm. He used five stimulus levels, each presented 100 times, as well as 300 flashes of zero luminance (blanks). The observer had to answer "seen", "not seen", or "possibly seen"; he never reported a blank as "seen", and among the 300 blanks reported only 3 as "possibly seen".

BARLOW plots two curves for this experiment, one to describe the "seens", the other the "seens" and "possibly seens". On the basis of his noise hypothesis, the author shows that the number of confusable events, x, per deg^2 and per 0.1 second (summation-area and summation-time limits) lies between 11 and 90, as a function of the fraction F of radiant energy impinging on the retina which is absorbed in the rods. (We should remember that quanta exist only during their emission and their absorption). The best fit is for $x = 19$, which would lead to a threshold of about 130 quanta at the cornea, i.e., a possible but quite high figure. Analyzing the results of HECHT *et al.*, and of VAN DER VELDEN, BARLOW finds that the former's observers should have shown a false-alarm rate of 0.04% (in fact, this rate was zero throughout these experiments), whereas the latter's data indicate a false-alarm rate of 3.83%. Analyzing HECHT'S results further, BARLOW finds that for a fraction $n/N = 0.10$ of absorbed quanta, N being the equivalent quantum number on the cornea, and n the number of quanta absorbed in the rods, the highest permissible value of x is 9.7. We note that BARLOW makes the transmission factor of the ocular media equal to 0.75, which is higher than the values measured by LUDVIGH and MACCARTHY and by SAÏD and WEALE. (See also RUDDOCK, chapter 17, this volume.)

BARLOW concludes by stating that noise in the optic pathways as a limiting factor in the sensitivity of the eye to visible radiation is a likely idea *a priori* in view of its sensitivity, that this idea is supported by the finding of noise signals in the optic nerve of animals, and that it explains quantitatively why the measured threshold is lowered by reducing the reliability of the oberver's responses.

BARLOW (1957) applies his hypothesis to results with low background luminances, by considering increment thresholds as signal/noise discriminations. He does not take into account the thesis of DE VRIES, who states that the increment threshold is at a level as low as is compatible with the variability of the number of photons absorbed in the receptor (see also ROSE). Indeed, AGUILAR and STILES (1954) had already shown that these theories cannot account quantitatively for the psychophysical data at supra-threshold levels. BARLOW'S aim is to present a unique theory of increment thresholds, including absolute thresholds, as the last of a series that covers the whole scotopic range of vision or at least an important part of this range. Such a theory must also explain Piper's law, which states that within certain limits the threshold luminance is inversely proportional to the square root of the angular diameter of the test stimulus.

BARLOW proposes two hypotheses that concern increment thresholds at low levels, including absolute thresholds:

a) If the signal/noise ratio (uncertainty of the response) is constant, it is probable that the fluctuation of additional quanta required for a threshold signal is proportional to $n^{1/2}$.

b) If additional "intrinsic noise" exists in the visual pathway, the increment ΔI should level off at the absolute threshold.

Let

N be the threshold incremental radiation expressed in quanta entering the eye,

X[3] "dark light", i.e., the background luminance that, because of the fluctuations in the number of quanta absorbed, would have the same effect on the incremental threshold as the intrinsic retinal noise itself,

F the fraction of radiation entering the eye that is absorbed by the rods,

α the retinal area within which background radiation (or retinal noise) is likely to be confused with the test stimulus,

τ the time (duration) during which the background light is likely to be confused with the stimulus,

K the reliability factor = signal/noise ratio of threshold responses.

If there is no stimulus, the mean number of events liable to be confused with the effective absorption of a quantum of light from a stimulus is $F\alpha\tau\ (I + X)$. If this number is fairly large, the normal distribution of the standard deviation, which is the square root of the mean, is a reasonable approximation of the Poisson distribution which really applies. At threshold, if $F \times \Delta N$ quanta are absorbed, then according to BARLOW's hypothesis:

$$F \cdot \Delta N = K\ [F\alpha\tau\ (I + X)^{1/2} \quad \text{or}$$

$$\Delta N = (I + X)^{1/2} \cdot K\ (\alpha\tau/F)^{1/2}.$$

The experimental conditions to test these hypotheses include: 1 observer, flash area 0.011 deg^2, flash duration 8.6 ms, $\lambda = 507$ nm, energy level I in quanta/second/deg^2. Thus in Fig. 3 of BARLOW's (1957) paper, the theoretical curve is fitted to the experimental points, and the slopes for the low energy part and for the higher energy part should show the transition at an abscissa value equal to X, as shown by a cross.

The lumped parameter $K\ (\alpha\tau/F)^{1/2}$ is found to be 3.3, and 2.95 for another observer whose experimental results are not given in the paper[4].

For subject 1, $X = 1260$, for subject 2, $X = 2500$. In Table 1, estimations of X based on experiments by AGUILAR and STILES and by BARLOW (1957) yield values of X that range from 200 to 3200. The experiments cited share the common condition (not true of the others shown in this table) that the test stimulus duration was less than or only slightly greater than τ. K seems to vary within narrow limits. Putting $K = 3$, one finds

$$3 \times 200^{1/2} \leq \Delta N \leq 3 \times 3200^{1/2}, \quad \text{or}$$

$$42 \leq \Delta N \leq 170,$$

[3] X is now used by BARLOW, instead of x as in his 1956 paper.

[4] Note that BARLOW puts $\alpha\tau/F = 1$; thus K is 3.3 or 2.95, respectively.

which is not very far from the values actually measured for the lowest threshold expressed in quanta at about 507 nm, and thus approximately compatible with this type of experiment.

BARLOW (1957, p. 480) notes that background radiation "usually" increases the threshold. He considers this an argument in favor of his explanation, since alternative hypotheses might lead one to expect that a faint background radiation might be able to decrease the threshold. The latter idea is described by him as "naive", but he did not test it himself, since he was persuaded that signal/noise theories alone are able to describe and to explain the experimental facts. In the last part of this chapter we shall discuss this point.

BARLOW (1957) does not exclude the possibility that later on in the chain of events that terminate in the subject either seeing or not seeing the stimulus, random fluctuation may be the factor that more or less limits the threshold. He obviously uses the idea of DENTON and PIRENNE – that thermal breakdown of rhodopsin could be considered to be threshold-limiting – as a simple possibility that is easier to handle than hypothetical intrinsic noise later on in the visual pathway.

BARLOW (1958a) discusses experiments in which "green" stimuli on a "red" background and "red" stimuli on a "green" background are presented more or less foveally. He shows that his noise theory applies when the test stimulus is of short duration and small area. Some other factors must enter in the case of stimuli of long duration and large area, and the author assumes that these factors might be responsible for the ubiquitous tendency for Weber's law to show up. He states finally that "the cone mechanisms have a dark light about 10^3 to 10^5 times as high as the rods", and he adds that "this is, of course, just another way of saying that cones are less sensitive than rods". In fact, BARLOW believes that cones are less sensitive than rods by $\sqrt{10^3}$ to $\sqrt{10^5}$, i.e., 31 to 310 times. We know from experiment that this view is erroneous.

The last paper of BARLOW (1958b) that we shall discuss in this chapter is concerned with temporal and spatial summation in vision at different background luminances. Two series of experiments are described, each with one observer. In the first series, temporal summation is measured as a function of background luminance. In one half-series, the author uses a stimulus of 0.011 deg², in the second half-series, the stimulus area is 27.6 deg².

As pointed out earlier, up to 100 ms there is no significant difference between the slopes of the functions for the two sizes (log threshold energy is plotted as a function of log stimulus duration). This interpretation is at variance with that of BRINDLEY (1960), who notes that "the greatest duration at which complete summation occurs (gradient -1) is slightly shorter . . . for large fields than for small".

Since we are not concerned here with background levels that are really suprathreshold, we may turn to the second series of experiments, where spatial summation is measured as a function of background luminance, for a short duration (0.0085 second) and for a long duration (0.93 second). For the short duration, complete summation holds up to a value somewhere between 0.2 and 0.6 deg² – there are no intermediate measurements – which is compatible with the results reported above.

To sum up briefly: BARLOW states that intrinsic noise is the limiting factor for threshold, and he is able to find parameters such that his formula fits some experimental results for limited values of A, t and E, but he does not propose a general relation covering an appreciably larger scale of values of A, t and E that are still within the scotopic range of vision.

TREISMAN (1964, 1966) and TREISMAN and WATTS (1966) use the concept of threshold limited by noise to treat the discrimination of brightnesses, Weber's law together with a square-root law for low stimulus luminances, the relation between signal detectability theories, and traditional procedures for measuring sensory thresholds. The most important paper of TREISMAN (1966) offers a complete statistical decision model for sensory discrimination that predicts Riccò's and Piper's laws, Bloch's law, and, finally, Weber's law.

TREISMAN makes the assumption that noise arises from the irreducible physical variability of light, from spontaneous neural firing, and from variations in transmission in the afferent visual pathways. His model is simulated on a computer and predicts the form of the Weber function and the features of spatial and temporal summation.

TREISMAN (1964) bases his theory on criterion selection. Related to this criterion is the term $z\,\sigma_E$, where σ_E is the standard deviation of the noise distribution, and z is the standardized normal deviate which assures that the Neyman-Pearson requirement is met (TREISMAN, 1967). He shows that the false-positive rate may change considerably as a function of σ_E and of z, but one does not know if and how σ_E is related to the value of z. Thus, if the false-positive rate alone is known, one cannot calculate σ_E nor the hypothetical intrinsic noise. In a personal communication, TREISMAN (1967) considers the case of observers who are supposed never to give false-positive answers. This was the case for three observers of HECHT *et al.*, and for two out of four observers of BAUMGARDT (1960). Considering experiments each including the presentation of 600 blank trials, he shows that the probability that a subject will give no false positives at all in such an experiment is only 0.02 when z has a value of 2.5, but that if this value increases to 3.5, the probability that the subject will give no false positives at all will rise to 0.87. Quite small variations in z could substantially influence the observer's reliability, independently of his internal noise level. Thus, z appears to be a personal criterion which would be expected to vary with reward and punishment, for instance. In TREISMAN's theory as well as in BARLOW's, the false-positive rate is closely linked to the threshold. It appears that high false-positive rates should result in anomalously low threshold measures. It will be seen later that this does not correspond to the results obtained by systematic research in this field.

TREISMAN (1966) formulates a general equation (1)[5] from which he derives two particular solutions:

$$\Delta I = \frac{z}{g}\sqrt{g^2 v^2 (I_1 + I_n)^2 + g(I_1 + I_n) + v^2 g(I_1 + I_n)} \qquad (1)$$

[5] At absolute threshold, $I_n = 0$. TREISMAN adopts the reasonable value of 0.1 for v (whose meaning cannot be explained here), g is the lumped parameter $f A t$, which is of the order of 0.01 at the absolute threshold, but about 0.5 for test stimuli of 8° in diameter and 0.1 second in duration.

a) For faint or zero background luminances, the threshold ΔI is a constant at absolute threshold, increases with the background luminance, and finally is approximately proportional to the square root of the background luminance.

b) For background luminances I high enough to permit the second and third terms of the general equation to be neglected, Weber's law results.

The author shows that an increase in any of the three quantities, A, t and I, causes an increase in ΔI, and this generally happens, but not always (see also under B. Critical discussion); the predicted increase of ΔI as a function of A seems to fit some data very approximately but not others. Indeed, for a test patch of 8 degrees in diameter, Piper's law holds quite well, but according to TREISMAN's general formula it should not.

B. Critical Discussion

In this last section, we will review critically the so-called "physical quantum theories" as well as the most representative signal/noise theories of absolute thresholds and increment thresholds on faint backgrounds.

As an example of physical quantum theory, we may cite HECHT *et al.* (1942). Their explanation takes into account only the random distribution of incident quanta in order to explain the uncertainty of threshold in dark adaptation. These authors do not try to explain either Piper's law (the square-root law) of spatial summation nor the corresponding temporal law.

VAN DER VELDEN (1944) and BOUMAN and VAN DER VELDEN (1947) developed the two-quanta theory which explains these laws but, as we showed above, their theory does not fit the experimental data, for the slopes of all probability-of-seeing curves (psychometric functions) measured by all authors, including their own, point to values greater than $n = 2$.

Independently of VAN DER VELDEN and using a different mathematical approach, BAUMGARDT (1949), too, proposed a two-quanta theory, but abandoned it later for a modified theory. BAUMGARDT (1952, 1953) showed that Piper's square-root law holds even when more than two quantum absorptions are needed for a target to become visible at absolute threshold. He made the assumption that a number u of two-quantum absorptions is needed, where u: 2, 3, ... The idea underlying this hypothesis is that two quantum absorptions but not one, can trigger an action potential, and that more than one action potential is needed to evoke a light sensation. This hypothesis also explains the temporal summation square-root law but, like all other threshold theories, "physical quantum theories" as well as "signal/noise theories", it cannot explain why this law breaks down somewhere between 1 and 3 seconds of test duration.

It should be emphasized here that BAUMGARDT only treats thresholds for complete dark adaptation. BRINDLEY (1960) discusses this several-quantum hypothesis. He comments that, although this hypothesis accounts for a wide range of observations and has not yet been disproved, it cannot account for increment thresholds of, say, ten times the absolute threshold. This is because "the number of quanta absorbed from these incremental stimuli must be very nearly ten times the number absorbed at absolute threshold, so that their detection cannot then depend on the scoring of twofold coincidences". He does not believe it very plausible to suppose that the same law of spatial and temporal summation depends on one mechanism at absolute threshold, but on an entirely different mechanism at increment thresholds. This criticism is entirely justified, but we now know with certainty from Rushton's many publications that one quantum absorption always excites the same rod response, whereas the weight of this local response in the nervous pool diminishes with light adaptation. We thus are led to a more sophisticated hypothesis, where the two-quantum coincidence becomes in fact a two "nervous event" coincidence. It is possible and even probable that between the "quantum bumps" of the rods which have been shown to exist in *Limulus* by Yeandle (1958), and the action potential leaving the ganglion cell towards the supra-retinal centers, there is a gain-control mechanism which may, at increment threshold, reduce the sum of the quantum bumps to two nervous events. There need be only two quantum bumps at the absolute threshold, but they would have to become more and more numerous as light adaptation progresses and sensitivity diminishes.

The partisans of the signal/noise hypothesis try to develop generalized theories covering a large range of values of the parameters A, t and I, including $I = 0$ and A and t small enough to reach the lowest possible absolute threshold, i.e., the smallest possible quantum number. A common aspect of these theories is that they reject any possibility of "summation" or "addition" of quanta contained in the background field and quanta contained in the test stimulus. The possibility of such "summation", which appears to Barlow (1957) to be a "naive" idea, has been tested by Baumgardt (1959) and by Baumgardt and Smith (1965). The later experiment was a repetition of the earlier one and employed 4 observers and a forced-choice method. Since 2 of their observers knew the reason for the experiment, they were careful to exclude factors that might influence the results. The results, which confirmed Baumgardt (1959), showed:

1) Addition of background quanta and test quanta occurred for 2 of the 4 observers, whereas Baumgardt (1959) using a "yes-no" method had found this for both of his observers. Baumgardt, however, did not use random stimulus presentation but blocks of equal intensity.

2) Neither of the 2 observers who showed no "addition" effect showed any variation of their threshold in the presence of a sub-threshold background. Calculation shows that this was a significant result, since the hypothetical threshold elevation calculated according to Barlow's (1957) theory was more than 3 σ, and thus would easily have been detected.

The background diameter in both experiments was just a little larger than the 1° test patch. The test stimulus duration was 1 second. It is evident that, to test whether or not there is "addition", one must choose conditions such that, if the effect exists, its relative value, i.e., the luminance as compared with the threshold luminance in complete dark adaptation, would be as different as possible. Furthermore, the time interval during which it is possible for background quanta to be added to the test quanta must be as long as possible, i.e., the test duration should be long. There is no reason why these conditions should weaken the value of the author's conclusions, as suggested by Pirenne (1962). Indeed, Barlow (1957) explicitly specifies that the intrinsic noise X that might be confused with the stimulus is the noise of the functional nervous unit(s) of the tested retinal spot. Thus, following BARLOW himself, the noise of units situated outside the tested area is not confusable with the test stimulus.

In BAUMGARDT and SMITH'S experiment, the test field was exposed between 7.6° and 10° peripherally. During two sessions, one of the authors (who did not himself show the addition effect) arranged the angular projection of the test field in such a way that it was no longer centered on the sub-threshold background, but 1.5° to the side of the latter. This arrangement was not revealed to the other observers who, naturally, could not become perceptually aware of it. Under these circumstances the addition effect was totally absent. This is supplementary proof for the cleanness of the effect and it shows that no "psychological" factor is responsible for it.

Since 1958, many studies have been reported by BARLOW, BARLOW and SPARROCK, and by RUSHTON and his co-workers, concerning intrinsic noise and its consequences, especially for Weber's law. These studies are generally concerned with high illumination levels, hence we shall not consider them here. It may interest the reader that Weber's law can be observed under appropriate conditions very near absolute threshold, as shown by CORNSWEET and PINSKER (1965). MUNTZ and NORTHMORE (1968), in a study of the turtle, observed a law of the type $\Delta I = K(I + X)$, where ΔI is also a function of temperature. They are not certain that they obtained measures of absolute threshold (MUNTZ, personal communication), but they believe they were quite near this point. As evidence for this, MUNTZ cites the form of the dotted curve in their Fig. 4. Since there are only 3 abscissa values in the figure, any curve form and any type of interpretation are possible, and the argument is weak insofar as threshold or near-threshold values are concerned.

The spontaneous activity of the ganglion cells is naturally one of the essential arguments invoked in order to explain intrinsic noise as threshold-limiting. Some authors consider this noise as linked to spontaneous receptor activity as well as to the presence of free opsins in previously light-adapted receptors during their dark adaptation. The experimental evidence is not conclusive with respect to these more or less speculative hypotheses. KUFFLER *et al.* (1957) describe maintained activity in the cat's retina in light and in darkness. HUGHES and MAFFEI (1965) do not find any relation between spontaneous ganglion cell discharge frequency and threshold during dark adaptation, and they conclude that, if the threshold is limited by intrinsic noise, the "noise" is not the ganglion cell discharge. ARDUINI and PINNEO (1962) show that the optic nerve activity diminishes in light adaptation, whereas RODIECK (1967) shows that chemical destruction of the receptors diminishes the spontaneous activity of the ganglion cells. When recording from isolated ganglion cells, he finds that light adaptation increases the ganglion cells' discharge. The frequency difference is only slight, but this result is at variance with ARDUINI and PINNEO'S finding. ERNST (1968) shows that a luminous background and the after-effect of light adaptation do not always act in the same manner on critical flicker frequency and rod threshold, and NAKA and RUSHTON (1968) find that a real light background affects the S-potential, but the equivalent background of bleaching does not. Thus they cannot both be represented by similar signals in the same pathway. These authors conclude: "... little is known of the background signal and nothing on the free-opsin signal".

It has been pointed out that signal/noise theories necessarily link the observer's reliability (false-positive rate) to his threshold, and also that any real background necessarily must increase the threshold. After BARLOW (1956) had tested the first point on a single observer in an experiment with a total of 300 blank trials. BITTINI and GLORIA (1968) tried to obtain a definitive answer to this really important question. They used 4 observers and collected a considerable amount of data. Their conclusion is that there is no strict correlation between the threshold data and the false-alarm rate. A decrease in threshold sometimes corresponds to an increase, and sometimes to a decrease in the false-alarm rate.

Finally, we mention BORNSCHEIN (1951) who studied dark-adapted threshold variation as a function of time. He found considerable intra-observer variation, but the particularly interesting point is that these variations were periodic in several of his observers and that their time constant was of the order of some minutes.

There is no doubt that we do not really know precisely what determines the absolute threshold under the best possible conditions. But many well-established facts are at variance with the signal/noise hypothesis as applied to absolute threshold. Moreover, BARLOW (1965) remarks that "As the background is increased above about 100 quanta sec^{-1} deg^{-2} at the cornea the increment threshold at first rises according to a square root law", even though signal/noise theories require that this rise must start as soon as any background is present, however weak. We are, therefore, coming to the conclusion that signal/noise theories do not apply at absolute threshold. Thus, for the time being and until new experiments enrich our knowledge, we should consider that quantum noise is the most importtant factor that limits absolute thresholds, which does not mean at all that it is the unique factor.

References

ADOLPH, A. R.: Spontaneous slow potential fluctuations in the *Limulus* photoreceptor. J. gen. Physiol. **48**, 297—322 (1964).

AGUILAR, M., STILES, W. S.: Saturation of the rod mechanism of the retina at high levels of stimulation. Optica Acta **1**, 59—66 (1954).

ARDUINI, A., PINNEO, L. R.: Properties of the retina in response to steady illumination. Arch. ital. Biol. **100**, 425—448 (1962).

BARLOW, H. B.: Retinal noise and absolute threshold. J. opt. Soc. Amer. **46**, 634—639 (1956).

— Increment thresholds at low intensities considered as signal/noise discriminations. J. Physiol. (Lond.) **136**, 469—488 (1957).

— Intrinsic noise of cones. In: Visual Problems of Colour. Vol. 2, pp. 615—630. London: H. M. Stationery Office 1958a.

— Temporal and spatial summation in human vision at different background intensities. J. Physiol. (Lond.) **141**, 337—350 (1958b).

— Optic nerve impulses and Weber's law. Cold Spr. Harb. Symp. quant. Biol. **30**, 539—546 (1965).

BARNES, R. B., CZERNY, M.: Läßt sich ein Schroteffekt der Photonen mit dem Auge beobachten? Z. Phys. **79**, 436—449 (1932).

BAUMGARDT, E.: Les théories photochimiques classiques et quantiques de la vision et l'inhibition nerveuse en vision liminaire. Revue opt. **28**, Partie théorique 453—479; Partie experimentale 661—690 (1949).

Baumgardt, E.: Sehmechanismus und Quantenstruktur des Lichtes. Naturwissenschaften **39**, 388—393 (1952).
— Seuils visuels et quanta lumineux. Précisions. Ann. Psychol. (Paris) **53**, 431—441 (1953).
— Sur le caractère aléatoire de l'absorption des photons. C. R. Acad. Sci. (Paris) **245**, 2236—2238 (1957).
— Visual spatial and temporal summation. Nature (Lond.) **184**, 1951—1952 (1959).
— La nature statistique et aléatoire des flux lumineux extrêmement faibles et leur incidence sur la vision de nuit. Publication du Comité International de l'Eclairage No 4, 78—89 (1960).
— Hillmann, B. M.: Duration and size as determinants of peripheral retinal response. J. opt. Soc. Amer. **51**, 340—344 (1961).
— Segal, J.: Un dispositif permettant de réaliser des stimuli lumineux de durée ultracourte et de forme quelconque, mais constante. C. R. Soc. Biol. (Paris) **104**, 255—257 (1946).
— Smith, S. W.: Facilitation effect of background light on target detection: a test of theories of absolute threshold. Vision Res. **5**, 299—312 (1965).
— — Comparaison de la sensibilité des cônes et des bâtonnets de l'oeil humain. C. R. Acad. Sci. (Paris) **264**, 3041—3044 (1967).
Bittini, M., Gloria, E. M.: On the correlation between absolute thresholds and false alarms. Atti Fond. G. Ronchi **23**, 487—514 (1968).
Blackwell, H. R.: Psychophysical thresholds: experimental studies of methods of measurement. The University of Michigan, Engineering Res. Inst. Bull. No. 36, pp. 227 (1953).
— Neural theories of simple visual discriminations. J. opt. Soc. Amer. **53**, 129—160 (1963).
Blakemore, C. B., Rushton, W. A. H.: Dark adaptation and increment threshold in a rod monochromat. J. Physiol. (Lond.) **181**, 612—628 (1965).
Bloch, A. M.: Expériences sur la vision. C. R. Soc. Biol. (Paris) **37**, 493—495 (1885).
Blondel, A. M., Rey, J.: Sur la perception des lumières brèves à la limite de leur portée. J. Phys. **1**, 530—550 (1911).
Bornschein, H.: Die absolute Lichtschwelle des menschlichen Auges. Eine experimentell-varianzanalytische Kritik ihrer subjektiven Bestimmungsmethoden. Graefes Arch. Ophthal. **151**, 446—475 (1951).
Borsellino, A., Fuortes, G. F.: Response to single photons in visual cells of *Limulus*. J. Physiol. (Lond.) **196**, 507—539 (1968).
Boswell, F. P.: Über die zur Erregung des Sehorgans in der Fovea erforderlichen Energiemengen. Z. Sinnesphysiol. **42**, 299—312 (1908).
Bouman, M. A., Blokhuis, E. W. M.: The visibility of black objects against an illuminated background. J. opt. Soc. Amer. **42**, 525—528 (1952).
— van den Brink, G.: On the integrate capacity in time and space of the human peripheral retina. J. opt. Soc. Amer. **42**, 617—620 (1952).
— van der Velden, H. A.: The two-quanta explanation of the dependence of the threshold values and visual acuity on the visual angle and the time of observation. J. opt. Soc. Amer. **37**, 908—919 (1947).
— — The two-quanta hypothesis as a general explanation of the behavior of the threshold values and visual acuity for the several receptors of the human eye. J. opt. Soc. Amer. **38**, 570—581 (1948).
Brindley, G. S.: The Bunsen-Roscoe law for the human eye at very short durations. J. Physiol. (Lond.) **118**, 135—139 (1952).
— Physiology of the Retina and the Visual Pathway. London: Arnold 1960.
Brown, K. T., Murakami, M.: A new receptor potential of the monkey retina with no detectable latency. Nature (Lond.) **201**, 626—628 (1964).
Clark, W. C., Blackwell, H. R.: Relations between visibility thresholds for single and double pulses. The University of Michigan, Willow Run Laboratories, Report of Project Michigan No 2, 144—343—T (1959).
Cone, R. A.: Early receptor potential: photoreversible charge displacement in rhodopsin. Science **155**, 1128—1131 (1967).
Cornsweet, T. N., Pinsker, H. M.: Luminance discrimination of brief flashes under various conditions of adaptation. J. Physiol. (Lond.) **176**, 294—310 (1965).
Crouzy, R.: La structure quantique de la lumière et la sensibilité différentielle de l'appareil visuel considéré comme un détecteur de signaux. Thesis, Paris 1963.
Davson, H.: The Eye (Vol. 2, 138—140). New-York-London: Academic Press 1962.

DE GROOT, S. G.: Seeing in the U.V. Nature (Lond.) **134**, 494 (1934).
DENTON, E. J., PIRENNE, M. H.: The absolute sensitivity and functional stability of the human eye. J. Physiol. (Lond.) **123**, 417—442 (1954).
DE VRIES, H.: The quantum character of light and its bearing upon the threshold of vision, the differential sensitivity and acuity of the eye. Physica **10**, 553—564 (1943).
DOWLING, J. E.: Discrete potentials in the dark-adapted eye of the crab *Limulus*. Nature (Lond.) **217**, 28—31 (1968).
ERNST, W.: The dependence of critical flicker frequency and the rod threshold on the state of adaptation of the eye. Vision Res. **8**, 889—900 (1968).
EYSTER, in VON KRIES: Über die zur Erregung des Sehorgans erforderlichen Energiemengen. Z. Sinnesphysiol. **41**, 373—394 (1907).
FECHNER, G. T.: Elemente der Psychophysik. Leipzig: Breitkopf & Härtel 1860.
GALIFRET, Y., PIÉRON, H.: La transmission intraretinienne de l'excitation lumineuse. Ann. Psychol. (Paris) **49**, 1—20 (1950).
GARLICK, G. F. J., WRIGHT, G. T.: Characteristics of scintillation counters. Proc. phys. Soc. (Lond.) B **65**, 415—421 (1952).
GRAHAM, C. H., MARGARIA, R.: Area and the intensity-time relation in peripheral retina. Amer. J. Physiol. **113**, 299—305 (1935).
GREEN, D. A., SWETS, J. A.: Signal Detection Theory and Psychophysics. New York: Wiley 1966.
GRIFFIN, D. R., HUBBARD, R., WALD, G.: The sensitivity of the human eye to infra-red radiation. J. opt. Soc. Amer. **37**, 546—554 (1947).
HALLETT, P. E.: Spatial summation. Vision Res. **3**, 9—24 (1963).
— MARRIOTT, F. H. C., RODGER, F. C.: The relationship of visual threshold to retinal position and area. J. Physiol. (Lond.) **160**, 364—373 (1962).
HECHT, S.: Energy and vision. In: Science in Progress, Series IV, 75—97. New Haven, Conn.: Yale University Press 1945.
— SHLAER, S., PIRENNE, M. H.: Energy, quanta, and vision. J. gen. Physiol. **25**, 819—840 (1942).
HERRICK, R. M.: Foveal luminance discrimination as a function of the duration of the decrement or increment in luminance. J. comp. physiol. Psychol. **49**, 437—443 (1956).
HILLMANN, B. M.: Relationship between stimulus size and threshold intensity in the fovea measured at four exposure times. J. opt. Soc. Amer. **48**, 422—428 (1958).
HUBBARD, R., KROPF, A.: The action of light on rhodopsin. Proc. nat. Acad. Sci. (Wash.) **44**, 130—139 (1958).
HUGHES, G. W., MAFFEI, L.: On the origin of dark discharge of retinal ganglion cells. Arch. ital. Biol. **103**, 45—59 (1965).
JOHNSON, E. P., BARTLETT, N. R.: Effect of stimulus duration on electrical responses of the human retina. J. opt. Soc. Amer. **46**, 167—170 (1956).
KECK, W.: Über die Summation unterschwelliger farbiger Lichtreize. Z. Sinnesphysiol. **57**, 159—174 (1937).
KUFFLER, S. W., FITZHUGH, R., BARLOW, H. B.: Maintained activity in the cat's retina in light and darkness. J. gen. Physiol. **40**, 683—702 (1957).
LUDVIGH, E., MCCARTHY, E. F.: Absorption of visible light by the refractive media of the human eye. Arch. Ophthal. **20**, 37—51 (1938).
MARRIOTT, F. H. C.: The foveal absolute threshold for short flashes and small fields. J. Physiol. (Lond.) **169**, 416—423 (1963).
— MORRIS, V. B., PIRENNE, M. H., The minimum flux of energy detectable by the human eye. J. Physiol. (Lond.) **145**, 369—373 (1959).
MILLER, N. D.: Foveal thresholds for small targets and various pupil diameters in absolute units of energy. J. opt. Soc. Amer. **49**, 502 (Abstr.) (1959).
MUNTZ, W. R. A., NORTHMORE, D. P. M.: Background light, temperature and visual noise in the turtle. Vision Res. **8**, 787—800 (1968).
NAKA, K. I., RUSHTON, W. A. H.: S-Potential and dark adaptation in fish. J. Physiol. (Lond.) **194**, 259—269 (1968).
ØSTERBERG, C.: Topography of the layer of rods and cones in the human retina. Acta Ophthal. Suppl. **6** (1935).

Peyrou, C., Piatier, H.: Emploi des méthodes statistiques dans l'étude de la sensibilité de l'oeil. C. R. Acad. Sci. (Paris) **223**, 589—591 (1946).

Piper, H.: Über die Abhängigkeit des Reizwertes leuchtender Objekte von ihrer Flächen- bezw. Winkelgröße. Z. Psych. Physiol. Sinnesorg. **32**, 98—112 (1903).

Pirenne, M. H.: Rods and cones, and Thomas Young's theory of colour vision. Nature (Lond.) **154**, 741—742 (1944).

— Quantum fluctuations at the absolute threshold. In: The Eye, Davson, H. (Ed.), Vol. 2, 155—156. New York-London: Academic Press 1962.

— Marriott, F. H. C.: The quantum theory of light and the psycho-physiology of vision. In: Psychology: A Study of a Science Vol. 1, pp. 288—361. Koch, S. (Ed.) New York: McGraw Hill 1959.

— — O'Doherty, E. F.: "Individual differences in night-vision efficiency", with a section on "The frequency of seeing at low illumination" by Hartline, H. K. and McDonald, P. R. Spec. Rep. Ser. Med. Res. Coun., London **294**, (1957).

Riccò, A.: Relazione fra il minimo angolo visuale e l'intensità luminosa. Ann. Ottal. **6**, 373—479 (1877).

Rodieck, R. W.: Maintained activity of cat retinal ganglion cells. J. Neurophysiol. **30**, 1043—1071 (1967).

Rose, A.: The sensitivity performance of the human eye on an absolute scale. J. opt. Soc. Amer. **38**, 196—208 (1948).

Rushton, W. A. H.: The rhodopsin density in the human rods. J. Physiol. (Lond.) **134**, 30—46 (1956).

Saïd, F. S,, Weale, R. A.: The variation with age of the spectral transmissivity of the living human crystalline lens. Gerontologia **3**, 213—231 (1959).

Scholes, J.: Discontinuity of the excitation process in Locust visual cells. Cold Spr. Harb. Symp. quant. Biol. **30**, 517—527 (1965).

Stiles, W. S.: The physical interpretation of the spectral sensitivity curve of the eye. In: Transactions of the Optical Convention of the Worshipful Company of Spectacle Makers, pp. 97—107. London: Spectacle Makers' Comp. 1948.

Swets, J. A.: Is there a sensory threshold? Science **134**, 169—177 (1961).

— Tanner, W. P., Birdsall, T. G.: Decision processes in perception. Psychol. Rev. **68**, 301—340 (1961).

Tanner, W. P., Swets, J. A.: A decision-making theory of visual detection. Psychol. Rev. **61**, 401—409 (1954).

Thomas, J. G.: Threshold measurements of Mach bands. J. opt. Soc. Amer. **55**, 521—524 (1965).

Treisman, M.: Noise and Weber's law: the discrimination of brightness and other dimensions. Psychol. Rev. **71**, 314—330 (1964).

— A statistical decision model for sensory discrimination which predicts Weber's law and other sensory laws: some results of a computer simulation. Perc. Psychophys. **1**, 203—230 (1966).

— Personal communication (1967).

— Watts, T. R.: Relation between signal detectability theory and the traditional procedures for measuring sensory thresholds: estimating d' from results given by the method of constant stimuli. Psychol. Bull. **66**, 438—454 (1966).

Van der Velden, H.: Over het antaal lichtquanta dat nodig es for en licht prickel bij dat menselyk oog. Physica **11**, 179—189 (1944).

Weale, R. A.: Retinal summation and human visual thresholds. Nature (Lond.) **181**, 154—156 (1958).

Weinstein, C., Arnulf, A.: Contribution à l'étude des seuils de perception de l'oeil. Comm. Inst. Opt. Paris **2**, 1—43 (1946).

Williams, T. P.: Rhodopsin bleaching: relative effectiveness of high and low intensity flashes. Vision Res. **5**, 633—638 (1965).

Yeandle, S.: Evidence of quantized slow potentials in the eye of *Limulus*. Amer. J. Ophthal. **46**, part 2, 82—87 (1958).

Zegers, R. T.: Photosensitization in relation to mean and standard deviation values. Psychol. Monogr., General and Applied **73**, No. 11, 1—25 (1959).

Chapter 3

Signal Detection Theory and its Application to Problems in Vision

By

JACOB NACHMIAS, Philadelphia, Pennsylvania (USA)

With 9 Figures

Contents

I. Introduction

We shall consider in this chapter a certain class of formal theory and its bearing on the understanding of visual problems. This class encompasses both signal detection theory (hereinafter abbreviated SDT) and various threshold theories. Although most experimenters assume, implicitly or explicitly, some form of threshold theory, most recent theoretical work has centered on SDT. The latter is a fusion of concepts drawn from two major sources: 1) that part of mathematical statistics that deals with the testing of statical hypotheses, and previously applied to psychological scaling by THURSTONE, and 2) that part of electrical engineering dealing with communications systems.

Because the latter concepts are more readily applied to acoustic stimuli, most of the psychophysical applications of SDT to date have been to hearing, though the first "modern" application was actually to luminance increment detection (TANNER and SWETS, 1954). Furthermore, several theoretical formulations of visual detection and discrimination, put forward both before (ROSE, 1948) and after (JONES, 1959; BARLOW, 1956 to date) the advent of "official" SDT, closely resemble it in substance if not in terminology.

II. Overview of the Theories

Detailed expositions of these theories and related experimental work in psychoacoustics can be found in LUCE *et al.* (1963) and GREEN and SWETS (1966). In this section, only a general and simplified overview of various theories of detection will be presented which will stress the relations among them.

Each theory consists of three component theories which are more or less well developed. The central component is the *theory of internal states* (or state theory); it specifies the number of distinct or distinguishable internal states (sensory events) that may be induced on repetition of nominally identical stimulus presentations, as well as the probability distribution of these states. In any experimental situation of interest, the different types of stimulus presentations give rise to distributions of internal states that overlap at least partially. Consequently the observer, who must base his discriminative responses on the internal states, is confronted with a statistical decision task. The decision rules he is assumed to adopt in the face of this task constitute the *response theory*. Since internal states are transformed to responses only by means of decision rules, a theory of internal states can be tested only in conjunction with some response theory. However, this does not imply that there is always a necessary connection between a given state theory and a particular response theory.

The third component of any complete theoretical account of detection or discrimination is a *stimulus theory*, which relates the parameters of the distributions of internal states to the parameters of the physical stimuli. To a considerable extent, stimulus theories on the one hand, and state and response theories on the other, can be tested independently of each other. Stimulus theories for vision will be treated in a later section.

The general interrelations among stimuli, states, and responses are diagrammatically represented below.

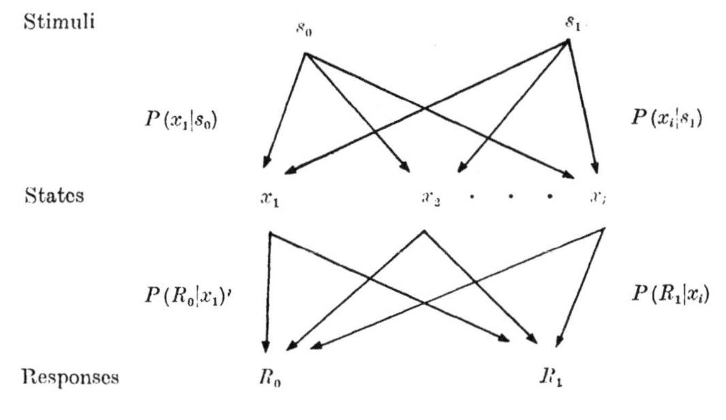

For simplicity, only two stimulus values s_0 and s_1 ($s_0 < s_1$), and two responses, R_0 and R_1, are shown. Some of the specific assumptions that have been put forward about these interrelations will be dealt with briefly in the paragraphs below.

A. Signal Detection Theory[1]

In SDT the internal states are represented by a continuous random variable, and the distribution functions associated with s_0 and s_1, $f(x|s_0)$ and $f(x|s_1)$, are usually assumed to be normal:

$$f(x|s_i) = (2\pi\sigma_i^2)^{-\frac{1}{2}} \exp\left[-\frac{(x-\mu_i)^2}{2\sigma_i^2}\right] = n(x;\, \mu_i, \sigma_i)\,. \tag{1}$$

This state theory is depicted in Fig. 1. By setting $\mu_0 = 0$ and $\sigma_0 = 1$, this theory can be specified by two free parameters: d', the mean difference between the two distributions, and $(1/b')$ the standard deviation of the distribution corresponding to s_1, in units of the standard deviation of the distribution corresponding to s_0. Note that since we are dealing with normal distributions, and consequently $n(x;\, \mu, \sigma) \neq 0$ for finite values of x, there are no excluded states in this theory: that is, any stimulus presentation can give rise to any internal state, with some non-zero probability.

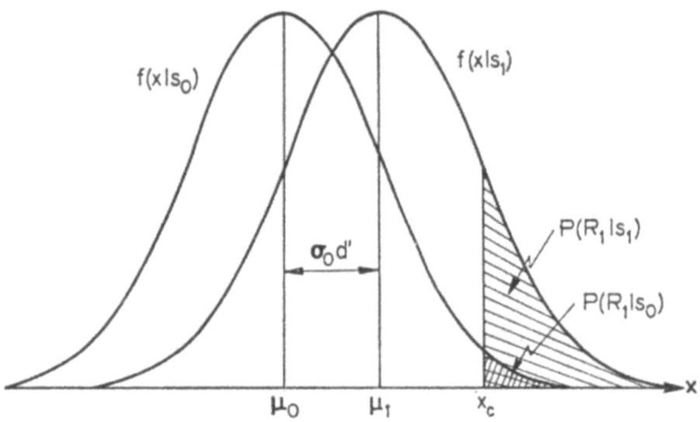

Fig. 1. Representation of the state and response theory components of SDT

There are specific stimulus theories (ideal detector theories for psychoacoustics) which give rise to normal distributions of internal states in certain circumstances. However, the assumption of normality can usually be justified by little else than mathematical convenience. Since many unimodal distributions are well approximated by normal distributions over most of their range, the assumption of normality is not a very risky one. For example, from stimulus theories for vision that are based on quantal fluctuations, x may be taken to be a Poisson-distributed discrete variable; but except where μ is small, x can be treated as a normally distributed continuous variable for all practical purposes.

The response theory component of SDT asserts that the observer adopts a deterministic response rule. On each trial, he compares the elicited value of the random variable representing the internal state, x', to a fixed criterion value, x_c,

[1] The likelihood ratio concept, extensively used by previous writers on SDT, will be omitted in the present discussion for the sake of simplicity of exposition.

and responds R_1 if $x' > x_c$ and R_0 otherwise. Any value of x_c fixes the values of all four response probabilities, two for the correct responses,

$$P(R_1|s_1) = \int_{x_c}^{\infty} f(x|s_1)\,dx \text{ and } P(R_0|s_0) = \int_{-\infty}^{x_c} f(x|s_0)\,dx\,,$$

and two for the incorrect responses, $P(R_0|s_1) = 1 - P(R_1|s_1)$ and $P(R_1|s_0) = 1 - P(R_0|s_0)$. The observer is presumed to adopt a particular criterion, or response threshold, in order to achieve some desired constraint on these response probabilities; the Neyman-Pearson criterion, $P(R_1|s_0) \leq k$, is one such constraint. Consequently, the observer's response criterion should depend on instructions, either in the form of explicit admonitions such as "reduce your false-alarm rate" or on information about the relative frequencies of s_0 and s_1 (presentation probability), and on the costs and values of correct and incorrect responses (payoff matrix).

On the other hand, instructions are supposed not to alter the probability distributions of internal states. Consequently the covariation of two of the response probabilities – the hit rate, $P(H) = P(R_1|s_1)$, and the false-alarm rate,

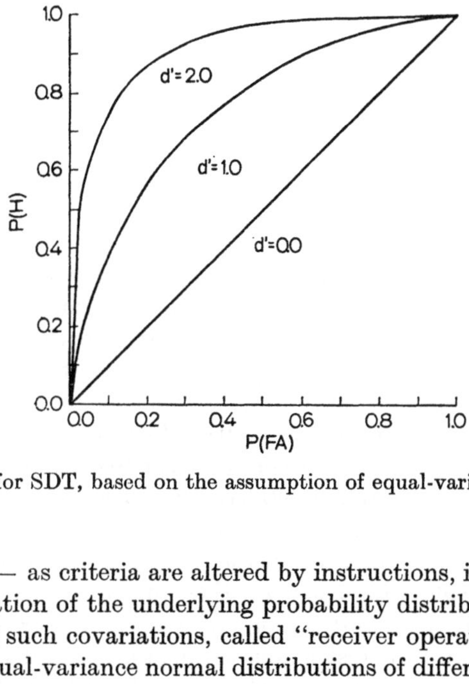

Fig. 2. ROC-curves for SDT, based on the assumption of equal-variance distributions

$P(FA) = P(R_1|s_0)$ – as criteria are altered by instructions, is dependent only on the form and separation of the underlying probability distributions. In Fig. 2 are plotted examples of such covariations, called "receiver operating characteristics" (ROC-curves) for equal-variance normal distributions of different separations. For normal distributions of equal or unequal variances, the normal deviates corresponding to the hit and false-alarm rates, $z(H)$ and $z(FA)$, are linearly related, as shown in Fig. 3. The general equation[2] for these ROC-curves is

$$z(H) = \frac{\sigma_0}{\sigma_1}\left[z(FA) - \frac{(\mu_1 - \mu_0)}{\sigma_0}\right] \tag{2a}$$

$$z(H) = b'\,[z(FA) - d']\,. \tag{2b}$$

[2] In the remainder of this chapter, b and d will be used as symbols for the slopes and horizontal intercepts of ROC-curves. For normal distributions only, $b \equiv b'$ and $d \equiv d'$.

With two stimulus values and two response categories, only one point on an ROC-curve can be obtained at a time. In rating-scale experiments where $n > 2$ response categories are allowed, the observer is assumed to adopt $n - 1$ hierarchical response thresholds simultaneously. In this way $n - 1$ points on an ROC-curve can be generated at a time.

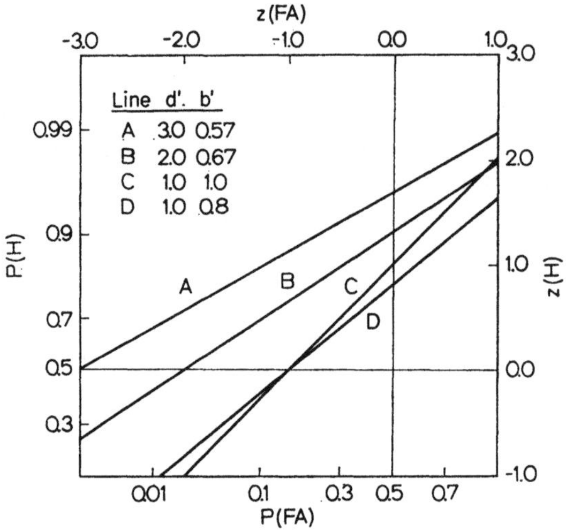

Fig. 3. ROC-curves for SDT plotted on double Gaussian coordinates

Signal detection theorists usually do not specify how an observer manages to adopt and maintain one or several criteria. The exception is SCHOEFFLER (1965), who has developed explicit models for criterion setting both with and without trial-to-trial feedback. One of the important predictions from this model is that, except when performance has reached asymptote without feedback, the observer should vary his response criterion from trial to trial. Criterion variability is implicitly assumed to be negligible in almost all work based on SDT. However, TANNER (1961), and in more detail, WICKELGREN (1968) have considered some of the consequences of appreciable criterion variability. For this purpose, it is convenient to treat x_c as a random variable rather than a constant. If x_c is normally distributed with variance σ_c^2 independent of its mean, μ_c, then the effects on ROC-curves can be represented succinctly by substituting $\sqrt{\sigma_c^2 + \sigma_0^2}$ and $\sqrt{\sigma_c^2 + \sigma_1^2}$ for σ_0 and σ_1 respectively in Eq. (2a). If no restrictions are placed on the distribution of x_c, then the ROC-curve could lie anywhere in the region bounded by the ROC-curve for $\sigma_c^2 = 0$ and the diagonal representing $d' = 0$.

B. Threshold Theories

Threshold theories may be regarded as restricted versions of SDT. The nature and extent of the restrictions differ among the theories.

The best developed of contemporary threshold theories for detection is that of LUCE (1963a, b). Following the neural quantum theory of BÉKÉSY (1930) and

STEVENS *et al.* (1941), LUCE makes the following assumptions: 1) Corresponding to each of at least some stimulus dimensions, there exists a discrete set of internal states. 2) For any particular value of s, all but a small number of states arise with negligible probability. 3) Furthermore, at least in simple detection experiments, where $s_0 = 0$, the observer groups this set of states into two subsets. In one statement of his theory, LUCE leaves open the possibility that the composition of the two subsets may depend upon the value of s_1 (LUCE, 1963b). 4) However, for any particular value of s_1, the observer does not discriminate between members of the resulting two subsets of states, referred to as D and $\bar{D}$, and responds to changes in instructions only by altering the response probabilities, t and u, conditioned on the states:

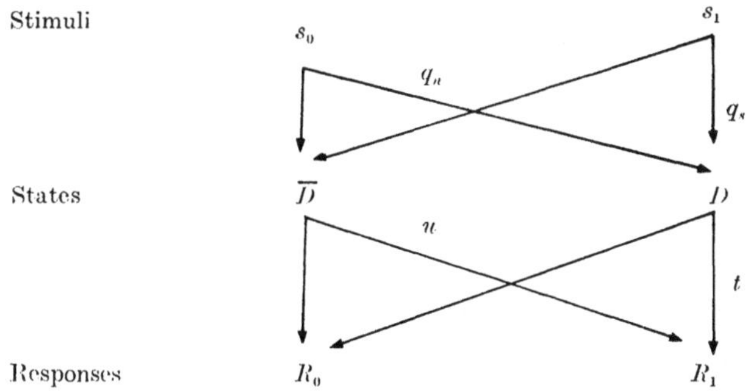

5) Over a significant range of instructions, he behaves in one of two ways: either he sets $t = 1$ and varies u, or he sets $u = 0$ and varies t. LUCE proposes an explicit learning model which predicts the asymptotic values of the biasing parameters, t and u.

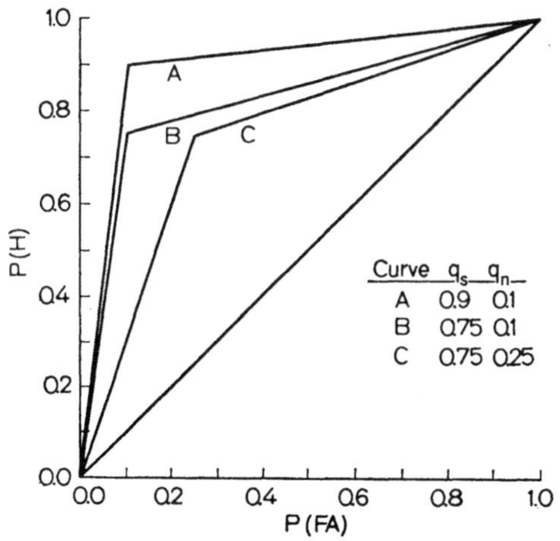

Fig. 4. ROC-curves for LUCE's threshold theory

The ROC-curve for this theory consists of two line segments, as shown in Fig. 4. The upper and lower limbs of the ROC-curve intersect at $[q_n, q_s]$. The value of q_s obviously must be a function of s_1; the value of q_n is a different function of s_1, if, as in LUCE (1963b), D and $\bar{D}$ are treated as two *subsets* of states rather than as two states.

An important additional assumption common to several threshold theories, though not to LUCE's, is that in simple detection situations certain internal states can be elicited only by $s_1 > 0$, and hence never by $s_0 = 0$. To put it more informally, the assumption is that the threshold of sensation is never exceeded in the absence of a signal. If one also assumes that the observer cannot discriminate between "subthreshold" excitations, one is led to a special case of LUCE's theory where $P(D|s_0) = q_n = 0$ for all values of s_1. These assumptions have been widely held for a long time, though not always explicitly, and form the basis for the standard "correction for guessing" applied to "yes-no" data: $q_s = [P(H) - P(FA)]/[1 - P(FA)]$. This form of threshold theory has also been recently discussed by BLACKWELL (1963), as well as by SWETS (1961) and others who refer to it as "high-threshold" theory to distinguish it from LUCE's "low-threshold" theory.

SWETS (1961) describes a different sort of "low-threshold" theory of detection, which is actually a hybrid form of SDT. In this version, the observer can move his response threshold in accord with instructions, but not below a "sensory threshold" located near the mean of $f(x|s_0)$. If pressed further, the observer resorts to the "upper limb" response strategy of LUCE's theory. The resulting ROC-curve, for equal variance, normal distributions, is displayed in Fig. 5.

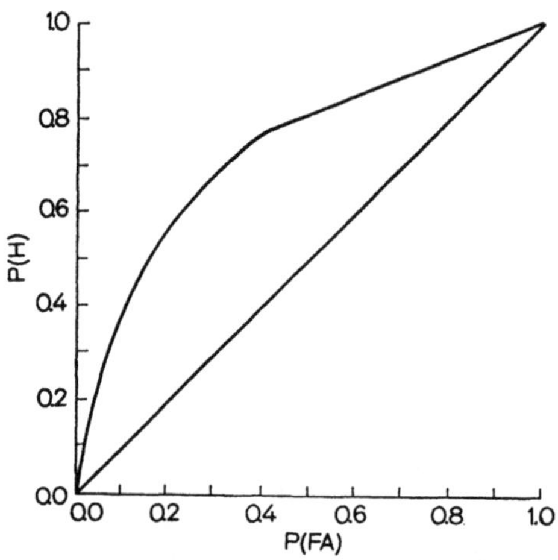

Fig. 5. ROC-curve for SWETS' low threshold theory. The sensory threshold is located slightly above the mean of $f(x/s_0)$

Finally, there are multi-state, multi-threshold theories (NORMAN, 1963; KRANTZ, 1969). In these theories, LUCE's assumptions 3) and 4) are dropped in favor of a response theory that is a hybrid between that of SDT and LUCE's assumption 5):

$$P(R_1|x_i) = \begin{bmatrix} 0 \\ t, 0 \leq t \leq 1 \\ 1 \end{bmatrix} \text{ for } i \begin{bmatrix} < \\ = \\ > \end{bmatrix} j. \qquad (3)$$

That is, response R_1, is given with probability t when state x_j occurs, but is either always or never given when any other state arises. The values of both j and t can be altered independently by instructions.

The ROC-curve for this theory is displayed in Fig. 6. The co-ordinates for each point of intersection between adjacent line segments are $[\sum_{i=j} P(x_i|s_0), \sum_{i=j} P(x_i|s_1)]$. In KRANTZ's version of multi-state theory, $i = 1, 2, 3$, and furthermore, $P(x_3|s_0) = 0$; that is, one of the states has a high threshold, in the sense that it is never exceeded when s_0 is presented (on catch trials).

Comparison of Figs. 2–6 will make it apparent why it has proved so difficult to choose among detection theories on the basis of experimentally determined ROC-curves.

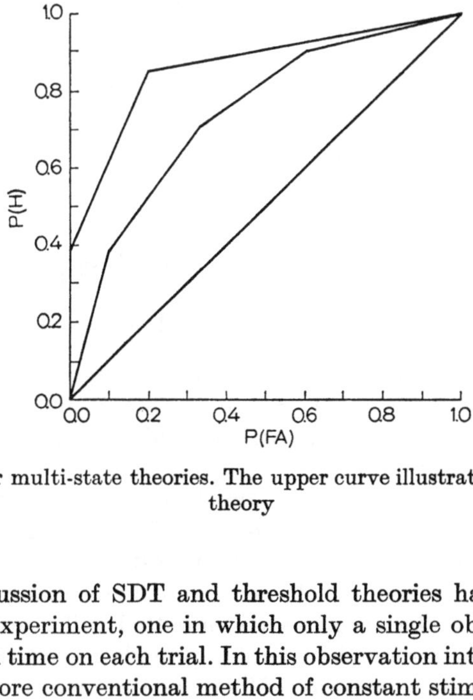

Fig. 6. ROC-curves for multi-state theories. The upper curve illustrates KRANTZ's three-state theory

So far, the discussion of SDT and threshold theories has considered only a particular type of experiment, one in which only a single observation interval is defined in space and time on each trial. In this observation interval, s_0 or s_1 may be presented. In the more conventional method of constant stimuli, the value of s_1 is varied randomly from trial to trial. (See TREISMAN and WATTS, 1966, for a discussion of this method in the light of SDT.)

C. Multiple Observation Intervals

Only a few of the experimental designs involving multiple observation intervals can be touched upon here. (See LUCE, 1963a, b, and GREEN and SWETS, 1966, for more complete treatments.) In the two-alternative, forced choice (2AFC) experiment, two observation intervals are defined in space or time on each trial, and either of two sequences, $\langle s_0\, s_1\rangle$ or $\langle s_1\, s_0\rangle$ is presented. According to two-state threshold theories, four possible sequences of internal states can arise, $\langle D\, \bar{D}\rangle$, $\langle \bar{D}\, D\rangle$, $\langle D\, D\rangle$ and $\langle \bar{D}\, \bar{D}\rangle$; the observer's selection of a response is governed by the bias parameter appropriate to the sequence of states aroused on that trial. According to SDT, the observer computes the difference between the values of x occurring in the two intervals of each trial, and makes his response by comparing this difference to a criterion value, which is usually assumed to be zero. Note that in SDT as well as in two-state threshold theories, the response theory components for 2AFC experiments are quite similar to those for one-interval experiments.

The treatment of 2AFC experiments by two-state theories presented above can be readily generalized to experiments with more than two observation intervals. The SDT treatment cannot be so generalized. An alternative formulation is required: the observer ranks the values of the internal states occurring in each interval and selects that interval which produced the highest value.

When there are more than two observation intervals per trial, the observer can also be asked to make a second choice as to the interval containing the signal. According to high-threshold theory, these second choices can only be pure guesses: in an n-alternative, forced choice experiment, the probability of a correct second choice preceded by an incorrect first choice, $P(C_2|\overline{C}_1)$, cannot exceed $1/(n-1)$, regardless of the probability of a correct first choice, $P(C_1)$. According to most other theories, $1/(n-1) \leqq P(C_2|\overline{C}_1) = g[P(C_1)]$, where g depends on the state and response parameters of the theory.

III. Results Bearing on State and Response Theories

A. Covariation of Hits and False Alarms

Detailed comparisons between models for detection and discrimination and results from psychoacoustics can be found in GREEN and SWETS (1966) and in LUCE *et al.* (1963). With few exceptions, the results discussed in this chapter will be from visual experiments.

The covariation of hits and false alarms has been examined in several yes-no experiments on luminance increment detection (TANNER and SWETS, 1954; SWETS *et al.*, 1961; HOHLE, 1965; NACHMIAS, 1968; MUNSINGER and GUMMERMAN, 1968). Different values of $\hat{P}(H)$[3] and $\hat{P}(FA)$ were obtained by changing the presentation probability of the signal, the payoff matrix, or both. In all cases, ROC-curves based on SDT and underlying normal distributions provide a good visual fit to the data. However, with the possible exception of TANNER and SWETS' data, the fit requires the assumption of unequal variance. In particular, σ appears to be a monotonically increasing function of s_1; for example, SWETS *et al.* used the relation, $\Delta\sigma = 1/4\Delta\mu$, which is equivalent to $\sigma_1 = \sigma_0\left[\frac{d'}{4} + 1\right]$.

In most of the results cited above, the dependence of $\hat{P}(H)$ on $\hat{P}(FA)$ for $\hat{P}(FA) \lesssim 0.15$ can be described just about as adequately by the "upper limb" segment (passing through $P(H) = P(FA) = 1.0$) of two-state theories. However, with the possible exception of the results from one of HOHLE's six observers, this same theoretical line clearly fails to fit points for which $\hat{P}(FA) \gtrsim 0.15$. For this reason, "high-threshold" theory, which underlies one of the common corrections

[3] In the remainder of this chapter, "hats", e.g. ($\hat{\mathrm{P}}$), will be used to designate estimates of parameters based on experimental data.

for guessing, must be rejected for the detection of luminance increments. LUCE's two-limbed ROC-curve fares much better and certainly cannot be rejected on the strength of these results alone.

The rating-scale procedure has been employed in several studies of luminance increment detection (BARLOW, 1956; SWETS *et al.*, 1961; NACHMIAS and STEINMAN, 1963; 1964; NACHMIAS, 1968; NACHMIAS and KOCHER, 1969); it has also been used in studies of luminance decrement detection (WICKELGREN, 1967), discrimination of highly detectable luminances (NACHMIAS and STEINMAN, 1965), and form discrimination (WEINTRAUB and HAKE, 1962; ULEHLA *et al.*, 1968). Only NACHMIAS and STEINMAN's data on luminance discrimination are incompatible with SDT and underlying normal distributions. On double-Gaussian co-ordinates, these data appear to be fitted better by downward concave curves rather than by straight lines. There are no other reported instances of systematic deviations from theoretical expectations. However, almost invariably, the underlying distributions of internal states appear to be of unequal variance: in the detection experiments, where $s_0 = 0, \hat{\sigma}_1^2 > \hat{\sigma}_0^2$ regardless of whether s_1 represented a luminance increment or decrement.

NACHMIAS and STEINMAN (1963) also used the results of their study of absolute detection by the rating-scale method to test LUCE's two-state threshold theory. To do so, they had to extend the response-theory component of LUCE's theory to cover the case of more than two response alternatives. In the most general case, $0 \leqq P(R_i|D) = t_i \leqq 1$, and $0 \leqq P(R_i|\bar{D}) = u_i \leqq 1$ for all R_i. However, NACHMIAS and STEINMAN reasoned that if two-state theory were true, their observers would be able to obey their instructions by using two of the response categories ("5" and "4") to report only on the D-state, and two others ("2" and "1") to report only on the $\bar{D}$-state; that is, they would be able to set $u_5 = u_4 = t_1 = t_2 = 0$. Generalized in this way, LUCE's theory is clearly contradicted by the results of this experiment which show that $\hat{P}(s_1|\text{"5"}) > \hat{P}(s_1|\text{"4"})$ and $\hat{P}(s_1|\text{"1"}) > \hat{P}(s_1|\text{"2"})$. However, as KRANTZ (1969) has pointed out, it would not take large departures from the simplifying assumptions just made about t_i und u_i to produce such results.

NACHMIAS and STEINMAN also calculated from their data the value of $\hat{q}_n$, the probability of the D-state on catch trials, and found it to be inversely related to the value of s_1. This result invalidates two-state theory, if the theory is taken to mean that q_n is the true probability that noise alone "passes" the threshold and that all $\bar{D}$ observations are actually indistinguishable (LUCE, 1963a). To be sure, the theory is not embarrassed by this finding if D and $\bar{D}$ are considered to be merely subsets of states whose membership varies with the value of s_1. On the other hand, this version of the theory would have to predict that the estimated location of the corner on the ROC-curve for a particular value of s_1 – even if the curve were generated in a "yes-no" experiment – could be altered by presenting some other value or values of s_1 on a random fraction of trials. This prediction from LUCE's theory has yet to be put to a thorough test, though EMMERICH (1968) reported some generally negative results from a psychoacoustic experiment.

Similar issues arise within SDT. In its simplest formulation, it assumes that a stimulus of constant nominal value is associated with a probability distribution of internal states whose parameters depend only on that stimulus and the visual system. State-parameters do not depend on such experimental variables as the presentation probability of that stimulus, the values of other stimuli presented in the same block, the payoff matrix, or the number of response alternatives available to the observer. Criterion-variability is also assumed to be independent of these same variables, or to be negligible in comparison to state-variability. It is precisely because of these assumptions that SDT holds out the promise of enabling us to extract pure measures of the sensory effects of stimuli from psychophysical results. To be sure, one cannot expect these assumptions to be strictly true; the question arises, however, whether they hold over a sufficiently wide range of irrelevant variables for the methods of SDT to be useful in the testing of stimulus theories.

All too few attempts have been made to investigate the effects of these extraneous variables. One study of luminance increment detection (NACHMIAS, 1968) revealed that hit and false-alarm rates generated by combing each of three presentation probabilities (0.25, 0.50, 0.75) with each of two numbers of response alternatives (2, 4) fall along the same ROC-curve. WEINTRAUB and HAKE (1962) reached a similar conclusion about the effect of varying the number of response alternatives between 2 and 4. In addition, they found that the ROC-curve for discrimination of two stimuli was unaffected by occasionally presenting a third one. NACHMIAS and KOCHER (1970) used three different luminance increments, s_A, s_B, s_C, where $0 \leqq s_A < s_B < s_C$, and studied the interrelations among the ROC-curves for discrimination of each of the three different pairings of these luminances: s_A and s_B, s_B and s_C, s_A and s_C. If the usual simplifying assumptions of SDT were true, one should be able to predict each set of results from the other two. In fact, in most cases, the predictions failed in a consistent manner: the predicted ROC-curve for discrimination of s_A from s_C (or detection of s_C, when $s_A = 0$) fell short of the empirically obtained points. Among the possible explanations for such discrepancies are: 1) Criterion variance is appreciable within blocks of trials and its value is greater when only very weak signals are presented; 2) The observer's uncertainty about the parameters of the signal is significantly greater when only weak signals are presented, so that effectively $f(x|s_B)$ is different when s_B is paired with s_C rather than with s_A. In psychoacoustics, there is an extensive theoretical and experimental literature on the effects of signal uncertainty (GREEN and SWETS, 1966). In vision, HOWARTH and LOWE (1966) and LOWE (1967) have investigated such effects, but their experiments leave many questions unanswered. The matter will be dealt with again later in this chapter when stimulus theories for vision are discussed.

B. Experiments with Multiple Observation Intervals

In forced-choice procedures, the observer's task on each trial is to select the one of the n-intervals most likely to contain the signal. These procedures have been deemed preferable to yes-no procedures by several visual investigators (BLACKWELL, 1952; CORNSWEET and PINSKER, 1965; BAUMGARDT and SMITH, 1965; among others). Forced-choice procedures are claimed to yield lower thresholds after correction for chance success, and the thresholds, moreover, are subject to less day-to-day variability and are less susceptible to extraneous influences. These claims may be empirically true, but it is hard to justify them theoretically, in view of the fact that for both SDT and threshold theories, the processes involved in n-interval experiments are the same whether or not $n = 1$.

Of course the comparison of empirical thresholds from yes-no and forced-choice procedures requires the application of some theory of the detection process in order to extract a measure of the pure sensory effects of stimuli. That such measures from the two procedures disagree may be due not to the inherent superiority of the forced-choice method, but rather to the incorrectness of the high-threshold theory which forms the basis for the standard corrections for guessing. Indeed, by applying SDT, TANNER and SWETS (1954) obtained quite comparable measures of detectability from the two procedures. Actually, as WICKELGREN (1968) has pointed out, their estimates depend on several simplifying assumptions which are not inherent in SDT. If instead some other assumptions were correct, the 2AFC method may appear to be better, or worse, than the yes-no method.

Further support for SDT comes from a 4-alternative, forced-choice experiment on luminance detection (SWETS *et al.*, 1961), in which observers were sometimes asked to make a second choice of the interval containing the signal. Contrary to high-threshold theory, these second choices were generally correct above chance level when they were made after an incorrect first choice. Furthermore, $\hat{P}(C_2 | \bar{C}_1)$ varied with $\hat{P}(C_1)$ in the manner predicted by SDT with the additional assumption of $\Delta\sigma_1 = 1/4\Delta\mu_1$. EIJKMAN and VENDRIK (1963) apparently repeated this experiment, and according to BLACKWELL (1963), so did KINCAID and HAMILTON. In both instances, results from the majority of observers failed to contradict high-threshold theory. Clearly, the matter requires further investigation.

IV. Stimulus Theories for Vision

We turn now to that component of any complete theoretical account of detection and discrimination which deals with the relation between the parameters of the distributions of internal states and the parameters of the physical stimuli. Most of the topics about to be discussed will also be found in other chapters of this volume. Their treatment here will stress primarily aspects closely related to the state and response theories presented in the earlier sections of this chapter.

A. Ideal Detectors and and Photon Fluctuations

The ideal detector of radiant energy is a device containing a noiseless photocell which counts every incident photon, and emits response R_1 whenever the total count exceeds some constant criterion value. The performance of such a device is limited by the noise inherent in any visual stimulus. Since the emission and absorption of photons is a Poisson process, the total number of photons counted, x, as a result of a stimulus delivering on the average s photons to the device is given by

$$f(x|s) = e^{-\mu}\mu^x/x! \equiv p(x;\mu) \tag{4}$$

where $\mu \equiv E[f(x|s)] = h(s)$. For this device, the psychometric function for absolute detection, Ψ, that is, $P(R_1|s)$ as a function of s, can be written as follows:

$$\Psi = \sum_{x=x_c}^{\infty} p([x; h(s)] = \Psi[h(s); x_c]\,. \tag{5}$$

In the case of the ideal photon detector, $h(s) = s$; therefore, $f(x|s) = p(x; s)$ and $\Psi = \Psi(s; x_c)$.

The ideal device's performance in discriminating between two stimuli, s_0 and s_1, is determined by the two density functions, $f(x|s_0)$ and $f(x|s_1)$, and the criterion value, x_c. The performance can be represented as the covariation of hits and false alarms, as in Fig. 7. Note that even for small values of μ_0 and μ_1, the theoretical

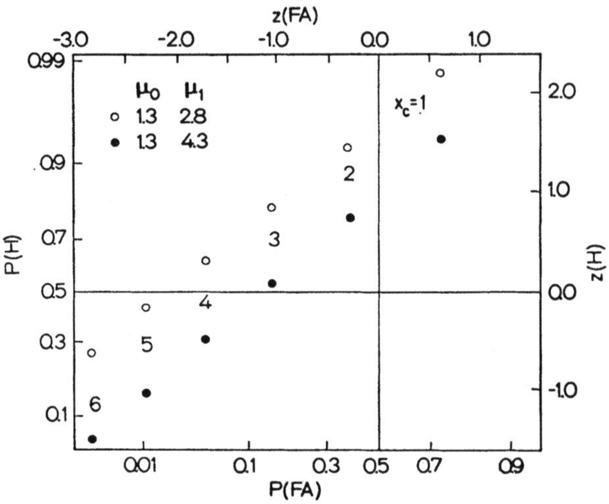

Fig. 7. The covariation of hits and false alarms for Poisson distributions

points fall along a straight line on double-Gaussian co-ordinates. For moderately large values of μ, the slope, b, and the horizontal intercept, d, of this line are approximately equal to b' and d' respectively:

$$b \approx b' = \frac{\sigma_0}{\sigma_1} = \sqrt{\frac{\mu_0}{\mu_1}}, \tag{6a}$$

$$d \approx d' = \frac{\mu_1 - \mu_0}{\sigma_0} = \frac{\mu_1 - \mu_0}{\sqrt{\mu_0}}. \tag{6b}$$

If we define $N \equiv s_0$ and $\Delta N \equiv s_1 - s_0$, we note that for a constant level of detectability, $d' = k$,

$$\Delta N = k\sqrt{N}. \tag{7}$$

Eq. (7) can be rewritten to explicitly contain the duration, t, and the area, a, of s_0 and s_1, by defining the quantities $I \equiv N/ta$ and $\Delta I \equiv \Delta N/ta$:

$$\Delta I = k\sqrt{I t^{-1} a^{-1}}. \tag{8}$$

In the discussion above, I and $I + \Delta I$ had the same duration and area. Suppose instead that $t_I \gg t_{I+\Delta I} = t$ and $a_I \gg a_{I+\Delta I} = a$; that is, I represents a large, continuously presented background which is incremented by ΔI for time t over area a. In this case, the ideal detector should start and stop counting photons whenever ΔI is expected to begin and end. If so, all the equations stated so far in this section continue to hold, except that now s_0 and s_1 must be reinterpreted to stand for the mean number of photons delivered in the time and space interval just defined. That is,

$$\mu_0 = s_0 = N = Ita\,, \tag{9a}$$

$$\text{and } \mu_1 = s_1 = N + \Delta N = (I + \Delta I)ta\,. \tag{9b}$$

B. Real and Ideal Detectors Compared

The performance of the ideal photon detector just described is limited by only one source of noise, that inherent in the visual stimulus itself. HECHT *et al.* (1942) put forward the claim that under certain experimental conditions – the detection of brief, small flashes delivered to the dark adapted peripheral retina – the human visual system approximates an ideal photon detector. However, every photon reaching the cornea bleaches a rhodopsin molecule only with probability F, $F < 1.0$. F, sometimes referred to as the quantum efficiency of the visual system, in this case represents attenuation by the ocular media, as well as the concentration and bleaching properties of rhodopsin. On this theory, $\mu = Fs$, and the psychometric function becomes

$$\Psi = \sum_{x=x_c}^{\infty} p(x; Fs) = \Psi(s; F, x_c)\,. \tag{10}$$

Note that since $p(x; 0) = 0$ for $x > 0$, we have here a special kind of high threshold theory.

The two parameters of the psychometric function, x_c and F, have usually been estimated from the empirical psychometric function plotted against log s. This is done by comparing the empirical function, $\Psi(s_1; 1.0, x_c)$, with respect to form and location along the horizontal axis, to the family of theoretical functions. (See Chapter 2 for details.) HECHT's theory is not grossly at variance with absolute detection data collected by himself or others (e.g., BAUMGARDT, 1959) and leads to estimates of x_c between 2 and 14, and of F in the order of 0.1.

The most straightforward extension of HECHT's theory to cover luminance increment detection and luminance discrimination – an extension which HECHT himself did not put forward – would lead to the following theoretical expectations:

$$d' = F^{\frac{1}{2}}\left(\frac{s_1 - s_0}{\sqrt{s_0}}\right), \tag{11a}$$

$$\Delta I = kF^{-\frac{1}{2}}\sqrt{It^{-1}a^{-1}}\,, \tag{11b}$$

where F is a constant quantum efficiency, and k is *a* constant detectability level.

These expectations are not borne out by experimental evidence. The value of $(\hat{k}/\hat{F})$ when obtained by means of Eq. (11b), turns out not to be a constant independent of I, t, and a, but rather is a u-shaped function of each of these experimental variables (JONES, 1959; BARLOW, 1965). Similarly, the application of a close relative of Eq. (11a) to luminance discrimination data shows that $\hat{F}$ varies with adapting luminance, as well as with the values of s_0 and s_1 (BARLOW, 1962a, b). The assumption of constant F and (k/F) is also incompatible with a vast body of other visual data which are not ordinarily used to test the assumption.

It is important to realize that these obtained variations in the values of $\hat{F}$ or of $(\hat{k}/\hat{F})$ do not necessarily imply that the concentration or bleaching properties of rhodopsin are changing in a similar manner. Rather, F should be interpreted much as η is in psychoacoustics, merely as a measure of the performance of a real detector, the human eye, relative to that of an ideal photon detector. At this writing, there is no complete stimulus theory for vision which accounts adequately for all the major observed discrepancies between real and ideal detectors. Some of the ingredients for such a theory will now be discussed.

C. Intrinsic Noise

In the most general sense, "intrinsic noise" can be taken to mean any source of variance, other than photon fluctuations, which limits the real observer's ability to detect and discriminate stimuli of different intensity. On this view, criterion variability which was discussed in section II B, is a source of additive intrinsic noise. All on its own, a constant value of σ_c^2 would tend to level off the theoretical ΔI vs. I function at small values of I, in accord with experimental evidence.

BARLOW (1956) revived an hypothesis about another possible source of intrinsic noise, namely that there is a significant amount of spontaneous decomposition of rhodopsin. If this spontaneous decomposition is treated as a Poisson process independent of that of photon absorption, then the number of molecular decompositions is still a Poisson-distributed random variable. However, μ, its mean and variance, is the sum of two components: μ', representing photon-induced decompositions (hence, $\mu' = Fs$), and μ'', representing spontaneous decompositions. An additional parameter is thus introduced into the equations for the psychometric function for absolute detection,

$$\Psi = \sum_{x=x_c}^{\infty} p(x; Fs + \mu'') = \Psi(s; F, x_c, \mu'') \tag{12}$$

and for ΔI at fixed d',

$$\Delta I = kF^{-\frac{1}{2}} \sqrt{(I + I_D)\, t^{-1} a^{-1}} \tag{13}$$

where I_D, sometimes referred to as "the dark light of the eye," is defined by the relation, $I_D \equiv \mu''/Fta$. Methods for estimating the magnitude of dark light can be found in two papers by BARLOW (1956, 1957). More recently, RUSHTON (1963) and BARLOW (1964b) hypothesized that rhodopsin in the bleached state also gives rise to dark light, and that the reduction of this dark light as rhodopsin is regenerated accounts for diverse phenomena of dark adaptation.

That dark light of some kind exists seems entirely likely for several reasons. One of them is that ganglion cells in the mammalian retina are spontaneously active, in the absence of external stimulation (KUFFLER *et al.*, 1957; FITZHUGH, 1957; RODIECK, 1967). Another reason for believing in the existence of dark light is the nature of the covariation of hits and false alarms in absolute detection (BARLOW, 1956; NACHMIAS and STEINMAN, 1963). However, it is less certain that dark light originates in the photoreceptors (HUBBARD, 1958; BARLOW, 1964b; RODIECK, 1967), and what role it plays in dark adaptation (ARDUINI, 1963).

D. The Transducer Function

The internal state on which psychophysical responses depend cannot be the bleaching of photopigments itself, but rather some neural activity in the brain which is modified by events initiated by photoreception. At each of the intervening stages in the visual system, an output is related to an input of some earlier stage by a transducer function. TREISMAN (1964, 1965, 1966) has written at length about the theoretical consequences for luminance detection of different possible transducer functions. This is a very complex topic which cannot be adequately summarized in brief at this point. However, it is of interest to review two quite different approaches to this problem.

One approach is to ascertain electrophysiologically the transducer function relating some measure of the neural output of a single retinal ganglion cell to the luminance of test flashes. FITZHUGH (1957) investigated this problem by measuring the total number of impulses generated by dark adapted cat's ganglion cells within a 30 msec interval following brief, small flashes of light of different luminance, as well as the spontaneous activity during similar intervals. He found that over a nine-fold range of luminance, the increase in the mean total number of impulses produced by a flash was roughly proportional to its luminance, whereas the variance was not systematically related to luminance. Over much greater ranges of luminance of test flashes superimposed on a large adapting field, neural activity appears to be a negatively accelerated function of test flash luminance (STONE and FABIAN, 1968).

The existence of small signal, incremental linearity is further established by some of the results of BARLOW and LEVICK (BARLOW, 1965; BARLOW and LEVICK, 1969) who recorded from retinal ganglion cells of the cat. They found that the transient change in firing rate, produced by briefly incrementing an adapting luminance, was directly proportional to the magnitude of the luminance increment, for increments up to four times "threshold magnitude." However, the value of the proportionality constant, the reciprocal of what they call "the quantum/spike ratio," turned out to be a monotonically decreasing function of the adapting luminance. The exact form of this function, and its relation to the steady-state transducer function, are still unclear. Further elucidation of these functions undoubtedly holds the key to the understanding of the discrepancy between ideal and real detectors discussed in Section IV B above. Nevertheless, it is already clear that the effect on luminance detection and discrimination of increasing the luminance of an adapting field may have relatively little to do with the increased variance of photon absorption from the adapting fieled. In fact, the variance of the steady-state firing rate depends little, if at all, upon the adapting luminance.

A totally different approach to the problem of the transducer function is to use psychophysics to assess the overall incremental transducer function, that is, the function relating the magnitude of luminance increments to the parameters of the density functions underlying detection and discrimination responses. Results from this approach and from the electrophysiological one just described do not at all resemble each other. Calculations based on detection data from 2AFC and from rating-scale detection experiments agree that $\hat{d}' = k(\Delta I)^p$, with estimates of p ranging between 1.5 and 3.3 (TANNER and SWETS, 1954; LESHOWITZ *et al.*, 1968;

NACHMIAS and KOCHER, 1970). Furthermore, as was stated in section III A, the slopes of ROC-curves for detection suggest that σ_1^2 is a monotonically increasing function of I.

Since p is greater than 1.0, we are led to a surprising prediction about the discriminability of two luminance increments, $\Delta' I$ and ΔI, where $\Delta I - \Delta' I = c > 0$. The expression for the discriminability index, $d'_{\Delta' I, \Delta I}$ turns out to be

$$d'_{\Delta' I, \Delta I} = \frac{\mu_{\Delta I} - \mu_{\Delta' I}}{\sigma_{\Delta' I}} = k \frac{\sigma_0}{\sigma_{\Delta I}} \left[(c + \Delta' I)^p - \Delta' I^p\right] . \tag{14}$$

Provided $(\sigma_0/\sigma_{\Delta' I}) = b'$ were essentially constant, $d'_{\Delta' I, \Delta I}$ would be a monotonically increasing function of $\Delta' I$ over the range of $\Delta' I$ for which $p > 1$.[4] In fact, this improvement in discriminability has been empirically obtained by LESHOWITZ *et al.* (1968) and by NACHMIAS and KOCHER (1970), and can also be seen in the results of BARLOW (1962b). The corresponding inverse relationship between $(\Delta I - \Delta' I)$ and $\Delta' I$ for constant $d'_{\Delta' I, \Delta I}$ can be found in the data of CORNSWEET and PINSKER (1965).

E. Multiple Sensory Channels[5]

Thus far, the results of electrophysiological and psychophysical approaches do not agree about the form of the transducer function. To be sure, in the first case we are dealing with the transducer function for the cat retina, in the other, with the overall transducer function for the entire human visual system. It is possible that results from electrophysiology of the human visual cortex would be in greater agreement with those from psychophysical experiments.

On the other hand, the key to the discrepancy may lie in the fact that whereas the electrophysiological investigators cited above were looking at only one retinal cell at a time, the human observer looks at a great many brain cells at a time. To be sure, in the detection experiments discussed thus far, all but one stimulus parameter is held constant and therefore the output of only a small fraction of all brain cells is likely to be affected, even on the average, by the presentation of the test flash. An ideal detector would ignore all but this fraction of cells. The human observer may not be able to do so. One possible reason for this inability is that in a situation in which the signal-to-noise ratio is low even for the most favored cells, it may not be easy to pick out those cells for which the signal-to-noise ratio is greater than zero. Consequently, the decision as to whether a signal is present probably depends on the output of many cells, some of which are never affected by the signal.

In what way are the outputs of many cells combined to determine the observer's response ? On this point there is little relevant experimental evidence and even less theory. One of the major blocks to theorizing here is the very large number of potentially important parameters. As yet it is far from clear what simplifying assumptions about these parameters are at all realistic, and how serious would be the theoretical consequences of making unrealistic assumptions. Nevertheless it

[4] However, as has been stated previously, $\hat{b}'$ is not a constant, but rather decreases as $\Delta' I$ increases. This factor would tend to reduce the anticipated amount of improvement in discriminability.

[5] The theory developed in this section also appears in NACHMIAS and KOCHER (1970).

may be of interest to pursue one set of assumptions about how information from many cells is combined. The development is based on theoretical work in another context (PETERSON *et al.*, 1954) whose applicability to vision was first suggested by TANNER (1961).

Consider m cells whose outputs, in the presence and absence of a signal increment, are independent Poisson random variables. For one of these cells, $f(x|s_0) = p(x;\mu_0)$ and $f(x|s_1) = p(x;\mu_1)$. For the remaining $m-1$ cells, $f(x|s_0) = f(x|s_1) = p(x;\mu_0)$. That is, only one of these cells is affected by the stimulus. On each trial of a yes-no experiment, the observer computes the quantity $(x - x_c)$, where $x_c = k$ is the criterion, separately for each cell, and responds R_1 if and only if that quantity is greater than zero for at least one cell. The resulting covariation of hits and false alarms is specified by the equations below:

$$P(H) = 1 - \left[\sum_{x=0}^{x_c} p(x;\mu_1)\right]\left[\sum_{x=0}^{x_c} p(x;\mu_0)\right]^{(m-1)} \tag{15a}$$

$$P(FA) = 1 - \left[\sum_{x=0}^{x_c} p(x;\mu_0)\right]^{m} . \tag{15b}$$

For $m = 1$, Eq. (15a) and (15b) reduce to Eq. (4) and (5).

Some of the properties of this theory are displayed in Figs. 8 and 9. In Fig. 8, $P(H)$ is plotted against $P(FA)$ on double-Gaussian coordinates for $\mu_0 = 40$,

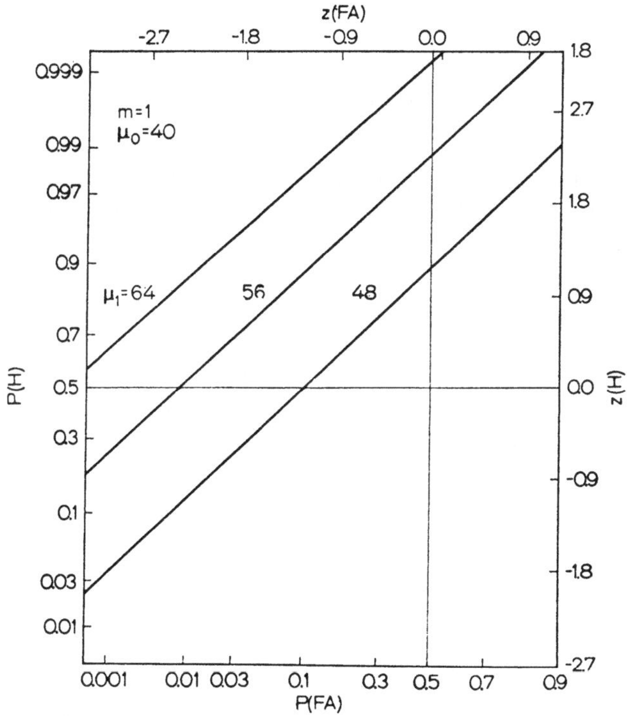

Fig. 8a. Continuous ROC-curves drawn through the values of $P(H)$ and $P(FA)$ generated by varying the value of x_c. Only the critical cell is monitored by the observer

$\mu_1 = 48, 56, 64$, and $m = 1, 16$. In Fig. 9, d is plotted against $\mu_1/\sqrt{\mu_0}$ on log-log coordinates for $m = 1, 4, 16$ and $\mu_0 = 1.3$ and 40. The theoretical curves for $m > 1$ show some important resemblances to experimental results on luminance detec-

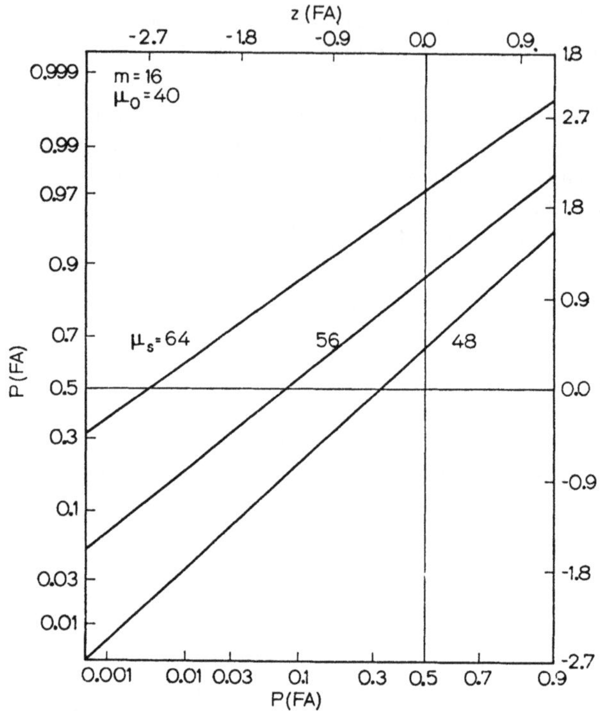

Fig. 8b. Continuous ROC-curves drawn through the values of $P(H)$ and $P(FA)$ generated by varying the value of x_c. Sixteen cells including the critical cell, are being monitored

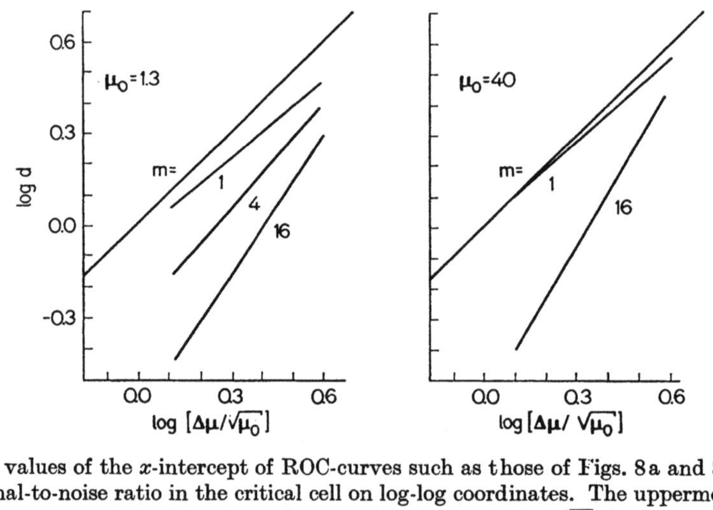

Fig. 9. The values of the x-intercept of ROC-curves such as those of Figs. 8a and 8b, plotted against signal-to-noise ratio in the critical cell on log-log coordinates. The uppermost curve in each panel represents the equation $d = \Delta\mu/\sqrt{\mu_0}$

tion: the slopes of the ROC-curves become appreciably shallower as d increases, and d appears to grow with signal strength raised to some power greater than 1.0. Whether or not these resemblances are coincidental remains to be seen.

Acknowledgement. This chapter was completed in January, 1969. Its preparation was supported in part by PHS Research Grant No. NB06050.

References

Arduini, A.: The tonic discharge of the retina and its central effects. In: Progress in Brain Research, Vol. 1. Moruzzi, G., Fessard, A., Jasper, H. H. (Eds.): Amsterdam: Elsevier 1963.

Barlow, H. B.: Retinal noise and absolute threshold. J. opt. Soc. Amer. **46**, 634—639 (1956).

— Increment thresholds at low intensities considered as signal/noise discriminations. J. Physiol. (Lond.) **136**, 469—488 (1957).

— Temporal and spatial summation in human vision at different background intensities. J. Physiol. (Lond.) **141**, 337—350 (1958).

— A method of determining the overall quantum efficiency of visual discrimination. J. Physiol. (Lond.) **160**, 155—168 (1962a).

— Measurements of quantum efficiency of discrimination in human scotopic vision. J. Physiol. (Lond.) **160**, 169—188 (1962b).

— The physical limits of visual discrimination. In: Photophysiology, Vol. 2. Giese, A. C. (Ed.): New York: Academic Press 1964a.

— Dark adaptation: a new hypothesis. Vision Res. **4**, 47—58 (1964b).

— Optic nerve impulses and Weber's Law. Cold Spr. Harb. Symp. quant. Biol. **30**, 539—546 (1965).

— Levick, W. R.: Three factors limiting the reliable detection of light by retinal ganglion cells of the cat. J. Physiol. (Lond.) **200**, 1—25 (1969).

Baumgardt, E.: La nature statistique et aléatoire des flux lumineaux extrêmement faibles et leur incidence sur la vision de nuit. C.I.E. Comptes Rendues, XIV Session, Bruxelles, 78—87 (1959).

— Smith, S. W.: Facilitation effect of background light on target detection: a test of theories of absolute threshold. Vision Res. **5**, 299—312 (1965).

Békésy, G. von: Über das Fechnersche Gesetz und seine Bedeutung für die Theorie der akustischen Beobachtungsfehler und die Theorie des Hörens. Ann. Phys. **7**, 329—359 (1930; translated in Békésy, 1960).

— Experiments in Hearing. New York: McGraw-Hill 1960.

Blackwell, H. R.: Studies of psychophysical methods for measuring visual thresholds. J. opt. Soc. Amer. **42**, 606—616 (1952).

— Neural theories of simple visual discriminations. J. opt. Soc. Amer. **53**, 129—160 (1963).

Cornsweet, T. N., Pinsker, H. M.: Luminance discrimination of brief flashes under various conditions of adaptation. J. Physiol. (Lond.) **176**, 294—310 (1965).

Eijkman, E., Vendrik, A. J. H.: Detection theory applied to the absolute sensitivity of sensory systems. Biophys. J. **3**, 65—78 (1963).

Emmerich, D. S.: ROCs obtained with two signal intensities presented in random order, and a comparison between yes-no and rating ROCs. Perc. Psychophys. **3**, 35—40 (1968).

Fitzhugh, R.: The statistical detection of threshold signals in the retina. J. gen. Physiol. **40**, 925—948 (1957).

Green, D. M., Swets, J. A.: Signal Detection Theory and Psychophysics. New York: Wiley 1966.

Hecht, S., Shlaer, S., Pirenne, M. H.: Energy, quanta, and vision. J. gen. Physiol. **25**, 819—840 (1942).

Hohle, R. H.: Detection of a visual signal with low background noise: an experimental comparison of two theories. J. exp. Psychol. **70**, 459—463 (1965).

HOWARTH, C. I., LOWE, G.: Statistical detection theory of Piper's Law. Nature (Lond.) **212**, 324—326 (1966).

HUBBARD, R.: The thermal stability of rhodopsin and opsin. J. gen. Physiol. **42**, 259—280 (1958).

JONES, R. C.: Quantum efficiency of human vision. J. opt. Soc. Amer. **49**, 645—653 (1959).

KRANTZ, D.: Threshold theories of signal detection. Psychol. Rev. **76**, 308—324 (1969).

KUFFLER, S. W., FITZHUGH, R., BARLOW, H. B.: Maintained activity in the cat's retina in light and darkness. J. gen. Physiol. **40**, 683—702 (1957).

LESHOWITZ, B., TAUB, H. B., RAAB, D. H.: Visual detection of signals in the presence of continuous and pulsed backgrounds. Perc. Psychophys. **4**, 207—213 (1968).

LOWE, G.: Interval of time uncertainty in visual detection. Perc. Psychophys. **2**, 278—280 (1967).

LUCE, R. D.: A threshold theory for simple detection. Psychol. Rev. **70**, 61—79 (1963a).

— Detection and recognition. In: Handbook of Mathematical Psychology, Vol. 1. LUCE, R. D., BUSH, R. R., and GALANTER, E. (Eds.): New York: Wiley 1963b.

— BUSH, R. R., GALANTER, E. (Eds.): Handbook of Mathematical Psychology. New York: Wiley 1963.

MUNSINGER, H., GUMMERMAN, K.: Simultaneous visual detection and recognition. Perc. Psychophys. **3**, 383—386 (1968).

NACHMIAS, J.: Effects of presentation probability and number of response alternatives on simple visual detection. Perc. Psychophys. **3**, 151—155 (1968).

— KOCHER, E.: Detection and discrimination of luminance increments. J. opt. Soc. Amer. **60**, 382—390 (1970).

— STEINMAN, R. M.: Study of absolute visual detection by the rating-scale method. J. opt. Soc. Amer. **53**, 1206—1213 (1963); **54**, 554E (1964).

— — Brightness and discriminability of light flashes. Vision Res. **5**, 545—557 (1965).

NORMAN, D. A.: Sensory thresholds and response bias. J. acoust. Soc. Amer. **35**, 1432—1441 (1963).

PETERSON, W. W., BIRDSALL, T. G., FOX, W. C.: The theory of signal detectability. Trans IRE PGIT-4, 171—212 (1954).

RODIECK, R. W.: Maintained activity of cat retinal ganglion cells. J. Neurophysiol. **30**, 1043—1071 (1967).

ROSE, A.: The sensitivity performance of the human eye on an absolute scale. J. opt. Soc. Amer. **38**, 196—208 (1948).

RUSHTON, W. A. H.: Increment threshold and dark adaptation. J. opt. Soc. Amer. **53**, 104—109 (1963).

SCHOEFFLER, M. S.: Theory of psychophysical learning. J. acoust. Soc. Amer. **37**, 1124—1133 (1965).

STEVENS, S. S., MORGAN, C. T., VOLKMANN, J.: Theory of the neural quantum in the discrimination of loudness and pitch. Amer. J. Psychol. **54**, 315—335 (1941).

STONE, J., FABIAN, M.: Summing properties of the cat's retinal ganglion cell. Vision Res. 8, 1023—1040 (1968).

SWETS, J. A.: Is there a sensory threshold? Science **134**, 168—177 (1961).

— TANNER, W. P., BIRDSALL, T. G.: Decision processes in perception. Psychol. Rev. **68**, 301—340 (1961).

TANNER, W. P.: Physiological implications of psychophysical data. Ann. N. Y. Acad. Sci. **89**, 752—765 (1961).

— SWETS, J. A.: A decision-making theory of visual detection. Psychol. Rev. **61**, 401—409 (1954).

TREISMAN, M.: Noise and Weber's Law: the discrimination of brightness and other dimensions. Psychol. Rev. **71**, 314—330 (1964).

— Statistical detection theory and Crozier's Law: derivation of a new sensory scaling procedure. J. math. Psychol. **2**, 205—218 (1965).

— A statistical decision model for sensory discrimination which predicts Weber's Law and other sensory laws: some results of a computer simulation. Perc. Psychophys. **1**, 203—230 (1966).

TREISMAN, M., WATTS, T. R.: Relation between statistical decision theory and the traditional procedures for measuring sensory thresholds. Psychol. Bull. **66**, 438—454 (1966).

ULEHLA, Z. J., HALPERN, J., CERF, A.: Integration of information in a visual discrimination task. Perc. Psychophys. **4**, 1—4 (1968).

WEINTRAUB, D. J., HAKE, H. W.: Visual discrimination, an interpretation in terms of detectability theory. J. opt. Soc. Amer. **52**, 1179—1184 (1962).

WICKELGREN, W. A.: Strength theories of disjunctive visual detection. Perc. Psychophys. **2**, 331—337 (1967).

— Unidimensional strength theory and component analysis of noise in absolute and comparative judgments. J. math. Psychol. **5**, 102—122 (1968).

Chapter 4

Luminance Difference Thresholds

By

H. RICHARD BLACKWELL, Columbus, Ohio (USA)

With 7 Figures

Contents

Introduction

Light, the physical stimulus to vision, may vary only in luminance, wavelength, and in its spatial and temporal distribution. Hence, it is not surprising that study of the operating characteristics of the visual system by psychophysical methods has long included study of luminance difference thresholds, along with studies of color-difference thresholds, acuity thresholds and flicker thresholds. Indeed, at one time or another luminance difference thresholds have played an important role in the elucidation of every known characteristic of the visual system. Let us begin by summarizing this illustrious history, then turn to a detailed consideration of the special place of luminance difference thresholds in contemporary visual psychophysics.

Historical Role of Luminance Difference Thresholds

Perhaps the earliest measurements of luminance difference thresholds were those of BOUGUER in 1760 (cited by VON HELMHOLTZ, 1909) who measured luminance difference thresholds at several different levels of luminance. The measurements had a practical purpose, BOUGUER being interested in the precision with which photometrists could set equality between two luminances. He found that experimental observers could discern a small percentage difference in luminance, the magnitude of which was independent of the absolute level of luminance. Bouguer believed that this psychophysical characteristic of human observers made them suitable for use in establishing photometric equivalences. Today we can perhaps agree that human observers make quite good null photometers without agreeing either that the magnitude of the luminance difference threshold is independent of the level of luminance or that, if true, this would be the only factor determining the precision of equivalence matches.

In 1832 Weber (cited in Boring, 1942) restudied luminance difference thresholds at different levels of luminance and reached the same conclusion, namely, that the luminance difference threshold is proportional to luminance. As is well known, Fechner in 1860 (cited by Boring, 1942) used this finding in establishing a scale of sensory brightness as a function of luminance. The method involved the assumption that apparent brightness could be scaled in terms of luminance difference units, Weber having shown these to be proportionally equal. The method proceeded as follows: A luminance just perceptibly brighter than zero was taken as the first just noticeable difference (jnd). Then a series of luminance differences was determined sequentially, each just one jnd greater in perceived brightness than the one before. The magnitude of sensed brightness corresponding to any given luminance was described by the number of jnd steps separating it from zero. Thus, a functional relation between the magnitude of brightness and luminance was established without requiring that experimental observers assess brightness directly, an operation Fechner believed them unable to perform. Of course, it is now well established that observers can assess the magnitude of brightness directly. Alternatively, various scaling operations can be performed in such a way that a reliable brightness scale can be established without the summation of jnd steps based upon luminance difference thresholds. Thus, this early use of luminance difference thresholds is no longer of great interest. (See Krantz, chapter 26, this volume.)

In 1845, Masson (cited by von Helmholtz, 1909) showed that $\overline{\Delta L}/L$, the luminance difference threshold expressed as a proportion of the luminance, was not independent of the value of L, but rather decreased as L increased. Subsequently, Koenig and Brodhun (1889) attempted to define a quantitative relation between $\overline{\Delta L}/L$ and L over a wide range of values of L. These authors found the value of $\overline{\Delta L}/L$ to decrease to a minimum value as L was increased, then to increase slightly as L was further increased. Subsequent work has shown that the secondary increase in the value of $\overline{\Delta L}/L$ at large values of L was artifactual. Steinhardt (1936) and Craik (1938) have shown that use of an inadequately extended field luminance increases $\overline{\Delta L}/L$ at large values of L. Keller (1941) has shown that, in addition, a secondary rise in $\overline{\Delta L}/L$ can occur for inappropriately selected values of exposure duration due to a complicating variation in the relation between $\overline{\Delta L}/L$ and exposure duration at different values of L.

Since Koenig and Brodhun, much attention has been devoted to the precise form of the relationship between $\overline{\Delta L}/L$ and L as a clue to the mechanisms involved in the response of the visual system to variations in luminance. Hecht (1935) used values of $\overline{\Delta L}/L$ as a function of L among other visual threshold data to test the validity of his photochemical theory of vision. According to this theory, detection of a threshold luminance difference corresponds to the presence of a fixed rate of decomposition of the visual photopigment, the concentration of which depends upon the magnitude of L. Hecht compared experimental values of $\overline{\Delta L}/L$ as a function of L with predictions based upon different rate constants and found the best conformity when bimolecular reactions were assumed. He predicted that Log $\overline{\Delta L}/L$ will relate to Log L in terms of a specific type of negative exponential function.

Crozier (1940) utilized data relating $\overline{\Delta L}/L$ to L to test his neural-statistical theory of vision. He conceptualized the visual system as consisting of a population of elements of neural effect, each having a different luminance threshold. Crozier deduced from extensive data on the critical flicker function of luminance that the magnitude of total sensory effect from all elements is related to Log L by a probability integral. Thus, the distribution of sensitivities of elements of neural effect is a normal frequency function of Log L. When the visual system is adapted to L, the total sensory effect represents effects from all those elements whose thresholds are reached or exceeded by L. Excitability to a luminance increment must therefore depend upon the number of elements of neural effect open to activation by the increment. Crozier predicted that $\frac{1}{\overline{\Delta L}}$ will be a declining normal probability integral in terms of Log L.

de Vries (1943) attempted to use values of $\overline{\Delta L}/L$ as a function of L to test his theory that luminance difference thresholds reflect only the operation of quantum variability in L. According to this view, the visual system attempts to detect the presence of an increment of light quanta, ΔN, added to a time-varying number of quanta having an average value, N. The time-variability in N is proportional to $N^{1/2}$. The threshold value of ΔN is directly proportional to the measure of time variability. Thus de Vries predicted that Log $\overline{\Delta L}/L$ will be related to Log L by a straight line of slope $-1/2$.

Still later, Bouman *et al.* (1963) developed a theoretical model of the visual system which combined quantum variability in the light stimulus with physiological fluctuations in the neural elements. This modification of the de Vries theory predicts that the relationship between Log $\overline{\Delta L}/L$ and Log L will be a continuous function passing through zones with slopes of -1, $-1/2$ and 0 as L is increased.

Blackwell (1963) developed a theoretical model of the visual system in terms of systems variability without identifying the sources of different components of the total variability. This theory assumes that the magnitude of sensory effect is related to luminance by a family of hyperbolas, each corresponding to one level of probability of occurrence. The assumption is made that discrimination of ΔL occurs whenever $\Delta L + L$ reaches or exceeds a level of sensory effect occurring from L alone with a fixed small probability. The theory explicitly assumes the existence of "dark light", that is, the presence of sensory effect in the absence of light stimulation. Blackwell predicts that Log $\overline{\Delta L}/L$ will be related to Log L by a continuous function passing smoothly between the limiting slopes of -1 and 0 as L is increased.

As we shall see, of these five theories, only the original de Vries theory can be rejected on the basis of currently-existing experimental data. Choice among the other theories must await definitive experiments designed to differentiate among them, or other lines of experimental evidence bearing on the general postulates of the different theories.

There is also a long history of use of luminance difference thresholds in studying the spatial and temporal operating characteristics of the visual system. With regard to spatial organization, RICCÒ (1877) studied the luminance difference threshold for circular light stimuli of varying diameter, showing that the threshold continued to decrease as stimulus diameter increased. GRAHAM *et al.* (1939) attributed this result to the operation of a spatial summative mechanism. The concept was that all points in a light stimulus contribute to the effect produced in the CNS, with points contributing increasingly less with increased separation from the center of the stimulus. These authors postulated the existence of a spatial summative effect which operates as a power function of the distance of a point from the stimulus center, and derived the exponent of the power function from experimental data. Subsequently, KINCAID, BLACKWELL, and KRISTOFFERSON (1960) formalized this conception in terms of a spatial isomorphic mapping system in which each point in the light stimulus produced a graded spatial distribution of effect in an hypothetical CNS space. The effects from different points in the light stimulus were assumed to be arithmetically additive. It was postulated that detection of the presence of the light stimulus requires that the sum of effects from different points in the stimulus reach a criterion value somewhere within the CNS map. On this basis, data on the luminance difference threshold for circular targets of varying diameter may be used to infer the form of the spatial point spread function.

A separate line of experimentation has suggested the existence of spatial inhibition. For example, BEITEL (1936) showed that a bright source of light in the vicinity of a light stimulus causes a rise in its luminance difference threshold. Whereas this effect could be the result of ocular stray light, FRY and BARTLEY (1935) had shown previously that a similar result could be obtained by adding a dark line near the vicinity of the edge of a test stimulus, a result contrary to the result to be expected from stray light.

BLOCH (1885) first studied the luminance difference threshold for light pulses varying in duration and showed that the luminance difference threshold was inversely related to pulse duration. GRAHAM and KEMP (1938) obtained more extensive data and postulated a temporal summative effect. The conception was that elements of light stimulation separated temporally produce additive effects to an extent dependent upon the time separation between them. It was suggested that all temporal events encompassed within the "integration time" of the visual system added algebraically, whereas those separated by more than the integration time of the system added not at all. This result was shown to be compatible with electrophysiological data such as those reported by HARTLINE (1934). Later, CLARK and BLACKWELL (reported by BLACKWELL, 1963) generalized this conception in terms of a temporal point spread function, analogous to the spatial point spread function mentioned above. Each momentary pulse of light stimulus was considered to produce a delayed and protracted graded distribution of effect across time. The effects from different momentary pulses were assumed to add algebraically. It was postulated that detection of the presence of a light stimulus occurs whenever the sum of all effects reaches a criterion value at some point in the time after stimulation during which the effects persist.

Hecht (1937) used luminance difference thresholds in large part to provide refined evidence in support of the "duplicity theory", the conception that the functional characteristics of the visual system depend upon the operation of two photosensitive receptor classes designated cones and rods. The existence of these two classes of receptors was inferred from a variety of experiments, depending upon differences in spectral sensitivity, differences in retinal location, and differences in the spatial and temporal operating characteristics of cones and rods.

Stiles (1939, 1947) used luminance difference thresholds to identify the operation of the rod photoreceptor system or of one or another of the cone photoreceptor systems. He first measured $\overline{\Delta L}$ as a function of L for cases in which the spectral composition of $\overline{\Delta L}$ and L was matched, (homochromatic increment thresholds), in which case the identity of the photoreceptor system could be defined with relative certainty in advance. Threshold ΔL was then measured as a function of L when $\overline{\Delta L}$ and L differed in spectral composition (heterochromatic increment thresholds). Identification of the operation of one or another of the photoreceptor systems was based upon a complex comparison of the relations between $\overline{\Delta L}$ and L for the heterochromatic and homochromatic increment cases. (See Enoch, chapter 21, this volume.)

Luminance difference thresholds have also been used as test probes of the level of effect produced by different spatial and temporal patterns of light stimulation. For example, Fiorentini *et al.* (1955) have used the luminance difference threshold for a point light probe to evaluate the effective luminance existing at various points within the Mach bands seen at the edges of certain luminance gradients. The effective luminance at a given point along the luminance gradient is given by the value of a field of uniform luminance for which the same threshold value of ΔL is obtained. The results reveal the existence of zones of reduced and enhanced effective luminance corresponding generally to the location of the dark and bright Mach bands. (See Fiorentini, chapter 8, this volume.)

Westheimer (1965, 1967) has applied this procedure to circular background fields of varying size. The fields are of uniform luminance and appear uniformly bright. The luminance difference thresholds for a point light probe reveal different effective luminances for fields of equal luminance but unequal size. Effective luminance increases as field size increases, then decreases as it is further increased. These results are taken to suggest the existence of point spread functions for L which involve both summative and inhibitive components. (See Westheimer, chapter 7, this volume.)

In the temporal domain, Crawford (1947) and Baker (1955) have used the luminance difference threshold to assess transient adaptive effects occurring when the visual system is exposed to first one then another level of luminance. The effective luminance may be inferred as in the spatial domain from luminance difference thresholds obtained with a continuously-exposed luminance. An unusually subtle version of this method was used by Boynton *et al.* (1961) who presented a momentary light probe on a background whose luminance varied periodically at a frequency above the critical fusion frequency. Thus, the background brightness appeared steady. However, the luminance difference thresholds obtained at different times relative to the periodic variation showed correlated periodic variations in effective luminance, demonstrating that the effect of the background was time-varying even though the brightness was not.

Luminance difference thresholds have also played an important role in the development of theories of the decision processes believed to be operative in psychophysical threshold measurements. In 1832 WEBER (cited in BORING, 1942) reported that the variability in successive determinations of the luminance difference threshold was directly proportional to the mean value of the threshold. CROZIER (1936) used this fact as the basis for a general theory of sensory discrimination, in which the psychophysical decision process was conceptualized as occurring in terms of the sensory effects of stimuli rather than the stimuli themselves. Subsequently CROZIER and his colleagues tested various implications of this theory by measuring luminance difference thresholds in humans as well as by other measurements of sensory response in many animal forms.

TANNER and SWETS (1954) used luminance difference thresholds in developing their statistical decision theory. This theory begins with CROZIER's conception that decision processes operate on the sensory effects of stimuli rather than on the stimuli themselves. It assumes the use of a criterion magnitude of effect which will be reached or exceeded by the effects due to $L + \Delta L$ on a certain fraction of the trials and the effects due to L alone on a different fraction of the trials. The observer may be induced to set this criterion magnitude at different values by rewards given to different classes of response. (See NACHMIAS, chapter 3, this volume.)

BLACKWELL (1963) reports an earlier decision theory based also upon luminance difference thresholds. This theory explains the proportionality between threshold variability and mean threshold first observed by WEBER (op. cit.), supported by more than 50 publications of CROZIER and his colleagues, and further supported by BLACKWELL (1946, 1963). The theory assumes that the visual system samples the time-variable effect produced by a fixed background luminance, L, and sets a criterion level of effect whose probability of occurrence is small. This criterion is then applied to presentations of $L + \Delta L$, and a detection occurs whenever the background plus increment produce a value of effect equal to or greater than the criterion. TANNER and SWETS argued for the replacement of this concept of a fixed criterion by the variable criterion described above. As BLACKWELL (1963) has pointed out, the predictions of the two theories are indistinguishable if the statistical decision theorists are allowed to assume a non-linear transfer function between stimulus magnitude and effect, as they do.

In very early times, such philosophers as HERBART (cited by BORING, 1942) believed that all sensory experiences related to luminance were constructed from luminance difference thresholds as building blocks. At a much more sophisticated level, HECHT and MINTZ (1939) used the photochemical equations inferred from luminance difference thresholds to describe the relation between visual acuity and luminance. These investigators used a simple conversion constant to go from luminance difference to acuity thresholds. Their procedure implies that the operating characteristics of the visual system are the same for the two classes of psychophysical discrimination.

Contemporary Role of Luminance Difference Thresholds

The historical survey presented in the last section reveals the important role luminance difference thresholds have played in the development of our knowledge in most areas of visual psychophysics. Of course, much the same could be said for such additional discrimination data as color-difference thresholds, and thresholds for visual acuity and flicker. Historically, data obtained by study of these different aspects of visual discrimination have entered a general pool of knowledge, and from this pool have come our conceptions of the operation of the visual system as a whole.

The more extensive data now available make it clear, however, that somewhat different operating characteristics of the visual system are revealed by studies of these different discriminatory processes. Let us examine the characteristics of the visual system revealed by the most precise luminance difference threshold data available today. As we shall see, the operating characteristics revealed by these data differ in important ways from those revealed by our most precise current data involving visual acuity and flicker discriminations.

Conditions Used in Measurement of Luminance Difference Thresholds

During the past two decades an extensive body of luminance difference threshold data have been collected under a standardized set of experimental conditions.

In the procedure utilized, test observers are presented with an extended field of uniform, controlled luminance which is designated the "background". They are instructed to direct their lines-of-sight toward some point or other within this field at all times during the experimental measurements, so that the adaptation of the visual system is presumed to be equilibrated. At scheduled intervals during the test period, the observers are required to direct their lines-of-sight to a particular point in the background field, at which the test stimuli were presented.

The test stimulus consists of a spatially-localized, temporally-controlled change in luminance, achieved by adding a luminance increment momentarily to the steady background luminance. The increment is designated the "target" with defined spatial and temporal characteristics.

In the experiments to be considered, a particular variant of the method of constant stimulus was used known as the "forced-choice" method (Blackwell, 1952). In this procedure, observers are required to indicate the presence of discrimination by correctly identifying some measurable aspect of the stimulus. The philosophy of the procedure involves limiting the decision task of the observers to an aspect of the experimental situation possessing little affective content, leaving the decision as to the threshold criterion to be deduced by the experimenter from the data obtained. In the experiments to be considered here, the "temporal" variant of the forced-choice method was used. With this method, the observers have to indicate in which of four time intervals the stimulus appeared, being forced to choose the most likely interval whether or not they believed that they had detected the presence of the target. Five values of the luminance increment were used to define the psychophysical curve. Luminance difference thresholds were calculated corresponding to 50% correct responses, allowance having been made for chance success, using a form of the probit analysis of FINNEY (1947) in which a normal ogive was fitted to the linear values of the luminance increment.

Observers were given periods of training of at least 20 hours before the initiation of data collection, and often used the method for more than 100 hours during a series of experiments. Retesting under identical conditions usually results in repeats of the threshold luminance increment within $\pm 5\%$. At the forced choice threshold, the practised observer rarely has any clear notion concerning either the spatial or temporal characteristics of the target. Thus, the data represent what is apparently the lowest possible level of information obtainable from a luminance increment, a level considerably below that involved in the classical luminance difference threshold established by the method of adjustment to jnd. This point should be borne in mind in interpretation of the data presented here.

The Effect of Luminance upon the Luminance Difference Threshold

Data collected by BLACKWELL and LAW (reported in BLACKWELL, 1963) will serve to illustrate the effect of the level of background luminance upon the luminance difference threshold. In these experiments, artificial stops were used to reduce the size of the observer's ocular pupils to 1 mm diameter, so that effects of luminance upon the pupillomotor mechanism would not complicate interpretation of the data obtained. Exposure duration was 0.01 second. Separate series of experiments were conducted with circular disc targets having diameters of 1 and 45 minutes of arc. The data take the form shown in Fig. 1, where the luminance difference threshold, $\overline{\Delta L}/L$ is plotted as a function of the level of background luminance, L, on a double logarithmic grid. Data for the two sizes of circular disc

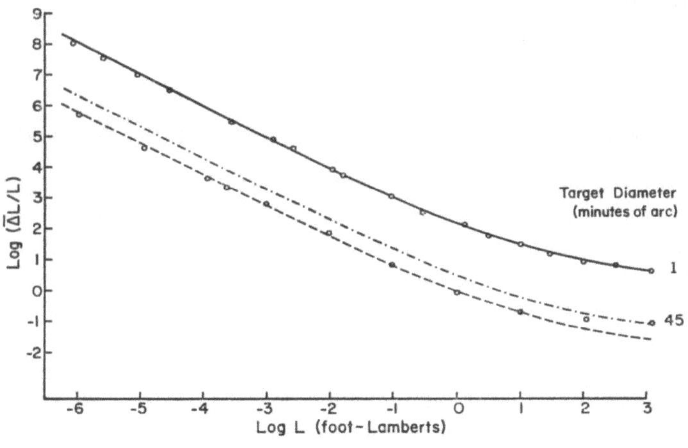

Fig. 1. Data of BLACKWELL and LAW (cited by BLACKWELL, 1963). The threshold luminance difference, $\overline{\Delta L}/L$, is shown as a function of the background luminance, L, for circular disc targets of two sizes. The solid curve is fitted to the data for the smaller target (1′). The dashed curves have the same form and are shown at two different ordinate positions for the data for the larger target (45′)

targets are plotted separately. We note that there is a continuous curve relating Log $\overline{\Delta L}/L$ to L with slopes varying from -1 to near zero. Of the five theories used to predict the $\overline{\Delta L}/L$ function of L, only the de Vries theory can be excluded. As noted, this theory predicts a straight line of slope $-1/2$ which can fit no more than three of the points on either curve.

(BLACKWELL and LAW conducted a special experiment to compare the value of $\overline{\Delta L}$ when L was zero, and when L had the smallest finite value studied, about 1×10^{-6} footlamberts. The values of $\overline{\Delta L}$ were equal, revealing that the classical distinction between the "absolute threshold" and the "difference threshold" has no significance for these conditions of measurement.)

In Fig. 1, the data for the 1-minute circular disc target have been fitted by an empirical curve, plotted as the solid line running through the data points. The curve fit appears very good. This empirical curve has also been drawn in comparison with the data points obtained with the 45-minute target. The upper dashed curve represents the fit of the empirical curve through the data point obtained at the highest value of L, whereas the lower dashed curve represents the fit of the same curve through data points obtained at the lower values of L. The empirical curve was fitted by simple adjustment along the ordinate scale. With a double logarithmic grid, this corresponds to fitting a curve having proportional values of $\overline{\Delta L}/L$ as a function of L. Note that the empirical curve fitted in this way fails to fit the data for the larger target. In terms of the upper dashed curve which is brought to agreement at the highest luminance level, the values of $\overline{\Delta L}/L$ for the larger target fall systematically below the curve at all the lower luminance levels, representing a proportionate increase in sensitivity at low luminances with respect to the level of sensitivity found at the highest level of luminance.

The construction of Fig. 1 suggests that the spatial organization of the visual system undergoes a progressive change as a function of luminance level, as has been suggested by BLACKWELL (1946, 1963). This idea will be developed further in the next section.

The Effect of Spatial Characteristics of the Target upon the Luminance Difference Threshold

Simplest to consider first will be data collected by KRISTOFFERSON and BLACKWELL (as reported by BLACKWELL, 1963). The luminance of the background, L, was fixed at 10 footlamberts. The observers used normal binocular vision, unencumbered by artificial pupils. Target exposure duration was fixed at 0.01 second. In the first series of experiments, circular disc targets of varying diameter were used. The values of the luminance difference threshold, $\overline{\Delta L}/L$, are presented in Fig. 2 as a function of target diameter on a double logarithmic grid. We see that the value of $\overline{\Delta L}/L$ decreases as target diameter increases. For very small values of target diameter, D, the empirical curve fitted through the data points is linear with a slope of -2, signifying that the product of $\overline{\Delta L}/L$ and D^2 is constant. For larger values of target diameter $\overline{\Delta L}/L$ continues to fall but at a progressively lesser rate of change. However, the condition where $\overline{\Delta L}/L$ is independent of D does not occur, even with a target whose diameter is 54 minutes of arc.

These data may be analyzed in terms of the spatial isomorphic mapping concept mentioned earlier. This conception begins with the map in the hypothetical CNS space produced by an infinitesimal area or point located in the target space, known as a point spread function.

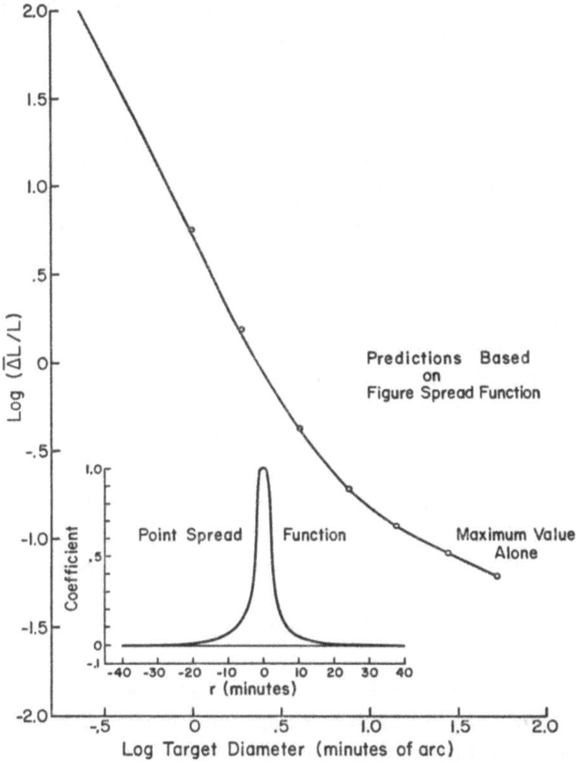

Fig. 2. Data of KRISTOFFERSON and BLACKWELL (cited by BLACKWELL, 1963). The threshold luminance difference, $\overline{\Delta L}/L$, is shown as a function of the diameter for circular disc targets. The solid curve represents expected values based on the point spread function shown, which was derived from the data

Describe a target in real space in terms of its "luminance profile", that is, the luminance distribution across the two dimensions of space in the target plane. Define a "figure spread function" as the map in the hypothetical CNS space obtained by a mathematical convolution of each point in the target luminance profile with the point spread function. Linearity and additivity are assumed in computing the figure spread function. Use as a metric for the hypothetical CNS space corresponding locations in the target space. It is possible to define criteria upon which a luminance difference threshold could be based in terms of quantifiable characteristics of the figure spread function existing in the CNS space. The usual form of the spatial summation concept implies that the basic requirement for a luminance difference threshold is that the maximum value of the figure spread function reach a criterion value, which is the same for targets of different spatial characteristics.

KINCAID, BLACKWELL, and KRISTOFFERSON (1960) showed that the point spread function could be inferred readily from experimental values of $\overline{\Delta L}/L$ as a function of diameter for circular disc targets. To do so, the point spread function must be assumed to have radial symmetry, and linearity and additivity must be assumed during the convolution process. It must also be assumed that the point spread function is identical in magnitude and shape for each point in the visual field over the area occupied by the largest target.

This assumption can be understood in the following way. The luminance difference threshold criterion is assumed to be expressible in terms of the spatial topologic map existing in the hypothetical CNS space. In effect, the experiment involves determining the level of luminance difference for a target in real space in order to produce a criterion value of the figure spread function at a particular site in the CNS space. As the target diameter increases, progressively less luminance difference is required, revealing the existence of a spatial summative effect from the perimeter to the center in the CNS space. Clearly we are studying the map of many points in target space upon one point in neural space, a process analogous to electrophysiological study of the receptive field of a ganglion cell. The point spread function, on the other hand, represents the map of one point in the target space upon many points in CNS space, expressed in terms of the metric of target space. These two maps, the many-to-one and the one-to-many, will be identical only if the point spread function is identical at every point within the limits of the spatial extent of the visual field covered by the largest target. As noted, we require that both the height and shape of the point spread function be equivalent from point to point. Equivalence of height corresponds to equal sensitivity whereas equivalence of shape corresponds to equality of the spatial extent and pattern of the summative effect.

Fig. 2 contains the data KRISTOFFERSON and BLACKWELL obtained, the empirical curve fitted to the data, and the point spread function derived from the smooth curve by trigonometric approximations. We note that the point spread function has a flat top at the center, with gradually smaller values as we move away from the center in either direction. The spatial topologic map of a point is fully represented by the three-dimensional figure obtained by rotating the point spread function through 180°. This construction reveals that a point in target space produces maximum effect at a number of points in CNS space, corresponding to points within the flat top of the three-dimensional figure, and produces a progressively lesser effect at points separated increasingly from the center of the site of maximum effect. The effect spreads a distance in CNS space corresponding to almost 30-minutes in each direction from the center as measured in the metric of target space, and the effects are never negative. This implies that we have a pure spatial summative process, without any inhibitory component, or that the inhibitory component is unmeasurable.

The point spread function in Fig. 2 was deduced from the solid curve in the figure. We may, of course, work in the other direction and "predict" the solid curve from the point spread function. In its full complexity, the process involves convolution of the luminance profile of each circular target by the point spread function. For circular disc targets, a trigonometric approximation may be used to compute the value of the figure spread function at its maximum. The value of $\overline{\Delta L}$

is proportional to the inverse of this maximum value. The maximum value of the figure spread function obtained from the smallest target is set as the required value for the luminance difference threshold. Then, the value of $\overline{\Delta L}$ for other targets is predicted as the target luminance difference required to produce the criterion value with the figure spread function of the target in question. When this process is carried out, we may say that our predictions of $\overline{\Delta L}$ are based upon the figure spread function computed for each target, and that the criterion depends upon the maximum value of the figure spread function alone. These remarks explain the legends used in Fig. 2.

Use of the prediction process for circular disc targets provides a consistency check on the calculational procedures. Maximum values of figure spread functions may also be used to predict thresholds for all noncircular targets, using the point spread function derived from circular disc targets for convolution with the luminance profile of each target. KRISTOFFERSON and BLACKWELL made predictions for a class of rectangular targets in this way, and then measured actual luminance difference thresholds for comparison, using the same observers. The full convolution was not made. Rather, trigonometric approximations were used to compute the value of the figure spread function for each target at its maximum. Rectangles varied in width with their length fixed at 51.1 minutes of arc. The predictions are shown as the solid curve in Fig. 3. The data points are plotted without adjustment. Agreement is generally good, but a systematic departure is noted, such that the rectangular targets in general yielded lower values of $\overline{\Delta L}/L$ than predicted.

Analogous studies of circular targets have been conducted at lower finite levels of background luminance and at zero background luminance (cited by BLACKWELL, 1963). The figure spread functions were shown to become progressively broader as luminance was decreased, with low finite luminances and zero luminance appearing to belong on a continuum. This characteristic is consistent with the form of the data for the two target sizes in Fig. 1. BLACKWELL and SMITH (cited by BLACKWELL, 1963) studied rectangular targets at zero background luminance, and predicted thresholds for these targets from the point spread function obtained with circular disc targets at the same luminance. In this case the predictions were more successful than those made for the finite background luminance level, but there was the same tendency for obtained values of $\overline{\Delta L}/L$ to fall below predicted values for narrow long rectangles.

KRISTOFFERSON and BLACKWELL, and BLACKWELL and SMITH also studied other classes of non-circular targets at the 10 footlambert and zero levels of background luminance. Predictions of $\overline{\Delta L}/L$ were very successful for large geometric forms. Multi-legged targets composed of long narrow rectangular elements, with and without circular centers, were also studied. Predicted values of $\overline{\Delta L}/L$ were generally successful but there was a definite trend for the obtained values to exceed predictions, opposite to the effect noted with rectangular targets.

All these related studies were restricted to one general class of targets, namely, targets for which the site of the maximum value of the figure spread could be identified in advance as the point in the CNS space corresponding to the precise center of the target in real space. It is intuitively obvious that the luminance profiles of circular disc targets will lead to maximum values at the centers of the figure spread functions obtained with monotonic, radially-symmetrical point spread functions such as shown in Fig. 2. The same is true of the rectangular and other targets studied by KRISTOFFERSON and BLACKWELL, and by BLACKWELL and SMITH. Thus, the trigonometric approximation to the full convolution process was acceptable for these targets. Of course, no information was provided as to the magnitude of the figure spread function at other points in the spatial topologic map, so that only the maximum value could be used as the threshold criterion.

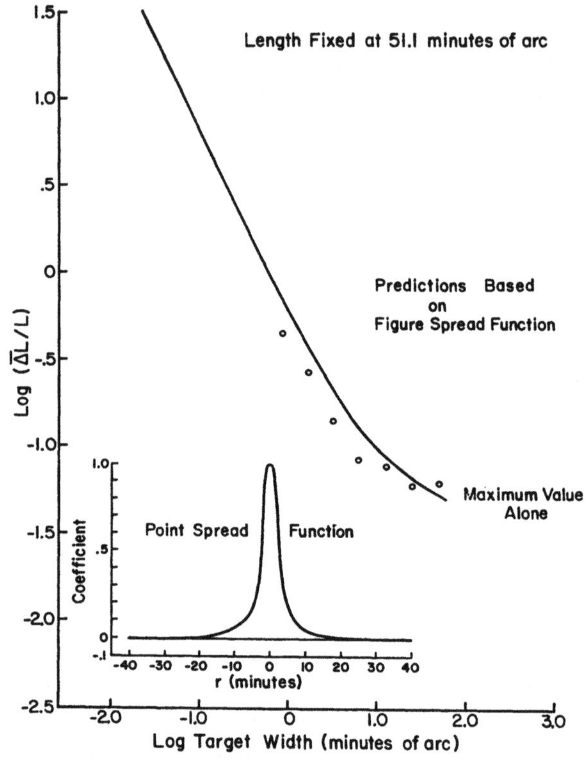

Fig. 3. Data of KRISTOFFERSON and BLACKWELL (cited by BLACKWELL, 1963). The threshold luminance difference, $\overline{\Delta L}/L$ is shown as a function of the width for rectangular targets of fixed length. The solid curve represents predicted values based on the point spread function derived from the data for circular disc targets as shown in Fig. 2

In principle, the digital computer provides us with the tool required to compute the full figure spread function resulting from convolution of the luminance profile of a target with the point spread function. Methods used recently to produce full figure spread functions with the digital computer are described by CLEAVER and BLACKWELL (in preparation). These methods do not require that the location of the maximum value of the figure spread function be known in advance. Rather, the maximum is located after performing the convolution. This makes it possible to predict values of $\overline{\Delta L}/L$ for classes of targets with unknown or more complex figure spread function maxima than those studied earlier by KRISTOFFERSON and BLACKWELL, and by BLACKWELL and SMITH.

CLEAVER and BLACKWELL have measured luminance difference thresholds for targets consisting of simple luminous annulae, and repetitive arrays of luminous bars separated by blank spaces. Circular disc targets were studied in addition so that appropriate point spread functions could be obtained. Normal binocular vision was used without artificial pupils. Exposure duration was 0.1 second. Background luminance was 10 footlamberts. The data are presented in Fig. 4. The data for the circular disc targets appear only in the form of the point spread function derived from them by essentially the same trigonometric calculational procedure as before. Note that, as before, the point spread function has only positive values, indicating the absence of spatial inhibitory effects.

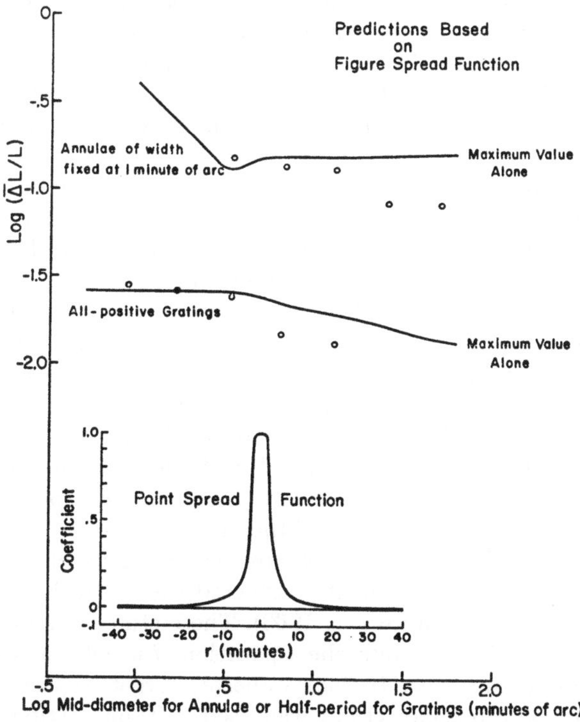

Fig. 4. Data of CLEAVER and BLACKWELL (in preparation). The threshold luminance difference, $\overline{\Delta L}/L$, is shown as a function of the mid-diameter of annulae and the half-period of all-positive squarewave gratings. The solid curves represent predicted values based on the point spread function shown, which was derived from related data for circular disc targets

The annulae had a fixed width of 1 minute of arc, and differed in the distance from the target center to the middle of each 1-minute annulus. Values of $\overline{\Delta L}/L$ are presented at the top in Fig. 4 for the annulae, expressed in terms of the mid-diameter, defined as the distance from the center of the annulus on one side to the center of the annulus on the other side. The values of $\overline{\Delta L}/L$ decrease as mid-diameter increases. The predicted values of $\overline{\Delta L}/L$ are shown by the solid curve plotted with the data points. Predictions show that $\overline{\Delta L/L}$ decreases at first as mid-diameter increases, reverses, and then approaches an asymptotic value. Agreement between the data points and predictions is good for the three smallest annulae, but the two largest annulae have considerably lower values of $\overline{\Delta L/L}$ than predicted. Analysis of the full figure spread functions, possible for the first time, revealed an interesting feature. When an annulus has a mid-diameter less than about 4 minutes of arc, the maximum in the figure spread function occurs at the center even though the target has no luminance at the center. As the annular mid-diameter is increased to 8 minutes of arc, the central maximum shifts into an annular ridge of maximum value, concentric about the target center. It is not until the annular mid-diameter reaches 64 minutes, however, that the location of the annular ridge of maximum value coincides with the location of the annular ring in the target. The reversal in the curve of predicted $\overline{\Delta L/L}$ as a function of mid-diameter is related to this shifting of the maximum from the center to an annular ridge.

The other targets studied by CLEAVER and BLACKWELL are designated "all-positive gratings". Each of these targets consisted of a series of bright rectangular bars. Bar length was fixed at 50 minutes of arc. Bar width varied, with the restriction that bar width was made equal to the blank space between bars. These targets were similar to square-wave gratings, except that only luminance increments were present in the form of arrays of bright bars. These gratings are described in terms of "half-periods", which are equal to the widths of individual bars or individual spaces. The data for these targets are presented as values of $\overline{\Delta L/L}$ as a function of half-period in the center of Fig. 4. Predictions are presented as the curve plotted with the data. As with the annulae, the data agree well with predictions for the smaller sizes. However, when the gratings become larger, the obtained values of $\overline{\Delta L/L}$ are again systematically smaller than predicted.

One aspect of these gratings deserves mention. The number of bars in the field of view was always an even number: 30, 16, 8, 4 and 2 for the different gratings. The figure spread functions always had twin maxima, corresponding generally to the sites of the two bars in the center of the array.

Before commenting further on the presumed significance of these results, let us consider the results of an experiment conducted earlier by KRISTOFFERSON and DEMBER (as reported by BLACKWELL, 1963). These studies involved targets consisting of two small luminous points, the separation of which was varied. The value of background luminance was 10 footlamberts; target exposure duration was 0.01 second. Normal binocular vision was used, without artificial pupils. Even though the targets consisted of two luminous points, the observers had only to correctly identify their time of occurrence in the temporal forced-choice sequence. Hence, the observers were not required to provide any information about the spatial characteristics of the targets.

It was obvious in advance that the site of the maximum value of the figure spread function for two-point targets will migrate from a central site to two separated sites as the two luminous points are moved apart. The value of $\overline{\Delta L/L}$ was measured for single points at various locations out from the foveal center to test the assumption that sensitivity was equal throughout the area of the visual field being tested with the different two-point targets. It was found that the value of $\overline{\Delta L/L}$ was lowest at the foveal center and increased somewhat as the target was removed from the center in any direction. This demonstrated that one of the basic assumptions required for derivation of the point spread function is not entirely justified. An approximate correction procedure was used to attempt to compensate for the non-homogeneity of sensitivity.

The data obtained by KRISTOFFERSON and DEMBER are presented in summary form in Fig. 5. The data for the circular disc targets appear only in terms of the point spread function derived from them. The data for the two-point targets are plotted in terms of $\overline{\Delta L}/L$ as a function of the total spatial extent of the target, consisting as it did of two points and a space between. (Each point measured 2.10 minutes in diameter so that the target extent was 2.10 minutes greater than the separation between centers of the two points.)

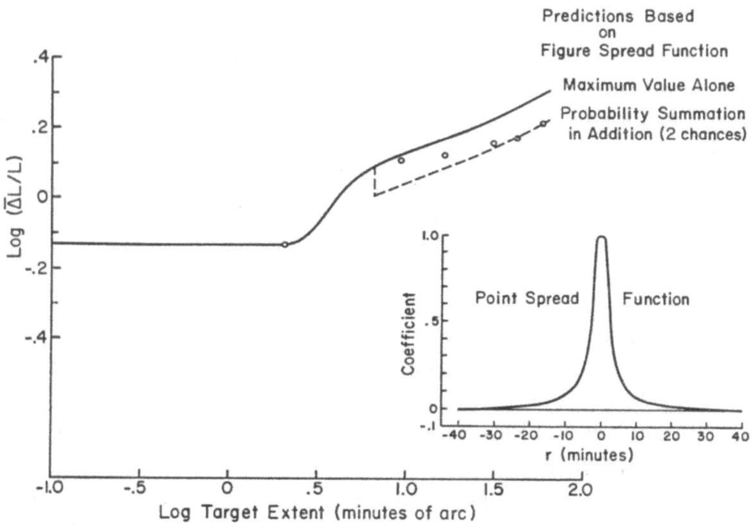

Fig. 5. Data of KRISTOFFERSON and DEMBER (cited by BLACKWELL, 1963). The threshold luminance difference, $\overline{\Delta L}/L$, is shown as a function of the spatial extent of targets composed of two points with a separation between. The solid curve represents predicted values based on the point spread function shown, which was derived from related data for circular disc targets. The dashed curve represents modified predictions to take account of multiple-site probability summation

Predictions were made by convolving the luminance profile of the two-point targets with the point spread function. In this case, the entire figure spread function was obtained even without the digital computer by assuming that the point elements in the two-point targets were small enough to be true points in terms of the gradient of the point spread function. First, predictions were made on the basis used before, namely that the luminance difference threshold is based upon the maximum in the figure spread function obtained with each target. Predictions made in this way are represented by the solid curve plotted with the data points in Fig. 5. The predicted value of $\overline{\Delta L}/L$ continues to rise as the target extent is increased because the maxima in the figure spread function continue to move farther from the foveal center and thus onto sites of ever-decreasing sensitivity. Only the data point for the smallest separation between the two stimulus points fits the predicted curve. All other experimental values of $\overline{\Delta L/L}$ fall below the predicted values.

Analysis of the figure spread functions for various two-point targets revealed that twin maxima appeared when the separation between the two points reached about 4.5 minutes in target space. Consideration of the probabilistic nature of the luminance-difference threshold suggested that each of these maxima represented a potential site at which the discrimination could occur. If the variability that gives rise to the probabilistic nature of the data is uncorrelated at the two sites, then probability summation should occur. That is, discrimination should occur whenever the figure spread function reaches the criterion value at either of the two sites of possible maxima. In probability terms

$$p_{1,2} = 1 - [(1 - p_1)(1 - p_2)] \tag{1}$$

where p_1 and p_2 are the probabilities of reaching the criterion level of the figure spread function at site 1 and site 2 respectively; and $p_{1,2}$ is the probability of reaching the criterion level at either site 1 or site 2, or both.

The concept of probability summation due to multiple independent sites has frequently been used in quantum theories of vision. PEYROU and PIATIER (1946) first suggested the existence of probability summation due to independent sites at which quanta might be absorbed in large targets. LAMAR *et al.* (1948) postulated the existence of probability summation due to large numbers of independent sites along the perimeters of targets at each of which quanta might be absorbed. VAN DEN BRINK and BOUMAN (1954) analyzed the luminance thresholds for pairs of points in terms of postulated probability summation of quantum absorption at twin sites. BLACKWELL (1963) was apparently the first to suggest multiple-site probability summation in the figure spread function.

The change in the expected values of $\overline{\Delta L/L}$ in the presence of this type of probability summation was computed from the parameters σ/M given by the probit analysis of the psychophysical data obtained with single-point targets. In this case, with probability summation $\overline{\Delta L/L}$ was reduced by 17% of the value obtained without probability summation. If we assume that probability summation occurs whenever two maxima were observed in the computed figure spread function, we may construct the dashed line in Fig. 5 to represent predictions based upon maximum value, modified by probability summation. Considering first the data points for the three largest spatial extents, we note that our modified predictions agree with the data points very well indeed, suggesting that evaluation both of the maximum value of the figure spread function and the probability summation afforded by the existence of two possible sites gives very good predictions for these targets. The data points for the targets with the two smallest spatial extents seem to show a transition from the solid line to the dashed line as separation is increased. This could be explained by assuming that variability correlation depends upon the separation between the two sites. When the sites are relatively close together, variability correlation is high and probability summation is small. It is only when the sites are sufficiently separated so that variability correlation is essentially zero that probability summation occurs fully.

It seems in order to invoke the probability summation process to explain the discrepancies between data and predictions found in the studies of annulae and gratings reported above. In the case of annulae, a localized annular ridge of maximum value occurred in the figure spread functions for the three largest targets, becoming more clear-cut for the two largest. Although it is not apparent how many possible sites exist in a continuous ridge of maximum value, there is no doubt that multiple sites do exist. Analysis of the degree of discrepancy between the obtained and predicted values of $\overline{\Delta L/L}$ suggests that at least six independent sites operated within the continuous annular ridge for each of the two largest annulae, whereas no more than two operated in the case of the third largest target. Such a result seems reasonable in terms of the spatial separation of the opposite sides of the annular ridge, considered in terms of the requirement that variability be uncorrelated in order for probability summation to occur.

In the case of all the gratings, equal maxima occurred in the two middle bars of each array. Furthermore, there were additional sites of equal or near equal magnitude along each of these bars, near the center. Thus, there were always at least two possible sites of maximum value, and usually more. The data for the three smallest gratings exhibit no probability summation. The data for the two largest gratings exhibit about the degree of probability summation to be expected from two independent sites. These results agree with the extent to which these potential sites might be expected to show uncorrelated variability due to their spatial separation.

It has been suggested (VAN DEN BRINK and BOUMAN, 1954) that multiple-site probability summation occurs also with circular disc targets, in which case this effect would be intertwined with the point spread functions reported here. Whereas this is a possibility, the present account would suggest that the effect, if present, would be smallest with circular disc targets. Such targets would have sites of maximum or near-maximum values of the figure spread function in close spatial proximity to the central maximum. In such cases, variability correlation would be high and probability summation would be small. For rectangular targets uncorrelated variability is more likely to occur at different sites within the figure spread function, thus producing probability summation. The inclusion of probability summation might explain the nature of the discrepancy between data and predictions shown for rectangular targets in Fig. 3. With the length fixed at 51.1 minutes, the three rectangles with the largest width would be most nearly circular and hence would have the least multiple-site probability summation compared to circular discs. These data points agree quite well with predictions. The long thin rectangular targets would have the greatest chance of multiple-site probability summation since their sites of maximum or near-maximum values of the figure spread function are farthest removed from the central site, and it is these targets which yield values of $\overline{\Delta L/L}$ farthest below predictions based on the maximum value alone.

This interpretation of the data for rectangular targets correctly explains the differences in the successfulness of predictions at different luminance levels. At lower luminance, the point spread functions are broader and hence there will be less chance for independent sites to occur which would lead to probability summation.

Perhaps the most interesting aspect of this account of the spatial organization of the visual system elucidated by luminance difference thresholds is the absence of any evidence for the spatial inhibitory processes found in so many physiological preparations, and suggested by other psychophysical data. The existence of an optimum spatial frequency for the resolution of sine-wave gratings, for example (Schade, 1956), implies the existence of a point spread function with both positive and negative values and is inconsistent with the all-positive point spread functions reported here. Similarly, the existence of Mach bands suggests (Ratliff, 1965) the existence of point spread functions with both positive and negative values. Thus, it appears evident that the visual system has quite different spatial operating properties under the different conditions involved in these different experiments. Perhaps, as has been suggested (for example, by Ratliff 1965) the presence of point spread functions with positive and negative values implies the existence of separate summative (facilitory) and inhibitory processes spreading across the visual field. If so, perhaps the luminance difference threshold experiments reported here involve only the spatial summative process whereas other experimental conditions involve this summative process and an additional inhibitory process. If this is the case, the luminance difference threshold experiments appear to offer a unique opportunity for study of the spatial summative process in isolation. Once the properties of the summative process are established, properties of the inhibitory process may be deduced by inference from experimental studies made under conditions in which both mechanisms operate. One interesting question concerns the number of data-processing stages in the visual system, and whether they are connected in series or in parallel.

The Effect of Temporal Characteristics of the Target upon the Luminance Difference Threshold

For our purposes here, we will select studies of the temporal domain carried out in analogy with the studies of the spatial domain described above. For convenience the language of point and figure spread functions will be applied to the temporal domain, as follows. Consider that a brief pulse of light generates an aftereffect with a time course involving a rise and fall of CNS effect. This will be called a point spread function in the time domain. Designate the time course of target luminance as the target luminance profile. Designate the convolution of the time course of target luminance with the point spread function as the figure spread function. Apply the criteria used in the spatial domain to the temporal domain. Thus, the simplest criterion for the luminance difference threshold involves a criterion value for the maximum of the figure spread function obtained with temporally-varying stimulation. Probability summation involves multiple sites in the course of time at which a maximum value of the figure spread function might occur. As in the case of the spatial domain, multiple-site probability summation can occur only if variability is uncorrelated between the sites.

Clark and Blackwell (as reported in Blackwell, 1963) studied luminance difference thresholds as a function of variations in the temporal characteristics of targets under the conditions for luminance-increment threshold experiments described above. Background luminance was 10 footlamberts. The target was a circular disc of diameter 18 minutes of arc. Consider first the data obtained with double-pulse targets, consisting of two pulses each of 0.0025 second duration with a variable separation between the pulses. The observers did not have to discriminate temporal characteristics of the targets but merely to select correctly that interval of the four in which the double-pulse target occurred.

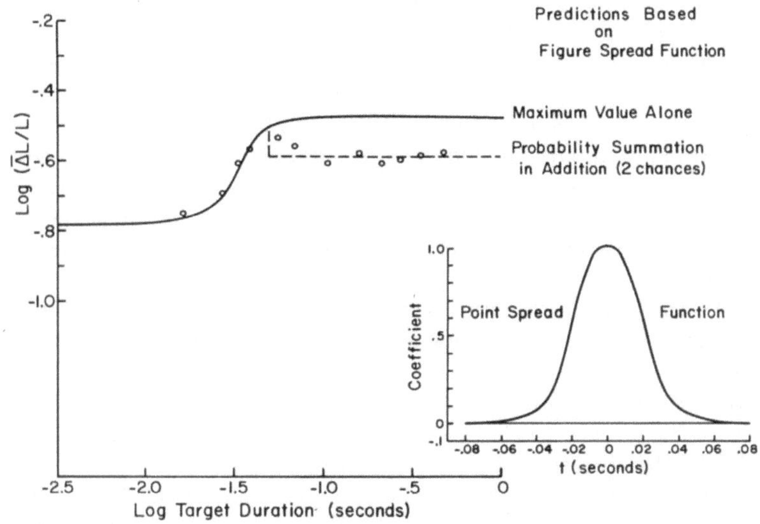

Fig. 6. Data of CLARK and BLACKWELL (cited by BLACKWELL, 1963). The threshold luminance difference, $\overline{\Delta L}/L$, is shown as a function of the temporal duration of targets composed of two pulses with a separation between. The solid curve represents expected values based on the point spread function shown, which was derived from the data. The dashed curve represents modified expectations to take account of multiple-site probability summation

The data are presented in Fig. 6. Target duration equals the temporal separation between the midpoints of the two pulses plus 0.0025 second. The theoretical predictions are analogous to those used in the spatial domain. In this case, the point spread function was derived from the double-pulse data, which was not the case in the spatial domain. The temporal case presents the difficulty that the exact time in the figure spread function at which the maximum value will occur cannot be known in advance. Since the digital computer program was not available to permit the calculation of the full figure spread function by convolution, the point spread function had to be derived from the double-pulse targets, assuming that each pulse was of infinitesimal duration compared to the time gradient of the point spread function. Symmetry of rise and fall of the temporal after-effects had to be assumed. Evidence from separate experiments with double-pulse targets of unequal luminance supported this assumption. The point spread function is shown in Fig. 6. It shows temporal aftereffects prolonged over a total of 0.160 second duration under the conditions of the experiment.

The solid curve plotted with the data points in Fig. 6 represents values of $\overline{\Delta L}/L$ predicted by reversing the calculational process. Thus the agreement of the four data points at shortest durations and the solid curve is trivial. However, the departure of the data points at the longer durations is meaningful. The dashed curve represents expectations based upon the existence of two possible sites in time at which the figure spread function maximum could have occurred. Complete figure spread functions were computed for different target durations and a discernible double peak was found to occur for a target duration of 0.0475 second. Thus, the multiple-site probability summation mechanism could be operative for target durations of that length and longer. The predicted magnitude of the probability summation effect was computed from the probability data for short single pulses as before. The value of $\overline{\Delta L}/L$ was found to be reduced by 22% when probability summation was assumed to operate. The data for the longer-duration double pulses agree very well with the modified predictions. Data for the shorter-duration double pulses in the region of possible probability summation show a gradual transition from the solid to the dashed curves, as would be expected from a gradually-reduced variability correlation as the two possible sites became further separated in time.

Data obtained with single pulses of varying length are presented in Fig. 7. The solid curve represents predicted values of $\overline{\Delta L}/L$ as a function of target duration based upon the point spread function derived from the double-pulse targets, using the criterion of a required maximum for the figure spread function. No adjustment was made on the data or predictions, so that the excellent agreement between data and prediction for durations less than 0.1 second is impressive.

At durations greater than 0.1 second, the data points fall below the predicted values and the magnitude of the discrepancy increases with duration. This

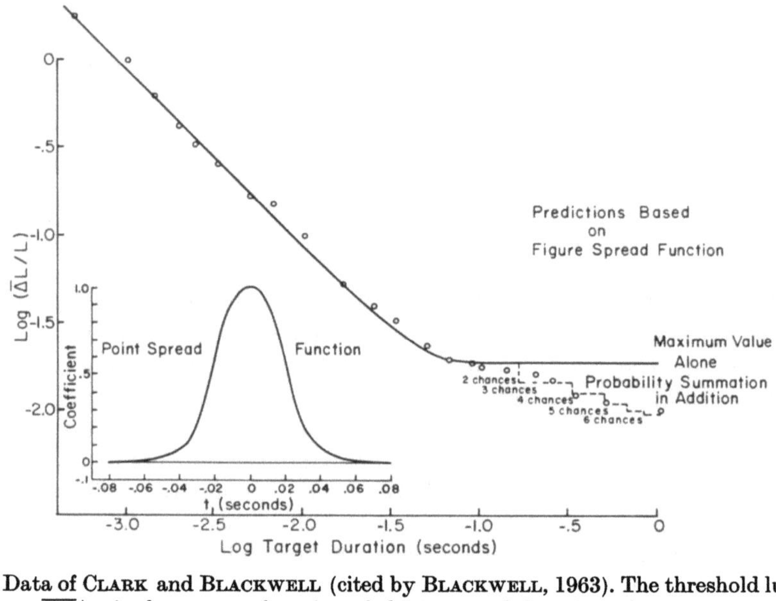

Fig. 7. Data of CLARK and BLACKWELL (cited by BLACKWELL, 1963). The threshold luminance difference, $\overline{\Delta L}/L$, is shown as a function of the temporal duration of targets composed of a single continuous pulse. The solid curve represents predicted values based on the point spread function shown, which was derived from the data for double-pulse targets as shown in Fig. 6. The dashed lines represent modified predictions to take account of probability summation due to a 6 cps cyclical scanning mechanism

departure can be explained quantitatively by assuming the existence of a CNS scanning mechanism which "cycles" six times per second. Each scan erases the effects from preceding scans, so that the continuously varying figure spread function produced by the longer pulses is considered to be broken into separate parts. Since the value of the figure spread function is at its maximum value beyond the duration of one scan, the scanner produces multiple sites for reaching the maximum value of the figure spread function, one per scan. The stair-steps in Fig. 7 represent the effects of multiple scans, derived from the relation:

$$p_{1,2\cdots n} = 1 - [(1 - p_1)(1 - p_2)\cdots(1 - p_n)] \tag{2}$$

where p_1, p_2, p_n are the probabilities of reaching the criterion level of the figure spread function at sites 1, 2, or n respectively; and $p_{1,2\cdots n}$ is the probability of reaching the criterion level at site 1, 2 or n or any combination thereof.

The quantitative reduction in $\overline{\Delta L/L}$ to be expected as the number of sites increases is computed from the probability data for a single short pulse as before. It appears that the data agree with modified predictions made on this basis to a very satisfactory degree. Thus, there appears to be evidence in the temporal domain for multiple-site probability summation for double-pulses in accordance with the analogy of the spatial domain, and a different type of multiple-site probability summation for single pulses which arises from the existence of a temporal scanner which has no analogy in the spatial domain.

Clark and Blackwell obtained analogous data at a zero level of background luminance. The temporal point spread function was broader than at 10 footlamberts but, otherwise, the nature of the data obtained and the mechanisms required to explain them were the same.

As in the spatial domain, we find that point spread functions inferred from luminance difference thresholds in the temporal domain have all positive values, corresponding to temporal summation alone. Here again, experiments with temporal sine-wave gratings suggest that there is an optimum temporal frequency (see for example deLange, 1954; also Kelly, chapter 11, this volume). As before, this implies the existence of a point spread function with both positive and negative values, and is inconsistent with the all-positive point spread functions reported here. Again, we may speculate that the luminance-difference threshold experiments give us the operating properties of a temporally summative process in isolation whereas other experiments give us the combined effects of temporally-summative and temporally-inhibitory processes. If this is the case, then luminance difference threshold experiments would seem to offer us an opportunity to study the temporally summative process in isolation also.

References

Baker, H. D.: Some direct comparisons between light and dark adaptation. J. opt. Soc. Amer. **45**, 839—844 (1955).

Beitel, R. J.: Inhibition of threshold excitation in the human eye. J. gen. Psychol. **14**, 31—61 (1936).

Blackwell, H. R.: Contrast thresholds of the human eye. J. opt. Soc. Amer. **36**, 624—643 (1946).

BLACKWELL, H. R.: Studies of psychophysical methods for measuring visual thresholds. J. opt. Soc. Amer. **42**, 606—616 (1952).
— Neural theories of simple visual discriminations. J. opt. Soc. Amer. **53**, 129—160 (1963).
BLOCH, A. M.: Expériences sur la vision. C. R. Soc. Biol. (Paris) **37**, 493—495 (1885).
BORING, E. G.: Sensation and Perception in the History of Experimental Psychology. New York: Appleton-Century 1942.
BOUMAN, M. A., VOS, J. J., WALRAVEN, P. L.: Fluctuation theory of luminance and chromaticity discrimination. J. opt. Soc. Amer. **53**, 121—128 (1963).
BOYNTON, R. M., STURR, J. F., IKEDA, M.: Study of flicker by increment threshold technique. J. opt. Soc. Amer. **51**, 196—201 (1961).
VAN DEN BRINK, G., BOUMAN, M. A.: Variation of integrative actions in the retinal system: An adaptational phenomenon. J. opt. Soc. Amer. **44**, 616—620 (1954).
CRAIK, K. J. W.: The effect of adaptation on differential brightness discrimination. J. Physiol. (Lond.) **92**, 406—421 (1938).
CRAWFORD, B. H.: Visual adaptation in relation to brief conditioning stimuli. Proc. roy. Soc. (Lond.) B **134**, 283—302 (1947).
CROZIER, W. J.: On the sensory discrimination of intensities. Proc. nat. Acad. Sci. (Wash.) **22**, 412—416 (1936).
— On the law for minimal discrimination of intensities. IV. ΔI as a function of intensity. Proc. nat. Acad. Sci. (Wash.) **26**, 382—389 (1940).
FINNEY, D. J.: Probit Analysis. Cambridge: Cambridge University Press 1947.
FIORENTINI, A., JEANNE, M., TORALDO DI FRANCIA, G.: Measurements of differential threshold in the presence of spatial illumination gradient. Atti Fond. G. Ronchi, **10**, 371—379 (1955).
FRY, G. A., BARTLEY, S. H.: The effect of one border in the visual field upon the threshold of another. Amer. J. Physiol. **112**, 414—421 (1935).
GRAHAM, C. H., BROWN, R. H., MOTE, F. A., JR.: The relation of size of stimulus and intensity in the human eye: I. Intensity thresholds for white light. J. exp. Psychol. **24**, 555—573 (1939).
— KEMP, E. H.: Brightness discrimination as a function of the duration of the increment in intensity. J. gen. Physiol. **21**, 635—650 (1938).
HARTLINE, H. K.: Intensity and duration in the excitation of single photoreceptor units. J. cell. comp. Physiol. **5**, 229—247 (1934).
HECHT, S.: A theory of visual intensity discrimination. J. gen. Physiol. **18**, 767—789 (1935).
— Rods, cones and the chemical basis of vision. Physiol. Rev. **17**, 239—290 (1937).
— MINTZ, E. U.: The visibility of single lines at various illuminations and the retinal basis of visual resolution. J. gen. Physiol. **22**, 593—612 (1939).
HELMHOLTZ, H. VON: Handbuch der Physiologischen Optik, 3rd. edit. vol. 2. Hamburg-Leipzig: Leopold Voss 1909.
KELLER, M.: The relation between the critical duration and intensity in brightness discrimination. J. exp. Psychol. **28**, 407—418 (1941).
KINCAID, W. M., BLACKWELL, H. R., KRISTOFFERSON, A. B.: Neural formulation of the effects of target size and shape upon visual detection. J. opt. Soc. Amer. **50**, 143—148 (1960).
KOENIG, A., BRODHUN, E.: Experimentelle Untersuchungen über die psychophysische Fundamentalformel in Bezug auf den Gesichtsinn. Sitzber. k. Akad. Wiss. (Berlin) **2**, 641—644 (1889).
LAMAR, E. S., HECHT, S., HENDLEY, C. D., SHLAER, S.: Size, shape, and contrast in detection of targets by daylight vision. II. Frequency of seeing and the quantum theory of cone vision. J. opt. Soc. Amer. **38**, 741—755 (1948).
DE LANGE, H.: Relationship between critical flicker-frequency and a set of low-frequency characteristics of the eye. J. opt. Soc. Amer. **44**, 380—389 (1954).
PEYROU, C., PIATIER, H.: Emploi de méthodes statistique dans l'étude de la sensibilité de l'oeil. C. R. Acad. Sci. (Paris) **223**, 589—591 (1946).
RATLIFF, F.: Mach Bands: Quantitative Studies on Neural Networks in the Retina. San Francisco: Holden-Day 1965.
RICCÒ, A.: Relazioni fra il minimo angolo visuale e l'intensità luminosa. Ann. Ottal. **6**, 373—479 (1877).

SCHADE, O. H., JR.: Optical and photoelectric analog of the eye. J. opt. Soc. Amer. **46**, 721—739 (1956).
STEINHARDT, J.: Intensity discrimination in the human eye. I. The relation of $\Delta I/I$ to intensity. J. gen. Physiol. **20**, 185—209 (1936).
STILES, W. S.: The directional sensitivity of the retina and the spectral sensitivities of the rods and cones. Proc. roy Soc. (Lond.) B **127**, 64—105 (1939).
— Increment thresholds and the mechanisms of colour vision. Documenta ophthal. **3**, 138—163 (1947).
TANNER, W. P., JR., SWETS, J. A.: A decision making theory of visual detection. Psychol. Rev. **61**, 401—409 (1954).
DE VRIES, HL.: The quantum character of light and its bearing upon threshold of vision, the differential sensitivity and visual acuity of the eye. Physica **10**, 553—564 (1943).
WESTHEIMER, G.: Spatial interaction in the human retina during scotopic vision. J. Physiol. (Lond.) **181**, 881—894 (1965).
— Spatial interaction in human cone vision. J. Physiol. (Lond.) **190**, 139—154 (1967).

Chapter 5

Visual Perimetry

By

E. AULHORN and H. HARMS, Tübingen (Germany)

With 33 Figures

Contents

I. Definitions

In this chapter the term "Perimetry" is used to include all kinds of investigations of visual fields. Before discussing perimetry we should explain what is meant by the "visual field". There are various definitions of this term:

According to TRAQUAIR (1927), the visual field is "that portion of space in which objects are visible at the same moment during steady fixation of the gaze in one direction".

According to TRENDELENBURG (1961) the visual field is "the totality of all objects which are perceived in a specific spatial arrangement with the gaze at rest".

SCHOBER (1958), following HERING and TSCHERMAK, differentiates three concepts:

the "object field" corresponding to the image area on the retina in objective space,

the "visual field" signifying physiological excitation,

the "seen field" signifying subjective perception.

These definitions relate the objective visible environment to that which is "seen", i.e., subjective perception. However, none of these definitions applies to that field which is determined and recorded by the ophthalmologist and which he calls the "visual field".

Perimetry is not, as a rule, merely concerned with qualitative determination of those areas of the external environment which are perceived, but with quantitative determination of the functional capacity of the visual system in the perceptual field. This is done by determining systematically the perceptibility of targets of different luminance, size and wavelength in various parts of the visual field. The functional capacity can be measured, for instance, by the increment-threshold luminance ΔL, the inverse of which, $1/\Delta L$, is usually called "sensitivity".

The field of functional capacity obtained and recorded by means of perimetry is what the ophthalmologist calls the "visual field".

Since this functional capacity is usually determined through perception of the target, i.e., through the subject's awareness, the findings are influenced by psychological as well as by physiological factors. The two components cannot be strictly differentiated. However, it is obvious that the more complicated the task assigned to the subject, the more psychological factors will influence the findings. On the other hand, there is reason for supposing that with simple tasks, such as "luminous target seen or not seen", the findings are mainly influenced by fundamental physiological processes in the visual system. Since in most cases it is the presence or absence of defects in the visual system that must be determined, it is preferable to do perimetry with simple test stimuli.

II. Development of Perimetry

The perimetric examination of patients suffering from eye diseases was introduced by the ophthalmologist ALBRECHT VON GRAEFE in 1856. A year later AUBERT and FOERSTER, with their fundamental studies on the distribution of space perception and color perception in the visual field, created a basis for the further development of perimetry. This method remained unchanged in principle over many decades.

In order to demonstrate the advances in perimetry achieved during the last 30 years, it is necessary to give a short synopsis of its evolution from the very beginning. From 1856 to about 1940 perimetry was almost exclusively based on the so-called kinetic examination technique. In this technique a target is moved from the outside towards the center of the visual field, or away from a scotoma, until it is just seen by the subject. The point where the target is first perceived in the tested field is then plotted in a diagram. By connecting in the diagram all those points where a particular target first appears, we get a line of equal vision which is called an isopter.

Initially, von Graefe examined the visual fields of his patients with only one and rarely with two different unspecified targets. But as early as 1857, through systematic research by Aubert and Forster, and by Aubert alone, the gradient of sensitivity of "space perception" and "color perception" in the visual field of normal eyes was ascertained. In this context Aubert already stressed the quantitative relation between these two functions, and he also surmised that there were similar relations with "light perception". This was the basis for clinical perimetry using several targets of different sizes and colors. At the same time, Aubert devised the first semicircular perimeter which could be used to measure spatially the limits and defects of the visual field.

Inspired by von Graefe, repeated efforts were made during the following decades to improve this method by doing perimetry at reduced illumination. But clearly these attempts failed, because the instability of vision, related to processes of local and general adaptation during the examination, was not taken into consideration.

Special attention was paid to the development of a most efficient method of perimetry with colored targets. Hess (1889) demanded invariable colors which were all to have the same luminance in the relatively color-blind periphery of the visual field. Engelking and Eckstein (1920) succeeded in producing such "periphery equalized" pigment colors. Ferree and Rand (1922, 1924), with their perimeter, exposed these colors briefly against a grey background of equal brightness, so that only the hue, and not the brightness influenced their perceptibility. This method of color perimetry is especially noteworthy, because it was devised exclusively with regard to the color sensitivity of the eye, completely disregarding the physical nature of the test stimulus.

Lauber (1932) and Hartinger (1936) introduced the projection of white and colored targets whose luminance could be varied by filters. This was mainly a technical improvement designed to keep the target at a constant level and to achieve noiseless movement of the target and automatic recording.

To sum up, we can state that until about 1940 visual field examinations were carried out by kinetic perimetry and that, generally speaking, the physical test conditions were controlled, if at all, in a very incomplete manner. The known relations between vision and state of adaptation of the eye were not considered in those methods of perimetry. In spite of Aubert's work, it was forgotten that all the separate visual functions occur in each part of the retina and to a characteristic degree, depending on the tested retinal area. No attention was paid to the fact that, in determining the functional capacity of the visual field, the functional relations might give rise to important discoveries.

Two significant innovations brought perimetry out of its clinical isolation and back into modern visual psychophysics. Goldmann (1945a, b) analysed the requirements for precise light-perception perimetry and devised a hemispheric perimeter that provided a constant and uniform state of light-adaptation in the whole visual field during the perimetric examination.

Sloan (1939) was the first to describe a method of determining differential light sensitivity at any point of the visual field by means of a stationary target. Using the same principle of "static perimetry", Harms (1940) investigated the pupillomotor thresholds in the visual field. These techniques resulted in "profile perimetry" providing for "vertical sections" located as desired across the visual field, for any state of adaptation and for every visual function.

The requirement of a constant state of adaptation during perimetry and the use of precise and finely graded series of targets in static perimetry, have made it possible to specify the physical test conditions with utmost precision. As a result, this examination technique has become a reliable and sensitive psychophysiological method of measurement, reaching beyond the traditional scope of clinical visual-field examination.

In this chapter we shall restrict our discussion to these new basic physiological aspects of perimetry. We shall not attempt to give a complete description of all customary clinical techniques or even of the diagnostic importance of perimetry to any specific disease.

III. New Techniques in Perimetry

A. Principles

Traquair (1927) superimposed the isopters of the visual field and thus created a three-dimensional representation of visual capacity. The extent of the base corresponds to the field of perception and the height above the base corresponds to the visual capacity at each position in the perceptual field. The peak of this visual field "hill" is equal to the highest visual capacity where targets of lowest intensity are seen, whereas in the lower parts of the "hill" only targets of higher intensity are seen. Thus target intensity is inversely proportional to the visual capacity (Fig. 1).

The visual capacity of any eye can be imagined as an individually shaped hill. In this hill, absolute or relative scotomata would be represented as deep craters reaching down to the bottom or as shallow depressions. It is then the task of perimetry to measure the surface of such a hill to discover irregularities and to record them in correct proportion.

For the discussion of different perimetric techniques it is useful to start with this picture of the hill of visual capacities, since with the measuring methods of perimetry we must solve problems similar to those in mountain cartography. If we imagine an underwater massif whose surface, with all its depressions, indentations and slopes, has to be measured, altimetry can be done either by soundings in a vertical direction or by bearings in a horizontal direction. In visual-field examinations, static perimetry is the method of sounding in a vertical direction resulting in profiles, and kinetic perimetry the method of bearings in a horizontal direction resulting in isopters[1] (Fig. 2). The best method of perimetry is that which gives maximum information about the hill of visual capacity within the shortest possible

[1] It is also possible to obtain isopters by means of static perimetry; but this method which is sometimes of clinical importance can be omitted in our main presentation.

period of time. Therefore, the two perimetric techniques should be studied and compared from this point of view.

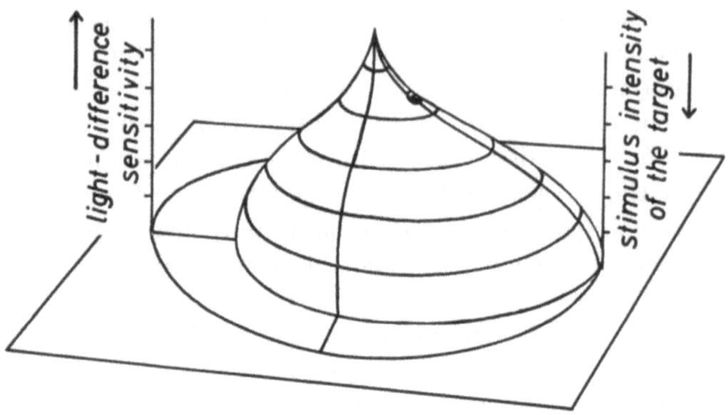

Fig. 1. Sketch of hill of vision. Bottom: field of perception. Height: visual capacity. Top: foveola with maximum light-difference sensitivity. The higher the light-difference sensitivity (L. H. ordinate), the lower the target intensity (R. H. ordinate) at which light-difference threshold is determined

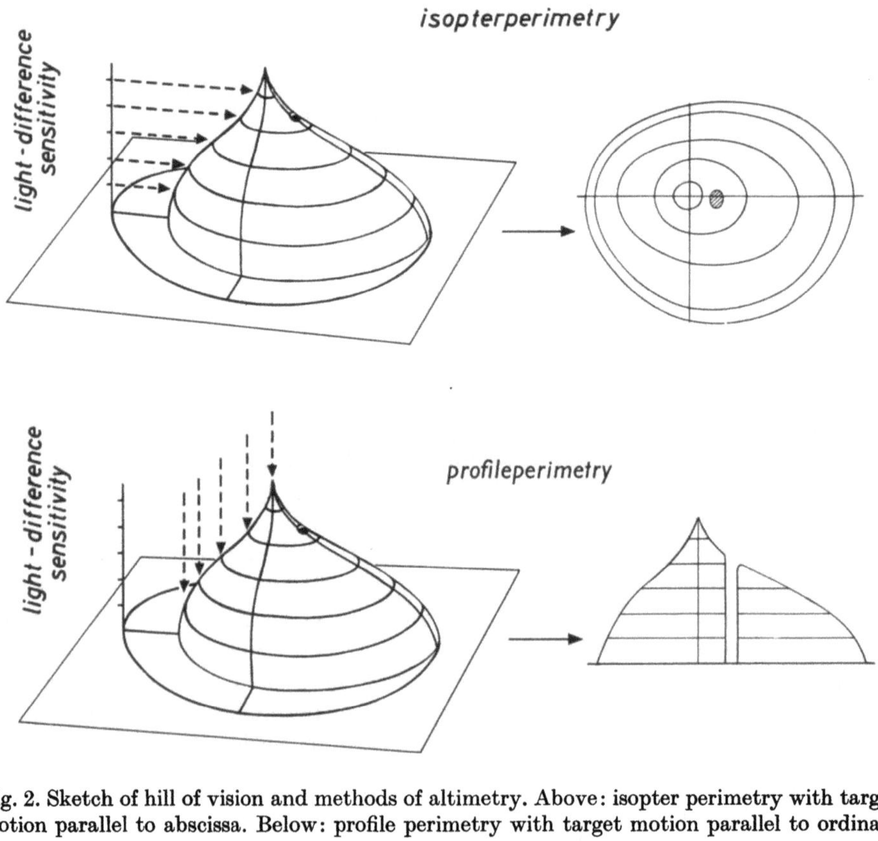

Fig. 2. Sketch of hill of vision and methods of altimetry. Above: isopter perimetry with target motion parallel to abscissa. Below: profile perimetry with target motion parallel to ordinate

1. Comparison of Profile Perimetry with Isopter Perimetry

Both methods are concerned with thresholds. However, there are characteristic differences which may be advantageous or disadvantageous according to the question asked. The most important difference lies in the fact that by isopter perimetry an approximate idea of the shape of the hill of visual capacity and also of large and deep depressions can be quickly obtained. Profile perimetry, on the other hand, makes precise altimetry of a hill of any shape possible, including very

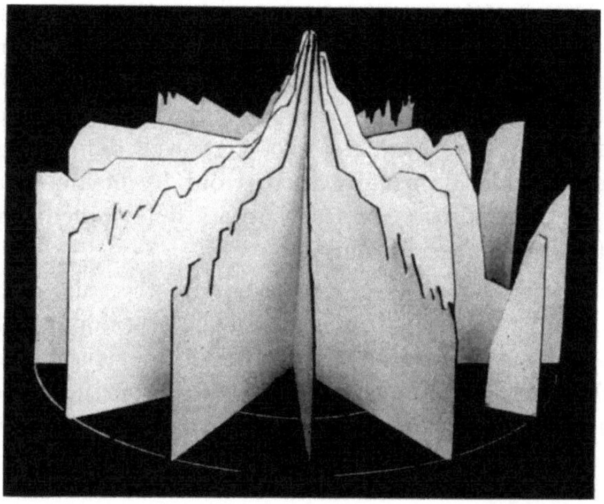

Fig. 3. Determination of the shape of hill of vision by profile perimetry in many meridians

small shallow depressions, but only along a particular meridian, arc, or straight line in the visual field. It would also be possible, of course, to obtain a survey of the whole hill shape with profile perimetry by means of a very large number of meridians (Fig. 3), and also to obtain an exact reproduction of the hill profile in all meridians by means of a large number of isopters. But this would take such a long time that both the examiner and the subject would be so exhausted that reliable results could no longer be expected. Therefore, it is more appropriate to choose the method which best suits the problem at hand.

a) Perimetry in Physiological Investigations. In physiological experiments normal eyes are investigated. In this case we have to count upon a nearly conical hill of visual capacity which, apart from the blind spot, does not show any depressions interrupting the smooth slope. The only deviation from radial symmetry is found in a somewhat steeper slope in the nasal, upper and lower periphery of the visual field, which is mainly due to the limitation of the field of view by the nose and the lower and upper orbital margins (Fig. 1). When such a uniform slope of the hill of visual capacity with approximate radial symmetry occurs, a survey of the shape of the whole hill is less important than measurements that are as precise as possible along one single meridian. From the height and shape of the profile obtained along this meridian, we can deduce the shape of the whole hill. Thus, for physiological investigations profile perimetry is the method of choice. With this method, it is possible to determine the dependence of vision upon slight changes in background luminance and color, as well as upon the color, shape, size and manner of presentation of the target. Also, local changes in retinal sensitivity, caused by local glare in a certain part of the retina or by successive or simultaneous luminance and color contrast in the visual field, can be assessed by measuring the sensitivity profile along a meridian which crosses this retinal area.

For various reasons, profile perimetry gives more exact and reproducible threshold values than does isopter perimetry:

1. It is carried out with a stationary target (static perimetry). Consequently the threshold can be determined independently of the temporal integration of the retina and of the patient's reaction time (compare with pages 127). Since threshold measurements in a profile curve are carried out with a target of constant size, spatial summation is always required to a very well defined degree. In isopter perimetry, however, which is usually carried out by means of a moving target (kinetic perimetry), the position of the isopters determined may be highly influenced by all three factors mentioned above.

2. Profile perimetry, more than isopter perimetry, allows the exact determination of any gradient, whereas in case of a shallow slope the horizontal direction of examination by isopter perimetry does not allow reliable threshold measurement (Fig. 4) (AULHORN, 1969). In such cases, the vertical direction of profile perimetry produces completely clear results. On the other hand, when a very steep

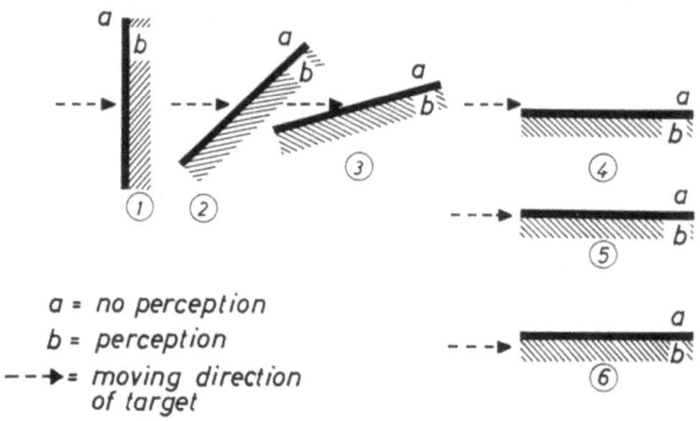

Fig. 4. Sketch of influence of slope on determination of light-sense thresholds by isopter perimetry. The flatter the slope, the less accurate the threshold measurement

slope occurs (Fig. 5), the vertical direction of examination, as a rule, is inferior to the horizontal direction. This disadvantage, however, is not significant in profile perimetry since thresholds are not measured at only one single retinal location, but also at adjacent areas which, in the case of a steep slope, naturally have very high or very low sensitivities. When such differences in sensitivity of contiguous retinal areas are determined, the sensitivity slope of the intermediate retinal area can be deduced by interpolation even if measurement of the sensitivity in this areas shows considerable scatter (Fig. 5).

3. Thanks to the vertical direction of examination, very accurate measurements of retinal sensitivity can be made through profile perimetry, even in regions of small, circumscribed scotomata, which may be caused, for instance, by experimental local blinding or by experimentally produced contrasts in the visual field.

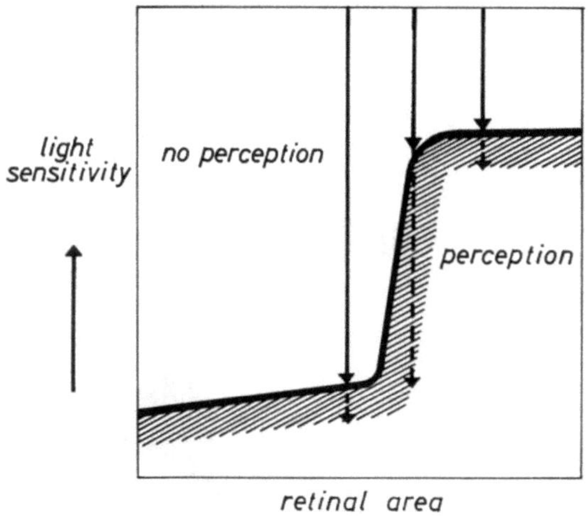

Fig. 5. Sketch of influence of slope or determination of light-sense thresholds by profile perimetry. The steeper the slope, the less accurate the threshold measurement

4. Since profile perimetry is carried out with stationary targets, thresholds can be determined in any retinal region in the very same way, even in the center of the visual field. Of course this is not possible with isopter perimetry.

Therefore, as regards scientific threshold measurements of the visual capacity of normal eyes, preference must be given to profile perimetry. We even believe that, in case of slight alterations in functional capacity in the visual field due to external or internal influences, such as changed background luminance, drugs, alcohol, fatigue, etc., only profile perimetry can give us reliable information on the existence and the extent of an altered functional capacity.

b) Perimetry as a Method of Clinical Diagnosis. The situation is very different if we want to determine pathological defects in the visual field exclusively by means of profile perimetry. At the outset, the shape of the hill of visual capacity is completely unknown. There could be a general reduction in height of the hill of vision as well as shallow depressions, deep indentations in the massif, or even steep slopes down to the base. Here, profile perimetry should be carried out along a large number of meridians in order to give complete and detailed information on the lack of, or existence and site of, pathological disturbances. This would be too time-consuming. For clinical purposes, therefore, it is very much more profitable first to get an approximate idea of possible defects in the visual field by determination of two or three isopters, and then to get details concerning site, shape and depth of the scotomata, by means of one or two sections across the pathologically altered areas of the visual field. With certain ocular diseases which are usually accompanied by visual field defects at characteristic locations (such as in glaucoma), it is also helpful to check the sensitivity profile along a meridian chosen across that area of the visual field, even if isopter perimetry does not show any pathological alteration. This means that with profile perimetry it is possible to detect slight, early defects which are still small enough to be "passed over" (i.e. remain undetected) by the moving test stimulus of isopter perimetry (Fig. 6).

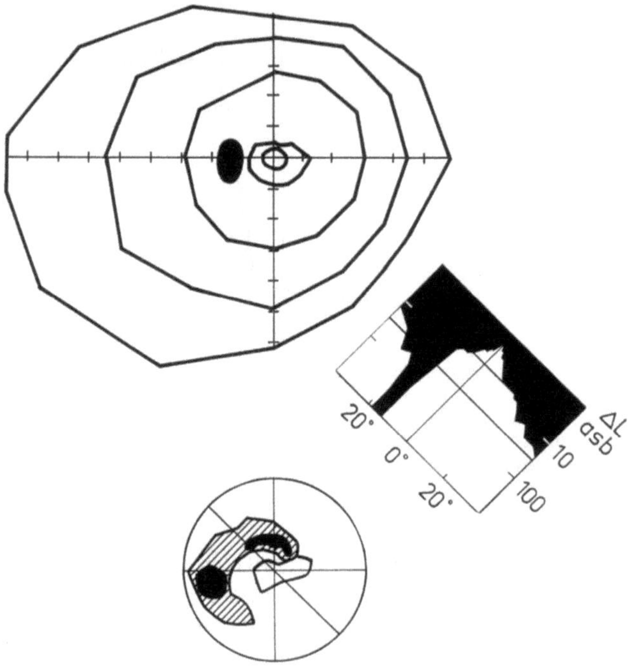

Fig. 6. Clinical perimetry in a case of a small pathological paracentral scotoma (glaucoma). Above: isopter perimetry of whole visual field, scotoma remaining undetected. Below (R. H.): profile perimetry clearly showing the shape of deep small scotoma. Below (L. H.): isopter perimetry in the central visual field after profile perimetry. Isopters now show the scotoma to its full extent. Profile perimetry in 135° meridian of visual field. Abscissa, therefore, parallel to that meridian. This profile curve can be thought of as situated vertically above the meridian in a three-dimensional way

Therefore, the most reliable method of detection and mapping of pathological alterations in the visual field, i.e., perimetry in ophthalmological practice, is a well-considered combination of isopter and profile perimetry. Modern perimeters (e.g., Goldmann's hemispherical perimeter, Tübinger perimeter) are adapted to both methods. It is advantageous to be able, if necessary, to switch quickly from one method to the other without any readjustment of the apparatus.

In summary, for psychophysiological investigations, profile perimetry is the method of choice, whereas for the detection and registration of pathological scotomata, the combination of both isopter and profile perimetry is recommended.

Since in this chapter perimetry is discussed mainly with regard to physiological questions, the following sections are chiefly concerned with profile perimetry.

2. The Influence of Practice on the Threshold Level

For inexperienced subjects differential light sensitivity is, on the average, somewhat lower than for experienced ones. But the effect of practice is not the same for all subjects (Fig. 7). Very attentive subjects who concentrate on the task give optimal threshold values from the outset. Because of the practice effect, experiments concerned with the effects of drugs, alcohol, fatigue, etc., can be carried out only after the subject is very well trained. Otherwise, changes in

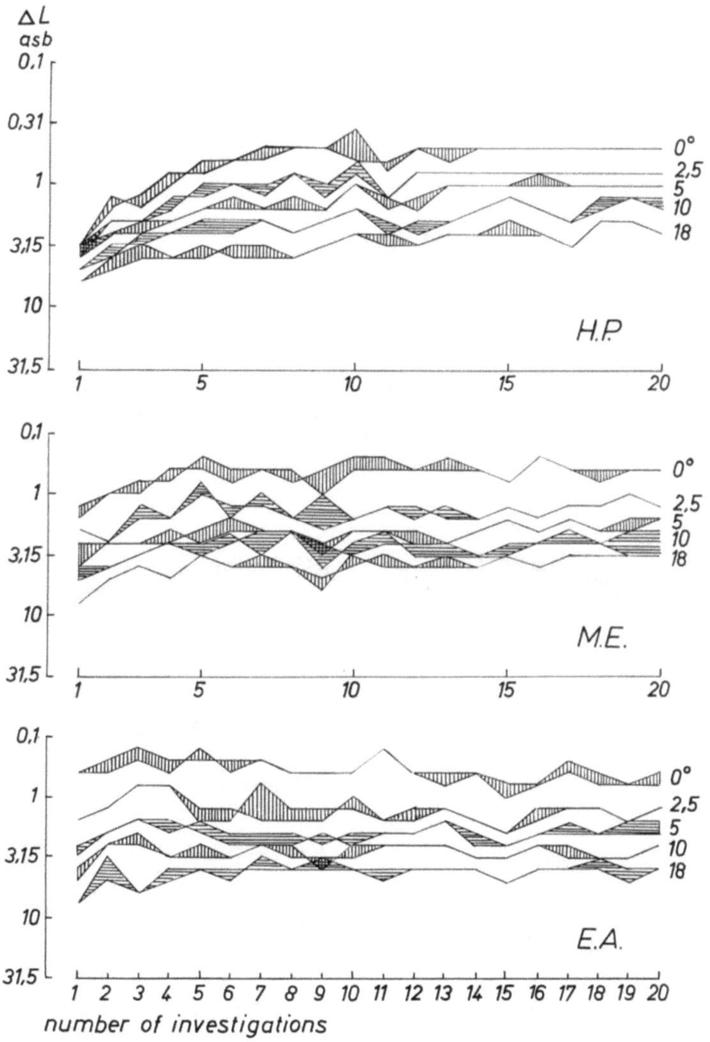

Fig. 7. Influence of training on determination of light-difference thresholds. Abscissa: number of investigations. Ordinate: target luminance ΔL in asb. Parameter: investigated retinal loci in the nasal part of 0° meridian. Thresholds determined by two measurements each (difference marked by hatching). Three subjects examined. Above: subject shows good training effect. Middle: subject shows little training effect. Below: subject shows no training effect

sensitivity that are actually due to practice might erroneously be attributed to the effect of drugs or fatigue.

3. Variability in Threshold Determinations

There are many reasons for intra-individual variability. Practice is an important factor, for inexperienced subjects show more scatter than experienced ones (Fig. 8). Moreover, mention must be made of the slight, almost imperceptible

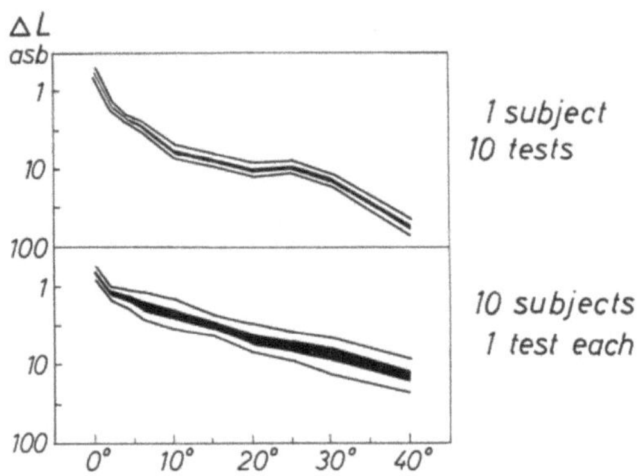

Fig. 8. Profile perimetry in 0° meridian of retina, nasal half; background und luminance: 10 asb. Abscissa: retinal locus. Ordinate: target luminance ΔL in asb. Standard deviation and mean error of average value

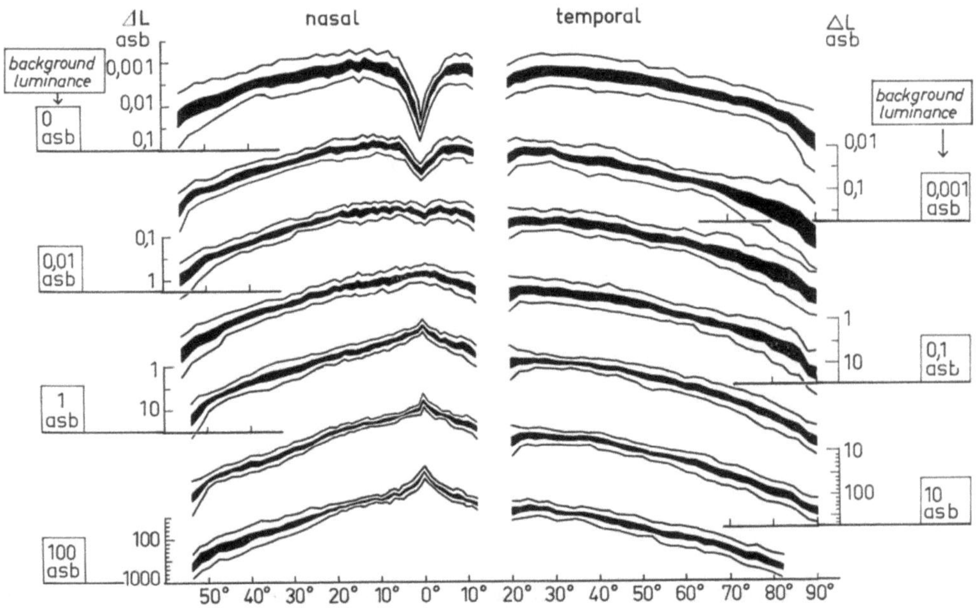

Fig. 9. Profile perimetry in 0° meridian of retina at 8 different background luminances. Coordinates: as in Fig. 8. Parameter: background luminance. Standard deviation and mean error of average value in 10 normal subjects

fluctuations in fixation, as well as slow rotational movements of the eye about the line of sight which can be measured by determination of the position of the blind spot. Even if both these movements are very slight, they are still large enough so that for one measurement, the target image might fall on a retinal blood vessel, and for the next measurement on an adjacent more sensitive area. The light-absorbing effect of the retinal vessel results in a higher threshold. This may perhaps explain why there is especially high variability in that part of the visual field corresponding to the retinal area which is particularly rich in blood vessels. Other sources of variability include real variations in sensitivity and the varying attention of subjects during threshold determination. (See also NACHMIAS, chapter 3, this volume).

Inter-individual variability exceeds intra-individual variability (Fig. 8). The inter-individual variability varies with the distance from the center of the visual field as well as with the state of adaptation, as shown in Fig. 9. For every level of adaptation the scatter range is smaller in the center of the visual field than in the periphery. It increases with reduction in background luminance which influences the adaptation of the eye.

4. The Influence of Refraction

If threshold measurement is to reflect optimal visual capacity, the target image must be well focused on the fundus of the eye. An uncorrected refractive error produces (because of the retinal blur circles) an enlarged blurred target image of reduced light intensity. According to Riccò's law, luminance and size of the test stimulus can substitute for each other under certain circumstances (see BAUMGARDT, chapter 2, this volume). But obviously this does not apply to retinal blur circles because of their unequal light-distribution in the retinal image, for any deviation from emmetropia exceeding one diopter causes a marked rise in increment threshold. This effect is usually most marked in the center of the visual field; it gradually decreases in paracentral regions and, depending on the refractive error, is very low or may not even exist in the periphery. This gives rise to the supposition that this phenomenon is due to spatial summation which increases towards the periphery, and which for its part is related to the enlargement of the receptive fields (Fig. 10).

In the periphery of the hill of vision only very large deviations from emmetropia result in a rise in thresholds. However, in the periphery, the retinal image of the test stimulus is, in any case, distorted and blurred. This is caused by the extremely oblique passage of the light rays through the refractive media. Therefore, a displacement of the image in front of or behind the retina, due to an uncorrected error of refraction, is not as important in this part of the visual field as in central and paracentral regions. For this reason, it is of little importance that the corrective effect of eyeglasses usually only extends to eccentric areas of 25° or 35° at the most. However, for examination of the central visual field within 25°, exact correction of the refractive error and also of presbyopia, calculated for the test distance, is necessary.

The correction needed for paracentral regions of the retina is not always equal to that needed for the retinal center. In such cases, with exact correction of the center, we find in other areas a measurable rise in thresholds. These show up in the

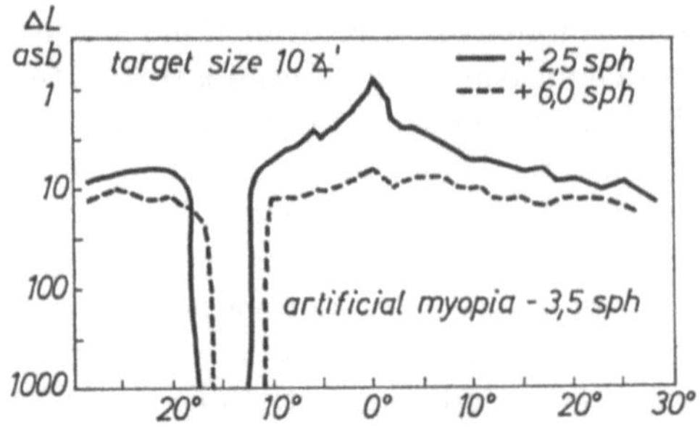

Fig. 10. Profile perimetry in 0° meridian of retina in hyperopic subject. Continuous curve: with full correction of refractive error. Dashed curve: with artificial myopia of 3.5 dptrs. Coordinates: as in Fig. 8

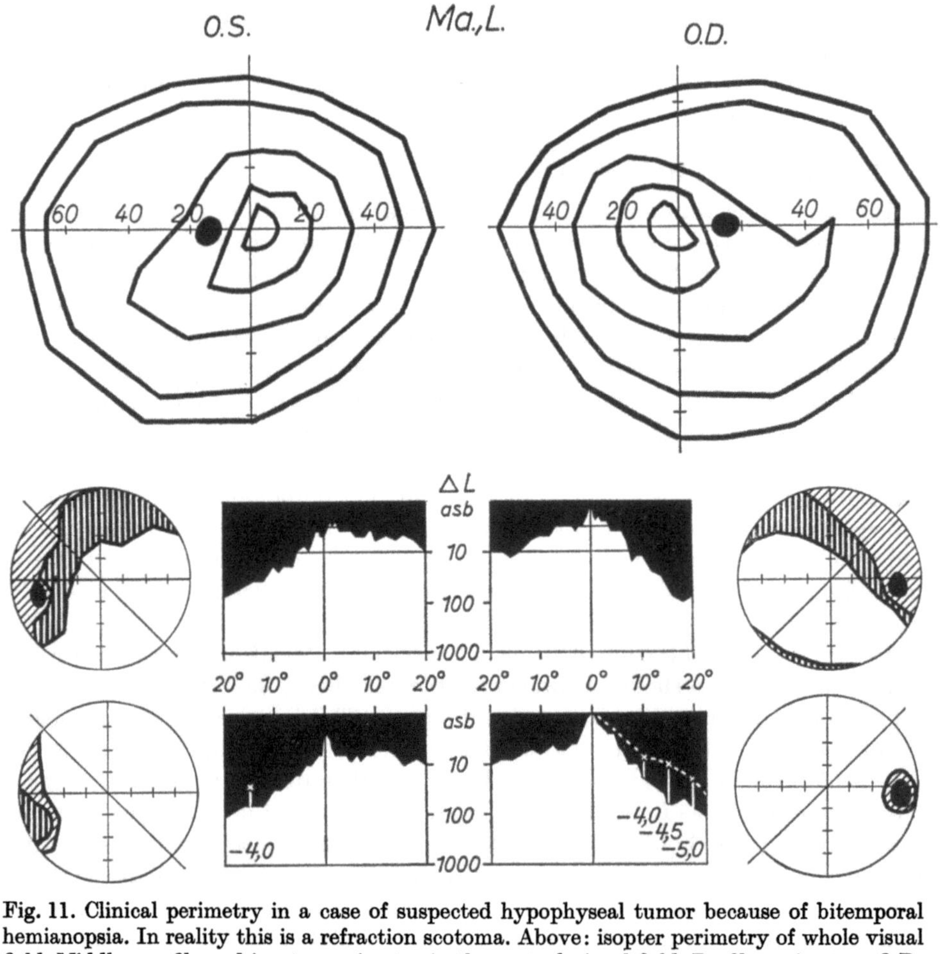

Fig. 11. Clinical perimetry in a case of suspected hypophyseal tumor because of bitemporal hemianopsia. In reality this is a refraction scotoma. Above: isopter perimetry of whole visual field. Middle: profile and isopter perimetry in the central visual field. Profile perimetry: O.D. in 45° meridian. O.S. in 135° meridian. Glasses corresponded to the correction needed for fovea. Below: Profile and isopter perimetry in the central visual field. Profile perimetry for 10°, 15° and 20° off the foveola with corrections needed for the respective retinal loci, isopter perimetriy with correction needed for 15° off the foveola

visual field as so-called refraction scotomata. They are mainly caused by deformations of the eyeball, i.e., they accompany any deviation from the spherical shape of the posterior segment of the eye (e.g., myopia), but they also exist in cases of bulges in the retina caused by tumours or edema. For the most part, refraction scotomata are found in both eyes in the temporal portion above the blind spot, sometimes giving rise to a false diagnosis of bitemporal hemianopsia which can then be erroneously interpreted as a chiasmal lesion.

As shown in Fig. 11, a refraction scotoma can be easily verified by means of static perimetry carried out in one or several parts of the scotoma, once without and once with additional corrective lenses. If the scotoma can be reduced or eliminated by eyeglasses, the existence of a refraction scotoma is proved.

B. Perimetry of Various Visual Functions

1. Introductory Remarks

In the preceding section we discussed visual capacity or retinal sensitivity as a criterion for vision in a general sense, since all factors mentioned so far apply to the same extent for each separate function of vision.

In the natural process of vision, all physiological visual functions, such as light sensitivity, visual acuity, color vision, adaptability, etc., and also the psychological visual functions, such as form perception, memory, etc., are invariably involved simultaneously. The experimental isolation of one separate function from the complex process of vision, achieved experimentally by keeping all but one physical variable constant, may produce an unnatural visual situation. We specify the separate function according to the nature of this one physical variable. During such experimental studies we try as much as possible to avoid psychological factors by producing a very simple test situation, so that the result is influenced exclusively by the physiological factor in question.

Among the various functions involved in the complex process of vision, the perception of differences in luminance and color plays an essential part. If in the visual field there is neither difference in luminance nor difference in hue, subjects will state that "they do not see anything", even if they are aware of a diffuse brightness. For this reason, we may consider the perception of differences in luminance or color as the basic function of vision which dominates all other functions, such as visual acuity, local adaptation, flicker-fusion frequency, and pupillomotor sensitivity.

In perimetry the investigation of this basic visual function is of utmost importance, as it probably gives the most exact information on disturbances of the physiological mechanism of vision. Because of its sensitivity and reproducibility, light-perception perimetry is at present the most important method and we shall analyze its physiological basis first.

2. Luminance-Difference Sensitivity as the Basic Function of Vision

a) Determination of Luminance-Difference Thresholds in the Visual Field. The functional capacity of the eye, as characterized by luminance-difference sensitivity, is measured by the reciprocal of threshold contrast. Photometric contrast can be expressed in three different ways as follows:

$$1.\quad \frac{L_2 - L_1}{L_1} = \frac{\Delta L}{L}$$

$$2.\quad \frac{L_2 - L_1}{L_2 + L_1}$$

$$3.\quad \frac{L_2}{L_1}$$

In perimetry $\Delta L/L$ is the measure most frequently used for the luminance-difference threshold, and its reciprocal $L/\Delta L$ the measure of differential sensitivity. If the absolute and not the relative luminance-difference sensitivity is to be represented, the correlation of threshold-luminance to background luminance can be neglected. In this case the ordinate only shows ΔL for absolute threshold luminance or $1/\Delta L$ for absolute luminance-difference sensitivity. If the test stimulus is projected on the illuminated background, as is usual with modern perimeters, ΔL is equal to the luminance of the target projected onto the background.

During threshold determination the eye must be fixed by looking steadily at a fixation point projected on the hemisphere or screen. The target is presented at the desired eccentricity. The position and size of the target are expressed in terms of visual angle. Threshold measurement proceeds as follows:

First the target is presented at sub-threshold luminance. Luminance is then gradually increased until the target is perceived. It is advisable to increase the luminance by steps of 0.1 log unit. Larger steps are too big to obtain an exact profile of the hill of sensitivity. Steps smaller than 0.1 log unit can be used only occasionally with particularly well-trained subjects and with a very high background luminance, but because of the increased scatter there is no gain in accuracy of the sensitivity profile. Luminance values are given in asb or better still in cd/m^2, where 1 cd/m^2 equals 3.14 asb.

Since test exposures reduce the sensitivity of the tested retinal area, interstimulus intervals of one to two seconds (cf. page 128) are required between exposures of constant duration. For the same reason continuous increase in luminance cannot be used. Once a threshold is located, the level can be verified by a repeated measurement. However, with well-trained subjects who give their full attention to the examination, no repetition is necessary, since sensitivity never varies by more than one or two steps in luminance (0.1 or 0.2 log unit). The next threshold determination is then made at the next point of the selected meridian, arc, or straight line.

Threshold values are recorded in a coordinate system in which light-difference threshold or sensitivity is plotted as ordinate, and the distance separating retinal test loci is plotted as abscissa and measured in visual angle. If the line of investigation is a meridian crossing the center of the visual field, the distance on the abscissa is measured relative to the fovea, i.e., the fixation point.

If the thresholds are determined by isopter perimetry, a target of constant size and given luminance difference relative to the background is moved from the periphery toward the center of the visual field until it is just perceived (Fig. 2, upper part). This means that the difference threshold for a given locus is not determined, but rather the locus is traced where a given luminance difference just exceeds the threshold. This investigation is repeated with targets of the same luminance moving in several directions from the periphery towards the center of the visual field. The determined threshold loci are then connected in a diagram. In this way we obtain an isopter. The relation between the threshold values of profile perimetry and those of isopter perimetry is demonstrated in Fig. 12.

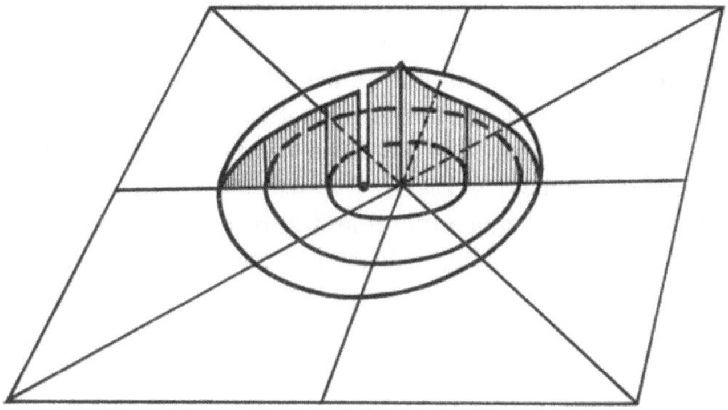

Fig. 12. Sketch of the relation between threshold values of profile perimetry and those of isopter perimetry

b) Profile Curves Obtained with Achromatic Targets for Different States of Adaptation. Prior to each perimetric investigation, the state of sensitivity must be stabilized by adaptation to the background luminance of the perimeter. The darker

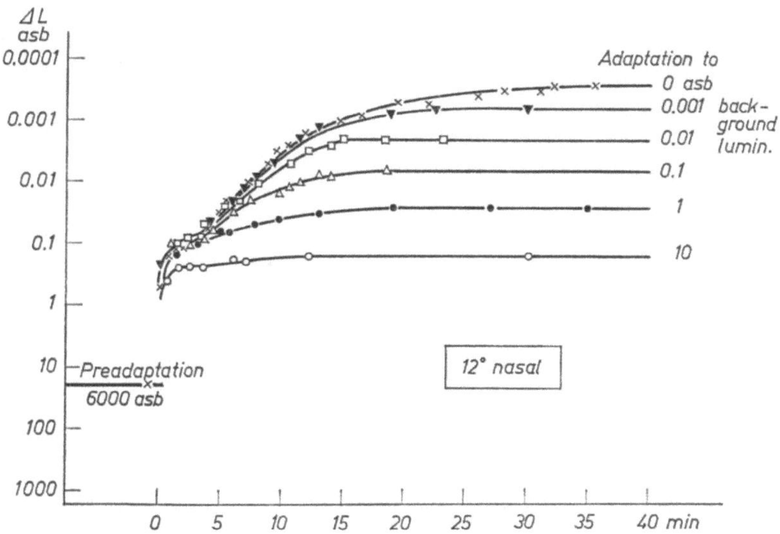

Fig. 13. Curves showing adaptation from 6000 asb to various lower background luminances. Abscissa: adaptation time in minutes. Ordinate: target luminance ΔL in asb. Parameter: background luminance. Investigated retinal locus: 10° nasally (according to MEYNER)

the background, the longer the time needed for adaptation before a perimetric investigation. According to Meyner (1962), an adaptation time of two minutes is needed for a background luminance of 100 asb. If the pre-adaptation luminance is 6,000 asb before perimetry, 12 minutes of adaptation are needed in case of a background luminance of 0.1 asb, and 60 minutes in case of an absolutely dark background (Fig. 13).

Fig. 14 shows on the left profile curves obtained with eight different levels of background luminance along the 0° meridian of the retina. Each point in the diagram is the average value of luminance-difference thresholds in 10 normal subjects. In this case, the ordinate gives target luminance ΔL or increment sensitivity $1/\Delta L$ respectively. Here the position of the curves is not determined by luminance difference sensitivity $L/\Delta L$, but by increment sensitivity for the different states of adaptation. Since increment threshold decreases with decrease in background luminance, increment sensitivity increases with the degree of dark adaptation.

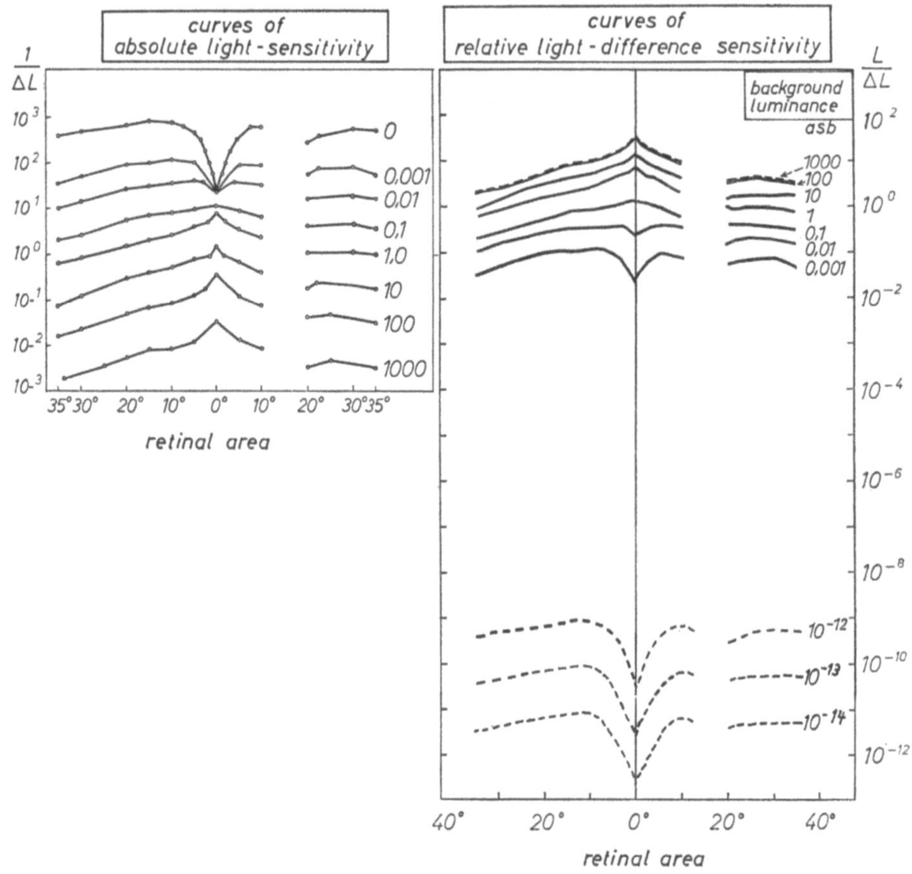

Fig. 14. Profile perimetry in 0° meridian for 8 different states of adaptation. Abscissa: retinal locus. Ordinate (left): absolute sensitivity $1/\Delta L$; (right): relative light-difference sensitivity $L/\Delta L$. Parameter: background luminance. Average values in 10 normal subjects. All thresholds obtained after completion of adaptation process

In Fig. 14 on the right the same results are shown in terms of luminance difference sensitivity $L/\Delta L$. The lower the background luminance during the test, the lower the curves obtained, since contrast sensitivity decreases proportionally as dark adaptation increases. This expression has the disadvantage that curves obtained at 0 asb cannot be plotted because the quotient $0/\Delta L$ equals 0. However, we can assume that there is a field luminance low enough to produce the same absolute light sensitivity as a completely dark background. We have tried to find such a background luminance in a series of experiments (AULHORN *et al.*, 1966). The influence of background luminance on the sensitivity threshold was tested in three different retinal areas (Fig. 15). It can be seen that with the lowest background luminance used (10^{-9} asb) in the two peripheral areas of the retina, maximum absolute sensitivity may indeed be nearly reached, but it still does not equal absolute sensitivity in complete darkness. This, of course, does not apply to the fovea. In the fovea, maximum absolute sensitivity is already reached with a background luminance of 10^{-3} asb. However, for the curves at the two peripheral

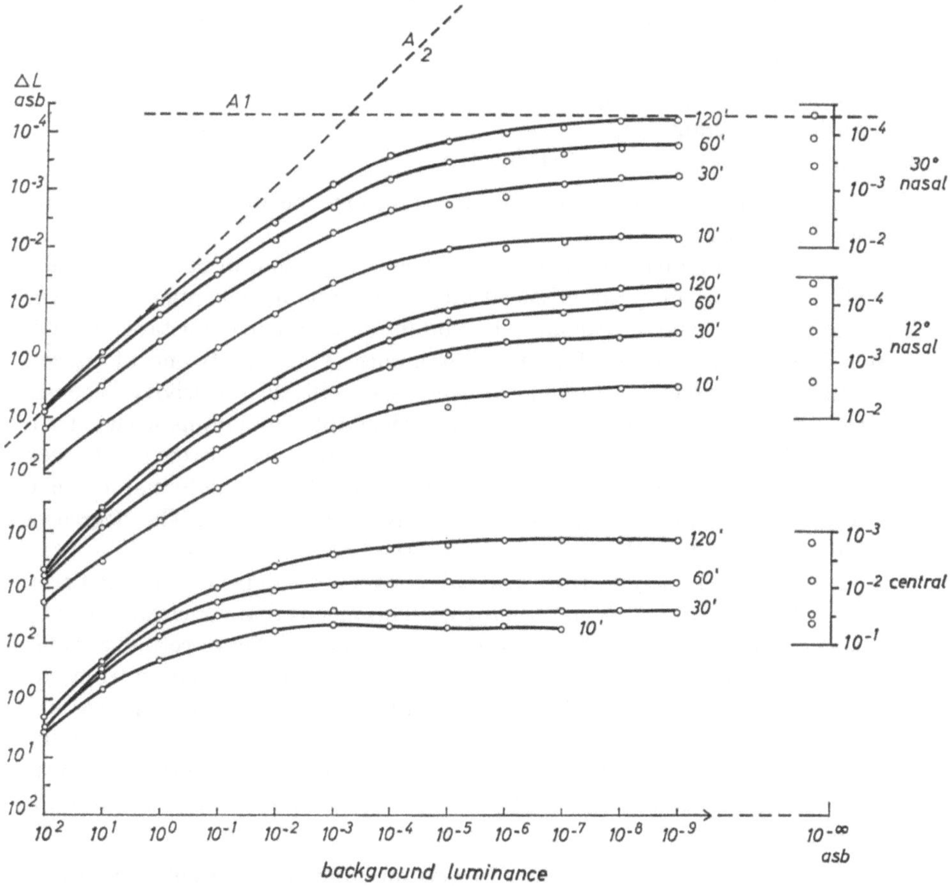

Fig. 15. Light-difference sensitivity for various states of adaptation in different retinal regions. Abscissa: background luminance in asb. Ordinate: target luminance ΔL in asb. Parameter: target size. Description of asymptotes A_1 and A_2 in the text

loci, interpolation between 10^{-9} and 0 asb background luminance is possible. With a background luminance of about 10^{-12} asb the result is the same absolute sensitivity as that reached with 0 asb. Therefore, this background luminance can be taken as "physiological darkness". Basing the calculation of light sensitivity on this background luminance, we obtain the curve shown in the lower part of Fig. 14.

The curves of increment sensitivity in Fig. 15 show a certain regularity, in that with very low background luminance they are parallel to the abscissa, and at very high background luminances they approach a slope of 45°. If we try to analyse the relationship between increment sensitivity or contrast sensitivity and adaptation luminance, we must attend to the extremes characteristic of these curves. The sensitivity curves have two asymptotes, A_1 and A_2. (In Fig. 15, these are shown for the uppermost curve.) Increment sensitivity at low adaptation luminance approximates asymptote A_1 ($\Delta L =$ constant), while the curve at high adaptation luminance approximates asymptote A_2 ($L/\Delta L =$ constant or $\Delta L/L =$ constant). Approximation of the curves to asymptote A_2 on the right and to asymptote A_1 on the left of the curve is about the same. Therefore, it is possible to express the sensitivity of a retinal locus, depending on the adaptation luminance, by means of three parameters:

1. location of asymptote A_1,
2. location of asymptote A_2,
3. approximation to A_1 and A_2 respectively.

The curve analysis shows the following relations between sensitivity and adaptation luminance:

An increase in adaptation luminance involves a reduction in increment sensitivity and an increase in contrast sensitivity. With adaptation luminance over 10^2 asb, contrast sensitivity reaches a maximum and remains constant, even if there is a further increase in adaptation luminance (Fig. 15, left end of curve). Proportionally, as adaptation luminance decreases, contrast sensitivity becomes poorer while increment sensitivity improves. With adaptation luminance less than 10^{-12} asb, maximum increment sensitivity is reached and remains constant, even if there is a further reduction in adaptation luminance. Thus, the human eye can adapt to any background luminance between 10^2 and 10^{-12} asb. The degree of adaptation is indicated by the convergence on the two asymptotes.

The curves in Fig. 15 demonstrate that this convergence depends on target size, as well as on the locus of the tested retinal area. This means that conclusions can be made about different spatial summation properties in the different retinal regions.

The smooth curve between the two asymptotes shows the transition from one state of adaptation to another. The curves approach the two asymptotes exponentially. It is of interest that the transition from constant contrast sensitivity to constant increment sensitivity occurs at about the same luminance that spectral luminosity changes from photopic V_λ to scotopic V'_λ. (See LEGRAND, chapter 15, this volume).

c) Profiles Obtained with Chromatic Targets for Different States of Adaptation.

Introductory Remarks. Thresholds can be measured with chromatic test stimuli on an achromatic background by the same method used for achromatic stimuli, i.e., by increase in test stimulus luminance. There are two different thresholds:

The target may appear colorless at the first threshold, with hue perceived only when luminance is further increased. The "photochromatic interval" between the two thresholds changes with wavelength, tested retinal area, target size, exposure time, and state of adaptation. The interval is minimal for long-wave test light, possibly equal to zero in the retinal center. For the first, "achromatic", threshold, the procedure and subject's task do not differ from threshold determinations for broad-band light, and variability and practice effects are about the same.

Chromatic Threshold Determinations. Determination of chromatic thresholds is more complicated. Although based on the same method (increase in luminance until the test stimulus color is recognized), the variability of threshold luminance is much greater than for achromatic thresholds. The threshold level depends strongly on the psychological test situation: if the subject knows that only two hues, e.g., red and green, are going to alternate in a random series, the thresholds for red and green will be much lower than if the subject knows that, of 10 different possible hues, the threshold for a particular green hue must be found. Even if the test luminance is high enough to give the impression that the stimulus is "green", the subject will wait for further luminance increase to be sure which green it is. Thus the subject has to answer a difficult question which depends on various psychological factors, whereas for determination of the achromatic threshold, just as in simple light perimetry with achromatic test stimuli, only the simple question: "Is the luminous spot visible or not?" has to be answered.

There are additional respects in which determination of chromatic thresholds cannot be equated with light-perception perimetry, for differences in hue can be recognized even if there is no difference in brightness between the two hues. If, therefore, for chromatic threshold determination, the same luminance is chosen for both test stimulus and background, this threshold determination means the determination of hue-difference sensitivity. For this reason, only achromatic thresholds are to be discussed in relation to light contrast sensitivity whereas chromatic thresholds, insofar as they concern perimetry, will be dealt with in section (d).

Specification of Stimulus Intensity Using Monochromatic Lights. When white test stimuli are used, the threshold can usefully be expressed in terms of luminance. This is not advisable, however, if we want to find out how sensitivity for monochromatic light changes in accordance with the degree of retinal eccentricity, since luminance is a measure based on the spectral sensitivity of the light-adapted fovea of the human eye (V_λ). However, since spectral light sensitivity is not the same in each part of the retina, the threshold stimulus level in perimetric measurements with monochromatic light should not be specified by luminance values. In this case, it is correct to use an objective physical definition for the intensity of a test stimulus which is independent of the sensitivity of the human eye, i.e., to use watts cm^2. In full agreement with this, DUBOIS-POULSEN (1952) writes in his monograph "Le Champ Visuel": "Devant de pareilles difficultés on est alors tenté de s'adresser à une spécification physique objective du test indépendant du sujet et l'on adopte l'énergie transmise par chaque radiation. Le seuil est caractérisé par la plus petite quantité d'energie nécessaire à la perception. Cette fois les travaux ont une base solide."

The Change in Profile Shape in Studies Using Test Stimuli of Different Wave-lengths. Achromatic threshold measurements in the visual field using exactly defined monochromatic light, corresponding to the requirements mentioned above, were carried out in 1930 by WENTWORTH in the laboratories of FERREE and RAND, and in 1962 by NOLTE in cooperation with AULHORN and HARMS. WENTWORTH projected spectral light directly into the subject's eye, whereas NOLTE projected spectral light for the test stimulus into the surface of the perimeter. Both authors

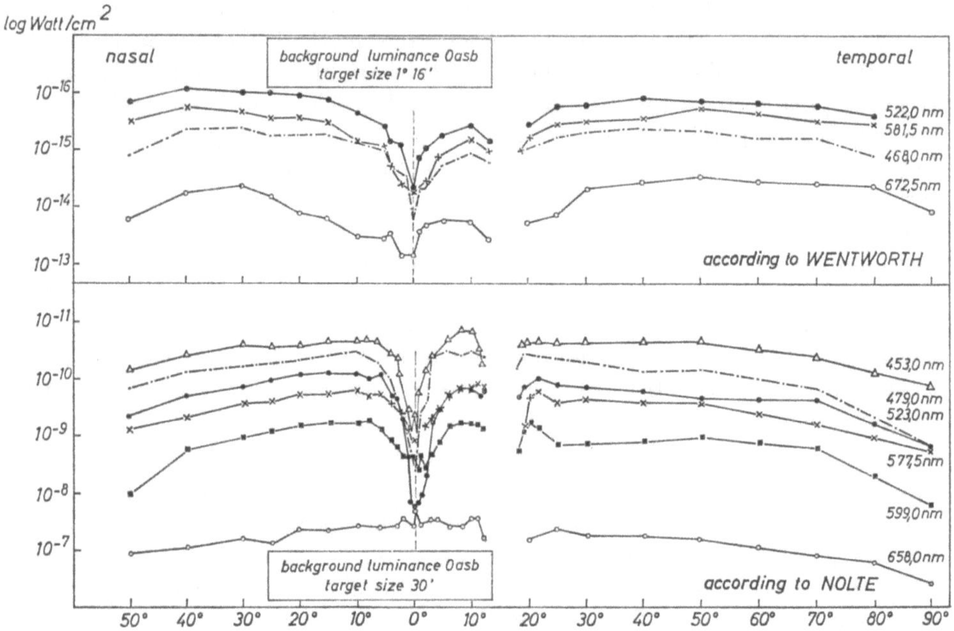

Fig. 16. Achromatic thresholds in 0° meridian of retina during complete dark adaptation. Above: according to WENTWORTH. Below: according to NOLTE. WENTWORTH's data points are entered in the same system of coordinates as NOLTE's. Abscissa: retinal locus in 0° meridian. Ordinate: target intensity in log Watt/cm². Parameter: wave-length of test stimuli

did their experiments in complete darkness. NOLTE did additional experiments with background luminances of 0.1 and 10 asb. In the latter experiments, where the test stimulus was projected onto an illuminated white background, there was some dilution of the spectral light stimulus. For this reason, the results obtained by the two authors are comparable only to a certain extent at the 0 asb background luminance (Fig. 16). Both studies show that the sensitivity profiles change considerably with change in wavelength. In both studies, the center of the retina shows a considerably deeper depression for short-wave light than for long-wave light. In NOLTE's studies, moreover, the depression disappears completely at 658 nm.

Fig. 17 shows NOLTE's results for four different wavelengths with three different background luminances. If we compare the curves for a given wavelength for three different states of adaptation, it is clear that not only the height, but also the form of the curves changes. The influence of adaptation varies considerably in the different regions of the retina, but there is a marked change in curve shape depending on the state of adaptation, as shown in Fig. 18 for the central area of the retina.

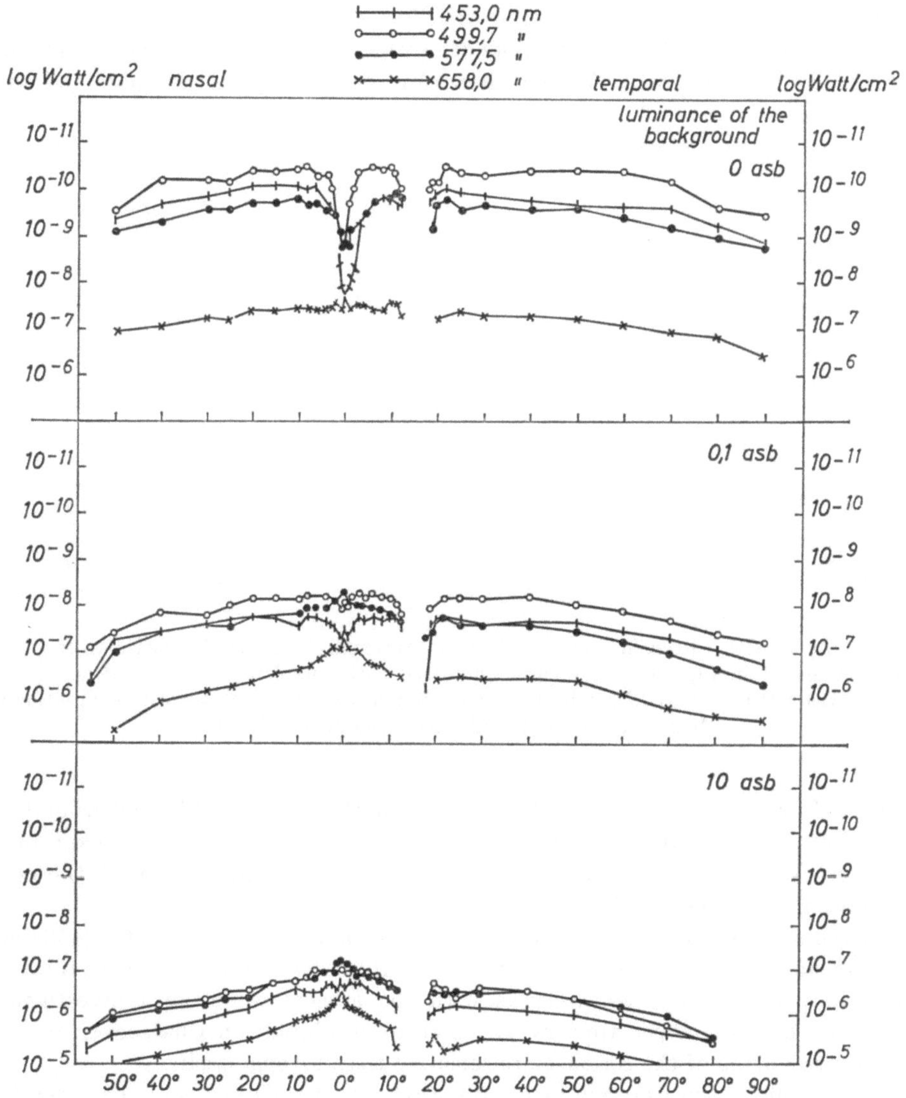

Fig. 17. Achromatic thresholds according to NOLTE for 3 different states of adaptation. Coordinates and parameters: as in Fig. 16

The family of curves in Fig. 18 is interesting in many respects. The upper set demonstrates that with a dark background the curve shape in the central area of the retina, as far as the depth of crater is concerned, changes in proportion to the change in wavelength. At 453 nm we have the deepest crater which becomes more and more shallow with increasing wavelength. At 658 nm there is no longer any crater. The sensitivity in the central retina is now as high as in paracentral areas. The crater diameter is approximately the same at every wavelength. It considerably exceeds the diameter of the macula lutea. In a state of mesopic adaptation (0.1 asb background luminance) there are slight craters only at short wavelengths. They disappear completely as wavelength increases and at long wavelengths they eventually become peaks. A very interesting curve shape is also obtained with

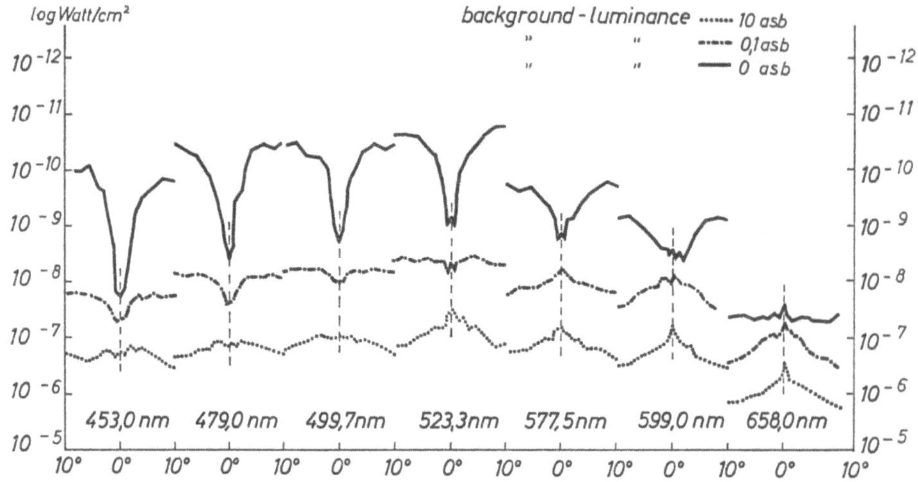

Fig. 18. Achromatic thresholds in the central and paracentral regions of 0° meridian of retina. Coordinates: as in Fig. 16. Upper curves obtained with complete dark adaptation, middle curves with adaptation to 0.1 asb background luminance and lower curves with adaptation to 10 asb background luminance (according to NOLTE)

light adaptation to a background luminance of 10 asb. With this background we never get a crater, but there is the same tendency as with a mesopic background: for short wavelengths there is no peak, but with increase in wavelength the peak becomes more pronounced.

To sum up, we can say that with the shortest wavelength investigated (453 nm), for any state of adaptation, there is never a higher sensitivity in the central retina than in paracentral areas, whereas with the longest wavelength investigated (658 nm), a crater never appears. In no state of adaptation whatsoever are the paracentral areas of the retina more sensitive than foveola itself.

The profile curves presented by WENTWORTH and NOLTE show considerable differences which are probably due to their different methods. Both studies contain interesting information on achromatic thresholds for monochromatic light. Because their results differ, however, their usefulness for speculations on the functional mechanism of color vision is limited. Nevertheless, both studies succeeded in demonstrating that the influence of adaptation on the change in spectral sensitivity varies in different retinal regions, so that one is not justified in describing a curve as scotopic spectral light sensitivity simply because it is based on values obtained in the peripheral retina.

d) The Value of Clinical Perimetry Using Colored Samples. Since their introduction by AUBERT (1857), colored samples have been used, among others, for the gradation of stimuli in clinical perimetry. It had been thought that the isolated constriction of a blue, red or green isopter might give some information on specific pathological alterations. Such disturbances were of particular interest to KÖLLNER (1912). He found that with choroidal or retinal diseases the usual sequence of isopters from outside to inside (i.e., blue, red, green) was often reversed, and that blue isopters became more constricted than red isopters, whereas disturbances in red-green perception prevailed in diseases of the optic nerve. Up to now, in fact, the idea still cannot be excluded that color perimetry, as compared to light-perception perimetry, might give additional diagnostic information. On the other hand, however, this hypothesis has not yet been confirmed for the following reasons:

1. The results of perimetry with colored samples obtained by various researchers at different hospitals can not be compared, since the colored samples differ in spectral composition depending on manufacture, storage, age, etc., and their subjective brightness, hue and saturation are not specified. DUBOIS-POULSEN writes in this context: "Les tests doivent être spécifiés d'une manière aussi rigoureuse que possible en ce qui concerne leur composition spectrale, sinon aucune conclusion valable ne peut être donnée. Ceci condamne irrémédiablement les méthodes cliniques utilisant des tests pigmentaires." Only the color perimetry devised by FERREE and RAND (1922; 1924) is done with a specified stimulus by equalizing the luminance of adaptation field, background and colored test stimulus. Thus, FERREE and RAND do not stress color-difference sensitivity and light-difference sensitivity simultaneously, as is customary in all other methods of isopter determination with colored samples. Theirs is a simple determination of color-difference sensitivity. However, their method was not adapted by the ophthalmologists for routine perimetry, mostly because of the complicated and repeated calibration of test stimuli that it requires.

2. With the usual method of color perimetry, the isopters for white, blue, red and green lie at different positions in the visual field. Constriction of a red isopter may be caused by a local disturbance in that part of the visual field, where the red isopter is usually found. A specific disturbance for red color could only be proved if an isopter obtained by other test colors in exactly the same part of the visual field failed to show any constriction.

3. As already discussed in section (c), chromatic threshold determination is inherently less exact than achromatic determination.

4. Colored test samples can be used only in isopter perimetry and only in four or five different stimulus gradations. Therefore, this method is not suitable for an exact picture of the often rather complex shape of a hill of visual capacity with pathological defects.

e) Spatial Summation. Within certain limits, the light-difference threshold, decreases as the test stimulus size increases. As shown in Figs. 15 and 19 (DANIEL, 1959), the influence of target size varies with retinal area and state of adaptation. A careful study of this index of spatial summation can give important information on the size of the receptive fields, depending on the retinal area and the state of adaptation.

DUBOIS-POULSEN and his associates (1959) have tried to develop a refined method of isopter perimetry on this basis. In their experiments two targets of different size and luminance are chosen so their two isopters coincide in the visual field of the normal eye. If in the diseased eye these isopters lie in different locations

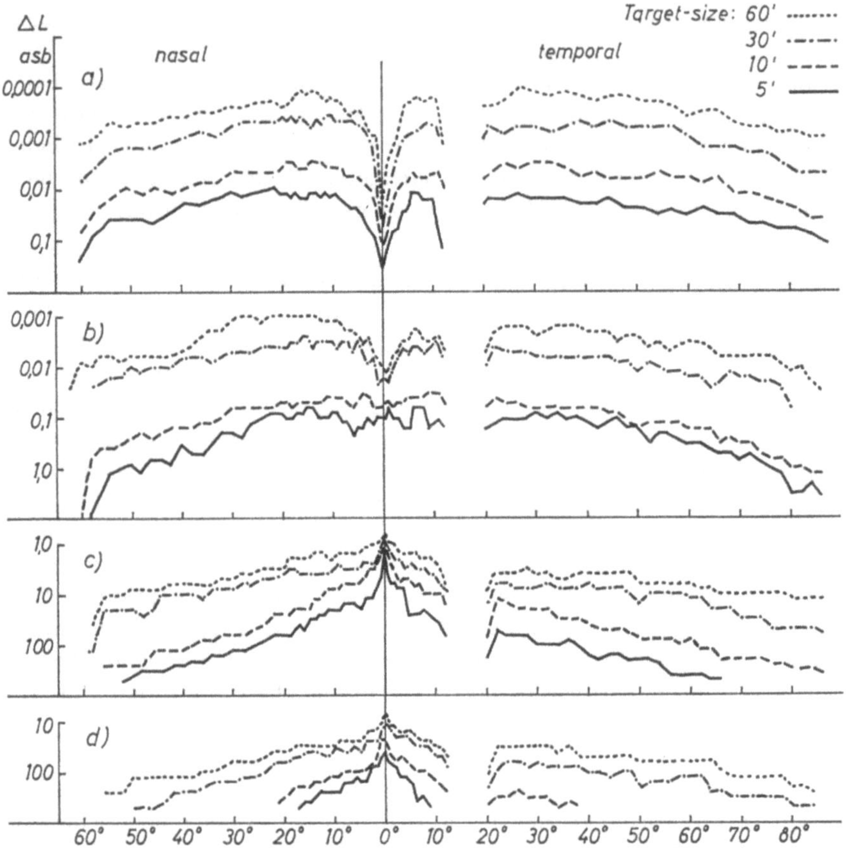

Fig. 19. Profile perimetry with various target sizes and 4 different states of adaptation. Coordinates: as in Fig. 8. Parameter: target size. a) complete dark adaptation, b) state of adaptation corresponding to 0.0063 asb background luminance, c) state of adaptation corresponding to 6.3 asb background lum., d) state of adaptation corresponding to 630 asb background lum.

in the visual field, it is called a "photometric disharmony". The latter is supposed to occur when there are changes in the eye, whereas it does not occur with disturbances in the optic tract.

In our opinion, however, it is very risky to investigate phenomena of summation, with which these experiments are concerned, with kinetic isopter perimetry. A safe statement about the summation ratio can only be made by investigating one and the same retinal area, which is only possible by means of profile perimetry. It would not be at all difficult to check the validity of photometric disharmony by means of profile perimetry.

f) Temporal Integration. The exposure time of a test stimulus can influence the level of the difference threshold. Bloch's law ($I \times T =$ constant) however, applies only to very small targets and very short exposures (see BAUMGARDT, chapter 2, this volume). Charpentier's law ($\sqrt{I \times T} =$ constant) is of limited validity. In 1953, DORFF made a detailed study of the influence of exposure duration using static perimetry (Fig. 20).

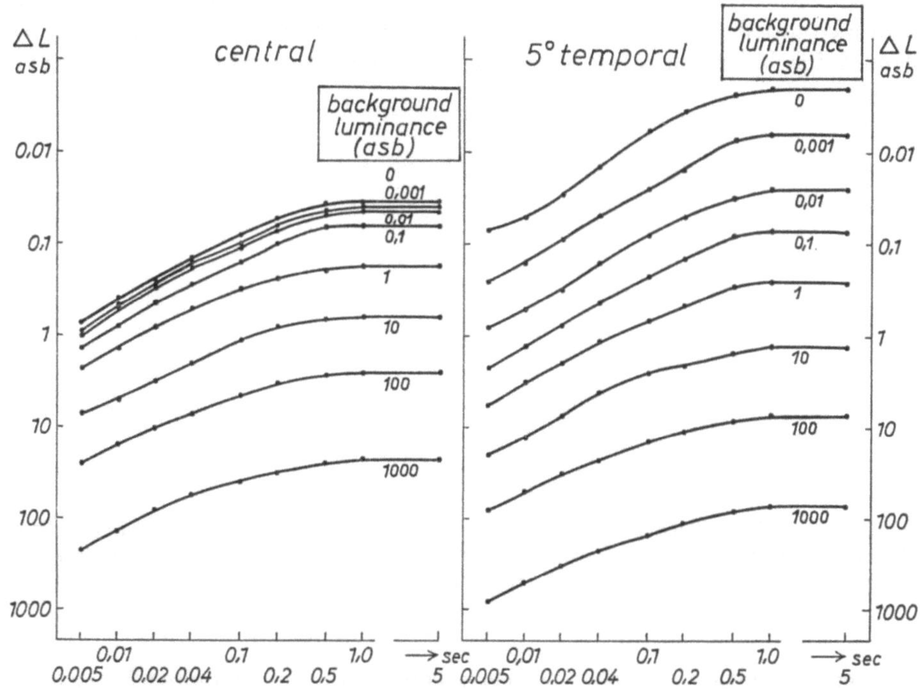

Fig. 20. Light-difference sensitivity with different exposure times of test stimulus and with 8 different states of adaptation. Abscissa: exposure time in sec. Ordinate: target luminance ΔL in asb. Parameter: background luminance in asb. L.H. group: investigation in retinal center. R.H. group: investigation 5° temporally off retinal center

In 10 normal subjects, luminance vs. duration curves were determined in four different regions of the visual field with eight different levels of background luminance. The results show that light-difference sensitivity reaches its maximum level in each tested retinal locus and at each background luminance with a stimulus duration of at least one second. Some preliminary tests on 10 eyes with defective vision due to various diseases gave the same result.

Therefore, if, for threshold determination with a stationary target, the minimal stimulus duration is not below one second, temporal integration is constant and light-difference sensitivity is also constant for the given conditions. In this way the time factor is, to a certain extent, eliminated in perimetry.

However, in isopter perimetry with moving targets, temporal integration influences the threshold level to an undetermined extent.

Likewise, we cannot fully exclude some influence of temporal integration on flicker-fusion frequency. The problem of perimetric determination of flicker-fusion frequency will be dealt with in a separate section.

g) Local Adaptation. If a test stimulus of supra-threshold luminance is imaged on a particular retinal area, the state of adaptation in this area changes in such a way that increment sensitivity ($1/\Delta L$) decreases, and relative light sensitivity or contrast sensitivity ($L/\Delta L$) increases, respectively. It is possible that due to this local adaptation, the test stimulus may become invisible after some time. The elapsed time before the target is no longer perceived is called the local-adaptation time.

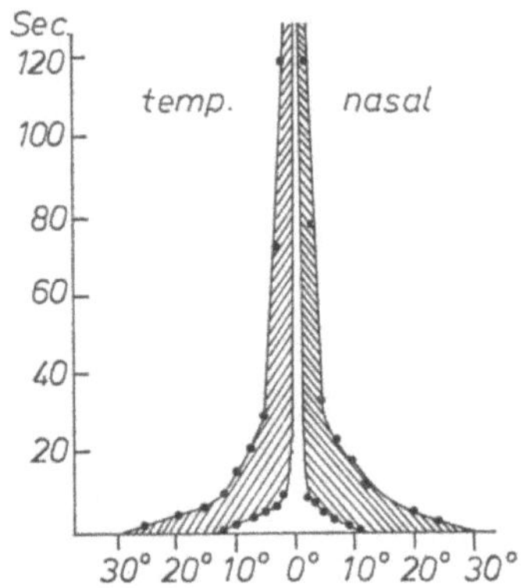

Fig. 21. Local-adaptation time in 0° meridian of retina with red stimulus according to CIBIS. Abscissa: retinal locus. Ordinate: local-adaptation time in sec. Hatched portions: scatter range between minimum and maximum values

Local-adaptation time does not correspond to the time required for changing over from the state of adaptation before stimulus exposure to the state of adaptation during stimulus exposure. If the field luminance on the tested retinal area is 10 asb before, and 20 asb during stimulus exposure, the center of the retina needs only a very short time (less than one second) for readaptation from 10 to 20 asb. In contrast to this, local-adaptation time based on the same luminance ratio in the retinal center is infinitely long: the target never becomes invisible. This proves that readaptation time and local-adaptation time are not the same.

Local adaptation occurs during stimulation with colorless and colored light, even if the colored stimuli have the same brightness as the background. Local adaptation, therefore, occurs not only with differences in brightness, but also with differences in hue. The disappearance of a colored light stimulus after prolonged exposure was described for the first time by TROXLER in 1802. In 1948, CIBIS studied local-adaptation time in normal and diseased eyes using colorless and colored light stimuli. For colored stimuli he used colored samples of equal brightness (Engelking-Eckstein's colors). Fig. 21 shows that local adaptation in the central retina, in experiments with colorless and colored stimuli, takes more than 120 seconds. Toward the retinal periphery, local-adaptation time becomes progressively shorter.

Because of the difficulty in maintaining steady fixation for a long time, HARMS (1954) suggested that the disappearance of the target itself should not be considered but rather the disappearance of the after-image produced by the stimulus exposure, in other words, that the time of local re-adaptation be measured. This method has the advantage that it is not necessary to maintain steady fixation for a long time, since stimulus exposure can be relatively brief, yet far above threshold. Steady fixation is thus necessary only during the brief exposure and not during observation of the after-image. The time for the after-image to disappear is much shorter than the time required for disappearance of the target itself. The method suggested by HARMS clearly reveals a local-adaptation process also, but it is by no means certain that this is in fact the same process. For this it would be necessary to make quantitative comparisons.

Local adaptation can be measured by static perimetry only, since retinal location should remain constant during determination of local-adaptation time. Because of the slight imperceptible unsteadiness of fixation, it is impossible to study local adaptation using very small targets. The target must at least be large enough to maintain the stimulus image within a circumscribed retinal area during the measurement, despite the nearly imperceptible unsteadiness of fixation.

Undoubtedly, it is possible through the measurement of local adaptation, to get some information on interesting physiological processes which have not been fully clarified so far. However, because of the difficulties in measuring, and the necessity to maintain very good, steady fixation, this method cannot be applied to the routine examination of patients. Moreover, since this method employs supra-threshold stimuli, the hill shape of the visual field of a diseased eye cannot be determined in detail and with the same accuracy as in light-perception perimetry using threshold stimuli only.

h) Profiles in Regions where Simultaneous Contrast Occurs. All the aforementioned methods of perimetry employ a background of homogeneous luminance. This is indispensable if each retinal area is to be in the same state of adaptation during perimetric examination. However, profile perimetry can be done equally well across retinal areas in different states of adaptation, if we want to obtain information on the behavior of light-difference sensitivity in this particular situation (HARMS and AULHORN, 1955; FIORENTINI and TORALDO DI FRANCIA, 1955; AULHORN and HARMS, 1956). For this purpose, the background should consist of several fields of unequal but exactly defined luminance. This not only results in different levels of sensitivity corresponding to the different states of adaptation, but also in a reduction in sensitivity on both sides of the border-line between the fields of different luminance. This phenomenon cannot be explained by the field luminance. It extends over an area of not more than half a degree on both sides of the border-line (Fig. 22). If two such zones of demarcation are put close together by presenting the field of different luminance as a narrow stripe, the reductions in sensitivity produced by the two zones of demarcation, are superimposed and intensified, so that even in the middle of the stripe we do not obtain the sensitivity we might expect from a broader stripe of the same luminance (Fig. 22, bottom curve).

The higher the contrast and the farther away from the retinal center the examination is carried out, the more distinct this phenomenon of lowered sensitivity

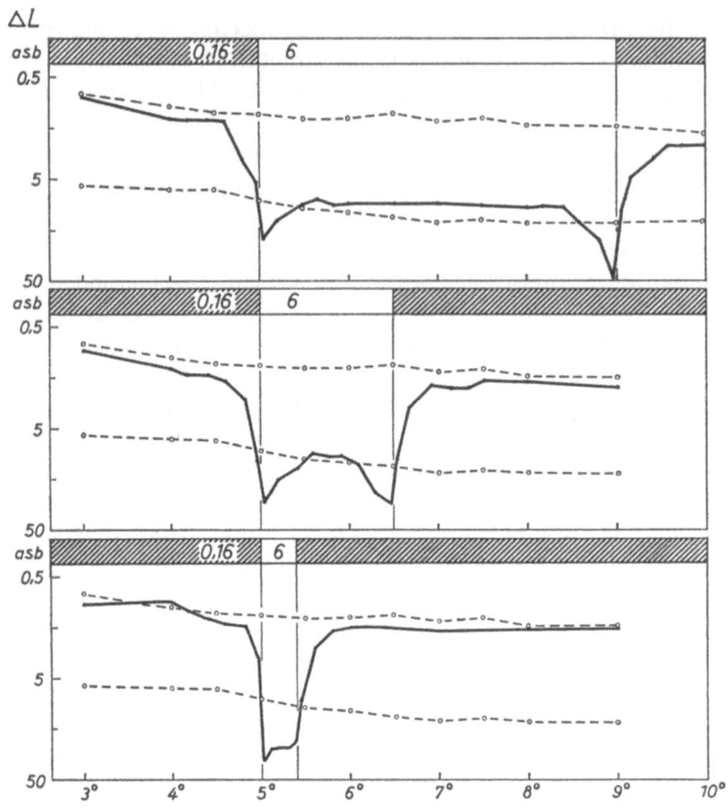

Fig. 22. Profile perimetry across retinal regions for different states of adaptation. Coordinates: as in Fig. 8. Numerals on the upper margin of graph: background luminance in asb, i.e., contrast in the zone of demarcation 1 : 37. Width of brighter portion of background luminance 4° in the upper curve, 2° in the middle curve and 25′ in the lower curve

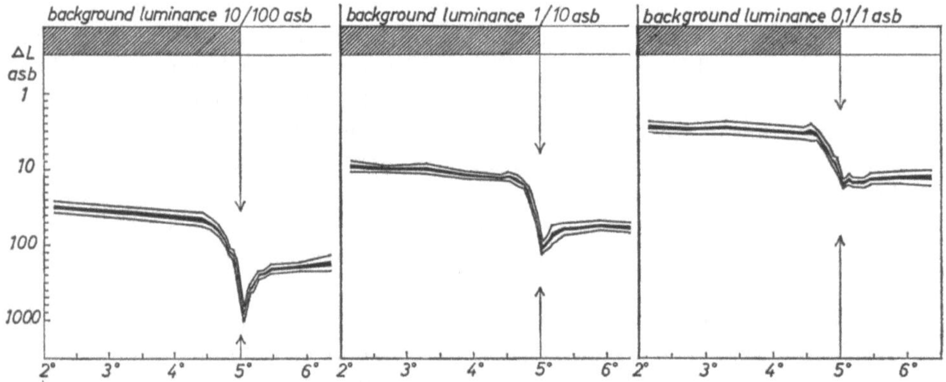

Fig. 23. Profile perimetry across retinal regions for different states of adaptation. Coordinates: as in Fig. 8. Relative luminance difference of background and always 1 : 10. Absolute luminance values given above the curves

in the zone of demarcation becomes. Another factor is the state of adaptation of the tested retinal areas: the most marked reduction in sensitivity is obtained if the different luminances are both within the range of photopic vision. The reduction in sensitivity in the zone of demarcation of the brighter field decreases and finally disappears as the two luminances of constant ratio approach scotopic levels. The reduction in sensitivity in the zone of demarcation of the darker field, however, remains constant (Fig. 23).

Obviously the reduction in sensitivity in the zone of demarcation can be related to so-called physiological simultaneous contrast. When two adjacent fields of different luminance are observed, the subject perceives a brightness distribution which does not correspond to the physical light distribution (Mach bands; see FIORENTINI, chapter 8, this volume).

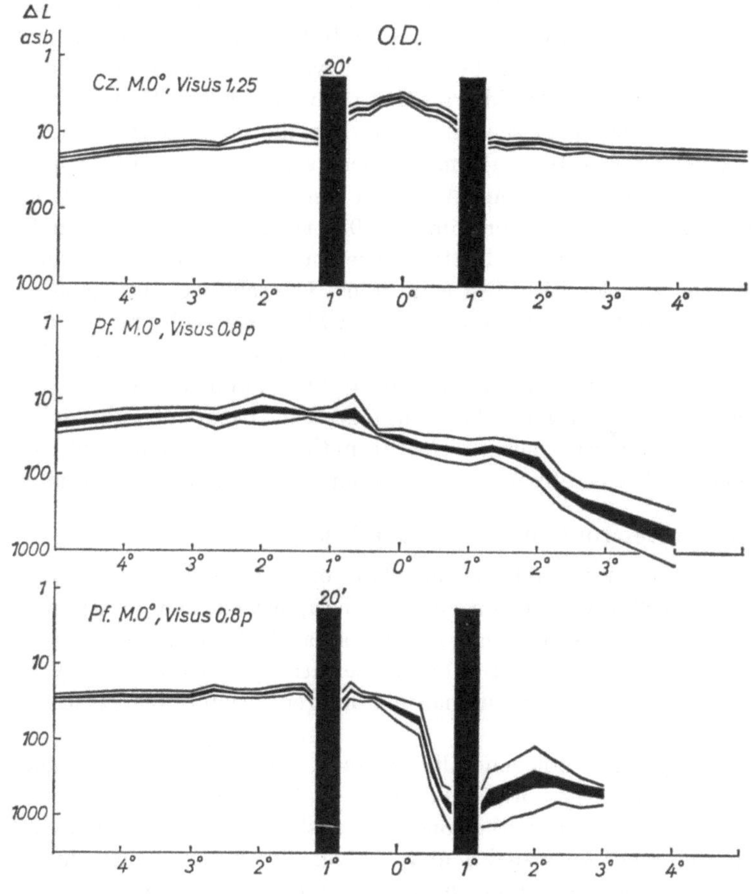

Fig. 24. Profile perimetry in 0° meridian of retinal background luminance: 10 asb with two dark stripes 20′ in width, each located 1° to the right and to the left of foveola. Coordinates: as in Fig. 8. Upper curve: light-difference thresholds in normal subject. Middle curve: light-difference thresholds in a case of strabismic amblyopia without dark stripes in the background. Lower curve: light-difference thresholds in the same amblyopic eye with dark stripes in the background

The reduction in sensitivity detected during perimetry, however, cannot be considered as the equivalent of the sensation produced by Mach bands. With a Mach band in the zone of demarcation of the darker field, a stripe becomes evident which seems to be darker than the remaining dark field, and in the zone of demarcation of the bright field one that seems to be brighter than the remaining bright field. If light-difference sensitivity across a border were a manifestation of the Mach-band phenomenon, only the zone of demarcation of the brighter field would show a reduction in sensitivity, whereas the zone of demarcation of the darker field would show an increase. But in fact there is a reduction in sensitivity in the zone of demarcation of the dark as well as of the bright field.

Without discussing in detail the results obtained from normal observers, we wish to demonstrate by a pathological case that profile perimetry across fields of different luminance can give important information on the pathology of specific diseases. The upper part of Fig. 24 shows a sensitivity profile obtained from a normal subject across two dark stripes. Only the sensitivity profile in the bright fields is shown. The break in the profile curves on the two outer borders of the black stripes shows on both sides a slight reduction in sensitivity, which is due to the stripes. The curves in the middle and in the lower part of the figure were obtained from a formerly strabismic patient suffering from amblyopia, who had lost his better eye in an accident. Although visual acuity in the amblyopic eye had risen after the accident to approximately 0.8, the patient was still unable to read. The middle curve was obtained without the black stripes and the lower curve with them, for otherwise identical test conditions. The region of the stripe on the right side shows a deep depression of sensitivity which exceeds by far the depression in the normal subject. This marked reduction in sensitivity on both sides of dark contours may account for the reading disability in amblyopia.

We cannot draw any general conclusions on the nature of amblyopia in strabismus from this single case, but it is clear from this example that results of scientific interest can be obtained by means of perimetry across fields of unequal luminance.

3. Perimetric Determination of Visual Acuity

In 1894 WERTHEIM published his chart of peripheral visual acuity on which HOFFMANN'S (1925) well-known curve of peripheral visual acuity is based. The more eccentric the site of the tested retinal area, the lower the visual acuity. There is a close relation between light-difference sensitivity and visual acuity, for without any perceptible difference in luminance a differentiation of perceived forms would not be at all possible.

The investigator is not generally aware of this relation since visual acuity is usually tested clinically with a difference in luminance between test-type and background that far exceeds the contrast threshold. Fig. 25 shows the influence of luminance difference on visual acuity. The arrows indicate the minimal level of luminance difference prevailing during the acuity tests. We see that, with this contrast, the optimal resolving power limited by the retinal structures is easily reached, so that either an increase or a moderate reduction in contrast cannot alter the visual acuity.

The reduction in visual acuity toward the periphery is not only manifested during the above-mentioned customary acuity test, using test-types of different sizes with supra-threshold contrast, this also becomes evident if we determine in each retinal area the minimal contrast required for optimal resolving power of the tested retinal area using constant size targets (Fig. 26). This method of acuity testing (AULHORN, 1960) gives more information on the nature of the reduction of visual acuity toward the periphery than the test using contrasts that exceed the threshold to such an extent that the contrast has no influence at all.

With this method there are two different ways of testing visual acuity in each area of the retina by means of profile perimetry, both of which result in the same threshold values. It is possible to increase the contrast in a given retinal area

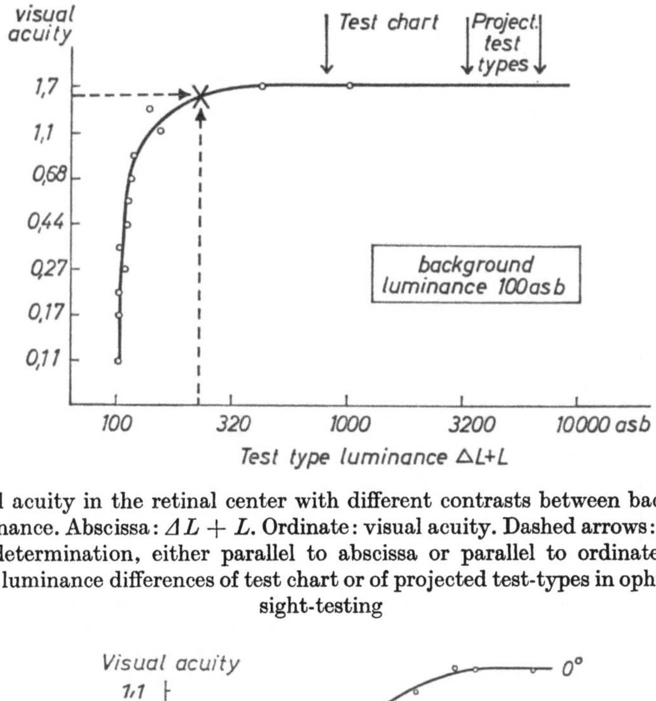

Fig. 25. Visual acuity in the retinal center with different contrasts between background and test-type luminance. Abscissa: $\Delta L + L$. Ordinate: visual acuity. Dashed arrows: two methods of threshold determination, either parallel to abscissa or parallel to ordinate. Continuous arrows: site of luminance differences of test chart or of projected test-types in ophthalmological sight-testing

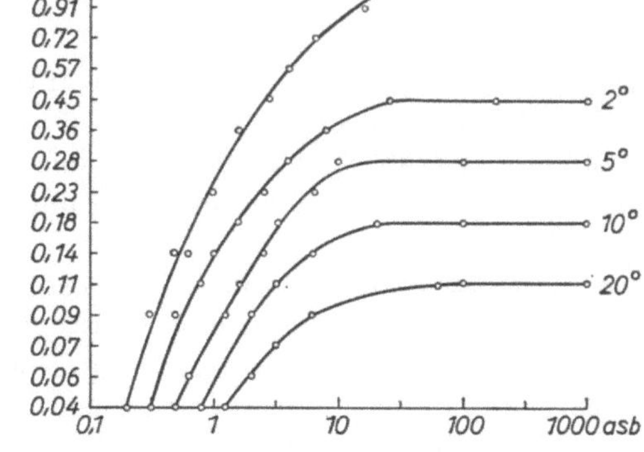

Fig. 26. Visual acuity in 5 different retinal regions. Abscissa: test-type luminance ΔL. Ordinate: visual acuity for square-circle test. Parameter: investigated retinal region. Background luminance: 10 asb

using a test-type of constant size until the test-type is recognized (direction of examination parallel to the abscissa; horizontal arrow in Fig. 26). On the other hand, it is also possible to maintain the contrast at a constant level, while the test-type increases in size until it is recognized (direction of examination parallel to the ordinate; vertical arrow in Fig. 26).

The method of contrast variation with test-types of constant size is closely related to the determination of light-difference thresholds, which is also done by

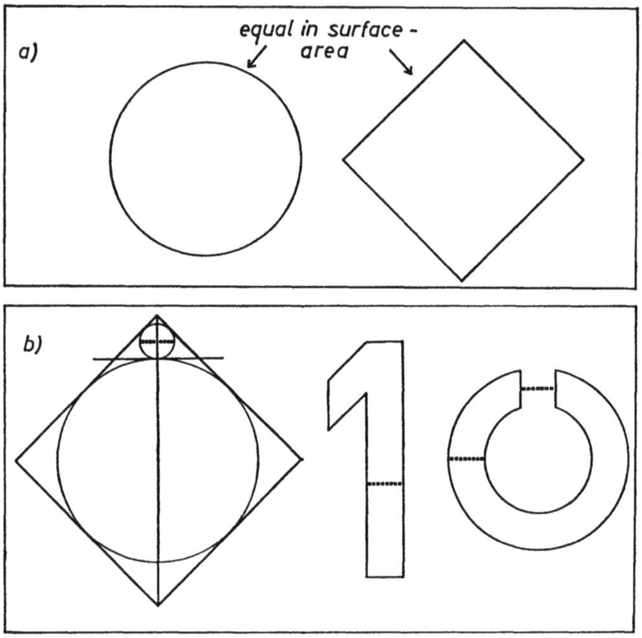

Fig. 27. a) Square-circle test-type for examination of visual acuity. b) Three test-types of equal visual acuity quotient. The "minimum separandum" is either the width of bars or width of opening or in the square the diameter of small circle which after insertion of an inner circle can be drawn in the remaining triangles

changing the contrast until a target of fixed size is seen. If the same test-types are used for determination of both light-difference sensitivity and visual acuity, the profile curves of both functions can be entered in the same system of coordinates, the difference between the two threshold curves giving important information on the functional behavior of the retina.

Such a combined examination of light-difference sensitivity and visual acuity of course cannot be carried out with ordinary acuity test-types, since they are not suitable for determination of light-difference sensitivity. Nor are they suitable for determination of visual acuity in the peripheral visual field. According to AULHORN (1960), suitable test objects for this combined examination are the square and circular test-figures (Fig. 27a). As soon as a subject can differentiate reliably between squares and circles of the same size presented in an irregular sequence, we can say that these test figures are recognized. The level of visual acuity obtained with these test-figures was empirically determined by comparison with test-types of known visual acuity levels. For this purpose 200 people were tested. Fig. 27b shows, in the square and in two other test-types, that size which is required for recognition.

In the combined experiment on light-difference sensitivity and visual acuity using square and circular test-figures, either the circle or the square is projected onto the field of the perimeter. Determination of light-difference sensitivity results in equal threshold values for both shapes, since the two are equal in area and similar in shape. It is most profitable to examine light-difference sensitivity

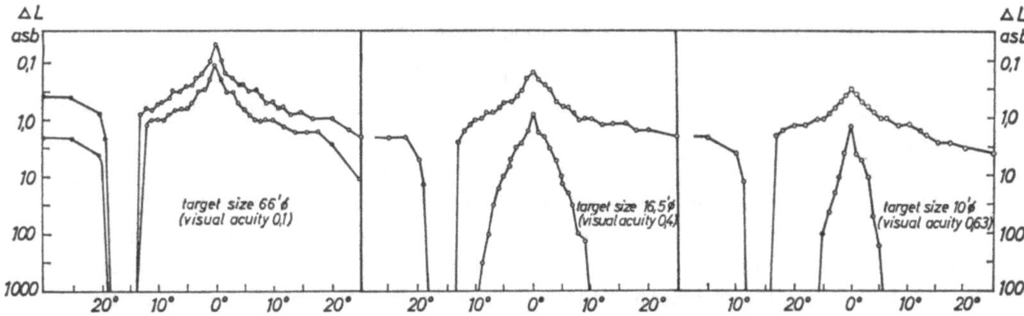

Fig. 28. Profile perimetry in 0° meridian of retina. Upper curve: light-difference threshold for target perception. Lower curve: light-difference threshold for visual acuity obtained by test-types of equal surface area (square-circle test-types). Coordinates: as in Fig. 8. L.H. curves: target size 66′ diam. corresponding to visual acuity 0.1. Middle curves: target size 16.5′ diam. corresponding to visual acuity 0.4. R.H. curves: target size 10′ diam. corresponding to visual acuity 0.63

in each retinal area first, and then to increase the difference in luminance until circles and squares, which are exposed to the same retinal area one after the other in random order, can be reliably differentiated.

In line with the difference between achromatic and chromatic thresholds that defines the photochromatic interval, the difference between detection threshold (light-difference sensitivity) and recognition thıeshold (visual acuity) could be considered as a photo-discriminating interval.

Fig. 28 shows the light-difference threshold for a combined light-perception and visual acuity experiment using test-figures of three different sizes. The smaller the test-figure, the closer to the retinal center and the more marked is the divergence of the two threshold curves. The basis for these typical curves is to be sought in the retinal structures.

It is a well-known fact that toward the periphery not only the summation capacity increases, but also the minimum and maximum size of receptive fields. The resolving power of the retina, i.e., visual acuity, depends upon the minimum size of receptive fields. The visual acuity profiles will drop off in that region of the periphery where the receptive fields become so large that resolution of the critical test elements is no longer possible. The curves of relative light-difference sensitivity, however, do not depend upon this minimum field size, since the target can be perceived even if it is smaller than the receptive field. But in this case, the target luminance must be high enough to stimulate the receptive field.

The combined examination of light-perception and visual acuity with the same test objects, as described above, is of clinical interest too, since the relation between reduction in visual acuity and reduction in light-difference sensitivity obviously varies in different diseases. For instance, in strabismus with amblyopia, visual acuity, as compared to light-difference sensitivity, is disproportionately reduced, whereas in pathological processes in the macula, both functions are subject to approximately the same reduction. Visual acuity perimetry can perhaps help to clarify the pathology of certain functional disturbances.

4. Perimetric Determination of Flicker-Fusion Frequency

Just as for acuity measures, a supra-threshold light difference between target and background is required for the observation and investigation of flicker phenomena.

Since flicker is treated in a separate chapter in this volume (see KELLY, chapter 11), we restrict ourselves here to those aspects related to perimetry.

In every area of the retina, flicker-fusion frequency changes with the luminance and size of the intermittently exposed test stimulus, and with the state of adaptation. We do not know whether these factors have direct influence on the speed of the excitatory process or whether they act indirectly by way of light-difference sensitivity. The latter possibility is easy to imagine because the factors mentioned determine how far the test stimulus used to determine flicker-fusion frequency lies above the light-difference threshold.

A reliable perimetric investigation of flicker-fusion frequency, i.e., investigation of various areas of the retina, can be carried out only in static perimetry, since in experiments with moving targets spatial and temporal summation might influence the flicker-fusion frequency to an uncontrollable extent.

The test stimulus luminance can be chosen according to two different principles (BEST, 1951; HARMS and AULHORN, 1959).

Either we use a test stimulus of constant luminance or we change the luminance for each tested retinal area, in such a way that the test stimulus exceeds the light-difference threshold by a fixed multiple. In the former case, we are indeed working with a physically constant test stimulus, but, on the other hand, the physiological stimulus, i.e., the supra-threshold luminance of the target, is different in each retinal area. As shown below, the two different methods result in a different gradient of flicker-fusion frequency in the visual field.

Fig. 29a and b show the flicker-fusion results in the nasal portion (0° meridian) of the visual fields of three and two subjects, respectively. Fig. 29a shows the results obtained with unchanged target luminance, whereas Fig. 29b demonstrates how flicker-fusion frequency changes if stimulus luminance is four or sixteen times higher than the threshold stimulus for light-difference sensitivity. This means that in Fig. 29b the influence of varying light-difference sensitivity in the tested retinal areas has been to a certain extent eliminated. We see that the gradient changes if a stimulus luminance related to the threshold is used instead of a constant stimulus luminance. In subject Ka., with a target luminance related to threshold stimulus, the slope becomes shallower. In subject Au. it even rises again toward the periphery. In both subjects the paracentral area of about 2–4° eccentricity shows a higher flicker-fusion frequency than the retinal center, whereas the results obtained with constant target luminance usually show highest sensitivity in the center.

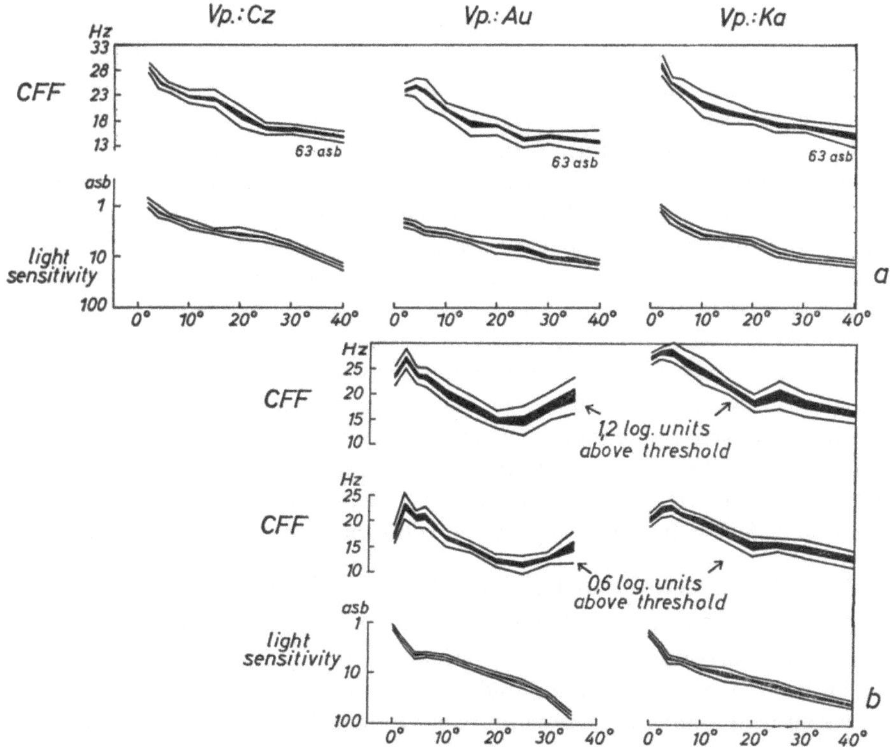

Fig. 29. Flicker-fusion frequency in three subjects in 0° meridian of retina, nasal half. a) Above: CFF with 63 asb target luminance. Below: light-difference thresholds. b) CFF with changing target luminance. Above: target luminance always 1.2 log. units above light-difference threshold. Middle: target luminance always 0.6 log. unit above light-difference threshold. Below: light-difference thresholds

From the curves in Figs. 29a and b, we must conclude that the characteristic fall in critical flicker-fusion toward the periphery is indeed influenced by the dependence of critical flicker-fusion on the degree to which the target luminance is above threshold. However, there is doubtless a further direct relation between the retinal area and critical flicker-fusion, that is evidently individually very variable. Only with target luminance related to threshold does it become clear that we are concerned with a special function of light-perception in critical flicker-fusion, that is determined by the period of time taken for the rise and fall of excitation.

The question, frequently raised in the last two decades, as to whether or not the determination of critical flicker-fusion is a better method of detecting a slight visual field abnormality than the determination of light-difference sensitivity, must clearly be answered in the negative, because of the marked dependence of critical flicker-fusion on the light-difference threshold. Only critical flicker-fusion determined with test luminance related to threshold would give additional diagnostic information. In order to determine threshold-related luminance, however, light-difference sensitivity would have to be measured first. This is absolutely necessary, especially for pathological defects in the visual field, since potential scotomata in the field of light-perception cannot be otherwise recognized, and consequently cannot be taken into consideration with regard to test-stimulus luminance in determination of critical flicker-fusion.

In our critical flicker-fusion curves, the ordinate scale is so chosen that CFF declines from the center toward the periphery in approximately the same proportion as the curves of light-difference sensitivity. When the measures are then compared, it becomes clear that the scatter is very much greater for CFF than for light-difference sensitivity. For this reason also, the determination of light-difference sensitivity is preferable as a clinical diagnostic method.

We reject flicker-fusion frequency as a routine clinical diagnostic method for the following reasons: other methods give more exact results and take less time, and also no isolated disturbance of flicker-fusion frequency in any pathological case has yet been demonstrated. However, it may be that specific disturbances occur in the excitatory process that can only be detected through supra-threshold flicker perimetry. If such disturbances should ever be demonstrated, the determination of flicker-fusion frequency too will form a part of clinical perimetry.

5. Perimetric Determination of Pupillomotor Excitability

It has long been known that the pupil contracts more on exposure to light if the stimulus falls on the center of the retina than on a peripheral locus. HESS (1908) stated that the area in which a pupillary light-reflex can be obtained is as large as the visual field and that there is probably a quantitative relation between light-sensitivity and pupillomotor excitability.

Pupillomotor perimetry is a threshold method comparable to light-perception perimetry. With this method, the target luminance in a specific retinal location is increased in steps until a pupillary contraction takes place.

This is the only perimetric method which is not based on statements made by the subject, but the investigator gets the necessary information about the subject's vision by observing his pupillary reaction (HARMS, 1940; HARMS and FRYDRYCHOWICZ, 1940a, b). Therefore, this method of "objective" perimetry is contrasted with the subjective perimetric methods.[2]

Pupillomotor perimetry raises problems of physiological interest (HARMS, 1949). We must assume at the outset that contraction of the pupils can only be elicited by a light stimulus that is clearly above the light-sensitivity threshold.

Precise determination of pupillomotor excitability is possible only in static perimetry. During exposure the target must not be shifted in the visual field, so that the pupillary reflex can give clear information on the sensitivity of a particular retinal locus. Exposure duration must remain constant and an interval of at

[2] Experiments are under way in several laboratories aiming to devise other objective methods of perimetry through electroretinography and electroencephalography. But the methods developed so far are not yet suitable for routine examinations.

least two seconds is necessary between successive exposures so that the sensitivity, altered by local adaptation, can regain its normal level before the next exposure. Observation of the pupil is possible either directly through the perimeter telescope, or by recording the pupillary movements with the aid of infra-red light reflected by the iris.

If we compare light-sensitivity with pupillomotor excitability in normals, following the procedures just mentioned, we see that the threshold stimuli for the

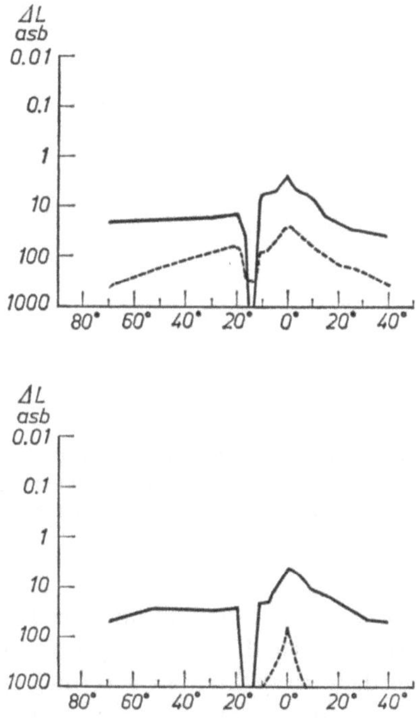

Fig. 30. Profile perimetry in 0° meridian of retina. Dotted curve: pupillomotor thresholds. Continuous curve: light-difference thresholds. Subject of upper curve shows high, subject of lower curve shows very low pupillomotor sensitivity. Coordinates: as in Fig. 8

two functions do not differ much from each other, and that the profile curves resemble each other to a great extent (Fig. 30).

However, the distance between the two profile curves and their divergence towards the periphery may show appreciable interindividual differences. The profile curves of light-difference sensitivity are very similar in all subjects, whereas the curves of pupillomotor excitability may be very different. There is no satisfactory explanation for such considerable interindividual variation in pupillomotor excitability. Perhaps these differences are due to the fact that the excitability of the motor nerve center for the sphincter pupillae is different in each individual. This hypothesis is supported by the observation that in one and the same individual, according to the state of health (i.e., probably according to the state of the autonomic nervous system) the size of the pupils and pupillomotor excitability vary considerably. Pupillomotor excitability increases with dark adaptation, i.e., it depends on the level of light sensitivity (Fig. 31).

If pupillomotor excitability is very low, its perimetric determination becomes rather difficult. The light of the test stimulus entering the eye is slightly dispersed on its passage through the refractive media, and much of it is then diffusely reflected from the wall of the eyeball. The resulting stray light in the interior of the eye remains below threshold for pupillomotor excitability as long as the test

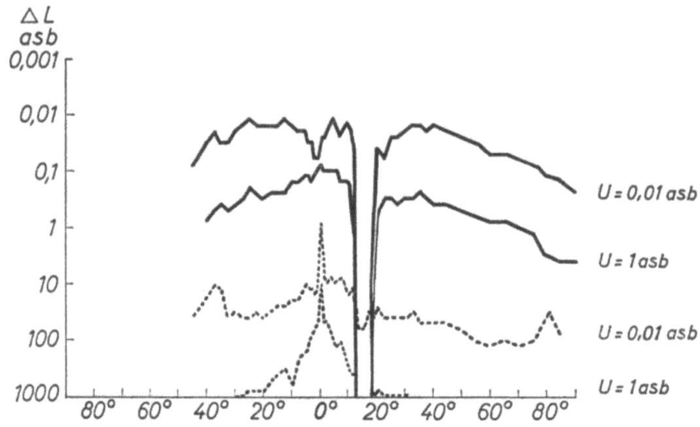

Fig. 31. Profile perimetry in 0° meridian of retina for two different background luminances. Dotted curves: pupillomotor thresholds. Continuous curves: light-difference thresholds. Coordinates: as in Fig. 8. Parameter: background luminance

stimulus itself is not too far above the perception threshold. If, however, pupillomotor excitability in the tested retinal area is very low, i.e., if a test stimulus of very high luminance is needed, stray light in a retinal area contiguous to that being tested increases to such an extent that it can cause a contraction of the pupils. In this case, pupillomotor examination lacks the main features of a perimetric method, since it does not then determine the functional capacity of the retinal region being tested, but rather shows the results of stimulation of another unspecified retinal locus.

This can be very simply checked. One can determine the target size and luminance which just elicits a contraction of the pupils if it is presented in the center of the blind spot in the visual field. This contraction can only be due to scattering of light in the eye and thus provides a measure of the stray light effective for pupillomotor excitability in the tested eye.

Another similar source of error is possible if a hemispheric perimeter is used. If a luminous target is projected onto a mat white hemisphere, the whole hemisphere is evenly illuminated by the light diffusely reflected from the bright spot. Provided it is of sufficient intensity, this illumination of the whole perimeter field can also produce a pupillary contraction. To eliminate this effect, the target is projected on the background outside the visual field of the subject, e.g., beyond the bridge of the nose, so that the stimulus light does not enter the eye. Then we determine the stimulus intensity required to just produce a pupillary reaction. At this stimulus intensity, the pupillary contraction must be brought about exclusively by the diffuse illumination of the perimeter background.

Only those pupillomotor reflexes that are obtained at a stimulus intensity lower than the "blind-spot" threshold and the "background" threshold, can be considered as a manifestation of pupillomotor sensitivity in the tested retinal area itself (HARMS, 1956).

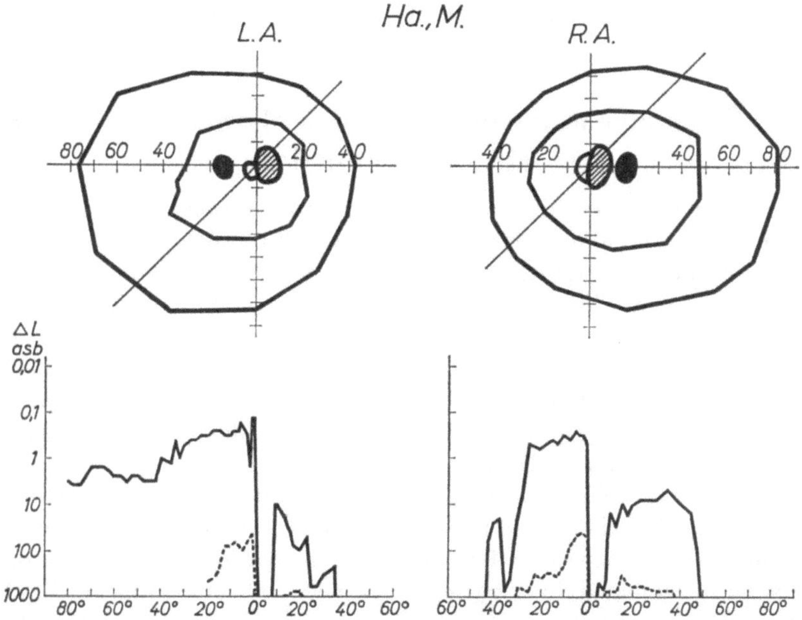

Fig. 32. Clinical perimetry in a case of small paracentral homonymous scotoma. Above: isopter perimetry. Below: profile perimetry in 135° meridian. Dotted curves: pupillomotor thresholds. Continuous curves: light-difference thresholds. Coordinates: as in Fig. 8

Defects in the visual field can be detected by pupillomotor perimetry. As shown in Fig. 32, a bilateral homonymous hemianopic central scotoma occured on the right due to a occipital lesion. The profile curves obtained in the 45° meridian show a complete loss of light sensitivity and pupillomotor sensitivity in the area of this hemianopic scotoma.

The clinical value of pupillomotor perimetry lies in the possibility of detecting simulation and exaggeration of disturbances in the visual field. Moreover, pupillomotor perimetry is of fundamental importance in so far as it questions the ideas prevailing up to now on the pathway of the pupillary light reflex.

It is generally supposed that the nerve fibres involved in the light-reflex reach the mesencephalon through the optic nerve and the tractus opticus and end in the pretectal region. From there the impulses are supposedly transmitted to the oculomotor nucleus Edinger-Westphal. If this hypothesis were true, with interruption of the visual tract above the lateral geniculate body, only a homonymous hemianopsia and no disturbance of light-reflex in the hemianopic defect of the visual field would occur (Wernicke, 1883; Wilbrand, 1881). But in the example of Fig. 32, and also in many other visual fields of patients suffering from occipital lesions (Harms, 1949, 1951), we find an absence of pupillary reflex in the visual field defect. This result is incompatible with the above-mentioned ideas on the pathway of the pupillary light-reflex. It points rather to a close connection between the optical and pupillomotor conduction paths, a connection which probably also exists in or is at least controlled by the visual cortex. As far as we know, there are still no neurophysiological experiments or neuroanatomical findings that explain these results.

C. Perimetry as a Comprehensive Method for Examing all Visual Functions

In discussing perimetric examination of the various separate functions of vision we have touched on almost every aspect of visual physiology. Aubert (1857), in his fundamental work, rightly said that there are quantitative relations between the different separate functions of vision in every area of the visual field. It is now up to us to find out the extent and nature of such quantitative relations and also to verify whether, as is repeatedly asserted, an isolated or preferential disturbance of one single separate function of vision is possible. The latter question could be of importance to an early diagnosis of pathological disturbances (Harms, 1950; Jayle *et al.*, 1958; Jayle, 1960).

To determine specific quantitative relations, or detect isolated disturbances of separate visual functions, it is necessary to make comparable investigations. In ophthalmological practice so far, however, the various visual functions have usually been examined by very different and non-comparable methods. Test results can only be compared if all of them are obtained under exactly the same physical conditions. With regard to visual field examination, this means that the various visual functions must be examined with the same apparatus, and for this purpose, it has been necessary to construct special perimeters as l'adaptocampimètre de Blet-Jayle (Dubois-Poulsen, 1952, p. 459) or Tübinger Perimeter (Aulhorn, 1960; Harms, 1960). The perimeter should make it possible to determine the following functions in any part of the visual field and for any state of adaptation:

light-difference threshold,
spatial summation,
temporal integration,
achromatic thresholds for monochromatic light,
visual acuity,
local adaptation,
pupillomotor excitability,
flicker-fusion frequency.

To be sure, quantitative comparisons are not possible to the same extent for all of the different visual functions. If the same background, the same target size and the same exposure time are used, difference thresholds for white and colored light, and for pupillomotor excitability thresholds can be entered in the same system of coordinates. In this case the abscissa corresponds to the tested retinal area and the ordinate represents the logarithm of stimulus luminance. However, for the examination of visual acuity with changing test-type size, for the determination of local adaptation, and for flicker-fusion frequency, the abscissa is the same, but the ordinates differ (e.g., size, time, frequency). Nevertheless, for these functions, too, it is always obvious whether, considered as a whole, they conform to the slope of the profile functions or whether they show characteristic deviations.

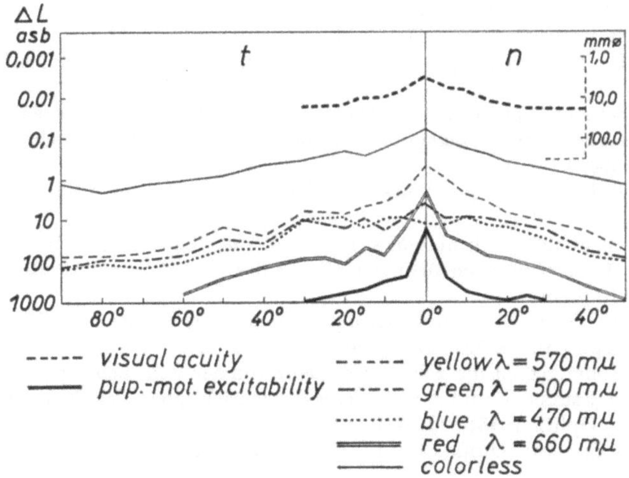

Fig. 33. Profile perimetry in 0° meridian of retina for visual acuity, pupillomotor sensitivity and light-difference thresholds for different wave-lengths and for colorless light. Coordinates: as in Fig. 8

Fig. 33 gives an example of how the results of such investigations can be compared with each other. From it we can deduce that there are some interesting relations between the different functions:

The gradient of visual acuity resembles to a great extent the difference sensitivity for white light.

The achromatic thresholds for red (660 nm) result in a profile curve quite similar to the thresholds of pupillomotor sensitivity.

The sensitivity for blue (470 nm) is relatively low in the center of the visual field. This relative scotoma far exceeds the diameter of the macula lutea.

All this applies when subjects are adapted to a background luminance of 1 asb.

Each of these findings gives rise to special considerations which cannot be pursued here, but they show that there are gaps in our knowledge of the distribution and linkage of visual functions in the different areas of the visual field. Our summary of the advances in perimetry is intended to show that, in its most recent development, this method which was originally intended only for clinical diagnosis, has gained importance for visual physiology. By modern perimetry it is possible not only to determine the relations between the various visual functions in the different areas of the visual field, but also to analyze very closely the way they are related through summation and inhibitory processes in the whole visual field

(Aulhorn and Harms, 1956; Harms, 1964). We are now able to make such investigations, but most of the work still lies ahead. As soon as we have succeeded in obtaining a complete and sound physiological basis for a comprehensive perimetry, we shall also be able to obtain full information on the nature of visual field disturbances in specific diseases.

References

Aubert, H.: Über die Gränzen der Farbenwahrnehmung auf den seitlichen Theilen der Retina. Graefes Arch. Ophthal. **3**, 38—67 (1857).
— Foerster, R.: Untersuchungen über den Raumsinn der Retina. Graefes Arch. Ophthal. **3**, 1—37 (1857).
Aulhorn, E.: Sehschärfeprüfung am Perimeter. Ber. dtsch. ophthal. Ges. **63**, 285—288 (1960).
— Psychophysische Gesetzmäßigkeiten des normalen Sehens. Ber. dtsch. ophthal. Ges. **66**, 144—161 (1964a).
— Über die Beziehung zwischen Lichtsinn und Sehschärfe. Graefes Arch. Ophthal. **167**, 4—74 (1964b).
— Glaukom-Gesichtsfeld. Ophthalmologica (Basel) **158**, 469—487 (1969).
— Harms, H.: Untersuchungen über das Wesen des Grenzkontrastes. Ber. dtsch. ophthal. Ges. **60**, 7—10 (1956).
— — Raabe, N.: Die Lichtunterschiedsempfindlichkeit als Funktion der Umfeldleuchtdichte. Documenta Ophthal. **20**, 527—556 (1966).
Best, W.: Die Abhängigkeit der Flimmerfrequenz von der Reizflächengröße und dem Ort der gereizten Netzhautstelle unter besonderer Berücksichtigung der Schwellenreizlichtstärke. Graefes Arch. Ophthal. **152**, 99—110 (1951).
Blet-Jayle, G. E.: In: Dubois-Poulsen, A.: Le Champ Visuel. Paris: Masson 1952. pp. 459—460.
Cibis, P.: Zur Pathologie der Lokaladaptation. Graefes Arch. Ophthal. **148**, 1—92 and 216—257 (1948).
Daniel, K.: Der Einfluß der Reizmarkengröße auf die Lichtunterschiedsempfindlichkeit der Netzhaut bei verschiedenen Adaptationszuständen. Inaugural dissertation. Tübingen (1959).
Dorff, W.: Der Einfluß des Zeitfaktors bei der Schwellenwertbestimmung des Lichtsinns des menschlichen Auges. Inaugural dissertation. Tübingen (1953).
Dubois-Poulsen, A.: Le Champ Visuel. Paris: Masson 1952.
— Magis, Cl., Ben-Mansour, Lanneau: La dysharmonie photométrique dans le champ visuel des glaucomateux. Documenta Ophthal. **13**, 286—302 (1959).
Engelking, E., Eckstein, A.: Physiologische Bestimmung von Musterfarben für die klinische Perimetrie. Klin. Mbl. Augenheilk. **64**, 88—106 (1920).
Ferree, C. E., Rand, G.: An illuminated perimeter with campimeter features. Amer. J. Ophthal. **5**, 455—465 (1922).
— — Effect of brightness of preexposure and surrounding field on breath and shape of the color fields for stimuli of different sizes. Amer. J. Ophthal. **7**, 843—850 (1924).
Fiorentini, A., Toraldo di Francia, G.: Mesures photométriques visuelles sur un champ à gradient d'éclairement variable. Optica Acta **1**, 192—193 (1955).
Goldmann, H.: Grundlagen exakter Perimetrie. Ophthalmologica (Basel) **109**, 57—70 (1945a).
— Ein selbstregistrierendes Projektionskugelperimeter. Ophthalmologica (Basel) **109**, 71—79 (1945b).
Graefe, A. von: Über die Untersuchung des Gesichtsfeldes bei amblyopischen Affektionen. Graefes Arch. Ophthal. **2**, 258—298 (1856).
Harms, H.: Objektive Perimetrie. Ber. dtsch. opthal. Ges. **53**, 63—70 (1940).
— Grundlagen, Methodik und Bedeutung der Pupillenperimetrie für die Physiologie und Pathologie des Sehorgans. Graefes Arch. Ophthal. **149**, 1—68 (1949).
— Entwicklungsmöglichkeiten der Perimetrie. Graefes Arch. Ophthal. **150**, 28—57 (1950).
— Hemianopische Pupillenstarre. Klin. Mbl. Augenheilk. **118**, 133—147 (1951).
— Neue Methoden der Perimetrie. In: Zeitfragen der Augenheilkunde. Leipzig: VEB Thieme 1954.

HARMS, H.: Möglichkeiten und Grenzen der pupillomotorischen Perimetrie. Klin. Mbl. Augenheilk. **129**, 518—534 (1956).
— Die Bedeutung einer einheitlichen Prüfweise aller Sehfunktionen. Ber. dtsch. ophthal. Ges. **63**, 281—285 (1960).
— Ort und Wesen der Bildhemmung bei Schielenden. Ber. dtsch. ophthal. Ges. **66**, 202—212 (1964).
— AULHORN, E.: Studien über den Grenzkontrast. Graefes Arch. Ophthal. **157**, 3—23 (1955).
— — Vergleichende Untersuchungen über den Wert der quantitativen Perimetrie, Skiaskotometrie und Verschmelzungsfrequenz für die Erkennung beginnender Gesichtsfeldstörungen beim Glaukom. Documenta Ophthal. **13**, 303—332 (1959).
— FRYDRYCHOWICZ, G.: Ergebnisse pupillomotorischer Untersuchungen bei Gesunden und Kranken. Ber. dtsch. ophthal. Ges. **53**, 71—79 (1940a).
— — Das pupillomotorische Perimeter. Ber. dtsch. ophthal. Ges. **53**, 326—329 (1940b).
HARTINGER, H.: Das Zeiss-Projektionsperimeter nach L. MAGGIORE. Z. ophthal. Opt. **24**, 39—52 (1936).
HESS, C.: Über den Farbensinn bei indirektem Sehen. Graefes Arch. Ophthal. **35**, (4) 1—62 (1889).
— Untersuchung zur Physiologie und Pathologie des Pupillenspieles. Arch. Augenheilk. **60**, 327—389 (1908).
JAYLE, G. E.: Méthodes et techniques nouvelles de périmétrie, de campimétrie et de mesure de l'acuité visuelle en clinique. Clermont-Ferrand: Edité par l'Institut Chibret 1960.
— AUBERT, L., VOLA, J.: Exploration du champ visual à l'explorateur universel de Jayle et Blet. Sommations et champ visual avec flicker du fond. Société d'Ophthalmologie du Midi, Toulouse, 7. 12. 1958.
KÖLLNER, H.: Die Störungen des Farbensinnes, ihre klinische Bedeutung und ihre Diagnose. Berlin: Karger 1912.
LAUBER, H.: Ein Lichtpunktwerfer für Perimetrie und Campimetrie. Ber. dtsch. ophthal. Ges. **49**, 487—488 (1932).
MEYER-GEHLEN, H.: Übungseinflüsse bei quantitativer Perimetrie. Klin. Mbl. Augenheilk. **129**, 850 (1956).
MEYNER, E. M.: Über die Bedeutung von Pupillenweite und Umfeldleuchtdichte bei der Prüfung des Adaptationsvermögens. Inaugural-Dissertation. Tübingen 1962.
NOLTE, W.: Bestimmung achromatischer Schwellen für verschiedene Spektrallichter. Inaugural-Dissertation. Tübingen 1962.
SCHOBER, H.: Das Sehen (2nd Ed.). Leipzig: Fachbuchverlag Leipzig 1958.
SLOAN, L. L.: Instruments and technics for the clinical testing of light sense. III. An apparatus for studying regional differences in light sense. Arch. Ophthal. **22**, 233—251 (1939).
TRAQUAIR, H. M.: An introduction to clinical perimetry. London: Kimpton 1927.
TRENDELENBURG, W.: Der Gesichtssinn (2nd Ed.). Berlin-Göttingen-Heidelberg: Springer 1961.
TROXLER, D.: Über das Verschwinden gegebener Gegenstände innerhalb unseres Gesichtskreises. Himly u. Schmidt's ophthalmologische Bibliothek **2**, 2 (1802).
WENTWORTH, H. A.: A quantitive study of achromatic and chromatic sensitivity from center to periphery of the visual field. Psychol. Monogr. **40** (3), Nr. 183. (Dissertation) 1930.
WERNICKE, C.: Amaurose mit erhaltener Pupillenreaktion bei einem Hirntumor. Z. klin. Med. **6**, 361 (1883).
WERTHEIM, TH.: Über die indirekte Sehschärfe. Z. Psychol. **7**, 174 (1894).
WILBRAND, H.: Über Hemianopie und ihre Verhältnis zur topischen Diagnose der Gehirnkrankheiten. Berlin: Hirschwald 1881.

Chapter 6

Simultaneous Brightness Induction

By

Eric G. Heinemann, New York, New York (USA)

With 15 Figures

Contents

Introduction

The term "brightness induction" refers to a change in the brightness of light imaged on one region of the retina caused by simultaneous illumination of other regions. The simplest experimental arrangement for studying induction effects uses two evenly illuminated fields called the *test field* and the *inducing field*. The inducing field may decrease or increase the brightness of the test field, or have no effect, depending on the relative luminances of the two fields and the geometric arrangement. Naturally, the test field may also have an effect on the brightness of the inducing field.

Under many conditions induction appears to increase the difference in the brightness of the test and inducing fields. This increase in the brightness difference between two areas is traditionally called "contrast," though the word "contrast" has been used in at least two other senses: (1) to refer to the ratio of the difference in the luminance of two adjacent areas to the lower or higher of these luminances, and (2) to refer to the depression of the brightness of a test field by an inducing field. In this chapter the term "luminance contrast" will be used when the first meaning is intended. The second usage is undesirable because the depression of the brightness of a test field does not necessarily indicate that the difference in the brightness of the test and inducing fields has been increased. By this definition, the common textbook illustrations, which show that a test patch on a background of high reflectance looks darker than an identical test patch on a background of lower reflectance, demonstrate induction but do not unambiguously demonstrate contrast.

Contrast in the traditional sense is difficult to measure because there is no generally accepted method for measuring brightness or brightness differences. Most measurements of induction effects are based on brightness matching. A comparison field, generally of the same size and shape as the test field, is presented in a way that eliminates or minimizes possible effects upon its brightness by the test and inducing fields. The luminance of the comparison field, L_c, is adjusted until the comparison and test fields have the same brightness. What is measured with this method is not brightness but the luminance L_c needed for a brightness match. To measure contrast the comparison field must be matched to the test field and to the inducing field when each is presented alone, and again when the two fields are presented simultaneously. If the brightness of either the test or the inducing fields is not affected by the simultaneous presence of the other, or if the brightness of the two fields changes in opposite directions, then it is possible to specify whether the difference in brightness between the two fields increased or decreased as a result of their interaction. However, if, as is often the case, each field depresses the brightness of the other, it is not possible to say how the brightness difference changed unless an assumption is made concerning the form of the relation between luminance and brightness (e. g., Fechner's Law or the Power Law).

Under some circumstances the interaction between the test and inducing fields might result in a decrease in the brightness difference between them. Effects of this type have been called "reverse contrast," "assimilation" and "equalization." Most discussions of such effects are based on illustrations published by BEZOLD (1874). These are colored strips overlaid with black arabesques in some regions and with white arabesques of the same design in other regions. Excellent reproductions of these patterns may be found in EVANS (1948), and BURNHAM (1953). Most observers say that the colored background looks darker in the region overlaid with the black design than in the region overlaid with the white one. This effect has been studied with a neutral background and a simplified overlay of straight lines by HELSON and ROHLES (1959) (see also HELSON, 1963). These investigators found that the relative darkening of the regions surrounding the black lines was most pronounced with thin closely spaced lines but was still noticeable when the lines were separated by angular distances of 1°3′. The effect also diminished as the lines were made wider, and for lines of sufficient width the area surrounding the white lines appeared darker than that surrounding the black lines. In these experiments and in viewing the BEZOLD patterns the judgments made concern the *relative* brightness of the regions surrounding the black and white lines. Whether the white and black lines produce similar effects upon their immediate backgrounds or whether the relative brightness change that is observed reflects the effects produced by only one class of lines is not known. Finally, it is not clear that the use of the word "equalization" or its synonyms is appropriate in describing these effects, because it has not been established that the brightness difference between the lines and the background is diminished as a result of their interaction.

The experiments to be considered in the following sections are concerned with the effect of various parameters of inducing fields upon the brightness of a test field and do not deal directly with the question of contrast or brightness differences.

Methods of Study

Several arrangements used in the study of induction are shown in Fig. 1. The letters *T*, *I* and *C* stand for test, inducing, and comparison fields, respectively. The subject may be required to fixate a point, usually between the test and comparison fields, or he may be permitted to shift his gaze back and forth. The brightness of the test and comparison fields can be matched by adjusting the luminance of either the test or the comparison field, or under some circumstances, by adjusting the luminance of the inducing field. The results do not depend on which luminance is adjusted (SCHOUTEN and ORNSTEIN, 1939; HEINEMANN, 1955).

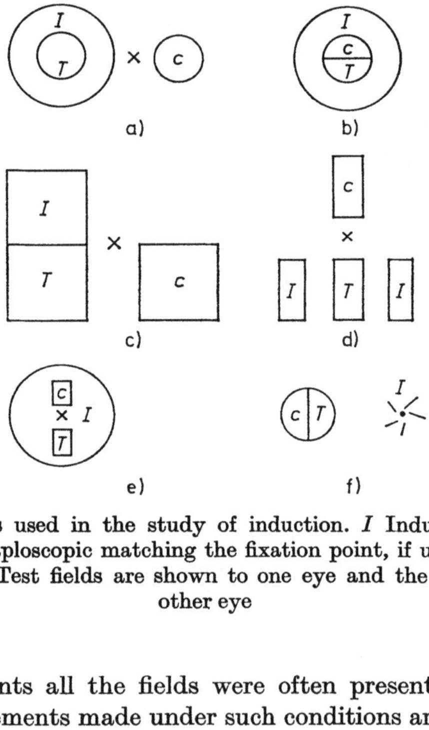

Fig. 1. Stimulus patterns used in the study of induction. *I* Inducing field, *T* Test field, *C* comparison field. In haploscopic matching the fixation point, if used, is presented to both eyes; the Inducing and Test fields are shown to one eye and the comparison field to the other eye

In early experiments all the fields were often presented simultaneously to the same eye. Measurements made under such conditions are difficult to interpret because of the many possible interactions among the three fields. To avoid this difficulty most recent experiments have used the binocular, or more correctly, haploscopic matching method in which the comparison field is presented to one eye and the test and inducing fields to the other eye. Provided the fields are imaged upon non-corresponding regions of the two eyes, interaction between fields presented to opposite eyes appears to be absent or negligible (SCHOUTEN and ORNSTEIN, 1939; DIAMOND, 1953). With arrangement *e* (Fig. 1) corresponding regions of the two retinas are stimulated by the inducing and comparison fields and some binocular summation has been found by FRY and ALPERN (1954); see also WHITTLE and CHALLANDS (1969). According to SAUNDERS (1968), slight binocular interaction occurs also with pattern *b* in which the edges of the test and comparison fields are contiguous in the binocular view.

DIAMOND *et al.* (1955) investigated the possible influence of the psychophysical method used in matching and found that the methods of adjustment, limits, and constant stimuli yield virtually identical results.

Effects of Test and Inducing Luminances

How the luminances of the test and inducing fields influence the brightness of the test field depends on many variables such as the sizes of the fields, their location on the retina, the distance between them, etc. In this section results obtained with adjacent test and inducing fields will be considered.

The matter was first thoroughly investigated by HESS and PRETORI (1894) who used test and comparison fields that were completely surrounded by inducing fields, with all fields presented simultaneously to the same eye. Similar experiments have been done with the haploscopic method by a number of later investigators. HEINEMANN (1955) used stimulus arrangement *a* (Fig. 1) with the following dimensions: diameter of test and comparison fields, 28′; outer diameter of the annulus, 55′; distance from the center of the test and comparison fields to the fixation point 52′. The results of one experiment are shown in Fig. 2. As the luminance of the inducing field, L_i, is increased, the curves at first rise slightly indicating that the brightness of the test field is increased. This initial rise in the brightness of the test field is slight but appears consistently in the results of three subjects who served in the experiment. For values of L_i greater than approximately half the luminance of the test field (L_t) the brightness of the test field is depressed. Near the point where $L_i = L_t$ small increases in L_i make necessary very large decreases in matching luminance, L_c, and when L_i exceeds L_t by only a few hundredths of a log unit the brightness of the test field is reduced so much that a match is no longer possible. Under these circumstances any comparison field that is visible at all appears brighter than the test field; in fact the test field may appear darker than the total absence of light. To measure the effect produced by higher inducing luminances it is necessary to darken the comparison field by also surrounding it with an inducing field. Curves *D*, *E*, and *F* in Fig. 3 show the measurements obtained by HEINEMANN when the comparison field was surrounded by an annulus of luminance $\log L = 1.05$ (mL). The curves are constant brightness contours, i. e., all test fields having luminances that lie on a single curve have the same brightness. (Curves *A*, *B*, and *C* represent measurements made under the conditions of the previous experiment, with the comparison field on a completely dark background.) The nearly linear portions of the curves have slopes near 1.0. This indicates that the brightness of the test field is almost constant when the ratio L_t/L_i is constant. It has been pointed out by many investigators that the dependence of test-field brightness on this

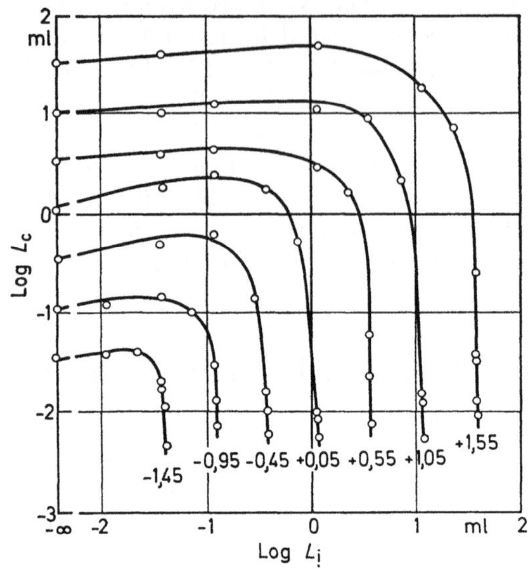

Fig. 2. The comparison-field luminances required for a brightness match between the comparison and test fields, as a function of inducing luminance. The parameters on the curves are the luminances of the test fields in Log mL. From HEINEMANN (1955)

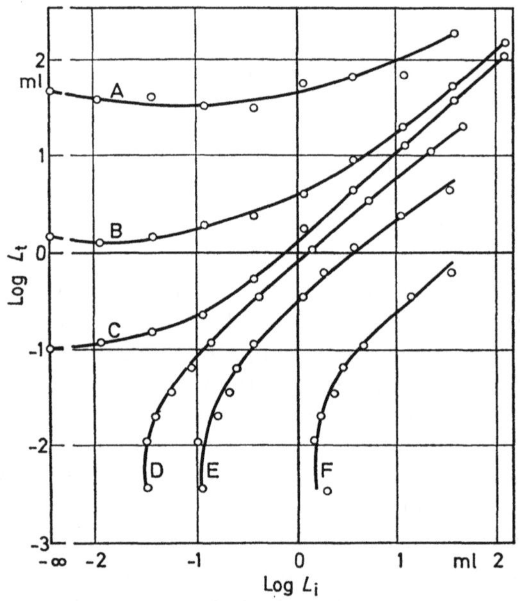

Fig. 3. The test field luminance needed to match a constant comparison field as function of the luminance of the inducing field. For curves A, B, and C, the comparison field was presented on a dark background; for curves D, E, and F, the comparison field was surrounded by an annulus of 1.05 log mL. From HEINEMANN (1955)

luminance ratio is largely responsible for the phenomenon of "brightness constancy" (cf. FREEMAN, 1967; HELSON, 1938, 1943; SAUNDERS, 1968; WALLACH, 1948). On the other hand, JAMESON and HURVICH (1961, 1964) have called attention to the fact that curves of the sort shown in Fig. 3 do not have slopes that are precisely identical and equal to 1.0, and they emphasize that "brightness constancy" is only approximate.

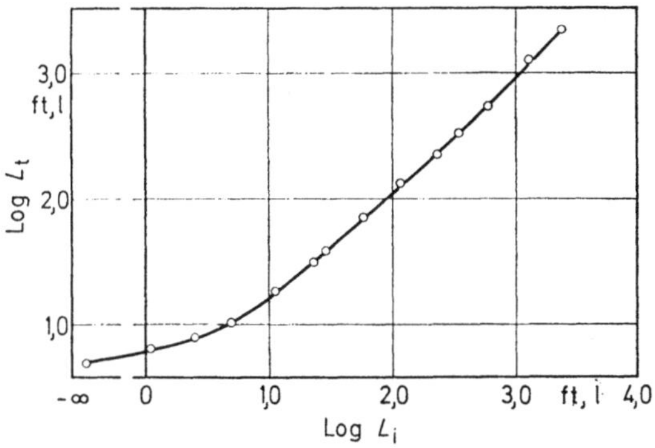

Fig. 4. The test field luminance needed to match a constant comparison field as a function of the luminance of the inducing field. Because the inducing field is superimposed on the test field, the test field luminance is the sum of the test and inducing luminances. Data from FRY and ALPERN (1953a)

Results similar to those of HEINEMANN have been obtained with the disk annulus pattern by HOREMAN (1965), SAUNDERS (1968), and TORII and UEMURA (1965). Although the depression of test-field brightness is greatest when the inducing luminance exceeds the test luminance, all the experimenters cited found that depression of test field brightness is also caused by inducing fields whose luminance is somewhat smaller than that of the test field. This fact is often overlooked in discussions of induction. It is of particular importance in interpreting the effects of glare on brightness (discussed in a later section) and has also been demonstrated by FRY and ALPERN (1953a, 1954), and by WHITTLE and CHALLANDS (1969). FRY and ALPERN used stimulus pattern *e* (Fig. 1) with the following dimensions: diameter of *I*, 9.5°; fields *C* and *T*, 0.5° × 2.5°, with a separation of 0.5° between the nearest edges of *C* and *T*. Field *C* was presented to one eye, fields *I* and *T* to the other eye. Field *I*, called the "veiling luminance" by FRY and ALPERN, was superimposed on field *T* so that the retinal illumination in the region stimulated by field *T* was always above that of the surrounding region. The subjects matched the brightness of *C* and *T* by adjusting the luminance of *T*, with the luminance of *I* as the independent variable. The constant brightness curve determined by this method (Fig. 4) is similar in form to those shown in Fig. 3 and also has a linear segment with a slope near 1.0.

When the inducing field does not completely surround the test field the induction effects are much weaker, as can be seen in the results of DIAMOND (Fig. 5). These results were obtained with pattern *c* (Fig. 1). The test, comparison, and inducing fields were 33′ × 33′ in angular size, and the distance from the nearest edge of the test and comparison fields to the fixation points was 21′. Under these conditions the inducing field appears to have little or no effect on the brightness of the test field when $L_i < L_t$. When $L_i > L_t$, increases in L_i require decreases in matching luminance, L_c, but the rate at which L_c changes with increases in L_i is smaller than found with a complete surround.

Horeman (1965) made similar measurements with patterns *b* and *d* (Fig. 1). The rate at which L_c changes with variations in L_i with these stimulus arrangements falls between that observed with the disk-annulus and adjacent-square patterns. Thus induction effects become more pronounced as the geometric arrangement approaches one in which the test field is completely surrounded by the inducing field.

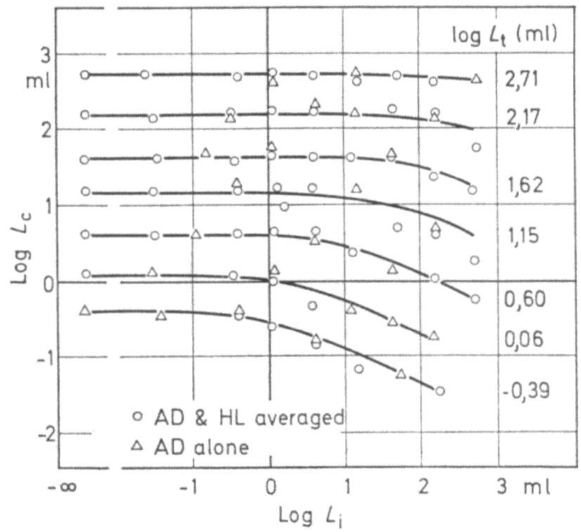

Fig. 5. The comparison-field luminances required for a brightness match between the comparison and test fields, as a function of inducing luminance. The parameters on the curves are the luminances of the test fields in log *mL*. From Diamond (1953)

Effects of Inducing-Field Size

The effect of varying the size of the inducing field in the disk-annulus arrangements has been investigated by Torii und Uemura (1965) under the following conditions: Diameter of the test and comparison fields, 36′; diameter of the inducing fields, 48′, 1° and 2°; distance from the center of the test and comparison fields to the fixation points, 1°24′. The inducing field was separated from the test field by a thin black line. The results for one subject are shown in Fig. 6. It can be seen that, for this subject, as the size of the inducing field is decreased the enhancement effect produced by inducing fields of luminance much below the test field luminance becomes smaller. Also the maximum enhancement appears to occur at progressively higher inducing luminances as the size of the inducing field is decreased. Under all conditions the brightness of the test field is depressed by inducing fields whose luminance is nearly equal to that of the test field or exceeds it, but the rate at which the matching luminance

Fig. 6 a—c. The comparison-field luminances required for a brightness match between the comparison and test fields, as a function of inducing luminance. Width of the annulus: (a) 6′, (b) 12′, (c) 42′. The parameters on the curves are the luminances of the test fields in log mL. From Torii and Uemura (1965)

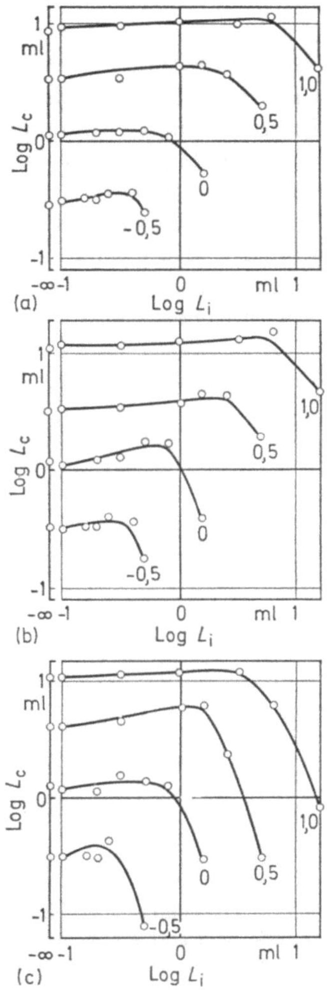

Fig. 7. The comparison-field luminances required for a brightness match between the comparison and test fields, as a function of inducing luminance. The parameters on the curves give the width of the annulus in minutes of arc. Heinemann, unpublished

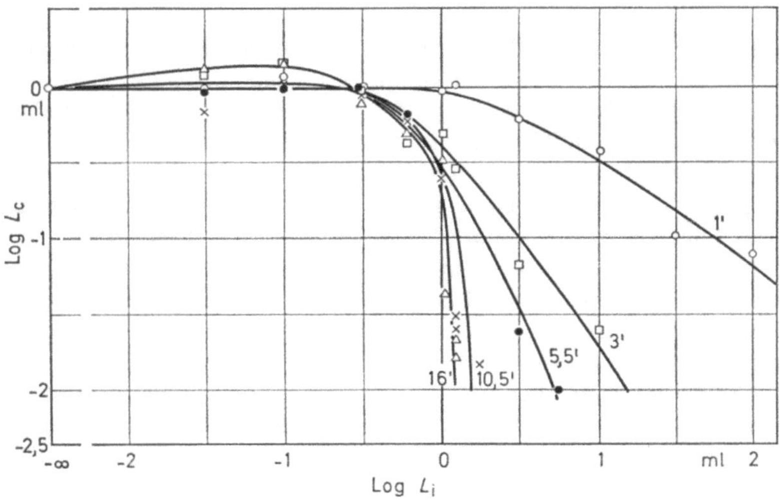

Fig. 7

decreases with increasing inducing luminance is greater for large inducing fields than for small ones. This change in the slope of the descending portions of the functions can be seen more clearly in Fig. 7 which represents measurements made by HEINEMANN under conditions identical to those of the experiment discussed previously (HEINEMANN, 1955) except that five inducing fields varying in outer diameter from 30′ to 60′ were used. The results in Fig. 7 indicate that the form of the induction curves changes rapidly as the width of the annulus is increased from 1′ to 10.5′, but that further increase in the width of the annulus has little effect.

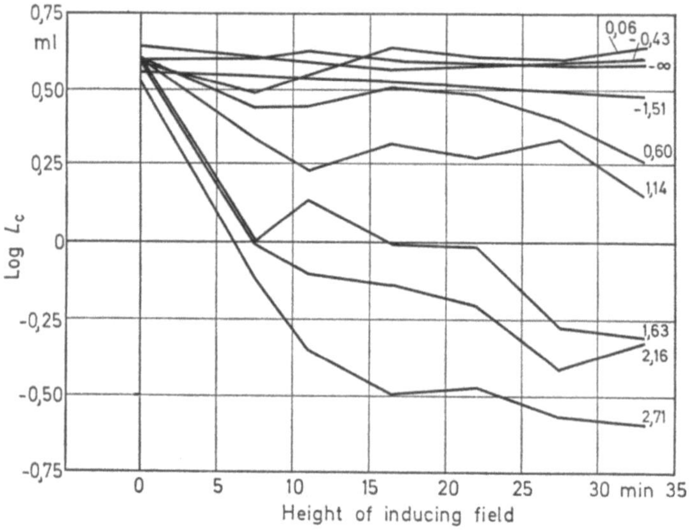

Fig. 8. The comparison-field luminances required for a brightness match between the comparison field and a test field of luminance 0.60 log *mL*, as a function of the height of the inducing field. The parameters on the curves are the luminances of the inducing field in log *mL*. From DIAMOND (1955)

In a similar experiment DIAMOND (1955) used contiguous rectangular test and inducing fields. The test- and comparison-fields were 33′ wide and 16.5′ high. The inducing field, 33′ wide and of variable height, was located above the test field. The other conditions were: distance of the fixation point from the nearest edges of the test and comparison fields, 21′, test field luminance constant at 0.60 log mL. The results for one subject are shown in Fig. 8. Inducing luminances less than the test luminance have little or no effect. At all inducing luminances that exceed the test luminance there is a depression of test field brightness. Successive increases in the height of the inducing field cause gradually diminishing increases in the size of the induction effects, and the form of the curves suggests that increases in the height of the inducing field beyond 33′ would not cause much further reduction in the brightness of the test field. If these results are plotted as in Fig. 5, the descending limbs of the functions become steeper with increasing inducing field area, as is the case for the disk-annulus pattern. In a second experiment DIAMOND (1955) measured the effect of varying the size of the inducing field when the distance from the center of the inducing field to the test field was held constant. Under this condition narrow inducing fields are separated from the test field by a black space and the effects are smaller than those found with adjacent inducing fields.

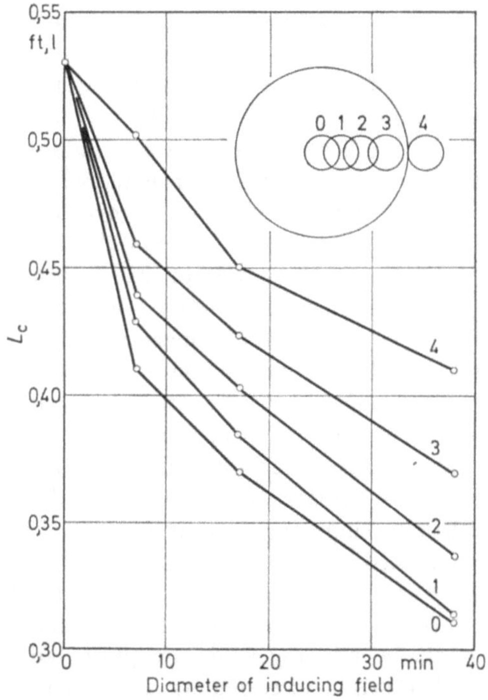

Fig. 9. The comparison-field luminance required for a brightness match between the comparison and test fields, as a function of the diameter of the inducing field. The numbers written next to each curve refer to the position of the inducing field as indicated in the inset (not drawn to scale). From results of STEWART (1959)

STEWART (1959) investigated the effect of varying the area of a small circular inducing field that was presented at various positions within a much larger circular test field. STEWART's arrangement is an elaboration of a well-known demonstration by GELB (1929) which shows that, if the rest of the visual field is totally dark, the introduction of a very small inducing field near the periphery of a large test disk of lesser luminance causes a dramatic depression of the brightness of the test disk. This demonstration has played an important role in treatments of "brightness constancy" (HURVICH and JAMESON, 1966; WOODWORTH and SCHLOSBERG, 1954). STEWART's experiment was done under the following conditions: Successive haploscopic matching, diameter of the test field 3°5'; diameter of the comparison field, 2°30'; diameters of the inducing fields, 7', 17', and 38'. The inducing field was presented in each of five different positions, viz., in the center of the test disk, at three progressively more eccentric positions within the test disk, and outside of the test disk with the outside edges of the test and inducing disks just in contact. The test and comparison fields were rotating black and white sector disks; luminances were computed by the present author on the basis of the Talbot-Plateau Law. The results (Fig. 9) show that the form of the curves relating the matching luminance to the diameter of the inducing field does not depend strongly on the position of the inducing field, and that inducing fields of fixed size depress the brightness of the test field more when they are located near its center.

Geometrically, one can, of course, treat an inducing field as composed of any number of elementary sub-areas. The possibility of formulating a simple rule for predicting the effects of a large inducing area by adding the effects produced by each of the elementary sub-areas has been explored by ALPERN and DAVID (1959) and THOMAS (1963). ALPERN and DAVID worked with a modification of pattern *d* (Fig. 1). In some of their experiments the two inducing fields that flank the test field were squares $150' \times 150'$ in size. In others the inducing fields were rectangles whose size and position in the visual field were such as would be obtained by dividing the $150' \times 150'$ square into two or more rectangular strips. Their analysis is based on a comparison of the induction effects produced by the various pairs of rectangles when presented alone with the induction effect produced by the two squares that are formed when all the rectangles are shown simultaneously. Let L_t and L_c be the luminances of the test and comparison fields, respectively, when they appear equally bright. Under ALPERN and DAVID's conditions $L_t = L_c$ when no inducing field is present. The magnitude of the induction effect ΔL, is defined as $\Delta L = L_t - L_c$. Effects were said to be additive if $\Delta L_s = \Delta L_1 + \Delta L_2 \ldots + \Delta L_n$, where $\Delta L_1, \Delta L_2, \ldots, \Delta L_n$ are the induction effects measured in the presence of each of n inducing fields, and ΔL_s is the induction effect measured when the n inducing fields are presented simultaneously. The results of ALPERN and DAVID's experiments show that the induction effect produced by several inducing fields presented simultaneously is smaller than the sum of the effects each field produces alone, with departures from additivity most pronounced at low inducing luminances.

A somewhat similar experiment by THOMAS (1963) used point source stimuli for all fields. Induction effects produced by each of two inducing fields when presented alone were compared with the effect produced when the two inducing fields were presented simultaneously. The inducing fields were not of constant intensity but were adjusted to have a constant brightness under the several conditions. Departing from the usage of ALPERN and DAVID, THOMAS defined the magnitude of the induction effect as the difference between the logarithms of the test and comparison field intensities required for a brightness match. This formulation also failed to yield a simple additivity principle. The results showed that the effect of the two inducing fields presented together is smaller than the sum of the effects of the single inducing fields.

Since definitions of the magnitude of the induction effects are quite arbitrary, the reported failures of additivity are not really surprising. The problem is further complicated by the fact that each of the inducing fields that are presented together may affect the ability of the others to influence the brightness of the test field. That such interaction among the inducing fields does occur was shown by ALPERN and DAVID (1959). Using a modification of pattern *d* (Fig. 1) they found that the induction effect of two rectangular fields that were separated from the test field by 105′ was reduced when two more inducing fields that were separated from the test field by 135′ were added to the stimulus pattern. The more peripheral inducing fields by themselves did not affect the test field, but they reduced the ability of their neighbors to do so. Very similar observations have been reported by MACKAVEY *et al.* (1962).

The theoretical treatment of brightness induction effects by JAMESON and HURVICH (1964) bases its quantitative predictions on systems of simultaneous equations to represent opponent interactions among all stimulated areas of the visual field. Also, MARSDEN's (1969) reformulation of their theory as an elemental, rather than integrated, one, is consistent with non-additive induction effects of the sort described above.

Effects of Test-Field Size

The influence of the size of the test field has been investigated by DIAMOND (1962a). The inducing field was a rectangle 33′ wide and 16.5′ high, located above the test field. The test field was 33′ wide and its height was varied from 5.5′ to 33′. The distance from the center of the test field to the inducing field was such that for a test-field height of 33′ the lower edge of the inducing field was contiguous with the upper edge of the test field. Test fields of lesser height were separated from the inducing field by varying distances. The comparison field was a 33′ × 33′ square in one experiment. In a second experiment the size of the comparison field was varied in the same way as the size of the test field. Measurements were made over a wide range of values of L_t and L_i, but no significant effect of the size of the test field upon its brightness was found under any of the conditions. When $L_i > L_t$ the decrease in test-inducing field separation that accompanied increases in the size of the test field might be expected to lead to a darkening of the test field (see next section). Perhaps such darkening occurred mainly in the portions of the test field nearest the inducing field and was disregarded by the subjects in assessing the overall brightness of the test field. That the darkening of the test field is most pronounced near the edge that is adjacent to the inducing field was noted by DIAMOND in an earlier report (DIAMOND, 1953).

Variation of test-field size over a larger range does cause some changes in brightness, at least if $L_i = 0$. WILLMER (1954) found that for test fields small enough to be considered point sources the intensity required to maintain constant brightness is inversely proportional to area (Riccò's Law). HANES (1951) who worked with circular test fields of diameters ranging from 9′ to 2°24′, found that at Log $L_t = -1$ and Log $L_t = 0$ brightness increased slightly with increasing area, whereas at Log $L_t = 2$ (mL) brightness decreased somewhat with increasing area. The measured changes in matching luminance did not exceed 0.4 log units. HANES presented the test and comparison fields simultaneously to both eyes. Similar experiments by DIAMOND (1962b) and TORII and UEMURA (1965) used the haploscopic matching method. DIAMOND found no effect of area on brightness with circular test fields of diameters ranging from 5.4′ to 54′ at luminances ranging from Log $L_t = 0.18$ to Log $L_t = 2.56$ (mL). TORII and UEMURA worked with circular test fields of diameters 36′ to 2° and luminance levels from Log $L_t = -0.5$ to Log $L_t = 1$ (mL). Over the range of sizes common to their experiment and DIAMOND's, TORII and UEMURA also found no significant effect of area on brightness; however, increases in the diameter of the field beyond 1° were associated with a progressive decrease in matching luminance at all levels of L_t. The maximum change in matching luminance was of the order of 0.4 log unit. The discrepancy between these findings and those of HANES for the lowest luminance levels has not been explained.

Except for point sources, the effects of size on brightness are in any case quite small. That they are so small seems inconsistent, at first thought, with the previously considered effects of surrounding a test field with an annulus of equal luminance. If $L_t = L_i$, the operation of surrounding the test field with an annulus is, of course, the same as the operation of increasing the size of the test field, but the effects found in the first case are much larger than those found in the second. It may be that the subject performs his task differently in the two situations. Viewed against a dark background and with rigid fixation, an evenly illuminated disk does not look uniform; most subjects say that there is a bright ring at the edge of the field and a dark blotch in the center, with a gradient of brightness in between. In experiments using the disk-annulus pattern the test field that the subject is instructed to match to the comparison field is the disk, i. e., the central region of the large field that is formed when $L_t = L_i$. Small differences in color or faint contours that can be observed even when $L_t = L_i$ probably help the subject to identify the region defined as the test field. In experiments designed to measure the effects of area on brightness, on the other hand, the test field is defined for the subject as the entire disk, whatever its size, and there is no reason why he should base his brightness assessment solely on the central region. In some further work that bears on this matter TORII and UEMURA (1965) used evenly illuminated circular fields of varying diameter on which a thin black circular line, a constant 36′ in diameter, marked off the region defined as the test field. The subjects were instructed to match the brightness of this test field to that of the comparison field. In all other respects the conditions were identical with those of their area-brightness experiment described in the previous paragraph, and the same subjects served in both experiments. The decreases in test-field brightness that resulted from increases in the total area in the experiment now under consideration were much larger than those found in the previous experiment.

Effects of the Distance between the Test and Inducing Fields

The effect an inducing field has on the brightness of a test field depends also on the distance that separates the two fields. The effects of changing this distance have been studied by LEIBOWITZ *et al.* (1953) with a stimulus pattern of type *c* (Fig. 1). The distance separating the nearest edges of the test and inducing fields was varied from 0 to 540 min of arc. The test, comparison, and inducing fields were squares, 30′ × 30′. The results (Fig. 10) show that the effect an inducing field of any particular luminance has on the brightness of the test field diminishes with increasing separation, and also that the rate at which the test field luminance must be increased to maintain constant brightness with increased inducing luminance is smaller for larger separations. The major changes occur over the range from 0′ to 30′. Measurements made at separations of 60′, 180′, 540′ did not differ consistently from those made at 30′.

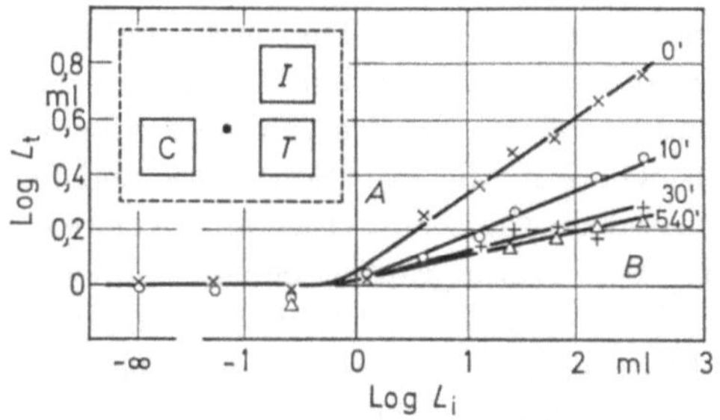

Fig. 10. The test-field luminance required for a brightness match with a comparison field of constant luminance (1 *mL*) as a function of the luminance of the inducing field. The parameters on the curves are the angular separations between the closest edges of the test and inducing fields in minutes of arc. From LEIBOWITZ *et al.* (1953)

FRY and ALPERN (1953a) conducted a similar experiment with pattern *d* (Fig. 1), varying the center to center distance between the test and inducing fields from 0.75 to 4.5 degrees. The angular size of each field was 0.5 degrees × 2.5 degrees. The results for various angular separations, θ, are shown in Fig. 11. FRY and ALPERN noted that an intense inducing field, sometimes called a "glare source," casts stray light over the whole retina; further, that in the presence of such an inducing field the retinal image of a test field is covered by a veil of stray light that should affect the brightness of the test field in the manner known from their direct measurement of the effect of veiling luminance (Fig. 4).

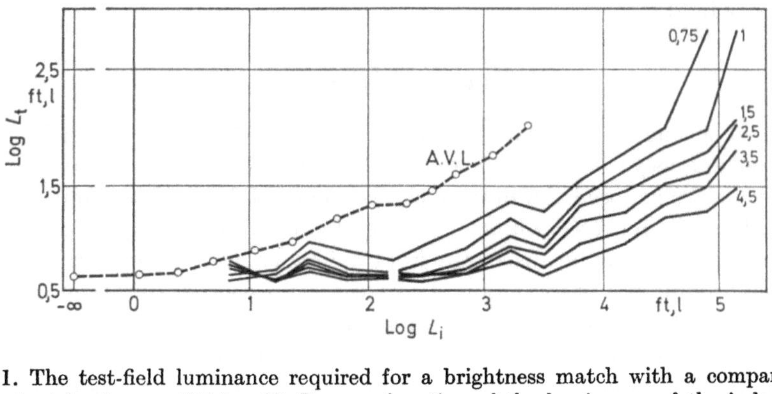

Fig. 11. The test-field luminance required for a brightness match with a comparison field of constant luminance (0.7 log *Ft. L*), as a function of the luminance of the inducing field. The curve labelled A. V. L. (artificial veiling luminance) is a replot of the data in Fig. 4. The parameters on the other curves represent the separations between centers of the test and inducing fields, in degrees. From FRY and ALPERN (1953a)

The stray light from an inducing field that falls on any point on the retina is a constant fraction of the light in the focussed image of the inducing field, and decreases with increasing distance from the inducing-field image. The data in Fig. 11 (including the direct measurements of the effect of a veiling luminance) can be made to fall along a single curve by subtracting a constant, whose value depends on θ, from all values of Log L_i. Thus the results of FRY and ALPERN are compatible with the assumption that the effects found were caused solely by stray light that surrounded the test field. That stray light can cause brightness depression is indicated also by the observation that a glare source imaged on the optic nerve head or "blind spot" of the eye produces effects similar to those of glare sources imaged elsewhere in the eye (SCHOUTEN and ORNSTEIN, 1939), as does a spot of light focussed on the sclera (FRY and ALPERN, 1953b).

The curves in Figure 10, however, cannot be superimposed on each other by moving them parallel to the x-axis. The fact that the form of these curves changes as the fields are moved farther apart probably means that the influence of the inducing field is transmitted through the nervous system. Interpreted in this way, the results of LEIBOWITZ *et al.*, indicate that the effects of the inducing field are transmitted physiologically over angular distances up to about 30′. Experiments reviewed in a previous section show that increases in the area of the inducing field have little further effect on the form of the induction curves when the distance between the test field and the farthest edge of the inducing field exceeds about 30′. The demonstration of interaction between inducing fields by ALPERN and DAVID (1959) also provides relevant information: the influence of the inducing fields that were nearer to the test field must have been transmitted physiologically because the effects of stray light are additive. The distance between the nearest edges of these fields and the test field was 1.5°, but it must be noted that the changes in the effects of the nearer fields caused by the introduction of the additional inducing fields were very small. It appears from these results that inducing fields may exert a physiologically transmitted influence upon a test field focussed on the fovea over angular distances of the order of 1.5° to 2°. More distant inducing fields probably exert their influence through stray light.

Effects of Time

In the experiments reviewed in the foregoing sections all the fields were exposed continuously. It is known that induction effects occur if the test and inducing fields are exposed simultaneously for very brief periods of time. Several early investigators reported observing them by the illumination provided by electric sparks produced by discharge from a Leyden jar. LEIBOWITZ and CHINETTE (1957) found strong induction effects with an exposure duration of 0.0002 sec, THOMAS (1963) found effects with a duration of 0.08 sec, and ALPERN (1953) with a duration of 0.005 sec. However, the influence of exposure duration on the magnitude of the induction effects has not been investigated systematically.

SCHOUTEN and ORNSTEIN (1939) studied how the magnitude of induction changes with the time elapsed since the onset of an inducing field. They used stimulus pattern *f* (Fig. 1). The semicircles were 2.9 degrees in diameter and were presented on the fovea; the distance of the inducing field or "glare source" from the test field was 10°. The eye was exposed to the glare source for varying periods of time and during the last 0.01 sec of this exposure the test and comparison fields were also presented. The experiment showed that the luminance required to match the test field drops gradually during the first 0.2 sec and thereafter remains at a nearly constant level, or even increases very slightly over larger intervals up to 10 min. Although lengthening the exposure of the inducing field beyond 0.2 sec has no effect on the brightness of a test field, the same operation has pronounced effects on subsequent recovery, measured by matching the test and comparison fields at various times after the extinction of the inducing field. According to SCHOUTEN and ORNSTEIN (1939), recovery functions measured in this fashion are very similar to those found after direct illumination of the foveal region. These findings led SCHOUTEN and ORNSTEIN to postulate two different adaptation processes, one called α adaptation responsible for the change in the brightness of a test field that occurs during the first 0.2 sec of exposure to the inducing field and then stops, the other, called β adaptation reflected in the differential effects of a much larger range of exposure durations upon the form of recovery curves.

If the inducing field is exposed very briefly, the phenomena following its extinction are more complicated than the term "recovery" implies. Measurements made by SCHOUTEN and ORNSTEIN with an inducing field exposed for 0.01 sec, followed after a variable interval by exposure of the test and comparison fields for an equal duration, show that the brightness of the test field is depressed progressively more as the interval between the exposures is increased up to 0.05 sec; thereafter the depression diminishes and is no longer noticeable after 0.15 sec. This observation has been confirmed by ALPERN (1953) and FRY and ALPERN (1953a). Inducing fields exposed after the test field has been extinguished can also have strong effects on the brightness of the test field. Such effects, often called "metacontrast," will not be considered in this chapter. (See WEISSTEIN, chapter 10, this volume.)

Brightness Phenomena in Non-Uniform Fields

As a result of inductive interaction, surfaces over which the light varies from point to point often show variations in brightness that differ greatly from the variations in luminance. These effects were discovered by MACH (1865) who investigated them with a very large number of different geometric distributions of luminance. The Mach band phenomena, and a number of recent experimental studies are treated elsewhere in this volume (see FIORENTINI, chapter 8, this volume.) Investigators have generally used patterns in which luminance changes along only one dimension; most often a rectangular field consisting of two uniform regions of different luminance with a continuous gradient of luminance in between. According to MACH, the basic phenomena observable in these simple patterns are as follows: the two uniform regions and the intervening region of graded luminance each appear relatively even in brightness, but a sharply defined bright band is seen at the position of the concave bend or flexion in the spatial luminance distribution curve, and a dark band is seen at the position of the convex flexion. Such bright and dark "Mach bands" can also be observed in distributions that have rounded corners in place of the sharp bends, but in that case the bands are less distinct.

The limiting case in which the transition between the two uniform regions is an abrupt step has been investigated by BÉKÉSY (1969) with a method of

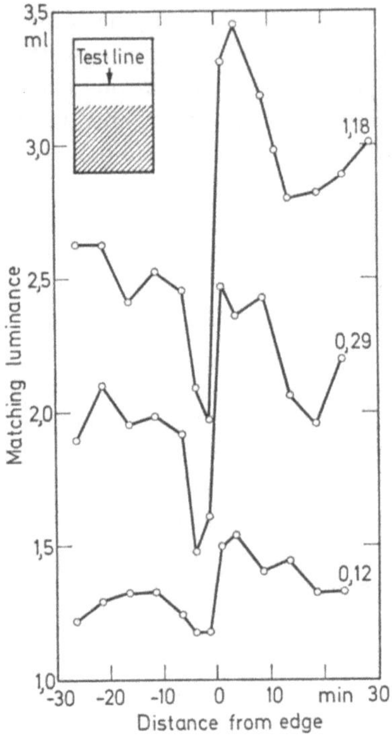

Fig. 12. Distribution of brightness across a bipartite field. The parameters on the curves represent the ratio of the luminance difference between the two sides of the field to the luminance of the dimmer side (luminance contrast). Luminance of the dimmer side: 2.72 *mL*. To avoid overlap, the middle curve has been lowered by 0.7 *mL*, and the bottom curve by 1.4 *mL*. From HEINEMANN, in preparation

flicker photometry, and by HEINEMANN with a method that has not been described in previous publications and is as follows: a thin line (width 1.3′) is placed at one of a series of positions in the bipartite field as shown in Fig. 12 (inset). The luminance of this "test line" will be called L_t, the luminance of the half-field that forms its background will be called L_i. L_t can be made less or greater than L_i, causing the line to appear, respectively, darker or brighter than its background. If $L_t = L_i$ the line simply constitutes part of the uniform field and is not visible as a line, of course. The bipartite field with the superimposed line was presented to one eye. With L_t adjusted to one of several values less or greater than L_i, the brightness of the test line was matched to that of a similar "comparison line" shown on an evenly illuminated background to the other eye. The results are used to construct a function showing the variation of matching luminance with L_t; and the match for the condition $L_t = L_i$, which represents a match made to a strip of the uniform field equal in width to the line, is found by interpolation on this function. The values of this match at various positions in the bipartite field are shown in Fig. 12 for three levels of luminance contrast. The form of the curves in Fig. 12 is quite similar to that found by Békésy (1969). In particular, the Mach band is quite broad in both experiments. For the curves in Fig. 12 the angular distance from the discontinuity in luminance to the point at which the brightness first levels off is of the order of 10′ to 15′; the comparable distance for Békésy's curve is 20′. The "width" of the Mach bands stated in this way, of course, cannot be compared with widths determined by pointer settings without knowing where along the continuous brightness curve the subject chooses to set the pointers.

The position of the peaks in Fig. 12 suggests that distinct bright and dark lines might be visible near the discontinuity, but this is contrary to reports by some investigators that such lines are not seen when the gradient is an abrupt step (cf. Ratliff, 1965, p. 60). Some qualitative observations suggest an extremely sharp peak very near the discontinuity, e. g., if a piece of white paper is viewed against a somewhat darker background its edge appears to have a bright "glow" even when a bright line of definite width is not seen. If there is such a sharp peak it would have escaped measurement in both of the experiments under consideration.

The curves in Fig. 12 show that brightness variations occur all through the physically uniform half-fields. This finding agrees with the often reported qualitative observation that evenly illuminated fields do not appear uniform in brightness. However, the problem of the appearance of uniform fields is complicated, for initial reports by subjects may be altered by special instructions and may disagree with the outcome of psychophysical measurement procedures. For example, Davidson (1966) presented subjects with a briefly exposed stripe of uniform luminance, somewhat greater than the luminance of its background. When asked, the subjects said that the stripe appeared uniform in brightness, but in a subsequent experiment in which the stripe was presented as one member of a series of patterns and the subjects were forced to say whether the center or the edge of each pattern appeared darker, the center of the physically uniform stripe was called "darker" on all trials. Under circumstances that permit the subject to control some conditions of stimulation, e. g., where and for how long to fixate, changes in conditions of stimulation may well be responsible for some of the changes in judgments. It seems certain, however, that the subjects can also use different criteria when assessing the brightness of an extended field. For example, they may base their judgment on the brightness at the edges, or at the center, or on the average brightness of the field. These considerations apply also to assessments of the brightness of non-uniform fields. A number of experiments have shown that, if the luminance of an extended field changes according to a function that does not produce Mach bands or contours, the field does not differ in appearance from a uniform one of the same average luminance (Cornsweet, 1970; Fry, 1931; Koffka, 1923).

Other experiments have shown that there are circumstances under which judgments of the relative brightness of two extended fields are governed largely by the nature of the transition or "edge" between them (O'Brien, 1958; Cornsweet, 1970). Some examples of effects observed by O'Brien with rotating disks are shown in Fig. 13, *a*—*c*. Part *a* schematizes the effects obtained with an abrupt transition between two regions; part *b* indicates that when the transition from one luminance level to another is very gradual no brightness change is seen. Part *c* is particularly noteworthy for it shows that the area to the right of the transition appears darker than that to the left, in spite of the fact that over most of its extent it has the higher luminance.

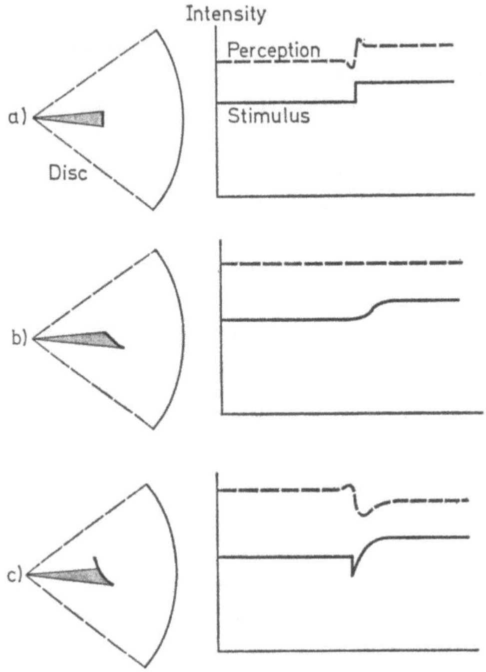

Fig. 13 a—c. Effect of the edge. (a) Sector. (b) Sector plus *S* shape. (c) Sector plus arrow shape. From O'Brien (1958)

Effects on Sensitivity to Luminance Differences

Inducing fields affect not only the brightness of nearby test fields, but also the detectability of temporal or spatial variations in their luminance. In a small foveally presented test field surrounded by an annular inducing field sensitivity to luminance changes is generally best when the luminances of the test and inducing fields are about equal. This has been reported for sensitivity evaluated by critical flicker frequency (Lythgoe and Tansley, 1929), acuity (Lythgoe, 1932), and luminance difference thresholds (Cobb, 1916; Dittmers, 1920; Heinemann, 1961). (See also Blackwell, chapter 4, this volume.)

It seems likely that, at least under the conditions of some detection experiments, when a subject reports that he notices a change in the luminance of a test field he bases this report upon a perceived change in brightness, while in others a change in the luminance of a test field may be detected by its effects on such characteristics of the field as its apparent duration, apparent time of onset, apparent size, etc. (CORNSWEET and PINSKER, 1965). When the detection is based on brightness changes it may be expected that the way inducing fields affect sensitivity to changes in the luminance of a test field will be closely related to the way they affect the amount by which the brightness of a test field changes as its luminance is changed. There are many complications, however. For example,

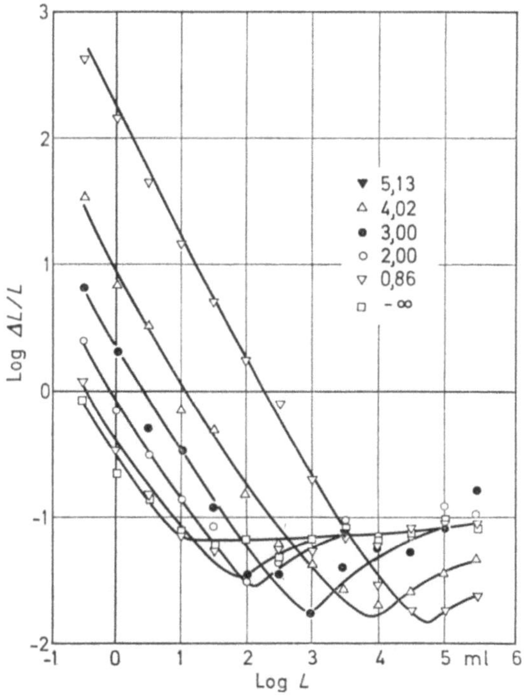

Fig. 14. The Weber-Fraction as a function of test-field luminance. The parameters are the luminances of the inducing field. From HEINEMANN (1961)

if a test field of constant luminance is presented repeatedly its brightness can be expected to vary somewhat from trial to trial, or if such a field is shown continuously, its brightness may vary from moment to moment. As emphasized in the theory of signal detection, (see NACHMIAS, chapter 3, this volume) the ability to discriminate between fields of different luminance must be affected by the extent of this variability; and inducing fields may affect this variability as well as the mean brightness.

A rather simple relationship between luminance difference sensitivity and brightness has been found in one situation by HEINEMANN (1961). The experiment was done with a stimulus pattern of type *a* (Fig. 1). The conditions differed in only minor ways from those described for an experiment with the same stimulus pattern (HEINEMANN, 1955) discussed in a previous section. In the first part of the (1961) experiment, the effect of induction on brightness was measured by haploscopic matching, with results very similar to those shown in Fig. 3. In the second part of the experiment, carried out under the same conditions as the first and with the same subjects, the increment in luminance needed to detect the presence of a small disk superimposed on the test field was measured. Each curve in Fig. 14 shows the variation in the value of the Weber fraction with changes in test field luminance, for a constant inducing luminance.

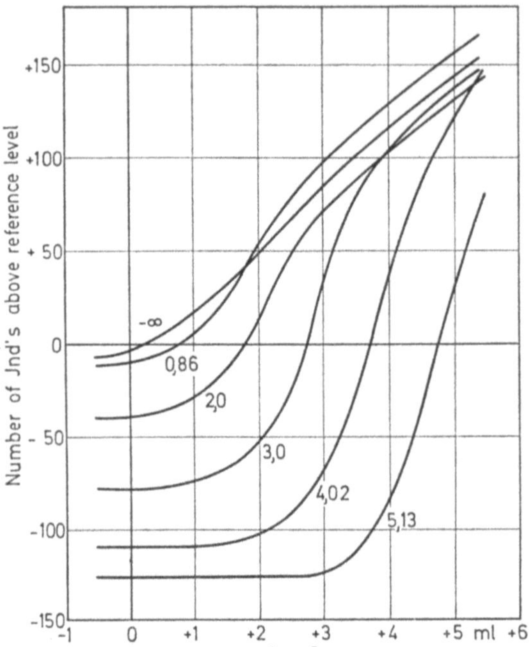

Fig. 15. Number of just-noticeable-difference steps above and below reference luminance L_r (see text). This is a replot of the data in Fig. 14. From HEINEMANN (1961)

To bring out the relation between the threshold measures and the brightness matches, the former are plotted differently in Fig. 15. As in Fig. 14, each curve represents the threshold measurements made in the presence of a constant inducing luminance. The variable on the ordinate axis is the number of just-noticeable-difference steps or "luminance steps" (cf. LE GRAND, 1957, p. 269), above or below a reference luminance, L_r, where L_r is different for each curve. The values of L_r used for each curve were read from an equal-brightness curve measured in the first part of the experiment. In other words, whatever the value of L_r, all fields of luminance L_r are of equal brightness. Fig. 15 then is so constructed that a horizontal line at an ordinate value of 0 represents a constant level of brightness. Analysis of the threshold and brightness measurements showed that horizontal lines at any other height also represent approximately constant levels of brightness, indicating that the JND axis of Fig. 15 is an ordinal scale of brightness.

Fig. 15 shows the effects of induction on brightness and on difference sensitivity in a rather fundamental way. The horizontal segment of the curves represents the lowest brightness that can be experienced with a given inducing luminance. As the inducing luminance is raised this horizontal segment is lowered and the range of brightness experience is thereby increased. One might say that induction increases the dynamic range of the visual system. On the other hand, the operating range, i. e. the range over which the different test-field luminances are associated with different brightnesses, is narrowed and shifted to higher luminances as the inducing luminance is increased. The slope of the curves at any point is $\frac{L}{\varDelta L}$, and is thus a measure of luminance difference sensitivity. If one were to assume, as FECHNER did, that all just-noticeable-difference steps are equal increments in brightness, the slope at any point of the curves would also represent the rate of change of brightness with log luminance. Since the results merely show that the JND scale is an *ordinal* scale of brightness, they justify only the weaker statement that the slopes of the various curves taken at points with equal ordinate values represent the relative rates at which the brightness of the various equally bright fields changes with log luminance. (For a fuller discussion of brightness scaling, see KRANTZ, chapter 26, this volume.)

References

ALPERN, M.: Metacontrast J. opt. Soc. Amer. **43**, 648—657 (1953).

ALPERN, M., DAVID, H.: The additivity of contrast in the human eye. J. gen. Physiol. **43**, 109—126 (1959).

BÉKÉSY, G. VON.: Brightness distribution across the Mach bands measured with flicker photometry, and the linearity of sensory nervous interaction. J. opt. Soc. Amer. **58**, 1—8 (1969).

BEZOLD, W. VON.: Die Farbenlehre. Brunswick: Westerman (1874).

BURNHAM, R. W.: Bezold's color-mixture effect. Amer. J. Psychol. **66**, 377—385 (1953).

COBB, P. W.: The effect on foveal vision of bright surroundings — IV. J. exp. Psychol. **1**, 540—566 (1916).

CORNSWEET, T. N.: Visual Perception. New York: Academic Press (1970).

— PINSKER, H. M.: Luminance discrimination of brief flashes under various conditions of adaptation. J. Physiol. (Lond.) **176**, 294—310 (1965).

DAVIDSON, M. L.: Perturbation approach to spatial brightness interaction in human vision. J. opt. Soc. Amer. **58**, 1300—1309 (1968).

DIAMOND, A. L.: Foveal simultaneous brightness contrast as a function of inducing- and test-field luminances. J. exp. Psychol. **45**, 304—314 (1953).

— Foveal simultaneous contrast as a function of inducing area. J. exp. Psychol. **50**, 144—152 (1955).

— Simultaneous contrast as a function of test-field area. J. exp. Psychol. **64**, 336—345 (1962a).

— Brightness of a field as a function of its area. J. opt. Soc. Amer. **52**, 700—706 (1962b).

— SCHEIBLE, H., SCHWARTZ, E., YOUNG, R.: A comparison of psychophysical methods in the investigation of foveal simultaneous brightness contrast. J. exp. Psychol. **50**, 171—174 (1955).

DITTMERS, F.: Über die Abhängigkeit der Unterschiedsschwelle für Helligkeiten von der antagonistischen Induktion. Z. Sinnesphysiol. **51**, 214—232 (1920).

EVANS, R. M.: An Introduction to Color. New York: Wiley 1948.

FREEMAN, R. B., JR.: Contrast interpretation of brightness constancy. Psychol. Bull. **67**, 165—187 (1967).

FRY, G. A.: The stimulus correlate of bulky color. Amer. J. Psychol. **43**, 618—622 (1931).

FRY, G. A., ALPERN, M.: The effect of a peripheral glare source upon the apparent brightness of an object. J. opt. Soc. Amer. **43**, 189—195 (1953a).

— — Effect on foveal vision produced by a spot of light on the sclera near the margin of the retina. J. opt. Soc. Amer. **43**, 187—188 (1953b).

— — The effect of veiling luminance upon the apparent brightness of an object. Amer. J. Optom. Monog. 165 (1954).

GELB, A.: Die „Farbenkonstanz" der Sehdinge. In: Handbuch der Normalen und Pathologischen Physiologie. Vol. 12/1, pp. 594—678. BETHE, A. *et al.* (Eds.). Berlin: Springer 1929.

HANES, R. M.: Suprathreshold area brightness relationships. J. opt. Soc. Amer. **41**, 28—31 (1951).

HEINEMANN, E. G.: Simultaneous brightness induction as a function of inducing- and test-field luminances. J. exp. Psychol. **50**, 89—96 (1955).

— The relation of apparent brightness to the threshold for differences in luminance. J. exp. Psychol. **61**, 389—399 (1961).

HELSON, H.: Fundamental problems in color vision. I. The principle governing changes in hue, saturation and lightness of non-selective samples in chromatic illumination. J. exp. Psychol. **23**, 439 (1938).

— Some factors and implications of color constancy. J. opt. Soc. Amer. **33**, 555—567 (1943).

— Studies of anomalous contrast and assimilation. J. opt. Soc. Amer. **53**, 179—184 (1963).

— ROHLES, F. H., JR.: A quantitative study of reversal of classical lightness contrast. Amer. J. Psychol. **72**, 530—538 (1959).

HESS, C., PRETORI, H.: Messende Untersuchungen über die Gesetzmässigkeit des simultanen Helligkeitskontrastes. Graefes Arch. Ophthal. **40**, 1—24 (1894).

HOREMAN, H. W.: Inductive brightness depression as influenced by configurational conditions. Vision Res. **3**, 121—130 (1963).

HURVICH, L. M., JAMESON, D.: The Perception of Brightness and Darkness. Boston: Allyn and Bacon 1966.

JAMESON, D., HURVICH, L. M.: Complexities of perceived brightness. Science **133**, 174—179 (1961).

— — Theory of brightness and color contrast in human vision. Vision Res. **4**, 135—154 (1964).

KOFFKA, K.: Über Feldbegrenzung und Felderfüllung. Psychol. Forsch. **4**, 176—203 (1923).

LE GRAND, Y.: Light, Colour and Vision. London: Chapman and Hall 1957.

LEIBOWITZ, H., CHINETTI, P.: Effect of reduced exposure duration on brightness constancy. J. exp. Psychol. **54**, 49—53 (1957).

— MOTE, F. A., THURLOW, W. R.: Simultaneous contrast as a function of separation between test- and inducing-fields. J. exp. Psychol. **46**, 453—456 (1953).

LYTHGOE, R. J.: The measurement of visual acuity. Med. Res. Coun. Spec. Rep. Ser. No. 173 London: H. M. Stationery Office 1932.

— TANSLEY, K.: The relation of the critical frequency of flicker to the adaptation of the eye. Proc. roy. Soc. (Lond.) B **105**, 60—92 (1929).

MACH, E.: Über die Wirkung der räumlichen Vertheilung des Lichtreizes auf die Netzhaut. S.-B. Akad. Wiss. Wien, math.-nat. Kl. **52**, II, 303—322 (1865).

MACKAVEY, W., BARTLEY, S. H., CASELLA, C.: Disinhibition in the human visual system. J. opt. Soc. Amer. **52**, 85—88 (1962).

MARSDEN, A. M.: An elemental theory of induction. Vision Res. **9**, 653—663 (1969).

O'BRIEN, V.: Contour perception, illusion and reality. J. opt. Soc. Amer. **48**, 112—119 (1958).

RATLIFF, F.: Mach Bands: Quantitative Studies on Neural Networks in the Retina. San Francisco: Holden-Day 1965.

SAUNDERS, J. E.: Adaptation, its effect on apparent brightness and contribution to the phenomenon of brightness constancy. Vision Res. **8**, 451—468 (1968).

SCHOUTEN, J. F., ORNSTEIN, L. S.: Measurements on direct and indirect adaptation by means of a binocular method. J. opt. Soc. Amer. **29**, 168—182 (1939).

STEWART, E. C.: The Gelb effect. J. exp. Psychol. **57**, 235—242 (1959).

THOMAS, J. P.: Relation of brightness contrast to inducing stimulus output. J. opt. Soc. Amer. **53**, 1033—1037 (1963).

TORII, S., UEMURA, Y.: Effects of inducing luminance and area upon the apparent brightness of test field. Jap. Psychol. Res. **7**, 86—100 (1965).

WALLACH, H.: Brightness constancy and the nature of achromatic colors. J. exp. Psychol. **38**, 310—324 (1948).

WILLMER, E. N.: Subjective brightness and size of field in the central fovea. J. Physiol. (Lond.) **123**, 315—323 (1954).

WHITTLE, P., CHALLANDS, P. D. C.: The effect of background luminance on the brightness of flashes. Vision Res. **9**, p. 1095 (1969).

WOODWORTH, R. S., SCHLOSBERG, H.: Experimental Psychology. New York: Holt 1954.

Chapter 7

Visual Acuity and Spatial Modulation Thresholds

By

G. Westheimer, Berkeley, California (USA)

With 5 Figures

Contents

Introduction

Seeing shapes and patterns is the major capacity inherent in our visual system. It depends, to be sure, on the ability to distinguish differences in light intensity and color, but this is not enough; they must be distinguished more or less simultaneously and identified as belonging to different areas of the visual field. Ultimately all this raises the question of the kind of spatial divisibility or capacity for spatial partitioning exhibited by the visual system. When taken to the limit of sensory threshold, this becomes the traditional topic of visual acuity or spatial resolving power of the visual apparatus.

In this chapter we will concern ourselves with measurements which have this in common: they identify a limit to visual sensory performance for which the threshold variable is distance in visual space. Occasionally the experimental procedure appears to be different, e.g., when a contrast threshold is determined, but the context into which such results are placed in our discussion is that of spatial rather than brightness discrimination.

A full description of the process of pattern recognition is not brought about by a study of visual acuity, though more so than by one of intensity discrimination alone. Yet thresholds are of abiding interest to physiologists and psychologists because they help to outline better than most other measurements what physical and anatomical-physiological factors underlie a given function. There is no better example of this than the case of visual acuity whose physical and anatomico-physiological bases have been relatively successfully identified.

To a vertebrate whose head and eyes are kept still, the outside world presents itself as a two-dimensional light distribution, spread over the receiving surface of the retina. Elaborate processes have evolved for retrieving information about the third spatial dimension, but each retinal image is only two dimensional. It has become convenient to express distances in terms of angles subtended by targets at the eye, rather than the distances along the retina, but this is not an important distinction because there is a unique relationship between the two.

The most appropriate reference point for object-sided angles is the center of the entrance pupil of the eye, for then it is immaterial whether the retinal image is in focus or not. In the human eye, the center of the entrance pupil is 3 mm behind the cornea. If an object subtends an angle θ at the center of the entrance pupil, its image will cover a linear distance on the retina given by

$$y = 20.3 \tan (0.82\,\theta)\ \text{mm}. \tag{1}$$

This equation is based on the assumption that in a typical emmetropic human eye the exit pupil is 20.3 mm in front of the retina, and that the ratio of the angle subtended by the image at the exit pupil to that subtended by the object at the entrance pupil is 0.82. Typically, a 1 min angle in object space becomes 4.7 μ on the retina. The relationship between object space and retinal distances needs, however, to be computed individually for each animal.

Behaviorally, the concept of visual acuity and its measurement is uncomplicated. Involved are a variable, typically distance in visual space (e.g. separation of two points, thickness of line, etc.), the subject's criterion (one point or two, seen or not seen), and the optimization of the experimental conditions. More than almost any other sensory threshold, visual acuity has been subjected to variation of all manners of experimental variables. Because a large number of these do, in fact, influence visual acuity, the elimination of interacting effects from unwanted factors is a mandatory prerequisite to a study relating visual acuity to changes in a given variable.

The itemization of the factors known to influence visual acuity is best left till later in this chapter because it will show that many of the effects fall readily into place once the optical, structural and functional bases of visual resolving power have been identified.

Optical Basis of Visual Resolving Power

In the limit no eye can do better than its optics. Neural processes of "image sharpening" can conceivably operate on the available information in the retinal image, but they cannot create information where the image does not contain any. As far as spatial vision is concerned, the optical apparatus of the eye is a linear filtering system. It transforms each luminous point in object space into a retinal light distribution called point-spread function. The latter depends on many factors and has been determined with some success in the human eye; but its virtue in the present discussion is that it permits the description of the image-sided light distribution for any kind of object, and *a fortiori*, the kind of objects that commonly constitute targets for visual acuity measurements. Each point on the object gives rise to this characteristic spread pattern on the retina, and the intensity contributions from all object points sum at each retinal point. The process of summing distance-weighted contributions from all object points into an image intensity configuration is called *convolution*. It is most easily illustrated for the classical case where the object consists of two stars. The image then consists of two point-spread patterns whose ordinates would be summed to show the energy delivered to each receptor. As the two object points are approached, more and more overlapping occurs of the two image spread patterns (Fig. 1). When the separation has been reduced to a

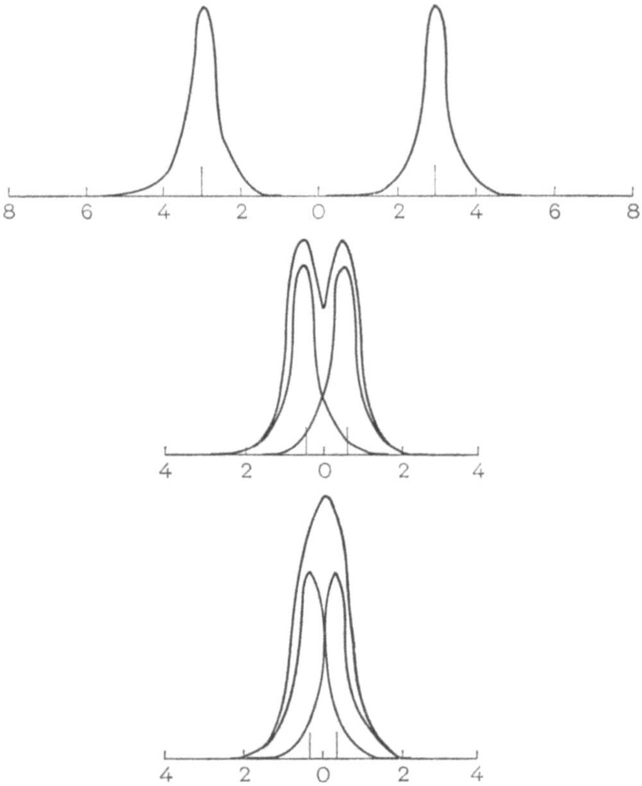

Fig. 1. Light spread in the images of two stars and summed intensity distribution as the two stars approach each other. The point-spread function used in this illustration is that from the most recent objective determination (GUBISCH, 1967) for a human eye in best focus with a 3 mm pupil diameter and white light. Scale is in minutes of arc, and cone diameter in center of fovea is about 1/2 min of arc

critical value, the two distributions have overlapped so thoroughly that their sum reveals only a single peak. When two stars are separated by a distance of the order of the size of their point-spread function, the resulting image contains no double hump. Traditionally, this constitutes the optical limitation of visual resolution. Superimposed on it are the anatomical and functional limitations to visual resolution, and the final decision is reached by the subject on the basis of prior probabilities and interacting sensory and perceptual factors.

The process of convolution illustrated in Fig. 1 is usually quite difficult to carry out when the target is complex, say, a letter of the alphabet. In their simplest form, however, visual acuity tests such as Snellen letters approach two-point discrimination, as for example in the discrimination between the letters *F* and *P*, or *C* and *O*. Black targets against a uniform bright background produce image-sided light distributions that are the complements of those of bright targets against black backgrounds. Thus the shape of the light-spread in the image of a black spot presented against a uniform bright background is the complement of the point-spread function. For the purpose of these considerations, light-spread functions must not be normalized for height at maximum, but should be normalized for

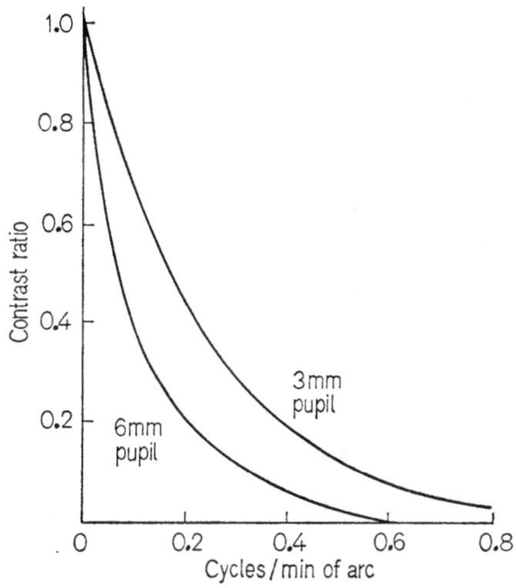

Fig. 2. Modulation transfer function of the optical system of the human eye in best focus for a 3 mm pupil (Campbell and Gubisch, 1966) and for a 6 mm pupil (Westheimer, 1963) based on objective measurements of light spread in ophthalmoscopic images

volume under the surface, since the total light reaching the retina is a constant which happens to be distributed according to the image defects of the system. In the same way, there is a given total light deficit when a small opaque disk that obscures a region of a uniform bright surface is imaged, but this light deficit is spread over an image region larger than the target with a result that not all image portions are totally devoid of light. In the extreme case of a wide point-spread function and a very small black point target, the image is merely a dimple in the expanse of a bright image field, and the detection problem is that of a small light decrement. This was shown by Hecht and Mintz in 1939, studying the visibility of a thin line, which can be seen when subtending an angle less than one second of arc.

A great deal of attention has recently been given to another way of specifying image/object relationships in optical systems, such as the eye. It is based on the proposition, which is always valid, that an object that is a sinusoidal grating, i.e., a grating with luminance variations that are sinusoidal with distance at right angles to the length of the grating lines, is imaged also as a sinusoidal grating, albeit with reduced contrast. This forms the basis for the description of optical imagery in terms of Fourier theory. The specification of the imaging characteristics of the eye, then, is in the graph showing the demodulation of sine wave gratings as a function of their spatial frequency, the so-called modulation transfer function. It contains the same information as the line-spread function, and these two functions are, in fact, Fourier transforms. It is common to give the modulation transfer function of an instrument like the eye (Fig. 2); it permits description in terms of a single parameter — the demodulation — of the image characteristics if the target is a sinusoidal grating. In a reasonably symmetrical optical system, there are no important phase shifts of the output sinusoids and only the amplitude need be considered. This is a great simplification over the complex statement of the shape of a point-spread function or the shape of the light-spread in a letter *C* which can be just distinguished from an *O*. The disadvantage of a sinusoidal grating is, however, that it says something about the properties of a large (theoretically an infinite) receiving surface, whereas the recognition of a break in a letter *O* refers specifically to a small and defined retinal region. This distinction is not confined to the topic of visual resolution; it is of wide significance in the physical sciences (BRILLOUIN, 1962) and also recently to those who regard the apparent distributedness of brain function as evidence for a special kind of organization underlying higher nervous processes.

Anatomical Factors in Visual Resolution

An inescapable fact is that the visual process is funnelled through individual receptors. Although a great deal can be said about the interaction of light from various object points at the site of the receptor, and the interaction of the output of the single receptors, there is general agreement that all receptive processes occurring in a given receptor are no longer divisible spatially. The analogy with fiber optics is, therefore, appropriate because there, too, we have a channelling into anatomically segregated pathways. Certain limitations to resolution are imposed through this receptor mosaic. Anatomical studies of receptor size, and resolution experiments bypassing the eye's optics by using interference fringes, both indicate that the human resolution at the fovea is essentially limited by the size of the receptors. As it happens, the optical performance of the eye is matched to this performance limit; but if it is artificially improved by an interference fringe method, the resolution limit is not concomitantly improved (LEGRAND, 1936; WESTHEIMER, 1959, 1960; ARNULF and DUPUY, 1960; CAMPBELL and GREEN, 1965). Other experiments, such as vernier acuity, show that neural processing of the output of receptors can sometimes help to retrieve some of the spatial information that is lost by the partitioning of the receptive layer into discrete cells.

The facts that the neural image can have a finer grain than the receptors, and that improving optical performance beyond that usually available in an eye does not improve visual resolution, suggest that at the fovea, the receptor grain sets the limit and that the eye's optics have evolved as far as necessary to match the receptor size. There are, however, a number of interacting factors which need attention simultaneously if the optics and receptor grain are to match and work optimally. Thus, if it were possible to have individually connected receptors half the cross-sectional diameter of those in the human fovea, and the axial eye length were retained, the eye's optics would have to be ideal (i.e., purely diffraction limited) not up to its present 2 mm pupil diameter, but up to a 4 mm pupil diameter. However, with such a change, there would be associated a greater susceptibility to chromatic aberration (correctable by achromatizing the eye's optics) and a smaller depth of focus (correctable by a better accommodative response). It is difficult to say what evolution could do to these factors, but it would not be surprising if receptor cell size is the real bottleneck.

The anatomical factors influencing visual acuity are, of course, not limited to the receptor size. Witness to this is the almost equal size and packing of cones in the fovea and of rods in the most densely populated periphery. Yet the resolution in these regions is vastly different (Fig. 3). The important difference here is the neural connectivity of the structures. Overall, there is a 150—200 fold reduction going from retinal receptors to optic nerve fibers. However, the foveal cones are matched by equal numbers of bipolar and ganglion cells and thus project individually to higher centers, whereas many peripheral receptors (up to several thousand) converge on each ganglion cell. The evidence for the convergence comes not only from anatomy but also from electrophysiology and psychophysics, where the concept of summation pool has been widely useful. Convergence need not merely be summation of similar signals from many receptors, but inhibitory signals

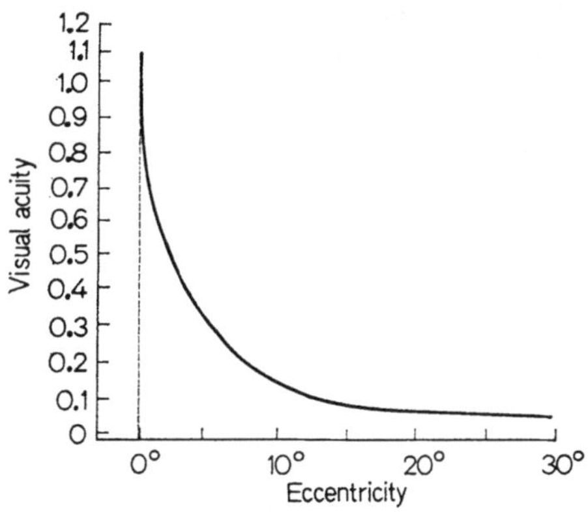

Fig. 3. Visual acuity measured along the horizontal meridian of the temporal retina at high luminance (from MANDELBAUM and SLOAN, 1947). Abscissa: eccentricity from fovea in degrees; ordinates: visual acuity normalized so that a minimum angle of resolution of 1 min of arc becomes unity

from surrounding areas are also fed in, again at a retinal level, probably at the horizontal cell layer. The result is that optic nerve fibers, while each clearly associated with a specific retinal region, conduct a complex signal made up of excitatory and inhibitory contributions from concentrically arranged summation pools. Thus the output of optic nerve fibers may be enhanced by a brightness difference in the corresponding receptive fields. One can readily conceive of a receptive system in which optic nerve fibers carry signals that may be regarded specifically as visual acuity information. Thus cells with of exquisitely balanced center-surround organized receptive fields would not change their output at all if a generalized lowering or raising of the illumination occurred, but would signal only *local* variation. Such a system would need considerable sophistication to act in a capacity other than a simple discontinuity detector without the intervention of a central processor. Complex detection systems, such as for target movement, exist in the retina in several animals, but resolution seems something that is universally reserved for higher levels of visual signal processing. It requires the simultaneous comparison of the incoming information from more than one channel. For example, at threshold visibility of a black wire against a uniform sky, a single row of receptive fields is stimulated at least a j.n.d. different from the adjacent ones. The detection implies a comparison between the three adjacent rows and the recognition that the middle one is at a different level of stimulation. There is no evidence that this comparison is made anywhere but centrally.

Physiological Considerations

The example just cited brings out the major functional aspects of visual acuity. For a spatial difference discrimination to be made, at least one channel in the afferent pathway has to be differentially stimulated. No such signal will be produced so long as the signal for the difference is below threshold. Thus even if the optical (image forming) and structural limitations to visual resolution are exceeded, so long as the stimulus does not reach, say, brightness or color discriminability it cannot yield a spatially differentiated sensation. This is the basis for the relative

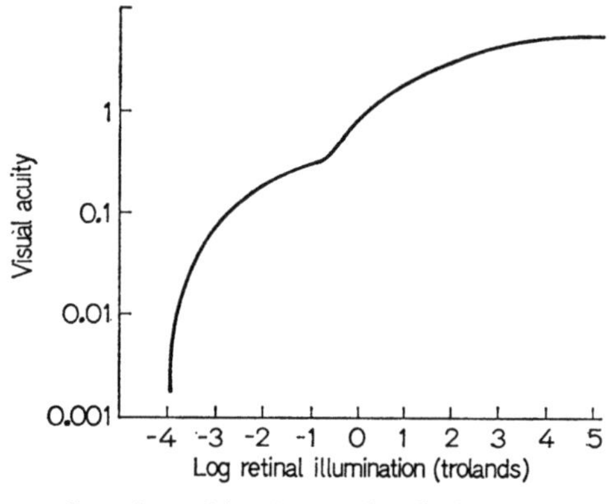

Fig. 4. Visual acuity as a function of luminance level (from PIRENNE, 1962). Rod and cone portion of the curve are clearly separate

independence of visual acuity on illumination: beyond a certain luminance level, the $\Delta I/I$ fraction remains constant and along with it the visual acuity (Fig. 4). Similarly, chromatic visual acuity depends on $\Delta\lambda$ thresholds. Temporal summation effects, including the Bunsen-Roscoe-Bloch law and the critical duration, are accurately reflected in visual acuity determinations, (GRAHAM and COOK, 1937; NIVEN and BROWN, 1944; KAHNEMAN, 1966) as are pre-adaptation (BROWN, 1954), dark adaptation (BROWN *et al.*, 1953) and spectral luminosity (BROWN *et al.*, 1960). In each of these cases, known retinal physiological effects provide a perfectly acceptable interpretation for the change in visual resolution with the variable.

Central Factors

It would be naive to assume that, so long as a spatially discriminable signal leaves the retina, a subject can immediately and reliably report it. Visual resolution measurement is a reductionist situation in which space perception has been pushed to the limit of a binary decision as to the presence or absence of a spatial difference. Even so, a great deal of central processing takes place, which, however, can be identified as such because of our detailed knowledge of the peripheral factors involved (*vide supra*). The following are some examples of visual resolution phenomena where there is good reason to believe that the mode of operation of some central factors are revealed.

It has long been known that there are meridional differences in visual acuity. Horizontal and vertical gratings are resolved better than oblique ones and this difference is not dependent on eye movements (NACHMIAS, 1960) exposure duration (HIGGINS and STULTZ, 1948, 1950) or illumination (LEIBOWITZ, 1953). Interference fringe experiments have shown that this difference is not caused by optical factors in the eye (MITCHELL *et al.*, 1967; CAMPBELL *et al.*, 1966). The anatomical lay-out of receptors, even if it did demonstrate a geometrical mosaic, would be expected to show meridional variations in 60° modules, not 90° modules, and the receptive fields of retinal neurons seem essentially circular. It may, therefore, be concluded that the better resolution for grating targets with horizontal and vertical lines is predicated upon a specialized connectivity in the higher visual pathways, a view that is borne out by more sophisticated perception experiments (ANDREWS, 1967).

Because there has never been any suggestion that a single receptor is anything but an indivisible entity, at least as far as its spatial value is concerned, the numerous visual tasks indicating a performance level much better than the width of a single receptor are of interest in that they can be regarded as manifestations of central processing. We have already alluded to one such threshold, the detection of a single line seen against a uniform background, which is of the order of a fraction of a second of arc. The fact that the threshold is so low is, of course, no real problem because the line-spread function is still of the order of magnitude of a single receptor, but that a straight rather than an irregular line is seen, must be regarded as significant, as was pointed out by HERING (1899).

There are, however, other thresholds which measure only a fraction of the diameter of a mosaic element and which clearly need a sophisticated central mechanism to achieve such a level of performance. VOLKMANN (1863) found that two distances of a few minutes of arc can be recognized as being unequal when they differed by as little as 12.4 seconds of arc. WÜLFING (1892) demonstrated that vernier acuity, i.e., the recognition of lateral displacement of two abutting line segments, is only about 10 seconds of arc. This has been repeatedly verified. Moreover, it has even been shown that the alignment of just three dots (not two lines) can be done with about the same precision (LUDVIGH, 1953). There is thus no doubt that there are spatial thresholds that are better than the size of the elements of the retinal mosaic. They imply that a central process is at work which recognizes the mean spatial value of the output of retinal mosaic elements to an accuracy of an order of magnitude better than the size of these elements. For a while it was thought that this kind of performance attended only line targets and that some kind of averaging of local sign along the length of a line accounted for the small threshold values. But the three dot experiment shows that lines are not the necessary prerequisite. When it is considered that a point of light in object space produces output graded with distance in dozens of receptors, the kind of neural connectivity necessary for this performance becomes recognizable. The situation is, unfortunately, not helped by the electrophysiological findings that the primary cortical projection system seems funnelled, even in the unanesthetized primate, through line units.

A further manifestation of higher level processing is seen in the effect of exposure duration on visual acuity. For exposures below the critical duration, the Bunsen-Roscoe-Bloch law holds. For slightly longer exposures there is the phenomenon of brightness enhancement or Broca-Sulzer effect, which may produce some non-monotonic behavior of threshold-duration behavior (BARTLEY *et al.*, 1963), but which nevertheless may fit into the known pattern of retinal physiology. Visual acuity, however, continues to improve for exposures lasting up to 2 seconds and perhaps even more. The minimum angle of resolution is lowered considerably as the exposure is increased from 100 to 800 msec, and this is not dependent on luminance (WESTHEIMER and BARON, unpublished). It is true that image movements occur when the exposure is as long as this, unless special precautions are taken to stabilize the retinal image, but this phenomenon is more in the nature of multiple "looks," something suggested by HECHT'S group years ago (LAMAR *et al.*, 1948), but never followed up. The kind of central processing that underlies this improvement with exposure duration has yet to be explored. It is likely that a similar phenomenon occurs when a target allows multiple decisions in space, such as gratings where recognition of spatial discontinuity can be made simultaneously at many locations.

Dynamic Visual Acuity

There is a suggestion of long standing that good visual acuity requires target movement across the retina (MARSHALL and TALBOT, 1942). The view was reinforced on the one hand by the discovery of what amounts to A.C. coupling of retinal neurons (HARTLINE, 1938), and on the other hand by the observations of continuous small movements of the eyeball even during "steady" fixation (DITCHBURN and GINSBORG, 1952; see also ALPERN, chapter 12, this volume). When it was found that stabilized retinal images fade (RIGGS *et al.*, 1953), this seemed a convincing case, except that the fading takes several seconds to be consummated, a period which allows ample time for the best visual resolution to be achieved. Many studies have now made it quite clear that image motion is not a prerequisite to good acuity (RATLIFF, 1952; KEESEY, 1960). Target motion at rates faster than eye-tracking can compensate for, produces a fall in resolution (LUDVIGH and MILLER, 1958). Some studies of visual resolution for moving targets, however, indicate a resistance of the resolution process to image motion that appears to need reconciliation with the simplistic notion of "one row of differentially stimulated receptors" developed earlier in this chapter.

Other Factors

Because visual acuity has been easily measureable for many years, an enormous literature has grown in which almost every conceivable variable has been tested. Much information can be found in more detailed reviews (DUKE-ELDER, 1942; PIRENNE, 1962; RIGGS, 1965; WESTHEIMER, 1965a; LIT, 1968) or appears in connection with studies of the variables involved. In most instances, the effect is easily reconciled with the general approach followed herein. To cite just two examples: refractive errors and pupil size affect visual acuity primarily through their influence on the optical image, and rod monochromats or normal subjects in low illumination demonstrate only scotopic acuity effects.

Occasionally, visual acuity measurements have been a valuable tool in the analysis of retinal function. An example of this is the demonstration of the separateness of color systems (STILES, 1949).

Modulation or Contrast Thresholds

The main emphasis has so far been on the standard techniques of visual acuity measurements. A given target configuration is spatially changed until a threshold is reached: two point targets are separated until they appear double (*minimum separabile*), a single black line is made wider until it becomes visible against a uniform background (*minimum visibile*) or two abutting line segments are shifted laterally until misalignment is recognized (*vernier acuity*). The determinations can be made, of course, by more elaborate procedures than the psychophysical method of adjustment implied in this description, and in fact the constant stimulus technique with forced guessing is ideally suited in that it yields a frequency-of-seeing curve. Moreover, in vernier acuity measurements the slope of the frequency-of-seeing curve is the parameter of choice.

That there is another, perhaps even better, way of looking at the problem is illustrated in Fig. 1. In general (although this is minimally so for vernier adjustments) the spatial manipulation required to bring the configuration to a criterion response confounds changes in the contrast and space parameters. For example, bringing two points together does not only vary the separation of the two peaks of the summed light distribution, it also varies the absolute luminance of the trough and the contrast ratio of the peaks to the trough. This situation is clearly the case also when a grating is made progressively finer in spatial frequency. In fact, the changes in contrast in the images of sine wave grating objects is one of the ways of specifying the quality of optical instruments. The contrast gets smaller and eventually reaches zero as the spatial frequency increases.

There is one experiment which clearly keeps contrast and spatial separation disconnected. It is the interference fringe method of bypassing the eye's optics and creating a fringe system on the retina with virtually 100% contrast.

The other approach is to keep the spatial pattern constant and vary just the contrast. This is in fact what is done when a line is made wider until it reaches visibility. Providing the line remains narrow compared with the eye's line-spread function, i.e., less than 1 min of arc in width, its retinal image will merely change in the scale of the ordinate and not in shape as the line width is increased.

Although there are some early experiments on the threshold contrast of small targets, the whole approach of varying contrast rather than spatial separation to reach threshold has only recently come into vogue. It had its major impetus from the prominent place that linear systems theory has found in modern technology. One of the standard methods in linear systems analysis is to subject the system to a sinusoidal input and record the output amplitude and phase as the frequency is varied. This gives the frequency response which can be graphed in various ways, of which the Bode plot (amplitude versus frequency, and phase versus frequency, both on rectilinear coordinates), is the most popular. When such analysis is restricted to linear systems, or at least to operating ranges over which the system is linear, it completely characterizes the operation of the system under investigation. This is so because, according to Fourier theory, all inputs are describable as sums of sine waves. The fate of each of the sinusoidal components of the input is specified in the Bode plot and this allows the prediction of the output corresponding to any input by Fourier synthesis of the amplitude and phase-weighted input sine-wave components.

Apart from the fact that a Bode plot provides a good visualization of the performance of a system, there is virtue in this approach in that it allows for easy specification of the total performance of cascaded systems, where the ordinates of the Bode amplitude plots of all the component systems need merely be multiplied.

It is important to be reminded of what is demanded of a system for the above technique to be rigorously applicable. The system needs to be linear, i.e., it must not suffer from such effects as saturation, intermodulation, etc. In the space domain, i.e., where the input is periodically varying with distance rather than with the more usual time, the concept of homogeneity becomes important in that it is necessary for the system's characteristics to be essentially invariant with location.

The advent of electro-optical devices, notably television systems, has made the application of spatial linear-systems analysis a matter of practical necessity and it has found excellent application particularly in instances where there are cascaded linear systems, as for example cameras, electro-optical transducers, amplifiers, etc. It was, therefore, inevitable that spatial Fourier analysis of the human visual system should be attempted, at about the same time as a similar analysis was carried out in the time domain (DELANGE, 1954; see KELLY, chapter 11, this volume).

The first of these spatial sine-wave experiments, and essentially the prototype of all subsequent ones, was published by SCHADE (1956). SCHADE created a grating pattern varying sinusoidally with distance on a television screen. He kept the spatial frequency constant and varied the modulation, i.e., he kept the average screen brightness constant and varied the height of the peaks and depth of the troughs which remained symmetrical about the mean screen brightness. Defining the modulation by the ratio

$$m = \frac{I_{\max} - I_{\min}}{I_{\max} + I_{\min}} \tag{2}$$

he determined the threshold modulation ratio for a variety of spatial frequencies of the pattern. By plotting the reciprocal of the threshold modulation ratio as a function of spatial frequency, one obtains a graph which is in many respects similar to a Bode plot. But it must be remembered that the modulation sensitivity function of the human visual system was obtained in the opposite way from the Bode plot of a physical system. In the latter, one keeps the input amplitude constant and measures output amplitude; in the former the input amplitude is varied until a subjective criterion — threshold visibility of the grating pattern — is reached. The linking hypothesis between the two methods is that threshold response corresponds to a constant output, and it would, of course, be permissible in a linear system to perform a Bode plot analysis by varying input amplitude for constant output and plotting the reciprocal of input amplitude versus frequency.

Two aspects of SCHADE's experimental results are interesting. The first relates to the fall-off of modulation sensitivity for high spatial frequencies. This is, of course, what could be expected from a knowledge of the eye's performance as an optical system, but what of the further stages of the visual process, e.g., receptor spacing, etc.? By using interference fringes I was able to demonstrate that a decrease down to zero of the threshold modulation occurs even if the eye's optics are bypassed (WESTHEIMER, 1960). The experiments have since been replicated (CAMPBELL and GREEN, 1965) and show that, as far as modulation response in the high spatial frequency range is concerned, the eye's optics and the rest of the visual system give somewhat parallel curves. There would, of course, have been no evolutionary advantage in a visual response in a spatial frequency range for which the retinal image has no information content. (Unlike electrical systems, optical systems have a cut-off spatial frequency at and beyond which the frequency response is zero.) The eye's optics and the rest of the visual system act, in systems theory parlance, as high-cut filters, meaning to say, they attenuate responses to high spatial frequencies.

The other interesting facet of SCHADE's curves was a response attenuation also at *low* spatial frequencies. This cannot be assigned to any optical effects in the eye, or, for that matter, to receptor grain, and must represent the manifestation of a

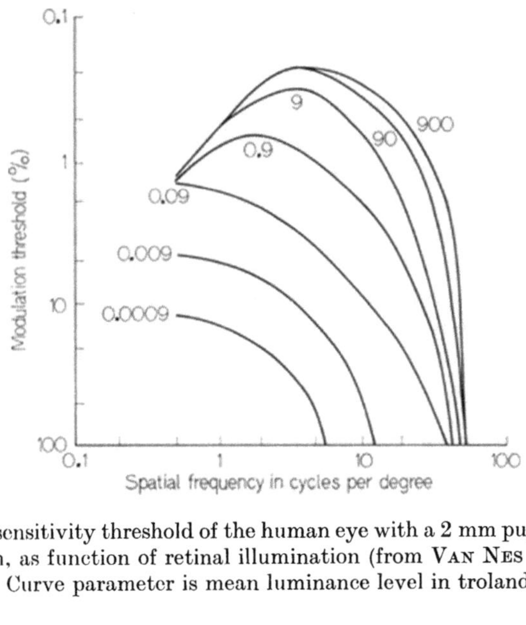

Fig. 5. Modulation sensitivity threshold of the human eye with a 2 mm pupil in monochromatic light of $\lambda = 525$ nm, as function of retinal illumination (from VAN NES and BOUMAN, 1967). Curve parameter is mean luminance level in trolands

property of visual processing. The total effect of the two kinds of filtering, high and low frequency, is to give the spatial frequency response of the eye the appearance of a band-pass filter, tuned to a center frequency of about 5 cycles/degree.

There have been many replications of the modulation threshold curves of the human visual system and several interesting parameters have been tested. For example, the curves are essentially unchanged by image stabilization (GILBERT and FENDER, 1969) which can, incidentally, be regarded as further evidence that the time-varying component of the visual receptor output, normally present because of small eye movements, does not improve visual acuity.

The effect of adaptation state on the shape of the modulation sensitivity curve was investigated in detail by ROBSON and CAMPBELL (1965), PATEL (1966), VAN NES and BOUMAN (1967), and DAITCH and GREEN (1969). They all showed that the low frequency attenuation does not occur at low luminance levels (Fig. 5). There the amount of modulation required for threshold is higher, i.e., the sensitivity lower, (as would be expected from all the other $\Delta I/I$ data; see BLACKWELL, chapter 4, this volume), but the modulation threshold curves stay flat down to at least 0.5 cycles/degree.

The influence of exposure duration on the modulation sensitivity function is another parameter that has been investigated. The two most thorough studies (SCHOBER and HILZ, 1965; NACHMIAS, 1967) were carried out with square-wave gratings, but there is no reason to suspect that the results would have been different with sinusoidal gratings. As the exposure duration is reduced to a few milliseconds, the low frequency attenuation disappears. But since all modulation thresholds are higher when the exposure is short it is not immediately apparent that the effects of mere shortage of light have been ruled out.

Of the two phases of the modulation threshold curve, the high and the low frequency attenuation, the former is the easier to relate to other findings of visual acuity. In fact, in the limit of 100% object modulation, the experiments are indistinguishable from ordinary grating acuity measurements and everything that has been said about the subject earlier in this chapter applies directly. Thus optical and anatomical limitations are of consequence at the high end of the spatial spectrum. The origin of the low frequency attenuation is less clear.

Depending on which way one wants to look at the shape of the modulation sensitivity curve, one can either say it shows a reduction of sensitivity as the D.C. end of the curve is approached, or that there is an enhanced sensitivity in a middle band of the spatial spectrum. The most likely explanation is the center-surround organization of retinal receptive fields which demonstrate a surround zone responding in the opposite way to that in the center. When one views gratings through such "Mexican hat" receptive fields, modulation sensitivity curves result that have the shapes illustrated. This has been clearly established through Fourier calculations by PATEL (1966). The size of the central excitatory zone, which would be of the order of 3 min of arc in diameter, fits in acceptably with the size obtained by direct measurement in the human fovea (WESTHEIMER, 1967). The effects of reduced light and exposure durations, which tend to eliminate the low-frequency attenuation, have also been demonstrated directly to reduce, or even eliminate, the contribution to receptive fields of inhibiting surround zones, both electrophysiologically in cat ganglion calls (BARLOW *et al.*, 1957) and psychophysically in the human rod

(Westheimer, 1965b) and cone systems (Westheimer, 1967). The simple interpretation of the low-frequency attenuation of the modulation sensitivity curve as being caused by lateral inhibition at the retinal level, is, however, not compatible with all observations.

Modulation sensitivity experiments are in effect increment-threshold experiments (see Enoch, chapter 21, this volume), albeit with extended and sophisticated targets. Comparable increment-threshold experiments with circular disk targets against uniform backgrounds have never demonstrated any effects that can be ascribed to the influence of inhibitory surrounds (Brindley, 1970). These should, in the threshold situation, tend to counteract the excitatory effect of light on the center and hence drive the threshold upward as target diameter is increased. Instead, the threshold luminance either remains unaffected by increases in target area beyond the range of application of Ricco's law, or in fact shows a small further reduction. If the modulation threshold curves derive their characteristic shape from surround inhibition at the retina, reconciliation with the universally accepted area-luminance curves is necessary.

On the whole, however, extrapolation from one threshold situation to a closely related one is a fairly successful procedure. This applies both to point-by-point analysis where the so-called excitation-contribution functions can be used (Graham *et al.*, 1939; Blackwell, 1963; and Blackwell, chapter 4, this volume) and to the sinusoidal kind of analysis where, for example, the threshold visibility of gratings of a variety of wave shapes (Campbell, 1965) can be predicted from the threshold visibility of their harmonic components.

Aside from its undoubted utility in describing the performance of optical instruments, is there a particular merit in the modulation sensitivity approach to the overall visual system? The answer to this question depends on whether the chosen signal is the appropriate one to expose the underlying mechanism of spatial discrimination. At the retinal level, signal processing is done within small areas. The light stimulus is funnelled through single receptors, subjected to a compressive transformation with light intensity and a differencing operation with respect to neighboring regions and other wavelength bands. Receptor population and neural connectivity vary with retinal location. Each area contains a mixture of detecting units with somewhat different receptive properties but whose receptive fields overlap and interlace. Thus the threshold in one situation may be given by a unit with a large receptive field and in another, by one with a smaller receptive field: the psychophysically determined function would then be the envelope of all the responsive units since the activation of any unit would yield a threshold sensation.

For these reasons it seems most helpful to have the primary analysis of spatial visual function carried out by means of localized rather than extended testing signals. For example, the acknowledged heterogeneity of retinal structure in the vicinity of the fovea makes the response to centrally fixated sinusoidal targets of period of 1/2 degree or more difficult to interpret. Just as a clear knowledge of retinal light distribution allows more definitive conclusions to be drawn about neural interaction at the retina, so a detailed knowledge of localized retinal spatial performance allows a less ambiguous specification of the properties of higher spatial analyzers.

Although the evidence at the retinal level all points the other way, and though the neural organization at the next two stages, the geniculate and the visual cortex, seems at present no more promising, there seems nevertheless to be an enhanced sensitivity to gratings somewhere at a higher level in the visual system (CAMPBELL and KULIKOWSKI, 1966; GILINSKY, 1968). Thus the visibility of gratings can be changed by masking (PANTLE and SEKULAR, 1968) or interocular transfer (GILINSKY and DOHERTY, 1969) and it can be made subject to fatigue (BLAKEMORE and CAMPBELL, 1969) or figural after-effects (BLAKEMORE and SUTTON, 1969). The exceedingly low modulation threshold in the best spatial region, of the order of 0.2 % (VAN NES, 1968), attests to a mechanism that is exquisitely attuned to such stimuli. Whether this is merely a question of probability summation of threshold being reached when many small regions are being stimulated near a spatial difference threshold, or whether we are here witnessing the operation of a mechanism with the specific properties of a spatial filter tuned to a frequency band, remains yet to be unequivocally demonstrated.

The extrapolation from threshold phenomena to suprathreshold phenomena is another step that needs support by more than the information now available. By definition, threshold phenomena concern themselves with the minimum energy exchange for any kind of response. The brightness distribution in patterns of suprathreshold luminance involves a great many additional factors, amongst which the transformations in the brightness domain (where there are logarithmic, hyperbolic tangential, and saturation nonlinearities) are only some. Changes and non-additive properties of excitatory and inhibitory spatial interaction, not always apparent for threshold phenomena, make temselves felt, so that results obtained depend strongly on the way a stimulus situation is approached. It is important to keep this in mind in connection with the modulation sensitivity functions, which are sometimes regarded as modulation transfer functions with the implied acceptance of the proposition that Fourier synthesis is a permissible operation.

Still, there are some similarities between the modulation sensitivity for threshold sinusoids and the apparent brightness contrasts in highly modulated sinusoidal gratings. Brightness matches were obtained between the brightest and dimmest parts of the sinusoidal patterns and contiguously placed lines (DEPALMA and LOWRY, 1962), or contiguous uniform fields on either side of the gratings (BRYNGDAHL, 1964, 1966). These techniques give a measure of the apparent contrast of the suprathreshold gratings, using Eq. (2) and substituting values of the luminance of the matching patches. Another experiment involved matches of contrast for sinusoidal gratings of adjacent spatial frequencies, where the modulation of one member of the pair was varied until they appeared equal in contrast (DAVIDSON, 1968). In all cases, a function of apparent contrast versus spatial frequency was obtained that resembles the modulation threshold curve. There are rather severe numerical discrepancies, but the overall shapes of threshold and suprathreshold curves are remarkably alike. This suggests that as a descriptive tool, the modulation sensitivity approach has a versatility that could only have been hoped for by those who took over the pleasing mathematical representation of Fourier analysis and synthesis from systems theory to visual physiology.

Acknowledgement. Preparation of this chapter was aided by grant EY 00220 from the National Eye Institute, U.S. Public Health Service.

References

ARNULF, A., DUPUY, O.: La transmission des contrastes par le système optique de l'oeil et les seuils de contrastes rétiniens. C. R. Acad. Sci. (Paris) **250**, 2757—2759 (1960).

ANDREWS, D. P.: Perception of contour orientation in the central fovea. Vision Res. **7**, 975—997 (1967).

BARLOW, H. B., FITZHUGH, R., KUFFLER, S. W.: Change of organization in the receptive fields of the cat's retina during dark adaptation. J. Physiol. (Lond.) **137**, 338—354 (1957).

BARTLEY, S. H., NELSON, T. M., SOULES, E. M.: Visual acuity under conditions of intermittent illumination productive of paradoxical brightness. J. Psychol. (Provincetown) **55**, 153—163 (1963).

BLACKWELL, H. R.: Neural theories of simple visual discrimination. J. opt. Soc. Amer. **53**, 129—160 (1963).

BLAKEMORE, C., CAMPBELL, F. W.: On the existence of neurones in the human visual system selectively sensitive to the orientation and size of retinal images. J. Physiol. (Lond.) **203**, 237—260 (1969).

— SUTTON, P.: Size adaptation: A new after effect. Science **166**, 245—247 (1969).

BRILLOUIN, L.: Science and Information Theory, 2nd Ed. New York-London: Academic Press 1962.

BRINDLEY, G. S.: Physiology of the Retina and Visual Pathway. 2nd Ed. London: Arnold (1970).

BROWN, J. L.: Effect of different preadapting luminances on the resolution of visual detail during dark adaptation. J. opt. Soc. Amer. **44**, 48—55 (1954).

— GRAHAM, C. H., LEIBOWITZ, H., RANKEN, H. B.: Luminance thresholds for the resolution of fine detail during dark adaptation. J. opt. Soc. Amer. **43**, 197—202 (1953).

— PHARES, L., FLETCHER, D. E.: Spectral energy thresholds for the resolution of acuity targets. J. opt. Soc. Amer. **50**, 950—960 (1960).

BRYNGDAHL, O.: Characteristics of the visual system: psychophysical measurements of the responses to spatial sine wave stimuli in the mesopic region. J. opt. Soc. Amer. **54**, 1152—1160 (1964).

— Characteristics of the visual system: psychophysical measurements of the response to spatial sine-wave stimuli in the photopic region. J. opt. Soc. Amer. **56**, 811—821 (1966).

CAMPBELL, F. W.: Visual acuity via linear analysis. In: Proceedings of the Symposium on Information Processing in Sight Sensory Systems. Pasadena: California Institute of Technology 1965.

— GREEN, D. G.: Optical and retinal factors affecting visual resolution. J. Physiol. (Lond.) **181**, 576—593 (1965).

— GUBISCH, R. W.: Optical quality of the human eye. J. Physiol. (Lond.) **186**, 558—578 (1966).

— KULIKOWSKI, J. J.: Orientational selectivity of the human visual system. J. Physiol. (Lond.) **187**, 437—445 (1966).

— — LEVINSON, J.: The effect of orientation on the visual resolution of gratings. J. Physiol. (Lond.) **187**, 427—436 (1966).

DAITCH, J. M., GREEN, D. G.: Contrast sensitivity of the human peripheral retina. Vision Res. **9**, 947—952 (1969).

DAVIDSON, M.: Perturbation approach to spatial brightness interaction in human vision. J. opt. Soc. Amer. **58**, 1300—1308 (1968).

DELANGE, H.: Relationship between critical flicker frequency and a set of low-frequency characteristics. J. opt. Soc. Amer. **44**, 380—389 (1954).

DEPALMA, J. J., LOWRY, E. M.: Sine-wave response of the visual system. II. Sine-wave and square-wave contrast sensitivity. J. opt. Soc. Amer. **52**, 328—335 (1962).

DITCHBURN, R. W., GINSBORG, B. L.: Vision with a stabilized retinal image. Nature (Lond.) **170**, 36—37 (1952).

DUKE-ELDER, W. S.: Textbook of Ophthalmology, Vol. 1, pp. 931—941. St. Louis: Mosby 1942.

GILBERT, D. S., FENDER, D. H.: Contrast thresholds measured with stabilized and non-stabilized sine wave gratings. Optica Acta **16**, 191—204 (1969).

Gilinsky, A. S.: Orientation-specific effects of patterns of adapting light on visual acuity. J. opt. Soc. Amer. **58**, 13—18 (1968).
— Doherty, R. S.: Interocular transfer of orientational effects. Science **164**, 454—455 (1969).
Graham, C. H., Brown, R. H., Mote, F. A.: The relation of size of stimulus and intensity in the human eye I. Intensity thresholds for white light. J. exp. Psychol. **24**, 555—573 (1939).
— Cook, C.: Visual acuity as a function of intensity and exposure time. Amer. J. Psychol. **49**, 654—661 (1937).
Gubisch, R. W.: Optical performance of the human eye. J. opt. Soc. Amer. **57**, 407—415 (1967).
Hartline, H. K.: The response of single optic nerve fibers of the vertebrate eye to illumination of the retina. Amer. J. Physiol. **121**, 400—415 (1938).
Hecht, S., Mintz, E. V.: The visibility of single lines at various illuminations and the retinal basis of visual resolution. J. gen. Physiol. **22**, 593—612 (1939).
Hering, E.: Über die Grenzen der Sehschärfe. Ber. math-phys. Cl. d. Königl. Sächs. Gesell. Wiss. Leipzig; Naturw. Teil, 16—24, 1899.
Higgins, G. C., Stultz, K.: Variations of visual acuity with various test object orientations and viewing conditions. J. opt. Soc. Amer. **40**, 135—137 (1950).
— — Visual acuity as measured with various orientations of a parallel-line test object. J. opt. Soc. Amer. **38**, 756—758 (1948).
Kahneman, D.: Time-intensity reciprocity in acuity as a function of luminance and figure-ground contrast. Vision Res. **6**, 207—216 (1966).
Keesey, U. K.: Effect of involuntary eye movements on visual acuity. J. opt. Soc. Amer. **50**, 769—774 (1960).
Lamar, E. S., Hecht, S., Hendley, C. D., Shlaer, S.: Size, shape and contrast in detection of targets by daylight vision. II. Frequency of seeing and the quantum theory of cone vision. J. opt. Soc. Amer. **38**, 741—755 (1948).
LeGrand, Y.: Réunions Inst. opt. 7ième Série, 6—11 (1936).
Leibowitz, H.: Some observations and theory on the variation of visual acuity with the orientation of the test object. J. opt. Soc. Amer. **43**, 902—905 (1953).
Lit, A.: Visual acuity. Ann. Rev. Psychol. **19**, 27—54 (1968).
Ludvigh, E.: Direction sense of the eye. Amer. J. Ophthal. **36**, 139—142 (1953).
— Miller, J. W.: Study of visual acuity during the ocular pursuit of moving test object. I. Introduction. J. opt. Soc. Amer. **48**, 799—802 (1958).
Mandelbaum, J., Sloan, L. L.: Peripheral visual acuity. Amer. J. Ophthal. **30**, 581—588 (1947).
Marshall, W. H., Talbot, S. A.: Recent evidence for neural mechanisms in vision leading to a general theory of sensory acuity. In: Biological Symposia, Vol. 8, pp. 117—164. Cattell, J., (Ed.) Lancaster, Pa.: Cattell Press 1942.
Mitchell, D. E., Freeman, R. D., Westheimer, G.: Effect of orientation on the modulation sensitivity for interference fringes on the retina. J. opt. Soc. Amer. **57**, 246—249 (1967).
Nachmias, J.: Meridional variations in visual acuity and eye movements during fixation. J. opt. Soc. Amer. **50**, 569—571 (1960).
— Effect of exposure duration on visual contrast sensitivity with square wave gratings. J. opt. Soc. Amer. **57**, 421—427 (1967).
Niven, J. I., Brown, R. H.: Visual resolution as a function of intensity and exposure time in the human fovea. J. opt. Soc. Amer. **34**, 738—743 (1944).
Pantle, A., Sekuler, R.: Size detecting mechanisms in human vision. Science **162**, 1146—1148 (1968).
Patel, A. S.: Spatial resolution by the human visual system. The effect of mean retinal illuminance. J. opt. Soc. Amer. **56**, 689—694 (1966).
Pirenne, M. H.: Visual acuity. In: The Eye, Vol. 2, pp. 175—195. Davson, H., (Ed.). New York: Academic Press 1962.
Ratliff, F.: The role of physiological nystagmus in monocular acuity. J. exp. Psychol. **43**, 163—172 (1952).
Riggs, L. A.: Visual acuity. In: Vision and Visual Perception. Graham, C. H. (Ed.) New York: Wiley & Sons 1965.

RIGGS, L. A., RATLIFF, F., CORNSWEET, J. C., CORNSWEET, T. N.: The disappearance of steadily fixated visual test objects. J. opt. Soc. Amer. **53**, 495—501 (1953).

ROBSON, J. G., CAMPBELL, F. W.: A threshold contrast function for the human visual system. In: The Physiological Basis for Form Discrimination. Symposium at W. S. Hunter Lab., Brown University, pp. 44—48, 1964.

SCHADE, O. H.: Optical and photoelectric analog of the eye. J. opt. Soc. Amer. **46**, 721—739 (1956).

SCHOBER, H. A. W., HILZ, R.: Contrast sensitivity of the human eye for square wave gratings. J. opt. Soc. Amer. **55**, 1086—1091 (1965).

STILES, W. S.: Increment thresholds and the mechanisms of colour vision. Documenta ophthal. **3**, 138—163 (1949).

VAN NES, F. L.: Experimental studies in spatio temporal contrast transfer by the human eye. Doctoral Thesis, Rijksuniversiteit Utrecht 1968.

— BOUMAN, M. A.: Spatial modulation transfer in the human eye. J. opt. Soc. Amer. **57**, 401—406 (1967).

VOLKMANN, A. W.: Physiologische Untersuchungen im Gebiete der Optik. Leipzig: Breitkopf & Härtel 1863.

WESTHEIMER, G.: A new method of measuring visual resolution at the retina. J. opt. Soc. Amer. **49**, 504 (1959).

— Modulation thresholds for sinusoidal light distributions on the retina. J. Physiol. (Lond.) **152**, 67—74 (1960).

— Optical and motor factors in the formation of the retinal image. J. opt. Soc. Amer. **53**, 86—93 (1963).

— Visual acuity. Ann. Rev. Psychol. **16**, 359—380 (1965a).

— Spatial interaction in the human retina during scotopic vision. J. Physiol. (Lond.) **181**, 881—894 (1965b).

— Spatial interaction in human cone vision. J. Physiol. (Lond.) **190**, 139—154 (1967).

WÜLFING, E. A.: Über den kleinsten Gesichtswinkel. Z. Biol. **29**, 199—202 (1892).

Chapter 8

Mach Band Phenomena

By

Adriana Fiorentini, Pisa (Italy)

With 5 Figures

Contents

Introduction

The Mach bands are bright or dark lines that are perceived near the boundary between a brightly illuminated region and a dimly illuminated region of the visual field (Fig. 1). The bands are a subjective contrast effect: they seem brighter or darker than their surroundings, although the physical distribution of light does not show any positive or negative peaks at the points where the bands are perceived.

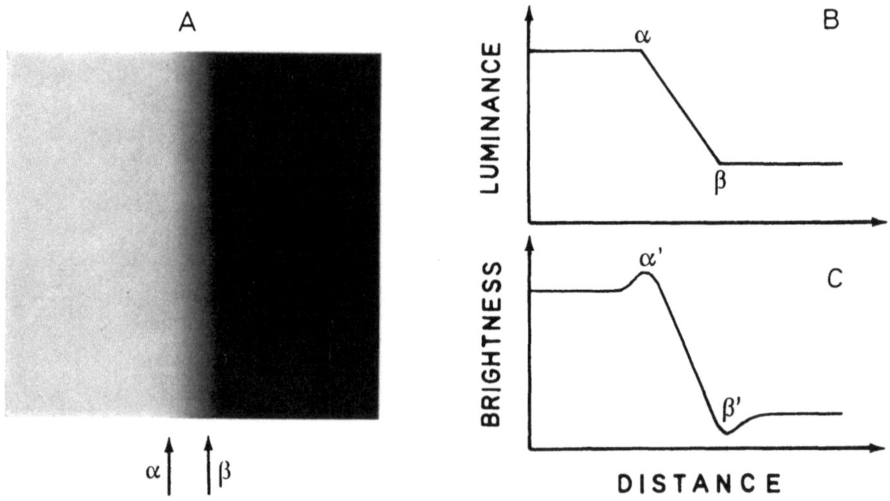

Fig. 1. In pattern *A* the luminance is constant in the vertical direction and varies horizontally according to diagram *B*. A bright Mach band appears at α and a dark band at β, so that the subjective brightness varies approximately as shown in *C*

In many cases the bands are rather faint and diffuse and may not be noticed, but under favourable conditions they appear so vividly as to be easily mistaken for real details of the light pattern.

The phenomenon, discovered by ERNST MACH a hundred years ago, is not a peculiarity of the visual system since there are similar effects in other sense organs (BÉKÉSY, 1967a and b). This indicates that the perception of Mach bands involves some general properties of the sensory systems. Indeed, as MACH suggested and recent electrophysiological experiments have shown, the subjective bright and dark lines result from reciprocal interactions among neighboring neurons in the retina and the brain. (See WEISSTEIN, chapter 10, and JAMESON and HURVICH, chapter 22, this volume.)

This is a striking example of the processes by which information contained in the pattern of retinal illumination is analyzed and elaborated in order to emphasize significant spatial features of the objective light distribution.

MACH gave an extensive description and a theoretical account of the phenomenon in a series of papers, the first of which appeared in 1865 (MACH, 1865, 1866a and b, 1868a and b, 1906. For an English translation of MACH'S papers, see RATLIFF, 1965).

He first noticed the bands while observing rotating figures of black and white paper (Fig. 2). When the disc of Fig. 2A is rapidly rotated the black and white sectors fuse, and the average luminance at a point on the disc is determined by the relative extents of the black and white sectors at that distance from the center. The brightness of the disc should decrease from the center to the edge, because of the increasing extent of the black sectors. The upper graph of Fig. 2A represents the average luminance distribution across the disc and illustrates qualitatively the brightness distribution that would be expected for uniform fields according to the Talbot-Plateau law. But the observed brightness distribution (bottom graph in Fig. 2A) is different: two bright rings appear at the positions β and γ (or two dark rings if the white figure on a black disc is replaced by a black figure on a white disc).

MACH described several other patterns that he used with rotating discs or cylinders which show similar effects. In the patterns used with rotating cylinders (Fig. 2B) the luminance varies in the direction parallel to the axis of rotation and is constant perpendicular to that direction. Although MACH also described and discussed more complicated patterns where the luminance varies in two directions, most of the later work on the Mach phenomenon has dealt with one-dimensional luminance distributions, like those obtained with rotating figures.

The bright and dark bands are not peculiar to rotating figures or to situations with intermittent illumination of the retina. Indeed, the bands appear very vividly in a photograph of the rotating disc of Fig. 2, even if the photograph is viewed under continuous illumination. (See also, e.g., Fig. 1.)

MACH pointed out that the phenomenon is related to the *spatial* distribution of luminance (curve B in Fig. 1) and more specifically that wherever the luminance curve has a flection, that particular place appears brighter or darker than its surroundings. In a one-dimensional pattern, bright bands appear at points of flection of the luminance distribution where the curve is convex from above (for instance, point α in Fig. 2B) and dark bands appear at flections where the curve is concave from above (point β in Fig. 2B).

If $I(x)$ represents the luminance of the viewed pattern along the direction x (supposing that the luminance is constant in the direction perpendicular to x), a band in the luminance curve corresponds to a high value of the second derivative of luminance with respect to the spatial variable. Thus, according to MACH, the bands are perceived at points where d^2I/dx^2 has a high absolute value, a bright

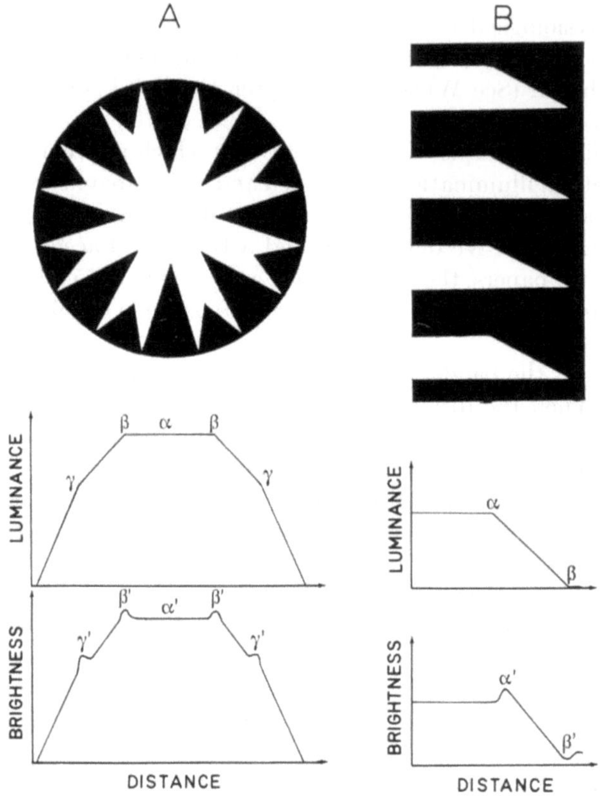

Fig. 2. Patterns used with rotating discs (A) or cylinders (B) to produce Mach bands. The Mach bands are perceived at points where the luminance curves bend (points β' and γ' of the disc diameter in A, and points α' and β' of the direction parallel to the axis of rotation of the cylinder in B)

band being associated with a negative sign of the second derivative (i.e. a convexity) and a dark band with a positive sign (i.e. a concavity). This holds true also for sharp edges (at which the second derivative has no finite value) when the luminance $I(x)$ of the external pattern is replaced by the corresponding retinal illumination $I'(x)$. The retinal image of an objectively sharp edge is not perfectly sharp because of imperfections in the optical imagery of the eye. (See WESTHEIMER, chapter 7, this volume.)

The retinal illumination cannot be measured *in vivo* without complex equipment, but under certain circumstances it can be computed with reasonable accuracy from a known light distribution at the object. This is true, for instance, for a distribution of monochromatic light viewed through a very small pupil. In this case the effects of diffraction largely exceed those of the optical aberrations or of other defects of the eye and the light distribution on the retina can be easily computed. Recent experiments with diffraction patterns have confirmed that the Mach bands are perceived with good approximation at points where the second derivative of retinal illumination is maximal or minimal (LUDVIGH, 1953; BURNHAM and JACKSON, 1955; WATRASIEWICZ, 1963).

Since the Mach phenomenon is related only to the spatial distribution of luminance, Mach bands will be produced by any suitable light distribution, no matter how it is obtained. For instance, it is very easy to see Mach bands in the shadows cast by an extended source, such as the sun: a dark band appears at the boundary between the full shadow and the half-shadow (at which the light curve has a concave flection) and a bright band at the boundary between the half-shadow and the region of full light (where the light curve has a convex flection). Producing Mach bands is not really a problem, and once they have been noticed it is very easy to identify them in all sorts of light distributions.

Lines and contours are very critical for the perception of luminance differences between adjacent regions of the visual field, as well as for the perception of shape, depth, etc. The very interesting point about Mach bands is the fact that lines and contours are perceived at positions where the light pattern does not show a sharp edge but only a smooth transition from a bright to a dim surface. The subjective lines enhance the border separating the two surfaces just as real lines would do.

The perception of Mach bands is usually accompanied by enhancement of the apparent contrast between the two surfaces separated by the diffuse boundary. It is even possible to produce a subjective contrast between two surfaces having the same luminance by modulating the light in a narrow strip between the two surfaces in such a way as to introduce a positive and/or a negative deflection in the otherwise homogeneous light distribution (O'BRIEN, 1958).

On the other hand, a non-homogeneous surface may appear quite uniform if the light distribution across that surface does not show any flections (BERGSTRÖM, 1966).

Psychophysical Measurement of Mach Bands

The first few works that followed the publication of MACH's papers (McDOUGALL, 1903; THOULESS, 1922; KOFFKA and HARROWER, 1931) were concerned mainly with the qualitative description of the phenomenon and with its theoretical implications.

More recently several attempts have been made to obtain quantitative measures of this phenomenon. The width, the position, and the brightness of Mach bands have been measured by psychophysical methods for a number of patterns.

The width of the bands varies from a few minutes of arc to 10–12 min or more depending on the shape of the light curve. In a one-dimensional light distribution consisting of a bright and a dim region and of an intermediate luminance gradient (as, for instance, Fig. 1) the width of the bright band decreases if either the highest luminance or the steepness of the gradient is increased (McCOLLOUGH, 1955;

Fiorentini and Radici, 1958). The dark band seems to be less influenced by a change in the slope of the light gradient.

In the patterns of Figs. 1 and 2 the Mach bands are approximately symmetrical about the points at which the light curve bends. But the position of the bands also depends on the absolute level of illumination and may be different for different subjects (McCollough, 1955; Watrasiewicz, 1966).

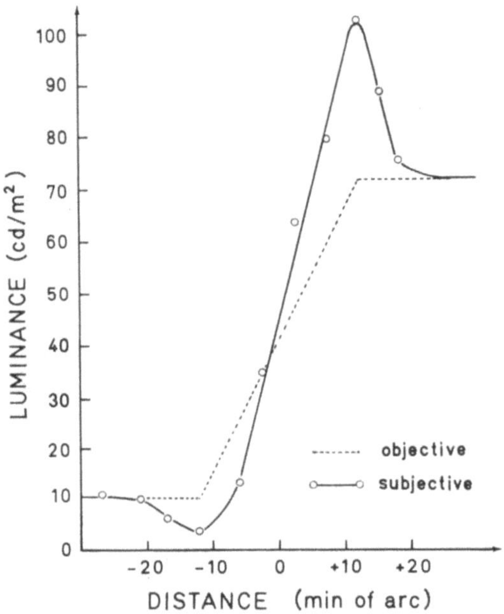

Fig. 3. Subjective brightness distribution (open circles) measured across the luminance distribution indicated by the broken line. (From Lowry and DePalma, 1961)

The subjective distribution of brightness across a pattern where Mach bands are perceived has been determined by various methods (Fiorentini and Radici, 1957; Lowry and DePalma, 1961; Bryngdahl, 1964; Charman and Watrasiewicz, 1964; Thomas, 1966; Békésy, 1968a). The curve obtained for a linear luminance gradient of about 24 min width is presented in Fig. 3 (Lowry and DePalma, 1961). Other curves, obtained from different experiments, are only approximately similar: the results seem to vary according to the experimental method by which they were obtained and also to differ widely from subject to subject. The asymmetry of the bright and dark bands, however, that is evident in Fig. 3, is common to most experimental curves. Another feature of Fig. 3 is typical of patterns with gradients of moderate slopes: in the region of the gradient the subjective curve is steeper than the objective curve. This indicates that the perception of Mach bands at a diffuse edge is accompanied by a subjective sharpening of the edge.

Obviously, the brightness of the Mach bands also depends on the geometrical and photometric parameters of the light distribution. For instance, in the pattern containing a linear gradient (Fig. 2B), the difference in brightness between the Mach bands and their surroundings increases (i.e. the bright band looks brighter and the dark band, darker) if the angular width of the gradient is decreased (HARTWIG, 1958; FIORENTINI and RADICI, 1958; THOMAS, 1966).

Where the angular width of the gradient is very small the phenomenon is more complicated and the bands may have a multiple structure (RONCHI, 1962; WATRASIEWICZ, 1963). The subjective appearance of an objectively sharp edge (luminance step) is even more variable and difficult to describe quantitatively, especially if the contrast is high. This must be due, at least in part, to eye movements: when fixation changes from one point to another in the region of the edge, the appearance of the pattern varies considerably (BÉKÉSY, 1968a) and transient bands may appear near the edge as an effect of successive contrast.

Even the presence of Mach bands at a sharp edge is controversial. Several investigators expressed the view that no Mach bands are present at a luminance step, while others decribe the bands at the step as being very narrow and rather unstable. A quantitative account of the Mach bands that may be perceived in a step pattern has been given recently by BÉKÉSY (1968a).

For a gradient of finite width, as we have seen above, the brightness of the Mach bands depends on the gradient width; and if the width exceeds a critical value no bands are perceived. Since this critical angle also depends on the contrast or luminance difference between the brighter and dimmer regions of the pattern, the threshold for the perception of the Mach bands may be better expressed in terms of the slope m of the gradient. (For a linear gradient, m is the luminance difference between two points of the gradient divided by the angular separation of the points.)

The threshold for a Mach band is found to vary with the local luminance level. If m is the critical slope of the gradient pattern and L is the luminance in the region of the edge, at high photopic levels m is proportional to L. Below about 50 trolands, the ratio m/L increases with decreasing L, and at mesopic or scotopic levels the bands are not visible even with a steep gradient (ERCOLES and FIORENTINI, 1959; CHARMAN and WATRASIEWICZ, 1964).

The observed relation calls to mind the dependence of the Weber-Fechner fraction upon the level of adaptation of the eye. And indeed it is not surprising that the threshold for the Mach phenomenon is affected by the local level of adaptation in the same way as the differential sensitivity of the eye.

The threshold for the Mach bands also depends on exposure duration. The bands can be perceived even when the eye is exposed for only 1 or 2 msec to the single gradient pattern, provided that the gradient is very steep (THOMAS, 1965; MATTHEWS, 1966). If the time of exposure is increased the critical slope of the gradient linearly decreases, as occurs for the absolute threshold (Bloch's law), for exposures up to about 50 msec (THOMAS, 1965).

Although eye movements and successive contrast modify the subjective appearance of the Mach bands, the basic phenomenon is not a successive contrast effect, as MACH (1865) demonstrated. He was able to observe the bands in his photographic patterns in electric spark flash illumination, and took this fact as evidence that the bands do not require eye movements.

Recent experiments have shown that the bands are visible in a light pattern whose image is stabilized on the retina and also in the after-image of the pattern (Riggs *et al.*, 1961; Ronchi and Ercoles, 1962). This provides further support for Mach's view that movements of the light pattern across the retina are not required for the perception of Mach bands. It does not mean, however, that motion of the pattern relative to the eye has no effect on the phenomenon. In fact, the bands appear more vividly when the pattern is oscillated at a few cycles per second in a direction perpendicular to the light-dark boundary (Fiorentini and Ercoles, 1957; Bittini *et al.*, 1960; Riggs *et al.*, 1961).

Similar results are obtained when a stationary pattern is flickered on and off; the bands are most prominent over a limited range of flicker rates (Békésy, 1968b). All this indicates that transients of the retinal illumination play an important role in the phenomenon, whether they are introduced by a movement of the pattern or by flickering the light on and off.

Mach bands that are obtained with a distribution of colored light do not differ in any important respect from those obtained with white light, at least when the spectral composition of light is the same at every point of the pattern and only the luminance varies from point to point. The bands have the same hue as the surrounding field, although the bright band may appear somewhat less saturated than its surroundings (Ercoles and Fiorentini, 1958). If the purity of light varies together with the luminance, then the Mach bands may differ in hue and/or saturation from their surroundings. Let us suppose, for instance, that a distribution like that shown in Fig. 1, but of red light, is superimposed on a uniform white background. The proportion of red light in the pattern decreases from left to right at the same rate as luminance. Then, the dark band that appears at point β is greenish (Mach, 1868a). In a step pattern where the darker region is yellow and the brighter region is white, the dark band is more saturated than the uniform yellow region (Békésy, 1968a).

A more controversial question is whether Mach bands can be produced by patterns where the chromaticity varies but the luminance is constant. Color contrast effects for large surfaces are similar to brightness contrast effects, and one could reasonably expect to find that a spatial variation in chromaticity is effective as a stimulus for the Mach phenomenon in the same way that a luminance variation is.

A linear gradient of chromaticity can be obtained for instance from a rotating pattern (Fig. 2B) where the black and white areas are replaced by areas of two different colors, say red and green. If the luminances of the red and green areas are equal, then the luminance of the rotating pattern is constant and only the chromaticity varies from one side to the other.

Most of both the early and the recent attempts to produce Mach bands with chromaticity gradients of this kind have given negative results (Thouless, 1922; Koffka and Harrower, 1931; Fry, 1948; Ercoles and Fiorentini, 1958; van der Horst and Bouman, 1967). However, some evidence has recently been reported which indicates that colored Mach bands can be produced even in the absence of any luminance variation (Daw, 1964; Jacobson and MacKinnon, 1969; Land, 1968). In one of these experiments, however, only three subjects out of six were able to see the Mach bands (Daw, 1964).

Thus at present we have no conclusive evidence in favor of the hypothesis that a change in the slope of the chromaticity color distribution alone is an effective stimulus for the Mach phenomenon.

Further information about the visual phenomena that occur in the region of a sharp edge may be derived from measurements of the increment threshold for a small test target (a bright line or a spot of light) that is superimposed on a step pattern of luminance at a variable distance from the edge. The increment threshold for the target is found to vary according to the distance of the target from the edge (Fig. 4A). For a sharp edge and high luminance contrast the increment threshold is highest when the target is superimposed on the edge and decreases on both sides, reaching steady values at some distance from the edge (HARMS and AULHORN, 1955; AULHORN and HARMS, 1956). The peak value of the threshold increases with the luminance difference of the step (HARMS and AULHORN, 1955; AULHORN and HARMS, 1956), or with the luminance of the brighter part of the field (FIORENTINI and ZOLI, 1966; BÉKÉSY, 1968a) but decreases when the time of presentation of the pattern is very short (NOVAK and SPERLING, 1963; MATTHEWS, 1966). No increase in threshold is found at the edge when the pattern is exposed for 10 msec or less. This fact is consistent with electrophysiological and other psychophysical findings which show that inhibition does not show up if excitatory and inhibitory regions are illuminated simultaneously with very short flashes (BARLOW *et al.*, 1957; SCHOBER and HILZ, 1965; NACHMIAS, 1966). Inhibitory mechanisms seem to take a longer time to build up their full activity than excitatory mechanisms. The increase in the threshold gradient for Mach bands with decreasing exposure would also result from the dependence of lateral interactions on exposure duration.

Similar results are found when the increment threshold is measured across a pattern with a linear gradient of light (FIORENTINI *et al.*, 1955; FIORENTINI, 1957; BURKHARDT, 1966). The threshold is highest in the region where the bright Mach band is perceived and the peak value of the threshold is greater when the gradient is steeper.

Increment sensitivity and subjective brightness are not necessarily related by any simple function. Thus there is no reason to expect that the increment threshold curve should reproduce the brightness distribution, with a positive peak of the threshold corresponding to the bright Mach band and a negative peak corresponding to the dark Mach band. In fact, increment thresholds measured across a gradient or an edge everywhere exceed the values that would be obtained if the target were viewed against homogeneous backgrounds having the corresponding luminances. The increase in threshold due to the patterning is found to be greatest in the regions where both the bright and dark Mach bands are perceived.

The elevation of the increment threshold increases with the contrast and the luminance of the step pattern more or less as does the brightness of the bright band (BÉKÉSY, 1968a) and this suggests that the two quantities are related. But even this relation between increment threshold and brightness of the bright Mach bands is relatively variable and complex (BURKHARDT, 1966).

With a step pattern of very low contrast the increment threshold measured across the edge undergoes an elevation on the dark side and an almost symmetrical depression on the bright side (Fig. 4B). In this case it is possible to make successful predictions based on the assumption of linearity of spatial interactions.

An example is given in Fig. 4. The bottom curve of the figure (C) was obtained by measuring the threshold for a bright line that was viewed at various angular separations from another line the luminance of which was just below threshold. The effect of varying the line separation on the threshold for the test line is evident: when the two lines are close to each other there is a facilitatory effect, whereas for a distance of 4–5 min of arc there is an inhibitory effect. At distances of 10 min of arc or more there is practically no interaction between the two lines.

If the threshold curve (C) is transformed into a sensitivity function by plotting the reciprocals of the threshold, a curve is obtained that may be assumed to

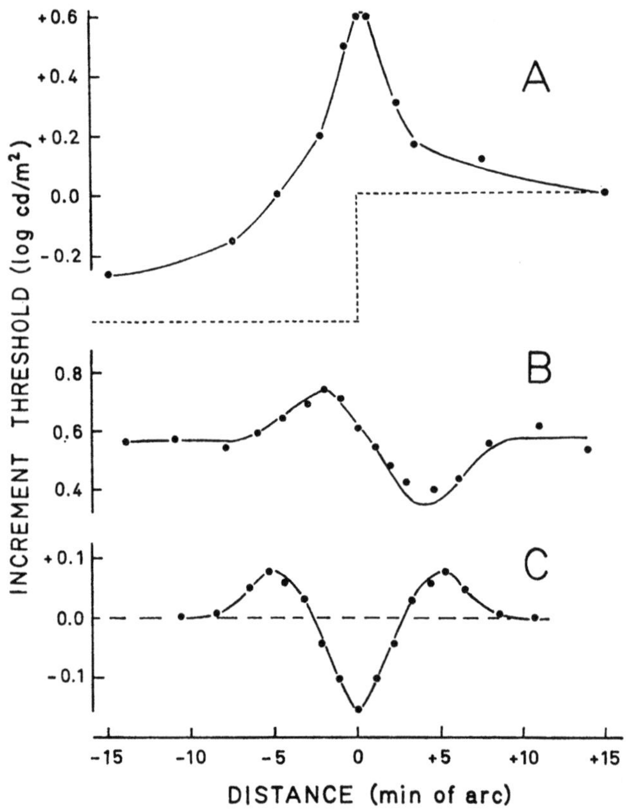

Fig. 4. Log increment threshold for a bright line superimposed on a step pattern of high contrast (*A*) or liminal contrast (*B*) plotted against distance of the line from the step. The luminance difference of step *A* (broken line) is 0.44 log unit. That of step *B* (not represented in the figure) is 0.005 log unit. Negative distances correspond to the dimmer region and positive distances to the brighter region of the pattern. (From A. Fiorentini and M. T. Zoli, Atti Fond. G. Ronchi **21**, 338—356 (1966) and **22**, 207—217 (1967)). (*C*) Log increment threshold for a bright line plotted against distance from a second bright line of just subliminal contrast. Background 15 cd/m². Line size: 0.5 × 30 min of arc. The curve in *B* was calculated from the data shown in (*C*), as explained in the text

represent the pattern of excitation and inhibition relevant for one-dimensional stimuli. The convolution of this curve with a step function, when plotted on a log scale, may be fitted with good approximation to the experimental points of curve B of Fig. 4, which are measurements of the increment threshold for a step pattern of low contrast.

A linear analysis thus approximately fits the behavior of the visual system under the restrictive conditions of this particular experiment, and the response to a step pattern may be derived straightforwardly from the function that describes the spatial interactions between two elementary stimuli. These results can be correlated with the electrophysiological findings that will be discussed in the next section.

In general the visual system cannot be considered as linear, however. For instance, the asymmetry of the bright and dark Mach bands that are produced by an objectively symmetrical distribution (Fig. 3) is indicative of nonlinearity (Marimont, 1963; Békésy, 1968a). Thus a completely general account of the Mach band phenomena can not be given by applying the methods of linear system analysis to the human visual system.

Lateral Inhibition and the Edge Response

Mach was the first to suggest that mutual interactions among the elements of the neural network in the retina were responsible for the maxima and minima in the subjective appearance of an edge. He supposed that the response of a single receptive unit of the retina was determined in part by the luminance of the light impinging on it and in part by the signals sent from neighboring cells to that unit. Mach's mathematical model can be interpreted in terms of excitatory and inhibitory components, in which the inhibitory effects are assumed both to increase with the stimulus luminance to the inhibiting cell and to decrease with increasing distance between the interacting cells. The inhibitory effects of different cells on the same unit are supposed to summate and the response of the first element to be inversely related to the sum of the inhibitory influences.

Mach's formulation of the lateral interactions in the nervous visual system accounts for the bright and dark bands that are perceived near a diffuse edge: the overshoot in the computed response to a light distribution with a linear gradient (Fig. 2B) is greater than the undershoot, in agreement with the observed brightness distributions (Fig. 3) (Ratliff, 1965).

An equivalent expression of the response of a single retinal unit can be given in terms of the spatial distribution of the stimulus luminance: the response at each retinal point is directly related to the square of the local illumination and inversely related to the sum of the local illumination plus a term proportional to the second derivative of luminance with respect to the spatial variable (Mach, 1868a). The significance of the second derivative of luminance for the Mach phenomenon is thus clear: lateral inhibition is strongest or weakest at points where the second derivative of the retinal illumination is maximal or minimal.

Several other models have been proposed more recently, each of which accounts for the Mach phenomenon at least in some respects. All the theoretical formulations can ultimately be reduced to the following basic assumption: the function that describes the response of each element of the neural network has an excitatory component, which depends on the luminance of the stimulus to that element, and an inhibitory component that depends on the luminance of the stimuli to the surrounding elements and on the distance of each of them from the first element. The various models differ as regards the mathematical expression of the excitatory and inhibitory functions and the way in which they are combined to yield the response function. For a review and comparative discussion of the various theoretical accounts of Mach bands, see RATLIFF (1965).

Evidence for the role played by lateral inhibition in the Mach phenomenon has been provided by electrophysiological recording of the responses to a step pattern in the eyes of invertebrates and of mammals (Fig. 5). In the lateral eye of *Limulus*, the sensory units inhibit each other by an amount that increases with the luminance of the light falling on the inhibiting unit and decreases with increasing distance between the interacting units. If the response of a single ommatidium is recorded while a step pattern is focused on the eye surface, the response is found to vary according to the distance of the edge in the pattern from that ommatidium. If the response is plotted as a function of distance, the curve shows an overshoot and an undershoot that are the obvious correlates of Mach bands. If however all the ommatidia that surround the responding unit are covered, so that they are prevented from exerting any inhibitory influence, the response function does not

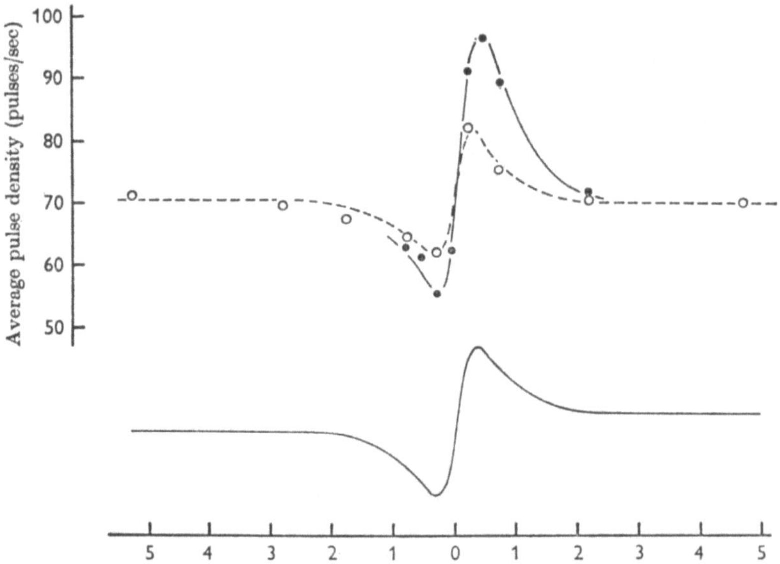

Fig. 5. Static response of an on-center ganglion cell of the cat to a contrast edge, for two different contrast levels (filled circles, 0.4; open circles, 0.2). The vertical edge was held stationary at different distances from the receptive field center and the contrast pattern was alternately introduced and removed, in such a way that the step pattern alternated with a homogeneous field of the same average luminance. The average pulse density was measured for each edge position. (From ENROTH-CUGELL and J. G. ROBSON, 1966). The solid line in the lower part of the figure is the edge sensitivity of the same cell calculated from the contrast sensitivity function obtained with sinusoidal gratings, assuming linearity of spatial summation

have any positive or negative peaks, but reproduces the stimulus pattern fairly well (RATLIFF and HARTLINE, 1959).

The mechanisms that underlie lateral interactions in the retina of vertebrates are more complex. However, the response of a ganglion cell of the cat to a step pattern that was located at various positions across the receptive field of the cell (ENROTH-CUGELL and ROBSON, 1966) has the familiar shape with the positive and negative peaks (Fig. 5) and looks very much like the response in *Limulus*. The similarity between these results and the psychophysical brightness distribution is striking. Unfortunately the comparison can only be qualitative because of the obvious differences between the retinae of the animals from which the electrophysiological responses are recorded and the visual system of human subjects.

Some recent psychophysical results, however, suggest that lateral interactions in the human visual system are spatially distributed according to a function that is similar to the distribution of excitation and inhibition in the receptive fields of cat retinal ganglion cells (WESTHEIMER, 1965 and 1967). These findings, together with those obtained from similar experiments (see, for instance, Fig. 4C) allow us at least to speculate about the possible sizes of receptive fields of the human visual system and on the relative extents of their excitatory and inhibitory regions.

Some of the quantitative data on Mach bands that have been reported in the previous section are in line with the most recent results relating to the receptive fields of the retina. Thus for instance, the minimal width of Mach bands seen with very steep gradients at high luminance levels is of the same order as the size of the excitatory region of the psychophysically inferred receptive field of the human fovea. The increase in width and decrease in apparent contrast of the Mach bands when the luminance decreases are consistent with the change in size of receptive fields in the cat that results from a decrease of the inhibitory peripheral influence at low luminances (BARLOW *et al.*, 1957). The absolute threshold for the perception of Mach bands presumably corresponds to a level at which the inhibitory component of the receptive units in the fovea is greatly reduced or practically ineffective.

On the whole, the structural organization of receptive fields in the neural visual system provides a good basis for the interpretation of the Mach phenomenon. Conversely, data on the Mach bands or on other similar contrast effects may supply information about the extent of elementary areas of excitation and inhibition (BÉKÉSY, 1960 and 1968b). But this is not the whole story. The electrophysiological response to a stationary stimulus (Fig. 5) or the psychophysical threshold for a steadily illuminated target (Fig. 4), do not supply any information about the effects of transients in retinal light stimulation which can play an important role in border contrast phenomena. Any realistic theory of the Mach phenomenon should account for the dynamic as well as for the stationary response to an edge.

The Mach bands are a complex phenomenon and it may not be an easy task for the physiologist to account for all the effects that have been described in this chapter. In the present state of knowledge other simpler and more basic aspects of visual perception seem to offer a more convenient approach to the study of neural interactions, both in the space and in the time domain. But the Mach bands still are among the most interesting and stimulating phenomena of sensory perception.

References

Aulhorn, E., Harms, H.: Untersuchungen über das Wesen des Grenzkontrastes. Ber. dtsch. ophthal. Ges. Heidelberg 1956.

Barlow, H. B., Fitzhugh, R., Kuffler, S. W.: Change of organization in the receptive fields of the cat's retina during dark adaptation. J. Physiol. (Lond.) **137**, 338—354 (1957).

Békésy, G. von: Neural inhibitory units of the eye and skin. Quantitative description of contrast phenomena. J. opt. Soc. Amer. **50**, 1060—1070 (1960).

— Mach band type lateral inhibition in different sense organs. J. gen. Physiol. **50**, 519—532 (1967a).

— Sensory Inhibition. Princeton, N.J.: Princeton University Press 1967b.

— Brightness distribution across the Mach bands measured with flicker photometry, and the linearity of sensory nervous interaction. J. opt. Soc. Amer. **58**, 1—8 (1968a).

— Mach- and Hering-type lateral inhibition in vision. Vision Res. **8**, 1483—1499 (1968b).

Bergström, S. S.: A paradox in the perception of luminance gradients. I. Scand. J. Psychol. **7**, 209—224 (1966).

Bittini, M., Ercoles, A. M., Fiorentini, A., Ronchi, L., Toraldo di Francia, G.: Enhanced contrast of an indefinitely contoured object by movement or intermittent illumination. Atti Fond. G. Ronchi **15**, 62—84 (1960).

Bryngdahl, O.: Visual transfer characteristics from Mach band measurements. Kybernetik **2**, 71—77 (1964).

Burkhardt, D. A.: Brightness and the increment threshold. J. opt. Soc. Amer. **56**, 979—981 (1966).

Burnham, R. W., Jackson, J. E.: Mach rings verified by numerical differentiation. Science **122**, 951—953 (1955).

Charman, W. N., Watrasiewicz, B. M.: Mach effect associated with microscope images. J. opt. Soc. Amer. **54**, 791—795 (1964).

Daw, N. W.: Visual response to gradients of varying colour and equal luminance. Nature (Lond.) **203**, 215—216 (1964).

Enroth-Cugell, C., Robson, J. G.: The contrast sensitivity of retinal ganglion cells of the cat. J. Physiol. (Lond.) **187**, 517—552 (1966).

Ercoles-Guzzoni, A. M., Fiorentini, A.: Simultaneous contrast effect produced by non uniform colored fields. Atti Fond. G. Ronchi **13**, 135—144 (1958).

Ercoles, A. M., Fiorentini, A.: Visibility of the Mach bands as a function of field luminance. Atti Fond. G. Ronchi **14**, 230—235 (1959).

Fiorentini, A.: Foveal and extrafoveal contrast threshold at a point of a non-uniform field. Atti Fond. G. Ronchi **12**, 180—186 (1957).

— Ercoles, A. M.: Vision of oscillating non-uniform fields. Optica Acta **4**, 150—157 (1957).

— Jeanne, M., Toraldo di Francia, G.: Measurements of differential threshold in the presence of a spatial illumination gradient. Atti Fond. G. Ronchi **10**, 371—379 (1955).

— Radici, T.: Binocular measurements of brightness on a field presenting a luminance gradient. Atti Fond. G. Ronchi **12**, 453—461 (1957).

— — Brightness, width and position of Mach bands as a function of the rate of variation of the luminance gradient. Atti Fond. G. Ronchi **13**, 145—155 (1958).

— Zoli, M. T.: Detection of a target superimposed to a step pattern of illumination. Atti Fond. G. Ronchi **21**, 338—356 (1966).

— — Detection of a target superimposed to a step pattern of illumination. II: Effects of a just-perceptible illumination step. Atti Fond. G. Ronchi **22**, 207—217 (1967).

Fry, G. A.: Mechanisms subserving simultaneous brightness contrast. Amer. J. Optom. and Arch. Amer. Acad. Optom. **25**, 162—178 (1948).

Harms, H., Aulhorn, E.: Studien über den Grenzkontrast. I. Mitteilung. Ein neues Grenzphänomen. Gräfes Arch. Ophthal. **157**, 3—23 (1955).

Hartwig, E.: Modelluntersuchungen zur qualitativen Erfassung von physiologischen Kontrastfehlern. Optik **15**, 414—421 (1958).

Horst, G. J. C. van der, Bouman, M. A.: On searching for Mach band type phenomena in colour vision. Vision Res. **7**, 1027—1029 (1967).

Jacobson, J. Z., MacKinnon, G. E.: Coloured Mach bands. Canad. J. Psychol. **23**, 56—65 (1969).

KOFFKA, K., HARROWER, M. R.: Colour and organization. Psychol. Forsch. **15**, 146—275 (1931).
LAND, E. H.: In: Report on O.S.A. Technical groups. J. opt. Soc. Amer. **58**, 441 (1968).
LOWRY, E. M., DEPALMA, J. J.: Sine-wave response of the visual system I. The Mach phenomenon. J. opt. Soc. Amer. **51**, 740—746 (1961).
LUDVIGH, E.: The perception of contours I. Introduction. Joint Project Report Number 4, U.S. Naval School of Aviation Medicine, Pensacola, Fla. 1953.
MACH, E.: Über die Wirkung der räumlichen Vertheilung des Lichtreizes auf die Netzhaut. I. S.-B. Akad. Wiss. Wien, math.-nat. Kl. **52**, 303—322 (1865).
— Über den Physiologischen Effect räumlich vertheilter Lichtreize. II. S.-B. Akad. Wiss. Wien, math.-nat. Kl. **54**, 131—144 (1866a).
— Über die physiologische Wirkung räumlich vertheilter Lichtreize. III. S.-B. Akad. Wiss. Wien, math.-nat. Kl. **54**, 393—408 (1866b).
— Über die physiologische Wirkung räumlich vertheilter Lichtreize. IV. S.-B. Akad. Wiss. Wien, math.-nat. Kl. **57**, 11—19 (1868a).
— Über die Abhängigkeit der Netzhautstellen voneinander. Vierteljahresschrift für Psychiatrie **2**, 38—51 (1868b).
— Über den Einfluß räumlich und zeitlich variierender Lichtreize auf die Gesichtswahrnehmung. S.-B. Akad. Wiss. Wien, math.-nat. Kl. **115**, 633—648 (1906).
MARIMONT, R. B.: Linearity and the Mach phenomenon. J. opt. Soc. Amer. **53**, 400—401 (1963).
MATTHEWS, M. L.: Appearance of Mach bands for short durations and at sharply focused contours. J. opt. Soc. Amer. **56**, 1401—1402 (1966).
MCCOLLOUGH, C.: The variation in width and position of Mach bands as a function of luminance. J. exp. Psychol. **49**, 141—152 (1955).
MCDOUGALL, W.: Intensification of visual sensation by smoothly gradual contrast. Proc. Physiol. Soc. **1**, 19—21 (1903).
NACHMIAS, J.: Effect of exposure duration on visual contrast sensitivity with square-wave gratings. J. opt. Soc. Amer. **57**, 421—427 (1967).
NOVAK, S., SPERLING, G.: Visual thresholds near a continuously or a briefly presented light-dark boundary. Optica Acta **10**, 187—191 (1963).
O'BRIEN, V.: Contour perception, illusion and reality. J. opt. Soc. Amer. **48**, 112—119 (1958).
RATLIFF, F.: Mach Bands: Quantitative Studies on Neural Networks in the Retina. San Francisco: Holden-Day 1965.
— HARTLINE, H. K.: The response of *Limulus* optic nerve fibers to patterns of illumination on the receptor mosaic. J. gen. Physiol. **42**, 1241—1255 (1959).
RIGGS, L. A., RATLIFF, F., KEESEY, U. T.: Appearance of Mach bands with a motionless retinal image. J. opt. Soc. Amer. **51**, 702—703 (1961).
RONCHI, L.: Quantitative aspects of the blur-to-sharp transition. Atti Fond. G. Ronchi **17**, 646—670 (1962).
— ERCOLES, A. M.: Adaptational effects at photopic and mesopic luminances as a function of contrast. Atti Fond. G. Ronchi **17**, 185—196 (1962).
SCHOBER, H. A. W., HILZ, R.: Contrast sensitivity of the human eye for square-wave gratings. J. opt. Soc. Amer. **55**, 1086—1091 (1965).
THOMAS, J. P.: Threshold measurements of Mach bands. J. opt. Soc. Amer. **55**, 521—524 (1965).
— Brightness variations in stimuli with ramp-like contours. J. opt. Soc. Amer. **56**, 238—242 (1966).
THOULESS, R. M.: Some observations on contrast effects in graded discs. Brit. J. Psychol. **13**, 301—307 (1922).
WATRASIEWICZ, B. M.: Measurements of the Mach effect in microscopy. Optica Acta **10**, 209—216 (1963).
— Some factors affecting the appearance of the Mach bands. J. opt. Soc. Amer. **56**, 499—503 (1966).
WESTHEIMER, G.: Spatial interaction in the human retina during scotopic vision. J. Physiol. (Lond.) **181**, 881—894 (1965).
— Spatial interaction in human cone vision. J. Physiol. (Lond.) **190**, 139—154 (1967).

Chapter 9

Discrimination of Homogeneous Double Pulses of Light

By

ROBERT M. BOYNTON, Rochester, New York (USA)

With 10 Figures

Contents

A. Introduction

When two pulses[1] of light are delivered successively to the same part of the retina, they may or may not be seen. If seen, they may appear as two flashes

[1] Following a suggestion of BARTLEY and WILKINSON (1953), we will use the term "pulse" to describe a brief physical stimulus, and the word "flash" to refer to the subjective appearance of a pulse or pulses.

separated by a definite dark interval, or they may be perceived instead as a single flash that seems to vary from bright to dim and back again to bright. Sometimes a single flash will be seen as having a subtle flickering appearance that barely suggests the temporal inhomogeneity of the double-pulse that produced it. At still other times the double-pulse may be indistinguishable from a single pulse, either because it appears as a distinctly unitary event, or because, under the given set of experimental conditions, a single pulse may itself sometimes be seen as a double flash.

This chapter will consider a variety of such two-pulse phenomena. We shall however restrict our attention to the special case where the pulses are spatially homogeneous, of the same color, and stimulate only a single region of the retina. This implies that no pattern or other cue has been provided to permit the discrimination of one pulse from the other; our concern is therefore limited to cases where the two pulses must be judged as a package. Many interesting topics are thereby excluded, because only when two pulses occupy different or partially-overlapping retinal locations can judgments be made with respect to each of the pulses individually.

B. Persistence of Vision

It has been recognized since PLATEAU'S doctoral thesis in 1829 that the sensation elicited by a brief pulse of light usually outlasts the duration of the stimulus. PLATEAU was not the first to notice this: according to a monograph published by him in 1877, persistence in the form of afterimages was first reported by ARISTOTLE more than three centuries B.C., and the fusion of colors on a rotating disc was described by PTOLEMY in the second century A.D. The first recorded observations of the luminous path traced by a rapidly-moving, glowing object are those of BOETHIUS (455–525 A.D.), later studied by SEGNER (1740) and quantified by D'ARCY (1773) who, by mounting his stimulus on a rotating wheel, found that the minimum time required to produce an apparent circle was 0.133 sec.[2]

The experiment of D'ARCY implies that the sensation produced by each element of the circular stimulus persists without noticeable diminution until the stimulus comes around again to provide reinforcement. Yet if D'Arcy's wheel were masked so that only a small portion of the luminous circle could be seen, only about seven or eight brief pulses per second would be delivered at his minimum time. These almost surely would be perceived as flickering. Modern results of VAN DEN BRINK (1957) and POLLACK (1953) also suggest that movement can somehow produce improved temporal integration in the eye. For pulses of light delivered to one retinal location, the upper limit of complete temporal integration, defining the so-called critical duration, is on the order of 100 msec, and frequently much less than this (see Section G). POLLACK found nearly complete reciprocity between luminance and exposure time at threshold, for conditions that included a 1-deg spot that required 400 msec to move 20 deg on the retina. BOUMAN and VAN DEN BRINK (1953) report only small departures from reciprocity for similarly long exposure times, for smaller spots moving shorter distances.

[2] ALLEN, F. (1926) describes these and many other observations in a monograph on "The Persistence of Vision."

C. Many Pulses vs. Two Pulses

Persistence of vision, as measured with the use of discrete pulses delivered successively to the same retinal area, has been studied in many hundreds of experiments concerned with flicker and the determination of critical flicker frequency (CFF). Most such studies (see the review by KELLY, chapter 11, this volume) employ a continuously oscillating luminance of the stimulus, and the observer is not expected to make his judgment until he has viewed the display for some time and his eye has come into equilibrium with respect to it.

There has also been some interest, though much less, in the study of flicker perception as a function of the number of pulses in the flicker train. Table 1 summarizes a number of such studies. Three of these are also summarized and discussed in PIÉRON'S (1961) monograph (translated by HURVICH and JAMESON, 1965). Despite a considerable variation in stimulus parameters, a general conclusion emerges from this work: the shorter the flash train, the longer must be the interval between pulses that is the required for flicker just to be perceived. Of specific interest here is the interstimulus interval (ISI[3]) for the limiting case of two flashes: PIÉRON concludes that ISI based on studies of just two flashes is about twice that obtained for a continuous series. He has suggested three factors to explain the apparent decrease of temporal resolution with decreasing number of pulses in the flicker train:

"The first is ... the facilitating influence of the increased duration of observation on perceptive discrimination ... The second ... is the progressive sinusoidal regularity of the wave of excitation potential whose own evolution becomes independent despite all dissymmetries of stimulation ... [and] a third factor ... is the progressive synchronization of periodic activities of a cellular ensemble ..."

A likely manifestation of the first factor is by way of probability summation: if we consider two separated pairs of pulses from a continuous flicker train and suppose that the chance of seeing flicker in either one of these is p, then the chance of seeing flicker in one or the other (or both) pairs increases to $1 - (1\text{-}p)^3$. With only two pulses there is only one chance to see flicker, while the probability of doing so increases with an increase in the number of chances afforded by progressively longer trains of pulses.

PIÉRON states that his second factor is the most important. This seems reasonable, particularly if the eye is relatively dark adapted before the flicker train is presented, which is true for all but one of the studies cited in Table 1. When the initial pulse is delivered to the dark-adapted eye, it may be expected to produce a large, and perhaps relatively long-lasting initial response, which should interfere with the response to the second pulse in the series. The repetitive series will eventually light-adapt the eye to the Talbot level (the mean luminance of the flickering stimulus) and regularize the responses to the individual pulses (see BOYNTON *et al.*, 1961). If the eye is light adapted prior to the onset of the flicker train, the effect should be greatly attenuated, although ANDERSON *et al.* find substantial improvement in temporal discrimination during the first 200 msec of exposure, even when the eye has pre-

[3] The "interstimulus interval" is the time elapsed between the offset of one pulse and the onset of the next.

viously been adapted to the level of the test pulses. A low-pass filter model such as that of LEVINSON (1968) (see his Fig. 7) shows that, with enough stages of filtering, this result is to be expected even when the eye has been initially light adapted to the Talbot level of the flicker train. PIÉRON'S third factor, although somewhat nebulous, does have a neurophysiological basis and has been particularly emphasized in the writings of BARTLEY (1941). (See also NELSON *et al.*, 1961.)

Table 1. *Studies of CFF as a function of the number of pulses in the flicker train, showing for a wide variety of conditions that flicker discrimination improves with increased numbers of pulses*

DUNLAP (1915)[b]
GRANIT and HAMMOND (1930)[a]
GRANIT and VON AMMON (1930)
BATTERSBY and JAFFEE (1953)[a, b]
MAHNEKE (1958b)[b]
NELSON, BARTLEY, and RANNEY (1961)[a]
NELSON, BARTLEY, and HARPER (1964)[a]
ANDERSON, HUNTINGTON, and SIMONSON (1966)[a]

[a] Studies for which detailed experimental conditions are listed by ANDERSON, HUNTINGTON, and SIMONSON (1966).
[b] Studies for which PIÉRON (1961) lists certain aspects of experimental conditions and results.

D. The Problem of Criterion in Two-Pulse Discrimination Experiments

1. Single Pulses Seen as Double

It has been recognized for a long time that a single pulse can sometimes be seen as double. DUNLAP (1915), in a study done in the old introspective tradition, remarked (p. 248) that a "... single flash is frequently seen as a succession of two, and although this 'twoness' may, under proper conditions, be discriminable from actual 'twoness,' these conditions are not easily actualized in quantitative work." Some of his results are shown in Table 2, where it will be noted that, for single pulses of 20 msec duration, double flashes were actually reported more often than single ones. Thus the fact that 15 of 20 double pulses of the same duration were seen "correctly" as double flashes when separated by 25 msec does not indicate that the subject could in fact usually distinguish two short pulses separated by this short interval: had only one of the pulses been presented, it would have been reported as double anyway, most of the time.

In a study concerned with "numerosity," CHEATHAM and WHITE (1952) presented flashes under light-adapted conditions and found that single flashes were *never* reported as double. When double flashes were presented, they obtained the results shown in Table 2. These data differ markedly from those of DUNLAP, particularly in that single flashes are much more often seen in response to double pulses at the shorter values of ISI.

Table 2. *Results of two studies of perceived number as a function of interpulse interval (ISI)*

Dunlap (1915): 2.5° centrally-fixated stimulus (dark adapted eye). Luminance 3 cd/m². Dark interval between double pulses = 25 msec.

Two pulses presented			One pulse presented		
pulse duration msec	No. flashes seen		pulse duration msec	No. flashes seen	
	double	single		double	single
50	26	4	106	3	23
50	16	4	80	4	16
30	18	2	60	2	18
20	15	5	40	4	16
10	15	5	20	11	9

Cheatham and White (1952): 25′ centrally-fixated stimulus (eye adapted to 1.8 ftL). Luminance: 1400 ftL. Flash duration: 11 msec.

Two pulses presented			One pulse presented		
ISI msec	No. flashes seen		pulse duration msec	No. flashes seen	
	double	single		double	single
88	50	0	11	0	200
55	45	5			
33	20	30			
22	6	44			

2. Criterion vs. Methodological Differences

A study by Bartley and Wilkinson (1953) helps somewhat to settle the issue of whether the differences between the two studies cited in Table 2 are attributable to differences of stimulus conditions, or to differences of the criterion adopted by the subjects for making their judgments. For a large combination of pulse durations and areas, Bartley and Wilkinson's subjects varied the intensity of a single pulse to determine a range within which two flashes were seen. With a stimulus area of 2-deg (similar to Dunlap's), double pulses were never seen, in agreement with Cheatham and White. Since Dunlap's subjects saw many double pulses under similar conditions, a criterion difference is suggested. Moreover, when using larger stimulus areas where double pulses could be seen, Bartley and Wilkinson found that shortening pulse duration reduced the probability of seeing the pulse as double – just the opposite of what Dunlap had found.

An alternative explanation of these differences makes use of the interpretation that Bartley and Wilkinson place upon their results. They conclude that the double flash phenomenon is attributable to simultaneous activation of the cone and rod systems. Because of a differential latency of the two systems, the cone signal is transmitted first, followed by that from rods. This interpretation seems plausible for their mesopic pulse luminances and larger areas, because the appropriate latency differences are known to exist between cone and rod vision. Failure to see double flashes for the 2-deg pulse could then be attributed to the negligible stimulation of rods by this relatively small, foveal stimulus. DUNLAP'S stimulus was not very much larger, being about 2.5-deg compared to BARTLEY and WILKINSON'S 2-deg. But the extra half degree of diameter increases stimulus area by more than fifty percent, and brings in an area of the retina that is much richer in rods. Further, it is possible that the control of fixation was more casual in the older work of DUNLAP. Provisionally, then, it may be concluded that double flashes will not be seen in response to single pulses, provided that care is taken to stimulate only the photopic (cone) system.

3. Forced Choice: Not a Solution

KIETZMAN and SUTTON (1968) attempted to clarify the criterion problem by using a forced choice technique. Subjects were presented with four stimuli, separated by one and one-half seconds. Three of these were single pulses lasting 4 msec each. The fourth, which could occur in any except the first temporal position, was a double pulse. Its two components, each lasting 2 msec, were separated by variable amounts. They found that the temporal forced choice permitted a correct discrimination 50 pct of the time (after chance correction) when the ISI was only about 30 msec, and this is less than half the interval required for the subject to report "two flashes" half the time using a subjective criterion of "oneness" vs. "twoness."

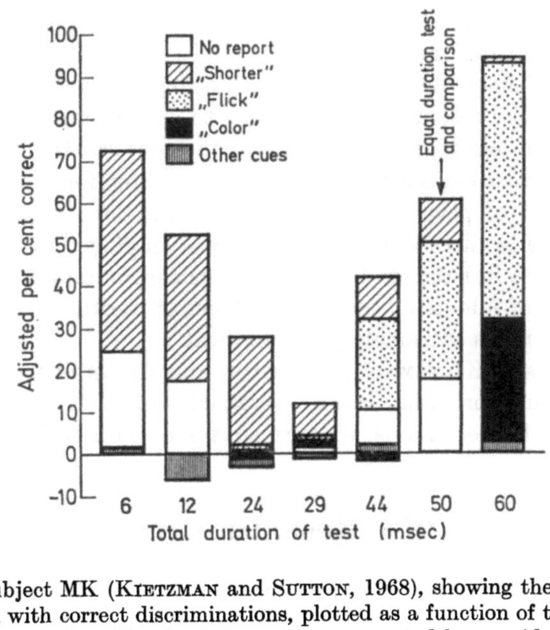

Fig. 1. Data of subject MK (KIETZMAN and SUTTON, 1968), showing the distribution of cue reports associated with correct discriminations, plotted as a function of the total duration of the two-pulse test stimulus. The shaded areas are computed by considering first just those trials on which a particular cue was reported (e.g., "flick") and then by determining what percentage of those trials was correctly reported. This value is then weighted according to the proportion of trials on which that cue was used, and a portion of the bar is shaded accordingly. Negative values indicate the use of a cue that is more often associated with incorrect than with correct responses. The adjusted percent correct is represented by the algebraic sum of the positive and negative heights

A difficulty with such forced choice experiments is that the cues used by the subject to make his discrimination are not necessarily the ones that the experimenter is interested in, or thinks that he is examining. A double-pulse package may differ from a single one because of a "double" appearance, but it may also appear as a single flash that flickers, is longer, brighter, or of different color than the comparison. To investigate this, KIETZMAN and SUTTON (1968) utilized cue reports. A 50 msec comparison stimulus was compared to equal-energy test stimulus pairs of 2 msec duration and variable temporal separation. Results for one subject are shown in Fig. 1, where the height of the bars represents the adjusted percent correct, and the shading depicts the distribution of cue reports associated with accurate discriminations. It will be seen that, for this subject, a condition does exist where almost all cues for discrimination are eliminated. This occurs when the two pulses are separated by 25 msec. Note that there are a number of correct discriminations for which no cue report is given: the subject discriminates somehow, but cannot report the basis of this discrimination.

4. Summary

KIETZMAN and SUTTON summarize their work with the discouraging observation (p. 300) that "... the presentation of two pulses of light separated by a brief and variable interpulse interval is not a sufficient set of operations to measure temporal resolution." The use of forced choice procedures, as we have seen, creates its own set of problems. Failure to use such procedures raises the spectre of uncontrolled variation in criterion from one subject and/or study to another, or even in the same subject at different times. ANLIKER (1966), who found systematic changes in the threshold for two-pulse resolution that seemed to depend upon the voltage of the alpha rhythm of the electroencephalogram, concludes (p. 318) that his findings "... indicate that great caution is required in controlling for the level of alertness in the measurement of psychological thresholds and in the assessment of performance, especially in cases where the procedures employed in the study tend to encourage drowsiness in subjects because of isolation, immobilization, and boredom. The absence of adequate controls on level of alertness renders the interpretation of such studies extremely problematical."

The admonitions of KIETZMAN and SUTTON and ANLIKER are well taken, and yet meaningful results probably can be obtained with well-trained subjects and sufficient numbers of observations. We turn next to a consideration of such studies.

E. Two-Pulse Resolution Thresholds

1. The Importance of Proper Measurement of the Time between Pulses

MAHNEKE (1958a) studied the shortest-perceptible dark interval between two easily-visible light pulses. His observers, who were light adapted for 10 minutes before the experiment started, observed the pulses within a 1-degree dark hole.

In the first of his experiments, the paired pulses were varied together in duration over a range from 1 to 300 msec. The results are shown in Fig. 2. The solid curve, which plots the data as MAHNEKE did, shows that the length of the just-perceptible dark interval (ISI) decreases monotonically over the range investigated. But a very different impression is gained from the same data if the onset-to-onset times (SOA)[4] are plotted instead (dotted curve). When this is done, there is only a slight change in SOA for the shorter durations, followed by a marked *increase* when pulse duration exceeds 20 msec.

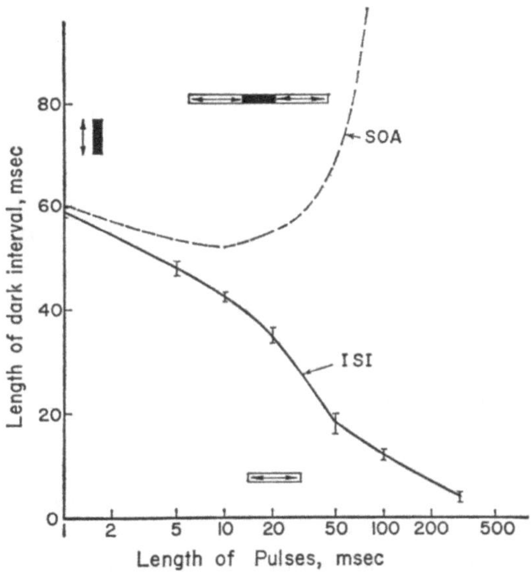

Fig. 2. The lower curve, after MAHNEKE (1958a), shows that the interstimulus interval (ISI), or dark period between two light pulses, decreases as the length of the pulses increases. (The two pulses are always of the same duration.) The same data may be plotted in terms of stimulus onset asynchrony (SOA), by adding the length of the pulse to that of the ISI required for two-pulse discrimination. When this is done, the upper curve results. An argument is presented in the text that, for the shorter pulse durations, the upper curve is a better index of two-pulse resolution than is the lower one. The vertical columns of the lower curve indicate twice the standard error of the mean; these values would be unchanged as applied to the the upper curve

Which measure should we accept as an estimate of the temporal resolving power of the eye? Does temporal resolution markedly improve as pulse duration is increased from 1 to 20 msec, as MAHNEKE concludes, or is it relatively constant, as the use of the SOA measure suggests? Beyond 20 msec, does temporal resolution get better, or worse?

For short pulses on the order of 20 msec or less, the following preliminary arguments can be marshalled in favor of using the SOA measure:

(1) The visual responses to these short pulses can be expected to have no distinct onset vs. offset, as would be true for longer pulses (see Section F). In MAHNEKE'S experiment, because the two pulses are equal in luminance and duration, each should produce the same response, except for possible adaptive and/or masking effects of the one upon the other. (Although such interactions are possible, they are probably not severe for the temporal separation of pulses that is required

[4] Meaning "stimulus onset asynchrony," a term introduced into the visual literature by KAHNEMAN (1968).

for their discrimination as "double.") If the two pulses do produce the same response, then the judgment of their timing must be with respect to some defining landmark that is common to each. Whatever this landmark is – onset, peak magnitude, or something else – SOA can be used to represent the asynchrony between any two such common landmarks of identical responses.

(2) If the two light pulses of the same duration are considered as the first pair of a flicker train, there will necessarily be a reciprocal relation between their SOA and the fundamental frequency of flicker as determined by Fourier analysis. If the light-dark-ratio (LDR) of the flickering stimulus is small, changing it will change the appearance of the stimulus very little, provided that luminance is adjusted to keep pulse energy (and thus the adaptive state of the eye) from varying with LDR. This is equivalent to saying that, if the adaptation level of the eye is controlled, then the fundamental frequency of the flickering stimulus (by Fourier analysis) predicts its appearance. This conception, first elucidated by De Lange (1954), has proved correct and has cleared up a great deal of ambiguity in the flicker literature which had been caused by measuring the characteristics of the stimulus in ways that obscured essential relationships. The use of ISI seems to have produced a similar problem in the case of two-pulse experiments. It is surprising, in a way, how the choice of metric can be so important. In one sense, the information is the same whether ISI or SOA is specified: after all, given one measure the other can easily be calculated from it. But in another sense, the information supplied is very different, since one way of looking at the problem may lead to insight while the other generates confusion. If the results of such an experiment were described in terms of the ISI between the first two pulses, this measure would change system-

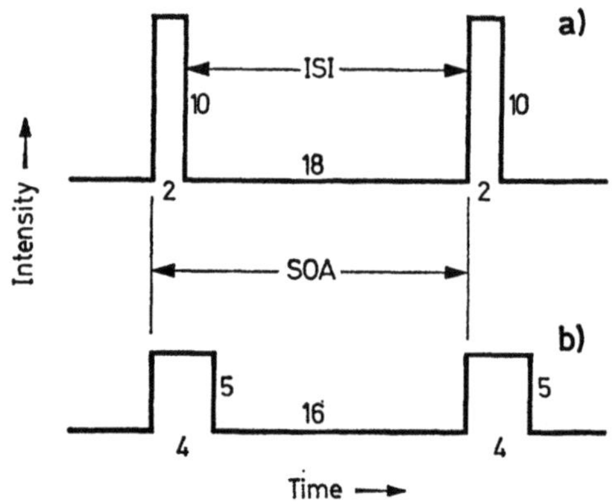

Fig. 3. Each of the pulses in the illustration has been drawn to contain 20 units of energy (intensity x time). The shorter pulses in (a), if considered as the first two pulses of a flicker train will (if near the threshold for flicker) resemble in appearance the two longer pulses in (b). This can be predicted after De Lange (1954) from a Fourier analysis of (a) and (b) which would yield the same steady-state component, the same fundamental frequency (50 Hz) and very nearly the same modulation amplitude. If stimulus-onset asynchrony (SOA) is used to describe the timing of the pulses, it will have the same value for (a) and (b) and will therefore correlate correctly with the very similar appearance of (a) and (b). On the other hand, if inter-stimulus interval (ISI) is used, the values will be different in the two cases (18 msec in (a) and only 16 msec in (b)), and if adjusted to have the same ISI, would produce a different appearance

atically with LDR although the sensation produced would not. SOA, being independent of LDR, therefore correlates much better with what is seen. This argument is illustrated with an example in Fig. 3.

Additional evidence in support of the two arguments just stated will be given in Section 6 where on- and off-responses will be considered in more detail.

2. Two Long Bright Pulses Become One Short Dark Pulse

For very long pairs of pulses MAHNEKE's use of ISI seems preferable to SOA. Consider, as a limiting example, a case where the first pulse has been present for a very long time, sufficient to allow the visual system to reach a steady-state of adaptation and a stable response. It will now make no difference exactly when the first stimulus was turned on, since that event will have happened so long ago that the only significant event will occur when it is turned *off*. What is now produced can best be characterized as a *dark pulse*, a momentary interruption of a prevailing adaptive state. Such a dark flash in many ways resembles a light flash of the same duration and amplitude, provided that the latter is superposed upon the same adapting level. BLACKWELL (1946) was the first to show clearly that positive and negative contrast thresholds, so defined, are nearly the same. HERRICK (1956) and CLARK and PICKETT (1959) found intensity-time reciprocity relations for dark pulses that turned out to be very similar to those for bright ones: moreover, RASHBASS (1970) has shown that, if a large field is used, one cannot even tell the difference between bright and dark pulses of the same low amplitude; he and IKEDA (1965) have independently shown that responses to bright and dark pulses differ mostly in their phase relationships (see Section G3, p. 225). Thus, the limiting case of MAHNEKE's experiment is actually concerned not with two pulses but with only one. MAHNEKE's intermediate conditions are, of course, the most difficult to analyze, as there must be some kind of gradual transition from the case of two positive pulses to that of a single negative one.

3. Effect of Pulse Duration

In a second experiment by MAHNEKE (1958a), instead of keeping the durations of the first and second pulses the same, he varied them in 36 combinations over a range from 1 to 50 msec. The results are given in Table 3, specified (as he did it) in terms of ISI. Values are also given for the same data, recalculated in terms of SOA (values in parentheses). A difficulty with this experiment is that, by keeping the luminance of all flashes the same, their energy content necessarily varies directly with duration. Arguments in favor of using SOA as a measure have already been advanced for the case of equal energy flashes, but it is less clear whether they apply with equal force to the case now being considered.

Table 3 includes a set of conditions similar to those used in MAHNEKE's first experiment, those along the upper-left to lower-right diagonal that embraces all cases where the two pulses were of the same duration. According to the arguments already advanced, these values should be about the same for SOA, but should vary much more for ISI. This is in fact the case: for ISI, the mean value is 39.10 and the standard deviation (SD) is 13.21, while for SOA, the mean is 53.68 and the SD is only 6.80.

Table 3. *Results of an experiment by* MAHNEKE *(1958a). Values given in the table represent threshold of temporal resolution in msec. Those not in parentheses are values of interstimulus interval (ISI) as given by* MAHNEKE; *those in parentheses are for stimulus onset asynchrony (SOA) and are obtained in each case by adding the duration of pulse 1 to the ISI value reported by* MAHNEKE

Duration of pulse 1, msec	Duration of pulse 2, msec: 1	2	5	10	20	50
1	53.6 (54.6)	53.7 (54.7)	53.3 (54.3)	53.2 (54.2)	52.8 (53.8)	51.4 (52.4)
2	52.0 (54.0)	49.3 (51.3)	48.2 (50.2)	45.6 (47.6)	46.0 (48.0)	49.9 (51.9)
5	56.5 (61.5)	48.0 (53.0)	42.3 (47.3)	42.9 (47.9)	41.2 (46.2)	39.2 (44.2)
10	65.3 (75.3)	51.0 (61.0)	41.0 (51.0)	38.5 (48.5)	41.2 (51.2)	36.6 (46.6)
20	71.8 (91.8)	60.4 (80.4)	41.2 (61.2)	38.3 (58.3)	34.8 (54.2)	32.3 (52.3)
50	64.1 (114.1)	55.4 (105.4)	36.5 (86.5)	29.3 (79.3)	23.7 (73.7)	16.1 (66.2)

Table 4. *Calculations from the results of* MAHNEKE'S *experiment (1958a), derived from the data given in Table* 3

Duration ratio of Pulse 1 : Pulse 2	Number of Cases	Mean values ISI	Mean values SOA	Standard deviations ISI	Standard deviations SOA
20 : 1	2	63.60	98.60	11.60	9.62
10 : 1	3	54.07	80.73	15.41	5.61
5 : 1	4	44.50	65.75	11.95	9.04
2 : 1	5	40.60	58.00	10.91	9.17
1 : 1	6	39.10	53.68	13.21	6.80
1 : 2	5	43.66	51.26	8.02	2.52
1 : 5	4	44.18	48.68	7.11	3.80
1 : 10	3	46.13	48.80	7.00	5.00
1 : 20	2	51.35	52.85	2.05	1.34

These ratios are not exactly the same along some of the diagonals of Table 1. 20 : 1 also includes 25 : 1, 2 : 1 includes 2.5 : 1, 1 : 2 includes 1 : 2.5; and 1 : 20 includes 1 : 25.

Other conditions also lend themselves to relevant analysis on the assumption that equal ratios of intensities produce similar visual effects. Moving up and to the right in the table, the next diagonal specifies conditions in which the second flash has about twice (in some cases, two and one-half times) as much duration and energy as the first. If SOA is again the more appropriate measure, and if there is no interaction between the two responses, SOA should once again be approximately the same for these conditions. In this case, the standard deviation for ISI is 8.02, for SOA, only 2.52.

Table 4 shows the complete matrix of SD's for the ISI and SOA measures. In every case, the SD is less for SOA than for ISI. It may also be noted that the means and SD's are larger, for both measures, when the longer flash precedes the shorter, compared to the converse. There appear to be at least two possible reasons for this, which are difficult to sort out. The first is that the more energetic first flash has an adaptive effect upon the weaker second one, and that the magnitude of this effect depends upon the energy contained in the first. The second possibility is that the first response lasts long enough to permit the development of an off-response to it. This could increase the persistence of the response to the first flash, requiring a longer interval, relative to first-flash onset, before the second flash could be perceived as such. When the longer flash comes second,this problem would be minimized. The data of Table 4 are consistent with the latter argument, but there is no way completely to rule out the first possibility. Finally, it appears that the variance calculated along any of the diagonals of the table is significantly greater than the error variance of the experiment, which can be estimated from the vertical bars of Fig. 1 as being between 1 and 2 msec.

In a more recent study, KIETZMAN (1967) also concluded that increasing pulse duration lowered resolution thresholds. He also used ISI as the dependent variable. The writer has done a reanalysis of KIETZMAN'S data, similar to that already reported in detail for MAHNEKE, with the same kind of result: if onset-to-onset (SOA) had been used instead of ISI, then the opposite conclusion would be drawn, namely that better temporal discrimination results from shorter, not longer, test pulses. For KIETZMAN'S shortest pulses of 4 and 27 msec, there was little difference between the threshold SOA's, as would be expected from the foregoing arguments.

LEWIS (1968), using a forced-choice procedure, has conducted systematic investigations of foveal two-pulse thresholds as a joint function of luminance and area. The pulses used were of 1 msec duration; the ranges covered were from 2 to 200 mL and from 5 to 30 min of arc. He found that thresholds decrease by approximately a factor of two with increasing luminance, with somewhat greater changes occurring for the larger areas. In an earlier study (LEWIS, 1967) large changes were also found for a 30-min pulse, when luminance was varied over a wider range (from 0.32 to 1000 mL). The largest part of the change occurred between 0.32 and 1.0 mL.

F. Experiments with Spatially Non-Contiguous Stimuli

1. Psychophysical Estimates of Responses to Light Pulses

Because the responses of the visual system certainly do not exactly copy the temporal characteristics of the stimulus, it is impossible to understand the phenomena being discussed in this chapter without making reference to *responses* of the visual system – whether real, imagined, or modeled – that are triggered by double-pulse stimuli. Reference to such responses has in fact already been made; the time has come to deal with them explicitly.

In this volume on visual psychophysics, it would be inappropriate to go into great detail concerning the relevant physiological evidence. Suffice it to say that, by using a wide variety of recording techniques, and by tapping into many stages of the visual system, responses are usually found which (1) have a definite latency between the presentation of the stimulus and the beginning of the response; (2) begin slowly, reach a peak frequency or amplitude, and then decline; (3) appear much the same in character if triggered by brief stimuli of differing duration but constant energy; (4) last longer than the pulses that produced them, particularly so when such pulses are brief.

It has often been assumed that physiological data will offer a more direct and easily interpretable record of such responses than could conceivably be obtained through psychophysical procedures alone. Reasonable as this sounds, it is not necessarily true.

Consider, as an example, the case of electrophysiological responses to flickering stimuli, that are recorded in the conventional electroretinogram (ERG). Numerous attempts have been made to show that a particular response is, or is not, capable of following the undulations of the stimulus. When it is found that the ERG is capable of following frequencies higher than CFF, one would immediately like to know whether the residual components of the ERG that follow the stimulus are actually in the direct chain of events leading to sensation, or whether the response is an epiphenomenon of some sort. On the other hand, if the response does *not* follow the stimulus, then one must ask whether a more sensitive recording technique, such as signal averaging, would be able to show following. Then if averaging techniques are used, even more stringent controls must be used to show that the recorded signal is not itself an artifact of some kind. There are other problems perhaps even more fundamental. Especially at those stages of the visual system where information is encoded in terms of spike frequency, it is wrong to assume that temporal variations in the stimulus will necessarily be encoded in some obvious way — for example, as similar variations in the running average of spike frequency — since a much more complex coding scheme may in fact be employed by the visual system. There is the further problem, in single-unit recording, of a very small sample of the much larger population of elements that must be contributing to the psychophysical result. Finally it must be emphasized that an electrophysiological record is never a sensation, and although it is also true that a verbal report of a sensation also should not be identified with the sensation itself, the verbal report does seem a step closer. The experimenter can, if he chooses, experience the sensation for himself and make the same reports as his other subjects, putting the same restrictions upon his verbalizations that have been applied to other subjects. If data from many subjects tend to agree with his own, then the experimenter is probably justified in concluding that, in some sense at least, the sensations of these other subjects probably were not very different from his own.

In any event, psychophysical inferences about responses to homogeneous double flashes will be emphasized in this section.

2. On- and Off-Responses

In 1947, Crawford published a now-classic study wherein he used a test stimulus (TS) as a probe to evaluate sensitivity changes in the visual system that were induced by a longer, larger, and brighter conditioning stimulus (CS). Boynton and Kandel (1957) attempted to show that this technique could be used to evaluate "on-responses" in the visual system. We argued that the record of log test-flash threshold, as this varied with time, resembled a physiological response in the visual system. We demonstrated that, in reaction to a CS of fixed luminance, such responses changed systematically as the adaptational state of the eye was manipulated. In another study, Onley and Boynton (1962) demonstrated that on-responses, so recorded, were of approximately equal magnitude when generated by equally-bright stimuli whose physical luminances, due to varying states of adaptation of the eye, were unequal. Although Sperling (1965) later analyzed these same data and showed that they could be accounted for equally as well in another way that made no use of the idea of on-responses, the concept has prevailed in our laboratory and has been applied to the study of stimuli that are relevant to the discussions of the present chapter.

3. Relative Latencies of Pulses Having Unequal Durations

BOYNTON and SIEGFRIED (1962) addressed themselves to the following questions: (1) Will the on-responses to a pair of brief CS pulses, each of the same energy but differing in duration, be of the same shape and magnitude? (The answer is yes.) (2) What is the relative "latency" of these responses? This second question is a difficult one to conceptualize properly. For one thing, the onset of the test stimulus used to record the psychophysical on-response begins *before* the onset of the background stimulus that influences it. This phenomenon, now known as "backward masking" has been verified in dozens of laboratories and had been clearly observed and explicitly discussed by CRAWFORD (1947). If only relative latencies are at issue, the problem can be circumvented, and it is best ignored for the moment.

It is possible to make psychophysical estimates of the time elapsed between the stimulus and the sensation induced. FRÖHLICH called this the "Empfindungszeit," and developed a method that was used in a careful study by MITA *et al.* (1950) to measure it as a function of state of adaptation and the part of the retina stimulated. The method makes use of the fact that, if a light is briefly flashed while the eyes are moving, it will be seen offset from its actual position, in the direction of the eye movement. (The phenomenon is quite easy to observe by sweeping the eyes across a television picture in a darkened room.) If the rate of eye movement is known, the Empfindungszeit can be calculated from the apparent location in visual space of the displaced image. The values obtained by MITA *et al.* ranged from about 60 to more than 300 msec. They were found to be independent of the speed of the eye movement that had been induced by using constant velocity stimuli that could be tracked. Values were lowest in the fovea, and increased, for stimuli of constant luminance, with light adaptation. Although the latter seems contrary to what is often reported in the electrophysiological literature for response latencies, the usual procedure in those cases is to increase the intensity of the stimulus, in the light adapted eye, until it produces the response of the same magnitude as that obtained under dark-adapted conditions. This is not what was done in the psychophysical experiment just described, as MITA *et al.* did not vary the intensity of their test stimulus. It seems very likely that the Empfindungszeit would decrease with increasing test intensity.

What is meant anyway by the relative latencies of responses to stimuli whose durations differ? Most workers seem to have uncritically accepted the onset of the stimulus as the proper point in time from which to make such a measurement, and yet upon reflection there seems to be no better basis for doing this than for using offset, midstimulus interval, or some other arbitrary criterion – each of which will of course yield a different answer[5].

---

[5] A very recent example is a study by GROSSBERG (1970), who was concerned specifically with the response latencies to double-pulse stimuli as assessed by reaction time measurements. Latency is not specifically defined in his abstract or in the legends to any of the figures; although clearly defined in his *Method* section as being measured from first-stimulus onset, no particular justification is given for the choice. Moreover, what is given on the graphs as "interflash interval" turns out to be, upon inspection, SOA. These facts are mentioned, not in criticism of GROSSBERG (whose experiment is very significant and will be discussed in Section G 2, p. 224) but to point up the fact that the matter of definition of temporal relationships, which is being given special attention in this chapter, seem not to have been widely pondered.

BOYNTON and SIEGFRIED reasoned that, if the records of identical on-responses to stimuli of unequal duration were superimposed, then the placement in time of the two stimuli would provide an indication, at least for the specific case under investigation, of the appropriate stimulus landmarks for measuring the latencies of responses to such stimuli. The answer, which is not a simple one, is illustrated in Fig. 4. With respect to the longer stimulus, the shorter one must be delayed to the intermediate extent shown, in order for the on-responses to superpose. Thus, if onset were used as the landmark, the response to the shorter stimulus would have the shorter latency, but if offset were used, that to the longer one would instead. This should be seen as very reminiscent of the problem of choosing between SOA and ISI that was discussed in Section E1, p. 208.

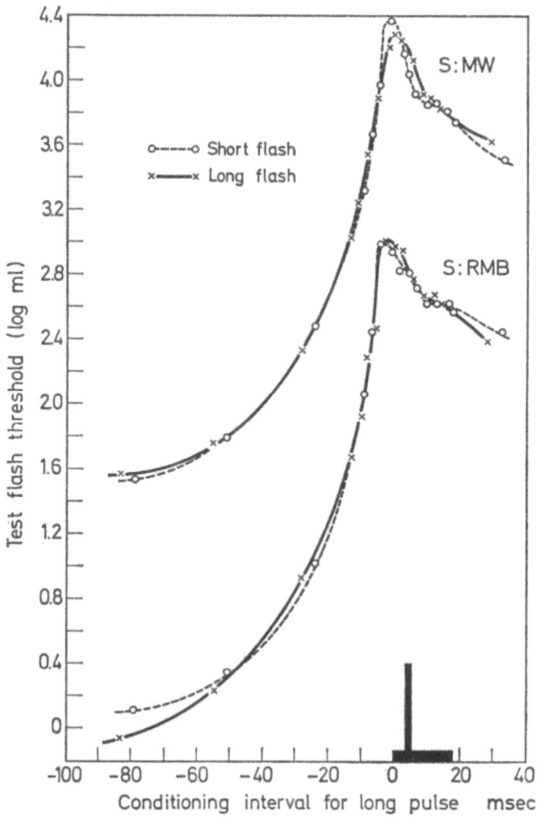

Fig. 4. In this experiment (BOYNTON and SIEGFRIED, 1962), "on responses" to brief stimuli of different duration but equal energy were assessed using the increment-threshold technique. The stimuli were cycled slowly enough to keep the eye in a relatively dark-adapted state. Luminance of a 1-deg foveal test pulse required for threshold visibility (ordinate) was determined upon each of the 2-deg conditioning pulses. The conditioning interval (abscissa) is the time elapsed between the onset of the longer conditioning pulse and the onset of the test pulse. The position of the threshold curve for the shorter conditioning pulse has been adjusted horizontally to superpose the two functions. The curves for subject MW have been raised one log unit to avoid overlapping of curves from the separate subjects.

For nearly a year before the BOYNTON and SIEGFRIED experiment was done the writer asked a large number of vision scientists to predict the outcome. Those questioned responded in the following ways: (a) Some did not understand the experiment, and/or failed to see why anyone would want to do it. (b) Some understood the experiment but honestly stated that they had no basis upon which to predict the outcome. (c) Most predicted that the stimuli would have simultaneous onsets. (d) A few opted for simultaneous offsets. (e) H. R. BLACKWELL correctly predicted that the shorter stimulus would have to be positioned about a third of the way between the beginning and the end of the longer one. BLACKWELL's prediction came from his temporal element theory (BLACKWELL, 1963), modified by a suspicion on his part that the elemental responses were probably not exactly symmetrical in time, as he had assumed for convenience in making his calculations.

In another study, BOYNTON *et al.* (1961) demonstrated that responses to a continuously flickering stimulus could also be measured in this way. An important demonstration in this experiment was that, under conditions where flicker was not clearly perceptible, the increment threshold continued to wax and wane with the light and dark stimulus phase, indicative of responses of the visual system which themselves were below the threshold of direct perception; yet these could be revealed by psychophysical investigation (see also BATTERSBY and STURR, 1970). For suprathreshold flickering stimuli, we also demonstrated that the first response to a train of stimuli following a dark interval was indeed inordinately large and tended to swamp the second response, and that these variations were themselves superposed upon a grosser wave of on-response, one that resembled what a steady light, presented after a dark interval, would produce. In other words, the system appears to integrate the effects of several successive pulses, while at the same time responding to some extent to the "fine grain" of temporal fluctuation produced by the individual pulses. IKEDA and BOYNTON (1965) carried this work a step further in a study designed to determine, among other things, how long a light must be left on before it is capable of producing an off-response. (Off-responses are observable in CRAWFORD's original data as a threshold rise that occurs just before a rapid threshold drop at the termination of the CS. BAKER (1953) later confirmed the phenomenon in studies of early dark adaptation.) IKEDA and BOYNTON found that a stimulus must remain on for at least 40 msec before it is capable of generating a discrete off-response. This is an important conclusion because it suggests that, for pulses of this duration or shorter (whose energy is more-or-less fully integrated by the eye), there really are not distinct on- and off-responses as such. There are simply responses. Although the response events last for a considerable time in excess of the stimuli that produced them, they nevertheless constitute unitary reactions to the total flux content of the pulse, and have an amplitude over time that carries no revelation of separable components for on vs. off. PIÉRON (1961) advanced a very similar argument in his monograph.

Using the psychophysical technique just described, STURR (1961) studied the responses of the eye to double pulses of light (each of 75 msec), as a function of the temporal separation between them. Some of his results are shown in Fig. 5 from which the following observations can be made. (1) For the longest separation used (125 msec), the response to the second flash appears identical in shape to that of the first, except that the temporal separation is not sufficient to allow a full return of the first response to the baseline. The peak (or any other landmark) of the second response occurs 200 msec after that of the first, which is the SOA rather than the

ISI, again suggesting that the SOA measure is the more appropriate, as argued in the previous section. (2) There appears to be no significant interaction between the two responses at this long interval, since the height and shapes of those parts of the responses that can be discriminated in the record are very nearly identical, and only where they overlap does the response appear to be determined by a weighted

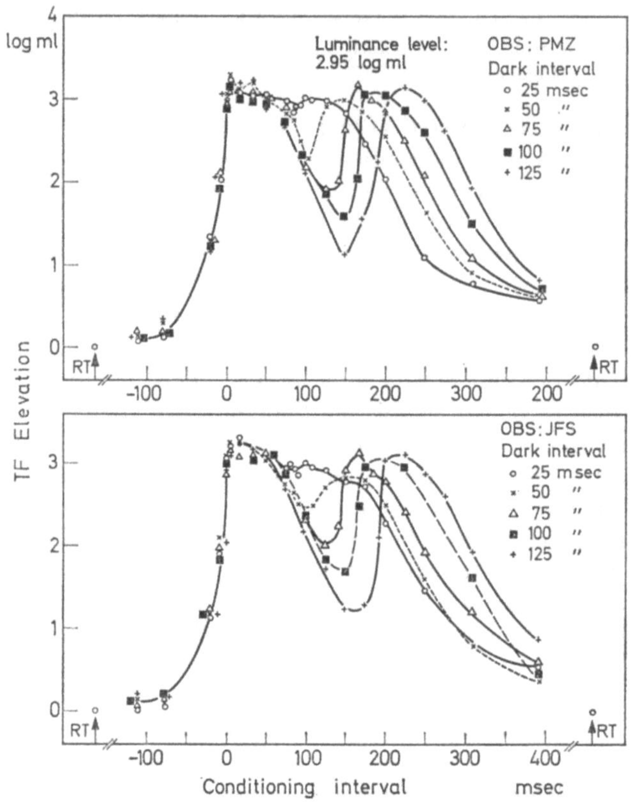

Fig. 5. Some results from the thesis of Sturr (1961). Threshold fluctuations (ordinate) are plotted as a function of the conditioning interval, defined as the time between the onset of the first pulse and the onset of the test probe. Two conditioning pulse were used: these were each of 75 msec duration and were separated by the dark interval indicated on the graph

sum of the two. (3) At an ISI of 150 msec, a very slight interaction appears to be developing: the peak of the second response is at about the same height as the first, but its shape is different, falling more abruptly on the descending side; the trough has begun to fill up and the basis for the discrimination of one flash vs. two has become a bit less. (4) This trend continues until finally, at the shortest separation used (ISI = 25 msec, SOA = 100 msec), there is only a trace of double quality about the response, and it would be expected that these flashes, and others more closely separated, would seem to last longer than the response to only one of the double pulses. It will be recalled from Section D 3, p. 207 that the cue of subjective duration was often employed in the forced-choice experiments of KIETZMAN and SUTTON in order to generate a "correct" response.

A number of studies have been done showing a dichoptic effect in visual masking with homogeneous flashes (WAGMAN and BATTERSBY, 1959; KANDEL, 1958; BATTERSBY *et al.*, 1964). This is a relatively small effect, capable of raising increment thresholds by a factor of two or three at the most. The dichoptic effect saturates at very low luminances of the conditioning stimulus, and the limits have never been properly established. This masking, presumably of cortical origin, probably adds to the retinal effect under monocular conditions. There is however no proper way to assess the quantitative contribution. It can be argued that it must be very small under most conditions because the threshold of the test flash, under monoptic conditions, is usually hundreds or even thousands of times higher than for the dichoptic case. Thus if the monoptic threshold flash were presented instead to the opposite eye it would appear very bright and it seems unlikely that the CS in the other eye would significantly alter its effectiveness.

4. A Possible Physiological Correlate

It has been implied in the preceding discussion that on-responses, as recorded psychophysically, reflect primarily activity that occurs early in the visual system and which therefore should provide input to more central stages where discrimination of oneness vs. twoness takes place. At the time this idea was originally proposed, little was known about the early stages of response in the primate eye, other than what had been inferred from the gross electroretinogram, which is a very complex record that is hard to interpret. The receptors themselves now seem to be a possible locus, because records from them, in the form of the late receptor potential (BROWN *et al.*, 1965), reflect the changing adaptive state of the eye which in turn limits the size of an increment response (BOYNTON and WHITTEN, 1970). Fig. 6 shows a record from BROWN *et al.* (1965) of late receptor potential of the cynomolgus macaque monkey in response to a very brief, bright flash. Note that, after 20 msec, it still has not quite returned to the baseline. Thus it represents a filtered version, at the receptor level, of the stimulus waveform. As a function of stimulus intensity, such receptor potentials do not vary in waveform, but only in amplitude. They are believed to represent the synchronized summation of many very tiny responses, each one the contribution of an individual receptor. Also shown in Fig. 6 is the impulse response as deduced psychophysically by SPERLING (1965), using very brief test and conditioning stimuli. Note that the psychophysical response also varies primarily in amplitude with changes in stimulus intensity. Whenever the responses to the conditioning and test stimuli overlap, there should be an adaptive effect of the conditioning stimulus upon the test, reducing its contribution to the total response. The maximum overlap will occur with simultaneous onset of the two stimuli, since only at that time will there be a complete coincidence in waveform. The total time interval over which SPERLING'S masking effect takes place is however greater than what would be expected on the basis of the temporal characteristics of the late receptor potential.

This analysis is not inconsistent with a similar one offered by SPERLING himself, provided that it can be demonstrated, as it has not yet been, that equal energy pulses of 40 to 50 msec or less all yield late receptor potentials of approximately the same size. Further research will also be needed to determine whether the timing relations found in the BOYNTON and SIEGFRIED experiment can be accounted for at this level, but this seems a likely possibility. The interpretation is also consistent with the temporal element contribution theory of BLACKWELL (1963).

Another argument in favor of a very peripheral basis for the psychophysical on-response is the unusually high precision of experiments of this type. Note, for example, the regularity and the high degree of agreement between the two sets of

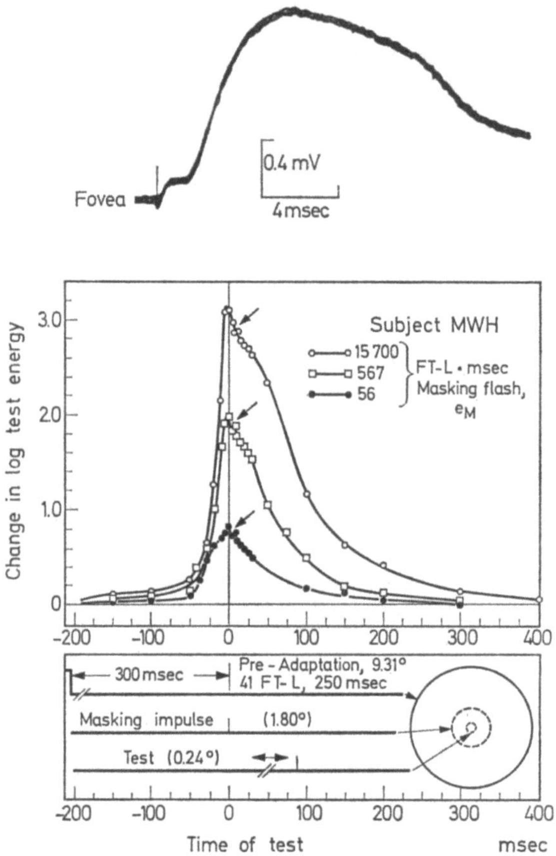

Fig. 6. (Bottom) Impulse masking functions as determined by SPERLING (1965) using very brief conditioning and test stimuli having the spatial configuration shown. (Top) Impulse response of the receptors of the cynomolgus macaque monkey (the late receptor potential) from BROWN *et al.* (1965)

data reported by BOYNTON and SIEGFRIED in Fig. 4, and by STURR in Fig. 5. Experiments by BATTERSBY and his colleagues and by SPERLING yield the same kind of highly reproducible results. Replications of findings between laboratories have also proved to be very easy, especially when compared with masking studies of the sort that involve patterned stimuli and more complex discriminations[6]. The

[6] For a review of the masking literature, which could not be covered here, see a book of readings by HABER (1969). Of particular relevance to this chapter is the paper by KAHNEMAN (1968), which is included in HABER's collection. (See also WEISSTEIN, chapter 10, this volume.)

precision of whatever is happening is nowhere better illustrated than during the rapidly rising phase of the on-response. For the conditions encountered in a study by KINTZ and BOYNTON (1969), the threshold rise of the test probe was found to be about 10 per cent per millisecond. In that study, we introduced double *test* pulses, and delivered them during the rising phase of the on-response to a single CS. The results indicated that, if the varying sensitivity of the eye, at the time of presentation of each pulse, were first taken into account, then the double test pulses summated exactly. This requirement for first weighting the responses very precisely according to the momentary sensitivity of the eye, before the responses can summate, would fit well with the idea that the weighting is done at the receptor level.

5. Simultaneity

EFRON (1970) did the following experiment. Two circular homogeneous fields, each about a degree and a half in diameter, were separated horizontally by 6° 16′. A fixation point bisected this distance. The two fields were pulsed in succession; the object of the experiment was to determine the ISI at which the *offset* of the first pulse appeared simultaneous with the *onset* of the second one. In the first of two studies of concern here, the duration of the first pulse was set at 500 msec while that of the second was varied systematically from 10 to 500 msec. In a second experiment, the first pulse was varied in duration while the second was fixed at 500 msec. The results are shown in Table 5, expressed in terms of ISI (as EFRON did it), and also for SOA, calculated from the ISI values reported by EFRON. The main point to be noted from the results of EFRON's first experiment is that the duration of the second stimulus is completely without effect upon ISI. This may be interpreted to mean that the subject was able to do as instructed, probably basing his judgment upon the separation between the off-response to pulse 1 and the on-response to pulse 2. In the second experiment, shortening the duration of

Table 5. *Results from the subjective simultaneity experiment of* EFRON *(1970). These results are from one subject; those from another subject are very similar in their main features, although the absolute values differ considerably*

Duration of variable	Experiment 1: second stimulus varied values in msec			Experiment 2: first stimulus varied values in mesec		
stimulus in msec	SOA	ISI	SD	SOA	ISI	SD
500	580.6	80.6	23.67	596.2	96.2	31.06
300	379.0	79.0	25.51	400.2	100.2	32.73
200	284.0	84.0	24.58	301.6	101.6	28.63
150	233.3	83.3	21.68	257.6	107.6	29.77
110	186.6	76.6	21.02	234.2	124.2	28.94
90	172.3	82.3	16.57	223.6	143.6	27.41
70	154.3	84.3	17.92	227.2	157.2	28.32
50	133.0	83.0	20.68	227.2	177.2	33.56
30	115.0	85.0	18.90	227.8	197.8	31.94
10	95.0	85.0	15.81	227.2	217.2	29.46

the first pulse had little effect upon ISI, provided that pulses were longer than about 150 msec. Again it may be inferred that the judgment was made on the same basis as in Experiment 1. For the shorter pulse durations, on the other hand, ISI decreases in direct proportion to the duration of the first pulse, meaning that SOA is constant over this range. This result may be interpreted to mean that the observer was no longer able to judge, as instructed, on the basis of an off-response to pulse 1. Based on the Boynton and Siegfried experiment, it could be argued that the SOA should have increased somewhat as pulse duration was shortened. But Efron did not compensate by increasing energy, and the small differences that would be predicted, even if he had, probably would be obscured by the intrinsic variance of simultaneity judgments, which is rather high.

The constant of ISI in Efron's first experiment might be taken to imply that the latency of the off-response to flash 1 was about 80 msec longer than that of the on-response to flash 2 which followed. It is not at all certain that this would be true for flashes of the same intensity and duration, if delivered to the same area of the retina. Efron did not control for possible differences in response speed for the two retinal locations used, and moreover the two flashes differed both in color and intensity. These considerations are not critical for the interpretation of his experiment offered here, nor for that matter for his own explanation which is quite different (as the title of his paper indicates, Efron was interested in the "Relationship between the duration of a stimulus and the duration of a perception").

G. Two-Pulse Interaction at Threshold

1. Single Pulses and Bloch's Law

In this final section, we turn our attention to the interaction of the responses to light pulses as they work together to determine a threshold probability of seeing. The most general form of such experiments permits the first and second pulses of the series to be varied both in sign and relative energy.

By "sign" is meant whether the pulse is positive-going or negative-going with respect to the adaptation level. In the two studies to be reviewed in detail in this section, Ikeda (1965) used test pulses that occupied only a small central part of the adapting field, whereas Rashbass (1970) eliminated the spatial cue entirely by utilizing, as Herrick (1956) had done earlier, a momentary variation in luminance of the entire field. Negative pulses of the sort that Ikeda used are technically difficult to produce, as it is not physically possible to superpose small decrements of light upon a background in the same easy way that works for increments. Many investigators today use the tachistoscope, wherein it is theoretically possible to produce negative pulses by momentarily replacing the adapting field with a test field of the same background luminance that has a dark spot in it. This is difficult — perhaps impossible — to do without artifact; some change in the background is often visible during the period of the interposed stimulus. Ikeda produced his negative pulses by starting with an annulus, then filling the hole with light from two other separate optical channels. By varying the ratio of the luminances of the latter, the removal of one component or the other produced a negative pulse of a pre-set and known amplitude. Some artifact was present in the form of a faint ring around the test area, but this was reduced well below the threshold of vision by superposing the entire pattern upon a much brighter fourth field. This technique was originally reported by Boynton *et al.* (1964), who used it to examine chromatic interactions at threshold between double pulses. Ikeda (1964) has subsequently extended this work on color which will not be reviewed here. An interesting study of the suprathreshold effect of color in the two-pulse situation is that of Keston (1965).

A limiting case of the two-pulse situation occurs as the energy of one of the pulses approaches zero. The single pulse that remains is often used as a reference condition against which thresholds for double pulses can be compared. A preliminary consideration of the behavior of single pulses at threshold is therefore useful as an introduction to this topic.

At threshold, Bloch's law (1885) of temporal summation has most often been tested with single, temporally-rectangular flashes. It is found that, within the so-called critical duration, $It = K$. (See BAUMGARDT, chapter 2, this volume.) The intensity term, I, relates to the rate of quantum incidence per unit area upon the region of the retina that is stimulated. If multiplied by the retinal area A and the duration t of the pulse, the resulting quantity is proportional to the total number of quanta in the pulse. Within certain limits, it makes no difference how the quanta are distributed in space or time, meaning that $IAt = K$. The limits over which this is true have been investigated with double pulses by VAN DEN BRINK and BOUMAN (1954). Within these limits, the eye acts as a quantum counter, and threshold appears to be reached when, for a given level of visual adaptation, some critical number of absorbed quanta is reached.

Although Bloch's law has often been identified with the Bunsen-Roscoe law that describes a similar behavior in photochemistry, this identification is misleading when applied to the visual case. BOYNTON (1961) and others have cited evidence showing that the photochemical events related to vision occur very rapidly, so that the rate of initial quantum absorption must follow the temporal configuration of the stimulus almost perfectly. Since the area of the stimulus may be varied considerably without altering the experimental result, it follows that the integration of response must occur somewhere beyond the receptor level, presumably as the result of some kind of neural summation. That the integration cannot generally occur in the receptors themselves is perhaps most obvious at the absolute threshold of vision, where the numbers of quanta are so small that the probability of a given receptor absorbing more than a single quantum is essentially zero (HECHT *et al.*, 1941).

Bloch's law has not yet been shown to have a lower limit. Three studies (BRINDLEY, 1952; GILMER, 1937; and BEAMS, 1934) have shown that there is no failure of the law (for a slightly suprathreshold criterion) at the shortest pulse durations that these experimenters could obtain, the shortest being 10^{-9} sec in GILMER's study. Failure of the law at still shorter durations is not to be expected on theoretical grounds, but no such tests seem to have been made, although the technical means for doing so are now available.

The upper limit of Bloch's law, which defines the critical duration, is much more controversial. The transition from complete to partial summation is a gradual one as pulse length increases. It is very hard to judge when a horizontal line describing It vs. t at threshold begins gently to depart from the baseline. In a classic study, GRAHAM and MARGARIA (1935) found the rate of such departure, and the critical duration as well, to be a marked function of the area of the test stimulus: critical duration dropped from about 100 msec to 1 msec as stimulus area was reduced from 3 deg to 2 min. BAUMGARDT and HILLMAN (1961) attempted to repeat the experiment but found very little difference as a function of area and attributed the GRAHAM and MARGARIA result to errors of filter calibration. IKEDA

(1964) has presented evidence to suggest that the critical duration differs for the different mechanisms of color vision. Sperling and Jolliffe (1965) confirmed Ikeda's finding and, like Baumgardt and Hillman, were unable to confirm the Graham and Margaria result where the effect of area was concerned. Wavelength dependence means that, in experiments using "white" light, results will depend upon the exact spectral distribution of the light used; this has varied from one experiment to another and is not usually specified.

The luminance of the adapting background against which the flash is presented also has an effect: the brighter the background, the less is the range over which temporal summation is observed (Graham and Kemp, 1938; Barlow, 1958; Sperling and Jolliffe, 1965). Although it is not uncommon to find complete temporal summation to intervals as long as 100 msec, significant departures occur in many studies for intervals as small as, or even less than, 20 msec. Excepting Graham and Margaria's large-area results, 20 msec can be taken as an interval within which nearly complete temporal summation will occur, no matter what the details of the experimental procedure. Pulse durations shorter than this have been used in all of the two-pulse studies to be considered next.

A very recent study by Battersby and Schuckman (1970) suggests that, for some conditions, the critical duration may be as small as 10 msec. It is quite possible that, for homogeneous pulses, there is no critical duration as such, but only a temporal range over which the summation of the impulse responses to two light pulses is sufficient to produce a summated response whose magnitude is not discriminably less than that to a single pulse of double luminance.

2. Double Pulses

Baumgardt and Segal (1946), working above threshold, found that two stimuli of 10 msec duration and equal luminance, if presented successively upon the same part of the retina, were additive in their effects only if the interval between them was very short. They also described an inhibitory action which lowered the brightness of both flashes, the inhibition being greatest when the interval between the flashes was on the order of 40–70 msec, and ceasing when the interval was greater than 100 msec.

At threshold, Davy (1952) appears to be the first to have shown, by presenting discrete pulses, that the distribution of flux within the critical duration made no difference. He tested this by using from 1 to 5 brief pulses. Davy's results for the two-pulse case are shown in Table 6, together with those from a number of other more recent experiments. These studies yield a critical duration that is based upon the period within which the energy of the two flashes is equally as effective, when spread in time, as when concentrated; the limit of SOA within which this is true defines another measure of the critical duration. The failure of summation to occur has been shown experimentally in various ways: as an increase in threshold energy of the second flash, with the first held at a constant value (Battersby and Defabaugh, 1968); as an increase in the total energy of the two flashes, with the energy of two flashes kept in a unit ratio (Blackwell, 1963); as a decrease in the probability of seeing with the total energy of the two flashes held constant (van den Brink and Bouman, 1964; Grossberg, 1970); or as an increase in the total energy at threshold of the two flashes, over a wide ratio of energies of the two

(IKEDA, 1965; RASHBASS, 1970). See Table 6 for a summary of two-pulse threshold experiments.

Of the various procedures just described, those of IKEDA and RASHBASS are the most general. Furthermore, IKEDA and RASHBASS worked with negative as well as positive pulses, extending the generality of their work still more. For these reasons, attention in the remainder of this section will be focused upon those two studies.

Table 6. *Summary of two-pulse threshold experiments*

Author	Pulse duration (msec)	Pulse geometry	Pulse λ	background	finding (τ = critical duration)
DAVY (1952)	10	2′ at 15°	white	dark	$\tau = 100$ msec
VAN DEN BRINK and BOUMAN (1954)	1	1′ at 0°, 2°, 4° 7° and 10°	red and green	widely variable	τ decreases as adaptation level increases $\tau = 80$ msec
BLACKWELL (1963)	2.5	1° at 0°	white	10 ftL	inhibition at 50 msec $\tau = 20$ msec
IKEDA (1965)	12.5	30′ at 0°	red	328 td 61.2 td	inhibition at 50—70 msec (excitation for $\pm$ pulses) $\tau = 10$ to 20 msec
BATTERSBY and DEFABAUGH (1968)	5	30′ at 6.5°	white	1 ml	$\tau = 10$ msec at most
GROSSBERG (1970)	2.5	0.5° at 0°	white	dark	$\tau = 10$ msec
RASHBASS (1970)	2	17° at 0°	green	700 td	like IKEDA

3. The Findings of IKEDA and RASHBASS

IKEDA (1965) used two pulses, each of 12.5 msec duration. The pulses were presented against backgrounds of either 328 or 61 trolands, over a range of SOA intervals varying from 0 to 100 msec. These use of negative as well as positive pulses allowed four possible sequences: ++, −−, +−, and −+. The experimental procedure first required the determination of the threshold of each of the component pulses to be employed in the two-pulse phase of the experiment. All stimulus levels were subsequently defined in terms of these reference thresholds, which were assigned an arbitrary value of unity. IKEDA called these "S-units," assigning the symbol S_1 to the strength of the first flash, and S_2 to the strength of the second flash, when these were used together. He then defined a "summation index" as $\sigma = 0.30 - \log(S_1 + S_2)$. The value of $S_1 + S_2$ is 1.0 when the combined level of the double flash at threshold is equal to the sum of the threshold levels of the components. This is the value to be expected for superposition, or within the critical duration if the pulses have the same sign. If there is less summation than this, then $S_1 + S_2$ will be greater than 1.0, implying that the two pulses are less efficient when spread in time than they would be if superposed. This will cause σ to become smaller. If σ reaches a value of zero, this implies that the effectiveness of the two flashes working together is the same as for either component working alone. If the two flashes are sufficiently separated in time to be treated as independent events, the summation index has a value of approximately 0.10, attributable to probability summation.

A summation index of less than zero or more than 0.3 is possible. Ikeda in fact found values of less than zero when positive and negative pulses were presented close together in time. For the case of simultaneous presentation, if the apparatus functions properly, the summation index would approach negative infinity, provided that the positive and negative pulses had the same thresholds (these were, in fact, slightly different). A summation index greater than 0.3 would mean that two flashes working together would be more efficient, when separated in time, than when superposed. This result was never obtained in Ikeda's experiment, nor has such a result ever been reported in any of the other temporal summation experiments in the literature. So the rule for two flashes of the same sign is that they are maximally effective when superposed in space and time, whereas separating them in either aspect, if sufficient to cause a change, reduces their joint effectiveness.

Ikeda's results, for one of his subjects, are shown in Fig. 7 for the two cases where the pulses have the same sign and are equal in strength. This curve applies to the special case of unit ratio of flash intensities. All of the functions have the same general shape: the summation index varies from 0.3 (complete summation)

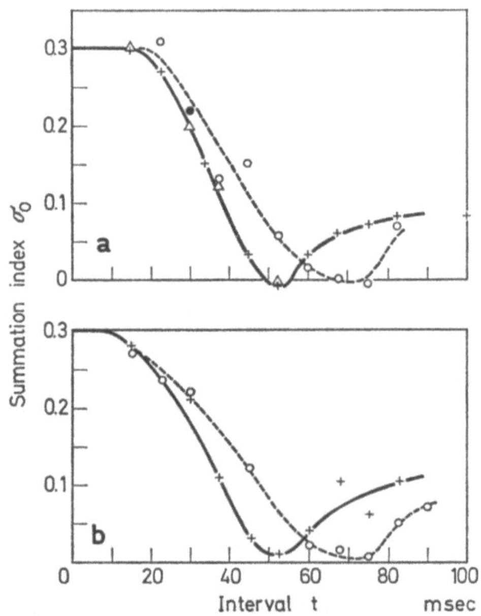

Fig. 7. Summation index (Ikeda, 1965) as a function of the interval (SOA) between two pulses, each of 12.5 msec duration, at two adaptation levels (crosses for 328 td and open circles for 61.2 td)

at short intervals, to zero at from 50 to 70 msec, depending upon adaptation level. It then rises again to a value of 0.1 for the longest separations used.

The result for the longest temporal separation is explained by probability summation. Evidence for this viewpoint exists in a recent experiment by GROSSBERG (1970), who measured the reaction time (from the onset of the first pulse) to double pulse stimuli. He found evidence, for the longer pulse separations, of a bimodal distribution of such reaction times, implying that the subject sometimes responds to the first pulse, but at other times does not see it and responds instead to the second one.

Although probability summation predicts $\sigma = 0.1$ in IKEDA'S experiment, it would be incorrect to suppose that such a value of σ necessarily implies probability summation. Note that the function for the high intensity case (solid line) also has this value for SOA of about 38 msec. Such flashes are much too close together in time to suppose that their effects are independent, and moreover this point on the function is part of a smooth transition from a condition of complete summation at 0 msec to a summation index value that, for whatever reason, reaches zero at about 50 msec.

The minimum value is of particular interest. In none of IKEDA'S work did this value fall significantly below zero. Insight into this matter can be gained by taking a closer look at IKEDA'S results for a condition that yields a summation index of zero. The value of $\sigma = 0$ holds only for the special case where the intensities of the pulse components are equal. Fig. 8 shows IKEDA'S results for other ratios of intensities that were used. On the abscissa is plotted log r, where r is the ratio of the intensity of pulse 2 to that of pulse 1. The lower panel of the figure shows how the summation index varies as a function of log r: it is not constant, but increases as the intensity ratio of the double pulse becomes imbalanced in

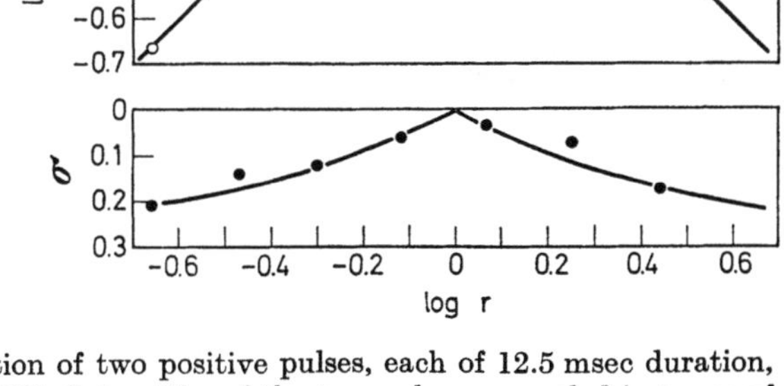

Fig. 8. Interaction of two positive pulses, each of 12.5 msec duration, at SOA = 52.5 msec, from IKEDA (1965). Intensities of the two pulses are scaled in terms of their threshold values when presented alone. The upper panel shows that the intensity of the weaker pulse has no effect upon the threshold, which is always determined by the stronger one. See text for an explanation of the lower panel

either direction. The upper panel of Fig. 1 helps to clarify the basis of this variation of σ. Plotted here is the log intensity value of the two components, each expressed in units of its own threshold intensity. These functions tell us that for all values of log r, the threshold to the double pulse is always obtained with a unit amount of the stronger pulse, whatever the relative intensity of the other (less intense) pulse.

If the two pulses act as independent events under this condition, the result of Fig. 8 could not occur. If the two pulses do not act as independent events, then there must be some kind of interaction between them. The nature of this interaction now seems rather clear: the response to the more intense pulse of the pair somehow completely inhibits the contribution of the less intense one.

For the case where one of the pulses is positive and the other is negative, Ikeda found nearly complete summation at the same intervals (50–70 msec) that had produced the inhibitory effect when the pulses were of the same sign. These results suggested to Ikeda that the visual system may, in response to a pulse of light, generate a bivalent response. For positive pulses this response would first become positive, and then go negative, before returning to the baseline. Negative pulses of light would produce similar responses, but initially negative-going and therefore out of phase with respect to the responses of positive pulses. Ikeda attempted to derive such bivalent response curves that could account for his data.

Ikeda's results have been confirmed in a detailed study by Rashbass (1970). The confirmation is particularly striking because there were enormous procedural differences between the two studies. Rashbass worked at a lower luminance level and caused the entire 18-deg field to alter its intensity to form a pulse, whereas

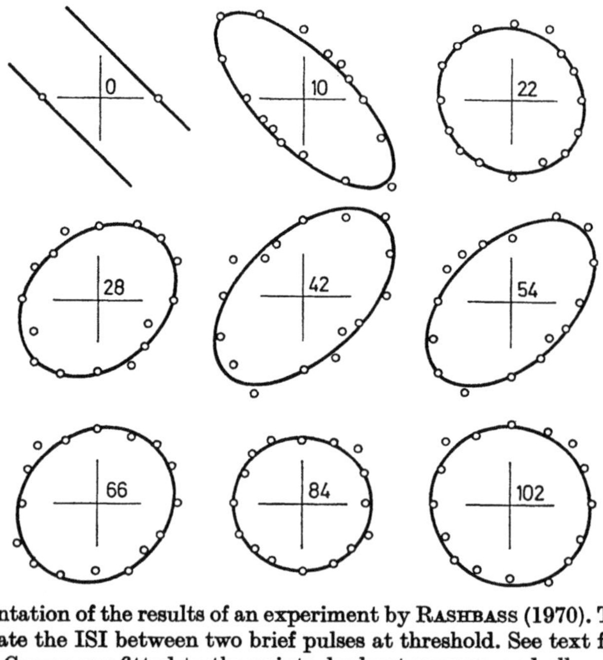

Fig. 9. A representation of the results of an experiment by Rashbass (1970). The numbers near the origins indicate the ISI between two brief pulses at threshold. See text for explanation of the data points. Curves are fitted to the points, by least squares, and all are ellipses. The one at the upper left has an infinitely long major axis

IKEDA had varied only the much-smaller central portion of an otherwise steady adapting field. RASHBASS developed a novel procedure for the display of his data. For each of the SOA values that he used, he plotted the threshold intensity of the first flash horizontally, and that of the second flash vertically, with positive flashes above and to the right of the origin, and negative flashes down and to the left. His results, as shown in Fig. 9, can all be fitted with ellipses. A model was proposed which supposes that the stimulus waveform first passes through a band-pass filter. It is supposed that a running average of the variance of the filter output is taken, with threshold being obtained when this average attains a certain criterion level. From the ellipses shown in Fig. 9, the function of Fig. 10 was derived, whose

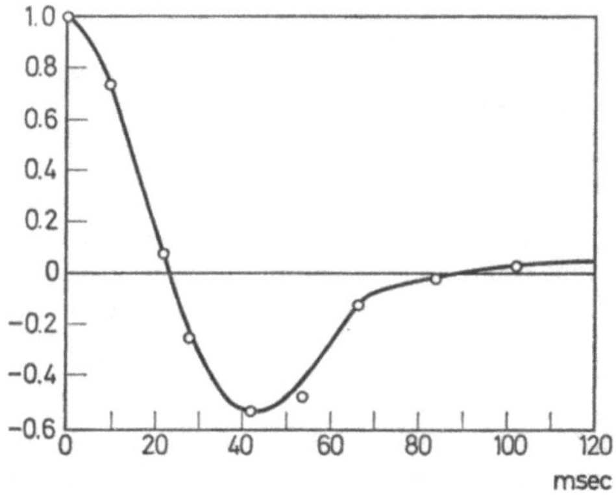

Fig. 10. In terms of RASHBASS's (1970) model, described in the text, this is the autocorrelation function of the impulse response function of the eye

ordinate is L_T, in the equation $A^2 + B^2 + L_T . 2\,A\,B = 1$, with time on the abscissa. (The greater the value of L_T, the greater is the departure of the ellipse from a circle.) In terms of the model proposed by RASHBASS, this function is the autocorrelation function of the impulse-response function of the system. RASHBASS explicitly makes the point that it is not possible to derive a unique impulse function from these data, as IKEDA tried to do. Nevertheless, it is clear that the impulse function, whatever its exact form, must be that of a bivalent response of the same general sort proposed by IKEDA. RASHBASS's model is one that should be taken very seriously, as he demonstrated its predictive power in a number of situations quite independent of that from which it was derived.

Acknowledgements. The writer wishes to express his special appreciation to Dr. ROBERT T. KINTZ, who assisted with the literature search, and to Mrs. MARJORIE SHANNON, who helped to track down references. I am also very much indebted to many of my former students for their help in the experiments in which we collaborated, and the original thinking that many of them brought to bear upon many of the topics discussed here. These are: Dr. JUDITH W. ONLEY, Dr. GILRAY KANDEL, Dr. JOHN B. SIEGFRIED, Dr. MILTON S. KATZ, Dr. JOSEPH B. STURR, and Dr. MITSUO IKEDA. The preparation of this manuscript, as well as all of the experiments at Rochester cited herein, have been supported by Grant No. EY00187 (formerly NB00624) from the National Institutes of Health, U.S. Public Health Service.

References

Allen, F.: The persistence of vision. Amer. J. physiol. Opt. **7**, 439—457 (1926).

Anderson, D. A., Huntington, J., Simonson, E.: Critical flicker frequency as a function of exposure time. J. opt. Soc. Amer. **56**, 1607—1611 (1966).

Anliker, J.: Simultaneous changes in visual separation threshold and voltage of cortical alpha rhythm. Science **153**, 316—318 (1966).

d'Arcy, C.: Sur la durée de la sensation de la vue. Mém. Acad. roy. Sci. (Paris) **37**, 700—718 (1773).

Baker, H. D.: The instantaneous threshold and early dark adaptation. J. opt. Soc. Amer. **43**, 798—803 (1953).

Bartley, S. H.: Vision: A study of its basis. New York: D. Van Nostrand, 1941.

— Wilkinson, F. W.: Certain factors in producing complexity of responses to a single pulse of light. J. Psychol. **9**, 299—306 (1953).

Barlow, H. B.: Temporal and spatial summation in human vision at different background intensities. J. Physiol. (Lond.) **141**, 337—350 (1958).

Battersby, W. S., Defabaugh, G. L.: Neural limitations of visual excitability: after-effects of subliminal stimulation. Vision Res. **9**, 757—768 (1969).

— Jaffe, R.: Temporal factors influencing the perception of visual flicker. J. exp. Psychol. **46**, 154—161 (1953).

— Oesterreich, R. E., Sturr, J. F.: Neural limitations of visual excitability. VII. Non-homonymous retrochiasmal interaction. Amer. J. Physiol. **206**, 1181—1188 (1964).

— Schuckman, H.: The time course of temporal summation. Vision Res. **10**, 263—272 (1970).

— Sturr, J. F.: Neural limitations of visual excitability. IX. Monocular and binocular changes of sensitivity during flicker stimulation. J. opt. Soc. Amer. **60**, 121—126 (1970).

Baumgardt, E., Hillman, B.: Duration and size as determinants of peripheral retinal response. J. opt. Soc. Amer. **51**, 340—344 (1961).

— Segal, J.: Un dispositif permettant de réaliser des stimuli lumineux de durée ultracourte et de forme quelconque, mais constante. C. R. Soc. Biol. (Paris) **140**, 231 (1946).

Beams, J. W.: The eye as an integrator of short light flashes. J. opt. Soc. Amer. **25**, 48 (1935).

Blackwell, H. R.: Contrast thresholds of the human eye. J. opt. Soc. Amer. **36**, 624—643 (1946).

— Neural theories of simple visual discrimination. J. opt. Soc. Amer. **53**, 129—160 (1963).

Bloch, A. M.: Experiences sur la vision. C. R. Soc. Biol. (Paris) **2**, 493—495 (1885).

Bouman, M. A., van den Brink, G.: Absolute thresholds for moving point sources. J. opt. Soc. Amer. **43**, 895—898 (1953).

Boynton, R. M.: Some temporal factors in vision. Chapter 37 in Sensory Communication, Rosenblith, W. (Ed.), pp. 739—756. New York: Wiley 1961.

— Kandel, G.: On-responses of the human visual system as a function of adaptation level. J. opt. Soc. Amer. **47**, 275—286 (1957).

— Siegfried, J.: Psychophysical estimates of on-responses to brief light flashes. J. opt. Soc. Amer. **52**, 720—721 (1962).

— Stiles, W. S., Ikeda, M.: Interactions among chromatic mechanisms as inferred from positive and negative increment thresholds. Vision Res. **4**, 87—117 (1964).

— Sturr, J. F., Ikeda, M.: Study of flicker by increment threshold technique. J. opt. Soc. Amer. **51**, 196—201 (1961).

— Whitten, D. N.: Visual adaptation in monkey cones: recordings of late receptor potentials. Science **170**, 1423—1426 (1970).

Brindley, G. S.: The Bunsen-Roscoe law for the human eye at very short durations. J. Physiol. (Lond.) **118**, 135—139 (1952).

Brown, K. T., Watanabe, K., Murakami, M.: The early and late receptor potentials of monkey cones and rods. Cold Spr. Harb. Symp. quant. Biol. **30**, 457—482 (1965).

Cheatham, P. G., White, C. T.: Temporal numerosity: I. Perceived number as a function of flash number and rate. J. exp. Psychol. **44**, 447—451 (1952).

Clark, W. C., Pickett, R.: Luminance required to detect the presence of a dark interval between two pulses of light. Amer. Psychologist **14**, 412 (1959).

CRAWFORD, B. H.: Visual adaptation in relation to brief conditioning stimuli. Proc. roy. Soc. (Lond.) B **134**, 283—302 (1947).

DAVY, E.: The intensity-time relation for multiple flashes of light in the peripheral retina. J. opt. Soc. Amer. **42**, 937—941 (1952).

DUNLAP, K.: The shortest perceptible time interval between two flashes of light. Psychol. Rev. **22**, 226—250 (1915).

EFRON, R.: The relationship between the duration of a stimulus and the duration of a perception. Neuropsychologia **8**, 37—55 (1970).

GILMER, T. E.: The integrating power of the eye for short flashes of light. J. opt. Soc. Amer. **27**, 386—388 (1937).

GRAHAM, C. H., KEMP, E. H.: Brightness discrimination as a function of the duration of the increment in intensity. J. gen. Physiol. **21**, 635—650 (1938).

— MARGARIA, R.: Area and the intensity-time relation in the peripheral retina. Amer. J. Physiol. **113**, 299—305 (1935).

GRANIT, R., HAMMOND, E. L.: The sensation-time curve and the fusion frequency of intermittent stimulation. Amer. J. Physiol. **98**, 654—663 (1931).

— AMMON, W. VON: Comparative studies on the peripheral and central retina. III. Some aspects of local adaptation. Amer. J. Physiol. **95**, 229—241 (1930).

GROSSBERG, M.: Frequencies and latencies in detecting two-flash stimuli. Perc. Psychophys. **7**, 377—380 (1970).

HABER, R. N.: Information-Processing Approaches to Visual Perception. New York: Holt, Rinehart and Winston 1969.

HECHT, S., SHLAER, S., PIRENNE, M. H.: Energy at the threshold of vision. Science **93**, 585—587 (1941).

HERRICK, R. M.: Foveal luminance discrimination as a function of the duration of the decrement or increment in luminance. J. comp. physiol. Psychol. **49**, 437—443 (1956).

HURVICH, L. M., JAMESON, D.: Vision in intermittent light. Translation of PIÉRON, H. (1961). La vision en lumière intermittente. In: Contributions to Sensory Physiology, Vol. 1. NEFF, W. D. (Ed.). New York: Academic Press 1965.

IKEDA, M.: Further use of the summation index for the study of color vision. J. opt. Soc. Amer. **54**, 84—94 (1964).

— Temporal summation of positive and negative flashes in the visual system. J. opt. Soc. Amer. **55**, 1527—1534 (1965).

— BOYNTON, R. M.: Negative flashes, positive flashes, and flicker examined by increment threshold technique. J. opt. Soc. Amer. **55**, 560—566 (1965).

KAHNEMAN, D.: Method, findings, and theory in studies of visual masking. Psychol. Bull. **70**, 404—425 (1968).

KANDEL, G.: A psychophysical study of some monocular and binocular factors in early adaptation. Ph. D. Dissertation, University of Rochester, 1958.

KESTON, R.: Temporal chromatic induction: the interaction of two successive pulses measured by subjective estimates. Amer. J. Psychol. **78**, 264—270 (1965).

KIETZMAN, M. L.: Two-pulse measures of temporal resolution as a function of stimulus energy. J. opt. Soc. Amer. **57**, 809—813 (1967).

KIETZMAN, M., SUTTON, S.: The interpretation of two-pulse measures of temporal resolution in vision. Vision Res. **8**, 287—302 (1968).

KINTZ, R. T., BOYNTON, R. M.: Temporal summation during backward visual masking. J. opt. Soc. Amer. **59**, 212—216 (199.

DE LANGE, H.: Relationship between critical flicker frequency and a set of low frequency characteristics of the eye. J. opt. Soc. Amer. **44**, 380—389 (1954).

LEVINSON, J.: Flicker fusion phenomena. Science **160**, 21—28 (1968).

LEWIS, M. F.: Two-flash thresholds as a function of luminance in the dark-adapted eye. J. opt. Soc. Amer. **57**, 814—815 (1967).

— Two-flash thresholds as a function of flash luminance and area. Perc. Psychophys. **4**, 241—244 (1968).

MAHNEKE, A.: Foveal discrimination measured with two successive light flashes: a psychophysical study. Acta ophthal. (Kbh.) **36**, 3—11 (1958a).

Mahneke, A.: Fusion thresholds of the human eye as measured with two or several light flashes. Acta ophthal. (Kbh.) **36**, 12—18 (1958b).

Mita, T., Hironaka, K., Koike, I.: The influence of retinal adaptation and location on the Empfindungszeit. Tohoku J. exp. Med. **52**, 397—405 (1950).

Nelson, T. M., Bartley, S. H., Ranney, J. E.: The sensory parallel of the reorganization period in the cortical response in intermittent retinal stimulation. J. Psychol. **52**, 137—147 (1961).

Nelson, T. N., Bartley, S. H., Harper, E. S.: Cf. for short trains of photic stimulation having various temporal distributions and separations. J. Psychol. **58**, 333—341 (1964).

Onley, J. W., Boynton, R. M.: Visual responses to equally-bright stimuli of unequal luminance. J. opt. Soc. Amer. **52**, 934—940 (1962).

Piéron, H.: La Vision en Lumière Intermittente. Monographes Françaises de Psychologie No. 8, Centre National de la Récherche Scientifique. Paris 1961.

Plateau, J.: Dissertation sur quelques propriétés des impressions produites par la lumière sur l'organe de la vue. 1—32. Liege: Dessain 1829.

Pollack, W. T.: The visibility of a target as a function of its speed of movement. J. exp. Psychol. **45**, 449—454 (1953).

Rashbass, C.: The visibility of transient changes of luminance. J. Physiol. (Lond.) **210**, 165—186 (1970).

Segner, J. A.: De raritate Luminis. 1—12. Göttingen: Vandenhoeck (1740).

Sperling, G.: Temporal and spatial visual masking. I. Masking by impulse flashes. J. opt. Soc. Amer. **55**, 541—559 (1965).

Sperling, H. G., Jolliffe, C. L.: Intensity-time relationship at threshold for spectral stimuli in human vision. J. opt. Soc. Amer. **55**, 191—199 (1965).

Sturr, J. F.: Psychophysical measures of on-responses to light flashes of unequal duration. Ph. D. Dissertation, University of Rochester, 1961.

van den Brink, G.: Retinal summation and the visibility of moving objects. Thesis, Utrecht, 1957. Report WW 1957—1959, Institute for Perception RVO-TNO, Soesterberg, Nether-Netherlands.

— Bouman, M. A.: Variation of integrative actions in the retinal system: an adaptational phenomenon. J. opt. Soc. Amer. **44**, 616—620 (1954).

Wagman, I. H., Battersby, W. S.: Neural limitations of visual excitability: II. Retrochiasmal interaction. Amer. J. Physiol. **197**, 1237—1242 (1959).

Chapter 10

Metacontrast

By

NAOMI WEISSTEIN, Chicago, Illinois (USA)

With 7 Figures

Contents

I. Introduction

A. Visual Masking

The term visual masking refers to events that occur when two or more stimuli are presented close to each other in time and space (see reviews by KAHNEMAN, 1968, and RAAB, 1963; also see BOYNTON, 1961, and BOYNTON, chapter 9, this volume). The threshold of one of the stimuli (the target) is raised, or, if the target presentation is suprathreshold, its appearance is changed, by the presence of another stimulus (the mask). The masking stimulus can be presented before, during, or after presentation of the target. What distinguishes masking from other psychophysical effects (such as brightness contrast) is that initial transients, as opposed to steady-state responses, are measured. Thus, target and/or masks are of brief duration, and the interval between their onsets is a small one. The term forward masking has been used when the mask onset precedes the target onset; the term backward masking has been used when the mask onset follows the target onset. The interval between target and mask onsets will be designated Δt; $-\Delta t$ will indicate forward masking, and $+\Delta t$ will indicate backward masking.

The decision to call one stimulus the mask and another the target is somewhat arbitrary since it is clear that most masking situations show mutual influences. However, the mask has usually been presented in such a way that its effect will be greater on the target than conversely; it has been bigger in size, or it has surrounded or flanked the target, or it has been of longer duration or more intensely illuminated.

The spatial requirements for masking are rather strict: masking occurs when the two stimuli are projected onto the same and/or adjacent retinal areas, or, for dichoptic masking, when the two stimuli are projected onto corresponding or closely similar retinal points.

The paradigms in which the mask and target are suprathreshold stimuli and are adjacent to one another, but in no way superimposed on the same retinal area, have been given special names: metacontrast and paracontrast (Stigler, 1910; 1913). Metacontrast refers to the backward masking case, or, at times, to both backward and forward masking; paracontrast refers to the forward masking case. There are two standard stimulus configurations which have been used in most metacontrast studies: a disc (target) surrounded by an annulus (mask); or a center rectangle (target) followed by two similar rectangles that flank it on each side.

This chapter will by and large restrict its attention to metacontrast, which has been studied much more extensively than paracontrast (see Alpern, 1953, and Kolers and Rosner, 1960, for studies of paracontrast as well as metacontrast).

B. Properties of Metacontrast

Metacontrast varies with stimulating conditions in the following ways.

1. When the mask surrounds the target, metacontrast can be obtained with a wide variety of target and mask shapes and sizes as long as the inner contours of the mask are similar to the outer contours of the target (Werner, 1935). When masks flank a target, metacontrast can be obtained in general provided that the shapes of the masks are similar to those of the targets (Uttal, 1970). Thus if two triangles flank a center triangle, metacontrast will be obtained, but if two rectangles flank a center triangle, metacontrast will be greatly reduced. Notice that this indicates considerable spatial non-linearities in metacontrast interactions.

2. As the distance between target and mask increases, masking decreases. In some instances, the metacontrast function is also translated towards the origin (Alpern, 1953), but this is not always the case (Weisstein and Growney, 1969).

3. Metacontrast can be obtained with dark stimuli on lighted backgrounds as well as with lighted stimuli on darker backgrounds.

4. The shape of the metacontrast function varies with stimulating conditions in different ways, depending on the response measure.

a) When the target energy is adjusted to some standard in order to obtain the response measure (e.g., a brightness match), the resulting metacontrast function is what has been called a U-shaped function of Δt. That is, maximum masking will occur at some $\Delta t > 0$. Fig. 7, p. 265 shows typical metacontrast (and paracontrast) functions (here, inverted U-shape) from ALPERN'S (1953) classic parametric study. The solid lines in both A and B are empirical functions obtained by adjusting the luminance of the target until it matched the brightness of a 10.6 ft L standard. The dotted lines are theoretical functions which will be discussed below.

b) With response measures in which the target and mask energy are constant (such as forced-choice or magnitude estimations) the target-to-mask energy ratio (T/M) will determine the shape of the function in the region $0 < T/M \leqq 1$. When T/M is near 1, U-shaped functions will be obtained; as $T/M \to 0$, the metacontrast functions will skew towards the origin, resembling a J more than a U, and masking will be obtained at greater values of Δt. For sufficiently low T/M (about $T/M = 0.09$, although this value varies from subject to subject, as will be discussed in section IV), the metacontrast function will be weak monotonic[1] with respect to $|\Delta t|$. This is illustrated in Fig. 6, p. 262—263. The solid, connected curves are empirical metacontrast functions for each of three subjects at T/M respectively of (1) 1.0, (2) 0.5, (3) 0.2, (4) 0.125, and (5) 0.0625. Notice paracontrast at small T/M – in general, paracontrast effects are much smaller than corresponding metacontrast effects, and become evident only when the target becomes much smaller in energy as compared to the mask. The vertical lines represent a computer simulation of the metacontrast functions; these will be discussed below.

In general, as target and mask are presented at greater and greater values above threshold, with $T/M \approx 1$ and a constant-stimulus response measure, the U of the metacontrast function becomes more pronounced (WEISSTEIN and GROWNEY, 1969).

c) Except when T/M and T are small, metacontrast functions appear to depend on the brightness rather than detection properties of the visual system. That is, given identical stimulating conditions with $T/M \approx 1$, and T and M high (above, perhaps, 1 ft L) detection generally remains at 100 % while the phenomenal appearance of the target changes according to a characteristic U-shape function. For instance, SCHILLER and SMITH (1966) showed that for $T/M = 1$, when a brightness match was required of a subject, a typical U-shaped function resulted, with complete occlusion of the target at $\Delta t = 65$ msec. However, when the subject was asked under identical conditions, to *detect* in which of two annuli the target had occurred, this could be done with 100 % accuracy. The same study successfully replicated an earlier finding of FEHRER and RAAB'S (1962) that under conditions in which U-shaped metacontrast functions were obtained, reaction times to the masked target were no greater than those to the unmasked target. (Metacontrast may in this respect be similar to brightness contrast in general: for instance,

[1] That is, for $|\Delta t_i|, |\Delta t_j| \in R$, if $\Delta t_i < \Delta t_j$, then $f(\Delta t_i) \leqq f(\Delta t_j)$, where R is the set of rational numbers, f is the metacontrast function, and Δt the interval between target and mask onsets.

Cornsweet and Teller, 1965, showed that while the brightness of a steadily presented disc varied, depending on the luminance of a steadily presented annulus, the increment threshold for a small briefly flashed spot in the center of the disc remained the same.) For T/M and T small, the situation changes. Here, both the phenomenal appearance and the detection of the target follow weak monotonic functions of Δt.

Unless otherwise noted, this chapter will follow the convention that metacontrast depends on the phenomenal appearance of the target. Thus, most metacontrast designs will have T and T/M in a moderate range (e.g., $T \geqq 1$ ft L, $T/M \geqq 0.01$), T suprathreshold, and the response indicator measuring a brightness or contrast change, or a reduction in discriminability of the target. (See below for a discussion of the experiment of Alpern, Rushton, and Torri, 1969, in this context.)

5. If target and mask are repeatedly presented with delays between presentations that are identical to delays within presentations the target will reappear (Schiller and Smith, 1966).

6. Metacontrast can be obtained dichoptically as well as monoptically. At small values of $+\Delta t$, dichoptic metacontrast is greater in magnitude than monoptic metacontrast; at large values of $+\Delta t$, the functions are similar in magnitude (Weisstein and Growney, 1969; Schiller and Smith, 1968). Most masking that involves patterns or nearby contours can be obtained with equal magnitude dichoptically (Kahneman, 1968); however, dichoptic non-metacontrast masking that involves contours well separated from each other is generally much smaller in magnitude than the corresponding monoptic effect (Boynton, 1961; Battersby and Wagman, 1962).

It has generally been assumed that U-shaped functions will be obtained only under metacontrast conditions, but this is not the case. For instance, concentric overlapping discs will yield U-shaped functions (Kolers, 1962; Schiller and Greenfield, 1969; Weisstein, 1971) if the discs are close to each other in size, and $T/M \approx 1$. But older work treated this result as an isolated phenomenon (e.g., see Schiller and Greenfield, 1969, where the U-shape is referred to as a reversal) and only recently has it been systematically related to metacontrast masking (Weisstein, 1971).

If the presence of the U indicates that a particular visual process has occurred, then it may be more fruitful to view the processes underlying metacontrast as more generally applicable to a class of masking paradigms including non-metacontrast where edges or contours of target and mask are close to each other. But this presages part of the theory that is being developed to explain metacontrast; a consideration of theory is thus in order.

II. Metacontrast and Theories of Visual Masking

Most explanations of metacontrast have been able either to predict U-shaped functions or to predict monotonic functions, but not both. Although two theories are less parsimonious than one, this in itself would not be sufficient grounds to reject either type of theory, since it is possible that two different mechanisms underlie metacontrast. However, theories that predict U-shaped functions do not handle adequately the behavior of these functions, and theories that predict monotonic functions predict them under conditions in which U-shaped functions are found. On the other hand, as will be discussed below, a theory that predicts both types of function may also be able to handle the behavior of each type of function under the conditions in which it is found.

A. Theories that Predict U-Shaped but not Monotonic Functions

1. Apparent Movement

The apparent movement hypothesis assumes that the more similar the metacontrast paradigm is to conditions which are effective for apparent movement, the greater the masking effect. According to this theory, the target either blends into the mask, thus reducing its own discriminability (FEHRER, 1966; SCHILLER and SMITH, 1966), or the target moves towards the mask in a way that is physically impossible and is, therefore, inadmissable to perception (KAHNEMAN, 1967).

Although it is clear that apparent movement is present in metacontrast paradigms, there are serious difficulties for the assumption that apparent movement is the basis of metacontrast. ERIKSEN and COLEGATE (1970) have shown that apparent movement alone (in two-stimulus designs) does not reduce discriminability of either stimulus. WEISSTEIN and GROWNEY (1969) showed that apparent movement is found over separations as great as 3°20′ between stimuli, whereas, for the same stimuli, there is a negligible metacontrast effect at such separations. Thus apparent movement by itself does not affect discriminability, and if "impossible" apparent movement (KAHNEMAN, 1967) were the basis of metacontrast, there should be metacontrast as long as there is apparent movement.

2. Replacement from Visual Storage

This explanation assumes that items are held in some temporary visual storage and "read in" one at a time. Before an item has been read in, another item can replace it. This theory predicts U-shaped functions. If the masking effect is assumed to increase as a function of the amount of "fading" of the temporary visual storage at the same time that the probability of any item having been read in is increasing, then a maximum masking effect would occur at some $\Delta t > 0$. The maximum effect will occur at some Δt when read-in has not proceeded very far but the image is faded enough so that there is a strong masking effect.

But the theory has difficulty in predicting why the maximum effect shifts with changes in stimulating conditions the way it does. If one assumes, as is implied in a general visual storage model (see, for example, SPERLING, 1963; RUMELHART, 1970) that the fading of this short-term store follows some uniform repeatable decay, then the maximum effect is fixed, or varies around some fixed value. (The maximum effect will hereafter be called Δt_m and will refer to the Δt at which maximum masking is obtained, or, if the maximum is obtained for more than one Δt, to the Δt at which the maximum begins, or, if this is at some negative value of Δt, to $\Delta t = 0$). However, Δt_m is not fixed: it decreases with increased spatial separation between target and mask (ALPERN, 1953); perhaps with increased size of mask although the data are conflicting here (see MAYZNER *et al.*, 1965; MATTESON, 1969), and with variations in the number of positions at which the target stimulus may be presented (WEISSTEIN, 1966). The read-in theory might counter this variation in Δt_m by assuming that the specific mechanisms of replacement are determined by the size, shape, and position of both target and mask. But this reduces to each different pattern having its own storage characteristic (e.g., its own decay time), in which case the theory is not at all parsimonious, especially as compared to a neural model, for instance. (See WEISSTEIN, 1969, for a general discussion of the preferability of neural models in perceptual theory.) A neural model would be able to predict differences in, say, decay characteristics for different patterns according to general principles.

Moreover, masking of one item alone occurs at rather large values of Δt, and short-term visual storage models do not predict this for two reasons. First, there should be nothing to store and thus nothing to mask. In other words, one would assume immediate read-in. However, even if storage were simply automatic, and occurred as well for one or two items, there should be no masking beyond about Δt of 20 msec, since read-in is assumed to be (and should be) a high-speed process. Estimates of read-in have been in the 10–20 msec range (AVERBACH, 1963; SPERLING, 1963), yet a typical value of Δt_m for one-target metacontrast is 60 msec. Thus, short-term visual storage explanations cannot account for single target metacontrast effects.

B. Theories that Predict Monotonic but not U-Shaped Functions

Theories that predict monotonic functions of Δt assume that although target and mask are not simultaneous in physical time, the response in the visual system sufficiently outlasts the physical stimulus so that for some duration, the responses to the two stimuli overlap (see KAHNEMAN, 1967, for a general statement of this assumption). It is during this period of overlap that masking is assumed to occur. General psychophysical explanations assume confusion of target with mask (KOLERS, 1968), luminance summation which reduces figure-ground differences for the target (ERIKSEN, 1966), or lowered signal-to-noise ratio (FRUMKES and STURR, 1968). All of these require $\Delta t_m = 0$, that is, only monotonic functions of Δt, under conditions in which U-shaped functions are actually found.

Some of these theories could be revised to account for U-shaped functions if some special assumptions were made. These special assumptions would, in effect, consist of hypotheses about specific neurophysiological mechanisms such as latency differences. But then, as was the case with visual storage explanations, it would seem more fruitful to develop theories that are built on these specific neurophysiological hypotheses. This is because the neurophysiological hypotheses provide *both* the underlying explanation for the general phenomena such as luminance summation as well as the basis for the special assumptions required to explain U-shaped functions in metacontrast.

Several neurophysiological mechanisms might be the basis of, or contribute to, general masking effects: the adaptation of responding elements after stimulation (which would explain a variety of forward masking effects); the saturation of responding elements such that no response to the target is possible since the elements are already responding at maximum frequency (see BOYNTON, 1958, for a different version of this hypothesis); or the inhibition of responding elements by nearby elements. All three such modifications of response to a target in the presence of a mask have been shown to occur in single units in the cat lateral geniculate nucleus (SCHILLER, 1968a and b). For the first two of these processes to occur, a mask must restimulate the elements that have responded to the target. In metacontrast, the mask stimulates elements adjacent to the target (except for the contribution of stray light). Thus lateral inhibition would seem the most likely mechanism to account for metacontrast because it involves interactions between adjacent areas.

But most explanations involving lateral inhibition would not predict U-shapes unless it were assumed that inhibition from the mask is faster than excitation from the target. If it is assumed, as it generally is, that inhibition is slower than excitation, then only paracontrast would be predicted for $T/M \approx 1$, and only weak monotonic functions for $T/M \ll 1$. If it is assumed that inhibition is as fast excitation, then for $T/M \approx 1$, $\Delta t_m = 0$; as T/M becomes small, the mask latency could become much shorter than that of the target, and one could predict a maximum at some $+\Delta t \neq 0$, and therefore, a U-shaped function. But the problem with metacontrast is that it is exactly when T/M is small that one does *not* obtain a U-shaped function.

So what is needed in order for a lateral inhibition explanation of metacontrast to predict U-shaped functions in accord with the data is the assumption of inhibition that is faster than excitation. Faster inhibition does not necessarily have to depend on latency or conduction time differences. If the rate constants of hyperpolarization were faster than those of depolarization at certain synapses, then inhibition would develop its maximum faster than would excitation, and maximum masking would occur at $+\Delta t \neq 0$. This is discussed further in section III.

C. A Theory that Predicts both U-Shaped and Monotonic Functions: Inhibition

With fast inhibition, both U-shaped and monotonic functions would be predicted. As the mask energy is increased in relation to the target energy, the inhibition would become greater and extend over longer periods of time. Metacontrast functions would then tend towards weak monotonic functions of Δt as T/M became small.

A possible difficulty with this theory may be the assumption of fast inhibition. It has generally been assumed that inhibition is slower than excitation, and, indeed, three kinds of studies do indicate that inhibition is slow compared to excitation. The Crawford overshoot (CRAWFORD, 1947; and see comments by MATTHEWS, 1971) does not disappear at long $-\Delta t$ values for small conditioning stimuli. Since it does disappear for large conditioning stimuli, this implies that inhibitory surrounds attenuate adaptation effects. However, since a steady-state value for adaptation in this type of situation takes some 300–500 msec to develop, this implies inhibition that is much slower than excitation. Impulse responses obtained from the inverse LaPlace or Fourier transforms of transfer functions obtained from flicker studies (see, for instance, Levinson's summary, 1968; Kelly, chapter 11, this volume and Kelly, 1971) generally have inhibition following excitation, that is, slower inhibitory time constants.

Lastly, the disappearance of Westheimer's sensitization effect (1965, 1967) for brief duration flashes also suggests slow inhibition.

However, both neurophysiological and psychophysical evidence is now accumulating that inhibition is not always slower than excitation. In many cases, inhibition may be at least as fast as, and, in one case (Licker, 1969) faster than excitation.

The neurophysiological evidence is as follows. Schiller (1968a) presented stimuli for 10 msec and recorded from single units in the cat optic nerve and lateral geniculate nucleus. He found, for on-center units, maximum suppression of response when disc targets and annulus masks of equal energy were presented simultaneously. Since he does not report responses at forward masking intervals, this result, by itself, does not show equality in rates; but it indicates similar temporal ranges. Nakayama (1968) recorded single unit output in the cat lateral geniculate nucleus and optic nerve for small diameter, 10 msec flashes masked either by larger diameter flashes or by annuli. (These flashes were very brief and very intense; however, they were equivalent in ERG amplitude to a 5 ft L, 20 msec stimulus.) He obtained decreased on-center single unit output for the large as opposed to the small diameter flashes; and he obtained decreased on-center single unit output for small flashes paired with large flashes or with annuli if the annuli were at least 1 log unit more intense than the luminance of the small flash. When he equated small flashes and annuli for energy (that is, luminance x duration), he obtained no reduction in output at all when they were presented together. Both backward and forward values of Δt were tested: maximum suppression occurred at $-$ 10 msec for small diameter flashes paired with annuli, and at $+$ 10 msec for small diameter flashes paired with larger flashes. This suggests that inhibition is within the same temporal range as excitation. Poggio *et al.* (1969), recording from single units in the cat lateral geniculate, and using as a measure of response suppression the average number of spikes, found, in general, maximum suppression of response in on-center units when stimuli to the surround were flashed 10 msec before stimuli to the center. However, since this measure obscures changes in the shape of the response, they also measured inhibition by the change in output at fixed intervals, measured from the onset of the excitatory flash and found, by this measure, that excitation and inhibition had nearly identical time courses. Finally, Licker (1969) found faster inhibition than excitation latencies in the frog retina.

Psychophysical non-metacontrast masking studies also suggest fast inhibitory responses. The Westheimer (1965, 1967) sensitization paradigm, for instance, when generalized to large (43′) targets (Frümkes and Sturr, 1968) is found for masking stimuli as short as 25 msec duration. Even with small probes as targets, Teller (1971) found that the threshold change at the onset of a mask consisting of a sensitizing annulus was no longer in latency than the threshold change to the onset of a mask consisting of a central disc. And in a recent replication of Westheimer's paradigm (Markoff, 1969) essentially the same type of sensitization was found for flashes that were as brief as 5 msec.

Most psychophysical studies that imply latencies for inhibition that are slower or equal to those for excitation appear to be testing visual system response at a subcortical level. For instance, the CRAWFORD (1947) effect shows only a minimal dichoptic component (BATTERSBY and WAGMAN, 1962). WESTHEIMER'S (1967) results were obtained monoptically but not dichoptically. (But see MARKOFF and STURR, 1971 for conflicting results when either brief masking flashes are used, or the stimuli are foveally centered.) Even frequency response functions obtained from flicker studies (which generally indicate slow inhibition), while presumably characterizing a total system response, may be measuring that response before the stage in the visual system where fast inhibition might be found. Moreover, the characterization rests on the assumption that the system is linear; but it is highly likely that elements active in metacontrast interactions simply are not activated in flicker paradigms.

If the metacontrast phenomena dealt with in this chapter have a central locus, then the psychophysical and neurophysiological studies that indicate slow or equal inhibition would not contradict a fast inhibition hypothesis, since the exclusive or major locus of the response in these studies appears to be subcortical.

And the metacontrast phenomena dealt with in this chapter do appear to have a central locus. Recall that this chapter defines as metacontrast those functions in which the response measure depends on the phenomenal appearance of the target. These are obtained in metacontrast designs in which T and T/M are in a moderate range, T is suprathreshold, and the response indicator measures a brightness or contrast change, or a reduction in target discriminability. In general it seems that a central response is reflected by these kinds of measures. This differs from detection measures, which seem to reflect largely peripheral responses. The most detailed argument for this can be given for the difference between apparent brightness and detection functions. When apparent brightness varies, detection remains constant if target energy is constant (CORNSWEET and TELLER, 1965; SCHILLER and SMITH, 1966). At the same time that apparent brightness varies and detection remains constant, the output from peripheral neurophysiological recordings also remains constant (DEVALOIS and PEASE, 1971; SCHILLER, 1968a; NAKAYAMA, 1968). On the other hand, under conditions where detection varies, recordings of neurophysiological output vary similarly (NAKAYAMA, 1968). Thus there is reason to associate detection with peripheral events; and there is no indication that a similar relation holds for apparent brightness.

There are additional lines of evidence that suggest that the metacontrast functions obtained with suprathreshold response measures – apparent brightness or others – reflect central events. The functions can be obtained dichoptically with equal or greater strength than monoptically, and they involve form and contour. In addition, for $T/M \approx 1$, not only is target suppression incomplete (as measured by detection or reaction time indicators), but the delay at which maximum masking occurs is often greater than the conduction time from periphery to visual cortex for T and M of that luminance (COBB and DAWSON, 1960). This suggests, at minimum, that there must be some cortical involvement in the change in appearance of the target.

It should be stressed that the metacontrast spatial arrangement in itself does not necessarily lead to responses that reflect cortical events: as stated, the decisive factors appear to be intensity of T, the size of T/M, and the response required of the subject. Thus, the work of ALPERN and his colleagues (for instance, ALPERN, 1965; ALPERN and RUSHTON, 1967; ALPERN *et al.*, 1969) utilizes a metacontrast spatial design and yet seems to be measuring retinal events. In ALPERN *et al.* (1969), the size of the rod signal is derived from annular inhibition. One would not expect to obtain such a derivation if the locus of inhibition were central. This work utilizes very small T and T/M and a detection response measure. Dichoptic transfer, and the shape of the function across Δt have yet to be determined for the paradigm used by ALPERN *et al.* (1969): some work in progress (ALEXANDER[2]) indicates that the functions are weak monotonic with a plateau from — 60 to + 150 msec Δt, and that although there is some dichoptic masking, the effect is much smaller than that obtained with monoptic masking, and for the range of annular intensities tested, occurs only with intermediate annulus luminances. It appears that this design measures a very different visual system response than the designs with which this chapter is concerned; in fact, ALPERN and his colleagues have used the term "contrast-flash" rather than metacontrast to describe their design.

In summary, according to this reasoning metacontrast as defined here is a cortical event and thus one would not expect to have obtained direct neurophysiological evidence for fast inhibition under conditions of metacontrast masking since the measurements were made subcortically. But there is some electrophysiological evidence that metacontrast does in fact involve inhibition. VAUGHN and SILVERSTEIN (1968) measured the visual evoked response (VER) during metacontrast. In non-metacontrast masking, the VER to superimposed masks and targets shows simply the response to the masking flash alone at intervals between target and mask where masking is obtained (DONCHIN and LINDSLEY, 1965). This finding is consistent with a saturation explanation of masking. If one measures VER's during metacontrast, the VER to the target remains clearly distinguishable but diminishes in amplitude. [SCHILLER and CHOROVER (1966) did not find an attenuation of the VER during metacontrast; however, as VAUGHN and SILVERSTEIN point out, this result may have been due to the presence of stray light.] VAUGHN and SILVERSTEIN obtained a very good correspondence between reduction of the target amplitude in the VER and reduction in apparent brightness; the reduction suggests a decrease in firing, which in turn, suggests an inhibition of response.

It might be reasonable to assume, then, in view of these data, a range of time constants such that at some stages in the visual system, for certain kinds of stimulus interactions, inhibition can be faster than excitation. Metacontrast occurring at some central locus would then be assumed to be such an interaction.[3]

In terms of a general theory about the way the visual system functions, two broad assumptions underlie the idea that fast inhibition occurs under some stimulating conditions and not others. The first is that there exist different channels in the visual system that respond independently of each other. This is well documented for spatial response (CAMPBELL and ROBSON, 1968; BLAKEMORE and CAMPBELL, 1969). The assumption of independent response channels implies nonlinearity (NACHMIAS *et al.*, 1969; but see CAMPBELL *et al.*, 1969). Different channels are turned on for different stimulus situations and are not on for others. In other words, different channels have characteristic thresholds.

[2] ALEXANDER, K. personal communication.

[3] ALPERN (1953) suggested several ways in which inhibition from the mask could be faster than excitation from the target. ALPERN'S suggestions, however, concerned retinal mechanisms, whereas the evidence indicates that metacontrast phenomena involve cortical levels of interaction.

The second assumption is that different channels have different rates of excitation and inhibition. This has been discussed above. For various kinds of stimulus interactions, various ranges of time constants for inhibition and excitation can occur.

These assumptions are congruent with a general information processing model of visual system response. Although not generally discussed in such terms, the typical information processing model of visual system response (e.g., KOLERS, 1968) implies both spatial and temporal channel independence. In particular, temporal channel independence would mean that at different loci in the visual system, or at the same loci at different times, different features of a stimulus are processed at different rates. Thus, for instance, for the most general classification, initial light adaptation can be considered a peripheral event, with its own temporal characteristics and the processing of pattern a central event, with its set of temporal characteristics. But central pattern processing would itself consist of many stages.[4] One such stage would be detected by metacontrast. The features processed at the stage detected by metacontrast do not have to be specified in order to make temporal assumptions (i.e., fast inhibition), although one would expect eventually to be able to characterize the processing and in fact such an expectation would be an important reason for studying metacontrast. Thus, the metacontrast interaction is assumed to measure a particular stage or temporal channel in pattern processing, and certain (spatial) pattern relations must be present in order for this stage to be activated.

WEISSTEIN (1971) reports some data that argue strongly for a temporal independence hypothesis. For disc-disc (non-metacontrast) masking, if the outer diameter of the mask equals that of an annulus which produces typical metacontrast functions, two types of functions will be obtained when T/M is high. With dichoptic presentations, U-shaped functions will be obtained that agree fairly well with functions obtained with annuli of the same outside diameter. With monoptic presentations, W-shaped functions are obtained that consist of a first trough resembling a simple masking-by-flashes paradigm, and a second trough that agrees fairly well with functions obtained with annuli of the same outside diameter. The W-shaped function in particular suggests strongly that different features of a stimulus are processed at different locations in the visual system and each processing operation has its own set of temporal characteristics.

In summary, then, if the idea of lateral inhibition is retained, and it is assumed to be a central effect involving fast inhibitory rate constants as compared to excitatory rate constants, then a plausible theory of metacontrast can be constructed that does not contradict the available data. This theory will then predict both monotone and U-shaped functions under the conditions found empirically, as well as many of the other characteristics of metacontrast (WEISSTEIN, 1968). The remainder of this chapter is devoted to presentation and discussion of the inhibition theory, quantified so that predictions can be tested as precisely as possible. It is hoped that this theory will suggest ways in which the difficulties in explaining metacontrast discussed above may be resolved. In addition, the inhibition theory is quantified in a way that appears generally applicable to neural theories of masking, that is, other neural theories of masking (saturation, slow inhibition, and so forth) can be easily put in quantitative form using this approach.

---

[4] Use of the term stages is not meant to imply a strictly serial process; the stages may occur simultaneously, or processing for many stages may overlap.

Thus it seems useful to describe in detail the method of construction of "neurons" (see below) which simulate a theoretical neural interaction, as well as to report the results of the particular quantification used to simulate metacontrast interactions.

III. Lateral Inhibition in a Network of Two-Factor Neurons

A. Assumptions

In the WEISSTEIN (1968) theory there were two assumptions. First, the metacontrast effect was assumed to involve single units receiving information about the whole target, from all overlapping receptive fields. This assumption puts virtually no constraints on spatial organization; however, it does imply that at some stage in the visual system one single unit must be summarizing all information about a stimulus. This assumption should be modified because, for instance, metacontrast could involve interaction between the edges of a target and mask, rather than the total stimulus (WEISSTEIN, 1969, 1970; BLAKEMORE and CAMPBELL, 1969). Indeed, in metacontrast interactions it is neither necessary nor likely that all traces of firing to the target be suppressed (FEHRER and RAAB, 1962; SCHILLER and SMITH, 1966; DEVALOIS and PEASE, 1971). But this first assumption is not necessary for a temporal model, which requires simply the notion of an inhibitory interaction. This can occur in a variety of ways, for a variety of kinds of units and numbers of units, without changing the temporal characteristics of the model.

It is the second assumption in WEISSTEIN (1968) that is necessary if the model is to explain metacontrast. Given equal energy stimuli, inhibition and excitation will develop at different rates. This was first suggested by LANDAHL (1967). In the general formulation, one assumes that the neurons that are excited by the target and by the mask mutually inhibit each other. Four effects are therefore possible, two corresponding to forward masking, and two corresponding to backward masking. For forward masking, the mask may be presented before the target and inhibit it; and the mask may be presented after the target and be inhibited. For backward masking, the mask may be presented after the target and inhibit it; and the mask may be presented before the target and be inhibited. All of these effects have been reported for adjacent targets and masks (KOLERS and ROSNER, 1960). The differences in amplitudes and periods of masking are assumed to result both from *stimulus* differences of energy and size, and neural *response* differences, given equal stimulus energies and sizes. These response differences involve differences in the asymptotes and rate constants of depolarization (leading to excitation) and hyperpolarization (leading to inhibition) at the synapse. This means that, depending on the stimuli and on the neurons stimulated, maximum masking can occur at plus and minus delays between two stimuli, as well as at zero delays between the two stimuli.

It is easily seen that differences in rate constants and asymptotes must be quantified if the model is to have predictive value. The Rashevsky two-factor neuron provides a general first approximation to the reponses of nerve cells or populations of nerve cells (RASHEVSKY, 1948). A network of these as suggested by LANDAHL (1962, 1967) results in quantification which can test predictions from a lateral inhibition theory of metacontrast.

Of those models that assume, as this one does, that the basic information carried by a neuron is its frequency of firing, the Rashevsky neuron is chosen because of its simplicity, flexibility, and generality. The Rashevsky neuron incorporates a number of approximations that are common in the neurophysiological literature (STEVENS, 1968). See CULL (1967) and HOUSEHOLDER (1944) for a discussion of the equivalence of other two-factor models to the Rashevsky model; see HARMON and LEWIS (1966) for an excellent review of neural modeling. A number of models that deal specifically with lateral inhibition are discussed in RATLIFF (1965); of these, two that have been tested empirically and that include temporal factors are briefly mentioned: those of LANGE and of STEVENS (in RATLIFF, 1965, pp. 116—117). These include a non-specific excitation function of time, and an explicit inhibition function of time which is equivalent to the j factor in the Rashevsky neuron. A class of models differing from the Rashevsky type assumes shunting inhibition rather than subtractive inhibition (e.g., FUORTES and HODGKIN, 1964; SPERLING and SONDHI, 1968). There is some dispute as to which kind of inhibition correctly describes neural interactions at a rather global level, for instance, at the level of ganglion cell output (see ENROTH-CUGELL and PINTO, 1970, for evidence of subtractive inhibition in cat ganglion cell output).

B. Formalization: The Rashevsky Two-Factor Neuron

Formalization of a two-factor neuron describes its firing frequency as a function of the difference between excitatory and inhibitory post-synaptic potentials which rise and decay exponentially with time. The firing frequency is limited at zero, and although this was not in the original formulation (WEISSTEIN, 1968) it should also be limited at some upper bound. This upper limit would correspond to the reciprocal of the refractory period of the neuron. The placement of this upper limit can determine the extent of saturation masking effects, and can also account for the extended energy range over which metacontrast effects are found. For instance, for $T/M \approx 1$, stimulus durations of 25 to 125 msec will yield metacontrast effects which are almost identical.

The derivation of equations from a description of neural response is given in WEISSTEIN (1968). These are usually written as the following first-order differential equations:

$$d\varepsilon_m/dt = \mathrm{A}F_{m-1}(t) - a\varepsilon_m$$
$$dj_m/dt = BF_{m-1}(t) - bj_m\,. \tag{1}$$

Here ε_m describes the depolarization at the synapse of a neuron in afferent order m (in terms of percentage change from resting potential), and j_m describes the hyperpolarization at the synapse (in terms of percentage change from resting potential). The input function $F_{m-1}(t)$ is assumed to be a frequency of firing from a neuron or population of neurons at afferent order $m-1$. (When different units are specified in a particular afferent order, this will be represented by ε_{nm}, j_{nm}, with n designating a unit in a particular layer, and m the afferent order.)

As discussed in WEISSTEIN (1968), ε_m and j_m can be viewed as generalized excitatory and inhibitory factors, respectively. The solution of the equation for the excitatory factor is the convolution integral:

$$\varepsilon_m(t) = \varepsilon_{m_0}\, e^{-at} + \int_0^t A\, e^{-a(t-\tau)} F_{m-1}(\tau)\, d\tau\,. \tag{2}$$

Thus $A e^{-a(t-\tau)}$ is an excitatory temporal weighting function, with A the proportionality constant, and $1/a$ the rate constant (ε_{m_0} is the initial condition).

Similarly for the inhibitory factor:

$$j_m(t) = j_{m_0} e^{-bt} + \int_0^t B e^{-b(t-\tau)} F_{m-1}(\tau)\, d\tau \tag{3}$$

and thus $Be^{-b(t-\tau)}$ is the inhibitory temporal weighting function, with B the proportionality constant, and $1/b$ the rate constant (j_{m_0} is the initial condition).

The output is $F_m(t) = l[\varepsilon_m(t), j_m(t)]$

$$l = \begin{cases} \varepsilon_m - j_m - h_m & \text{if } h_m \leqq \varepsilon_m - j_m < \lambda_m \\ 0 & \text{if } h > \varepsilon_m - j_m \\ \lambda_m & \text{if } \varepsilon_m - j_m \geqq \lambda_m \end{cases} \tag{4}$$

l expresses the non-linearities: if $\varepsilon_m - j_m$ is between h_m and λ_m, then the neuron fires at a frequency proportional to $\varepsilon_m - j_m - h_m$. Otherwise the neuron does not fire, or it fires at frequency λ_m. Thus h_m is the threshold, and λ_m the asymptote.

Equations (2) and (3) appear analytically quite similar to a linear system consisting of one RC stage. The two-factor neuron $(\varepsilon_m - j_m)$ resembles two RC stages in cascade. However, the differences ($A \neq B$; A, $B \neq k/(b-a)$, [where k is some constant]) lead to some very marked differences in the behavior of the neurons, especially when they are put together in a network. For instance, as the number of cascaded RC stages increases, the impulse response tends to "spread out", but with different A and B as well as different a and b, the impulse response can remain sharp, with a maximum near $t = 0$, over many stages (see Fig. 1, the mask line). What this means is that, in general, the Rashevsky two-factor neuron is a very flexible formulation, and can simulate a number of elementary temporal responses of neurons (such as "on" and "off" responses) depending on the ratios A/a to B/b, and of the relation between a and b.

Viewed as a neuron, A and B represent the receptive field contributions of an excitatory and inhibitory region, respectively, if the regions are fully stimulated. Thus, there is an implicit spatial factor in each neuron. The rate constants $1/a$ and $1/b$ represent the rate at which excitatory and inhibitory post-synaptic potentials develop. Viewed as a generalization to a population of neurons, $1/a$ and $1/b$ would represent typical or characteristic excitatory and inhibitory rate constants, and A and B would represent the integrals of weighting functions describing the spatial characteristics of neurons involved in the metacontrast interaction at layer m.

1. Construction of the Neural Net from Two-factor Neurons

A two-factor neuron then consists of a responding element that combines excitatory with inhibitory processes; if the result is above threshold, the neuron will fire at a frequency proportional to its excitation. The neural net constructed to simulate metacontrast consists of these two-factor neurons, combined in such a way that a target stimulus alone results in more excitation than inhibition, a masking stimulus alone results in more excitation than inhibition, and a target and masking stimulus together results in increased inhibition to the target stimulus. The general principle behind the construction of this net is the parameterization of neurons whose firing frequencies increase at different rates, and whose effects are inhibitory as well as excitatory. Whether the metacontrast effect involves a few single units or populations of single units, its temporal properties can be represented by a small network of units. If populations of neurons are involved, this network represents a characteristic temporal response.

The net to be described uses five neurons. Two of these are identical neurons representing transmission in the periphery: one conveys messages about the mask, the other conveys messages about the target. The other three are central neurons: an inhibitory collateral from the neuron conveying information about the mask, a second-order neuron continuing the conveyance of information about the target, and a "decision" neuron, whose strength of response is translated into some psychophysical response measure (see below). Empirical reasons motivate the construction of identical peripheral neurons. A stimulus within some given spatial range can either serve as a mask or be masked, depending on the other stimulus in the visual field. Thus, a symmetrical net is required; the visual system should not "know" which is going to be target and which is going to be mask.

2. The Responses of Neurons in the Net

A solution for each neuron in this net involves four parameters: A and a, proportionality and rate constants, respectively, for the excitatory factor; and B and b, proportionality and rate constants, respectively, for the inhibitory factor. The choice of these four constants determines the rate at which the neuron will fire and the shape of changes in this rate with time.

The four parameters for each neuron are listed in Table 1. All subsequent theoretical figures are generated with these parameter values, with the exception of the Schiller and Smith (1966) simulation, as noted below. A fuller explanation of how these parameters are derived, what they mean and a discussion of how these particular values were chosen is given in Weisstein (1968).

Table 1. *Parameter values for the neural net*

Parameter	Neuron				
	n_{11}	n_{21}	n_{12}	n_{22}	n_{13}
A	1.5	1.5	1.2	1.6	0.2
a	0.025	0.025	0.03	0.3	0.009
B	1.5	1.5	2.4	6.4	0
b	0.1	0.1	0.09	0.6	0
h	0	0	0	0	0

a, b in terms of milliseconds; $1/a$, $1/b$ are time constants.

The net from which calculations are made consists of the neurons displayed in Fig. 1. In this figure, the firing frequency of each neuron is plotted from the onset of the target stimulus, that is, from $t = 0$. The neurons are indexed according to their typical presentation order. Target neurons have the index n_1k and mask neurons have the index n_2k. Whereas k indicates prior and subsequent afferent orders, the numbers 1, 2, and 3 refer to elements in the net, rather than actual afferent orders.

The condition of simultaneous presentation ($\Delta t = 0$) is illustrated. The target stimulus, S_1, is presented ($S_1 = k \log I + c$, where I is the stimulus luminance in ft $L's$, k and c are constants, and S_1 is in volts) and n_{11} simultaneously begins to fire. Similarly, a masking stimulus S_2 is presented (again, $S_2 = k \log I + c$, with k and c the same constants) and n_{21} simultaneously begins to fire. The rate of impulses from each neuron varies with time as shown in Fig. 1. Here (*a*) represents the

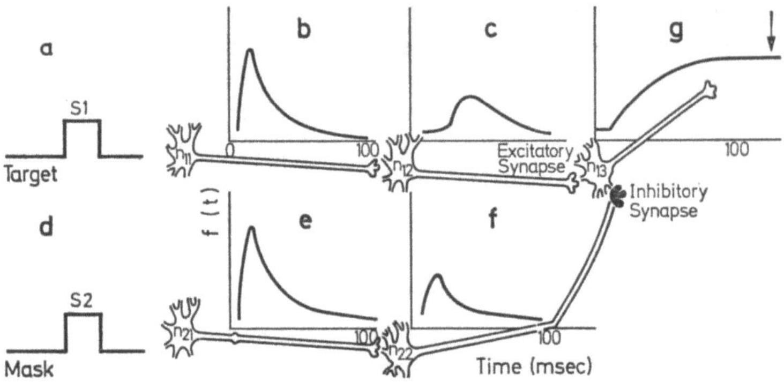

Fig. 1. The neural network from which calculations were made. Functions (b), (c), (g), (e), and (f) represent the frequency of firing of each individual neuron. Each function begins at $t = 0$. Functions (a) and (d) represent the stimulus input. The neurons n_{11} and n_{21} are "peripheral"; n_{12}, n_{22}, and n_{13}, central. The inhibitory collateral, n_{22}, is algebraically added to the excitation from the neuron in the target line, n_{12}, and this sum is responded to by the decision neuron, n_{13}, whose maximum cumulative frequency of firing is then translated into some response measure, e.g., per cent detection, or magnitude estimation

transformed stimulus energy and (*b*) represents the frequency of firing of n_{11} as it varies with time. Neuron n_{11} synapses with n_{12}, which in turn begins to fire porportionately to the building up of a de- and hyperpolarization at its dendrites, that is, polarizations proportional to the rate of firing of n_{11}. The frequency of firing of n_{12} is shown in Fig. 1 (*c*). The situation is similar with the masking stimulus. Curve (*d*) represents the transformed masking energy. Both n_{11} and n_{21} have the same parameters. Neuron n_{22}, the inhibitory collateral, is displayed in (*f*). Functions (*c*) and ($-f$) are algebraically added; if their sum is above zero, as it is in this example, then n_{13} begins to fire.

The maximum cumulative frequency at which n_{13} fires [see arrow in (g)] is transformed into an empirical response measure in the following ways. With response measures in which the target and mask energies remain constant, the computer output is simply scaled to match the empirical function. For a per cent detection measure (e.g., the comparison to the WEISSTEIN and HABER, reference function, Fig. 2) the maximum cumulative n_{13} value, that is $\left[\int_0^{400} f_{13}(t)\,dt\right]$ in the absence of the mask is considered 0 errors in response. Each successively lower value is subtracted from this maximum value and the resulting percentage of the maximum is set equal to the percentage of error in response. For magnitude estimation comparisons (e.g., Fig. 6), the computer output is scaled so that the minimum to maximum equals the minimum to maximum for the empirical function at $T/M = 1$. For comparison to response measures in which the target energy is adjusted to some standard, the target voltage is increased until $\left[\int_0^{400} f_{13}(t)\,dt\right]$ under the metacontrast conditions for each Δt matches $\left[\int_0^{400} f_{13}(t)\,dt\right]$ to the unmasked standard. Then I, the luminance in ft L's, is found from the adjusted target voltage, that is, $I = \log^{-1}(S_1/k + c/k)$.

This is obviously a shorthand net for purposes of calculation. A net that gives a fuller simulation would specify functions which transform luminance into the logarithm of the luminance, determine latencies of response to different stimulus energies, and set light patterns on dark grounds or black patterns on white grounds into equivalent stimuli for contrast and contour detectors. No process by which any of these transformations come about is incorporated into the net. Instead, a simple crude assumption is made that either light patterns on dark grounds or dark patterns on light grounds result centrally in an excitatory response that is proportional to the logarithm of the luminance in the visual field. The convention that both kinds of stimuli will result in a central excitatory response assumes tentatively as a mechanism peripheral "on" neurons mediating the response to light stimuli, and "off" neurons mediating the response to black stimuli, as suggested, for instance, by Baumgartner (1961). A fuller net, in addition, would depict cross-inhibition, with an inhibitory collateral from target to mask, and an independent decision neuron for discrimination of the mask. But since perception of the mask is not studied here, the cross-inhibition is not included in the net. The output — the maximum cumulative response of n_{13} — is the quantity sought. This gives the amount of excitation as a result of presenting S_1 (target) and S_2 (mask) at different times.

The net has been programmed on the University of Chicago Beckman EASE analog computer (Rothberg, 1968) with results described in the following section.

IV. The Network's Prediction Compared with Empirical Data

A. The Fundamental Network Output

Fig. 2 shows five metacontrast functions as they appear from a machine readout. The insert shows the way in which these functions are related to Fig. 1. Each function is plotted in the insert from $t = 0$, showing how the response of each neuron in the net overlaps. The mask (d) is presented 20 msec after the target (a). These are the square pulses in the insert. Their heights correspond to the transformation of ft L's into a proportional logarithmic value, and their widths are the equivalent in the computer time scale of 16 msec duration. The initial neurons are n_{11} and n_{12} [dashed lines (b) and (e)], the central neurons are n_{21} and n_{22} [solid lines (c) and (f)], and the decision neuron is n_{13} [solid line (g)]. Lines (f) and (e) are inverted to indicate inhibitory action. Each vertical line in functions 1–5 represents the cumulative value of n_{13} after 400 msec of computation time. The set of lines that comprise each of the functions (1) through (5) are generated by repeatedly changing the delay between the onset of the target and mask by 10 msec and calculating the cumulative value of n_{13} for that delay.

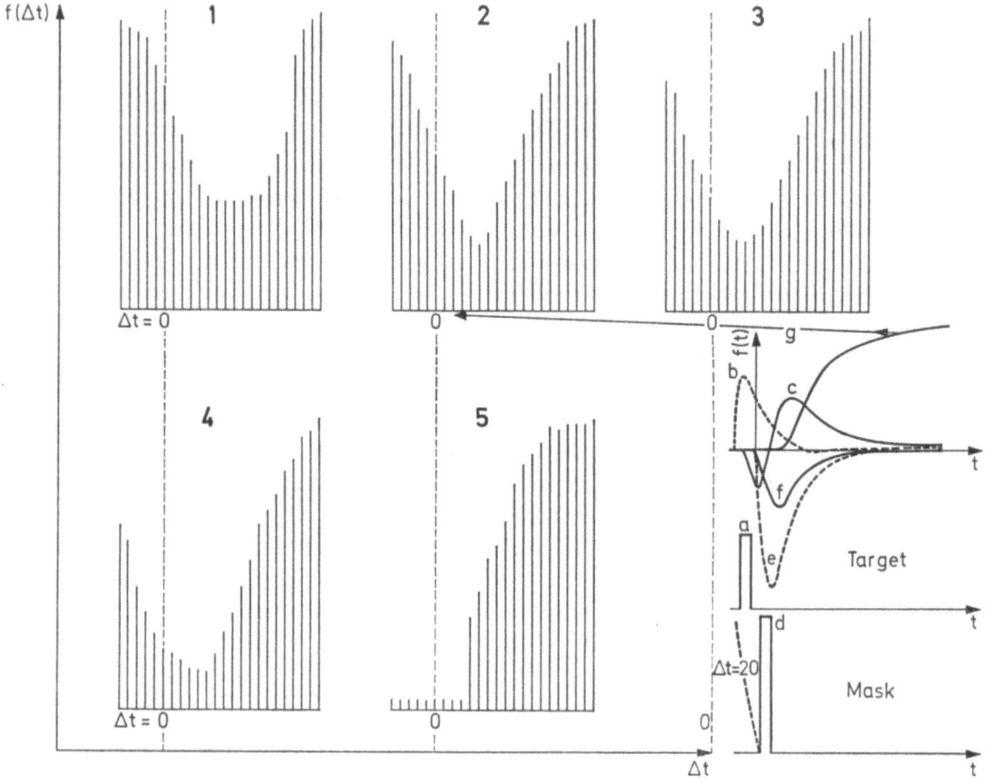

Fig. 2. The fundamental network output. Each vertical line is the maximum cumulative frequency of firing of n_{13}. Each function is the output obtained to a different T/M. Details are in the text

As noted, the constants A_{ik}, B_{ik}, a_{ik} and b_{ik} that generate each function are the same. What is changing is the T/M ratio, which is, in order: 1) 1, 2) 0.5, 3) 0.2, 4) 0.125 and 5) 0.0625. Target luminance is decreased and mask luminance is held constant; the functions are then normalized so that each has the same maximum target excitation value. Their shapes can then be compared. Each of the set of functions (1) through (5) begins with −50 msec Δt. A dashed vertical line has been drawn at $\Delta t = 0$ and a possible explanation for a central issue in metacontrast, that of monotonic vs. U-shaped functions, is apparent. The explanation is that the same process (fast inhibition) will result in differently shaped metacontrast functions, depending on the size and duration of the inhibitory masking signal, as compared to that of the excitatory signal. (Notice also the following secondary shape changes as $T/M \to 0.0625$: the metacontrast function becomes narrower and deeper, then begins to widen as it skews toward the origin.) The point at which maximum masking occurs is determined by the region in which there is maximum overlap of target excitation and mask inhibition [(c) and $(-f)$ in the insert, Fig. 2]. This region is itself determined by how fast and how high the frequency of firing climbs for each individual neuron. Thus, for instance, for a long duration high intensity masking stimulus, the individual inhibition function will peak at a relatively late time [see Fig. 2, insert, neuron (f)]; to maintain a steady U-shaped function, the target stimulus must be similarly extended. This dependence of the shape of the metacontrast function on the overlap of the responses to target and mask has been noticed by KAHNEMAN (1967). His analysis was qualitative, however, and did not extend to the shape of the individual responses as determined by their rate constants. This is a necessary inclusion if *both* U-shaped *and* monotonic functions are to be predicted. The rate constants (Table 1) to the target are slower than to the mask collaterals. Thus, for equal energy stimuli, maximum overlap between (c) and $(-f)$ occurs at some nonzero delay between target and mask, and U-shaped masking functions are obtained. If the mask energy is increased, the waveforms of excitation and inhibition will coincide so that a complete target-mask overlap will occur at any short interval of Δt, and a monotonic masking function will result.

Are the predicted changes in shape found empirically?

B. The Reference Function

The parameters used to generate the functions obtained in Fig. 2 are the same as those reported in WEISSTEIN (1968). These parameters were chosen to fit a particular empirical function (WEISSTEIN and HABER, 1965). The fit is shown in Fig. 3. The dotted line is the theoretical function; the solid line an empirical function which is an arithmetic mean of four subjects. The fit is generally within $\pm 0.5\,\sigma$, as drawn on the figure. It can be readily seen that from 0 to 100 msec the fit is everywhere well within one standard deviation. After 100 msec there seems to be a slight steady rate of error in the WEISSTEIN and HABER function, or perhaps even a rise in the function; the theoretical function, however, returns to zero.

It was not clear whether this error at long delays represented the steady-state rate for detection under conditions used in the WEISSTEIN and HABER study, or represented a second slight peak of masking. No attempt was made to fit the WEISSTEIN and HABER study at delays after 100 msec. The constants in the net were fit to a specific study, one using black patterns on white grounds: two letters of the alphabet which appeared in any of four positions. Does this setting of parameters to a specific, somewhat idiosyncratic design now afford a neural network from which general predictions of metacontrast can be confirmed? The preliminary answer is that the literature provides very striking confirmation of the predictions from this fixed net, although, with the exception perhaps of the MAYZNER *et al.* (1965) replication of WEISSTEIN and HABER (1965), no two studies in the metacontrast literature, used the same size, color, type of illumination, distance from fovea, or angle between target and mask, for their stimulus presentations, nor the same illumination or duration values, notation, and/or response indicators. First, consider the distinctions between U-shaped and monotonic functions in metacontrast.

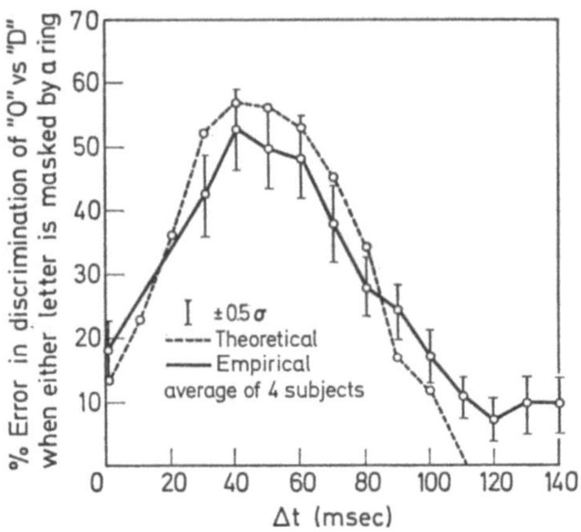

Fig. 3. A comparison of metacontrast as predicted by the neural net with metacontrast as obtained by WEISSTEIN and HABER (1965). A guessing correction has been made for the empirical function

C. Monotonic vs. U-Shaped Functions in Metacontrast

The network predicts that Δt_m depends primarily on the ratio of the target energy to the mask energy (with T/M_a indicating the ratio of target luminance to mask luminance, and T/M_d indicating the ratio of target duration to mask duration). The ratio relationships are illustrated by the surface in Fig. 4. Here, the x-axis represents T/M_d and the y-axis represents T/M_a. The z-axis represents $L(\Delta t_m)$, that is, a function only in the first octant, so that all $\Delta t_m < 0$ are represented and treated in the subsequent discussion as $\Delta t_m = 0$. The surface is fit to points generated by the analog computer. It is not symmetrical with respect to the diagonal plane. Hence, intensity x time reciprocity does not hold. That is, reciprocity holds for the two parallel plane portions of the surface (at $z = 0$, the striped portion, and at $z = 40$, the defined region) but not for the region between them. So, for instance, the slope at $T/M_a = 1$, T/M_d varying is different from the slope at $T/M_d = 1$, T/M_a varying.

Although reciprocity does not strictly hold, a convenient rule of thumb for the function could be summarized very roughly by:

$$z = L(\Delta t_m) = \left\{ \begin{array}{l} 0 \text{ if } xy \leqq 0.09 \\ \qquad > 0 \text{ and } < 40 \text{ if } 0.09 < xy < 0.4 \\ 40 \text{ if } xy \geqq 0.4 \\ (\text{for } \{x,y|\ 0 < x,y, \leqq 1\}) \end{array} \right\} \tag{5}$$

The surface summarizes Δt_m predictions. The $z = 0$ plane (diagonal lines) indicates those T/M at which weak monotonic functions will be obtained. The white area, the part of the surface where $\Delta t_m > 0$, indicates those T/M at which U-shaped functions will be obtained. Notice that for T/M_d and $T/M_a > 0.4$, Δt_m becomes constant at 40 msec. This value actually varies between 40 and 60 msec, depending on the absolute value of the duration and luminance. This secondary variation is indicated by a dotted line.

The predictions (the surface) are compared to studies from the literature in Fig. 4 in the following way. Arrows represent those x and y values and Δt_m for each condition for each study reported. Different conditions from the same study are indicated by letters; the studies themselves are indicated by numbers. The network's predictions in terms of the U/monotone dichotomy are contradicted only once (a result not later replicated [see below]). The differences between specific values of predicted and observed Δt_m vary from one study to the next. A detailed discussion of predicted and observed Δt_m and the correspondance of the

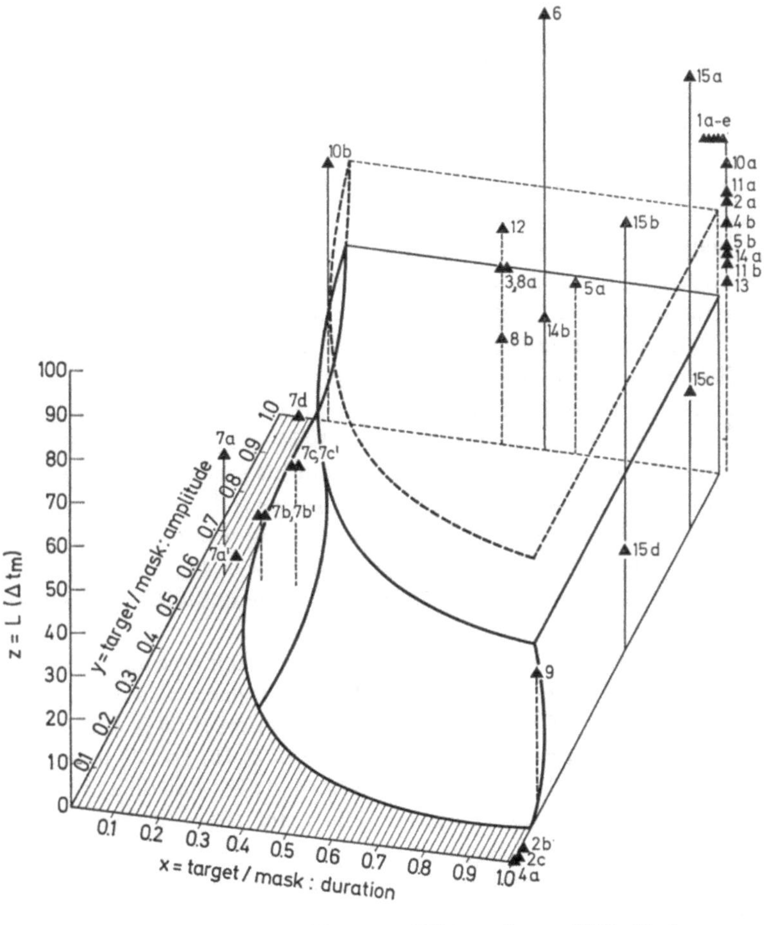

Fig. 4. $L(\Delta t_m)$ as predicted by two variables: $x = T/M_d$, and $y = T/M_a$. Each arrow represents a point reported in the literature. Arrows on the hatched $z = 0$ plane represent monotonic functions; those on the $z > 0$ portion of the surface or above it, U-shaped functions. Exact fits to U-minima are represented by arrowheads attached only to dotted lines; if attached to a solid line, the prediction deviates by the length of the line from the empirical finding

general shape of the predicted function to that of the observed function is therefore in order.

KAHNEMAN (1967) used an illuminated square outline as a target, and two flanking square outlines as masks, with varying durations of target and mask but always with $T/M_d = 1$ and $T/M_a = 1$. Viewing was binocular. He obtained a Δt_m between $\Delta t = 50$ and $\Delta t = 75$ msec; this is indicated by Arrows 1a, b, c, d, and e. The prediction of the net is thus confirmed for his study. Clearly, for constant Δt_m the absolute values of the durations do not matter; what is constant in their presentation is the ratio between them. Similarly, when SCHILLER and SMITH (1966) used a lighted disc and ring as target and mask, respectively, each at a luminance of 43 ft L, and a duration of 5 msec they obtained a Δt_m at about 65 msec; this is indicated by Arrow 2a. Here again, with T/M_a and $T/M_d = 1$, Δt_m is as predicted. Moreover, when they decreased T/M_a to 0.01 and 0.001 (Arrows 2b and 2c, respectively), they obtained monotonic detection functions. Viewing was monoptic in all conditions. WEISSTEIN and HABER (1965) used $T/M_a = 1$, $T/M_d = 0.4$ with binocular viewing. Their data are included for reference since their function provides the basis for the other predictions. They obtained $\Delta t_m = 40$ msec (Arrow 3). Viewing was binocular. FEHRER and SMITH (1962) used $T/M_d = 1$, $T/M_a = 0.005$ (Arrow 4a) and 1 (Arrow 4b) with monoptic viewing. They obtained, respectively, $\Delta t_m = 0$ (monotonic function) and Δt_m at an unspecified $\Delta t > 0$ (U-shaped function). Viewing was monoptic. KOLERS and ROSNER (1960) used dichoptic presentations, a black disc to one eye, and a black ring to the other. With $T/M_a = 1$, $T/M_d = 0.57$ to 2.3, they obtained U-shaped functions with Δt_m from 40–120 msec. Arrow 5a represents the point for $T/M_d = 0.57$ and Δt_m no later than 40 msec; 5b, for $T/M_a = 1$ and Δt_m no later than 55 msec. The other points in this study involve $T/M_d > 1$, and thus are not represented here. In his 1962 study, KOLERS used as a response measure the duration at which the target reached threshold. This means that T/M_d was constantly varying and thus valuable data from his study cannot be represented on this surface[5] except for one experiment, where he used a probability of detection measure. Here, $T/M_a = 1$, and $T/M_d = 0.5$. Viewing was monoptic. He obtained $\Delta t_m = 100$ msec which is quite above the 40–60 msec Δt_m predicted by the net, although the correct shape of the function — U vs. monotonic — is predicted. This is indicated by Arrow 6.

HECKENMUELLER and DEMBER (1965a) used a black disc and ring on a white ground and a white disc and ring on a black ground, each with a disc field illumination (reflected) of 15 ft L and a ring field illumination of 25 ft L, at a steady ring duration of 100 msec and variable disc durations of 5, 15, and 25 msec. They used interstimulus intervals (ISI's), which differ from Δt in that delays are measured from target *offset* to mask onset. Thus, in effect, for ISI = 0, their Δt's are 5, 15, and 25 msec, respectively. Except for the 5 msec black disc, which showed a slightly more pronounced minimum at 30 msec Δt, (Arrow 7a), they obtained minima at ISI = 0 ($\Delta t \leq 5$, 15, and 25 msec; Arrows 7a′, 7b and 7b′, and 7c and

[5] Similarly ALPERN's (1953) careful work on metacontrast cannot be represented on this surface since the response measure (adjustment of luminance of target so that it matches a comparison stimulus) confounds T/M_a; so does MATTESON's (1969) study. However, ALPERN's data will be discussed more fully below.

7c′). Thus, except for 7a ($\Delta t_m = 30$ msec), no prediction from the model is inconsistent with their findings. However, measurement at shorter values of Δt are needed to substantiate any predictions. The 5 msec condition (7a) is inconsistent with predictions. However, in another study, they used a black disc and ring each illuminated by a 25 ft L lamp, again with a disc duration of 5 msec and a ring duration of 100 msec and got a monotonic function, failing to replicate the earlier finding (Arrow d). Viewing in all conditions was binocular.

When black targets and masks are used, a difference in background illumination has been assumed to be a difference in stimulus intensity, and the amplitude of neural response is set proportional to the logarithm of the background illumination. This can only be a rough approximation. Another difficulty of amplitude interpretation applies to the MAYZNER *et al.* (1965) study (Arrows 8a and 8b). They used the same stimulus conditions as did WEISSTEIN and HABER (1965), except that in one experiment they varied ring size. With the same ring size as WEISSTEIN and HABER (1965), they obtained the same $\Delta t_m = 40$ msec. But with a masking ring five times as thick, the Δt_m shifted to 20 msec. In terms of the model, a decrease in T/M would be needed in order to shift Δt_m toward the origin. Does an increase in the thickness of a black ring qualify for areal reciprocity and, therefore, for a decrease in T/M_a? Probably not. Sensitization data (e.g., WESTHEIMER, 1967; MATTHEWS, 1971) predict peripheral attenuation of lighted masks as their width increases, and "disinhibition" data (ROBINSON, 1966; DEMBER and PURCELL, 1967; SCHILLER and GREENFIELD, 1969) imply attenuation of the mask signal which may be peripheral or may be central. Both would result, for this net, in a small inhibitory signal, and thus a reduction in the amplitude of masking as well as either a shift *away* from the origin, or a steady value for Δt_m, depending on whether or not Δt_m was already at its upper limit. The amplitude of masking is reduced in MAYZNER *et al.* (1965) in accord with an attenuation hypothesis, but there is a shift in Δt_m toward the origin.

In the network, attenuation either shifts Δt_m away from the origin, or does not influence it at all (if T/M is in the limiting regions). On the other hand, a more elaborate network might predict that attenuation would result in slower conduction times (i.e., longer inhibition latencies). Thus mask width increases that produce attenuation would result in longer latencies, and Δt_m would shift toward the origin. Latencies would be longer because the signal amplitude is lowered (e.g., see KUFFLER, 1953, for latency increases with decreases in stimulus intensity). Latencies might also be longer if the mask signal had to travel over a greater distance to get to the site at which it interacts with the target, but such distance assumptions are based on a certain class of spatial models (see below) and do not necessarily have to be made. In any case, a shift in Δt_m toward the origin as mask width increases might provide indirect support for the basic fast inhibition hypothesis, namely, that as inhibition became slower Δt_m would decrease.[6]

[6] MATTESON (1969) found no shifts in Δt_m when the widths of lighted annuli were varied relative to a fixed target disc; however, he found no attenuation of masking, either. This may indicate that black stimuli (as in MAYZNER *et al.*) are processed differently from lighted stimuli; however, since predictions of Δt_m shifts based on increases in mask width involve an implicit spatial model, further discussion of this is deferred until Section V. In the same study, MATTESON failed to confirm a temporal prediction: he varied annulus luminance and found no Δt_m shifts.

However, the network makes no provision for latency shifts and no provision for spatial factors and thus while such an argument reasonably supports the fundamental idea of fast inhibition, it is not a prediction from the network as it stands. Hence Δt_m in the second condition (Arrow 8b) differs from prediction.[7]

Difficulties both in amplitude interpretation and in the definition of monotone functions arise with the ERIKSEN *et al.* (1967) data. They used targets and masks of equal contrast with T/M_d and $T/M_a = 1$ under binocular conditions. When they observed masking both at $\Delta t = 0$ and $\Delta t \approx 36$ msec, they found $\Delta t_m \approx 36$ msec (target durations varied for each individual subject, and 36 msec corresponds to a mean duration for an ISI of 0). It is not entirely clear where the neural net Δt_m should be (Arrow 9), since the mask was many times as thick as the target. As with MAYZNER *et al.* (1965), this probably indicates a beginning of maximum masking at a Δt somewhat less than 40 msec. From their data, it is evident that Δt_m is somewhere between $\Delta t = 0$ and $\Delta t \approx 36$, but clearly at $\Delta t > 0$. The prediction of the model is thus not inconsistent with the empirical findings, but measurement at earlier values of Δt would be needed to substantiate any prediction. However, there is a curious controversy here. The authors seem to think that they obtained a monotone function. They note that "contrary to Weisstein's findings, masking was a monotonic decreasing function of ISI for both 1 and 6 form displays [p. 500]." But they used ISI's, and a 0 msec. ISI corresponds, in their study, to a Δt of about 36 msec. If 0 msec ISI were the first point that they observed, then it would be understandable that they would conclude that they had a monotone function. But what is inexplicable is that although they also observed masking at ISI $= -36$ ($\Delta t = 0$), and found it to be considerably less than at ISI $= 0$ ($\Delta t = 36$), they do not connect these two points in their masking function (p. 503). They explain that the methodologies used to collect the data at these two points differed, and thus the points are not comparable. This explanation has merit; but because they prefer not to use the $\Delta t = 0$ point does not mean that they have substantiated a claim for having obtained a monotonic decreasing function for metacontrast. Thus, although it is not entirely clear where the predicted value would be, it is clear that their study does not contradict the shape of the function predicted by the net.

Later studies by ERIKSEN and his colleagues (ERIKSEN and MARSHALL, 1969; ERIKSEN *et al.*, 1970) have attempted to replicate studies of other investigators in which U-shaped metacontrast functions were found, but with a change in the response measure to a forced-choice indicator. Other, "subjective" response indicators that have been used, they argue, are invalid. KAHNEMAN (1968) answers

---

While no provision for latency has been made in the neural network, one would expect, given a fast inhibition hypothesis, that decreases in annulus luminance would increase its latency, and thus Δt_m would shift towards the origin. But the response measure that MATTESON used (adjustment of target luminance until it matches a standard) may obscure latency differences, since, as the annulus decreases in luminance, so does the target in order for a match to the standard to occur. So if latency increases are predicted for the annulus, they should hold equally for the target. Hence, latency shifts would be predicted for both target and mask in the same direction; a relatively constant Δt_m might result.

[7] This differs from WEISSTEIN (1968), where a leftward Δt_m shift was predicted on the basis of increase in ring size.

this argument at length. Briefly, the question is: valid for what? For metacontrast, most of the "objective" response indicators devised yield results with a large amount of variance (e.g., ERIKSEN *et al.*, 1970), whereas "subjective" response indicators, such as magnitude estimations, yield highly consistent results with little intertrial variance. For instance, in WEISSTEIN *et al.* (1970) ten magnitude estimations were required for each subject at each of 27 Δt's, presented in random order; yet the resulting functions were remarkably smooth, and the residual variance low, especially as compared to the forced-choice response from the same subjects in similar conditions. Even with only *five* magnitude estimations at each of 27 Δt's (see Figure 6), functions are quite smooth. In any case, these later studies of ERIKSEN and his colleagues do not avoid the difficulty presented in the study considered above, namely, determination of the $\Delta t = 0$ point; in fact, in the later studies, a $\Delta t = 0$ point is not even included in the observations. Thus these later studies cannot be represented on this surface.

The results of FEHRER and RAAB (1962) support the predictions in the case where a monoptically viewed center lighted square target was flanked on both sides by masking squares at $T/M_d = 1$, $T/M_a = 1$ (Arrow 10a). There were no response measures taken of the amplitude of masking at each of the Δt's used; however, a qualitative account of the masking function was given, and maximum masking occurred at about 75 msec. In a second condition, however, where T/M_d was changed to 0.1, although there was now a noticeable darkening at $\Delta t = 0$, the target was reported to have disappeared more completely at Δt's corresponding to the first condition (Arrow 10b). The net predicts, on the other hand, a masking minimum starting at about 15–20 msec Δt. In view of the qualitative nature of the FEHRER and RAAB function, it is not clear whether or not this second finding is a contradiction.

The twenty-five data points that have been discussed so far are those reviewed by WEISSTEIN (1968). Since then, some additional studies have been reported.

SCHILLER and SMITH (1968) presented a lighted disc and ring with $T/M_a = 1$, $T/M_d = 1$ and duration of stimuli 5 msec.[8] With monoptic viewing, $\Delta t_m = 65$ msec; with dichoptic viewing, $\Delta t_m = 45$ msec. Neither function contradicts the U vs. monotone dichotomy, and the minima are within the range predicted by the net (Arrows 11a and 11b).

STEWART and PURCELL (1970) presented dark letters (targets) and dark rings (masks) on lighted grounds in three different experiments. For all of them, $T/M_d = 0.4$ and $T/M_a = 1$. In the first experiment, they varied the target and mask over five different retinal positions. Except for central fixation, where they did not obtain masking, they reported $\Delta t_m = 50$ msec. This point is within the predicted range, but since they only tested Δt's of 0, 50, and 110 msec, not much significance can be attached to the agreement. In a second experiment, they added Δt's of 0, 25, 30, 40, 50, and 90 msec. Here, for the letters *O* and *D* and the letters *A* and *T*, they obtained Δt_m at 50 msec; for the letter *C*, $\Delta t_m = 30$ msec. Except for the letter *C*, then, the study places Δt_m in the 50 to 90 msec region. Finally, in a third experiment, using *O* and *D* and Δt's of 22.5, 25, 30, 40, 60 and 90 msec, they report $\Delta t_m = 50$ msec for both dark and light interstimulus intervals. Thus,

[8] Personal communication from PETER H. SCHILLER (duration was not specified in the published report).

50 msec (Arrow 12) seems an accurate estimate of their Δt_m. This agrees with predictions.

WEISSTEIN *et al.* (1970) presented lighted targets consisting either of a disc or of a *C* in one of four orientations. Masks were lighted annuli of equal energy or lighted annuli with four gaps corresponding to the gap in the *C* at each orientation. Viewing was dichoptic. They compared forced-choice responses (the orientation of the *C*) with magnitude estimations (the disc). In all cases, U-shaped functions were obtained. Subjects varied considerably both in similarity of the functions when measured these two different ways, and in Δt_m. One subject had almost identical functions, whereas for another subject, the function obtained with the forced-choice measure shifted to the right by 60 msec. If Δt_m is averaged across subjects and across response measures (without weighting by amplitudes which vary considerably for each subject and for each type of measure), the average Δt_m is 40 msec, which is again in agreement with the network's predictions (Arrow 13).

BLANC-GARIN (1968) presented white discs or half discs on black grounds, followed by white annuli, and asked subjects to rate the apparent brightness, duration and size of the discs, under varying mask durations and viewing conditions. Masking functions differed depending on the judgment required. In general, as the mask increased in duration, Δt_m shifted toward the origin for ratings of apparent brightness, but not for ratings of apparent duration. For $T/M_a = 1$, $T/M_d = 1$; and $T/M_a = 1$, and $T/M_d = 0.5$, for apparent brightness, $\Delta t_m = 50$ and $\Delta t_m = 30$, respectively (Arrows 14a and 14b). For both conditions, $\Delta t_m = 75$ msec for apparent duration. For the other experiments in this study, Δt_m was in this range, which agrees generally with predictions from the network, although there were some small departures from prediction.

Finally, WEISSTEIN (1971) compared two kinds of masks: lighted discs, and lighted annuli of equal outside diameter. Targets were lighted smaller discs. T/M was varied in several ways. Luminance ratios were varied with duration ratios held constant at 1, duration ratios were varied with luminance ratios held constant at 1, or both luminance and duration were varied. The Δt_m did not change with these different ways of varying energy ratios. Although U-shaped functions (or W-shaped functions if monoptic presentation is used) were obtained for both types of masks, only results for annuli will be considered in this section. For the monoptic function (an average of three subjects), $\Delta t_m = 100$ msec for $T/M = 0.875$; and $\Delta t_m = 90$ msec for $T/M = 0.5$. For the dichoptic function, $\Delta t_m = 30$ msec for $T/M = 0.875$; and $\Delta t_m = 20$ msec for $T/M = 0.5$. Monoptic viewing produces Δt_m larger than predicted (Arrows 15a and b). Dichoptic viewing produces Δt_m smaller than predicted (Arrows 15c and d).

In all, thirty-five points are considered. Only one of these contradicts the U/monotone dichotomy, and this was not replicated in a later study (HECKENMUELLER and DEMBER, 1965a; 1965b). It seems from this, then, that a general prediction from the fast inhibition hypothesis holds, namely that the network accurately predicts the shape of the metacontrast function.

On the other hand, seven other points varied enough from the predicted Δt_m range to suggest that there were systematic variations which the network did not account for. While intersubject variance is high, and this accounts for much of the variation (e.g., see WEISSTEIN *et al.*, 1970) there are at least two other factors that systematically influence Δt_m: viewing conditions, and size of masks. In particular, monoptic viewing conditions produce Δt_m values that are generally higher than those obtained under dichoptic conditions. The constants in the net were fit to a function obtained under binocular conditions. Four of the points considerably higher than predicted (KOLERS, 1962, Arrow 6; WEISSTEIN, 1971, Arrows 14a and b; FEHRER and RAAB, 1962, Arrow 10b) were from functions obtained under monocular conditions. Two points lower than predicted (WEISSTEIN, 1971, Arrows 14c and d) were from functions obtained under dichoptic conditions. If functions obtained under binocular viewing conditions reflect both monoptic and dichoptic contributions, then it would be reasonable that the network would underpredict monoptic metacontrast, and overpredict dichoptic metacontrast.

Finally, with other conditions equal, a mask five times as thick moved Δt_m 20 msec closer to the origin (MAYZNER *et al.*, 1965, Arrow 8b). As discussed above (and below, Section V) an inverse relationship between Δt_m and width of mask may, in fact, support the basic fast inhibition hypothesis. But such a relationship involves spatial factors, and these are yet to be incorporated into the network.

Before exploring these systematic variations in more detail (see below) another general prediction from the fast inhibition hypothesis will be discussed. This is that, as a target-mask sequence is recycled, in other words, as the response to the sequence (target-mask-target-mask- . . .-target-mask) approaches steady state, the target will increase in apparent brightness.

D. Steady-State Conditions

SCHILLER and SMITH (1966) found, using a lighted 43 ft L disc and ring as target and mask, respectively, that if a target-mask combination is "cycled," that is, if the target is presented, then the mask presented after a delay at which maximum masking occurs, then the target presented again after another delay equal to the first, and so forth, up to six target-mask cycles, the target reappears with a particular apparent brightness which matches that of a 21.5 ft L disc presented for 5 msec.

The reappearance of a target under these circumstances is predicted very naturally from the fast inhibition hypothesis.

Each new target presentation builds upon a pre-existing level of decaying excitation; each new masking presentation must build up inhibition from an almost zero level of inhibition. This is because the inhibition has a much faster time constant than the excitation; it builds up more rapidly, and it decays more rapidly. That the inhibition has a much faster time constant means that a maximum metacontrast suppression will occur at some nonzero delay between target and mask. In other words, this fast time constant is a crucial factor: it determines both that the metacontrast function will be U-shaped for certain stimulus combinations, and that cycling a target and mask will lead to the reappearence of the target. Specific predictions concerning the value of apparent brightness to which this excitation will return are extremely difficult, however. SCHILLER and SMITH used lighted discs and rings, presented to a dark-adapted eye, and WEISSTEIN and HABER used black targets and masks presented to a light-adapted eye. The model at present provides no mechanism for dark and light adaptation nor for the difference between dark and lighted stimuli. Thus no corrections can be made for possible differences in the size of the neural response that may result from these differences in stimulating conditions.

Nevertheless, the question of whether the rise in excitation approaches the level reported in SCHILLER and SMITH is such an interesting one in light of the predictions possible from this model that a preliminary investigation was undertaken. Since masking increased in SCHILLER and SMITH (apparent brightness decreased over a $2^1/_2$ log unit range in SCHILLER and SMITH, as compared to a discrimination decrease of less than 1 log unit in WEISSTEIN and HABER), it was assumed that the neural inhibitory response had increased. Thus, a parameter change was made which increased the size of the response to the mask in the second neuron in the masking line, and thus increased the amount of inhibition that the mask exerted. The value of B_{22}, the inhibitory proportionality constant, was increased. (This is, in effect, a scaling change. Alternately, A_{21} could have been increased or A_{11} or A_{12} decreased. That is, the parameter change does not involve changing time constants; it merely involves a correction for the size of mask inhibition as compared to target excitation.)With this change, the output of n_{13} at the sixth target-mask cycle matches the output of n_{13} to a 21.5 ft L stimulus presented for 5 msec. This is shown in the machine readout, Fig. 5b. In addition, it is possible to describe the machine masking function using apparent brightness as the response measure. The masking function thus obtained is compared to the SCHILLER and SMITH function in Fig. 5a. A change in one parameter value is made, and thus the fit is *ad hoc*. While this restricts the generality of the prediction, it is nevertheless interesting that with this fit, a "cycled" target reappears at the value found empirically.

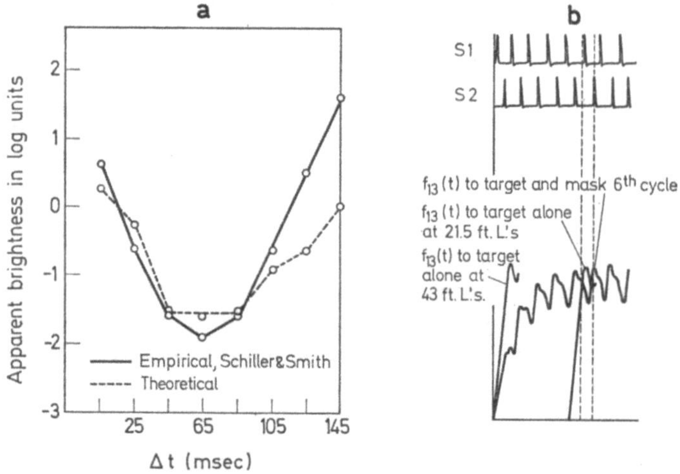

Fig. 5. A masked disc of light will reappear if the target-mask sequence is repeated six times in succession, with the delay between mask and repeated target = delay between target and mask = Δt at which maximum masking occurs. [This is shown in b), a machine read-out: the output from n_{13} rises to a value which would be obtained if a light of 21.5 ft L had been presented; this matches the apparent brightness value at which the target reappears in the Schiller and Smith study. In a) is a comparison with the Schiller and Smith (1966) data of the backward masking function as predicted by the net. This fit is *ad hoc*, since the proportionality constant, B_{22}, has been increased for this simulation]

E. Specific Shape Predictions

In summary, general consequences of the fast inhibition hypothesis are in accord with empirical data. However, in order to move toward strong validation of this hypothesis,[9] specific shapes of the metacontrast functions must be compared to predicted shapes and shown to vary in the same way.

Similar difficulties to those discussed above in attempting a specific fit to the SCHILLER and SMITH function were encountered in almost every metacontrast study reviewed in WEISSTEIN (1968). Precise function fitting was thus not attempted in that paper, since each study varied from every other study with regard to stimulus shapes, sizes, types of illumination and background, response indicators, viewing conditions and subjects.

Intersubject variance in particular presents a problem. In general, it appears unwise to average subjects. While this was done in the WEISSTEIN (1968) fit to the WEISSTEIN and HABER (1965) function, it is clear from that study and subsequent ones that each subject in metacontrast should be considered individually. It is a perhaps unfortunate, but nevertheless persistent fact that there is a great deal of variation among subjects in metacontrast (WEISSTEIN *et al.*, 1970) and indeed, in many psychophysical paradigms (e.g., MATTHEWS, 1971; TELLER and LINDSAY, 1970). In the WEISSTEIN and HABER study (1965), if the four subjects are considered individually, large differences are apparent: amplitudes of masking at maximum vary between 40 to 80% incorrect response; Δt_m's range from 40 to 70 msec. In the WEISSTEIN (1968) model the original neural net was fit to an average from WEISSTEIN and HABER (1965). While there appeared to be departures from predicted Δt_m which were based on systematic factors, and while specific shape comparisons between empirical data and network output had to be compared, clearly the factors responsible for departures from prediction could not be sorted out with certainty until subjects themselves were held constant across conditions.

Some of these factors can now be compared, since two subjects have subsequently been run on an extensive series of parametric experiments[10]; and a third on most of them). These subjects do differ considerably in Δt_m; on the other hand, the behavior of the metacontrast function obtained for each subject changes in the *same* way with changes in stimulating conditions, and the subjects remain internally consistent: their differences are stable over many trials and many experiments.

Both dichoptic and monoptic viewing conditions have been tested. A major difference between functions obtained under these two conditions is that although dichoptic functions are skewed towards the origin at any T/M, $\Delta t_m = 0$ occurs at a lower T/M than that predicted by the network. It is not entirely clear why this is so, although there are a number of plausible explanations. For instance, it is possible that binocularly driven neural units occur at higher afferent orders than monocularly driven units (HUBEL and WIESEL, 1968). If an extra layer

---

[9] See WEISSTEIN (1968) and WEISSTEIN (1969) for discussions of criteria for acceptance or rejection of these types of models.

[10] WEISSTEIN, N.: Some further elaborations of the Rashevsky-Landahl neural net in light of parametric metacontrast studies. In preparation.

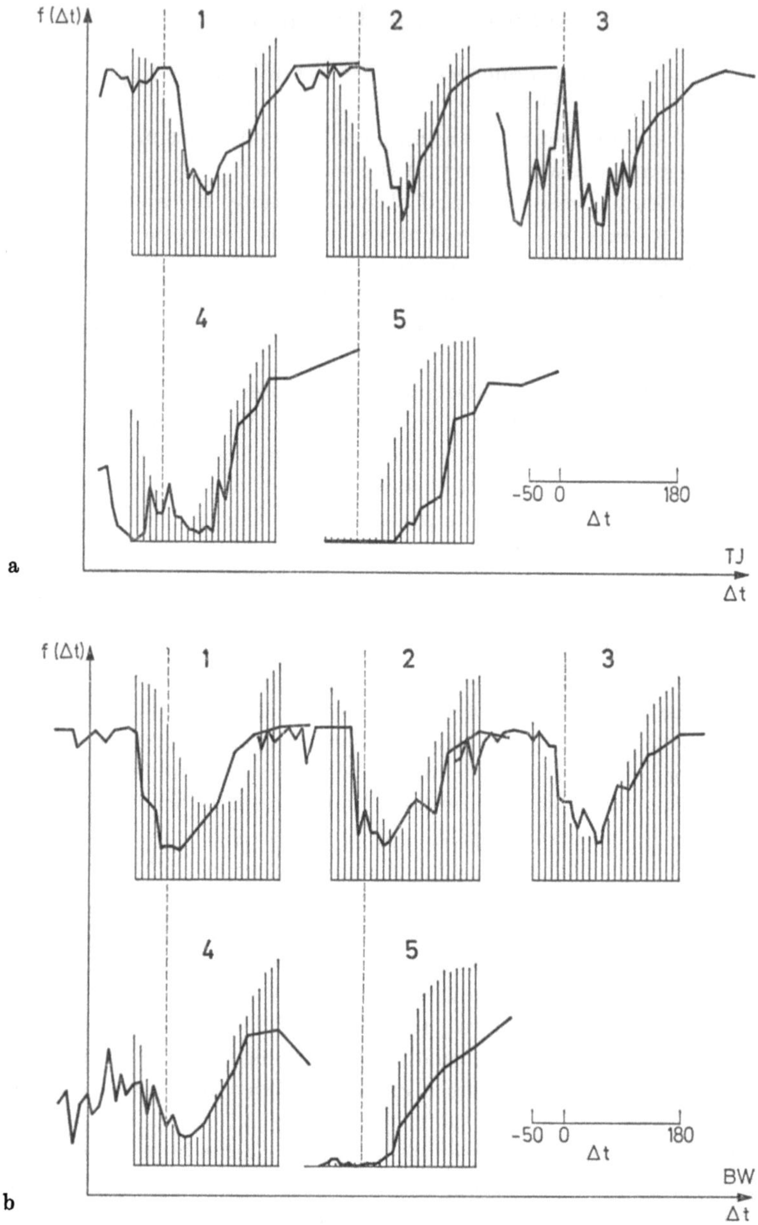

Fig. 6. Monoptic metacontrast for each of three subjects as compared with the fundamental network output. The solid connected curves are empirical metacontrast functions obtained by presenting a lighted 16 msec. 1° disc whose luminance varied, and a lighted 16 msec, 16 ft L annulus with a 1° 1′ inside diameter and a 1° 23′ outside diameter. Each point on the solid curves represents a geometric mean of five magnitude estimations at each of 27 Δt's, beginning with $\Delta t = -100$ and proceeding in 10 msec increments to $\Delta t = +100$; in 25 msec increments to $\Delta t = +200$; and 250 and 300 msec. Dotted vertical lines indicate $\Delta t = 0$ for each function. For each target luminance, the unmasked target was assigned a modulus of 10. As the target luminance varied, T/M_a was respectively (1) 1.0, (2) 0.5, (3) 0.2, (4) 0.125, and (5) 0.0625. Each vertical line represents the maximum cumulative frequency of firing of n_{13} at Δt's in 10 msec increments beginning with —50 msec, as in Fig. 2

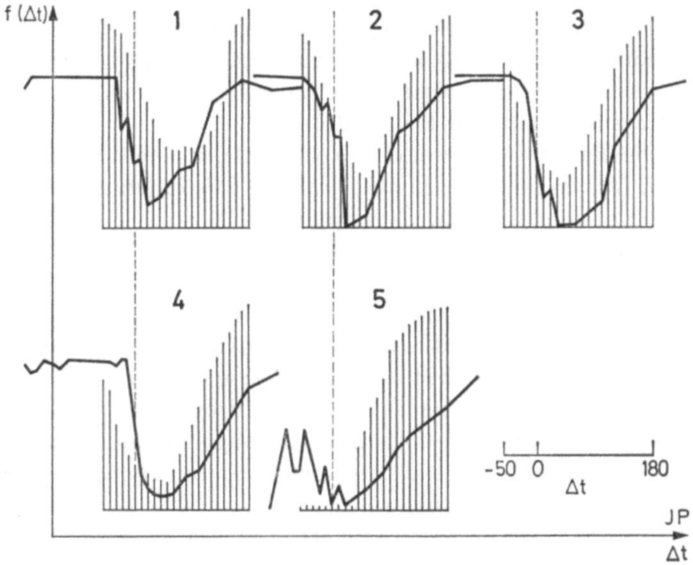

Fig. 6c

is added to the network, with approximately the same parameters as n_{12} and n_{22}, then the network will undergo much less rapid changes in shape with changes in T/M. On the other hand, this also shifts Δt_m to the right. However, the righward shift might be obscured by binocular rivalry. SCHILLER and SMITH (1968) suggested that binocular rivalry enters into dichoptic metacontrast and that the resulting masking function reflects this interaction. For instance, the small Δt_m may be a consequence of this interaction, as would be the skewing toward the origin at any T/M. The monoptic vs. dichoptic functions obtained by SCHILLER and SMITH (1968) support this interpretation. Dichoptic masking is much greater at early Δt; at later Δt, the dichoptic function coincides with the monoptic masking function.

On the other hand, the monoptic functions follow closely the predictions of the network (if they are corrected, in two out of three subjects, for a rightward shift in Δt_m at all T/M). A comparison of the phase shift and shape changes in the fundamental network output with monoptic masking functions from the three subjects mentioned above follows.

A lighted target disc was presented, 1° visual angle, preceded, followed, or simultaneous with a lighted annulus, 1° 1′ inside diameter and 1° 23′ outside diameter, whose centers were 1° from a lighted 4 ft L, 4′ central fixation cross. The mask was kept constant at 16 ft L's; the target luminance was varied so that T/M_a was 1) 1.0, 2) 0.5, 3) 0.2, 4) 0.125, and 5) 0.0625. Target and mask durations were both 16 msec. Each subject made 5 magnitude estimations at each of 27 Δt's, from -100 to $+100$ in 10 msec increments; from $+100$ to $+200$ in 25 msec increments; and at 250 and 300 msec. For each different target luminance, the subject used the same modulus; thus, in effect, each metacontrast curve was normalized, and their shapes could be compared.

Fig. 6 shows the results for TJ, BW and JP, superimposed on the computer readout (the fundamental network output) shown in Fig. 2.

For TJ (Fig. 6a), notice the following striking similarities: in (2), the function narrows and becomes deeper; in (3) and (4) the function skews towards the origin; and in (5) the function becomes weak monotonic. There are some dissimilarities:

1. Paracontrast is obtained at low T/M_a.

2. Δt_m is to the left of the network's output in (1), and to the right of the network's output in (2), (3), and (4); in other words, TJ's functions do not shift as rapidly to the left as does the network output.

3. TJ's function in (5) recovers more slowly at larger Δt than the network output.

As for the first dissimilarity, the network was not designed to predict paracontrast. The other two dissimilarities are interesting in that they may indicate an interaction between a left phase shift due to reduction in T/M_a, and a right phase shift due to longer target latencies as luminance drops from 16 to 1 ft L. The rightward movement in TJ's functions then, although in disagreement with the network output, might, in fact, tend to support the underlying hypothesis of a difference in excitation and inhibition rates.

In order to compare the functions for JP and BW (Fig. 6b and 6c) each empirical function was translated 70 msec to the left. (A translation was required because the network underpredicts monoptic functions.) In other words, Δt_m for JP at the highest T/M_a tested is actually 90 msec; for BW, 60 msec. It would be better to fit new constants for JP and BW than simply to shift the functions, since, as Δt_m increases, T/M at which $\Delta t_m = 0$ decreases. For JP, whose unshifted Δt_m was highest, 90 msec, (as compared to an unshifted Δt_m of 60 msec for BW), the need for new constants is clearly noticeable at (4) and (5). It is only at (5), in fact, that the function shows the characteristic skewing toward the origin. It was decided to continue to use the same set of constants as in WEISSTEIN (1968), however, to show that although subjects differ, the fundamental similarities in the behavior of metacontrast functions over decrease in T/M does not.

Functions for subjects JP and BW illustrate both the leftward (predicted) and rightward (not predicted but in agreement with underlying hypothesis) motion of the metacontrast functions as T/M decreases. Notice again, for JP, the narrowing of the function at (2), and the gradual widening of the functions in both directions, especially at (5). At (5), the empirical curve is not weak monotonic with respect to Δt, but resembles more the network output for (4). As discussed previously, given an initial Δt_m of 90 msec, the T/M at which $\Delta t_m = 0$ is less, which is consistent with the model's output.

The functions for BW do not show a narrowing at (2), but at (3); and starting with (3), the functions closely follow the computer readout, with the exception, again, of a much slower recovery at (5) for large Δt's.

There is wide variation in Δt_m between subjects; however, what is striking about these data is that the shapes of the functions follow so closely the shapes generated by the computer. In two of the three subjects (although not always the same two) the functions narrow and lengthen at (2), become asymmetrical and skew at (4), and drop to weak monotonic at (5). For the subject where narrowing does not occur at (2), it occurs at (3); for the subject where skewing does not occur at (4) it occurs at (5). Thus, these departures from prediction are regular and related to the particular rate constants of each subject.

Although it seems clear that hereafter each subject should be fit individually, a specific shape prediction from the WEISSTEIN (1968) constants should be made for one more study: that of ALPERN (1953). His classic study has been a notable omission in this discussion of the metacontrast literature so far, as well as in WEISSTEIN (1968). His study could not be represented on the surface predicted by the network (Fig. 4), since his response measure involved continual changes in T/M. In addition, no attempt was made at that time to fit individually the functions he obtained, for the reasons discussed on p. 261. On the other hand, if it is assumed that values of Δt_m obtained with monoptic viewing are underpredicted by the network, then there is a reasonable basis upon which to adjust the network's predictions to the functions obtained in ALPERN'S study: namely, to translate the network's predicted function to the right.

Predictions to compare with ALPERN'S design can be generated by the network using the same constants as in all other predictions (except the SCHILLER and SMITH, 1966 "cycling" discussed above) and by obtaining a response measure by varying target voltage for each Δt until it matches a standard output from

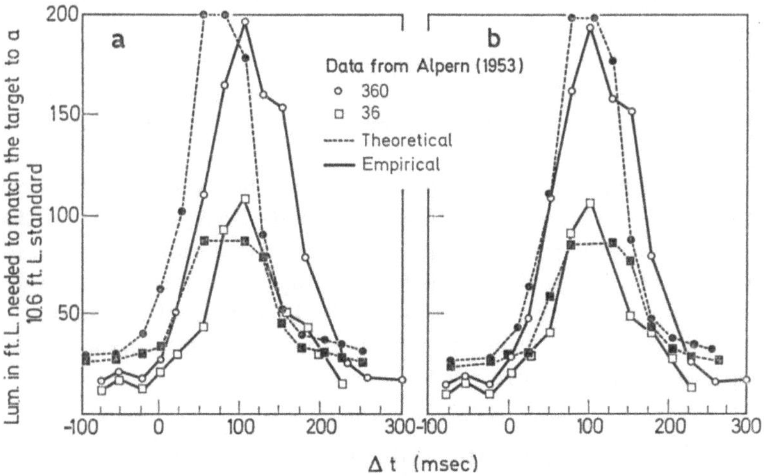

Fig. 7. A comparison of two of the metacontrast functions for subject R.V.H. obtained by ALPERN (1953) with those predicted by the neural net. The solid lines are the empirical functions obtained by adjusting the luminance of the target (a center rectangle) until it matched the apparent brightness of a 10.6 ft L standard. Functions are shown for masks (flanking rectangles) of 36 and 360 ft L (squares and circles, respectively). All flashes: 5 msec. The dotted lines are the network functions: in a) as predicted by the net; in b) as predicted by the net except translated 25 msec to the right

the network, i.e., the network's response to a 10.6 ft L, 5 msec pulse. This voltage is then converted into its luminance value, that is, into $\log^{-1}(S_1/k + c/k)$. Fig. 7 shows matches for two masking luminances: 36 ft L and 360 ft L. In 7a, the dotted line represents the function generated from the neural net and the solid line represents ALPERN'S data. Following the reasoning above (monoptic functions have higher Δt_m), the theoretical functions have been translated by 25 msec in 7b. The fit then becomes rather good. There are departures to the right for predictions using the 360 ft L mask, and departures to the left for predictions using the 36 ft L mask. A possible explanation for this is individual subject variation.

In summary, the agreement between the model's predictions and the empirical data is very good. In WEISSTEIN (1968), general consequences of the fast inhibition hypothesis were in accord with empirical data; data against which to compare specific shape predictions were not available. Since then, such data have been collected, and as shown in the section above, the agreement is striking. There are departures from prediction: subjects vary, and metacontrast functions at small T/M recover more slowly than predicted. But if this slow recovery is due to increase in target latency, although not provided for by the model, such a departure from prediction may, in fact, support the fast inhibition hypothesis.

Thus, the notion of fast inhibitory rate constants and slow excitatory rate constants provides a working temporal model that makes a number of basic predictions that agree with empirical findings. For response measures in which stimulus energy is constant, the reappearance of the target in steady-state is predicted, as well as the monotone/U dichotomy, and the narrowing and subsequent skewing of functions as T/M decreases. In addition, although not incorporated into the network, the suggestion of further increases in Δt at which masking will be obtained due to possible longer target latencies is in accord with a fast inhibition hypothesis. For response measures in which target energy is adjusted to match a standard, the model also predicts the general shape of the function under different masking energies.

But there is a final variation in Δt_m which must be considered: the decrease in Δt_m with increase in width of mask (MAYZNER *et al.*, 1965; see above, p. 225). This involves not only considerations of latency, but also an implicit spatial model. The neural network was designed to predict only temporal factors, and thus the MAYZNER *et al.* results, although in accord with the basic idea of fast inhibition, were not an explicit prediction from the model. However, spatial modeling is clearly the next priority if metacontrast is to be explained.

V. Elaboration: Space as Well as Time

In some ways, development of a spatial model is a more difficult task than of a temporal model, because of essential non-linearities such as form-specific effects (UTTAL, 1970). If the goal is to account for metacontrast in terms of neural response and organization, then a spatial model must describe receptive fields for units or populations of units involved in metacontrast interactions. But this is a difficult task because different estimates for receptive fields are obtained, depending on what stimuli are used (see below). The difficulty is no doubt related to the central locus of the metacontrast effect. Higher-order analyses occurring in the visual system may classify different stimuli in such a way that either different units are involved in metacontrast, depending on the stimuli, or different stimuli are processed in such a way that their input to constant units involved in metacontrast is entirely different, and thus receptive field estimates vary. The task becomes then to describe higher-order processing as a precondition for specifying higher-order structure. Work on a spatial model has only begun although a few preliminary remarks can be made about what such a model may have to look like.

Because of the essential non-linearity of spatial metacontrast interactions, it is clear that simple homogeneous or composite neural layer models will not work. (See RATLIFF, 1965, for a description of such models; also see LYUBINSKII *et al.*, 1968, for a derivation of some properties of such models.) This is true whether the models are based on receptive fields as described by neurophysiologists for the retina, lateral geniculate nucleus, or even Area 17 of the visual cortex (e.g., HUBEL and WIESEL, 1968), or whether they are based on weighting functions (impulse responses) derived from frequency response or other psychophysical measures. Nevertheless, it is instructive to begin with predictions from such models.

The integral over the region of the target stimulus of a weighting function derived either from the inverse Fourier transform of a contrast sensitivity curve (e.g., CAMPBELL *et al.*, 1969), or from other techniques (THOMAS, 1968), convoluted with a metacontrast paradigm consisting essentially of edges (three 1′ or 3′ vertical lines) at various spatial separations from each other will not predict an empirical metacontrast function obtained using the same stimuli[11]. Empirically, the inhibitory region is much larger than predicted. Inhibitory effects are predicted up to, but not beyond, separations of 15′ between target and mask; empirically, they are found at separations of 2° to 3°. ALPERN (1953), using much larger rectangles, found effects up to, but not including, a 2° separation.

However, if instead of measuring the extent of inhibitory effects by varying the separation between targets and masks, the stimuli are kept at the same separation (45″ visual angle), and the width of the mask is increased in small increments, then the weighting function derived from the empirical metacontrast function closely resembles the weighting function mentioned above (GROWNEY and WEISSTEIN, 1971). In other words, inhibitory effects increase with increase in mask width through a width of about 10′; then the masking amplitudes are constant as mask widths increase further.

Thus, for most subjects and most designs, an essential non-linearity occurs. The effect can be obtained over a fairly large separation between target and mask (2° to 3°, depending on the study and stimuli used), but increasing widths of masks over this range while keeping the edge-to-edge separation between target and mask constant, does not produce increases in masking amplitude.

An initial hypothesis to explain this is that one type of metacontrast effect primarily involves interaction with the nearest edge of a stimulus, perhaps up to 10′ of width, and that masks beyond that width contribute little to the effect except for the near-edge information. No mechanism by which a near edge is involved in the interaction while a far edge is ignored is proposed at this time. The near edge, however, may resemble what one would predict as output from a prior convolution of a weighting function (e.g., the inverse Fourier transform of the CAMPBELL *et al.*, 1969 contrast sensitivity function) with a gate function, except that disinhibition or attenuation is not invariably obtained. Attenuation would be expected because as masks increase beyond the width of the positive region of the weighting function, the "edges" formed as neural output to the mask are lower in amplitude than the neural output to masks of smaller widths. Then any linear neural layer model with a weighting function that consists of both positive and

[11] COX, S., GROWNEY, R., and WEISSTEIN, N.: Determination of weighting functions inferred from metacontrast interactions. In preparation.

negative components will predict disinhibition due to prior attenuation for more than one layer. The Mayzner *et al.* results with wide black rings (see above, Section IV) conforms to this prediction of disinhibition; so do the results for one subject in Growney and Weisstein (1971) and, apparently, all subjects in Dember and Purcell (1967). In the Dember and Purcell study, as in Mayzner *et al.* (1965), black stimuli were used; this may have something to do with the fact that disinhibition was obtained. But other studies (Matteson, 1969; the two remaining subjects in Growney and Weisstein, 1971) do not show disinhibition. The amplitude of masking levels off at some width (10′ in Growney and Weisstein, 1971; between $37^1/_2{}'$ to $1^1/_2{}^\circ$ in Matteson, 1969); it does not decrease beyond that width.

Because results between subjects within studies and results between studies vary with regard to disinhibition, no attempt will be made at this time to explain in detail the failure to find it in several instances. However, there are certain spatial models for which disinhibition would not be predicted.

For instance Sperling (1970) discusses the failure to observe threshold minima for discs at a predicted optimum radius. Although his discussion is based on predictions from a neural model which involves shunting inhibition, and his threshold criteria are different from the response criteria assumed for metacontrast, the arguments he presents might hold for the failure to find disinhibition with wide masks in metacontrast. In particular, if the input to the metacontrast interaction is assumed to be some function (such as an average) of an output from a subset of independent detectors, each with a threshold and asymptote, rather than the convolution of initial input with a single, broad-band weighting function (independent detectors have been suggested for different reasons, by Campbell and Robson, 1968; Blakemore and Campbell, 1969), then one might expect increase in amplitude of masking with increase in the width of a mask up to a certain width, and no further decreases in masking beyond that width. The maximum output of a single detector with a receptive field similar to the weighting function mentioned above occurs at different separations from the target given increasing widths of masks, first increasing in separation, and later jumping back to a fixed separation. This may interact with metacontrast weighting to produce less attenuation for wide masks. Then, if there were a number of independent detectors, each turned on at a different mask width, a more or less steady output might result. With very wide masks, there would be some attenuation, but it would be sufficiently small so as to be hard to detect with psychophysical measures.

It is interesting, in connection with a "near-edge" hypothesis, that Uttal (1970) did find masking when two adjacent rectangles flanked two vertical lines, even though, otherwise, flanks and center had to be identical.

One support for a "near-edge" hypothesis would be if an inside edge and a single edge acted somewhat in the same manner. That is, if metacontrast, or one type of metacontrast, depended primarily on the nearest edge, then one should be able to obtain similar U-shaped functions with disc-disc masking as with disc-annulus masking. With disc-disc masking, however, as the masking disc increases in diameter the results should resemble more what one obtains when target and mask are at increasing separations from each other.

U-shaped functions can be obtained with disc-disc masking (this was mentioned in the introduction p. 236; Schiller and Greenfield, 1969; Weisstein, 1971). There is not much information on this yet, and since there is considerable variation between studies, not much weight can be attached to a single study. But it does appear from the Schiller and Greenfield study (1969) that as lighted masking discs increase in diameter, the masking function both attenuates and shifts phase toward the origin. These results are in accord both with spatial and temporal predictions.

In some ways then, if one is to look for receptive field characteristics of units or populations of units involved in metacontrast interactions, one must devise ways to measure spatial metacontrast weighting functions and this will necessarily involve understanding the kind of preprocessing that has occurred at afferent orders prior to the locus of the metacontrast effect. That is, the preprocessing itself will have to be described. It is possible that the nature of this preprocessing may become clearer by using designs whereby both adjacent and superimposed masks are used, so that two-edge stimuli may be compared to stimuli containing only one edge.

In summary: work on a spatial model involves discovering the mechanisms that produce the essential non-linearities found in metacontrast and relating these mechanisms to organization or receptive field characteristics of units or populations of units involved in higher-order visual processing.

VI. Conclusion

Although metacontrast paradigms resemble other masking paradigms, the results exhibit some interesting properties that cannot be explained on the basis of either temporal or spatial peripheral neural models. Yet there is considerable heuristic value in attempting neurophysiological modeling of the effect. Masking models based on neural interactions can be easily constructed, using Rashevsky two-factor neurons as components. The predictions from a network of such neurons can then be tested against the empirical evidence.

A network of five two-factor neurons constructed to simulate the temporal aspects of metacontrast produces results that are in very good accord with empirical data. Thus, there is a strong basis for agreement with the assumption that metacontrast involves fast inhibitory interaction at some central locus.

If this is assumed, as indeed this chapter suggests that it should be, there is an obvious next question: what is the spatial nature of this inhibitory interaction? Here, there are a number of essential non-linearities. These are, no doubt, related to the central locus of the effect, and the kind of processing that occurs at such a locus. At more central locations, neural units and populations of units respond in feature-specific ways to stimuli. Thus, the edge and form-specific properties of metacontrast do not preclude interpretation in primarily neurophysiological terms; rather, a satisfactory neurophysiological explanation of both the spatial and the temporal properties of metacontrast would contribute immeasurably to our understanding of higher-order visual processing. There is no reason why such higher-order visual processing cannot be understood in the basic terms of sensory physiology. An analysis of the processes involved in the metacontrast effect may contribute greatly to this understanding.

Acknowledgements. This work was supported in part by Grants PHS 8-RO1-EY-00143-03 to the author, and PHS 2-RO1-CA-06475 to Dr. L. Skaggs, Principal Investigator, Department of Radiology. The University of Chicago.

This chapter is an updating, revision, and expansion of "A Rashevsky-Landahl Neural Net: Simulation of Metacontrast", which appeared in Psychol. Rev. **75**, 494—521 (1968). Some material from that paper has been incorporated directly into this text. I wish to thank SUE COX, RONALD GROWNEY, and PAUL WACHOWIAK for their careful and critical readings of this text.

References

ALPERN, M.: Metacontrast. J. opt. Soc. Amer. **43**, 648—657 (1953).

— Rod-cone independence in the after-flash effect. J. Physiol. (Lond.) **176**, 462—472 (1965).

— RUSHTON, W. A. H.: The nature of the rise in threshold produced by contrast-flashes. J. Physiol. (Lond.) **189**, 519—534 (1967).

— — TORRI, S.: Encoding of nerve signals from retinal rods. Nature (Lond.) **223**, 1171—1172 (1969).

AVERBACH, E.: The span of apprehension as a function of exposure duration. J. verb. Learning and verb. Beh. **2**, 60—64 (1963).

BATTERSBY, W. S., WAGMAN, I. H.: Neural limitations of visual excitability. IV. Spatial determinants of retrochiasmal interaction. Amer. J. Psychol. **203**, 359—365 (1962).

BAUMGARTNER, R.: Kontrastlichteffekte an retinalen Ganglienzellen: Ableitungen vom Tractus opticus der Katze. In: The Visual System: Neurophysiology and Psychophysics. JUNG, R., KORNHUBER, H. (Eds.). Berlin-Göttingen-Heidelberg: Springer 1961.

BLAKEMORE, C., CAMPBELL, F. W.: On the existence of neurones in the human visual system selectively sensitive to the orientation and size of retinal images. J. Physiol. (Lond.) **203**, 237—260 (1969).

BLANC-GARIN, J.: Divers aspects de l'interférence dans le phénomène de masquage latéral. Vision Res. **8**, 509—523 (1968).

BOYNTON, R. M.: On-responses in the human visual system as inferred from psychophysical studies of rapid adaptation. Arch. Ophthal. **60**, 800—810 (1958).

— Some temporal factors in vision. In: Sensory Communication. ROSENBLITH, W. A. (Ed.). Cambridge: M.I.T. Press 1961.

CAMPBELL, F. W., CARPENTER, R. H. S., LEVINSON, J. Z.: Visibility of aperiodic patterns compared with that of sinusoidal gratings. J. Physiol. (Lond.) **204**, 283—308 (1969).

— ROBSON, J. G.: Application of Fourier analysis to the visibility of gratings. J. Physiol. (Lond.) **197**, 551—566 (1968).

COBB, W. A., DAWSON, G. D.: The latency and form in man of the occipital potentials evoked by bright flashes. J. Physiol. (Lond.) **152**, 108—121 (1960).

CORNSWEET, T., TELLER, D. Y.: Relation of increment thresholds to brightness and luminance. J. opt. Soc. Amer. **55**, 1303—1308 (1965).

CRAWFORD, B. E.: Visual adaptation to brief conditioning stimuli. Proc. roy. Soc. B **134**, 283—302 (1947).

CULL, P.: General two factor models. Bull. math. Biophys. **29**, 405 (1967).

DEMBER, W. N., PURCELL, D. G.: Recovery of masked visual targets by inhibition of the masking stimulus. Science **157**, 1335—1336 (1967).

DEVALOIS, R. L., PEASE, P. L.: Contours and contrast: Responses of monkey lateral geniculate nucleus cells to luminance and color figures. Science **171**, 694—696 (1971).

DONCHIN, E., LINDSLEY, D.: Visual evoked response correlates of perceptual masking and enhancement. Electroenceph. clin. Neurophysiol. **19**, 325—335 (1965).

ENROTH-CUGELL, C., PINTO, L.: Algebraic summation of centre and surround inputs to retinal ganglion cells of the cat. Nature (Lond.) **226**, 458—459 (1970).

ERIKSEN, C.: Temporal luminance summation effects in forward and backward masking. Perc. Psychophys. **1**, 87—92 (1966).

— BECKER, B. B., HOFFMAN, J. E.: Safari to masking land: A hunt for the elusive U. Perc. Psychophys. **8**, 245—250 (1970).

— COLEGATE, R. L.: Identification of forms at brief durations when seen in apparent motion. J. exp. Psychol. **84**, 137—140 (1970).

— COLLINS, J. F., GREENSPON, T. S.: An analysis of certain factors responsible for non-monotonic backward masking functions. J. exp. Psychol. **75**, 500—507 (1967).

— MARSHALL, P. H.: Failure to replicate a reported U-shaped visual masking function. Psychon. Sci. **15**, 195—196 (1969).

FEHRER, E.: Effect of stimulus on retroactive masking. J. exp. Psychol. **71**, 612—615 (1966).
— RAAB, D. H.: Reaction time to stimuli masked by metacontrast. J. exp. Psychol. **63**, 143—147 (1962).
— SMITH, E.: Effect of luminance ratio on masking. Perc. mot. Skills **14**, 243—253 (1962).
FRUMKES, T. E., STURR, J. F.: Spatial and luminance factors determining visual excitability. J. opt. Soc. Amer. **58**, 1657—1662 (1968).
FUORTES, M. G. F., HODGKIN, A. L.: Changes in time scale and sensitivity in the ommatidia of Limulus. J. Physiol. (Lond.) **172**, 239—263 (1964).
GROWNEY, R. L., WEISSTEIN, N.: Metacontrast and some spatial characteristics of human visual receptive fields. Paper delivered at meetings of Midwestern Psychological Association, 1971.
HARMON, L. D., LEWIS, K.: Neural modeling. Physiol. Rev. **46**, 513—591 (1966).
HECKENMUELLER, E., DEMBER, W. N.: A forced-choice indicator for use with Werner's disc-ring pattern in studies of backward masking. Psychon. Sci. **3**, 167—168 (1965a).
— — Paradoxical brightening of a masked black disc. Psychon. Sci. **3**, 457—458 (1965b).
HOUSEHOLDER, A. S.: Equivalence of the theories of nervous excitation of Hill, Monnier, and Rashevsky. Bull. math. Biophys. **6**, 79—81 (1944).
HUBEL, D. H., WIESEL, T. N.: Receptive fields and functional architecture of monkey striate cortex. J. Physiol. (Lond.) **195**, 215—243 (1968).
KAHNEMANN, D.: An onset-onset law for one case of apparent motion and metacontrast. Perc. Psychophys. **2**, 577—584 (1967).
— Method, findings, and theory in studies of visual masking. Psychol. Bull. **70**, 404—425 (1968).
KELLY, D. H.: Theory of Flicker and Transient Responses, I. Uniform Fields. J. opt. Soc. Amer. **61**, 537—546 (1971).
KOLERS, P. A.: Intensity and contour effects in visual masking. Vision Res. **2**, 277—294 (1962).
— Some psychological aspects of pattern recognition. In: Recognizing Patterns: Studies in Living and Automatic Systems. KOLERS, P. A., EDEN, M. (Eds.). Cambridge: M.I.T. Press 1968.
— ROSNER, B.: On visual masking (metacontrast): Dichoptic observation. Amer. J. Psychol. **73**, 2—21 (1960).
KUFFLER, S.: Discharge patterns and functional organization of mammalian retina. J. Neurophysiol. **16**, 37—68 (1953).
LANDAHL, H. D.: Mathematical models of neurone interaction. AIEE Special Publication S-134 (Switching Circuit Theory and Logical Design) 1962.
— A neural net model for masking phenomena. Bull. math. Biophys. **29**, 227—232 (1967).
LEVINSON, J. Z.: Flicker fusion phenomena. Science **160**, 21—28 (1968).
LICKER, M. D.: Early inhibition and excitation of the retinal ganglion cells. Vision Res. **9**, 25—36 (1969).
LYUBINSKII, I. A., POZIN, N. V., YAKHNO, V. P.: An analysis of models of a homogeneous neuron layer with lateral connections. Automation and Remote Control **28**, 1565—1576 (1968).
MARKOFF, J. I.: Thesis, Syracuse University, Syracuse. New York 1969.
— STURR, J. F.: Spatial and luminance determinants of the increment threshold under monoptic and dichoptic viewing. Abstract. J. opt. Soc. Amer. **59**, 1543 (1969).
MATTESON, H. H.: Effects of surround size and luminance on metacontrast. J. opt. Soc. Amer. **59**, 1461—1468 (1969).
MATTHEWS, M. L.: Spatial and temporal factors in masking by edges and disks. Perc. Psychophys. **9** (1 A), 15—21 (1971).
MAYZNER, M. S., BLATT, M. H., BUCHSBAUM, W. H., FRIEDEL, R. T., GOODWIN, P. E., KANON, D., KELEMAN, A., NILSSON, W. D.: A U-shaped backward masking function in vision: A partial replication of the Weisstein and Haber study with two ring sizes. Psychon. Sci. **3**, 79—80 (1965).
NACHMIAS, J., SACHS, M. B., ROBSON, J. G.: Independent spatial-frequency channels in human vision. J. opt. Soc. Amer. **59**, 1538 (1969).
NAKAYAMA, K.: Analysis of visual masking in terms of unit responses in the optic nerve and lateral geniculate body of the cat. Ph. D. Thesis, University of California (1968).
POGGIO, G. F., BAKER, F. H., LAMARRE, Y., RIVA, SANSEVERINO, E.: Afferent inhibition at inputs to visual cortex of cat. J. Neurophys. **32**, 892—925 (1969).
RAAB, D. H.: Backward masking. Psychol. Bull. **60**, 118—129 (1963).

RATLIFF, F.: Mach Bands: Quantitative Studies on Neural Networks in the Retina. San Francisco: Holden Day 1965.
RASHEVSKY, N.: Mathematical Biophysics. (Rev. ed.) Chicago: University of Chicago Press 1948.
ROBINSON, D. N.: Disinhibition of visually masked stimuli. Science **154**, 157—158 (1966).
ROTHBERG, J. M.: Simulation of neural nets with some applications to visual information processing. Computers and biomed. Res. **1**, 435—451 (1968).
RUMELHART, D. E.: A multicomponent theory if the perception of briefly exposed visual displays. J. math. Psychol. **7**, 191—218 (1970).
SCHILLER, P. H.: Single unit analysis of backward visual masking and metacontrast in the cat lateral geniculate nucleus. Vision Res. **8**, 855—866 (1968a).
— Single unit analysis of backward and forward masking in the cat lateral geniculate nucleus. Proc. 76th Ann. Conv. Amer. Psychol. Assn. **3**, 319—320 (1968b).
— CHOROVER, S. L.: Metacontrast: Its relation to evoked potentials. Science **153**, 1398—1401 (1966).
— GREENFIELD, A.: Visual masking and the recovery phenomenon. Perc. Psychophys. **6**, 182—184 (1969).
— SMITH, M.: Detection in metacontrast. J. exp. Psychol. **71**, 32—46 (1966).
— — Monoptic and dichoptic metacontrast. Perc. Psychophys. **3**, 237—239 (1968).
SPERLING, G.: A model for visual memory tasks. Hum. Factors **5**, 19—31 (1963).
— Model of visual adaptation and contrast detection. Perc. Psychophys. **8** (3), 143—157 (1970).
— SONDHI, M. M.: Model for visual luminance discrimination and flicker detection. J. opt. Soc. Amer. **58**, 1133—1145 (1968).
STEVENS, C. F.: Synaptic Physiology. Proc. IEEE **56**, 916—930 (1968).
STEWART, A. L., PURCELL, D. G.: U-shaped masking functions in visual backward masking: Effects of target configuration and retinal position. Perc. Psychophys. **7**, 253—256 (1970).
STIGLER, R.: Chronophotische Studien über den Umgebungskontrast. Arch. ges. Physiol. **134**, 365—435 (1910).
— Metacontrast (demonstration). Arch. int. Physiol. **14**, 78 (1913).
TELLER, D. Y.: Sensitization by annular surrounds: temporal (masking) transients. Vision Res. in press (1971).
— LINDSEY, B.: Sensitization by annular surrounds: Individual differences. Vision Res. **10**, 1045—1056 (1970).
THOMAS, J. P.: Linearity of spatial integrations involving inhibitory interactions. Vision Res. **8**, 49—60 (1968).
UTTAL, W. R.: On the physiological basis of masking with dotted visual noise. Perc. Psychophys. **7** (6), 321—327 (1970).
VAUGHN, H. G., JR., SILVERSTEIN, L.: Metacontrast and evoked potentials: A reappraisal. Science **160**, 207—208 (1968).
WEISSTEIN, N.: Backward masking and models of preceptual processing. J. exp. Psychol. **72**, 232—240 (1966).
— A Rashevsky-Landahl neural net: Simulation of metacontrast. Psychol. Rev. **75**, 494—521 (1968).
— What the frog's eye tells the human brain: Single cell analyzers in the human visual system. Psychol. Bull. **72**, 157—176 (1969).
— Neural symbolic activity: A psychophysical measure. Science **168**, 1489—1491 (1970).
— W-shaped and U-shaped functions obtained for monoptic and dichoptic disk-disk masking. Perc. Psychophys. **9** (3A), 275—278 (1971),
— GROWNEY, R. L.: Apparent movement and metacontrast: A note on Kahneman's formulation. Perc. Psychophys. **5**, 321—328 (1969).
— HABER, R. N.: A U-shaped backward masking function in vision. Psychon. Sci. **2**, 75—76 (1965).
— JURKENS, T., ONDERISIN, T.: Effect of forced-choice vs. magnitude-estimation measures on the waveform of metacontrast functions. J. opt. Soc. Amer. **60**, 978—980 (1970).
WERNER, H.: Studies on contour: I. Qualitative analyses. Amer. J. Psychol. **47**, 40—64 (1935).
WESTHEIMER, G.: Spatial interaction in the human retina during scotopic vision. J. Physiol. (Lond.) **181**, 881—894 (1965).
— Spatial interaction in human cone vision. J. Physiol. (Lond.) **190**, 139—154 (1967).

Chapter 11

Flicker

By

D. H. Kelly, Menlo Park, California (USA)

With 26 Figures

Contents

I. Introduction

The phenomena of visual flicker have been studied for more than two centuries. During the last several years, however, it has become apparent that most of the resulting data and theories can be simplified by the principles of Fourier analysis (mathematical relations that have been widely used in the physical sciences for more than a century). This analytic trend is the main theme of the present review; selected experimental results (psychophysical and electrophysiological) are emphasized primarily to clarify the underlying rationale.

This review covers only experiments on achromatic flicker sensitivity. Some flicker studies help to elucidate the mechanisms of color vision (Kelly, 1962; Green, 1969) or spatial-pattern processing in the retina (Ratliff *et al.*, 1967; Kelly, 1969), but these interactions among the variables of the visual process are not included here. Even experiments with transient stimuli and recent developments in flicker theory are mentioned only briefly in Secs. III and VII.

Several previous reviews of the field are available. The reader who wants a survey of the traditional literature on flicker can refer to an extensive, annotated bibliography by Landis (1953). Also, a classic monograph by Piéron (1961) is now available in English translation (1965); Piéron attempts a synthesis of the last half-century of flicker experiments. More recent work, up to 1963, is generally covered in a competent review by Brown (1965). The proceedings of the 1963 Amsterdam symposium on flicker (Henkes and Van der Tweel, 1964) should also be consulted for this period. A more recent review article by Levinson (1968) is excellent but narrower in scope; it is primarily concerned with a group of experiments that bear on a particular model.

A cautionary note to begin with: Despite its importance, mathematical analysis of the stimulus alone does not constitute a theory. Some current investigators seem to regard Fourier analysis itself as a model of the visual process (which they call "the Fourier model"), but this is erroneous. Fourier analysis has the same status as vector analysis, matrix analysis, or any other branch of mathematics; it is one of many tools that are useful for constructing models. But there is usually more to constructing a good theory than just using the right tools.

A detailed discussion of Fourier series and integral-transform techniques cannot be given here; the interested reader is referred to any text or handbook of engineering mathematics. But it is essential to understand that most physically realizable waveforms can be analyzed into (and hence synthesized out of) sinusoidal components. An infinite series of these sinusoidal elementary functions is generally required for periodic waveforms, and a continuous integral for transient pulses.

The simplest non-trivial model one can make for flicker responses is shown in Fig. 1. Here $f(t)$ represents a stimulus waveform (in units of, e.g., trolands or w/cm^2 at the retina) and $h(t)$ is the corresponding "output" waveform, at some point in the retina or central nervous system. (Certain mathematical restrictions apply to these inputs and outputs, but they permit all the types of pulses and periodic waveforms of interest here.) The key postulate of this model is the principle of superposition, which states that the output corresponding to the sum of two given inputs is equal to the sum of the two corresponding outputs. If superposition holds, then the output corresponding to any admissible input can be calculated from a knowledge of the transfer function, $G(\omega)$.

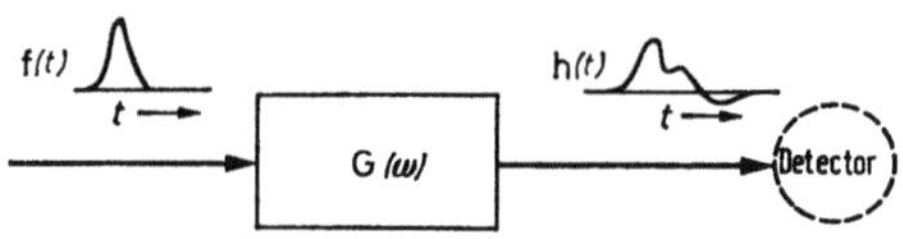

Fig. 1. Schematic representation of the linear model of flicker sensitivity, governed by the transfer function, $G(\omega)$

Although no real system obeys linear superposition under all possible conditions, many do so over a usefully large range of input values, and most are linear to a good approximation for sufficiently small perturbations of the input. Thus, linear models are widely used in many fields. Moreover, the describing function, a generalization of the transfer function, is used to characterize certain well-behaved types of nonlinear systems. For all such models, the analysis of input waveforms into their elementary sinusoidal components is an essential step in the theoretical prediction process.

The transfer function is generally complex, or it may be treated as two real functions representing the amplitude and phase response of the model. In principle, $G(\omega)$ can always be derived from the linear, integro-differential equation of the system, if it is known; hence, the term "linear system". But sometimes the transfer function can also be measured empirically; even if the differential equation is unknown, $G(\omega)$ still provides a complete description of any system for which superposition holds.

An equivalent description of such a linear system is also given by its impulse response, which in this model is the output obtained when the input is a very brief flash of light. The transfer function and the impulse response contain exactly the same information, since one is the Fourier transform of the other. (But in a given experimental situation, it may be possible to measure one and not the other.)

The threshold predictions of any visual model also depend on the assumed behavior of the detector. The latter is shown in dashed lines in Fig. 1, because this assumption varies with the type of data being collected. In electrophysiological experiments, there is usually a measurable output (e.g., receptor potential, impulse train, etc.); hence, the detector is part of the measuring equipment and its properties are known. But in a psychophysical experiment, where the detector is actually part of the organism, it must still be regarded as also part of the measuring apparatus. Some assumption about its behavior must therefore be made by any theory that purports to account for psychophysical thresholds, and in this case, the detector cannot be linear. For example, one might assume that the detector responds to the maximum excursion (peak-to-trough amplitude) of the output, $h(t)$, and that flicker is reported whenever this output amplitude exceeds a certain fixed threshold value. This turns out to be a rather good assumption for high-frequency flicker thresholds.

When appropriate values for the amplitude sensitivity or modulus of $G(\omega)$ are derived from sine-wave flicker experiments of the type described in Sec. II, the model shown in Fig. 1 can account for essentially all the traditional flicker-fusion data; examples of such predictions are treated in detail in Sec. IV. Moreover, by augmenting $G(\omega)$ with some type of nonlinearity which can make the gain at low frequencies inversely proportional to the dc component of the input (i.e., logarithmic response), this model can be generalized to predict not only low-frequency flicker thresholds, but also flash and increment thresholds.

However, these ideas had no influence on flicker studies until the experiments described in Sec. II were undertaken. Earlier flicker experiments were usually conducted with the square-wave stimulus shown in Fig. 2, primarily for reasons of expedience. With very simple apparatus, a sectored "chopper" disc can be arranged to intercept a beam of light in such a way that its luminance will change from zero to maximum in a more or less rectangular waveform. The speed of the disc can then be varied to find the flicker-fusion point, usually known as the critical flicker frequency (CFF). In literally hundreds of these studies, the actual frequency content of such a square-wave stimulus was never considered.

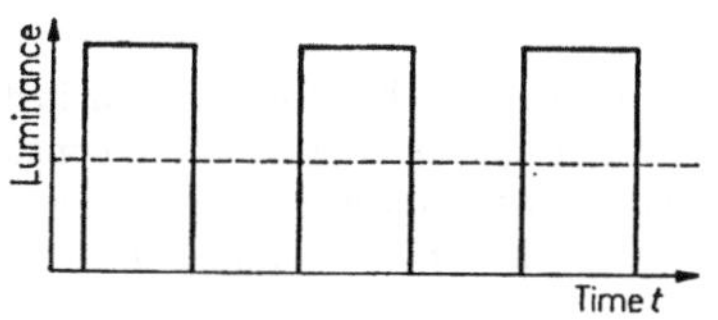

Fig. 2. Periodic rectangular waveform used in traditional flicker experiments. The dotted line represents the time-average luminance of the stimulus

Two important results emerged from the traditional experiments. First, it was found that over a considerable range, the CFF varied approximately as the logarithm of the stimulus *amplitude* (the Ferry-Porter Law). It was once believed that this relation applied to the adaptation level (time-average luminance) of the stimulus, but this is erroneous. As shown in Sec. IV, if the peak-to-trough amplitude is held constant, the CFF actually *decreases* when the time-average luminance of the flickering waveform is increased (Kelly, 1964).

Second, for all frequencies above fusion, it was found that the apparent brightness of the periodic stimulus closely matched that of a steady stimulus of the same time-average luminance (the Talbot-Plateau Law). A match of this kind is shown by the dashed line in Fig. 2, at one-half the maximum luminance of the square-wave stimulus. Such perfect integration at high frequencies is a necessary property of a low-pass, linear system; but the reverse implication is not necessarily true (see Sec. III). Arguing from flicker threshold measurements, Van der Tweel (1961) has shown that at high frequencies, the attenuation represented by $G(\omega)$ is more than enough to conceal the presence of a subsequent logarithmic nonlinearity, even if the Talbot-Plateau Law could be verified with three times the precision usually obtained in brightness-matching experiments.

II. Sine-Wave Flicker Measurements

The transfer function of the linear model described in Sec. I can be expressed in the form

$$G(\omega) \equiv A e^{j\varphi}, \tag{1}$$

where t is time, and $A \sin(\omega t + \varphi)$ is the output obtained when the input is $\sin \omega t$. Both the amplitude, A, and the phase, φ, are functions of ω, the (radian) frequency of the input. We cannot generate $\sin \omega t$ as a visual stimulus (it has negative values, and radiant power is a non-negative quantity); but we can obtain the closely-related waveform,

$$f(t) = L(1 + m \sin \omega t), \tag{2}$$

shown in Fig. 3. This is the sum of a steady component of luminance L, and a sine wave of luminance amplitude mL, where $0 < m < 1$. Since L is now the time-average value of the waveform, it governs the subject's adaptation level. The dimensionless ratio of the "ac" and "dc" components, m, is usually called the "modulation."

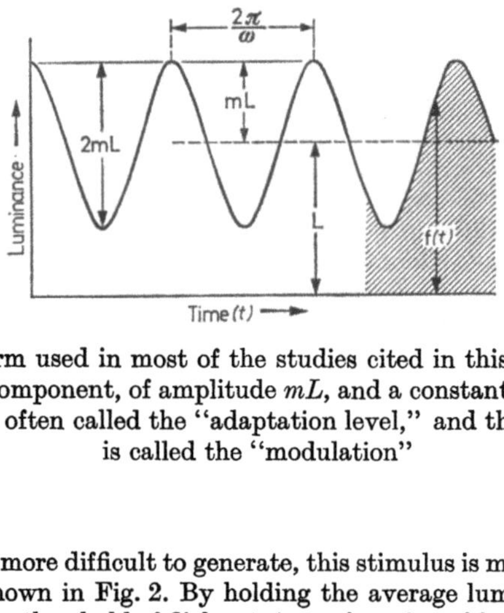

Fig. 3. Stimulus waveform used in most of the studies cited in this review. This waveform is the sum of a sinusoidal component, of amplitude mL, and a constant component, L. The time-average luminance, L, is often called the "adaptation level," and the dimensionless ratio, m, is called the "modulation"

Although sometimes more difficult to generate, this stimulus is much more generally useful than the square wave shown in Fig. 2. By holding the average luminance (L) constant, and measuring the modulation threshold of flicker (m) as a function of frequency (ω), one obtains a complete amplitude sensitivity or "frequency response" curve at any desired adaptation level (compared to the single point obtained at the CFF by earlier methods). Phase information has also been obtained psychophysically in certain experiments (see Sec. V), but not as directly as amplitude thresholds are measured.

The earliest data of this type known to the author were taken by Dow (1907), for the purpose of determining the precision of a flicker photometer consisting of a grease spot on a spinning disc of blotting paper, viewed through a low-power telescope. This instrument did not provide a uniform field or a perfect sinusoidal waveform, and Dow's curves cover a rather limited frequency range in the region of maximum sensitivity, as shown in Fig. 4. Nevertheless, his results are very similar to the more recent modulation-sensitivity data described below.

The next sine-wave flicker data were obtained at scotopic levels, by IVES (1922a, 1922b). IVES showed for the first time that high-frequency flicker thresholds for certain other waveforms could be predicted from the sine-wave flicker thresholds, but his work was also ignored by students of flicker for the next 30 years, except for some comments by COBB (1934).

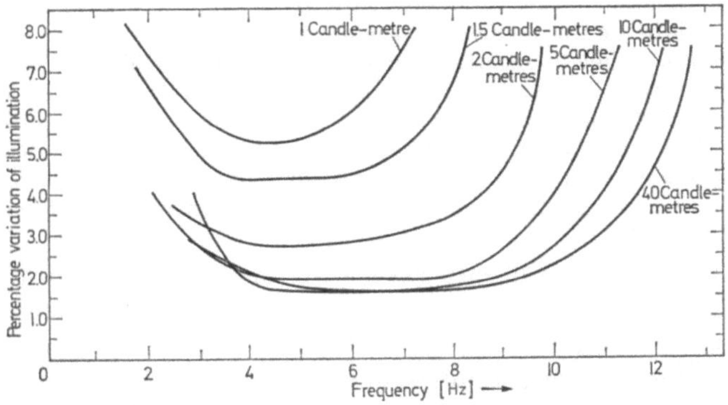

Fig. 4. Some early modulation threshold data, obtained with a grease-spot flicker photometer (Dow, 1907)

Then in 1952, DELANGE undertook to explore the sensitivity to sine-wave flicker at photopic adaptation levels over a broad frequency range, with the results shown in Fig. 5. At photopic levels, these modulation threshold curves show a peak of sensitivity in the frequency range between 5 and 10 Hz, with a gradual decrease of sensitivity at lower frequencies, and a very sharp decrease at higher

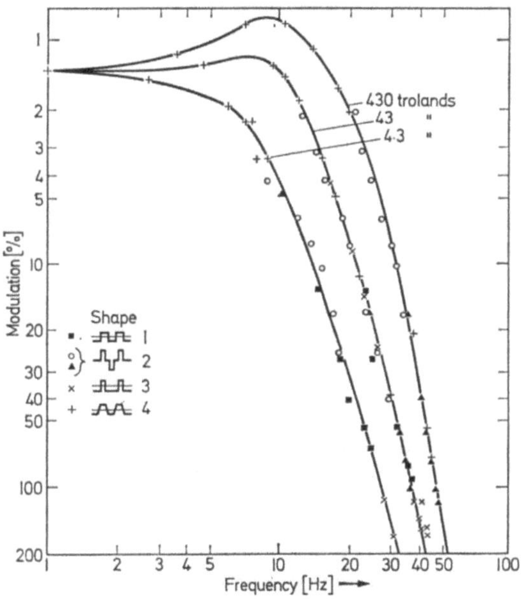

Fig. 5. Small-field flicker sensitivity curves, showing the Fourier equivalence of various waveforms at frequencies above 10 Hz (DELANGE, 1958a)

frequencies. At lower adaptation levels, the peak disappears and the high-frequency cutoff shifts toward lower frequencies. Similar results were obtained by JONES (1957) and VAN DER TWEEL (1961).

DELANGE also tried various non-sinusoidal waveforms, as indicated in Fig. 5, and confirmed that their high-frequency flicker thresholds for a given adaptation level could be predicted from the amplitude of the first Fourier component (the "fundamental") of the waveform (1952, 1954). These results led him to undertake a more elaborate study (1957, 1958a, 1958b), testing other observers, exploring a greater range of adaptation levels, and investigating certain chromatic effects. DELANGE's work provided the stimulus for many of the subsequent flicker studies reviewed in this chapter, both psychophysical and electrophysiological. In 1963, an international symposium was held in his honor at Amsterdam. The proceedings of this symposium provide an excellent cross-section of the work in progress at that time (HENKES and VAN DER TWEEL, 1964).

Most such flicker experiments have used small fields. DE LANGE's data, for example, were taken with a 2° flickering field and a large (60°), steady surround. The luminance of this surround was held at the average level (i.e., the "Talbot brightness") of the flickering stimulus, in order to control the subject's adaptation level. In 1959, however, KELLY obtained a sine-wave flicker curve with a very large (65°), uniformly flickering field. This wide-field stimulus shifted the high-frequency cutoff slightly toward higher frequencies, but its main effect was a decrease in the sensitivity to low frequencies, and a correspondingly steeper slope at frequencies below the peak sensitivity (see Fig. 6).

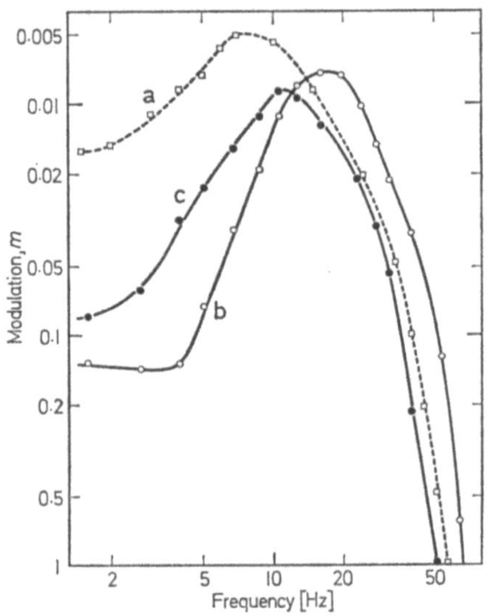

Fig. 6. Small-field *vs.* large-field flicker sensitivity at 10^3 trolands. (a) 2° sharp-edged field with steady surround, (b) 65° flickering field with blurred edges, and (c) 4° sharp-edged field with dark surround (KELLY, 1959)

KELLY (1959) suggested that eye-movements may play an essential role in this effect of target size on low-frequency flicker. However, a stabilized-image experiment performed by TULUNAY-KEESEY to test this hypothesis gave negative results (KELLY, 1964; see also WEST, 1968). Another related experiment was performed by LEVINSON (1964), with a very small (40′)

flickering field, surrounded by a 2° annulus. The annulus was also flickered sinusoidally, at various phases relative to the phase of the central test spot. Keeping the waveform of the annulus at a fixed fraction of its threshold amplitude, LEVINSON found that the modulation threshold in the central spot varied with the relative phase of the annulus in such a way as to indicate that this subliminal annular stimulus inhibits the low-frequency flicker response in the central spot.

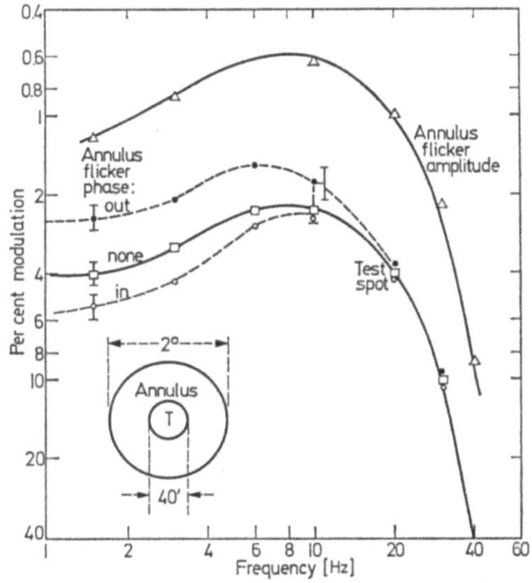

Fig. 7. Effect of a subliminally flickering annulus on the flicker sensitivity with a very small test spot (LEVINSON, 1964)

As shown in Fig. 7, the inhibiting effect is large, and has the proper sign and frequency range to account for the major difference between DELANGE's and KELLY's data. This alone would not eliminate the eye-movement hypothesis, since LEVINSON's stimulus was not stabilized. But under certain conditions, the inhibiting effect also showed a linear phase shift, corresponding to a fixed time-delay of about 10 milliseconds (independent of frequency), which argues for a neural explanation.

More recently, KELLY (1969) explored a large variety of flickering patterns and found two components underlying the differences shown in Fig. 6: Increasing the size of the flickering area raises the modulation sensitivity at all frequencies, while the number or sharpness of edges affects the sensitivity only at frequencies below 10 Hz. On this basis, he hypothesized that lateral inhibition becomes ineffective at frequencies above 10 Hz.

RATLIFF *et al.* (1967) have demonstrated similar effects in the electrical responses to sine-wave stimulation of the horseshoe crab, *Limulus*; here, the results can be unequivocally related to lateral inhibition. Other neurophysiological data which bear on the low-frequency inhibition of the flicker response are discussed in Sec. VI.

These electrophysiological results suggest a close relation between the threshold frequency-response data and the frequency response of the visual system above threshold. In addition, some supra-threshold psychophysical data are available from the flicker-matching experiments of VERINGA (1958). Using a sinusoidal waveform, VERINGA asked his subject to adjust the modulation at various frequencies to match the apparent modulation depth of a standard, supra-threshold sine wave. His results are shown in Fig. 8, together with a fusion threshold curve (from DELANGE) for the same adaptation level. Even with modulations as great as 10 or 20 times threshold, the flicker-matching curves at 1000 trolands are very similar to the fusion curves at lower adaptation levels.

It is important to know whether the inhibition of sensitivity at frequencies below 10 Hz in, e.g., Fig. 6, also occurs under supra-threshold conditions. This cannot be determined from VERINGA's (1958) data, since he used a small field and his curves do not extend to sufficiently low frequencies. However, the electrophysiological data indicate that this low-frequency behavior also persists well above the modulation threshold (see Sec. VI).

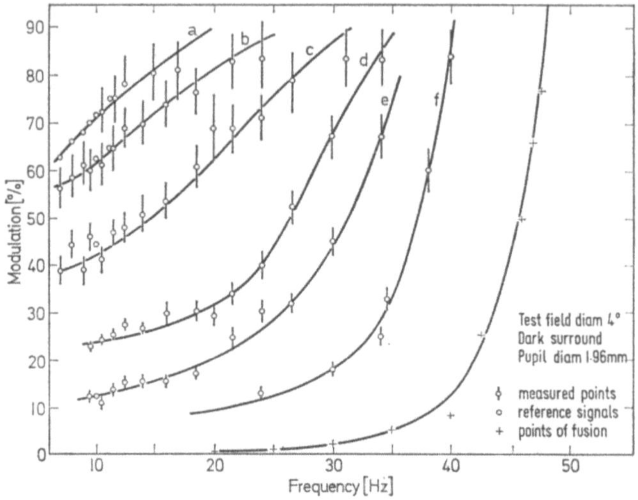

Fig. 8. Modulation amplitudes for subjectively equivalent flicker at 10^3 trolands for six standard amounts of flicker (curves *a*—*f*). Lowest curve represents the flicker threshold (VERINGA, 1958)

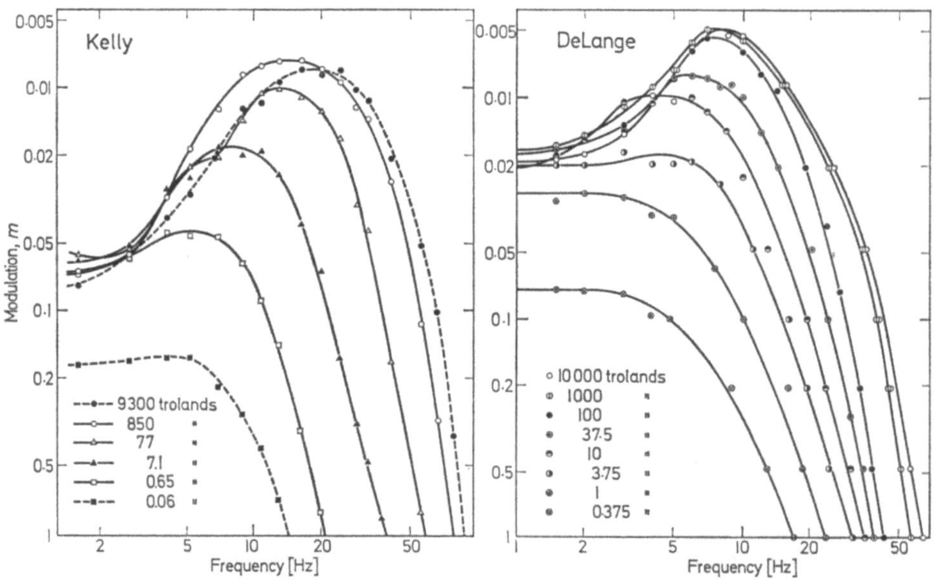

Fig. 9. Photopic modulation sensitivity data. The curves on the left were obtained with a large flickering field; those on the right with a small flickering spot on a steady surround (KELLY, 1961 a; DELANGE, 1958 a)

Like DeLange, Kelly obtained modulation threshold curves at various levels of retinal illuminance; but he used a wide field throughout. Typical results from Kelly (1961a) and from DeLange (1958a) are compared in Fig. 9 over a range of adaptation levels. In both sets of data, the curves for all retinal illuminance levels tend to converge to a common value at the lowest frequencies. Since the modulation, m, is analogous to the Weber fraction, this low-frequency behavior is in accord with the Weber-Fechner Law. However, the value of the low-frequency modulation threshold is quite different for the two field sizes: less than 2 percent in the small-field case, but more than 6 percent in the wide-field data. The sensitivity peak also occurs at slightly higher frequencies in the wide-field data; but at frequencies greater than 10 or 20 Hz, the two experiments gave very similar results at all adaptation levels.

Kelly (1961a, 1964) also extended the Ives-DeLange waveform analysis to a broader class of stimuli, in the following sense. DeLange had shown that flicker thresholds for many traditional waveforms could be predicted from the sine-wave thresholds, provided both were measured at the same adaptation level, but Kelly eliminated the latter restriction. He pointed out that if the high-frequency flicker thresholds are really governed by a linear filtering process (as DeLange's Fourier-component tests indicate), then the response to the ac component of the stimulus must be independent of the dc component (i.e., of the adaptation level). To test this hypothesis, Kelly plotted his data in terms of the absolute amplitude of the sine wave (i.e., in trolands) as shown in Fig. 10 (Kelly, 1961a). This means multiplying each threshold modulation value, m, by the retinal illuminance, L, at which it was obtained (or in log coordinates, simply translating each curve in Fig. 9 downward by an amount proportional to log L).

Now if the threshold values of the absolute amplitude, mL, are indeed independent of L, then all the curves should be superimposed at high frequencies. Fig. 10 shows that this is true, over a remarkably wide range of adaptation levels, for all modulation values greater than a

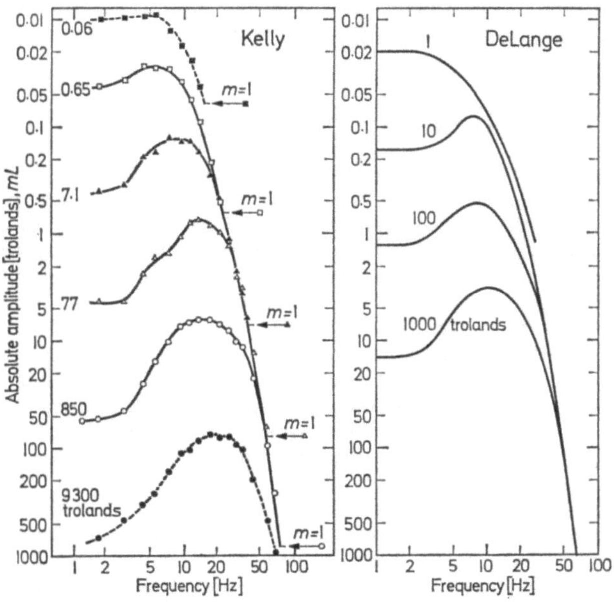

Fig. 10. The flicker thresholds from Fig. 9 replotted in terms of absolute retinal illuminance amplitude, mL (trolands). The wide-field data are again on the left and the small-spot data on the right (Kelly, 1961a; Levinson and Harmon, 1961)

few percent (i.e., just where the first Fourier component governs most other waveform thresholds). DELANGE's data were replotted in the same way by LEVINSON and HARMON (1961); as shown in Fig. 10, they also have the same property. This figure, like the previous one, shows that the small-field and the wide-field flicker thresholds are practically identical at high frequencies (and systematically different at low frequencies).

Regardless of field size, the amplitude thresholds in Fig. 10 are independent of the adaptation level at high frequencies (linear behavior), but they are approximately proportional to it at low frequencies (Weber-Fechner Law). Between these two extremes lies a frequency region of maximum sensitivity (minimum threshold), and this sensitivity peak shifts toward higher frequencies as the absolute amplitude of the stimulus increases.

The fact that all the flicker data of Fig. 10 fall on the same curve for large values of m is of fundamental importance, since it represents the range of stimulus conditions under which the linear model appears to govern flicker thresholds, as described in Sec. IV. This result also indicates that the traditional formulation of the Ferry-Porter Law is erroneous. The stimulus frequency along the common asymptote in Fig. 10 is approximately proportional to the logarithm of the absolute amplitude threshold; but this means that the Ferry-Porter Law, correctly understood, does not involve the adaptation level of the stimulus. The CFF does not increase with the adaptation level (dc component) of the stimulus but rather with its absolute amplitude (ac component). It is merely an accidental artifact that these two quantities were usually related by a constant factor (e.g., $4/\pi$ for the traditional square-wave stimuli). Direct tests confirm that the CFF remains constant as the adaptation level is increased with a fixed stimulus amplitude; or if this process is carried far enough, the CFF actually decreases (see Sec. IV). This reformulation of the Ferry-Porter Law also has important theoretical ramifications, which are discussed in Sec. VII.

III. Relation to Transient Data

Since $G(\omega)$ in the linear model is sufficient to predict the output for any periodic or transient input, and Fig. 10 indicates that flicker thresholds obey this model under certain conditions, one might expect that these steady-state data could be used to predict transient visual phenomena, such as flash or increment thresholds. However, the amplitude sensitivity data of Sec. II are not measurements of the complete transfer function but only of its modulus. In order to deduce the impulse response of the model, the necessary phase information must be obtained by some other means (see Secs. V and VI).

Even without knowing the exact form of the impulse response at any given adaptation level, however, one can predict from the data of Sec. II many of the classical transient threshold data. A thorough discussion of this topic is beyond the scope of the present review. However, ROUFS has shown that the threshold for a rectangular pulse of varying duration as a function of either adaptation level or field size can be predicted from flicker data similar to those of Fig. 10 (ROUFS, 1966; ROUFS and MEULENBRUGGE, 1967).

In a sense, this is the reverse of PIÉRON's (1961) attempt to predict flicker thresholds from flash data by assuming that the CFF should be inversely proportional to the "critical time," τ (defined as the longest duration for which single-flash thresholds depend only on the total energy of the flash). But PIÉRON's hypothesis apparently was based on the erroneous belief that the CFF varied with adaptation level, rather than stimulus amplitude (as discussed in the previous section), and he ignored the effects of waveform and modulation depth. In the special case where the waveform and the modulation are both held constant, the stimulus amplitude becomes proportional to the adaptation level, and then τ^{-1} is approximately proportional to the CFF, since τ^{-1} varies logarithmically with the adaptation level (MATIN, 1968) while the CFF varies logarithmically with the stimulus amplitude. But for other modulation levels or other waveforms in general, flicker thresholds cannot be predicted in this way.

On the other hand, Bloch's Law can readily be deduced from the linear flicker model, since shortening the duration of a constant-energy flash leaves its Fourier analysis unchanged except for the addition of some higher frequencies. Now, if the original duration of the flash was already negligible compared to the total length of the impulse response (PIÉRON's "utilization time"), then these added frequencies are beyond the frequency range of the transfer function and cannot be detected; hence, Bloch's Law is obeyed for all constant-energy flashes of greater bandwidth than $G(\omega)$.

If the stimulus pulse is longer than the critical time, its low-frequency content predominates, and then the increment threshold behaves nonlinearly (obeying the Weber-Fechner Law). But even in this region, according to ROUFS (1966), the increment threshold is directly proportional to the minimum amplitude threshold of the sine-wave flicker curve over a large range of adaptation levels, and the critical time is inversely proportional to the frequency at which the amplitude threshold has increased by a factor of 2 over its minimum value. (Unlike the CFF, this "dominant frequency" of ROUFS does vary with adaptation level.) He also found that the increment threshold and critical time could be predicted from the sine-wave data in this way for various test field sizes from a few minutes of arc up to the entire visual field (ROUFS and MEULENBRUGGE, 1967).

This suggests that the same threshold-detecting mechanism must be in operation for both continuous flicker and single pulses; ROUFS postulated a simple peak detector for both (see Sec. I). If this is the case, then the same threshold values should be obtained for a decremental ("negative") flash as for an incremental ("positive") flash. With a 1° test field, ROUFS *et al.* (1967) found no significant difference between positive and negative flashes, in either critical time or sensitivity.

More complex types of threshold data result from attempts to probe the transient response directly. For example, consider the threshold energy of a short test flash superimposed on a positive- or negative-going step-function of luminance (e.g., BAKER, 1953; BOYNTON and KANDEL, 1957). (See BOYNTON, Chapter 9, this volume.) No matter how short the flash, the corresponding linear output consists of the entire impulse response, superimposed on the step-response waveform with the appropriate delay (positive or negative). Thus a peak-to-trough detector could detect only the maximum excursion of this composite waveform as a function of the delay (a function which could readily be predicted from the impulse response, but not vice versa.)

The same experimental technique has been used with various other waveforms, including double flashes, positive and negative (IKEDA, 1965), pulse trains (IKEDA and BOYNTON, 1965) and continuous square-wave flicker (BOYNTON *et al.*, 1961). The resulting threshold functions can be qualitatively explained by assuming that the impulse response is diphasic (IKEDA, 1965), which is also implied by the sine-wave flicker data (KELLY, 1961b). But no psychophysical technique has yet provided a quantitative measurement of the impulse response (or of its time-integral, the step response); this remains the prerogative of electrophysiology.

IV. Fourier Equivalence Calculations

The common asymptote of the flicker data of Fig. 10 permits the Fourier technique of IVES and DELANGE to be generalized in the following way. According to DELANGE, the waveforms in any horizontal row of Fig. 11 are equivalent, because they have the same first-component modulation, m_1, and average illuminance, L. But according to KELLY (1964), every waveform in this figure is equivalent to every other one (at high frequencies), since they all have the same value of the product, $m_1 L$. (Where m_1 increases from 50 percent to 150 percent in Fig. 11, L decreases from 60 to 20 trolands, keeping the absolute amplitude equal to that of a 30-troland sine wave.)

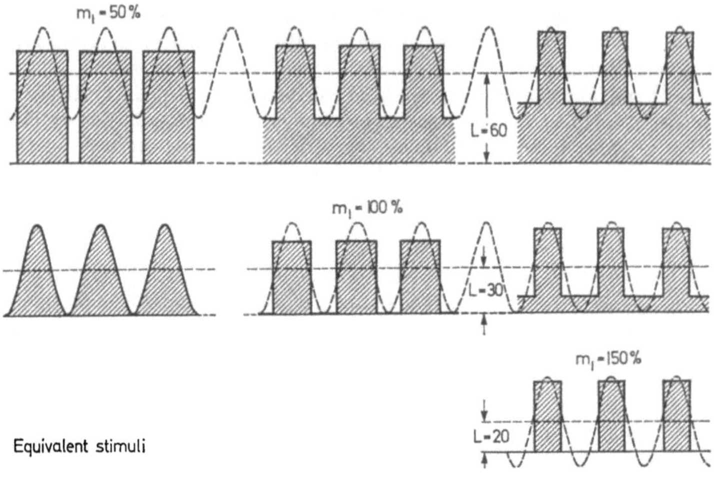

Fig. 11. Fourier-equivalent flicker waveforms. By DELANGE's rule, the waveforms in any horizontal row are equivalent because m_1 and L have the same values. But by KELLY's rule, all the waveforms in this figure are equivalent because $m_1 L$ is constant (KELLY, 1964)

Note also that every non-negative waveform has a maximum realizable modulation, which may have any value between 0 and 200 percent, depending upon the shape of the given waveform. The maximum modulations obtainable with the three rectangular waveforms shown in Fig. 11 are 50 percent, 100 percent, and 150 percent, respectively.

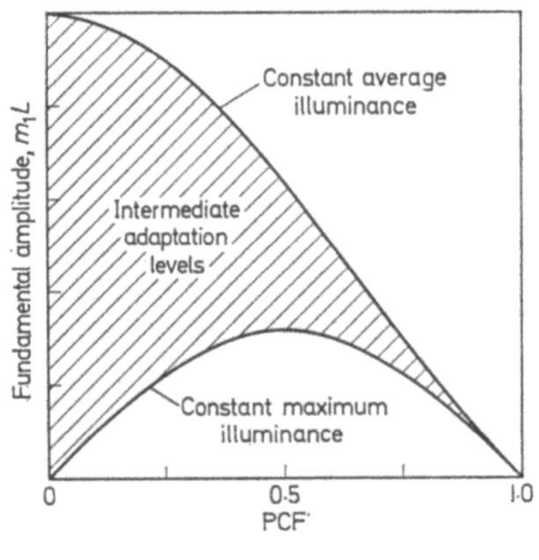

Fig. 12. Upper and lower bounds for the first-harmonic retinal illuminance amplitude of the rectangular-wave stimulus with variable pulse-to-cycle-fraction (PCF), when natural pupils are used. The upper curve represents the extreme case of complete pupillary adaptation to maintain a fixed time-average illuminance; the lower one, no adaptation, i.e., a small artificial pupil (KELLY, 1961c)

Along the diagonal from upper left to lower right of Fig. 11 are three maximum-modulation waveforms that belong to a family of stimuli much used in traditional flicker-fusion studies of the pulse-to-cycle fraction (duty cycle or on-time) of the stimulus. This type of waveform was not usually adjusted to keep the absolute amplitude constant with varying PCF, as it is in Fig. 11. But it is a simple matter to calculate the relevant parameters of these waveforms, and the PCF experiments provide a large body of data to test their Fourier equivalence to the sine-wave thresholds.

The first-component modulation of such a waveform is given by

$$m_1 = \frac{2}{\pi R} \sin \pi R \,. \tag{3}$$

The variation of m_1 with the pulse-to-cycle fraction, R, is shown by the upper curve in Fig. 12. The lower curve shows the absolute amplitude, $m_1 L$, where L is the average retinal illuminance. IVES (1922a) made some calculations of this type, and DELANGE (1954) pointed out that duty-cycle effects can be explained on the basis of the curves in Fig. 12, if either the average or the maximum retinal illuminance of the rectangular waveform is held constant. The procedure is as follows:

If the *maximum* luminance is held constant and an artificial pupil is used, then the appropriate amplitude is read off from the lower curve of Fig. 12 and the corresponding CFF of the equivalent stimulus is determined from the absolute amplitude threshold curve of Fig. 10. On the other hand, a natural pupil attempts to keep the *average* retinal illuminance, L, constant; if it did this perfectly, the upper curve in Fig. 12 would be the appropriate one to use (regardless of the maximum luminance). Thus the amplitude threshold curve for the natural pupil actually falls somewhere within the intermediate shaded area of Fig. 12, depending on just how the pupil varies with adaptation level. Fortunately for the analysis of natural-pupil experiments, the CFF changes slowly enough with stimulus amplitude to make the duty-cycle threshold predictions about the same for any reasonable law of pupil adaptation.

Nevertheless, for several years after DELANGE (1954), various workers continued to ignore his Fourier-equivalence data and attempted to endow PCF thresholds with some deeper significance (see PIÉRON, 1961). Next, KELLY carried out a similar waveform analysis of some typical PCF data obtained by BARTLEY and NELSON (1961), showing that their results could also be accounted for on this basis (KELLY, 1961c). Fig. 13 shows his CFF predictions for one stimulus level, based on Fourier equivalence (and the assumption that the effective area of the pupil varies as the —0.6 power of the average luminance). Also shown are the extremes of BARTLEY and NELSON's data for several subjects, which bracket most

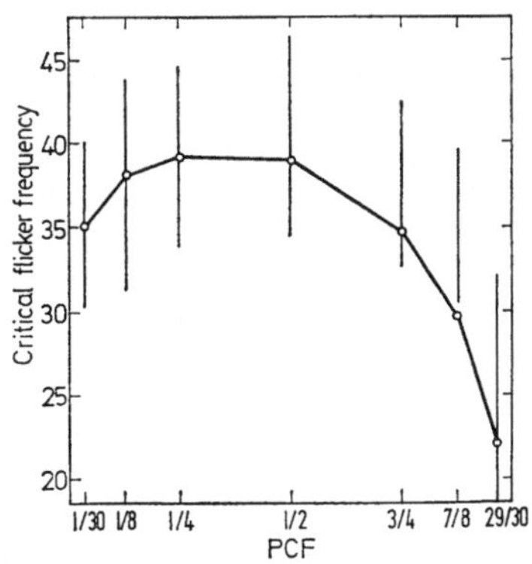

Fig. 13. Prediction of PCF effects from sine-wave flicker data. The points were calculated from Fig. 12 and the sine-wave data, as described in the text. The vertical lines represent the total spread of BARTLEY and NELSON's (1961) PCF data for five observers (KELLY, 1961c)

of the theoretical points. Finally, a third analysis of duty-cycle effects was made by GIBBINS and HOWARTH (1961), with similar results. Evidently, the effect of the pulse-to-cycle fraction on the CFF is entirely predictable from the sine-wave flicker thresholds.

A similar mathematical analysis was made by LEVINSON (1959) to explain the results obtained by FORSYTH and BROWN (1959) with the flickering waveform shown in Fig. 14. This analysis was subsequently elaborated by BROWN (1962). The waveform used by FORSYTH and BROWN consisted of alternating pulses of different lengths, $A/2$ and $B/2$, each followed by a dark period of the same length as the preceding pulse. Keeping interval A constant, they varied interval B until the subjective frequency of this waveform appeared to match that of a standard stimulus consisting of a single-period square wave of some fixed frequency. Interval A was then set to a new value and the criterion value of B was again found; thus, curves of A vs. B were constructed as shown in Fig. 15. A similar curve of A vs. B was also obtained for the criterion of fusion.

The fundamental frequency of such a waveform is obviously $(A + B)^{-1}$. The relative modulation due to this first Fourier component varies with A and B in accord with:

$$m_1 = \frac{4}{\pi} \cos \left[\pi \frac{A}{A+B}\right]; \tag{4}$$

while the modulation due to the second Fourier component is given by

$$m_2 = \frac{4}{\pi} \sin^2 \left[\pi \frac{A}{A+B}\right]. \tag{5}$$

Since frequencies below 15 Hz were not present, LEVINSON (1959) was able to approximate the sine-wave flicker data by the equation

$$m = k f^N, \tag{6}$$

where f is the frequency of the sinusoidal waveform, m is the threshold modulation, and k and N are constants. Setting each of the Fourier components of the stimulus, m_1 and m_2 in turn, equal to this threshold expression given two functional relations between the intervals A and B, at which fusion may be expected to occur if each component acts independently of the other. For the fusion thresholds, this is a reasonably good assumption, as shown by the results in Fig. 14.

In order to make similar predictions for FORSYTH and BROWN's (1959) flicker-matching results, BROWN (1962) repeated LEVINSON's analysis using the supra-threshold sine-wave data of VERINGA (1958). As might be expected, the fit is not as good in this case, mainly because the assumption that the two Fourier components act independently breaks down in the region where they are about equally effective. BROWN's predicted curves are shown in Fig. 15 on one side of the line $A = B$, the experimental ones on the other. Both sets of curves are symmetrical about this line.

FORSYTH and BROWN (1961) also experimented with a waveform consisting of two alternating trains of square-wave pulses of two different repetition rates, either of which would be fused alone (see Fig. 16). These two rapid pulse trains were alternately presented at the rate of 12.5 alternations per second. Holding the repetition rate of one of the rapid pulse trains constant, FORSYTH and BROWN (1961) varied the repetition rate of the other to determine the fusion point. It was subsequently shown by LEVINSON and KELLY (see FORSYTH and BROWN, 1962) that the modulation due to the first Fourier component of this waveform (i.e., at 12.5 Hz) is

$$m_1 = \frac{1}{\pi}\left(\tan\frac{\pi}{4\,n_1} - \tan\frac{\pi}{4\,n_2}\right). \tag{7}$$

where n_1 and n_2 are the number of pulses in each of the two alternating pulse trains. Setting m_1 equal to the sine-wave flicker threshold at 12.5 Hz, LEVINSON and KELLY were able to predict FORSYTH and BROWN's (1961) results quite satisfactorily (FORSYTH and BROWN, 1962). The same result was obtained by MATIN (1962), who repeated the analysis.

FORSYTH (1960) also studied the four different waveforms shown in Fig. 17. The first waveform consists of square pulses of three different lengths, $A/2$, $B/2$, and $C/2$, each followed

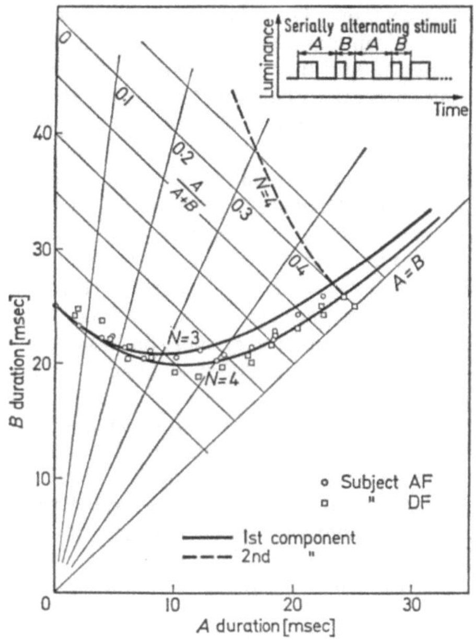

Fig. 14

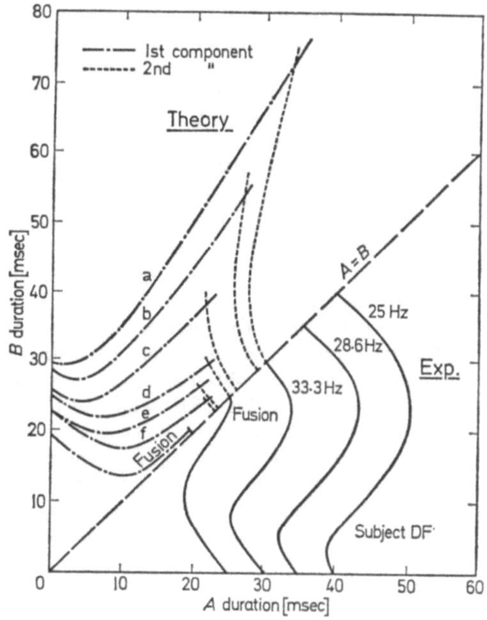

Fig. 15

Fig. 14. Prediction of thresholds for rectangular pulses of alternating duration from sine-wave flicker data. The points represent Forsyth and Brown's (1959) rectangular-pulse thresholds. The curves were derived from the sine-wave data as described in the text (Levinson, 1959)

Fig. 15. Prediction of Forsyth and Brown's supra-threshold flicker-matching data for rectangular pulses of alternating duration, from Veringa's (1958) supra-threshold sine-wave flicker data, by the same method used in Fig. 14 (Brown, 1962). Theoretical and experimental curves are symmetrical about line $A = B$

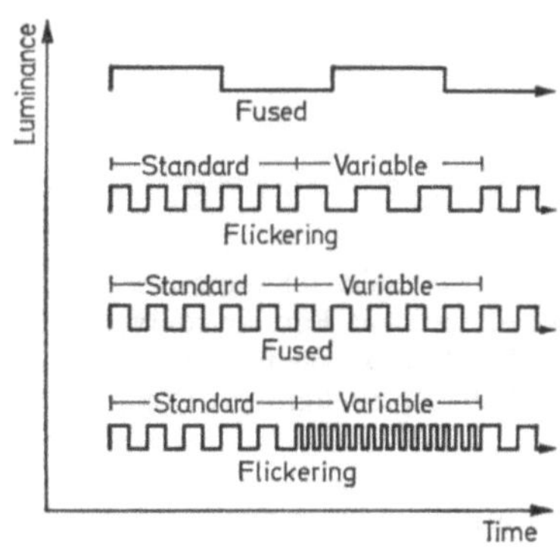

Fig. 16

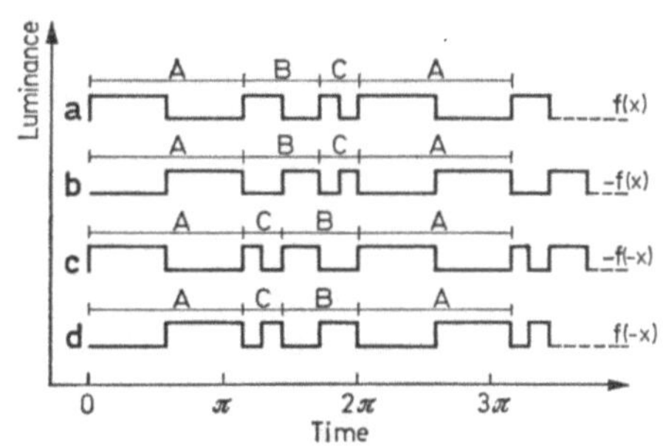

Fig. 17

Fig. 16. Alternating trains of rectangular pulses used as stimuli by Forsyth and Brown (1961). The thresholds for these waveforms are also predictable from the sine-wave data as described in the text

Fig. 17. Four types of flickering waveforms used by Forsyth (1960). The thresholds for these waveforms are again predictable from the sine-wave data

by a dark interval of the same length arranged in an arbitrary order. The other three waveforms were derived by turning the first waveform upside down, running it backward, or both. In each case, the intervals A, B, and C were separately varied to find the fusion threshold for the entire waveform. Using a large quantity of data from six observers, FORSYTH (1960) calculated the first Fourier component of all these threshold waveforms, and found that this technique "... adequately handles the experimental data ...."

In predicting the CFF from the first Fourier component of such a stimulus, one can ignore the higher harmonics primarily because they will be greatly attenuated by the steep, high-frequency cutoff of the sine-wave flicker sensitivity curve. However, for most of the rectangular waveforms that have been used, the amplitude of the first Fourier component is usually greater than that of any other harmonic even before attenuation. Therefore, KELLY (1964) measured the CFF for a waveform in which the amplitude of the second component (and all higher components) is the same as the first; namely, a periodic train of very short flashes. For such a flash train, the equivalent sine-wave modulation, m_1, equals 200% (which is the maximum value of m_1 obtainable with any non-negative waveform).

KELLY compared his CFF values to the (absolute amplitude) sine-wave thresholds, and found that even this extreme waveform was no exception to the first-component prediction rule, as shown in Fig. 18. Using the same waveform, he also confirmed that its dc level could be changed over a large range by adding a steady background luminance, without affecting the CFF (KELLY, 1964). As shown in Fig. 19, this linear behavior breaks down at small modulation values, which in this experiment involve very high adaptation levels (e.g., 10^4 trolands). But for $L < 10^3$ trolands (and $m_1 > 10\%$), the CFF is nearly independent of adaptation level.

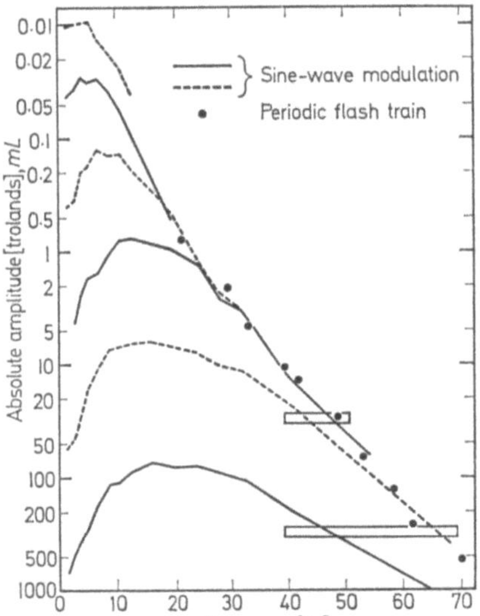

Fig. 18

Fig. 18. Wide-field data from Fig. 10 replotted on a linear frequency scale. Filled circles represent flicker thresholds for submillisecond periodic flashes plotted in terms of their Fourier-equivalent (first-harmonic) amplitudes. Note that in these coordinates the Ferry-Porter Law would be a straight line (KELLY, 1964)

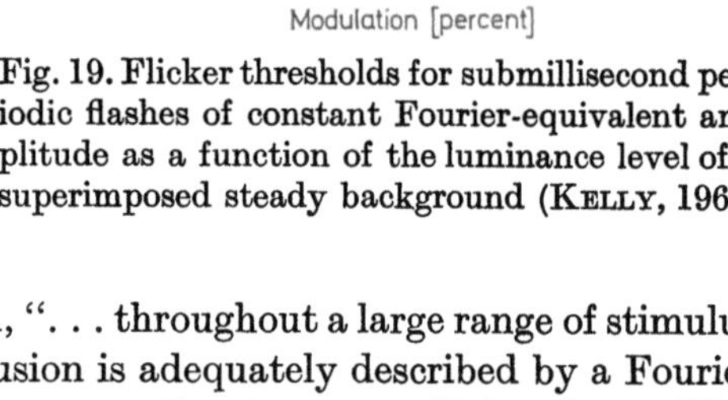

Fig. 19. Flicker thresholds for submillisecond periodic flashes of constant Fourier-equivalent amplitude as a function of the luminance level of a superimposed steady background (KELLY, 1964)

As FORSYTH (1960) finally concluded, "... throughout a large range of stimulus conditions, the response of the eye at fusion is adequately described by a Fourier analysis of the stimulus ..." (and, of course, the sine-wave flicker data). This conclusion is particularly relevant to experiments that are undertaken with a view to model-making or theorizing about the visual process. Data from a complicated experiment that can be explained in terms of data from a simpler experiment contribute nothing to the theorist, since they do not call for any new inferences which the simpler data did not require.

V. Two-Component Experiments

It is of course possible for two or more frequency components of the stimulus waveform to contribute to the flicker threshold, but the waveform must be carefully designed for this purpose if its fundamental is much above 10 Hz. For example, in BROWN's (1962) analysis of the FORSYTH and BROWN (1959) results shown in Fig. 15, the assumption that the first and second Fourier components act independently broke down only in the region where they were both about equally effective.

A more critical test of this assumption was carried out by LEVINSON (1960), using stimuli composed of two pure sinusoidal components at frequencies f and $2f$, controllably phase-locked. First he set the amplitudes of these two frequency components to subjective equality, by measuring the modulation threshold for each component separately. Thereafter, the amplitude of the sum was varied to find the modulation threshold for the composite waveform, as a function of the phase difference between the two components (see Fig. 20).

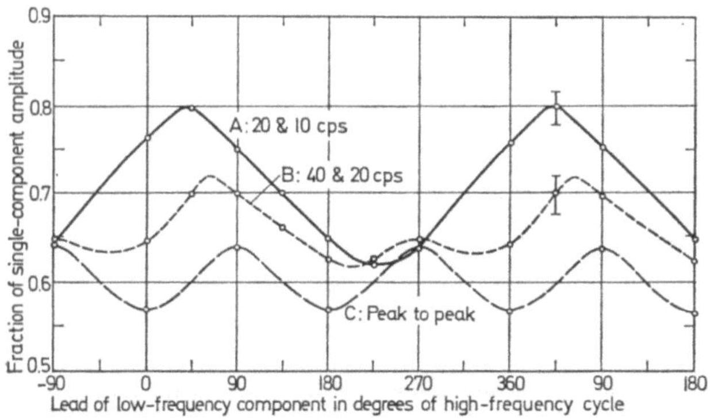

Fig. 20. Threshold amplitudes for a flickering waveform consisting of two coherent sinusoidal components, as a function of the phase difference between the components (LEVINSON, 1960)

LEVINSON found that, even though the relative amplitudes of the individual sinusoidal components remain constant, the modulation threshold under these conditions depends on the shape of the stimulus waveform (i.e., on the phase difference between the two components), as would be expected. But in general, this threshold variation does not follow the peak-to-peak amplitude of the composite waveform. For example, at the phase marked 180° in Fig. 20, the waveform is the same as the one at 0° but turned upside down; note that there is a difference of a few percent in the modulation thresholds at these two phases, even when the lowest frequency present is 20 Hz.

As LEVINSON points out, these phase effects are small, although the stimulus was chosen to maximize them. But at low frequencies, they apparently violate the peak-detector assumption that accounts for all the CFF data discussed in Sec. IV (as well as the transient experiments of Sec. III).

The flicker-detecting mechanism may respond to the maximum excursion of the output waveform at frequencies near the CFF, but LEVINSON's experiment indicates that this rule does not hold at lower frequencies. This conclusion does not depend on assuming a particular attenuation or phase-shift of the two components by the linear part of the visual system: Changes in the relative phase of the stimulus components will produce identical changes in the relative phase of the output components, regardless of the phase-shift within the system. But in spite of the theoretical importance of understanding this flicker-detecting mechanism, there are few other psychophysical data which bear directly on the problem.

Using nonsinusoidal waveforms, BOYNTON *et al.* (1961) varied the phase of a test flash superimposed on a flickering square wave, with the results shown in Fig. 21. Note that their criterion was the detection of the test flash on the flickering background, not flicker detection. For the reasons discussed in Sec. III, these increment threshold curves cannot be regarded as output waveforms (neither can the data of Fig. 20, of course). But their sinusoidal shape at 30 Hz is again consistent with the assumption of a linear, low-pass filter. On the other hand, the extremely distorted waveform obtained at 15 Hz seems to be clear evidence of at least a supra-threshold nonlinearity (regardless of the shape or duration of the threshold impulse response).

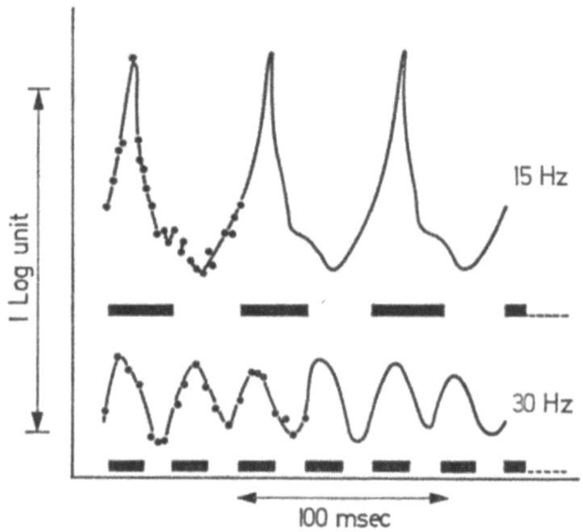

Fig. 21. Increment threshold as a function of test-flash phase, relative to square-wave stimuli of 15 and 30 Hz. Background on at times indicated by solid horizontal bars. (BOYNTON *et al.*, 1961)

Using the same phase-locked, double-frequency waveform described above, LEVINSON also attempted to investigate low-frequency nonlinearities by means of supra-threshold changes in the subjective flicker *frequency* as the relative amplitudes of the two components were changed (LEVINSON, 1964). In the frequency range from 4 to 14 Hz (for the fundamental component), he was able to obtain a clear-cut subjective transition point as the amplitude of the higher frequency component was increased. This subjective frequency-transition amplitude varied periodically with the relative phase of the two components (but quantitatively not in the same way as the fusion threshold of Fig. 20). To account for these results, LEVINSON hypothesized that the frequency perception mechanism performs a count of just those waveform minima which fall below the time-average luminance. His data also indicate that this effect depends only on the shape of the waveform, being relatively independent of amplitude and changing very slowly with increasing frequency compared to the rapid increase of the sine-wave flicker threshold. Evidently, frequency perception and flicker detection are not governed by the same mechanism.

A quite different type of experiment involves the direct, psychophysical measurement of phase-shift, by comparing luminous flicker with the visual response to electrical stimulation of the eye (the "phosphene" phenomenon). For this purpose, one must assume that electrical stimulation enters the visual system at a point that is beyond the linear filter being measured (e.g., at the bipolar cells). Since electrical frequencies higher than 200 Hz can produce visual effects (even though the maximum CFF is usually lower than 100 Hz), this seems to be a plausible assumption.

Using sinusoidal waveforms of both luminous and electrical stimulation, VERINGA (1964) determined the relative phase at which the luminous and electrical waveforms most nearly cancel each other. Measured in this way, the phase lag increases smoothly with frequency, reaching a full cycle between 30 and 40 Hz (at photopic luminance levels), as shown in Fig. 22; this corresponds to a delay of about 30 msec.

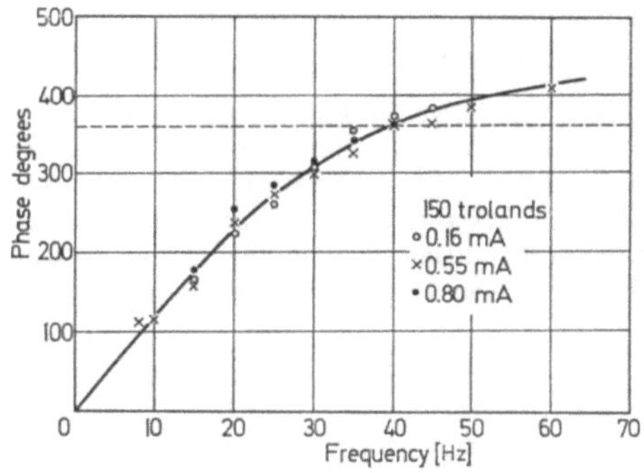

Fig. 22. Phase shift between electrical and optical sine-wave stimulation to maintain maximum subjective flicker. Maximum and minimum flicker settings were invariably 180° apart (VERINGA, 1964)

The first such data were obtained by BRINDLEY (1962), in a study of the interaction between square-wave flicker and short electrical pulses. But BRINDLEY missed the first cycle of phase-shift; since he did not take any data below 40 Hz, his values were too small by 360° (VERINGA, 1963). When this correction is made, BRINDLEY's data are confirmed by VERINGA's sinusoidal amplitude and phase measurements, and extended down to about 1 Hz. In this low-frequency region, the phase varies approximately as the square root of frequency (VERINGA and ROELOFS, 1966).

As VERINGA remarks, this electro-optical technique would seem to provide a bridge between the methods of psychophysics and those of electrophysiology. Moreover, the phase characteristic obtained in this way is not unreasonable when compared to the amplitude data of Sec. II.

VI. Physiological Data

Only a small sample of the large body of recent work on electrophysiological responses of the visual system will be mentioned here. A general review of this area is given by RIGGS (1965). The studies described below were chosen particularly for their relevance to the psychophysical results discussed in previous sections.

A direct application of the linear model to electrophysiological flicker data was made by DEVOE (1961, 1962, 1963, 1964), who analyzed the retinal action potentials evoked in the wolf-spider, *Lycosa*, by various stimulus waveforms. Since there seem to be no synapses or ganglia among the retinal cells of this spider, the electric potential measured at its cornea probably represents the pre-synaptic depolarization of receptor cells (DEVOE, 1961).

With sine-wave stimuli at a fixed adaptation level (about 1270 footcandles at the spider cornea), DEVOE found that the harmonic distortion of the output was negligible, and that its amplitude was directly proportional to the input modulation (over a range from 10 to 100 microvolts at 10 and 25 Hz). Using rectangular waveforms, he varied the pulse-to-cycle fraction, and found the exact response predicted by Fourier equivalence (as discussed in Sec. IV). He also conducted additivity tests (with flash and step responses), and confirmed that the principle of superposition held to within the accuracy of the measurements. Finally, he measured complete transfer functions (amplitude and phase) under various conditions.

For example, the measurements shown in Fig. 23 were obtained by varying the input modulation to obtain a constant output of 10 microvolts, and are thus analogous to psychophysical flicker thresholds. Except for a slightly flatter peak and broader bandwidth, these amplitude and phase characteristics are remarkably similar to the human data (e.g., Fig. 9). With increasing frequency, the amplitude sensitivity increases up to a maximum in the region between 5 and 10 Hz, and then decreases very rapidly at frequencies above 20 Hz.

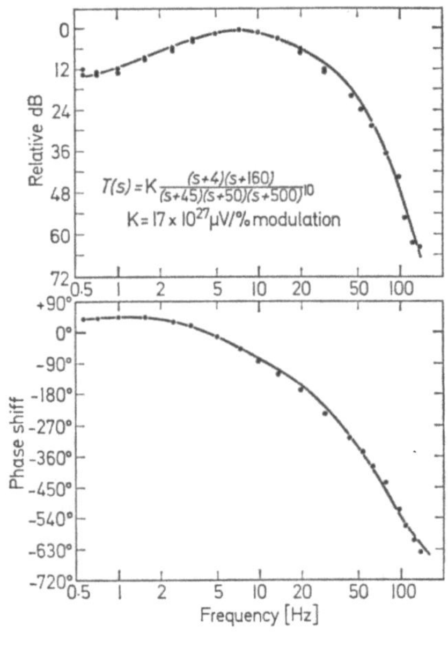

Fig. 23. Criterion amplitude and phase characteristics of wolf-spider eye, with sine-wave stimulation. These stimulus amplitudes elicited a 10 μV response with an average illumination of 1270 footcandles on the spider eye (DEVOE, 1964)

The phase characteristic in Fig. 23 is also much like the human phase-shift measurements obtained by the phosphene method described in the previous section (Fig. 22). The spider phase-shift data are roughly approximated by a fixed delay of about 20 milliseconds. But at frequencies above 4 Hz, some of these data (e.g., DEVOE, 1963) are well fitted by a square-root phase function, as proposed by VERINGA and ROELOFS (1966) for the phosphene data.

From his transfer functions, DeVoe also calculated the theoretical transient responses to impulse and increment-step inputs, and showed that by this method the actual responses could be predicted quite accurately for positive or negative increments up to 8 %. Larger deviations from the fixed level at which the transfer function was determined, however, led to increasingly nonlinear adaptation effects.

Similar small-signal linearity was demonstrated by Pinter (1966) in the generator potential of the horseshoe crab, *Limulus*. One of his tests involved measuring the impulse response, calculating from it a theoretical transfer function, and then comparing the latter with the measured amplitude and phase response, as shown in Fig. 24. Note that the bandwidth of the *Limulus* response is much narrower than that of the light-adapted human response. Some of Pinter's data show a rather flat sensitivity maximum in the region of 5 Hz; sharper peaks have been obtained by Ratliff *et al.* (1967). As in the wolf-spider, the linear model is adequate in *Limulus* only at a fixed adaptation level, since the generator potential is approximately a logarithmic function of the stimulus at very low frequencies. A quantitative treatment of the transient behavior of this nonlinearity was given by Fuortes and Hodgkin (1964).

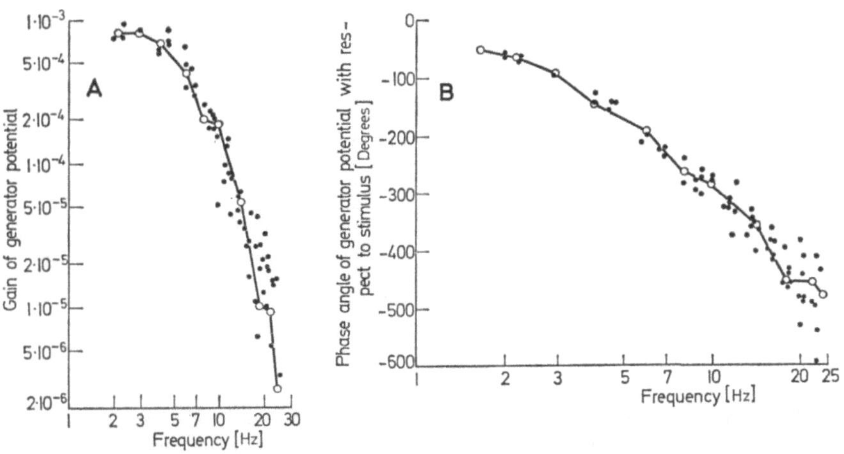

Fig. 24. Amplitude and phase response of *Limulus* eye at an illumination level of 9500 lm/m². Open circles represent measured output for sinusoidal stimulation at constant 30 % modulation. Filled circles represent amplitude and phase characteristics calculated from impulse response measurements at the same adaptation level (Pinter, 1966)

There is considerable literature on the flicker responses of ganglion cells in the cat (which has a predominantly rod retina). Enroth (1952) showed that the spikes generated by these cells occur in bursts that are phase-locked to the flicker waveform. At fusion, this "frequency modulation" of the impulse train ceases; i.e., the pulse intervals become random, uncorrelated with the stimulus frequency. These square-wave results were extended and refined by Ogawa *et al.* (1966).

Using a very small spot of light (< 1°), Cleland and Enroth-Cugell (1966) obtained modulation sensitivity (constant-output) measurements, as well as amplitude and phase response curves not unlike those of Figs. 23 and 24, from ganglion cells having both on-center and off-center receptive fields. The "output" for such measurements is usually obtained by counting the number of pulses in a fixed interval of time or by integrating the pulse train with a suitable filter. CLELAND and ENROTH-CUGELL found considerable waveform distortion by either method.

Other recent results in the cat are contained in a series of papers by MAFFEI and his collaborators, who recorded several types of electrical responses to uniform sinusoidal stimulation over a 12° or 15° field. Recording massed electrical responses (ERG) from the dark-adapated retina, MAFFEI and POPPELE (1968) demonstrated small-signal linearity both for what appeared to be late receptor potentials (BROWN, 1968), and for the "b-wave" responses of the inner nuclear layer (probably from bipolar and/or horizontal cells). They also found a linear relation between the receptor potentials and the b-wave over a considerable range of scotopic adaptation levels. No peak of amplitude response (or low-frequency inhibition) was found in either case; these preganglion-cell responses seem to be mediated by a simple, low-pass filter, representing one stage of integration with a corner frequency of about 10 or 20 Hz.

From retinal ganglion-cell impulse trains in the cat, HUGHES and MAFFEI (1966) obtained amplitude and phase characteristics such as those shown in Fig. 25. This cell had an off-center receptive field; data from other ganglion-cell types were similar, but the low-frequency phase shift of on-center cells leads that of off-center

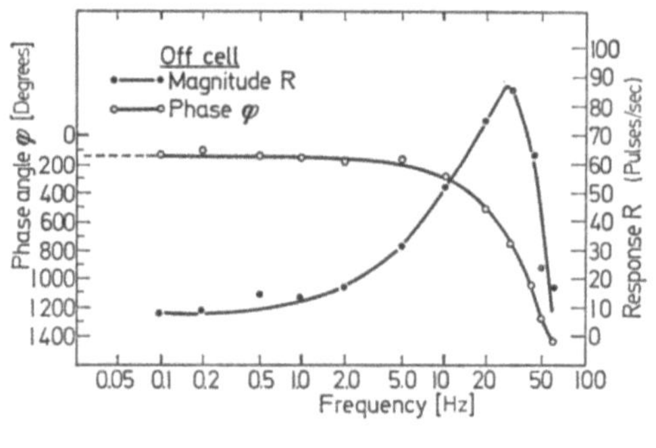

Fig. 25. Amplitude and phase response of an off-center ganglion cell in the cat. Sinusoidal stimulus waveform, output measured in terms of the firing rate of the ganglion cell (HUGHES and MAFFEI, 1966)

cells by about 180°. The most striking feature of these responses is the sharp peak of sensitivity at about 20 Hz. (Even if plotted in log coordinates, this peak would still be significantly sharper than the spider or *Limulus* sensitivity peaks shown in the two previous figures.) HUGHES and MAFFEI also found that linearity could not be assumed at the ganglion-cell output, except for small signals at frequencies below 1 Hz (where the output varied approximately as the 0.7 power of the stimulus modulation); harmonic distortion increased considerably at higher frequencies. Another type of nonlinearity affected the dc component of the output pulse frequency, which varied with both the frequency and amplitude of the input.

Since these ganglion-cell outputs are inhibited by inputs to some receptor cells and facilitated by others, it seems likely that the amplitude response of Fig. 25 could be simply the difference between two low-pass filter characteristics of different bandwidth. Dynamic interaction of this kind has recently been observed at frequencies below 10 Hz within the receptive fields of the cat (ENROTH-CUGELL and ROBSON, 1966; MAFFEI and CERVETTO, 1968). Without knowing whether the broader or narrower passband pertains to the center of the field, one cannot determine which part of the amplitude response curve in Fig. 25 represents the inhibiting influence and which part, the facilitating one. But in either case, the increasing response at low frequencies would correspond to the narrow-band (receptor and/or bipolar-cell) characteristic, while the decreasing response at higher frequencies would correspond to the broad-band characteristic. On this hypothesis, the exact frequency at which the sharp peak occurs is not a property of the ganglion cell, and might vary considerably from cell to cell. HUGHES and MAFFEI did not report on a large enough sample of ganglion cells to determine whether this is the case.

Finally, MAFFEI and RIZZOLATTI (1967) made similar recordings from post-synaptic neurons of the lateral geniculate body (LGB). Here the output varied as the 0.5 power of the input modulation depth, while the frequency response showed a much flatter 20-Hz peak. By comparing these results with the ganglion cell outputs just described, they concluded that the LGB response peak could be entirely accounted for by the properties of the retinal system (as measured at the ganglion cell), leaving the effect of the lateral geniculate as a simple, low-pass filter with a corner frequency of about 10 Hz (like the receptor potentials).

From these and other experiments, it seems plausible to infer that the characteristic shape of the human flicker threshold curves (including the prominent low-frequency "differentiating" behavior) is not a result of photochemistry, nor a property of individual cells, but instead is mediated by the inhibiting synaptic interconnections of the inner nuclear layer (which also produce lateral inhibition of spatial responses at the retinal level). This conclusion is also in accord with the results of LEVINSON (1964) and of RATLIFF *et al.* (1967) mentioned in Sec. II.

Micro-electrode studies usually depend on repetitive stimulation (sinusoidal or otherwise), in order to take advantage of various forms of data processing. Similar techniques are also being used to obtain electrophysiological data with much improved signal/noise characteristics in humans, but the interpretation of these data is by no means as clear-cut as that of the micro-electrode results. With the notable exception of one set of recordings obtained from imbedded cortical electrodes (KAMP *et al.*, (1960), the human flicker data consist of either massed retinal responses (ERG), or massed cortical responses (VECP). (See RIGGS and WOOTEN, Chapter 27, this volume.)

GOURAS and GUNKEL (1964) explored both light- and dark-adapted ERG responses to (fully-modulated) sinusoidal flicker over a 68° field with monochromatic light (e.g., 502 nm). They obtained a photopic sensitivity peak in the region of 15 to 25 Hz, which shifted to lower frequencies at lower adaptation levels (as in the psychophysical data). They also noted low-frequency nonlinearities in the photopic ERG, including a double-frequency response (second-harmonic component) in the region of 4 to 8 Hz. Using a spatial alternation technique, RIGGS and his co-workers obtained large-amplitude photopic flicker reponses from the human ERG at about 5 Hz; they have used these mainly to elucidate chromatic effects (RIGGS *et al.*, 1966). Recent work in cats and monkeys has assigned various components of the mammalian electro-retinogram to specific retinal structures, not all of which contribute to the sensation of vision; these results were reviewed by BROWN (1968).

According to TROELSTRA and SCHWEITZER (1964), the ERG can be fairly well modeled in the dark-adapted state by a memory-dependent nonlinearity, followed by a linear filter. Their predictions, like those of FUORTES and HODGKIN (1964) for *Limulus*, are considerably better for transients than for the steady-state case. Even an elaborate nonlinear analysis (cf. TROELSTRA, 1964) does not provide a very good prediction of the ERG flicker response from the flash response, when compared to the results of, e.g., DEVOE (1961) in the spider or PINTER (1966) in *Limulus*. Since the human ERG seems to be an admixture of potentials from receptors, higher-order neurons, and even the pigment epithelium, TROELSTRA'S (1964) results are probably as consistent as can be expected.

The earliest attempts to study the superficial cortical potentials evoked by sinusoidal flicker were made by VAN DER TWEEL (1961, 1964) and his collaborators. These massed electrical responses of the visual cortex are so complex that their amplitude and phase characteristics alone are not very informative. After some 250 experiments on 20 subjects over a period of 2 years, VAN DER TWEEL and LUNEL (1965) concluded that "the subjective flicker threshold curves bear no clear relation to either the size or shape of these responses." Such experiments must also deal with the spontaneous, quasi-periodic, occipital potentials that occur even in the absence of stimulation (e.g., the 10-Hz "alpha" waves).

Nevertheless, with sinusoidal modulation of a large, uniform field and bipolar, midline electrodes, VAN DER TWEEL and LUNEL found the spontaneous potentials to be essentially independent of the response to small-amplitude periodic stimulation; careful frequency analysis showed that the two outputs are additive, in contrast to the photic driving and "synchronization" effects obtained with very bright, repetitive flashes. Although there are large individual differences, some subjects show a very sharply peaked amplitude response (e.g., $Q = 15$) in the region of 10 Hz. This is intriguing because white noise passed through such a sharply tuned filter would closely resemble the alpha rhythm.

In the frequency range from 9 to 15 Hz, the sine-wave responses consist mainly of the fundamental frequency. But at lower or higher stimulus frequencies, the VECP may contain only the second harmonic; e.g., a 5-Hz input yields a 10-Hz output, even at very small stimulus modulations. This frequency-doubling effect seems to have no counterpart in the subjective response. Both the fundamental and the second-harmonic amplitudes increase with field size, and both saturate at modulations of 40% or less under all conditions. Hence with flash stimuli, the VECP is probably always nonlinear. Stimulating the two eyes in opposite phase suppresses the cortical response to a 10-Hz stimulus, but not to a 5-Hz one.

The frequency-doubling effect was studied extensively by SPEKREIJSE and VAN DER TWEEL (1965, 1966), who found that the distorted responses could be linearized by adding either random noise or a periodic auxiliary signal to the stimulus waveform. This behavior is characteristic of a memoryless, asymmetrical rectifier. From the effect of the auxiliary signal on the second-harmonic amplitude, SPEKREIJSE (1966) inferred the amplitude response of a linear process preceding this rectifying nonlinearity. As shown in Fig. 26, the results are very similar to the psychophysical flicker data described in Sec. II, but remarkably independent of adaptation level.

Although a large value of noise power is required (e.g., 10 times the signal power) to suppress completely the double-frequency component of the VECP, the fundamental-frequency outputs remain essentially unchanged under these conditions. However, if the random noise is not added directly to the sinusoidal stimulus, but the two waveforms are instead presented to opposite eyes, there is no linearizing effect. This suggests that frequency doubling occurs at a precortical level.

Finally, the double-frequency output can be greatly enhanced for input frequencies below 12 Hz by flickering a sharp-edged checkerboard pattern in counterphase, the luminance of any given square being maximum when that of its immediate neighbors is minimum (SPEKREIJSE, 1966). The greatest effect is obtained with squares about 15′ on a side, which agrees with microelectrode measures of receptive-field size in monkeys (HUBEL and WIESEL, 1968); the resulting amplitudes are large enough to be recorded without signal-averaging (e.g., 20 μvolts). These low-frequency pattern responses and various other flicker effects in the VECP were reviewed by VAN DER TWEEL and SPEKREIJSE (1968).

Another promising experimental technique is synchronous detection of the VECP, introduced by REGAN (1966a, b). His apparatus generated sine and cosine electrical waveforms, phase-locked to the sinusoidally flickering stimulus. Each of these synchronous waveforms was then multiplied by the VECP and integrated to obtain the steady-state amplitude and phase response at a given frequency. This cross-correlation technique gives no direct indication of the response waveform, but it provides greater precision than signal-averaging, particularly in the case of phase measurements.

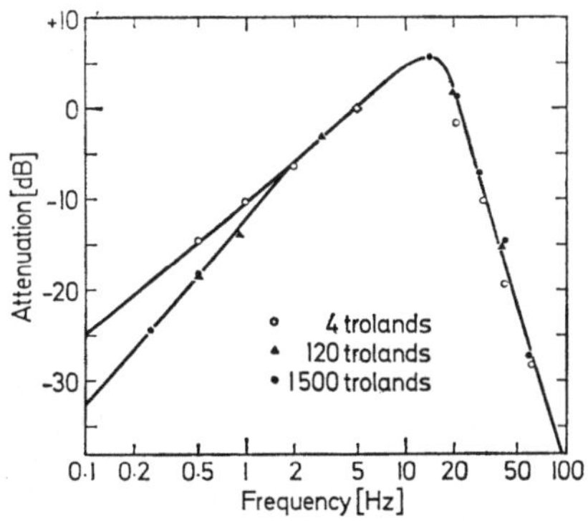

Fig. 26. Pre-rectification response of the VECP, calculated from the behavior of the double-frequency output in the presence of an auxiliary signal (SPEKREIJSE, 1966)

Although REGAN used this technique primarily to explore chromatic effects (1966b, 1968a), he also confirmed that the white-light amplitude response is sharply peaked near 10 Hz, but is essentially independent of spontaneous potentials. Another maximum appears at about 50 Hz (REGAN, 1968b), and persists even under conditions where there is no subjective response. This peak was also found by SPEKREIJSE. Finally, by cross-correlating with sine and cosine waves of twice the stimulus frequency, synchronous detection can also measure the frequency-doubling phenomena (REGAN, 1968b); still higher harmonics can be detected in a similar fashion.

VII. Theoretical Models

As a result of the experimental studies reviewed in the preceding sections. flicker theory is currently in a state of ferment. New models abound, but none seems very durable. The classic flicker theories (e.g., of HECHT, CROZIER or PIÉRON) cannot predict the sine-wave modulation thresholds. But this is the first criterion a good flicker theory should meet, since a model that can explain the sine-wave data can also account for all the classic flicker data (by determining the first Fourier component of the stimulus, regardless of its waveform, as shown in Sec. IV).

For this purpose, a low-pass, linear-filter model with the right high-frequency asymptote is sufficient.

However, in order to account for the photopic sensitivity peak at 10 to 15 Hz and the logarithmic (Weber-Law) behavior of the modulation sensitivity at frequencies below 3 Hz, some kind of nonlinearity must be added to the model. This step is also necessary to predict the transient responses of most species, and it is included in many recent flicker models.

The first attempt to account for the sine-wave data was made by IVES (1922b), who proposed a model based on ionic diffusion. KELLY (1961b) suggested a second-order, linear filter, followed by a nonlinear stage simulating refractory neural behavior. Earlier, DELANGE (1952, 1961) had proposed an electrical analog that consisted of several (identical but isolated) stages of low-pass, exponential (RC) filtering in cascade. The DE LANGE model was modified by FUORTES and HODGKIN (1964), who added feedback control of the gains and time constants of all stages from the output. With this nonlinear feature, they were able to fit fairly well the transient response of *Limulus*, and PINTER (1966) was able to fit its steady-state response. A similar control of gain (but not time-constant) had been used by TROELSTRA (1964) to fit human ERG responses at scotopic levels. MARIMONT (1965) improved the fit of the Fuortes-Hodgkin model to the *Limulus* data, by taking the feedback signal from the penultimate stage, rather than from the final output. Replacing the feedback gain control by a nonlinear element (e.g., a thermistor) DEVOE (1966, 1967) was able to fit both transient and steady-state responses of the wolf-spider with a similar multi-stage model. LEVINSON (1966), noting the formal identity of the Fuortes-Hodgkin equation to the Poisson distribution, abandoned the multi-stage interpretation in favor of a more plausible, single-stage, multiple-event, statistical process (i.e., photon detection). Still more elaborate treatments have recently appeared, in which variations of the Fuortes-Hodgkin model are applied to the human flicker data and other psychophysical thresholds (MATIN, 1968; SPERLING and SONDHI, 1968).

It seems possible that these increasingly complex explanations may not be necessary to fit the relatively simple facts about flicker thresholds. Furthermore, the multi-stage, RC-filter models have not yielded a firm value for N, the number of stages, particularly for the human data. Values of 9 or 10 are often assumed, but the range is from 4 to 12 in the literature just cited. This ambiguity in the model is made slightly more plausible, but not eliminated, by LEVINSON's statistical interpretation.

If the N-stage filter model is applicable to human flicker sensitivity, then the value of N must equal the slope of the high-frequency asymptote of the sine-wave data plotted in log-log coordinates; i.e., the high-frequency thresholds shown in Fig. 10 must vary as an integral power of the frequency. However, the value of N cannot be determined unambiguously from these psychophysical data. Perhaps this is because the data are not precise enough in this region, but careful inspection of Fig. 10 suggests that the high-frequency envelope of these flicker thresholds is continously downward-curving, and hence cannot be fitted by a straight line of any slope.

As discussed in Sec. II, this high-frequency envelope depends on the absolute amplitude of the first Fourier component of the stimulus, not on its average luminance level. But according to the Ferry-Porter Law, it then follows that the CFF increases as the logarithm of this amplitude; i.e., that the amplitude sensitivity varies as an exponential function of frequency, *not* a power function. Thus, to the extent that the Ferry-Porter law is correct, no rectilinear asymptote exists for the sine-wave flicker data. Since the slope of an exponential function increases continuously in log-log coordinates, all N-stage models of the Fuortes-Hodgkin type are logically excluded by the Ferry-Porter Law (and vice versa).

Now consider instead a model that rigorously obeys the Ferry-Porter Law; i.e., one with the amplitude sensitivity function

$$|G(\omega)| = e^{-k|\omega|} \tag{8}$$

as the modulus of its transfer function (where $\omega/2\pi$ is the flicker frequency and k is a constant). With the assumption of zero phase-shift, this formally transforms to the impulse response,

$$g(t) = \frac{2k}{k^2 + t^2}\,. \tag{9}$$

But this response is not physically realizable in the time domain, since $g(t)$ does not equal 0 for $t < 0$ (i.e., the effect would precede the cause). Worse, $e^{-k|\omega|}$ does not obey the Paley-Wiener criterion, which means there is *no* phase function that can make this modulus correspond to a physically realizable impulse response (e.g., see Mason and Zimmerman, 1960, Sec. 7.14).

The inevitable conclusion is that, although the high-frequency envelope of the sine-wave flicker data is not a power function, it is not exactly an exponential either; i.e., at least to the extent that the CFF is governed by a linear process, the Ferry-Porter Law cannot be rigorously true.

If high-frequency linearity is assumed, this non-realizability of the Ferry-Porter Law must also be taken into account to obtain a plausible model. In order to yield a physically realizable response, $|G(\omega)|$ must be slightly concave upward relative to the Ferry-Porter Law; and this trend seems to be present in the psychophysical data (see Fig. 18). Thus, it is an urgent task of current flicker theory to find some other analytically simple function that fits these data better than a power function. Obviously the desired relation must be close to the Ferry-Porter Law, but not so close that it fails on grounds of physical realizability.

References

Baker, H. D.: Instantaneous threshold and early dark adaptation. J. opt. Soc. Amer. **43**, 798—803 (1953).

Bartley, S. H., Nelson, T. M.: A further study of pulse-to-cycle fraction and critical flicker frequency. A decisive theoretical test. J. opt. Soc. Amer. **51**, 41—45 (1961).

Boynton, R. M., Kandel, G.: On responses in the human visual system as a function of adaptation level. J. opt. Soc. Amer. **47**, 275—286 (1957).

— Sturr, J. F., Ikeda, M.: Study of flicker by increment threshold technique. J. opt. Soc. Amer. **51**, 196—201 (1961).

Brindley, G. S.: Beats produced by simultaneous stimulation of the human eye with intermittent light and intermittent or alternating electric current. J. Physiol. (Lond.) **164**, 157—167 (1962).

Brown, J. L.: Harmonic analysis of visual stimuli below fusion frequency. Science **137**, 686—688 (1962).

— Flicker and intermittent stimulation. Ch. 10. In: Vision and Visual Perception. Graham, C.H. (Ed.). New York: Wiley 1965.

Brown, K. T.: The electroretinogram: Its components and their origins. Vision Res. 8, 633—677 (1968).

Cleland, B., Enroth-Cugell, C.: Cat retinal ganglion cell responses to changing light intensities: Sinusoidal modulation in the time domain. Acta physiol. scand. **68**, 365—381 (1966).

Cobb, P. W.: Some comments on the Ives theory of flicker. J. opt. Soc. Amer. **24**, 91—98 (1934).
De Lange, H.: Experiments on flicker and some calculations on an electrical analogue of the foveal systems. Physica **18**, 935—950 (1952).
— Relationship between critical flicker frequency and a set of low-frequency characteristics of the eye. J. opt. Soc. Amer. **44**, 380—389 (1954).
— Attenuation characteristics and phase-shift characteristics of the human fovea-cortex systems in relation to flicker-fusion phenomena. Doctoral dissertation, Technical University, Delft (1957).
— Research into the dynamic nature of the human fovea-cortex systems with intermittent and modulated light. I. Attenuation characteristics with white and colored light. J. opt. Soc. Amer. **48**, 777—784 (1958a).
— Research into the dynamic nature of the human fovea-cortex systems with intermittent and modulated light. II. Phase shift in brightness and delay in color perception. J. opt. Soc. Amer. **48**, 784—789 (1958b).
— Eye's response at flicker fusion to square-wave modulation of a test field surrounded by a large steady field of equal mean luminance. J. opt. Soc. Amer. **51**, 415—421 (1961).
De Voe, R. D.: Electrical responses to flicker in the eye of the wolf spider, *Lycosa baltimoriana*. Doctoral dissertation. The Rockefeller Institute, New York (1961).
— Linear superposition of retinal action potentials to predict electrical flicker responses from the eye of the wolf spider, *Lycosa baltimoriana* (Keyserling). J. gen. Physiol. **46**, 75—96 (1962).
— Linear relations between stimulus amplitudes and amplitudes of retinal action potentials from the eye of the wolf spider. J. gen. Physiol. **47**, 13—32 (1963).
— Linear electrical flicker responses from the eye of the wolf spider. Documenta ophthal. **18**, 128—136 (1964).
— A nonlinear model of sensory adaptation in the eye of the wolf spider. In: The Functional Organization of the Compound Eye. Bernhard, C. G. (Ed.), pp. 309—328. Oxford: Pergamon 1966.
— A nonlinear model for transient responses from light-adapted wolf spider eyes. J. gen. Physiol. **50**, 1993—2030 (1967).
Dow, J. S.: The speed of flicker photometers. Electrician **59**, 255—257 (1907).
Enroth, C.: The mechanism of flicker and fusion studied on single retinal elements in the dark-adapted eye of the cat. Acta physiol. scand. **27**, Suppl. 100 (1952).
Enroth-Cugell, C., Robson, J. G.: The contrast sensitivity of the retinal ganglion cell of the cat. J. Physiol. (Lond.) **187**, 517—532 (1966).
Forsyth, D. M.: Use of a Fourier model in describing the fusion of complex visual stimuli. J. opt. Soc. Amer. **50**, 337—341 (1960).
— Brown, C. R.: Flicker for intermittent photic stimuli of alternating duration. J. opt. Soc. Amer. **49**, 760—763 (1959).
— — Nonlinear property of the visual system at fusion. Science **134**, 612—614 (1961).
— — Visual system at fusion. Science **135**, 794—795 (1962).
Fuortes, M. G. F., Hodgkin, A. L.: Changes in time scale and sensitivity in the ommatidia of *Limulus*. J. Physiol. (Lond.) **172**, 239—263 (1964).
Gibbins, K., Howarth, C. I.: Prediction of the effect of the light-time fraction on the critical flicker frequency; an insight from Fourier analysis. Nature (Lond.) **190**, 330—331 (1961).
Gouras, P., Gunkel, R. D.: The frequency response of normal, rod achromat and nyctalope ERGS to sinusoidal monochromatic light stimulation. Documenta ophthal. **18**, 137—150 (1964).
Green, D. G.: Sinusoidal flicker characteristics of the color-sensitive mechanisms of the eye. Vision Res. **9**, 591—601 (1969).
Henkes, H. E., van der Tweel, L. H. (Eds.): Flicker (Documenta Ophthalmologica, Vol. XVIII). Hague: Dr. W. Junk 1964.
Hubel, D. H., Wiesel, T. N.: Receptive fields and functional architecture of monkey striate cortex. J. Physiol. (Lond.) **195**, 215—243 (1968).
Hughes, G. W., Maffei, L.: Retinal ganglion cell response to sinusoidal light stimulation. J. Neurophysiol. **29**, 333—352 (1966).

IKEDA, M.: Temporal summation of positive and negative flashes in the visual system. J. opt. Soc. Amer. **55**, 1527—1534 (1965).
— BOYNTON, R. M.: Negative flashes, positive flashes, and flicker examined by increment threshold technique. J. opt. Soc. Amer. **55**, 560—566 (1965).
IVES, H. E.: Critical frequency relations in scotopic vision. J. opt. Soc. Amer. and Rev. sci. Instr. **6**, 254—268 (1922a).
— A theory of intermittent vision. J. opt. Soc. Amer. and Rev. sci. Instr. **6**, 343—361 (1922b).
JONES, R. C.: On the quantum efficiency of scotopic and photopic vision. J. Wash. Acad. Sci. **47**, 100—108 (1957).
KAMP, A., SEM-JACOBSEN, C. W., VAN LEEUWEN, W. S., VAN DER TWEEL, L. H.: Cortical responses to modulated light in the human subject. Acta physiol. scand. **48**, 1—12 (1960).
KELLY, D. H.: Effects of sharp edges in a flickering field. J. opt. Soc. Amer. **49**, 730—732 (1959).
— Visual responses to time-dependent stimuli. I. Amplitude sensitivity measurements. J. opt. Soc. Amer. **51**, 422—429 (1961a).
— Visual responses to time-dependent stimuli. II. Single-channel model of the photopic visual system. J. opt. Soc. Amer. **51**, 747—754 (1961b).
— Flicker fusion and harmonic analysis. J. opt. Soc. Amer. **51**, 917—918 (1961c).
— Visual responses to time-dependent stimuli. IV. Effects of chromatic adaptation. J. opt. Soc. Amer. **52**, 940—947 (1962).
— Sine waves and flicker fusion. Documenta ophthal. **18**, 16—35 (1964).
— Flickering patterns and lateral inhibition. J. opt. Soc. Amer. **59**, 1361—1370 (1969).
LANDIS, C.: An annotated bibliography of flicker fusion phenomena, covering the period of 1740—1952. Ann Arbor: Armed Forces -Nat. Res. Council (1953).
LEVINSON, J.: Fusion of complex flicker. Science **130**, 919—921 (1959).
— Fusion of complex flicker II. Science **131**, 1438—1440 (1960).
— Nonlinear and spatial effects in the perception of flicker. Documenta ophthal. **18**, 36—55 (1964).
— One-stage model for visual temporal integration. J. opt. Soc. Amer. **56**, 95—97 (1966).
— Flicker fusion phenomena. Science **160**, 21—28 (1968).
— HARMON, L. D.: Studies with artificial neurons, III: Mechanisms of flicker-fusion. Kybernetik **1**, 107—117 (1961).
MAFFEI, L., CERVETTO, L.: Dynamical interactions in retinal receptive fields. Vision Res. **8**, 1299—1303 (1968).
— POPPELE, R. E.: Transient and steady-state electroretinal responses. Vision Res. **8**, 229—246 (1968).
— RIZZOLATTI, G.: Transfer properties of the lateral geniculate body. J. Neurophysiol. **30**, 333—340 (1967).
MARIMONT, R. B.: Numerical studies of the Fuortes-Hodgkin Limulus model. J. Physiol. (Lond.) **179**, 489—497 (1965).
MASON, S. T., ZIMMERMAN, H. J.: Electronic Circuits, Signals and Systems. New York: Wiley 1960 (see Sec. 7.14).
MATIN, L.: Fourier treatment of some experiments in visual flicker. Science **136**, 983—985 (1962).
— Critical duration, the differential luminance threshold, critical flicker frequency, and visual adaptation: a theoretical treatment. J. opt. Soc. Amer. **58**, 404—415 (1968).
OGAWA, T., BISHOP, P. O., LEVICK, W. R.: Temporal characteristics of responses to photic stimulation by single ganglion cells in the unopened eye of the cat. J. Neurophysiol. **29**, 1—30 (1966).
PIÉRON, H.: La vision en lumière intermittente (Monographies Francaises de Psychologie No. 8). Paris: Centre National de la Récherche Scientifique 1961.
— Vision in intermittent light. In: Contributions to Sensory Physiology, NEFF, W. D. (Ed.). New York: Academic Press 1965.
PINTER, R. B.: Sinusoidal and delta function responses of visual cells of the Limulus eye. J. gen. Physiol. **49**, 565—593 (1966).
RATLIFF, F., KNIGHT, B. W., TOYODA, J., HARTLINE, H. K.: Enhancement of flicker by lateral inhibition. Science **158**, 392—393 (1967).

Regan, D.: Some characteristics of average steady-state and transient responses evoked by modulated light. Electroenceph. clin. Neurophysiol. **20**, 238—248 (1966a).
— An effect of stimulus colour on average steady-state potentials evoked in man. Nature (Lond.) **210**, 1056—1057 (1966b).
— Chromatic adaptation and steady-state evoked potentials. Vision Res. 8, 149—158 (1968a).
— A high frequency mechanism which underlies visual evoked potentials. Electroenceph. clin. Neurophysiol. **25**, 231—237 (1968b).
Riggs, L. A.: Electrophysiology of vision. Ch. 5. In: Vision and Visual Perception. Graham, C. H. (Ed.). New York: Wiley 1965.
— Johnson, E. P., Schick, A. M. L.: Electrical responses of the human eye to moving stimulus patterns. Science **144**, 567 (1964).
— — — Electrical responses of the human eye to changes in wavelength of the stimulating light. J. opt. Soc. Amer. **56**, 1621—1627 (1966).
Roufs, J. A. J.: On the relation between the threshold of short flashes, the flicker fusion frequency and the visual latency. In: IPO Annual Progress Report No. 1. Eindhoven: Institute for Perception Research 1966.
— Lammers, J. T. H., Siemons, J. A.: Positive and negative flashes. In: IPO Annual Progress Report No. 2. Eindhoven: Institute for Perception Research 1967.
— Meulenbrugge, H. J.: The quantitative relation between flash threshold and the flicker-fusion boundary for centrally fixated fields. In: IPO Annual Progress Report No. 2. Eindhoven: Institute for Perception Research 1967.
Spekreijse, H.: Analysis of EEG responses in man evoked by sine wave modulated light. Doctoral dissertation, University of Amsterdam (1966).
— Van der Tweel, L. H.: Linearization of evoked responses to sine wave modulated light by noise. Nature (Lond.) **205**, 913 (1965).
— — Flicker and noise. In: Clinical Electroretinography Symp. 1964, Vision Res. Suppl. 1, pp. 275—280. Oxford: Pergamon 1966.
Sperling, G., Sondhi, M. M.: Model for visual luminance discrimination and flicker detection. J. opt. Soc. Amer. 58, 1133—1145 (1968).
Troelstra, A.: Nonlinear systems analysis in electroretinography. Soesterberg: Institute for Perception RVO-TNO 1964.
— Schweitzer, N. M. J.: On the relation between the single flash ERG and the ERG elicited by more complex stimuli. Documenta ophthal. 18, 114—127 (1964).
Tweel, L. H. van der: Some problems in vision regarded with respect to linearity and frequency response. Ann. N. Y. Acad. sci. **89**, 829—856 (1961).
— Relation between psychophysics and electrophysiology of flicker. Documenta ophthal. 18, 287—304 (1964).
— Spekreijse, H.: Visual evoked responses. In: The Clinical Value of Electroretinography, ISCERG Symp. Ghent 1966, pp. 83—94. Basel: Karger 1968.
— Verduyn Lunel, H. F. E.: Human visual responses to sinusoidally modulated light. Electroenceph. clin. Neurophysiol. 18, 587—598 (1965).
Veringa, F.: On some properties of nonthreshold flicker. J. opt. Soc. Amer. 48, 500—502 (1958).
— Phase shifts in the human retina. Nature (Lond.) **197**, 998—999 (1963).
— Electro-optical stimulation of the human retina as a research technique. Documenta ophthal. 18, 72—82 (1964).
— Roelofs, J.: Electro-optical interaction in the retina. Nature (Lond.) **211**, 321—322 (1966).
West, D. C.: Flicker and the stabilized retinal image. Vision Res. 8, 719—745 (1968).

Chapter 12

Eye Movements

By

MATHEW ALPERN, Ann Arbor, Michigan (USA)

With 3 Figures

Contents

The eye, a spatial frequency analyzer par excellence, is enormously sensitive to very small differences in visual angle. For human psychophysics, at least, the problems of eye movements are intimately related to the fact that the retina has outstanding spatial sensitivity only for a very small area (around 20′ diameter) in the center of the fovea. For the rest, spatial sensitivity is extremely poor. Hence only an insignificant fraction of total retinal area is concerned with almost all of high luminance level acute vision. What makes this paradox possible is not only a visual cortex with large magnification of the linear extent concerned with the fovea (almost 7 mm/degree of visual angle) compared with that related to the rest of the retina (about 1/3 mm/degree, 20° from the fovea, for example), (DANIEL and WHITTERIDGE, 1961) but also twelve extraocular muscles (six attached to each eye) and a neurological control system which gives the two eyes very great mobility, pointing their sensitive foveas in rapid succession at one object of regard after another. It is towards the understanding of this mobility that the present chapter is directed. Little if anything will be said, because little if anything is known, as to how the eyes, or rather the perceiver, pieces together from successive oculocentric isomorphs (in cortical area 17), each radically different from its predecessor, and successor, a map of immobile egocentric objects whose fine detail if not everywhere apparent is at least not at all conspicuous in its absence.

Steady Fixation

Even when exerting every effort to fixate steadily, it is a fact that the two eyes are constantly moving (MARX and TRENDELENBURG, 1911; ADLER and FLIEGELMAN, 1934; LORD and WRIGHT, 1948; RATLIFF and RIGGS, 1950; BARLOW, 1952; DITCHBURN and GINSBORG, 1952; HIGGINS and STULTZ, 1953; CORNSWEET, 1956; YARBUS, 1967; KRAUSKOPF *et al.*, 1960; NACHMIAS, 1959, 1961; STEINMAN, 1965; CUNITZ and STEINMAN, 1969; DITCHBURN and FOLEY-FISHER, 1967; WEST and BOYCE, 1968; ST. CYR and FENDER, 1969, among others). The literature is extensive and a summary has been given elsewhere (ALPERN, 1970) so only the major features will be discussed here.

1. Flicks, or Microsaccades. These are very rapid, irregularly occuring movements, binocularly synchronized (exactly so according to YARBUS, 1967, but not according to FENDER and JULESZ, 1967, and ST. CYR and FENDER, 1969, and only approximately so according to KRAUSKOPF *et al.*, 1960) which range in amplitude from about 2′ to a maximum of 40–50′ though they rarely exceed 20′. The mean value is about 5.6′ (STEINMAN *et al.*, 1967) (median of 4.5′). Their duration (DITCHBURN and FOLEY-FISHER, 1967), depending on amplitude, is typically 10 to 20 msec. The peak velocity of the flicks (v_{max}) is linearly related to the amplitude α by the equation

$$v_{max} = 82.4\,\alpha, \qquad (1)$$

which is reasonably accurate not only for the flicks of steady fixation but for somewhat larger saccadic eye movements as well. For values of $\alpha \geq 3.3°$, Eq. (1) breaks down, however, and the relationship becomes highly non-linear (WESTHEIMER, 1954a; ZUBER *et al.*, 1965). Flicks are commonly referred to as "involuntary" largely because their occurrence among subjects instructed to "fixate" as accurately as possible seems to be a random event, not under control of the "fixater". But STEINMAN *et al.* (1967) have now shown that this may be an artifact of the instruction "fixate", since subjects instructed to "hold the eye steady" were able to reduce the microsaccade rate to zero throughout a 9.8 second trial. This occurred whether or not the sphincture of the iris and the parasympathetically innervated ciliary muscle fibers were paralyzed with 2% cyclopentolate hydrochloride, a parasympathetic blocking agent (which however leaves iris dilator and sympathetically controlled ciliary muscle fibers unaffected) (STEINMAN *et al.*, 1969).

2. High Frequency Tremors. These have the mean amplitude of from 1 to 1.5 foveal cone diameters (20–30 seconds of arc) according to YARBUS (1967) though DITCHBURN's (1955) estimate is smaller (5–15 seconds for horizontal and vertical movements and 45 seconds for torsional tremor). The major frequency component is 70–90 Hz, a frequency above critical flicker frequency (CFF) as YARBUS emphasizes. Its small amplitude makes a precise study of tremor difficult because of potential artifacts from head movements and apparatus vibration. Almost nothing is known about their physiology (for example the extent to which they are binocularly synchronized), though there can no longer be any question that they are valid eye movements. They are moreover a constant feature of the third variety of eye movements of steady fixation, namely:

3. Slow Drifts. These movements of the two eyes occur quite independently. In the literature, the measure of drift amplitude ranges from 0.8 to about 6.0 min of arc with the median for all subjects (16) about 2.5 min (DITCHBURN and FOLEY-FISHER, 1967). Drifts are always accompanied by tremors. The drift of the line of sight during steady fixation is an irregular movement during which the retinal image of the fixation point remains nonetheless inside the fovea. The velocity is about 6′/sec; hence the retinal image of the fixation point covers from 10–15 cone diameters a second during the drift (YARBUS, 1967).

CORNSWEET (1956) advanced the idea that microsaccades brought the retinal image of the fixation point back to some "optimal locus" from which it had strayed as a consequence of the drifts. This proposal was in agreement with a number of facts including (in some subjects) the high negative correlation found between the direction of the microsaccade and that of the immediately preceding drifts. Individual differences among subjects are wide, however; many subjects show no such correlation (PROSKURIAKOVA and SHAKHNOVICH, 1968). Furthermore the variability of eye positions under instruction to "hold eyes steady" (when microsaccade frequency can go to zero) is no larger than that found under "fixate" instruction when microsaccades occur at regular intervals. Drifts in and of themselves do not carry the eyes farther from an "optimal locus" than when they are interspersed with allegedly correcting microsaccades (STEINMAN *et al.*, 1967).

What is the function of microsaccades? Although it has been suggested from time to time, they cannot function to improve visual acuity or the ability to see straight lines as straight. CUNITZ and STEINMAN (1969) suggest that they, like large saccadic eye movements (cf. below), function to scan the visual field (in this case only in the neighborhood of the fixation point). The idea that microsaccades are exactly the same in their physiology as macrosaccadic eye movements is in agreement with a number of observations, including the finding (ZUBER *et al.*, 1965) that the relationship between amplitude of the microsaccade and its maximum velocity could be predicted by extrapolation given this relationship for macrosaccades 3° or smaller. Moreover it is in agreement with the finding of CUNITZ and STEINMAN (1969) that the frequency of occurrence of microsaccades during the fixation pauses of normal reading is greatly reduced compared to the frequency during steady fixation. There seems to be one essential difference between large and small saccades besides the amplitude of the movement. Macrosaccades (but not microsaccades) can be evoked by a "position error" signal; the threshold angular separation for this effect is about 15 min of arc (RASHBASS, 1961).

Although one cannot doubt the general similarity between large and small saccadic eye movements, it is now evident that there is no similar analog in large eye movements to the slow drifts of steady fixation. The idea that the drifts are analogous to smooth pursuit movements (cf. below) is seductive, but two considerations show that such an inference is spurious: (1) The drifts of the two eyes are quite independent (YARBUS, 1967) while in smooth pursuit movements the two eyes move synchronously in conjugation. (2) The stimulus for smooth pursuit movement is a discrepancy between the velocity of the target to be fixated and the velocity of the eye. No analagous stimulus can be demonstrated for the drifts. This independence of the drifts for two eyes also excludes the possibility that drifts are analogous to vergence movements.

What is then the function of the slow drifts and the tremor? As to the latter no clear answer can be given, but the answer to the former opens one of the most exciting chapters in modern retinal physiology. It begins with the hypothesis (first disproved by RATLIFF, 1952) of WEYMOUTH *et al.* (1923), MARSHALL and TALBOT (1942), JONES and HIGGINS (1947, 1948) that the eye movements of steady fixation were responsible for the ability of the retina to resolve (in, say, a vernier acuity task) fine detail of angular subtense about one third to one fifth the diameter of a foveal cone. To test this possibility RIGGS *et al.* (1953) devised a method of holding the specific retinal receptors stimulated by the different parts of the image of a target always the same, independent of the eye movement of "steady" fixation. It was found that, for short exposures of the test target (less than 0.2 secs), acuity under "stabilized" conditions was no poorer than acuity under normal viewing (KEESEY, 1960). If however the observer continued to view for longer periods under stabilized conditions all detail in the visual field faded away! (RIGGS *et al.*, 1953; DITCHBURN and GINSBORG, 1952; YARBUS, 1957b; PRITCHARD *et al.*, 1960; BARLOW, 1963).

The time characteristics of this phenomenon are much too slow to attribute the failure of its occurrence in steady fixation to tremor. Saccades cause a decrement (rather than increment) in visibility of the target, and when they are not made, targets do not disappear. Apparently it is the function of slow drifts to prevent the fading of targets that is observed when retinal images are stabilized. The resolving power of the eye and the color appearance of objects are held relatively constant during fixation as a result of slow drifts (YARBUS, 1967). YARBUS found that in the presence of a sharp retinal image of a border, a single drift of the eye was capable of preventing the formation of an empty visual field over the whole retina. On the other hand no effect of tremor was found. [The artificial "tremor" imposed by DITCHBURN *et al.* (1959) which hindered fading was quite unphysiological, as YARBUS (1967) has emphasized.] Further experiments are required to exclude the possibility that tremor, particularly in combination with slow drifts, which they always accompany, may not play some role in preventing fading. But the available evidence suggests that the role is unlikely to be large.

Vision with Stabilized Retinal Image

Besides the slow drifts (and possibly the tremors) other conditions can oppose the fading of a "stabilized" image, among them head movements, accommodation defocus, pupil size fluctuation and variable transcleral illumination as well as eyelid blinks. Such effects are not always given close attention when the fading of the stabilized image is studied. This is undoubtedly part of the reason for the large differences in the literature as to the details of subjective appearances of stabilized images (Barlow, 1963).

The details of these reports of subjective appearances by the various investigators are so different it becomes difficult to evaluate the extent to which the discrepancies are due to various artifacts of their techniques that lead to incomplete stabilization, to other experimental differences, or to genuine individual differences among observers. Experimental evaluation of the stability of the retinal image by any given method is straightforward (Barlow, 1963), but so far it has not been extensively employed (for an exception cf. Riggs and Schick, 1968).

Most careful investigators agree that there is loss of vision of high contrast test targets within a few seconds after the onset of viewing of a stabilized image. The exception to this appears to be Fender and his co-workers (Beeler *et al.*, 1964; Fender and Julesz, 1967). Since these reports are so much at variance with those described by the remaining groups, concrete evidence of the sort mustered by Barlow (1963) is necessary to demonstrate that their method, in fact, produced stable images. Yarbus (1967) describes a true fading of all details into an "empty visual field" within 1–3 sec after onset of viewing the stabilized image. The intermittent resurgence of visibility of high contrast targets described by others (Ditchburn *et al.*, 1959; Pritchard, 1964) were attributed by Yarbus to artifacts of imperfect stabilization. Barlow (1963) confirms this in most details but does not agree that with perfect stability luminance discrimination within the stabilized field reduces to zero. For Barlow the target appears with full clarity only for the first few seconds, the details and high contrast of the original are then lost. For the following minute there is a fluctuation of the appearance which dies out leaving a stable appearance of gray fog with poorly defined light and dark clouds in it corresponding to the black and white parts of the original. This final appearance is a blurred low contrast version of the original which persists as long as conditions are unchanged. Turning off the background causes the negative of the original to appear without fine detail. Resurgence can then be initiated by turning the light on again. A good deal of interest has been centered on the optimum rate of intermittent exposure necessary for best visibility (Cornsweet, 1956; Fiorentini and Ercoles, 1960; Pritchard, 1964; West, 1968; Keesey, 1969, to name only a few). In general these reports are in agreement that optimum visibility is obtained when the intermittent rate is considerably below the CFF. Cortical neurons in cat (PRITCHARD, 1964) appear to be optimally sensitive to black-white borders oscillating at these same frequencies when they are viewed by the immobilized retina. In man the most recent work gives maximum visibility at 5 Hz (WEST, 1968), and 2.5–7.0 Hz (KEESEY, 1969). Lower values than this are found in earlier experiments (CORNSWEET, 1956). Differences may well be due to slight differences in experimental designs. Frequencies higher than 15 Hz are not effective in maintaining visibility of the target though the flicker in the empty field continues to be visible.

CAMPBELL and ROBSON (1961), using the entoptic view of retinal capillaries, found that only the spatial (not the temporal) component of stimulation was effective in improving visibility of their target; a result which perhaps differs from those described above because the contrast of retinal capillaries is relatively low compared with that of good targets prepared for view in the conventional optical devices (say a "suck-on" contact lens).

YARBUS (1967) measured the rate of change of illumination necessary to maintain visibility of the stabilized image of a black line on a bright background. The threshold rate dI/dt was found to depend upon the background luminance I:

$$dI/dt = 0.3125\, I. \tag{2}$$

WEST (1967) has examined many factors which influence one's ability to discriminate luminance differences with a stabilized image. Although his "visibility time" is large according to YARBUS, and hence many indicate imperfect stability (due to contact lens slippage), his results, even if quantitatively inappropriate for the perfectly immobilized retinal image, are nonetheless suggestive. Visibility time decreases as eccentricity from the fovea is increased, as target blur increases, as the length of the boundary decreases. For red and green, "receptive field size" in the fovea is of the order of twice the diameter of a foveal cone. For blue it is much larger. Once fading occurs, sharp spatial displacements as small as 2 min restore vision (DITCHBURN *et al*, 1959).

It is generally agreed that the fading of stabilized images emphasizes the importance of on and off cells in maintaining continuous vision of details during normal viewing. (RIGGS *et al.*, 1953; DITCHBURN, 1955; YARBUS, 1967, to cite only the principle sources.) Experiments in which a disk of one color is surrounded by an annulus of another in stabilized viewing show that, when the outer edge of the annulus was destabilized, the border between the disk and the annulus fades and the disk which results always has the color of the annulus (KRAUSKOPF, 1964). The fact that fine detail is lost very soon after stabilization signified to BARLOW (1963) that the mechanism responsible for signalling high spatial frequencies was incapable of signalling low temporal frequencies. Spatial-temporal differentials and spatial averages are signalled but not actual local luminances, nor are spatial averages of temporal differentials, nor temporal averages of spatial differentials. BARLOW proposed a two-channel hypothesis similar in some respects to the hypothesis of YARBUS (1967) and of WEST (1967). The rapidly adapting channel signals an approximation to the spatio-temporal derivative of the light $-\partial(\partial^2 I + \partial^2 I/\partial y^2)\, \partial t$ from a local region with properties similar to the on-center and the off-center units of the cat retina. The loss of fine detail in stabilized images is attributed to the rapid adaptation of these channels. A slowly adapting or nonadapting channel, which has large receptive fields, signals the "dim clouds" that appear after prolonged stabilization and are correctly related to the luminance of different parts of the field. It is possible that these slow adapting channels drive the photopupil response, and it is therefore of some interest to know the extent to which the photopupil response "fades" with a stabilized retinal image.

Stabilized Images without Attachments to the Eye

Although it is not widely appreciated, many incidental features of ocular structure make it possible to view the characteristics of stabilized retinal images without attachments to the globe (Ratliff, 1958; Campbell and Robson, 1961). These include the shadows of the retinal arteries and veins, of its capillaries, Haidinger's brushes, Maxwell's spot, the blue arcs of the retina, and the yellowgreen splotches of Shurcliff (1959). Many of these effects are described in standard texts (Adler, 1965). They all have in common that they fade but can be made to regenerate by alterations in the viewing conditions. Working with macular capillaries, Campbell and Robson (1961) found that only the spatial component in the "renewal" stimulus was responsible for improving visibility, a result which can account for resurgence of visibility of Haidinger's brushes viewed through a rotating polaroid, but not Barlow's (1963) result and those of others (Keesey, 1969) who used attachments to the globe. These differences are probably due to the low contrast of retinal capillaries (Maxwell's spot can certainly be kept visible by only temporal, and not spatial, changes in stimulation.)

A commonly overlooked stabilized image is the after-image. If an after-image of a very fine grating is viewed against a white homogeneous surface, it fades with characteristics similar to other stabilized images. The details of the grating disappear first (Brindley, 1962). But closing the eyes briefly or turning the background off, and then on, can cause it to reappear and the whole cycle can be repeated many times. One aspect of the fading of stabilized after-images which has so far received little or no attention is that duration of time that the fine detail in the after-image of (say) a Xenon flash tube is visible depends upon the luminance of the background against which it is viewed. If care is taken to avoid blinks or obvious eye movements, the after-image viewed against a very bright uniform background quite likely loses all its detail in the 1–3 sec that Yarbus found for real images. For backgrounds of 63 cd/m^2, I found the detail fading in about 11 sec, but it could be made to reappear by a very slight blink or eye movement to a nonuniform part of the background. Viewed against the backgrounds of 10 cd/m^2 that Brindley (1962) used, the fading was slower and the detail remained visible for 25 sec. On the other hand, in total darkness the details could be seen for a full minute. Why should this detail in after-images seen in the dark be visible for a duration 20 times as long as that obtained with real images? It might be imaged that this is because the equivalent background of the bleach (B) is changing as the visual pigments regenerate at a rate faster than required by Eq. (2). However, for the foveal "red" and "green" cone pigments, this process follows the time course

$$-t_0 dB/dt = B + (B/B_0)^2 \qquad (3)$$

where t_0 is the time constant of regeneration of the pigments (about 120 secs.), and B_0 is the equivalent background at which half the pigment has regenerated. For $B < B_0$, the higher order term in (3) can be neglected and this equation becomes similar to (2) except that this constant is almost 40 times *slower* (rather than faster) than that obtained in YARBUS' experiment. YARBUS (1967) recognized this difficulty and assigns the fading of after-images to a slow process associated with retinal adaptation. But what sort of channels are these which are capable of signalling the fine detail in a positive after-image viewed in the dark and incapable of signalling similar detail in a real image?

Viewing the negative after-image against a uniform screen of 10 cd/m^2, BRINDLEY found that following very bright red and green flashes the finest detail (about 1 min of arc grating) was visible after 20 seconds in the dark. Blurring begins after about 2 min in the dark (which for a full bleach of the cone pigments chlorlabe or erythrolabe would be a time when 37% of the pigment was still unregenerated). After 2 minutes in the dark, the visual acuity for the after-image (the finest grating which could be resolved in the after-image) decreases at a rate of 4.1 min of arc/60 sec for the green flash. Perceptible after-images persisted for 15–20 min in the dark, though virtually all "red" and "green" cone pigments have regenerated by six minutes after a full bleach.

The phenomenon described in the last paragraphs is due not to the fading of the stabilized image but to more peripheral effects related to diffusion of photochemical products of the bleaching flash, as BRINDLEY's experiments clearly show. It has been investigated at some length by RUSHTON and BAKER (1963) who designate it as the Θ effect. The disappearance of after-images in the Θ effect is much slower than the pigment regeneration. This seems to be a peculiarity of flash bleaching.

RUSHTON and BAKER (1963) have demonstrated that when cone pigments are fully bleached (not by very brief flashes but by prolonged exposures, say, about 10 sec) the after-images disappear as the pigments regenerate and as sensitivity improves. There is now a direct proportion between the log threshold and amount of pigment regenerated after a full bleach. BARLOW and SPARROCK (1964) showed that the after-image resulting from the bleach under such circumstances acts as an "equivalent background" and elevates the threshold (in both the rods and the cones) for the full 30 minutes in the dark in which sensitivity changes can be measured. The way in which this occurs is one of the fundamental problems in current visual theory, but the major issues are foreign to the subject of this chapter. It is mentioned here to emphasize that it was the stabilized-image property of the after-image, i. e. fading, that obscured its role in dark adaptation for so long. It was only by measuring after-image brightness by matching it to the luminance of an adjacent stabilized real background that BARLOW and SPARROCK were able to document that the stabilized after-image was the equivalent background of the bleach. One paradox stemming from this work should be mentioned because it may ultimately shed light on the character of after-image fading. It is this: Just before the break in the dark adaptation curve, the "dark light" of the rods is very high and falling very rapidly, but at this time the equivalent luminance of the after-image is constant and determined apparently by the dimmer "dark light" from the cones. Similarly just after the break, the "dark light" from the cone is presumably constant and brighter than that of the rods which in turn is still falling rapidly; now the equivalent luminance of the after-image is matched to the dark light of the rods. Thus in each of these cases and in fact in every other moment during dark adaptation, it is the dimmer (not the brighter) dark light which determines the brightness of the after-image. The brighter dark light is ignored! This is a very curious result for which no satisfying explanation exists (see BARLOW, chapter 1, this volume, for discussion of dark adaptation).

Large Eye Movements

The literature on large eye movements is vast and space limitations preclude in-depth analysis of each aspect of the subject. Fortunately a number of recent reviews (ALPERN, 1970; ROBINSON, 1968 a, b) cover this ground and the proceedings of a very recent symposium on *Control of Eye Movements* should be available in the near future. An earlier symposium (BENDER, 1964) emphasizes anatomy and physiology more than the newer developments in human psychophysics. In what follows I have attempted a broad survey of the work directly related to human psychophysics. Anatomy and physiology, if discussed at all, are brought in only when they succeed in clarifying normal (as distinct from pathological) human eye movements. As it turns out, that is not too often. Where the discussion becomes deep rather than broad it is because the problems have not been treated to my satisfaction elsewhere.

Classification of Eye Movements

A fundamental property of large eye movements in man is their binocular coordination. The eyes nearly always move synchronously together. Corresponding muscles of each eye normally receive equal innervation so that for any shift of gaze the muscles of the two eyes are yoked together. In eyes with normal muscles the result is that, independent of the degree or direction of movement, the two eyes always move exactly in the same way and exactly the same amount. This is true (except in accommodation convergence) even if one of the two eyes is occluded. If, however, there is a fresh paralysis of a muscle of one eye resulting in strabismus, then a consequence of this law of equal innervation to yoked muscles of the two eyes is that the amount of strabismus is greater when the eye with the paralyzed muscle fixates than when the other eye fixates, for it takes a greater innervation to the paralyzed muscle of the former to bring this eye on to fixation than will be needed when the normal eye fixates. This law, formalized in 1868 by EWALD HERING, is known as Hering's Law of equal innervation to the yoked muscles of the two eyes.

The fact that the visual fields of the two eyes overlap to a considerable extent requires a special kind of binocular coordination. Visual space is three (rather than two) dimensional, and retinal images are two (rather than three) dimensional. To allow the lines of sight of the two eyes to intersect any object in three dimensional space while simultaneously following Hering's Law, two basically different kinds of eye-movement patterns have evolved. These are (a) versions and (b) vergences. This is not the only possible way that bifoveal fixation might have been achieved, but the fact that no other is used even in severe pathology testifies to the fundamental importance of Hering's Law.

Versions constitute all eye movements in which the angle that the lines of sight of the two eyes make with each other does not change during the movement. Vergences constitute eye movements in which this angle changes. Except under laboratory conditions, eye movements rarely are either purely versions or purely vergences; usually a given shift of gaze contains both components. Vergence movements are always very slow (reaching at best a maximum velocity of the order of 15°/sec). The slowness of the movement is apparently due to the slow buildup of active state tension (which finds no parallel in the muscle electromyogram) rather than to differences in orbital impedance during this movement (compared with that in faster movements) (ROBINSON, 1966). Versions may be either very fast or slow. In the case of a combined movement with a fast version component, the large differences in velocity of the components allows ready evaluation of the contribution of each to the movement. A good example of this is illustrated in Fig. 1. The observer's task is to change his fixation from a far to a near plumb line which have been carefully aligned on the line of sight of the right eye. Obviously this task requires only nasal rotation of the left eye

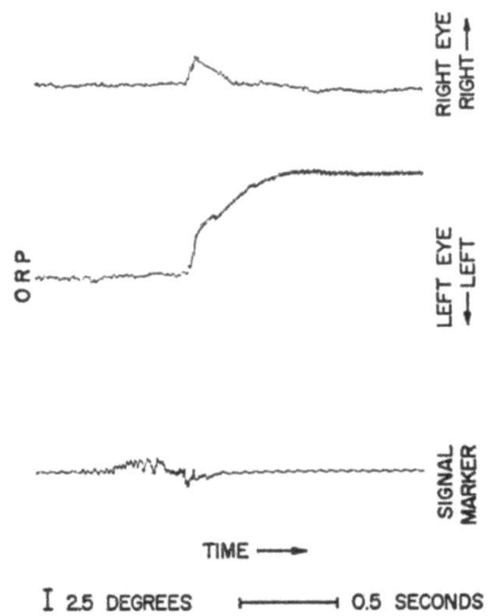

Fig. 1. Record of eye position in asymmetric binocular convergence. The signal marker is a voice record of the signal for the subject to change fixation from a far to a near object (two-plumb lines) along the line of sight of the right eye. The difference in fixation distances is equivalent to five diopters accommodation stimulus change. The eyes move according to Hering's Law. Electrooculographic record by ALPERN and ELLEN (1956a)

(the right eye holding itself steady), but it is impossible for the eyes to complete this shift of gaze in that way. Both eyes move and they move nearly the same amount. The movement follows Hering's Law of equal innervation. In the example shown in Fig. 1 (although not invariably, see ZUBER and STARK, 1968) dextro versions and convergence begin together. Since the former is much faster and hence completed sooner than the latter – the total amplitude of the movement of the right eye is somewhat less than 1/2 that of the left (the convergence component of the right eye movement begins immediately to neutralize its dextro version component). Since both versions and vergence components follow Hering's Law in this single shift of gaze, it needs emphasis that the medial rectus muscle of the right eye is, during this movements, yoked to two different muscles of the left eye (the medial and lateral recti) which are themselves antagonistic.

Besides versions and vergences, large eye movements have been classified, according to their neurology, as reflex and non-reflex, difficult as it is to drive an unequivocal operational wedge between them. The stimuli for reflex movements include adequate excitation of the head and neck muscles, the semicircular canals, the otoliths and basilar membrane of the inner ear. All these elicit version movements, and they represent the oldest and most primitive and hence most universal varieties of eye movements. According to WALLS (1962) they evolved in order to hold the retinal image of the environment fixed as vertebrates began to move about. Vergences appear much "higher" or "later" in the animal world as the eyes migrate to the front and overlapping visual fields in the two eyes emerge.

Vergence Movements

Vergence movements were classified by HOFMANN and BIELSCHOWSKY (1900) as "psycho-optical reflex" movements, implying by the term "reflex" automaticity, and by "psycho", nerve pathways which must include visual cortex. Vergence movements can be classified by the direction of the movement or by the stimulus which evokes them. One major stimulus which evokes a vergence movement is egocentric disparity, i. e. a disparity in the egocentric localization of the visual field of one eye with respect to that of the other. Vergence movements evoked by egocentric disparity are called fusional vergence movements or simply fusional movements, and they can occur in either the horizontal or the vertical direction. The problem of cyclofusional movements presents a special difficulty and will be discussed below.

Fusional Movements

Good quantitative data on the dynamic characteristics of fusional movements all concern horizontal movements. Why this is so is difficult to answer since horizontal fusional movements can be altered, perhaps subtly, with an undescribed and perhaps undetected contribution from an accommodative vergence component, and this is not the case for vertical fusional movements. The definitive paper on fusional movements is by RASHBASS and WESTHEIMER (1961a). The reaction time is fast, around 160 msec. The movement begins with a steady velocity which is a function of the amplitude of the egocentric disparity. The eyes approach their final position asymptotically, the total movement duration being about 0.8 secs. Convergence is slightly more rapid than divergence (ZUBER and STARK, 1968). Such movements can be modified during their course if the disparity is suddenly changed, since the disparity error is continuously monitored. The movement can be described by the equation

$$dr/dt = ka_{(t-\tau)} \qquad (4)$$

in which r is the eye vergence, a the disparity, τ (150 msecs.) the reaction time, and k is a constant (about 10°/sec). In addition to responding to the disparity itself, the vergence system attempts to predict the future course of the disparity, apparently by monitoring the first derivative of the disparity with respect to time.

The extent to which fusional movements can follow sine wave disparity changes of increasing frequencies is controversial. RASHBASS and WESTHEIMER (1961 a) found that disparity changes of 1 Hz were followed for only a few cycles, but YOSHIDA and WATANABE (1969) (quoted by ZUBER, 1970) obtained responses up to 2 Hz, and ZUBER and STARK (1968) up to 4 Hz. The extent to which these reports represent individual differences, or peculiarities specific to the stimulus arrangement, needs elucidation. ZUBER and STARK (1968) succeeded in inducing instability oscillations at 2.5 Hz by artificially increasing the loop gain of the systems (by an unspecified amount).

Vertical fusional movements have been studied extensively by ELLERBROCK (1949 a, b; 1952) but he used subjective methods and these only under steady state viewing conditions. Little is known about how their time characteristics compare to those of horizontal fusional movements.

Disparity

It has been pointed out that the stimulus for fusional movements is disparity in egocentric localizations in the two eyes. By this is meant that the observer localizes the visual fields seen by his two eyes in different places. If the disparity is large, double vision (diplopia) results, but even disparities too small to evoke diplopia nonetheless evoke fusional movements. A disparity of this kind needs to be sharply differentiated from the disparity in oculocentric localization of a given point in the visual fields of the two eyes. By oculocentric localization is meant the localization of an object in the visual field with respect to the fixation point. Horizontal oculocentric localization disparities of an object in space for the two eyes provides the stimulus for the stereoscopic perception of depth of that object (i. e. the object is seen either nearer to, or farther from, the observer than the fixation point depending upon whether the disparity is "crossed" or "uncrossed" respectively). Vertical disparity in oculocentric localization provides no similar signal for stereoscopic depth since the two eyes are laterally, rather than vertically, separated in the head. However they can, and do, provide signals for equivalent compensatory changes in the relative magnification of the images seen by the two eyes of an object whose (asymmetric) position in space makes it significantly closer to one eye than to the other (OGLE, 1950).

The distinction between oculocentric and egocentric disparity is important in analyzing the one case in which physically it cannot validly be drawn: Imagine the visual field of one eye twisted through a small angle around its line of sight. To keep it simple, suppose that the visual field consists entirely of a single black vertical line without ends seen against a bright homogeneous background. (The arrangement, in fact, is not as difficult to manage as it may seem). The disparity produced by the twisting can be conceptualized either as a disparity in oculocentric localization, in which case the vertical line appears tilted (say with its top nearer and its bottom farther than at the midpoint upon which the two eyes are fixating), or as a disparity in egocentric localization. In the latter case it acts as a stimulus for a (cyclo) fusional movement, which should have the consequence of reducing the disparity to zero and the perceptual result that the line continues to be seen as vertical. Since either disparity evokes responses which increase in magnitude as an increasing function of the disparity, these alternatives are by no means mutually exclusive, and in fact the responses actually obtained in this situation are as if they were in part a result of the oculocentric disparity and in part a consequence of the egocentric disparity (OGLE and ELLERBROCK, 1946; OGLE, 1950; ELLERBROCK, 1954). Clearly, though the physical distinction between these two disparities is contrived in this case, the fact that the organism nonetheless responds precisely with this distinction is a powerful argument for its physiological importance.

Cyclofusional Movements

The experiments described in the preceding paragraph were carried out using subjective methods to measure the magnitude of cyclofusional movements. Typically, geared meridional size lenses were introduced before the two eyes to produce declination of the images and two small intermittently illuminated lights which the subject aligned to appear vertical, were used to measure "eye position". One inferred cyclofusional movements from the amount the points of light had to be tilted in order to appear vertical. The possibility that the organism possessed other methods of compensating for rotational disparities in egocentric localization besides cyclofusional movements cannot be excluded in this way, though at the time the measurements were made there seemed to be no obvious reason for entertaining it. However KERTESZ (1969) has now raised exactly this issue in an experimental effort to demonstrate cyclofusional movements objectively which yielded a clear negative result. KERTESZ' method of measuring eye position was capable of detecting cycloversions smaller than 1/2°, and in fact did detect movements of this kind about five times as large in response to rotating discs (as described originally by BRECHER, 1934). Observers responded to cyclo-egocentric localization disparities (since the stimulus line was horizontal no oculocentric disparity compensation was possible) with immediate unification even when the disparity was as large as $\pm 5.0°$. But no cyclofusional movement of the eyes was detected! These same observers could, however, make typical and quite unequivocal fusional movements in response to horizontal disparities in egocentric localization.

This baffling result raises more questions than it answers. If an observer were not equipped to make any fusional movement on the one hand, or alternatively, if he were unable to rotate his eyes about their lines of sight, then it might be reasonable to imagine that he would develop some other (central?) mechanism for nullifying cyclo disparities in egocentric localization. But KERTESZ' subjects could do both! What is the physiology of such a (central?) mechanism for nullifying egocentric disparity? What makes it necessary? How has it evolved and what is its survival value? Does it also function in the horizontal and vertical directions?

With regard to the last question it will be recalled that no good objective measurements of vertical fusional movements have ever been made, but the literature on horizontal fusional movements is replete with examples of objective indexes of eye position which failed to match (by as much as 1° or 2°) their stimulus, though unification persisted (see for example, WESTHEIMER and MITCHELL, 1956; TANI *et al.*, 1956; ALPERN, 1957a, among others). As the result of the close relation between disparity and movement demonstrated by RIGGS and NIEHL (1960) and RASHBASS and WESTHEIMER (1961a), we have tended to regard such examples as spurious results due to various artifacts in the indication of eye position (mainly the failure to separate translational shifts of the eye in the orbit from rotations). But KERTESZ' result reminds us that the matter is by no means settled, even in the horizontal meridian (ALPERN, 1957a). Neither RIGGS and NIEHL nor RASHBASS and WESTHEIMER have tested how carefully eye position matched stimulus disparity near the limits of the amplitude of fusional movements where all known examples (spurious and/or real) suggest that the mismatch must be greatest. Further evidence for a mismatch of eye position and target disparity after horizontal and vertical fusional movements comes from very recent experiments of FENDER and JULESZ (1967) whose subjects viewed random dot patterns in sterograms under binocular stabilized image conditions, thereby nullifying the effects of fusional movements. Once unification occurred, egocentric disparities larger than 2° (horizontally) or 20 min (vertically) could be introduced and tolerated without diplopia.

The Fender-Julesz results are suggestive rather than unequivocal, however, because the stabilized images were apparently continuously visible. We know from YARBUS (1967) that whenever perfect stabilization is achieved retinal images fade. Since FENDER and JULESZ (1967) make on mention of fading we must entertain the possibility that their stabilization was incomplete, and if their stabilization was incomplete we have no way of being certain how much of their measured disparity was compensated by fusional movements.

Disparity Detection

If egocentric disparity evokes fusional movements, horizontal oculocentric disparity stereoscopic depth, and vertical oculocentric disparity compensation for magnification differences in the two eyes, to what extent are these various stimulus disparities effective in evoking responses at cellular levels of the visual central nervous system? The answer to this question (BARLOW *et al.*, 1967; NIKARA *et al.*, 1968; PETTIGREW *et al.*, 1968; HUBEL and WIESEL, 1970) by microelectrode studies of single neurons in cat and monkey visual cortex has opened up an exciting new chapter in the neurophysiology of binocular vision.

The details are beyond the scope of this review particularly in view of the excellent summary by P. O. BISHOP in Volume VII/3 of this Handbook. Here we are concerned only with the cellular basis for fusional movements. The early work has shown abundant examples of "simple" cortical cells whose responses are exquisitely sensitive to binocular disparity. None of the investigators has made the distinction drawn here between egocentric and oculocentric disparity, but from the context it is clear that the disparity they are thinking of is an oculocentric one, though the best documentation that it is, in fact, oculocentric is sparse (Fig. 3 of BISHOP's chapter which is Fig. 6 of NIKARA *et al.*, 1968). Granting for the moment that these simple cortical cells are driven by disparities of oculocentric localization, how are we to imagine that the two eyes properly align themselves so that such a stimulus can prove effective? BISHOP's answer is that "...the eyes are directed towards a particular fixation point when the maximal number of binocular receptive fields are in correspondence at that point", which is satisfactory as far as it goes. But how do we know when this has been achieved, and what mechanisms detect the situation in which less than the maximum number are in correspondence (i. e., the disparity in egocentric localization), and consequently drive the fusional movements that continuously monitor not only the disparity but its rate of change, as RASHBASS and WESTHEIMER's (1961a) experiment suggests they must? We do not know. One possibility so far unrecognized is provided by a complex cortical cell (cat) described by PETTIGREW *et al.* (1968). This cell (Fig. 8, p. 403 of PETTIGREW *et al.*) had a very large receptive field (about 6°) and yet was sensitive to a very small disparity. Complex cells are best understood as being driven by a large number of simple cortical cells all with much smaller (about 1°) receptive fields (HUBEL and WIESEL, 1962). If that is the case here, then the simple cells which drive this complex cell are all sensitive to the same oculocentric disparity. Hence perhaps this cell is detecting egocentric disparity and functions to align the two eyes for optical correspondence by driving fusional movements. Even more intriguing is the possibility raised by KERTESZ' result, that this cell is the starting point for some "central" mechanism of compensation for egocentric disparity! If such a cell is an egocentric disparity detector, one expects "spatial summation" or "recruitment" in that a large number of identical disparities within the 6° receptive field would be much more effective in firing this cell than only a few. A test for this has yet to be made.

Other Varieties of Vergence Movements

Egocentric disparity is the most compelling, but by no means the only stimulus for vergence movements, particularly horizontal vergence movements. In fact some ten per cent of the population lack normal stereoscopic binocular vision, have no trace of the conventional kind of fusional movements (described above), but nevertheless show clear evidence for vergence movements in response to other stimuli. MADDOX (1886) provided the most useful distinction among the varieties of stimuli that can evoke horizontal vergence movements. These have been analyzed in some detail elsewhere (ALPERN, 1970), and I will only mention them here: (a) tonic (b) proximal (c) accommodative. Even this list is not exhaustive since, for example, changes in stimulus size can produce vergence changes (ALPERN, 1958) and undoubtedly there are other, more psychologically relevant, stimulus variables which can also cause the eyes to converge or diverge. MADDOX regarded the total vergence as the linear algebraic sum of the responses to each of these stimuli called "components".

Accommodation Vergence

Of all these "components" of horizontal vergence movements the most extensively analyzed is accommodation vergence, though theoretical treatments are neither as satisfying nor as exhaustive as are those for other kinds of eye movements. The movement is evoked by a change in accommodation stimulus. It is studied most easily by occluding one eye and changing the point of fixation from a distant to a near object aligned on the line of sight of the viewing eye, which, in a flagrant violation of Hering's Law of equal innervation (in fact, the only unequivocally documented instance), remains quite motionless (ALPERN and ELLEN, 1956 a and b). The occluded eye makes a smooth nasal vergence movement with time characteristics not obviously different from those of horizontal fusional movements (Fig. 2). The vexing problem as to whether such movements are relevant for responses to accommodation stimulus changes in binocular viewing is only partially answered in the affirmative from experiments on fixation disparity (OGLE, 1950; OGLE and MARTENS, 1957; OGLE *et al.*, 1967), because these experiments looked only at eye position in the steady state. A particular puzzle is the way accommodative vergence movements are nulled in

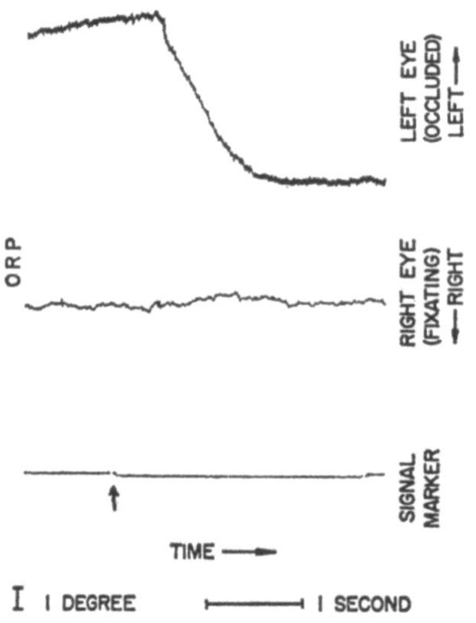

Fig. 2. Record of eye position with change in fixation from a far to a near object along the line of sight of the right eye. (The left eye is occluded.) The far object is a plumb line, the near target a thin horizontal thread. The right eye fixates the intersection of the two lines and at the signal (arrow) changes focus from the vertical to the horizontal line. The stimulus change in this case is 5 diopters. Note only the occluded eye moves. This violates Hering's Law (the only known example). Record of ALPERN and ELLEN (1956a)

binocular viewing when the stimulus to accommodation (and no doubt the accommodation response) is changed, but the egocentric disparity is not (ALPERN, 1957b). Evidently disparity and accommodation drive the same output channel and nullification must occur prior to the final common path. Where and how remain very much unanswered questions. Furthermore, if the output channels in fusional and accommodation vergences are identical, how does it happen that step inputs to the latter (Fig. 2) – but never to the former (Fig. 1) – can cause eye movements which are not in accord with Hering's Law?

The most reasonable interpretation of accommodation convergence is that a stimulus for accommodation evokes innervation to increase accommodation, and a linear relation exists between this innervation, the innervation to increase vergence, and the innervation to miosis (the narrowing of the pupil accompanying near viewing). The details are described elsewhere (ALPERN, 1970).

For those interested in individual differences, a useful measurement is the AC/A, i. e., the amount of accommodation vergence (AC) associated with a unit change in the accommodation response (A). It is sometimes inconvenient to measure accommodation response, in which case changes in accommodation stimulus will suffice, if care is taken to require exact focus on a target with fine detail. The response AC/A is a characteristic of an individual which remains remarkably uninfluenced by age, occupation, reading habits and so on. Drugs (such as atropine, phospholine iodide, DFP, eserine) which alter the accommodation control system at the ciliary body, and perhaps extraocular muscle surgery (which might interfere in a somewhat similar way with vergence control at a peripheral level), will change the AC/A in a straightforward way predicted according to the above theory. Certain other drugs (alcohol, COHEN and ALPERN, 1969; amphetamine and barbiturates, WESTHEIMER, 1963) apparently influence AC/A by selective effects on the central nervous system, since very mild doses produce unequivocal effects, while other aspects of peripheral control remain unaffected.

Unique as AC/A is for a given individual, there are large differences from one individual to the next. Although correlations with personality characteristics have not been studied, performances in a variety of industrial tasks have been sorted out according to AC/A: Low AC/A among good batters in baseball; high AC/A among good pitchers; high AC/A among good vacuum-tube assemblers; low AC/A among good transistor assemblers; camera assemblers and skilled tradesmen are best when AC/A is moderate and are more apt to do poorly if AC/A is either very high or very low; but the productivity of telephone typists is best if AC/A is high (DAVIS and JOBE, 1957).

"Nearness" Effects

Much less regular than the vergence changes evoked by accommodation changes are horizontal vergences evoked by perceived nearness and by changes in both perceived and retinal image size (ITTLESON and AMES, 1950; HOFSTETTER, 1950; ALPERN, 1958). Size changes produce vergence changes and vergence changes also produce size changes (HEINEMANN *et al.*, 1959), though the relative capacities of the various vergence "components" in this latter respect have never been systematically analyzed. Once more, individual differences are large and these phenomena are probably much more closely related to such psychological variables as past experience, motivation, cognitive processes and psychodynamics than are other aspects of the vergence oculomotor system.

Version Movements

Version movements by definition are conjugated. It is still an open question whether, as suggested by ALPERN and WOLTER (1956), the final common path for vergence movements is different from that used for versions. The best evidence for this suggestion (RASHBASS and WESTHEIMER, 1961b; ROBINSON, 1966) is of necessity quite indirect. However this may be, it seems quite unlikely that the two types of version movements, the saccades and the smooth pursuit, though they also are organized independently, use different final common paths. The best evidence – it comes from human extraocular muscle electromyography (BJÖRK, 1955; MOMOSSE, 1958; MILLER, 1958; TAMLER *et al.*, 1959a and b; BREININ, 1962) – is that these two modes of version eye movements differ in the same way, and for the same reasons, that two varieties of movements produced by ordinary striped muscles (ballistic and slow tension movements) differ (STETSON and MCDILL, 1923; HARTSON, 1939).

The present discussion is devoted only to primates (mostly man). EASTER (1971) presents a fascinating analysis of visually evoked versions (and vergences!) in fish.

Saccadic Eye Movements

One of the simplest of all eye movements is the sudden shift of gaze between two points equally distant from the observer. This is a saccade. Saccadic eye movements are extremely fast (WESTHEIMER, 1954a); the eyes can achieve a peak velocity of the order of 830°/sec near the middle of a large movement (HYDE, 1959). The movement is nearly perfectly conjugate in man (but see ROBINSON, 1964, for suggestion of slower nasal than temporal movement), if not in fish (EASTER, 1970), and remarkably stereotyped (WESTHEIMER, 1954a; ROBINSON, 1964). Its reaction time (about 200 msec) is, however, shortened by practice effects (SASLOW, 1967a; 1967b), and square-wave eye-tracking quickly becomes predictive (RASHBASS, 1961). At about 5 Hz, the eyes actually soon learn to lead the target by about 50 msec (DALLOS and JONES, 1963). Whether or not monkeys learn predictive tracking is uncertain. FUCHS (1967b) reports that they do not. The stimulus for saccadic eye movement is a retinal position error (RASHBASS, 1961), though there is a "dead zone" of about 15 min of arc in the very center of the fovea. The retina remains sensitive and vision persists during a saccade (YARBUS, 1967; UTTAL and SMITH, 1968), but the ability of an observer to detect or resolve a target (VOLKMANN, 1962; LATOUR, 1962, 1966) even with foveal vision (VOLKMANN *et al.*, 1968) is measurably reduced, as is the photopupil response (ZUBER *et al.*, 1966). Extraocular muscle electromyograms during saccadic eye movements (BJÖRK, 1955; MILLER, 1958; BREININ, 1958a and b; TAMLER *et al.*, 1959b) show high frequency bursts of activity in the agonist and complete inhibition of firing in the antagonist that last throughout the movement. There is no convincing evidence for active checking at termination, and ROBINSON (1964) suggests that deceleration is achieved by the very high viscosity of the orbital contents, including the muscles themselves. Mechanical changes in the orbit persist for about 250 msec after the eye has come to rest. A pulse of the full force of the muscle (about 150 gms) is called upon to produce each saccade. It is needed to achieve the incredibly high instantaneous velocity for a few milliseconds, not to hold the eye in a steady (deviated) position. Larger saccades last longer and so does the duration of application of this pulse of full reserve of muscle force (ROBINSON, 1964, 1968b). It is probable that these phenomena are causally related.

Saccades (and only saccades) are evoked by electrical excitation of the frontal eye fields of the awake monkey (ROBINSON and FUCHS, 1969), Though BIZZI, 1968, has evidence for activity in this area during smooth pursuit movements. The saccades evoked by cortical stimulation are essentially identical to spontaneous saccades. Nor are such movements very different from the quick return of the optokinetic nystagmus, the return eye movement following deviation produced by electrical stimulation of ampullary nerves (GOTO *et al.*, 1968), the quick position-error correction in eye-tracking of a moving target, and the rapid eye movements (REM) of sleep. The latter supposedly reveal fixation of different aspects of the visual "image" during dreams (DEMENT, 1955, 1964). Other kinds of eye movements also occur during REM sleep including one unique to this condition, FUCHS and RON (1968).

The retina apparently monitors position errors for the saccadic system with a discrete or semi-discrete, sampling process. Hence a position error briefly introduced and then eliminated within the reaction time of a saccade evokes nonetheless two saccades separated by a 200 msec reaction time, the first quite inappropriate at the time it was made, the second returning the eyes to the starting point (WESTHEIMER, 1954a). The concept of a sampled data model for the monitoring of eye-position errors (YOUNG and STARK, 1963; STARK, 1968) is only approximately applicable, because once a position error has been introduced, subsequent changes in both target velocity and position can influence the amplitude of the forthcoming saccade. The probability that they will do so decreases with increasing time between the initial sample and the final response (ROBINSON, 1965; WHEELESS *et al.*, 1966).

Smooth Pursuit Movements

Smooth pursuit movements are evoked by error in the matching of eye velocity and target velocity (RASHBASS, 1961). Their latent period is about 125 msec, considerably faster than that of saccades, but not so fast that in a typical smooth pursuit response to a target suddenly moving in the field the eye and the target can be initially perfectly matched both in velocity and position (WESTHEIMER, 1954b; RASHBASS, 1961). The position error is corrected by a saccade which in these circumstances occurs at a quite irregular (unpredictable) moment and with only imperfect success in eliminating the position error. The eye velocity at the end of the saccade will be a closer match to the target velocity than before, and if both position and velocity errors have been nulled, the eye will continue to follow the target. If not, further saccades may be required, though velocity correction is occasionally effected during the smooth pursuit movement as well. To study the smooth pursuit movement uncontaminated by saccades, RASHBASS (1961) designed a method of presenting a target in such a way that the position error was zero, at about the moment of onset of the smooth pursuit movement. The target was suddenly displaced in one direction and immediately began moving with a constant velocity in the opposite direction. If the size of the step (in degrees) is about 1/5 of the velocity (deg/sec), the target will recross its original position in 200 msec and the eye will make a pure, smooth pursuit response. Smooth pursuit movements succeed in correctly matching target velocities provided the latter are less than 20–30 deg/sec (WESTHEIMER, 1954b; ROBINSON, 1965), though the maximum velocity of the eye in smooth pursuit can on occasion be three to five times as large as these upper limits. The tracking limitation seems to be in the velocity detection system in the retina rather than in the final common path. Eye-tracking of a target that is oscillating at, say, 4 Hz is so poor the target is blurred; but fixation is quite exact for the same (now steady) target, and it continues to be seen sharply when the head is oscillating at 4 Hz (ROBINSON, 1968a). Smooth pursuit movements are evoked by moving targets and almost exclusively by moving targets (though they occur in REM sleep – FUCHS and RON, 1968 – and an occasional subject can learn to make them in the absence of a moving stimulus, WESTHEIMER and CONOVER, 1954).

Electromyographic records of the responses of the eye muscles during smooth pursuit movement show that both the agonist and antagonist are active. Apparently only a very small difference in muscle tension rotates the globe (MOMOSSE, 1957, 1958).

The smooth pursuit system appears to be driven by continuous monitoring of target velocity. In this way it differs from the saccadic system. The two movements are also differently affected by drugs such as barbiturates (RASHBASS, 1961) and by certain diseases such as multiple sclerosis (VON NOORDEN and PREZIOSI, 1966) which paralyze only the smooth pursuit system. Under such conditions eye-tracking of a sinewave oscillating target becomes a series of successive saccades (called barbiturate nystagmus).

Another way of differentiating the smooth pursuit from the saccadic control system is to change the "feedback loop". In simple terms this means to make the target viewing-system electrically or optically capable of being altered by the subject's eye position, as for example in stabilized image experiments. Ordinarily (closed loop) the eye movements act to reduce target position and velocity errors to zero. (Net feedback gain is 1.0). In stabilized image experiments the net feedback gain is 0. If sufficient external feedback is added, control systems and eye movements oscillate (FENDER and NYE, 1961). For the saccadic system, the net feedback gain must be at least 5.0, and the frequency of oscillation produced is 2.0 Hz, whereas smooth pursuit oscillates at 3.3 Hz but requires a gain of more than 8.0 to produce the oscillation (ROBINSON, 1965).

Reflex Movement

Changes in position and acceleration of the head are capable of exciting eye movements by the stimulation of receptors of the vestibular apparatus, as well as head and neck muscle proprioceptors. The excitation of eye movements by changes in head position is a useful clinical tool in diagnosis of supra nuclear lesions of the oculomotor control system. Thus there can be no doubt of the existence of the phenomenon in man, though careful analysis of the physiology in normal humans is a very neglected subject. Apparently both the otoliths of the vestibular apparatus (the macula of the saccula and utricle) and the stretch receptors of the muscles of the head and neck cooperate to produce the eye movement responses. Neither the muscle receptors nor the vestibular receptors are essential, but without either the eyes fail to respond to changes in head position. The influence on eye movements by gravitational excitation of the macula of the saccule and utricle (independent of the effects of head and neck muscle afferents) has been carefully analyzed by WOELLNER and GRAYBIEL (1959), and MILLER (1962) in normal man, and by MILLER and GRAYBIEL (1962) in labryinthine defective subjects. In normal man change in head position of 90° produces counter-rolling of about 7°. The effect is absent among bilateral labryinthine defectives.

The semicircular canals evoke eye-movement responses to acceleration of the head and body. Ordinarily these inputs are very transitory, but to study them in the laboratory (and the clinic) repetitive stimulation of the semicircular canals (hot or cold water in the ears, rotation in a Barany chair) is employed, and the result is a rhythmical beating motion of the eyes, a slow movement away from the direction of head acceleration and a rapid saccadic (GOTO *et al.*, 1968) return – so called vestibular nystagmus (MCCABE, 1965). The semicircular canals behave as an integrating accelerometer over a range of frequencies of head movement (0.017 to 17 Hz according to ROBINSON (1968 a, b). A second integration of signals from the canals occurs in the nervous system before these signals are transmitted to eye muscles. Three neurone arcs connect each semicircular canal to a different pair of yoked muscles (one for each eye) (SZENTAGOTHAI, 1950). The remarkable thing about this arrangement is that it lays down the basic pattern for Hering's Law in animals whose visual fields scarcely overlap.

The "Plant"

All of these varieties of eye-movement control have as end result the rotation of the globes of the two eyes within their respective orbits. There is a good deal of viscosity, inertia, and elasticity in both the passive (optic nerve, orbital fat, conjunctiva, TENON's capsule) and active (muscles and rotating globe) tissues concerned with eye movement which have recently come under experimental analysis (ROBINSON, 1964; CHILDRESS and JONES, 1967; THOMAS, 1967, 1969, to name but a few), stimulated no doubt by WESTHEIMER's (1954a) theoretical treatment of saccadic eye movements. The mechanics of these structures is still controversial and a summary at this time can only be regarded as tentative. In the material presented here I have closely followed ROBINSON (1968a, b). A slightly different view is held by THOMAS (1967, 1969).

Fig. 3 illustrates a scheme describing the mechanics of the globe and one antagonistic pair of extraocular muscles. The passive tissues of the orbit, the ligament of LOCKWOOD, Tenon's capsule, the conjunctiva, the orbital fat, the optic nerve and check ligaments represented by the springs and dashpots of the passive viscoelastic components (POVE) hold the globe of moment of inertia (J)

in place. Each muscle also has passive elements as well as an active portion composed of a contractile component subdivided into an active state tension generator (F_1, F_2) which displays a length tension relation (LTR) and an element with a force velocity relationship (FVR). The active portion also has a series elastic component. When the eyes look straight ahead both muscles exert a tonic force of about 14 grams. In deviation, the force in the agonist increases (up to 50 gm) and decreases in the antagonist until the difference just balances the restraining forces of the passive tissues. In a saccade, the sudden transitory build up of a pulse of active state tension which is needed to rotate the globe reaches its maximum (for a duration which increases as the amplitude of the saccade) and falls to the steady value in a way that has already been described. This is shown in Fig. 3 (a); F represents the isometric force of the muscles and M represents the eye movement. In the illustrated case the position error is not nulled by the initial movement and a second saccade is needed to bring the eye on to target. It occurs only a full saccade reaction time after completion of the first saccade. Fig. 3 (b) shows similar tracing of isometric force and eye movement in a smooth pursuit movement. Here the eye is initially accelerated by a rate of rise of force twice as large as that needed to maintain velocity in

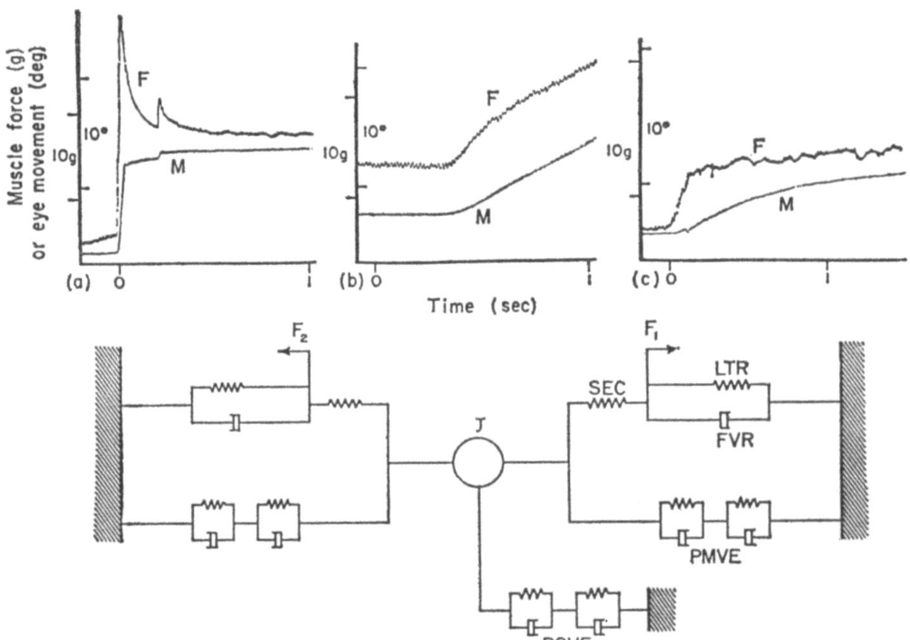

Fig. 3. The lower figure is a model of the oculomotor "plant". The eyeball with a moment of inertia J has attached to it two (horizontal) rectus muscles. The globe is held in the orbit by passive orbital viscoelastic elements (POVE). Each muscle also has passive viscoelastic elements (PMVE) and an active portion composed of a series elastic component (SEC) and a contractile component subdivided into an element with a force-velocity relationship (FVR) and an active state tension relationship (LTR). The upper sets of figures show the net isometric force (F) and the eye rotation (M) for the three kinds of large eye movements (a) saccades (b) smooth pursuit and (c) accommodation vergence. From Robinson (1968b)

the steady state. This extra force is used to overcome the viscoelastic properties of the "plant" (globe and eye muscles). In Fig. 3 (c) the isometric force and movement of the occluded eye in accommodative vergence are shown. The muscles apply a slightly lagged step-function of force in response to a step stimuls. There seems to be a very low gain "integrator" in the forward loop. This gain is so low that time constant of the movement is little – if at all – better than the 500 msec time constant of the plant alone.

Summary

Given two eyes in the same head with overlapping visual fields and single binocular vision the various kinds of large eye movements described above fulfill the following roles: The vergence system assures successive binocular alignment on targets at different distances through an exquisite organization pattern, one major feature of which is Hering's Law. The versions correct for errors in target position (through the saccadic system) and velocity (through the smooth pursuit system) for objects at the same distance from the observer. The vestibular ocular reflex system insures that the alignment is maintained with changes in position and velocity of the head.

Small eye movements of steady fixation, particularly the binocularly uncoordinated drifts, insure continuous visibility of our world (by discontinuous excitation of "on" center and "off" center cells?) though the functions of the fine tremor and microsaccades are uncertain. Images perfectly stabilized on the retina fade – though vague clouds of average luminance differences persist. Faded images are revitalized by spatial and temporal changes in the retinal image light distribution.

Acknowledgement. Assisted by grant EY-00197-12 from the National Eye Institute.

References

ADLER, F. H.: Physiology of the Eye. 4th Ed., pp. 351—548. St. Louis: Mosby 1965.

— FLIEGELMAN, M.: Influence of fixation on the visual acuity. Arch. Ophthal. **12**, 475—483 (1934).

ALPERN, M.: The position of the eyes during prism vergence. Arch. Ophthal. **57**, 345—353 (1957a).

— Does relative accommodation exist? (abstract). Amer. J. Ophthal. **43**, 464 (1957b).

— Vergence and accommodation. I. Can change in size induce vergence movements? Arch. Ophthal. **60**, 355—357 (1958).

— Muscular mechanisms. In: The Eye, 2nd Ed., vol. 3. pp. 1—252. DAVSON, H. (Ed.). New York: Academic Press 1970.

— ELLEN, P.: A quantitative analysis of the horizontal movements of the eyes in the experiment of Johannes Müller. I. Method and results. Amer. J. Ophthal. **42**, 289—296 (1956a).

— — A quantitative analysis of the horizontal movements of the eyes in the experiment of Johannes Müller. II. Effect of variation in target separation. Amer. J. Ophthal. **42**, 296—303 (1956b).

— WOLTER, J. R.: The relation of horizontal saccadic and vergence movements. Arch. Ophthal. **56**, 685—690 (1956).

BARLOW, H. B.: Eye movements during fixation. J. Physiol. (Lond.) **116**, 290—306 (1952).
— Slippage of contact lenses and other artefacts in relation to fading and regeneration of supposedly stable retinal images. Quart. J. exp. Psychol. **15**, 36—51 (1963).
— BLAKEMORE, C., PETTIGREW, J. D.: The neural mechanism of binocular depth discrimination. J. Physiol. (Lond.) **193**, 327—342 (1967).
— SPARROCK, J. M. B.: The role of afterimages in dark adaptation. Science **144**, 1309—1314 (1964).
BEELER, G. W., FENDER, D. H., NOBEL, P. S., EVANS, C. R.: Perception of pattern and colour in the stabilized retinal image. Nature (Lond.) **203**, 1200 (1964).
BENDER, M. B.: The Oculomotor System. New York: Harper & Row 1964.
BIZZI, E.: Discharge of frontal eye field neurons during saccadic and following eye movements in unanesthetized monkeys. Exp. Brain Res. **6**, 69—80 (1968).
BJÖRK, A.: The electromyogram of the extraocular muscles in optico-kinetic nystagmus and in reading. Acta Ophthal. (Kbh.) **33**, 437—454 (1955).
BRECHER, G. A.: Die optokinetische Auslösung von Augenrollung und rotatorischem Nystagmus. Pflügers. Arch. ges. Physiol. **234**, 13—28 (1934).
BREININ, G. M.: Analytic studies of the electromyogram of human extraocular muscle. Amer. J. Ophthal. **46**, 123—142 (1958a).
— Electromyography: a tool in ocular and neurologic diagnosis. III. Supranuclear mechanisms. Arch. Ophthal. **59**, 177—187 (1958b).
— The Electrophysiology of Extraocular Muscle. Toronto: University of Toronto Press 1962.
BRINDLEY, G. S.: Two new properties of foveal after-images and a photochemical hypothesis to explain them. J. Physiol. (Lond.) **164**, 168—179 (1962).
CAMPBELL, F. W., ROBSON, J. G.: A fresh approach to stabilized retinal images. J. Physiol. (Lond.) **158**, 11 (1961).
CHILDRESS, D. S., JONES, R. W.: Mechanics of horizontal movement of the human eye. J. Physiol. (Lond.) **188**, 273—284 (1967).
COHEN, M. M., ALPERN, M.: Vergence and Accommodation. VI. The influence of ethanol on the AC/A ratio. Arch. Ophthal. **81**, 518—525 (1969).
CORNSWEET, T. N.: Determination of the stimuli for involuntary drifts and saccadic eye movements. J. opt. Soc. Amer. **46**, 987—993 (1956).
CUNITZ, R. J., STEINMAN, R. M.: Comparison of saccadic eye movements during fixation and reading. Vision Res. **9**, 683—693 (1969).
DALLOS, P. J., JONES, R. W.: Learning behavior of the eye fixation control system. IEEE Trans. Auto. Control. AC-8, 218—227 (1963).
DANIEL, P. M., WHITTERIDGE, D.: The representation of the visual field on the cerebral cortex in monkeys. J. Physiol. (Lond.) **159**, 203—221 (1961).
DAVIS, C. J., JOBE, F. W.: Further studies on the A.C.A. ratio as measured on the orthorater. Amer. J. Optom. **34**, 16—25 (1957).
DEMENT, W.: Dream recall and eye movements during sleep in schizophrenics and normals. J. nerv. and ment. Dis. **122**, 263—269 (1955).
— Eye Movements during Sleep. In: The Oculomotor System. BENDER, M. B. (Ed.), pp. 366—416. New York: Harper & Row 1964.
DITCHBURN, R. W.: Eye-movements in relation to retinal action. Optica Acta **1**, 171—176 (1955).
— FENDER, D. H., MAYNE, S.: Vision with controlled movements of the retinal image. J. Physiol. (Lond.) **145**, 98—107 (1959).
— FOLEY-FISHER, J. A.: Assembled data in eye movements. Optica Acta **14**, 113—118 (1967).
— GINSBORG, B. L.: Vision with a stabilized retinal image. Nature (Lond.) **170**, 36—37 (1952).
EASTER, S. S. TR.: Spontaneous eye movements in restrained goldfish. Vision Res. **11**, 333—342 (1971).
ELLERBROCK, V. J.: Experimental investigation of vertical fusional movements, Amer. J. Optom. **26**, 327—337 (1949a).
— Experimental investigation of vertical fusional movements. Amer. J. Optom. **26**, 388—399 (1949b).

Ellerbrock, V. J.: The effect of aniseikonia on the amplitude of vertical divergence. Amer. J. Optom. **29**, 403—415 (1952).

— Inducement of cyclofusional movements. Amer. J. Optom. **31**, 553—566 (1954).

Fender, D., Julesz, B.: Extension of Panum's fusional area in binocularly stabilized vision. J. opt. Soc. Amer. **57**, 819—830 (1967).

— Nye, P. W.: An investigation of the mechanisms of eye movements control. Kybernetik **1**, 81—88 (1961).

Fiorentini, A., Ercoles, A. M.: Vision with stabilized images and intermittent illumination. Atti Fond. G. Ronchi **15**, 618—633 (1960).

Fuchs, A. F.: Saccadic and smooth pursuit eye movements in the monkey. J. Physiol. (Lond.) **191**, 609—631 (1967a).

— Periodic eye tracking in the monkey. J. Physiol. (Lond.) **193**, 161—171 (1967b).

— Ron, S.: An analysis of rapid eye movements of sleep in the monkey. Electroenceph. clin. Neurophysiol. **25**, 244—251 (1968).

Goto, K., Tokumasu, K., Cohen, B.: Return eye movements, saccadic movements, and the quick phase of nystagmus. Acta oto-laryng. **65**, 426—440 (1968).

Hartson, L. D.: Contrasting approaches to the analysis of skilled movements. J. gen. Psychol. **20**, 263—293 (1939).

Heinemann, E. G., Tulving, E., Nachmias, J.: The effect of oculo-motor adjustments on apparent size. Amer. J. Psychol. **72**, 32—45 (1959).

Hering, E.: Die Lehre vom binocularen Sehen, S. 92—102. Leipzig: W. Engelmann 1868.

Higgins, G. G., Stultz, K. F.: Frequency and amplitude of ocular tremor. J. opt. Soc. Amer. **43**, 1136—1140 (1953).

Hofmann, F. B., Bielschowsky, A.: Über die willkür entzogenen Fusionsbewegungen der Augen. Pflügers Arch. ges. Physiol. **80**, 1—40 (1900).

Hofstetter, H. W.: Accommodation, convergence, and their relation to apparent distance: a criticism. J. Psychol. **30**, 393—394 (1950).

Hubel, D. H., Wiesel, T. N.: Receptive fields, binocular interaction and functional architecture in the cat's visual cortex. J. Physiol. (Lond.) **160**, 106—154 (1962).

— — Cells sensitive to binocular depth in area 18 of the macaque monkey cortex. Nature (Lond.) **225**, 41—42 (1970).

Hyde, J. E.: Some characteristics of voluntary human ocular movements in the horizontal plane. Amer. J. Ophthal. **48**, 85—94 (1959).

Ittleson, W. H., Ames, A., Jr.: Accommodation, convergence, and their relation to apparent distance. J. Psychol. **30**, 43—62 (1950).

Jones, L. A., Higgins, G. C.: Photographic granularity and graininess. III. Some characteristics of the visual system of importance in evaluation of graininess and granularity. J. opt. Soc. Amer. **37**, 217—263 (1947).

— — Photographic granularity and graininess. IV. Visual acuity thresholds; dynamic versus static assumptions. J. opt. Soc. Amer. **38**, 398—405 (1948).

Keesey, U. T.: Effects of involuntary eye movements on visual acuity. J. opt. Soc. Amer. **50**, 769—774 (1960).

— Visibility of a stabilized target as a function of frequency and amplitude of luminance variation. J. opt. Soc. Amer. **59**, 604—610 (1969).

Kertesz, A. E.: Analysis and measurement of human torsional eye movements. Ph. D. thesis, Northwestern Univ., June, 1969.

Krauskopf, J.: Experiments with colored stabilized images. In: The physiological basis for form discrimination. (Brown University Symposium, Providence, R. I.) 114—116 (1964).

— Cornsweet, T. N., Riggs, L. A.: Analysis of eye movements during monocular and binocular fixation. J. opt. Soc. Amer. **50**, 572—578 (1960).

Latour, P. L.: Visual threshold during eye movements. Vision Res. **2**, 261—262 (1962).

— Cortical control of eye movements. Thesis, Institute for Perception, RVO-TNO, Soesterberg: (1966).

Lord, M. P., Wright, W. D.: Eye movements during monocular fixation. Nature (Lond.) **162**, 25—26 (1948).

Maddox, E. E.: Investigations in the relation between convergence and accommodation of the eyes. J. Anat. **20**, 475—508; 565—584 (1886).

MARSHALL, W. H., TALBOT, S. A.: Recent evidence for neural mechanisms in vision leading to a general theory of sensory acuity. Biol. Symp. **7**, 117—164 (1942).

MARX, E., TRENDELENBURG, W.: Über die Genauigkeit der Einstellung des Auges beim Fixieren. Z. Psychol. **45**, 88—102 (1911).

MCCABE, B. F.: The quick component of nystagmus. Laryngoscope **75**, 1619—1641 (1965).

MILLER, E. F., 2d: Counterrolling of the human eyes produced by head tilt with respect to gravity. Acta oto-laryng. **54**, 479—501 (1962).

— GRAYBIEL, A.: A comparison of ocular counterrolling movements between normal persons and deaf subjects with bilateral labyrinthine defects. U. S. Nav. Sch. Aviat. Med. Res. Rep. **68**, 1—9 (1962).

MILLER, J. E.: Electromyographic pattern of saccadic eye movements. Amer. J. Ophthal. **46**, 183—186 (1958).

MOMOSSE, H.: Application of an integrator in the analysis of ocular muscle movements by electromyography. Behavior of the horizontal and vertical muscles in monocular movements. Acta Soc. ophthal. jap. **61**, 1570—1593 (1957).

— Studies on the action of the extraocular muscles in monocular movements by means of quantification of integrated EMG. Jap. J. Ophthal. **2**, 108—122 (1958).

NACHMIAS, J.: Two-dimensional motion of the retinal image during monocular fixation. J. opt. Soc. Amer. **49**, 901—908 (1959).

— Determiners of the drift of the eye during monocular fixation. J. opt. Soc. Amer. **51**, 761—766 (1961).

NIKARA, T., BISHOP, P. O., PETTIGREW, J. D.: Analysis of retinal correspondence by studying receptive fields of binocular single units in cat striate cortex. Exp. Brain Res. **6**, 353—372 (1968).

OGLE, K. N.: Researches in Binocular Vision. Philadelphia: Saunders 1950.

— ELLERBROCK, V. J.: Cyclofusional movements. Arch. Ophthal. **36**, 700—735 (1946).

— MARTENS, T. G.: On the accommodative convergence and the proximal convergence. Arch. Ophthal. **57**, 702—715 (1957).

— — DYER, J. A.: Oculomotor Imbalance in Binocular Vision and Fixation Disparity. Philadelphia: Lea and Febiger 1967.

PETTIGREW, J. D., NIKARA, T., BISHOP, P. O.: Binocular interaction on single units in cat striate cortex: simultaneous stimulation by single moving slit with receptive fields in correspondence. Exp. Brain Res. **6**, 391—410 (1968).

PRITCHARD, R. M.: Physiological Nystagmus and Vision. In: The Oculomotor System. BENDER, M. B. (Ed.), pp. 321—331. New York: Harper & Row 1964.

— HERON, W., HEBB, D. O.: Visual perception approached by the method of stabilized images. Canad. J. Psychol. **14**, 67—77 (1960).

PROSKURIAKOVA, N. G., SHAKHNOVICH, A. R.: Quantitative characteristics of fixational micromovements of the eye. Biofizika **13**, 117—126 (1968).

RASHBASS, C.: The relationship between saccadic and smooth tracking eye movements. J. Physiol. (Lond.) **159**, 326—338 (1961).

— WESTHEIMER, G.: Disjunctive eye movements. J. Physiol. (Lond.) **159**, 339—360 (1961 a).

— — Independence of conjugate and disjunctive eye movements. J. Physiol. (Lond.) **159**, 361—364 (1961 b).

RATLIFF, F.: The role of physiological nystagmus in monocular acuity. J. exp. Psychol. **43**, 163—172 (1952).

— Stationary retinal image requiring no attachments to the eye. J. opt. Soc. Amer. **48**, 274—275 (1958).

— RIGGS, L. A.: Involuntary motions of the eye during monocular fixation. J. exp. Psychol. **40**, 687—701 (1950).

RIGGS, L. A., NIEHL, E. W.: Eye movements recorded during convergence and divergence. J. opt. Soc. Amer. **50**, 913—920 (1960).

— RATLIFF, F., CORNSWEET, J. C., CORNSWEET, T. N.: The disappearance of steadily fixated visual test objects. J. opt. Soc. Amer. **43**, 495—501 (1953).

— SCHICK, A. M. L.: Accuracy of retinal image stabilization achieved with a plane mirror on a tightly fitting contact lens. Vision Res. **8**, 159—169 (1968).

ROBINSON, D. A.: The mechanics of human saccadic eye movement. J. Physiol. (Lond.) **174**, 245—264 (1964).
— The mechanics of human smooth pursuit eye movement. J. Physiol. (Lond.) **180**, 569—591 (1965).
— The mechanics of human vergence eye movements. J. Pediat. Ophthal. **3**, 31—37 (1966).
— The oculomotor control system: a review. Proc. Inst. elec. electron. Engrs. **56**, 1032—1049 (1968a).
— Eye movement control in primates. Science **161**, 1219—1224 (1968b).
— FUCHS, A. F.: Eye movements evoked by stimulation of frontal eye fields. J. Neurophysiol. **32**, 637—648 (1969).
RUSHTON, W. A. H., BAKER, H. D.: Effect of a very bright flash on cone vision and cone pigments in man. Nature (Lond.) **200**, 421—423 (1963).
SASLOW, M. G.: Effects of components of displacement-step stimuli upon latency for saccadic eye movements. J. opt. Soc. Amer. **57**, 1024—1029 (1967a).
— Latency for saccadic eye movement. J. opt. Soc. Amer. **57**, 1030—1033 (1967b).
SHURCLIFF, W. A.: New visual phenomenon: The greenish-yellow blotch. J. opt. Soc. Amer. **49**, 1041—1048 (1959).
STARK, L. S.: Neurological Control Systems; Studies in Bioengineering. New York: Plenum Press 1968.
ST. CYR, G. J., FENDER, D. H.: The interplay of drifts and flicks in binocular fixation. Vision Res. **9**, 245—265 (1969).
STEINMAN, R. M.: Effect of target size, luminance, color on monocular fixation. J. opt. Soc. Amer. **55**, 1158—1165 (1965).
— CUNITZ, R. J., TIMBERLAKE, G. T., HERMAN, M.: Voluntary control of microsaccades during maintained monocular fixation. Science **155**, 1577—1579 (1967).
— SKAVENSKI, A. A., SANSBURY, R. V.: Voluntary control of smooth pursuit velocity. Vision Res. **9**, 1167—1171 (1969).
STETSON, R. H., MCDILL, J. A.: Mechanism of the different types of movement with a preliminary report of experimental data. Psychol. Monogr. **32**, No. 3, 18—40 (1923).
SZENTÁGOTHAI, J.: The elementary vestibulo-ocular reflex arc. J. Neurophysiol. **13**, 395—407 (1950).
TAMLER, E., MARG, E., JAMPOLSKY, A.: Electromyographic study of coactivity of human extraocular muscles in following movements. Arch. Ophthal. **61**, 270—273 (1959).
— — NAWRATZKI, I.: Electromyography of human saccadic eye movements. Arch. Ophthal. **62**, 657—661 (1959).
TANI, G. T., OGLE, K. N., WEAVER, R. W., MARTENS, T. G.: On the precise objective determination of eye movements. Arch. Ophthal. **55**, 174—185 (1956).
THOMAS, J. G.: The torque-angle transfer function of the human eye. Kybernetik **3**, 254—263 (1967).
— The dynamics of small saccadic eye movements. J. Physiol. (Lond.) **200**, 109—127 (1969).
UTTAL, W. R., SMITH, P.: Recognition of alphabetic characters during voluntary eye movements. Perc. Psychophys. **3**, 257—264 (1968).
VOLKMANN, F. C.: Vision during voluntary saccadic eye movements. J. opt. Soc. Amer. **52**, 571—578 (1962).
— SCHICK, A. M. L., RIGGS, L. A.: Time course of visual inhibition during voluntary saccades. J. opt. Soc. Amer. **58**, 562—569 (1968).
VON NOORDEN, G. K., PREZIOSI, T. J.: Eye movement recordings in neurological disorders. Arch. Ophthal. **76**, 162—171 (1966).
WALLS, G. L.: The evolutionary history of eye movements. Vision Res. **2**, 69—80 (1962).
WEST, D. C.: Brightness discrimination with a stabilized retinal image. Vision Res. **7**, 949—974 (1967).
— BOYCE, P. R.: The effect of flicker on eye movements. Vision Res. 8, 171—192 (1968).
WESTHEIMER, G.: Mechanism of saccadic eye movements. Arch. Ophthal. **52**, 710—724 (1954a).
— Eye movement responses to horizontally moving visual stimulus. Arch. Ophthal. **52**, 932—941 (1954b).

WESTHEIMER, G.: Amphetamine, barbiturates, and accommodation-convergence. Arch. Ophthal. **70**, 830—836 (1963).
— CONOVER, D. W.: Smooth eye movements in the absence of a moving visual stimulus. J. exp. Psychol. **47**, 283—284 (1954).
— MITCHELL, A. M.: Eye movement responses to convergence stimuli. Arch. Ophthal. **55**, 848—856 (1956).
WEYMOUTH, F. W., ANDERSEN, E. E., AVERILL, H. L.: Retinal mean local sign; a new view of the relation of the retinal mosaic to visual perception. Amer. J. Physiol. **63**, 410—411 (1923).
WHEELESS, L. L., JR., BOYNTON, R. M., COHEN, G. H.: Eye-movement responses to step and pulse-step stimuli. J. opt. Soc. Amer. **56**, 956—960 (1966).
WOELLNER, R. C., GRAYBIEL, A.: Counterrolling of the eyes and its dependence on the magnitude of gravitational or inertial forces acting laterally on the body. J. appl. Physiol. **14**, 632—634 (1959).
YARBUS, A. L.: Motion of the eye on interchanging fixation points at rest in space. Biophysics **2**, 679—683. (Translated from Biofizika **2**, 698—702) (1957a).
— The perception of an image fixed with respect to the retina. Biophysics **2**, 683—690. (Translated from Biofizika **2**, 703—712) (1957b).
— Eye Movements and Vision. New York: Plenum Press 1967.
YOSHIDA, T., WATANABE, A.: Analysis of interaction between accommodation and vergence feedback control systems of human eyes. Bull. N.H.K. Broadcasting Sci. Res. Lab. **3**, 72—80 (1969).
YOUNG, L. R., STARK, L.: Variable feedback experiments testing a sampled data model for eye tracking movements. IEEE Trans. Human Fact Electronics **HFE-4**, 38—51 (1963).
ZUBER, B. L.: Control of Vergence Eye Movements. (In press.) 1970.
— STARK, L.: Dynamical characteristics of the fusional vergence eye-movement system. IEEE Trans. Sys. Sci. Cyber. **SSC-4**, 72—79 (1968).
— — COOK, G.: Microsaccades and the velocity-amplitude relationship for saccadic eye movements. Science **150**, 1459—1460 (1965).
— — LORBER, M.: Saccadic suppression of the pupillary light reflex. Exp. Neurol. **14**, 351—370 (1966).

Chapter 13

Eye Movements and Perceived Visual Direction

By

LEONARD MATIN, New York, New York (USA)

With 19 Figures

Contents

I. Introduction

The implicit assumption that visual perception is not susceptible to influences from extraretinal sources[1] has held extremely well in the areas of color vision, contour perception, and intensity discrimination. It has permitted the development of theoretical models of considerable generality for treatment of psychophysical phenomena in these areas that are based essentially on reasonable inferences from present knowledge regarding the neurophysiology, photochemistry, and neuroanatomy of the primary visual projection system. As will be indicated below, where this assumption can be reasonably made in the area of space perception some progress has taken place in a search for physiologically-based theoretical mechanisms for treatment of psychophysical data.

On the other hand, many of the most significant phenomena in space perception suggest a relation between visual perception and retinal stimulation that is susceptible to inputs from sources other than light to the retina, and here there is as yet relatively little physiological information to help with the main problems. Perhaps the clearest simple example of such susceptibility is the visual perception of the vertical, where turning an observer's head and body from an upright position to the horizontal in a frontal plane in complete darkness results in an offset of perceived from physical vertical by no more than 10°–15° (cf., AUBERT, 1861; MÜLLER, 1916; WITKIN and ASCH, 1948; BAUERMEISTER, 1964). Allowing a liberal 10° for uncompensated ocular torsion (cf. WOELLNER and GRAYBIEL, 1958; MILLER, 1962; SCHONE, 1962)[2] leaves a rotation of at least 65° between the orientation of a retinal stimulus and its perceived orientation in a frontal plane consequent to head and body turning. At one time or another it has been suggested that influences on visually perceived orientation, motion, direction, position, size or distance – as well as analogous spatial perceptions regarding the body or parts of the body – derive from afferent signals (from extraocular, neck, or trunk musculature, the intrinsic eye muscles, or the vestibular system), or from signals paralleling those which control the relevant muscles.

Closely intertwined with questions of extraretinal influence on visual space perception are the converse questions regarding the influence of visual stimulation on nonvisual perceptions of the body. In addition problems regarding intermodal discrimination (e.g., perception of the relative spatial locations of a visually presented target and an auditorily presented target), and the influence of visual stimulation on control of bodily movement (e.g., manually pointing to a visually presented target) point us toward questions regarding the genesis and nature of relations between the spatial metrics involved in the different avenues by which communication with the environment is carried out.

Limitations of space prevent a comprehensive treatment of all of these problems. Instead, this chapter will center on a treatment of some aspects of visual

[1] The terms extraretinal source, signal or influence are intended to refer to any channel in which information is not derived from stimulation of the retina by light.

[2] This is a "worse case" calculation; it is not intended to imply that visually perceived orientation does not involve compensation for ocular torsion. If torsion does not occur or is compensated the disparity between orientation of the retinal stimulus and its perceived orientation consequent to head turning alone would be even greater.

discriminations of spatial relations in the frontal plane. Even here the treatment will not be comprehensive, but rather the focus will be on the relation between perceived visual direction and stimulated retinal locus and on some of the ways in which this relation may be modified.

It will be useful to consider first some material regarding local sign in relation to discriminations that are not susceptible to extraretinal influences, at least to a first approximation.

II. Local Signs — Some Basic Considerations

A. Mean Retinal Local Sign

Perhaps the most elementary fact of visual space perception is that the spatial order of stimulus points in the environment remains correctly preserved in perception. Around this central fact has developed the general viewpoint that the visual perception of direction is mediated in the visual neurosensory pathway by a system of local signs that topographically maps locations of retinal stimuli into values of perceived direction. In essence this viewpoint assumes that a foveally fixated point is perceived as lying in what may be called the principal visual direction; an object whose image strikes any other retinal point is then perceived at a distance to the left, right, above, or below this principal direction in accordance with the retinal signal, i.e., the direction and distance values of the stimulated retinal point relative to the fovea (HERING, 1879; LOTZE, 1886). Quite apart from any considerations regarding the neuroanatomical, genetic or developmental basis of such a mapping or its modifiability we shall refer to the perceived visual direction associated with stimulation of a particular retinal point under any particular set of conditions as its local sign.

HERING's (1879) original suggestion regarding local signs attached the spatial quality to the single photoreceptor. However, on this basis alone sensitivity to position could not be finer than a visual angle corresponding to the separation between two adjacent receptors. Since discrimination of vernier offset of two vertical straight lines (Fig. 1a) yields thresholds as small as 1″ to 2″ of arc in the central fovea (AVERILL and WEYMOUTH, 1925; BERRY, 1948; BERRY, RIGGS, and DUNCAN, 1950) – a dimension that is less than 1/10 the width of a single foveal cone – some further theoretical developments were called for. It was thus suggested that the vernier discrimination is based on the ability of subjects to detect a difference in the mean retinal positional local sign between the two lines[3] (HERING, 1899; ANDERSEN and WEYMOUTH, 1923; WEYMOUTH, ANDERSEN, and AVERILL,

[3] HERING's (1899) suggestion regarding a mean local sign basis for vernier acuity presumed a regularity of the mosaic of cones and stability of the retinal image which later work showed did not hold. Nevertheless, the assumption that the local signs associated with particular single receptors can "interact" in determining the perceived location of a stimulus is an important precursor to WEYMOUTH's and to MARSHALL and TALBOT's (1942) later mean local sign "scanning" theory of vernier acuity as well as the theoretical suggestions described below. It is worth emphasizing also that these earlier theories assume that the discrimination underlying the report in the vernier task is one of position. WALLS (1943) has taken a similar point of view: "one does not discriminate the gap or offset between the ends of the line, but the difference in *spatial locations* of the lines" (1943, p. 497).

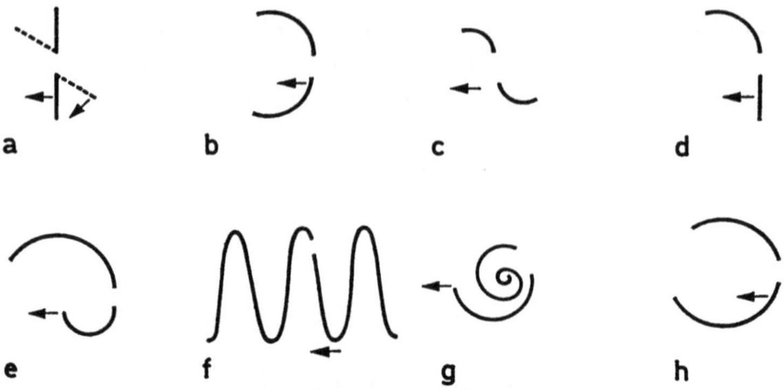

Fig. 1. Some target patterns in which the subject is required to report on alignment of two lines. The arrow in each pattern indicates the dimension along which the experimenter varies the location of the test line during psychophysical experimentation. In (*a*) the solid lines and dashed lines form two separate vernier target patterns. Only one is presented at a time in a given experimental trial; they have been superimposed here for comparison by the reader only (see text). In *a*, *b*, *c*, *d*, and *e* a smooth continuous line can be formed by "filling the gap" with a straight line when the test line is located appropriately. In *h* only a curved line of uniform curvature in the gap will yield a smooth continuous line; in *f* and *g* only a curved line with variable curvature will do so

1923; AVERILL and WEYMOUTH, 1925). This concept assumes that the subject can average over the length of each line the local sign from each cone stimulated at a given moment, and can further average over time the signals from different receptor arrays successively stimulated by the stimulus pattern as a result of the continuous occurrence of involuntary eye movements.

This view of local signs is supported by the fact that vernier acuity improves with increase in line length (AVERILL and WEYMOUTH, 1925; FENDER and NYE, 1962) and increasing exposure duration (AVERILL and WEYMOUTH, 1925; BAKER, 1949; KEESEY, 1960) (Fig. 2). Further, during attempts at steady fixation the median horizontal excursion of the eye in a given time interval grows linearly with interval duration up to at least 1 second, at which point it is about 3′ of arc (RIGGS, ARMINGTON, and RATLIFF, 1954) (Fig. 3). This is roughly six cone diameters, and thus considerable opportunity for temporal averaging over different arrays is possible.

The vernier task is not unique among monocular spatial discriminations in its high precision. For example, thresholds as low as 7″ for the discrimination of width of two narrow rectangles have been reported (VOLKMANN, 1863); [4,5] in addition

[4] For sufficiently narrow rectangles it is possible that subjects may be making the discrimination on the basis of differences in apparent brightness since stimulus area and luminance have similar influences on apparent brightness.

[5] VOLKMANN (1863, quoted in HELMHOLTZ, 1866) has reported that the average error for discriminating differences in distances between pairs of narrowly spaced parallel vertical lines is proportional to the standard distance over a range from 0.7° to 16.7° $\left(\text{constant of proportionality was between } \frac{1}{80} \text{ and } \frac{1}{100}\right)$; for smaller standard distances (between 2′ and 14′) the average error approaches an asymptote of about 4″. VENIAR (1948) also finds Weber's law to hold for the discrimination of large squares. No information appears to be available on the influence of exposure duration on width discrimination.

when a subject is required to discriminate whether two lines are parallel or not (Fig. 4a) values of Θ (Fig. 4b) as small as 0.1–0.2° have been reported for thresholds of relative tilt (SULZER, 1954; ROCHLIN, 1955; ANDREWS, 1967a, b). These reduce to values of differential retinal offset ($W_1 - W_2$, Fig. 4b) as small as 4.5″ (calculated

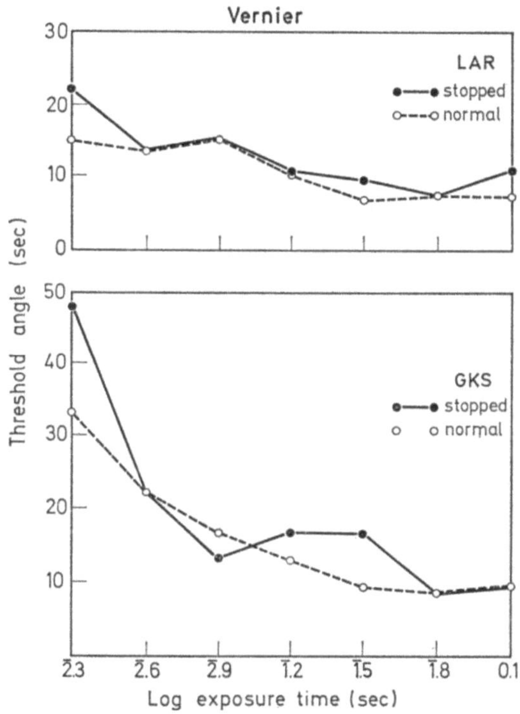

Fig. 2. Threshold curves for vernier discrimination as a function of log exposure time under normal viewing and viewing with a stabilized image for two subjects. (From KEESEY, 1960)

from ANDREWS' 1967b data) and 7″ (calculated from the data of SULZER, 1954 and ROCHLIN, 1955)[6]. Decreased thresholds for the discrimination of parallelness result from increased exposure duration (ANDREWS, 1967b) and decreased interline separation (SULZER, 1954; ROCHLIN, 1955; ANDREWS, 1967b) as for the vernier task. Increased line length results in a U-shaped function for threshold differential retinal offsets ($W_1 - W_2$) for parallelness (Fig. 5), which is the reverse of the vernier

[6] It is worth noting that the stimulus pattern employed for the discrimination of parallelness allows the subject to base his response on a discrimination of length. Thus, for example in the pattern : : the subject may report that the vertical line connecting the two righthand points is tilted counterclockwise relative to the line connecting the two lefthand points when he perceives the horizontal distance between the upper endpoints as smaller than the horizontal distance between the lower endpoints. Similarly, every length discrimination for the horizontal distances with such a pattern could be based on a relative orientation discrimination between the verticals. The point-line and three-point measures of orientation discrimination and partition measurement of length discrimination do not contain this ambiguity.

situation for lines longer than 8′.[7] A reasonable interpretation leaves these results susceptible to a treatment in terms of mean retinal local signs:

The vernier threshold increases approximately linearly with retinal eccentricity of the stimulus (WEYMOUTH, 1958). The major portion of the critical detail for discrimination of vernier offset is in the neighborhood of the gap. For a foveally centered vernier pattern increase

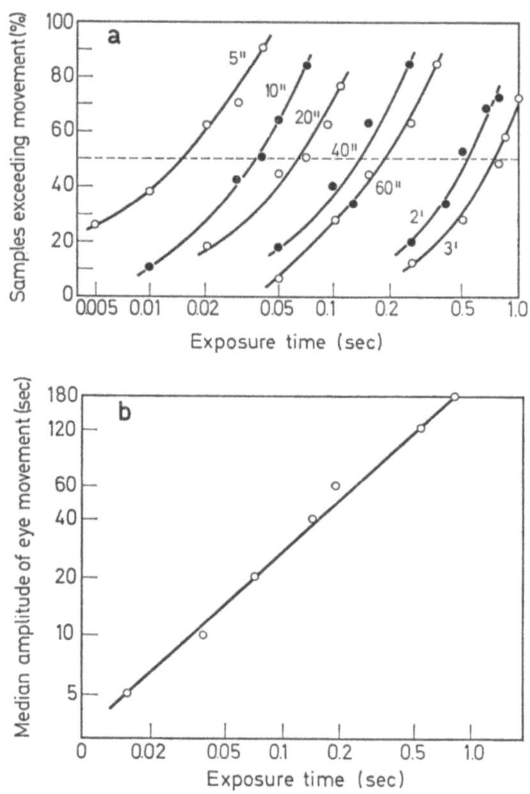

Fig. 3. a) Percentage of eye movement records showing given amounts of motion as a function of the length of the record during attempts at steady fixation. Each experimental point is the result of measuring 50 sample eye-movement records having one particular duration. b) The median extent of motion of the retinal image as a function of exposure time. Medians computed from data in a). (From RIGGS, ARMINGTON, and RATLIFF, 1954)

in line length leaves the critical detail in the same retinal region — the central fovea — while variability in perceived *angle* of orientation of the two lines decreases. Since variability of perceived orientation of the target lines would be expected to contribute to the variance of vernier discrimination (see below), it would also be expected that the discrimination would improve with line length. On the other hand, since the major portion of the critical detail for the discrimination of parallelness lies at the ends of the lines and increase in line length brings these ends into more eccentric retinal regions where offset discrimination is poorer, the threshold differential retinal offset for parallelness increases with line length.

[7] Plotted in a different way the same data (ANDREWS, 1967b) shows a monotonic decrease in threshold Θ with increase in line length. This agrees with previous reports (SULZER, 1954; ROCHLIN, 1955).

However, although the concept of a mean local sign for position appears reasonable there are compelling reasons for requiring some further development.

B. Difficulties with the Traditional Version of Mean Retinal Local Sign

Although vernier acuity improves with increased stimulus duration, no differences are obtained between acuities measured under normal and stabilized viewing conditions for stimulus durations up to at least 1.28 seconds[8] (KEESEY, 1960; see Fig. 2), indicating that the improvement consequent on increased exposure duration is *not* due to the fact that from moment to moment *different* receptor arrays look at the image. This result does not comment directly on the assumption of averaging over time or over space, since an average may still be taken, whether over the same spatial array from moment to moment (stabilized viewing) or over different arrays (normal viewing). It is thus not appropriate to conclude from this result either that temporal factors are of lesser importance than spatial ones or that averaging of positional local signs is not involved in the vernier discrimination. The result does however establish that "scanning", which is a central feature of dynamic theories (ANDERSEN and WEYMOUTH, 1923; WEYMOUTH, ANDERSEN, and AVERILL, 1923; AVERILL and WEYMOUTH, 1925; MARSHALL and TALBOT, 1942), is not required for maximizing acuity in the interval from stimulus onset until disappearance sets in.

FENDER and NYE (1962) report no difference in the ratio of magnitudes of horizontal to vertical eye movements between conditions in which vertically and horizontally oriented stabilized vernier targets are being set to alignment. This result adds further evidence against "scanning" theories of acuity by indicating that meridional variations in involuntary eye movements are not produced by variations in line orientation. The result does not comment directly on the converse relation — the influence of meridional variations in eye movements on meridional variations in acuity. In line with these results showing that ocular scanning is not required for localization are GILBERT's (1969) experiments in which distance comparisons within the frontal plane were made with stabilized and non stabilized viewing. No significant differences in either mean values or variability were found.

Results for stereoscopic acuity are similar to those for vernier acuity: Although stereoscopic acuity is about as fine as vernier acuity (BERRY, 1948) and improves with stimulus duration (OGLE and WEIL, 1958; SHORTESS and KRAUSKOPF, 1961), no significant threshold differences are found between stabilized and normal viewing conditions for durations up to 1.0 second (SHORTESS and KRAUSKOPF, 1961).

To look more closely at the concept of "averaging" over the spatial array of cones stimulated at a given moment, LUDVIGH (1953) required subjects to report on whether a point placed midway between two other vertically oriented points appeared to lie to the left or right of alignment with the two points (Fig. 4e).

[8] A retinally stabilized image begins to fade and disappear shortly after stimulus onset — generally after at least one or two seconds (RIGGS, RATLIFF, CORNSWEET, and CORNSWEET, 1953; DITCHBURN and GINSBORG, 1952). Since the vernier threshold in both normal and stabilized viewing begins to asymptote at a stimulus duration of about 0.2 seconds, continued stimulation beyond this duration may not influence the report on any given trial (KEESEY, 1960). Thus, even should disappearance take place for the longer stimulations, the report has already been determined by the earlier portion of the stimulation.

Precision in this task is as fine as in vernier discrimination. LUDVIGH (1953) points out that since only three bundles of a few cones each are involved in this three-point task, serious questions are raised about whether averaging of positional local signs goes on at all in the vernier task.

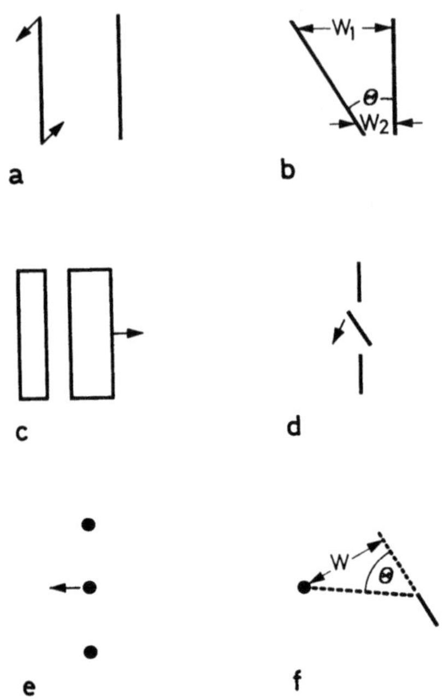

Fig. 4. Some target patterns employed to measure spatial discrimination. a) The discrimination of parallelness can be measured as shown in b) by the angle of tilt between the two lines, Θ, or by W_1—W_2, the visual angle difference between horizontal offsets between the tops of the two lines and between the bottoms of the two lines; c) discrimination of rectangle width; d) a configuration sometimes employed for orientation discrimination; e) the three point task in which the subject is required to report on the offset of the center dot relative to the imaginary straight line connecting the two other dots. Threshold can be given in terms of visual angle offset of dot from this line or in terms of tilt angle Θ between the two lines formed by the three points; other measures are also possible; f) the point/line measure of orientation discrimination

The three-point task, however, differs from the vernier task. It may be viewed as measuring the ability of subjects to discriminate orientations in the frontal plane of the two imaginary lines connecting the three points. Viewed in this way the discrimination in the three-point experiment would appear to be more closely related to the discrimination of parallelness than to the discrimination of vernier offset.

The similarity of the functions shown in Fig. 5 for the three-point and parallelness discriminations supports this view. In addition, some results with the situation in Fig. 4f provide a bridge between the three-point experiment and the parallelness discrimination and make somewhat more feasible the above view that the three-point experiment is primarily concerned with orientation discrimination. Thus BOUMA and ANDRIESSEN (1968) have found no difference under comparable conditions between thresholds for the discrimination of differences in orientation in this (Fig. 4f) point/line situation and in a situation in which the two endpoints of the line replaced the line itself; the latter is in effect identical to the three-point experiment of LUDVIGH with the exception of employing different distances between the center point and the two outer reference points. From his point/line threshold data I calculate 7″ to be the smallest threshold retinal offset of the far end of the line from the projection of the (imaginary) line connecting the point with the near end of the line (W in Fig. 4); this 7″ threshold was obtained for a distance of 5.7° between point and line and a line length of 14′.

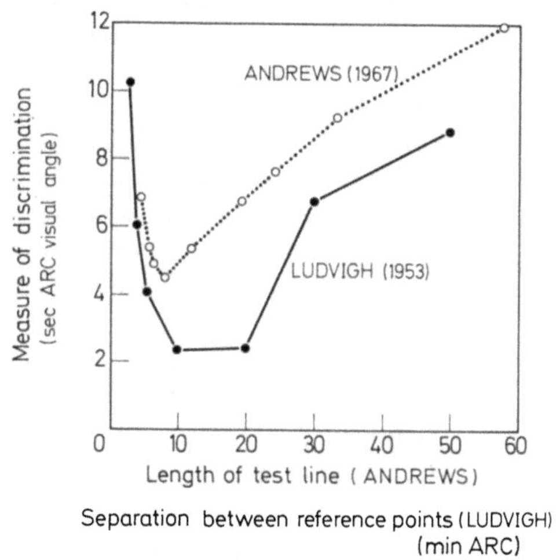

Fig. 5. LUDVIGH's (1953) data for three-point discrimination (Fig. 4e) are plotted as offset of center dot needed for 75% correct subject's report (ordinate) as a function of separation between the reference points (abscissa). ANDREWS' (1967b) data for discrimination of parallelness (Fig. 4a and 4b) plotted as threshold differential retinal offset W_1—W_2 (see Fig. 4b) as a function of line length; values of W_1—W_2 calculated from ANDREWS' values of threshold Θ by the present author

Although acuity for orientation appears to be involved in the vernier task, the critical detail itself is not orientation. Thus the cogency of LUDVIGH's point regarding the need for "averaging" over line length might appear to be somewhat diluted in reference to the vernier task. BOUMA and ANDRIESSEN's (1968) finding that thresholds for a variant of the three-point task are indistinguishable from the point/line task suggests that two points "define" a linear direction in the frontal plane as well as does an entire line filling the space between the points,[9] and LUDVIGH's point might thus at least apply to the discrimination of orientation. In fact, however, the final satisfactory setting of alignment in both orientation (three-point or point/line) and vernier tasks yields an identical appearance — that of a straight line. This would be particularly clear if each task employed two lines. There is thus good reason to expect that vernier acuity would be as good if a pair of points at the extremities of each line were to replace the lines themselves. This would justify LUDVIGH's doubt about the need for spatial averaging in vernier discrimination.

However we regard LUDVIGH's argument against a concept that involves averaging of positional local signs over the array of photoreceptors stimulated, further difficulties arise from some considerations of discriminations involving curved lines. The thresholds for all four of the configurations in Fig. 1a–1d are

[9] Constant errors were not the same for point/line and three-point situations in BOUMA and ANDRIESSEN's data, but this does not influence the above conclusion. Also see SULZER (1954).

essentially the same as are the PSEs (MATIN, unpublished data). Use of straight lines is thus not necessary for precision in the vernier task. The results further imply that the precision of discrimination cannot be critically dependent on averaging of positional local signs over each of the arrays if photoreceptors stimulated and comparing average horizontal location or any other frontal plane dimension (particularly compare Figs 1b and 1c). Instead the subject's setting not only makes use of information regarding visual direction, but also *change* of visual direction between points composing the line (i.e., the derivatives[10] of the line in the viewing plane); at alignment he requires that the relative position of the two lines be such that a continuation across the gap by a straight[11] line would yield a smooth continuous contour[12]. In effect, this implies that in his discrimination the subject is making use of the frontal plane directions of each of the two lines at their adjacent endpoints. This description is reminiscent of the gestalt "principle of good continuation" and suggests that the vernier task, as well as the three-point and point/line tasks, lie very much in the realm of form or contour discrimination.[13]

C. Contours and Cortical Local Sign

MARSHALL and TALBOT'S (1942) theory of sensory acuity provided an important advance in our thinking on this problem by moving the locus of HERING'S local signs up to the visual cortex. They pointed out that the cortical representation of the fovea was sufficiently fine-grained to deal with the fineness of vernier discrimination. The details of connectivity and interaction in their model of the projection system require considerable revision as a result of more modern work, particularly our increased knowledge regarding the role of peripheral inhibition. But their model yielded the concept that the perceived localization of a point on a contour is correlated with the location of the peak of a spatial distribution of cortical response, in effect, a principle by means of which a mean retinal local sign was obtained as the calculated output of a cortical neuron. The details of the appropriate spread function and the method of its production aside, the general principle appears to be applicable over a broad range of phenomena and across sensory systems (VON BÉKÉSY, 1957, 1960, 1967; RATLIFF, 1965). Incorporated into more complex models of interaction and adaptation in the primary visual projection system, it permits reasonable interpretations (OSGOOD and HEYER, 1952; GANZ, 1966) of figural aftereffect phenomena (KÖHLER and WALLACH, 1944)

[10] The derivative is the tangent to the curve at the point. Note that in Figs. 1b and 1c the subject cannot align the targets by "filling" the gap with a curve with curvature identical to the two shown in each figure.

[11] The "simplest" line which would physically satisfy a requirement of smoothness in Figs. 1a—e would be the straight line that would be the common tangent to the two curves at their adjacent tips.

[12] In Figs. 1a—e the curvature of each line is uniform and "requires" a straight line in the gap. It remains to be seen whether thresholds are equally small in alignment tasks such as Fig. 1h where smoothness requires a curved line of uniform curvature in the gap, and in Figs. 1f and 1g where only curved lines of varying curvature will do.

[13] It should be clear that anything we say about the *appearance* of shape of the line "filling" the gap (e.g. "the line appears straight") is a matter of inference on the part of the experimenter and depends at some point on a definition by the experimenter.

based on the assumption that although retinal local sign has been modified cortical local sign has not.

This approach to localization and orientation has now been taken a step further. The presence in cat and monkey of cortical cells selectively sensitive to line stimulation over a restricted range of orientations and locations of the retinal stimulus (HUBEL and WIESEL, 1962, 1968) implies special kinds of selectivity in the determination of connections between retinal ganglion cells and cortical cells as well as between cortical cells themselves. A variety of psychophysical experiments have given evidence of their presence in man (e.g., McCOLLOUGH, 1965; CAMPBELL and KULIKOWSKI, 1966; SEKULER, RUBIN, and CUSHMAN, 1968; WEISSTEIN, 1969). Most of these experiments involved measuring differential sensitivity to contours differently oriented in the frontal plane following an adaptation period with contours in one orientation. Determinations of either a loss in sensitivity at the orientation employed during adaptation or other orientationally selective aftereffects were generally effected by requiring the subject to report the orientation of a particular aspect of the test stimulus which he could resolve, or the existence of some phenomenal aspect of the stimulus when the latter was presented in different orientations. As such, the tasks were concerned with either resolution or detection acuities rather than with the discriminability of orientation.

ANDREWS (1965, 1967a, b) and BOUMA and ANDRIESSON (1968), however, have attempted to account for data on the discrimination of relative orientation by means of models which employ such "line detectors" as their elements. Here, instead of assuming neural elements with spatial response distributions to point stimuli as in the models discussed above, the assumption is made that each "line detector element" has a gaussian distribution of response magnitude with variation of orientation over a narrow range. ANDREWS assumes that units with peak responses near the horizontal or vertical orientation are more finely tuned than those with response peaks to other orientations, thus accounting for the finding that sensitivity to orientation is greatest near the horizontal and vertical dimensions (ROCHLIN, 1955; ANDREWS, 1967; BOUMA and ANDRIESSEN, 1968). However, BOUMA and ANDRIESSEN point out that this assumption predicts that perceived orientation (PSEs in the point/line situation) will be biased away from the nearest vertical or horizontal in contradiction to the measured variations. They propose instead greater densities of units in the horizontal and vertical dimensions with tuning that is equal in width to those units that have peaks in other meridians. Although the model has not yet been developed in quantitative detail, it predicts the observed variations in both sensitivity and bias for orientation discrimination as a function of orientation.[14]

---

[14] The influence of orientation in the frontal plane on threshold is quite similar for vernier discrimination (LEIBOWITZ, 1953; MATIN, POLA, and McCONCHIE, unpublished data), the discrimination of parallelness (ROCHLIN, 1955), the point/line situation (BOUMA and ANDRIESSEN, 1968), the three line orientation task (ANDREWS, 1967a), and the discrimination of perpendicularity (ONLEY and VOLKMANN, 1958). Threshold is lowest for vertical and horizontal lines and increases symmetrically to reach maxima at tilts of about 45°. Such effects could be due to basic properties of the ocular dioptrics (WEYMOUTH, 1959) or to combinations of astigmatic and accommodative peculiarities. However, a similar effect of orientation on grating (HAMBLIN and WINSOR, 1927; HIGGINS and STULZ, 1950) and fine line (OGILVIE and TAYLOR, 1958; NACHMIAS, 1960) acuities has been obtained. Although changes in the astigmatic

The employment of such hypothetical characteristics and distributions of line detectors for handling psychophysical data has so far involved assuming that their outputs combine in an uncomplicated way, in effect by some averaging process over a selected set of cortical neurons. So again a "mean local sign" is an implied feature of these more recent models, although so far the treatment has been concerned only with "mean cortical local sign for orientation of straight lines." The approach also appears to have some utility in dealing with some of the geometrical illusions of space (BOUMA and ANDRIESSEN, 1970), which are of particular interest in the present context since they are instances of modifications of visual direction induced by simultaneously viewed lines.

Moreover, the results with the three-point experiment do not appear to be at all intractable to such a theoretical approach to orientation since it does not seem unreasonable to assume that a group of units selectively tuned for orientation will be adequately stimulated by three points, leaving units that are inappropriately tuned unstimulated. Since the topographical organization of such cortical "line detectors" preserves the retinal organization by means of selective connectivity of cells between the two layers, an approach that assumes averaging of positional local signs of a subpopulation of cortical cells tuned for orientation also appears to provide a reasonable way of handling the vernier data. In addition, larger numbers of directionally-tuned elements have been observed near the vertical and horizontal in rabbit retina (OYSTER and BARLOW, 1967) and in cat striate cortex (PETTIGREW *et al.*, 1968) — as postulated by BOUMA and ANDRIESSEN in man — although not as yet in monkey. Nevertheless, difficult problems remain for solution for the presently-prevailing view of hierarchically-organized feature detectors: For example, it is clear that the "direction-tagged" outputs of "straight line detectors" cannot be averaged in any simple fashion to deal with dicrimination of offset with curved lines. Neither are "principles" of selectivity available by which curvature could be derived from the output of such detectors.

III. Flexible Local Signs

Combinations of eye, head, and bodily movements continually bring about variations in the retinal loci of images corresponding to stationary objects, and questions of how we perceive these objects in stable positions and do not confuse them with moving objects are thus central to any understanding of space perception and sensorimotor coordination. In this section we shall be primarily concerned with modifications of local sign by extraretinal signals normally associated with

properties of normal eyes with changes in the accommodative stimulus can produce changes in the variation of grating acuity with orientation (ARNULF and DUPUY, 1960; BECK, 1965), the effect on grating resolution remains when a technique of stimulus production is used that bypasses the effects of the ocular dioptrics in forming the retinal image (CAMPBELL, KULIKOWSKI, and LEVINSON, 1966). Thus, for grating acuity at least — and very likely for the other acuities as well — the influence of orientation depends on factors beyond the ocular dioptrics, although the effects can be influenced by the dioptrics. The influence of ocular factors on variation of bias (the point of subjective equality) as a function of target orientation has not yet been determined for any of the alignment tasks (see PEARCE and MATIN, 1969 on this point).

eye movements. These problems will be considered here quite apart from the genesis of the mechanisms in either innate processes or past experience.

Voluntary changes of the direction of gaze are generally thought to be carried out solely by means of saccadic eye movements when the observer views a field of stationary objects (see Fig. 6a); slow voluntary movements on the other hand are generally considered possible only when an observer visually pursues a moving

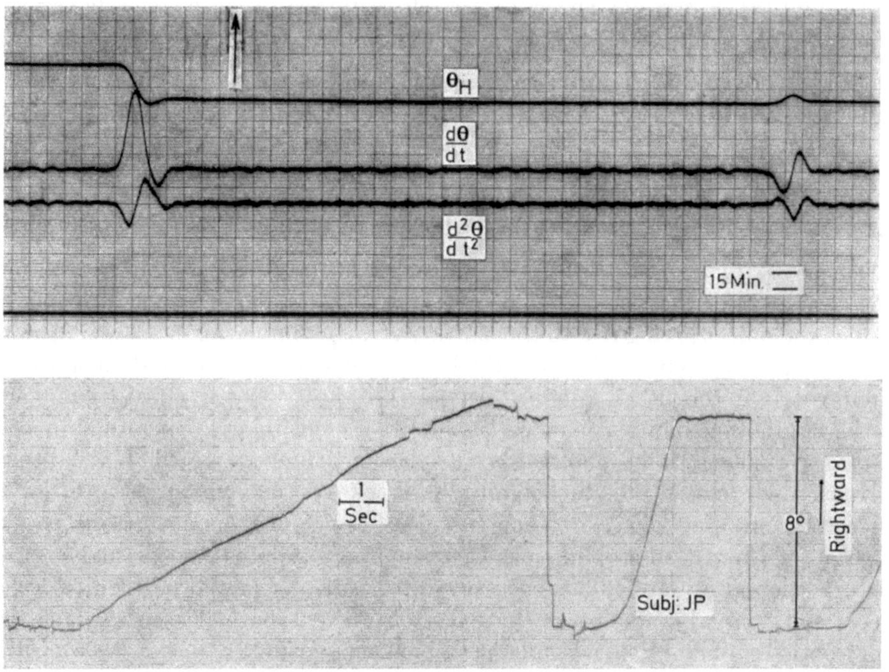

Fig. 6. a) Recording of a voluntary horizontal saccade (near left of figure) made by a subject changing his direction of gaze from one 4′ target to a second one located 39.3′ to the right of the first. Upper trace records change of eye position, middle trace records first derivative of eye position change (velocity), and lower trace records second derivative of eye position change (acceleration). Small oscillations on middle and lower traces (about one per time line) are a measure of velocity and acceleration of involuntary fine ocular tremor. ("grass" on middle and lower traces is amplifier noise). Time lines are separated by 10 msec intervals; major horizontal separations correspond to 15′ of arc for upper trace, 13 deg/sec for middle trace, and 6500 deg/sec² for lower trace. The actual saccade length undershot intertarget distance and is about 35′. Saccade velocity normally scales up for increasing saccade lengths; increase is a negatively accelerated function of saccade length (cf., involuntary saccade toward right of figure). (Recording is from MATIN and PEARCE, 1964). b) Recording of slow horizontal eye movements in the absence of any moving visual stimulus. Two stationary, continuously illuminated circular 3.5′ targets horizontally separated by 8° were the only visual stimuli present. These were employed only to define for the subject the endpoints of the eye movements; essentially identical movements are made by this subject without any visible stimulus. The different velocities of the two slow movements in the figure are under voluntary control of the subject who is able to produce velocities even slower than the one on the left of the figure, and can in a graded series of such movements produce velocities almost up to the speed of saccades. He can, in addition, produce these velocities with the eye moving in either direction, although only slow movement from left to right is shown in the figure with return via saccades. (Unpublished recording is by POLA, MATIN, and MATIN)

target. Although this does not hold as a generalization (see Fig. 6b), it is undoubtedly true that saccades are usually the means by which voluntary changes of the direction of gaze are achieved when viewing stationary fields.

That slow movements cannot be carried out voluntarily in the absence of a moving stimulus is explicitly stated by numerous authors, and implied equally frequently. Occasional reports of slow movements in the absence of a moving stimulus have appeared. They have perhaps failed to be convincing either because eye movements were not directly measured (GERTZ, 1916), the measuring technique was not sufficiently sensitive to discriminate a smooth movement from a chain of small saccades (DECKART, 1964), or the velocity of the movement does not appear to be sufficiently different from a saccade of equal length (WESTHEIMER and CONOVER, 1954). Recordings obtained with a contact-lens technique leave no further room for doubt (see Fig. 6b).

A. Voluntary Saccades

1. Existence of Saccade-Contingent Extraretinal Signals

During steady fixation a shift of the retinal locus stimulated is normally a sufficient condition for the visual perception of target movement and displacement. If the object giving rise to the shifting retinal stimulation is viewed against a stationary background, relative retinal displacement of object and background is involved. On the other hand, when the observer's eye is turned from one location to another in a stationary visual field, the entire array of retinal images undergoes an essentially undistorted displacement on the retina (in degrees of visual angle) equal to the magnitude of the eye movement (in degrees of ocular rotation) (see Fig. 7). It has therefore been questioned whether an explanation of perceptual stability of visual direction requires extraretinal sources of information at all, and it has been suggested that the spatial relation between objects and "visual frameworks" provide a sufficient basis for an explanation of perceptual stability and visually perceived movement (KOFFKA, 1935). Such contextual influences are of importance in determining where we localize seen objects. However, two well-known observations strongly implicate extraretinal processes, and thus invalidate any explanation which relies on the influence of visual context alone: (1) When the eye is moved by an external object (e.g., pushed by the finger) during an attempt at steady fixation, movement of the visual field is perceived in a direction that would be appropriate to the direction of retinal image shift were the latter generated by physical displacement of the entire visual field with the eye held steady (HELMHOLTZ, 1866). In addition, when the entire visual field is displaced as a unit during an attempt at steady fixation, movement of the field may be perceived. (2) When the eye is immobilized – as a result either of extraocular muscle paralysis or by mechanical restriction of the normal eye – and a voluntary eye movement attempted, motion of the visual field is observed in the direction of the attempted ocular rotation although no motion of the retinal image has occurred (HELMHOLTZ, 1866). Although both situations are "physiologically abnormal" in the sense that the normal linkages between attempted eye movement, actual eye movement, and retinal image shift are severed, the latter observation shows that relative stimulus motion or change of location of objects within the field is not necessary to the perception of movement or change of visual direction. Thus extraretinal influences are effective producers of perceived motion or visual direction change. The observation that a uniform displacement of the entire retinal array need not result in perceptual stability shows that a stable visual framework is not sufficient for perceived stability.

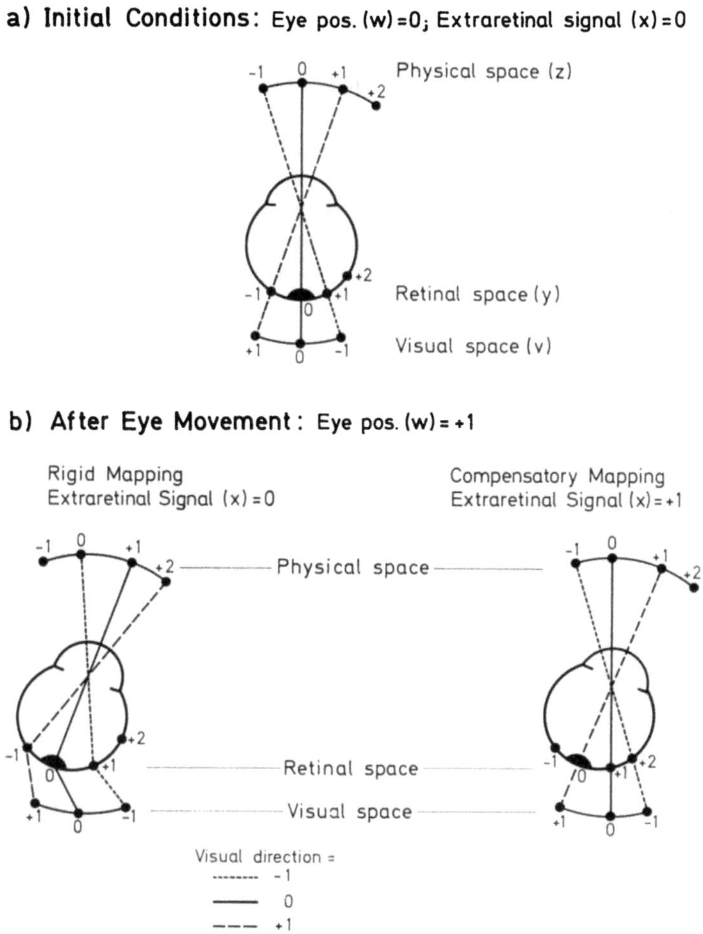

Fig. 7. View of an eye from above (a) while gaze is in some initial direction, and (b) following an eye movement which rotates the direction of gaze 1° to the right. The dark patch at the back of the eye represents the fovea. The figures show the relations between angular distances in the stimulus domain ("physical space"), at the retina ("retinal space") and visually perceived directions psychophysically measured ("visual space") prior to the eye movement (a), and following the eye movement for two cases: no change has occurred in the relation between retinal locus stimulated and perceived visual direction (b, "rigid mapping"); the magnitude of change in the relation between retinal locus stimulated and perceived visual direction exactly compensates the magnitude of the eye movement (b, "compensatory mapping"). The solid, dashed, and dotted lines connecting points in the three spaces are each anchored to a different visual direction and connect to the coordinated points in physical and retinal space. Although angular relations between the three spaces is accurate, angular distances are not drawn to scale

2. Quantitative Properties of Extraretinal Signals Associated with Voluntary Saccades

a) Temporal Development. The extraretinal signal itself, however, although involved in the mechanism underlying the perceived stability of stationary objects when voluntary saccades occur, does not provide a sufficient basis for its explanation. This conclusion derives from a series of experiments in which the influence on visual direction of the saccade-contingent extraretinal signal has been isolated from influences resulting from variations in visual stimulation produced by the saccade (MATIN and PEARCE, 1965; MATIN, 1968; MATIN, MATIN, POLA, and PEARCE, 1968; MATIN, MATIN and PEARCE, 1969; MATIN, MATIN, and POLA, 1970, also in preparation). In these experiments subjects reported on the visual direction of a brief flash presented at various times either before, during, or after a voluntary saccade relative to the visual direction of a fixation target viewed and extinguished prior to the saccade (see Fig. 8). The stimuli in these experiments were presented in complete darkness; thus the possibility of influences on dis-

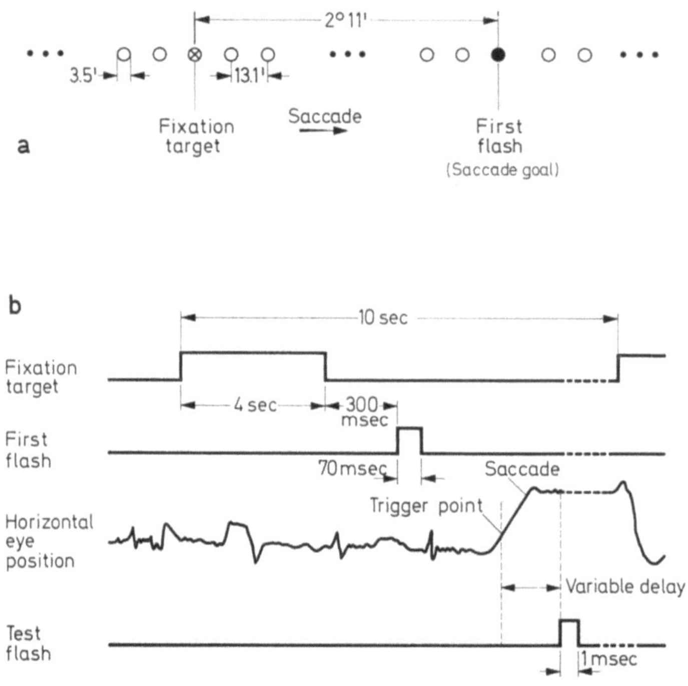

Fig. 8. a) Spatial array of stimuli employed in experiments measuring the relation of visual direction of a flash presented either before, during, or after a voluntary horizontal saccade to that of the previously-viewed fixation target; any target in the array could be used as a test flash. b) Temporal sequence of stimuli. For test flashes produced during the saccade the variable delay was zero; different trigger points within the saccade were employed. Test flashes presented before the saccade were initiated at a fixed duration following first flash onset (350 msec for observer JP and 300 msec for EM); test flash — saccade interval could not be set beforehand as a consequence of the variable reaction time, and was thus measured during each trial. Test flashes during the saccade were 1 msec as shown; test flashes before and after the saccade (when the eye was moving more slowly) were 2 msec

crimination arising from extraneous visual context was completely eliminated. Low intensity but easily visible stimuli were employed and the presentations of the two stimuli whose visual direction were compared were separated by at least 500 msec; thus the influence of afterimages and other similar short-term "visually persistent" consequences of the presentation of the fixation target, which could make the discrimination one of "simultaneously viewed" stimuli, were minimized or eliminated. In addition, the use of a brief flash when the eye was in motion during a saccade essentially eliminated the "smearing" of the retinal image which occurs in continuously illuminated environments.

The experiments provided measurements of the location of a flash that appeared in the same location as the previously-viewed fixation target (target point of subjective equality or target PSE) as a function of time of test flash presentation measured from the beginning of the saccade. These values are shown in Fig. 9b. From simultaneous measurements of eye position obtained by means

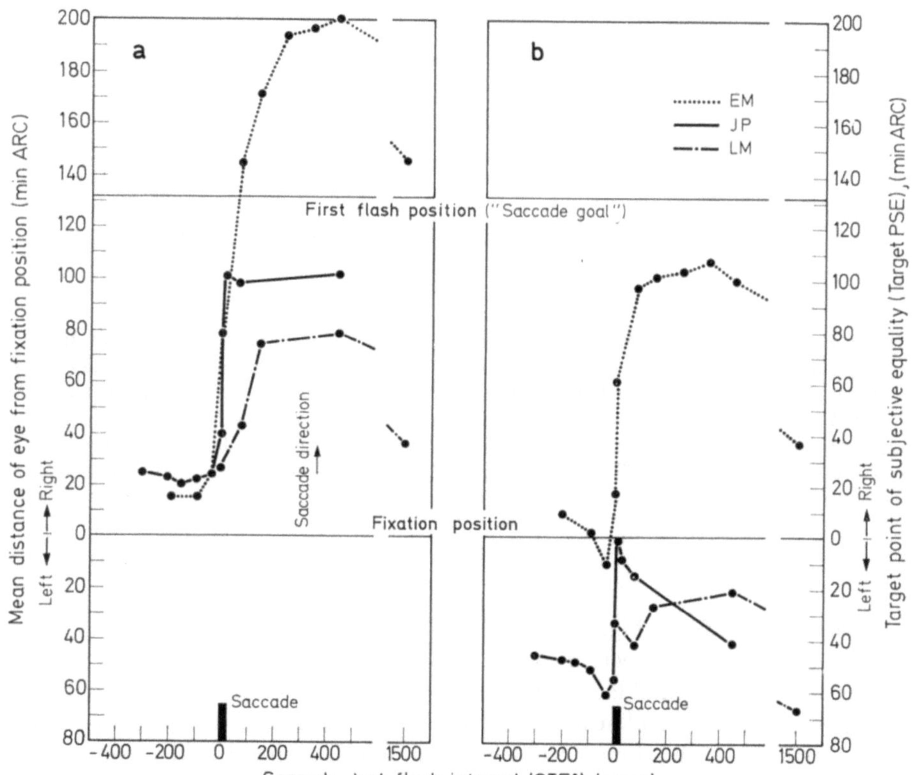

Fig. 9. a) Mean eye position at times before, during and after saccade when test flashes were presented. b) Points of subjective equality at the stimulus array determined from subject's report of horizontal visual direction of test flash relative to previously-viewed fixation target. Negative values of STFI refer to trials in which test flash was presented before the saccade. It was not possible to reproduce on this graph all of the points during the saccade; only one or two are shown here. Presaccadic data for EM are for leftgoing saccades; all the rest are for rightgoing saccades as shown. (Graph compiled from data in MATIN *et al.*, 1969, 1970, also in preparation)

of a contact-lens technique employing invisible (infrared) measuring beams (MATIN, 1964; MATIN and PEARCE, 1964), determinations were made of the variations of retinal locus at which the target PSEs were imaged (see Fig. 7). These values (retinal PSEs) are shown in Fig. 10.

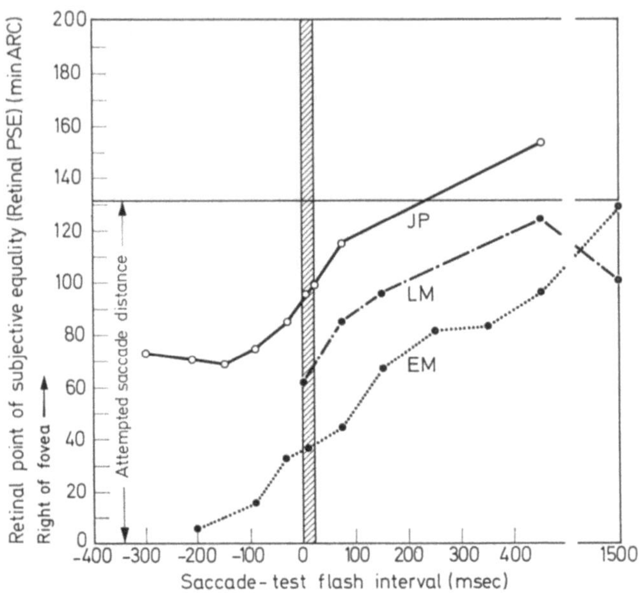

Fig. 10. Points of subjective equality for the fixation target measured as horizontal distances at the retina. These are plotted as a function of time relative to saccade onset. The data are from the same experiments as Fig. 9. Although there is a close correspondence between the retinal PSEs and the differences between mean eye position and target PSEs at corresponding values of STFI, it is not exact; this is mainly a result of the fact that distributions of eye positions at fixed values of STFI were frequently skewed. Each retinal PSE was calculated directly from the distribution of retinal distances and psychophysical responses over trials at a given value of STFI

It is apparent from Fig. 10 that the mapping of visual direction into retinal locus changes in the time period associated with the saccade (i.e., there is a saccade-contingent shift in retinal local signs). Since this shift in local signs occurred in the absence of ongoing visual stimulation, it may be attributed to the growth of an extraretinal signal whose magnitude is monotonically related to the magnitude of local sign shift. However, it is also apparent from Fig. 10 that the growth of extraretinal signal is very much slower and more prolonged than the saccade itself, beginning to grow considerably before the saccade begins, changing only slightly when measured with flashes presented during the saccade, and showing considerable growth both before the saccade and for some time after the saccade is completed. In these experiments the peripherally presented target was 2° 11′ from the fixation target. Essentially similar results have been obtained with separations of 4° 22′ for flashes presented during the saccade (MATIN, MATIN, and

PEARCE, 1969), and with separations of 5° and 8° for flashes presented during and after the saccade (POLA, 1971).

The comparison of the time courses of extraretinal signal growth and of the saccade itself shows that a saccade-contingent extraretinal signal cannot be the sole factor responsible for the production of perceived stability when saccades occur. Quite apart from the specific details of any theory regarding the nature of the extraretinal signal or the mechanism by which it influences perceived visual direction, if its operation were to be the sole means by which stability of perceived visual direction is produced, the shift of local signs could follow only one time course. It would have to parallel the eye movement exactly; if it did not, variations of the perceived visual direction of stationary targets would result. Clearly such a time course was not followed.

b) Determination of Extraretinal Signal Magnitude by Time, Eye Position, Saccade Length, and Distance of the Saccade's Goal. Since eye position changed systematically with time in the saccadic period (Fig. 9), it follows that the variation in local signs with time shown in Fig. 10 implies a variation with eye position. But this is not an incidental relation; even at a specific time the local sign shift is a function of eye position. This was determined by making use of the considerable trial-to-trial variability in saccade length and in eye position at a given time[15]. Sensitivity of this shift was about 0.5 minute of arc shift in local signs per minute of arc change in eye position at 75 msec following the saccade (MATIN, MATIN, and POLA, in preparation). Since saccade length and eye position at a given time after the saccade are highly correlated it is not yet known which is the more significant.

In further work, POLA (1971) has extended these findings to 8° saccades. In addition, by preconditioning a reduction in saccade length he has been able to extend the range of positions assumed by the eye on different trials at particular times during and following the saccade.

The preconditioning was carried out by a technique based on a finding by MCLAUGHLIN (1967). During a saccade to a target 10° removed from a fixation target, MCLAUGHLIN displaced the distant target 1° toward the original point of fixation. This resulted in an overshoot of the saccade with respect to the new target position. When this was repeated several times, the saccade's length was reduced to nearly 9°. By a variant of this procedure the saccades of POLA's subjects were reduced from 8° to nearly 5° in preconditioning over 100 trials. Sessions in which reduction in saccade length was preconditioned were mixed with those in which saccade length reduction was not preconditioned, thus extending the total range of saccade lengths obtained.

[15] Repeated saccades between two given points in a continuously-illuminated environment are extremely uniform. Hence the eye reaches a given point in every saccade at virtually the same interval after saccade initiation. In the experiments referred to above the peripheral target toward which the saccade was aimed was presented as a 70 msec flash. Since the subject did not turn his eye to look at the peripheral flash until it appeared, it was extinguished before the saccade had begun. This mode of presentation precisely localized the retinal location of the peripheral flash and prevented its image from being dispersed over the retina at successive moments during an eye movement as it would were the stimulus presented for a longer duration. It also permitted the employment of a stimulus sequence in which no two stimuli were simultaneously presented. However, when the eye saccades to a target that is no longer present in a dark field, as in the above experiments, there results considerable inaccuracy and variability in saccade length, more frequent occurrences of multiple saccades on a single trial (most frequently two), and particularly for the longer saccades some variability in saccade shape and duration. (See also BECKER and FUCHS, 1969).

POLA reports that at a given duration not only is the local sign shift linear with eye position but that sensitivity is the same when saccade length is experimentally reduced and when it is not. In addition, he finds that the distance of the peripheral target eliciting the saccade may be a less potent variable in determining visual direction than is the actual distance that the eye travels. Thus, although the temporal development of the local sign shift consequent to saccade elicitation by a target 5° in the periphery is roughly a scaled down version of the 8° function, a substantial portion of this difference is due to the fact that a 5° target typically elicited a smaller saccade than a target 8° in the periphery.

c) Summary of Characteristics of Growth of the Saccade-Contingent Extraretinal Signal. The change in retinal locus associated with a given visual direction prior to, during, and following a voluntary saccade is much slower and more extended in time than the saccade itself, beginning at least 100 msec before the saccade and growing monotonically until at least 300 msec following saccade completion. Although the shift is in a direction that is compensatory for the actual saccade, and reaches a magnitude that is close to the distance between the peripheral target calling out the saccade and the prior fixation target, considerable inaccuracy is manifested in reporting the visual direction of flashes before, during, or after the saccade relative to a previously-viewed fixation target. Three variables are connected with the growth of extraretinal signal guiding the shift of local signs: (1) time relative to saccade beginning, (2) either saccade length or position of the eye at the moment the test flash is presented, (3) either distance of the peripheral target eliciting the saccade or the "attempted saccade magnitude." The two alternatives for each of variables (2) and (3) have not yet been separated.

The experiments on which these conclusions are based were carried out under conditions of visual stimulation that differ from normal viewing: (1) the fixation target, the standard target in the comparison, was removed before the saccade had begun; (2) the comparison target was presented as a brief flash; (3) a stable visual background was absent; (4) the target toward which the saccade was aimed was extinguished before the saccade had begun. If the influence of the extraretinal signal on perceived visual direction were to be sufficient to account for perceptual stability, however, its operation should be tied to either the position of the eye or the subject's intention to move it, and independent of the details of the visual stimulation per se. Hence these conclusions regarding extraretinal signal influence should be applicable to more normal viewing situations. Since, then, the growth of extraretinal signal does not parallel the change in eye position, it cannot by itself be sufficient to explain the stability of visual direction in the presence of voluntary saccades. The following section will also indicate some restrictions placed on the operation of the extraretinal signal by conditions of visual stimulation.

3. Influence of Visual Stimulation on Visual Direction in the Presence of Voluntary Saccades

Two aspects of the spatiotemporal pattern of visual stimulation have been shown to have substantial influences on the relation of visual direction and retinal locus when voluntary saccades occur. These are: (1) the time interval between stimulations whose visual directions are being compared and (2) factors related to visual masking.

a) Failure of the Extraretinal Signal to Mediate Relative Visual Direction during Brief Time Intervals. In the experiments described above there was a minimum time interval of about 500 msec between stimulations from the two targets whose visual directions were compared (see Fig. 8). Quite different results were obtained with shorter time intervals (MATIN and PEARCE, 1965; MATIN, MATIN, POLA, and BOWEN, 1971), although the dependence of visual direction on this temporal variable has not yet been determined in detail for short intervals. In an experiment in which a flash was presented when the eye was at each of two different positions during a single 8° horizontal saccade (approximately 30 msec between presentation of the two flashes), it was necessary for the two successive flashes to strike very nearly the same horizontal retinal coordinate in order for the flashes to appear in the same visual direction (Fig. 11). This result could not be predicted from an extraretinal signal function for 8° saccades obtained for this subject in a way similar to the one in Fig. 10. Thus, although the target PSE for the previously-viewed fixation target was 3° to the left of the fixation target when the test flash was delivered with the eye 1° into the saccade, and 1/3° to the right of the fixation target when the eye was 6° into the saccade (Fig. 11), there was a failure of transitivity between the outcome of these comparisons and the direct comparison to each other of the directions of flashes from the two targets corresponding to the target PSEs (Fig. 11). The difference between the target PSEs for the fixation target

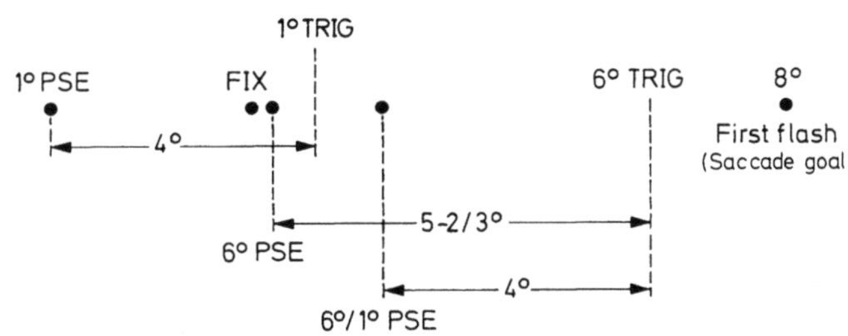

Fig. 11. Points of subjective equality (PSEs) were measured for the fixation target under two conditions: (1) Test flashes were presented when the eye crossed a point (1° trig) 1° from the fixation target (measured value indicated at 1° PSE); (2) On other trials test flashes were presented when the eye crossed a point (6° trig) 6° from the fixation target (measured value indicated at 6° PSE). On each of another set of trials a first flash was presented from the target at "1° PSE" when the eye crossed 1° trig, and a second flash was presented when the eye crossed 6° trig from a target whose location was randomly varied. The subject reported the location of the second flash relative to the first; the PSE is indicated at "6°/1° PSE." (From MATIN, MATIN, POLA, and BOWEN, 1971)

determined when the eye is at the two different points in the saccade corresponds to a difference of $1-2/3°$ at the retina. But when the visual direction of a flash presented as the eye crosses the 6° point was compared to a flash presented when the eye crossed the 1° point the required retinal distance was reduced to near zero.

Further indication of the failure of saccade-contingent extraretinal signals to differentially influence the visually perceived directions associated with visual events that are sufficiently close to each other in time may be derived from the following: When an entire visual scene is presented as a brief flash during a saccade, spatial relations within the scene appear undistorted. Yet, it is well known that dimmer stimulus intensities result in visual responses with longer latencies, and that a substantial portion of these differences are already present at the level of the optic nerve and thus presumably prior to influence by extraretinal signals. Influence on visual direction by a saccade-contingent extraretinal signal whose magnitude grows with time (such as in Fig. 10) would then be expected to yield distortions in the briefly-flashed visual scene that are related to local intensity variations in the scene.[16] Failure to observe distortion in brief flashes has been confirmed in a formal experiment in which detection of horizontal vernier offset was measured for two vertical lines differing by 2 log units in stimulus intensity that were simultaneously presented in a 1 msec flash during a horizontal saccade (Matin, Matin, Pola, and Bowen, 1971).

It has been possible to measure distortion when parts of a "scene" were sequentially presented. In an experiment which employed the stimulus configuration and temporal sequencing shown in Fig. 8, the subject was required to report whether the randomly-located test flash (presented when the eye was at a point near the middle of the saccade) lay to the left of the fixation target, between the fixation target and the flash target defining the goal of the saccade, or to the right of the latter target (Matin and Pearce, 1965). PSEs for each of the comparison targets are illustrated in Fig. 12.[17] In this case the test flash was presented

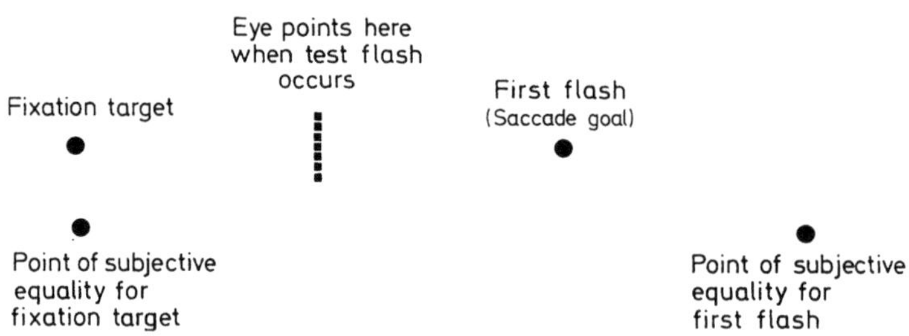

Fig. 12. An experiment in which Points of Subjective Equality (PSEs) for two targets viewed before the saccade were simultaneously determined by use of test flashes presented during the saccade (see text). PSEs were actually on same horizontal line as targets and are vertically displaced in the figure only for clarity. (From Matin and Pearce, 1965)

more than 500 msec following fixation target extinction (300 msec + reaction time to the flash from the target which constituted the "saccade's goal"), but only about 200 msec (the subject's reaction time alone) following onset of the flash from the saccade's goal. The results indicate that the comparison of visual direction of the test flash to that of the fixation target was influenced by an extraretinal signal of substantial magnitude, but that the comparison of the test flash to the flash

[16] The consideration that variation of latency with intensity might be sufficient to generate distortion is in fact much too simplistic; for example, it neglects the fact that more intense stimuli also generate longer lasting discharges in the optic nerve.

[17] Exact PSE values could not be meaningfully calculated since the eye position during the saccade at the moment of test flash presentation was not held constant over trials. The error in estimating the PSEs due to this factor would not have exceeded 5′, however.

from the target constituting the saccade's goal was not – thus requiring rough identity of retinal locus in order to be seen in the same visual direction.

The phenomena described in this section suggests that the influence of a saccade-contingent extraretinal signal on relative visual direction of different stimuli is severely restricted unless a "sufficiently" long time interval separates their presentations. Relative visual directions of successive stimulations presented at shorter time intervals appear to be essentially judged on the basis of relative retinal location alone as in the steadily fixating eye. The short interval effects evidently depend on whether the neural consequences of the earlier stimulation can persist into the time period during which the second stimulus is being processed. This peristence will undoubtedly depend on variables such as state of light adaptation and stimulus intensity.

The general picture that emerges so far suggests that we may conceive of two storage "registers": a "short-term" memory storage and a "long-term" storage. When a saccade occurs, the extraretinal signal associated with it may influence the relation of visual directions of two targets only if the neural process corresponding to one of them exists in the long-term storage when the other one is seen. It is not likely that the movement of a memory from short to long term storage is abrupt. Rather it is more likely that the memory of direction of a given target will have one foot in short term and the second in long term memory for some time and that as more of it moves into the long-term memory the susceptibility to extraretinal influence of a discrimination of this target against a more recently presented one increases.

b) Suppression. When voluntary saccades are carried out in a normally illuminated environment we generally do not perceive stimulation available to the eye during the movement. Dodge (1900, 1905) originally suggested that the effect was a consequence of the close temporal adjacency of different images at a given retinal region resulting from the sweep of the retina across the image plane of the eye, and that the observer had learned to disregard the resulting blur. Holt (1903) suggested that a "central anesthesia" accompanied voluntary saccades. The latter suggestion has received support from several studies in which a diminished sensitivity to very brief flashes has been shown to have a time course synchronized to the saccade (Volkmann, 1962; Latour, 1962; Volkmann, Schick, and Riggs, 1968; Zuber and Stark, 1966; Richards, 1969; Pearce and Porter, 1970). Since this increase in threshold is only about 0.5 log unit it is not sufficient by itself to account for the fact that in normally illuminated environments we generally do not perceive stimulation during the saccade. However in a recent report (Matin, Matin, Pola, and Kowal, 1969) evidence was presented for a suppression mechanism which would be sufficient. That mechanism is backward lateral inhibition or metacontrast. The experiment that led to this suggestion was the following:

When a small target is presented for 0.5 msec against a background of complete darkness shortly after the onset of a horizontal saccade, it is seen as a small spot. If on subsequent trials the flash onset again follows the onset of the saccade but the flash duration is extended so that it is present during more of the saccade, the appearance is of a horizontally extended "smear" whose length increases with stimulus duration. Maximum smear length appears to be reached when the flash is extinguished at about the time the saccade terminates. Further increases in flash duration result in *decreasing* length of the "smear" and finally, if the stimulus is left on for a sufficiently long period of time, no smear is seen and the appearance of the target reverts to that of a small spot. This phenomenon has now been studied as a function of flash luminance and duration against a dark background with 4° horizontal saccades (Fig. 13, MATIN, CLYMER, and MATIN, in preparation). Similar observations were made at other values of luminance, contrast, and saccade length.

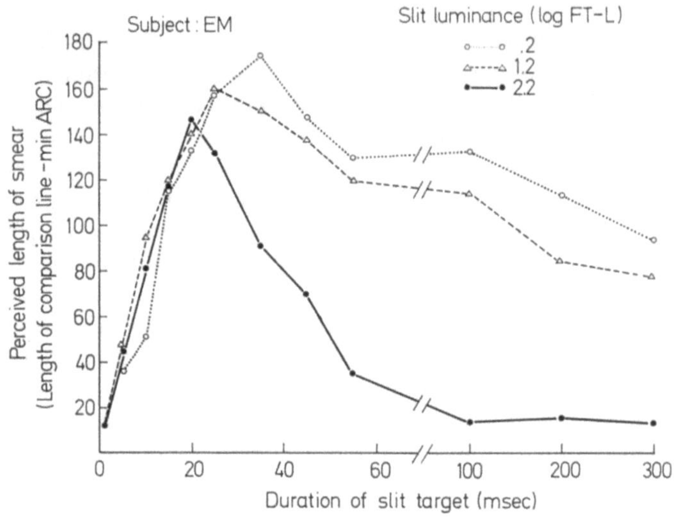

Fig. 13. Perceived length of a 2′ wide slit illuminated when the eye had traveled 1° into a 4° horizontal saccade. The slit remained illuminated for the duration indicated on the abscissa. Saccade duration was approximately 36 msec. A variable length 3.2 ft. L. comparison line was presented for 2 msec 350 msec following onset of the slit and was located 1.5° above the slit; since this presentation was in the postsaccadic period the eye was virtually steady. (MATIN, E., MATIN, L., CLYMER, A., in preparation)

The increase in perceived smear length with stimulus duration until length reaches a maximum correlates well with the retinal energy distribution.[18] However, the diminution in perceived smear length for increasing stimulus durations after the maximum length is reached strongly suggests inhibitory interactions like those generally classified as metacontrast i.e., masking produced by subsequent

[18] SMITH (1969a, b) has determined relations for the dark-adapted steadily-fixated eye among luminance, velocity, wavelength, target diameter, eccentricity, and arc length for a target moving with constant angular velocity in a circle around a fixation point in order for a stimulus to appear as a continuous fused arc (to appear as an evenly illuminated band in all parts of the field at once). She finds that for parametric values similar to those employed in dealing with smears during saccades (above), a target traveling over 1.7° of visual angle will appear as a fused arc if it remains in the field as long as about 75 msec (traveling at a velocity of about 22.7° of visual angle per second). Targets traveling for shorter duration (higher velocities) over the same arc length all appear fused. Thus increasing smear length with increasing stimulus duration up to duration of the saccade (36 msec) might be expected for a stationary eye and identical spatiotemporal energy distribution across the retina [However, note the nonuniformity of ocular velocity during the saccade (see Fig. 6a) and consequent nonuniform spatial energy distribution over the retina].

stimulation to retinal areas adjacent to those whose threshold is being measured (cf., STIGLER, 1910; WERNER, 1935; ALPERN, 1953; KOLERS and ROSNER, 1960; KOLERS, 1962; RAAB, 1963; KAHNEMAN, 1968; see WEISSTEIN, chapter 10, this volume). This interpretation is particularly suggested by the fact that the diminution in length begins at about the time the saccade ends and subsequent stimulus energy all "piles up" on a restricted retinal locus. Threshold increase for a test flash in a metacontrast situation also is an increasing function of energy with a fixed duration masking flash. The detailed relation to parametrically measured influences in metacontrast phenomena has not yet been worked out although the characteristics of smear shortening do appear consistent with them.

Thus, for example, it has generally been found (KOLERS, 1962) that threshold increase produced at any given temporal interval between test and masking flashes is maximum when the two share a common border and that the effect decreases monotonically with angular separation. In the present case with increasing stimulus duration the smear begins to disappear first at its tail, i.e., the portion that is further away from the retinal region at which the increased energy accruing from increased stimulus duration piles up. But the retinal region at which the tail of the smear would exist was also the first to be stimulated by the prolonged flash, and so the tail would have preceded the beginning of "energy pileup" by the longest time. Therefore, the decrease in smear length could be caused by a type B temporal metacontrast function (KOLERS, 1962), in which the threshold decrease produced by a subsequent fixed duration flash at a given angular separation increases with increased temporal separation of test and masking flashes up to intervals of 20—100 msec. The disappearance of the tail of the smear first is thus consistent with presently available data on metacontrast.

In the present context it is worth noting that MACKAY (1970) has reported decreased sensitivity with a steadily-fixating eye when a uniformly-illuminated, circular 10° background was horizontally-displaced by 3.06° at various times relative to the presentation of a 100 ms test flash (background displacement was completed in 10 ms after displacement onset); the retinal area under test was homogeneously stimulated by the background throughout; the moving contour was never less than 1.8° away from the retinal area tested.

Whatever the details of the mechanism underlying the decrease in smear length with increased stimulus duration beyond that corresponding to the saccade, its significance for spatial localization is clear. If we neglect for the moment the existence of visual stimulation from a stationary scene present before the saccade begins, the perception of the smear produced by the saccade that corresponds to each point in the scene will have been masked by stimulation from that same point after the eye "comes to rest" at the end of the saccade, and the entire "blur" will thus not be seen. Of course stimulation of a given retinal locus by many points in the scene complicates this point-by-point analogy to the observations on smear length and remains to be worked out. If postsaccadic stimulation from a stationary scene also has masking effects on presaccadic stimulation as well as on stimulation during the saccade, it should hasten the removal of the persistent effects of prior stimulation. As noted above these persisting effects tend to pull discriminations of visual direction toward one based on retinal identity alone; operation of the extraretinal signal requires removal of these persisting effects.

B. Pursuit Eye Movements

1. Existence of Extraretinal Signals Related to Pursuit Eye Movements

When a subject visually tracks a target moving sufficiently slowly with uniform linear motion the target appears to move. Such movement is perceived whether the target moves in complete darkness or against a visible background. If tracking were perfectly accurate so that the retinal locus of the tracked target was stabilized the appearance of movement of the target in complete darkness would imply an extraretinal basis for the perceived movement.

But if tracking were perfectly accurate what basis would the oculomotor system have for tracking at all? Some "retinal error signal" appears to be necessary if ocular velocity is to have any relation at all to stimulus velocity. This is even more obvious in the tracking of a target oscillating in one dimension of the frontal plane with sinusoidal motion; here not only are target position and eye position changing with time but velocity and acceleration as well. Reports of the characteristics of pursuit eye movements have tended to emphasize that a brief time after the target begins to move, the eye catches up to the target with a brief saccade and then for target velocities up to 20°/sec — 40°/sec, ocular velocity matches target velocity (WESTHEIMER, 1954; RASHBASS, 1961; DODGE, TRAVIS, and FOX, 1930; STARK, VOSSIUS, and YOUNG, 1962; ROBINSON, 1965). BARMACK (1970) has also reported accurate velocity matching up to 90°/sec for brief periods. Some authors, however, report that the eye continues to lag the target even at very low velocities (FENDER and NYE, 1961; ST-CYR and FENDER, 1969; PUCKETT and STEINMAN, 1969). What aspects of the motion of the stimulus are significant in controlling the pursuit velocity of the eye is not yet clear but it seems clear *a priori* that some characteristic of the deviation of the target's image at the *retina* must be involved. Whether this "retinal slip" is primarily or secondarily involved in the perception of motion during target pursuit is not yet known.

Some information is derived from viewing afterimages (which are of necessity retinally stabilized). Afterimages viewed in a completely dark background appear to move in the direction of the eye movement when voluntary eye movements are made (HELMHOLTZ, 1866). These apparent movements consist of a series of jerks that suggests synchronization with the voluntary saccades (GREGORY, 1958) although no direct evidence exists on the matter. The apparent movement of the afterimage appears to be converted to smooth motion when the observer attempts to visually track the "proprioceptive locus" of his own moving hand in complete darkness (GREGORY, 1958). When a subject turns his eye slowly in darkness (Fig. 6b) while viewing an afterimage it also appears to move slowly (POLA and MATIN, unpublished observations). Attempts at fixating an afterimage of a small target eccentrically located on the retina also result in a series of jerky apparent movements in the direction of the "fixation movements" if the eccentricity is large; if eccentricity is of the order of 0.5°, however, attempts at fixation may result in smooth apparent motion (CRONE and LUNEL, 1969). Attempts at fixating a well-centered stabilized image may reduce apparent motion (MATIN and MACKINNON, 1964). Although more work is needed here, these observations suggest that an extraretinal signal influential in determination of visual motion and direction is associated with slow pursuit-type eye movements. The latter observation also suggests that the "error signal" guiding the slow motion may be a retinal *positional* error and the prior two observations suggest that the error signal need not simply be a retinal signal (see however RASHBASS, 1961).

2. Some Relations between Perceived Motion and Pursuit Eye Movements

Although experiments have not yet been reported in which pursuit eye movements and perceived visual direction or motion have been measured simultaneously so that direct determinations of the retinal stimulus could be obtained, absolute velocity thresholds for motion of a luminous target moving in darkness have been found to be 10–20 min/sec when the subject attempts to maintain fixation on the moving target (AUBERT, 1886; BOURDON, 1902). In attempting to maintain fixation during actual target movement, pursuit movement would necessarily have been engendered. Both of these workers noted the unavoidable occurrence of autokinetic movement and its possible disturbing influences on their measurements. PEARCE and MATIN (1966) have measured velocity thresholds for the detection of target motion in complete darkness in a direction opposite to the direction of ongoing autokinetic movement during attempted steady fixation. Immediately following the subject's initial directional report of autokinetic movement while viewing a spatially fixed oscilloscope spot, a step of uniform linear motion in a direction opposite to the reported autokinetic movement was imposed on the target for 3 seconds followed by target extinction. The velocity of target movement was varied between trials, and reports of reversal or no-reversal of motion were obtained. Threshold velocities for reversal of 20′/sec were obtained with fixation in the primary position (involving displacements of 1° during the three second period of target movement) and 40′/sec with fixation in extreme secondary or tertiary fixation positions. These reversal thresholds may be considered objective measures of the speed of autokinetic movement as well as absolute motion thresholds, and thus are in agreement with previous reports of increased speed and unidirectionality of autokinetic movement for extreme fixation positions (CARR, 1910; ADAMS, 1912; MATIN, PEARCE and MACKINNON, 1963).[19] These absolute thresholds are an order of magnitude higher than minimum thresholds obtained for a moving target against a visible background (AUBERT, 1886; BOURDON, 1902; GRAHAM, 1968; HENDERSON, 1971). But since involuntary fixation patterns show standard deviations of 3′–5′ of ocular motion (see Fig. 3), such thresholds for visual motion of a target must be considered very fine indeed. Whether they are simply a result of "retinal slip" during pursuit or of an extraretinal signal or of some combination of these influences remains to be determined.

Such involuntary movements would constitute a noisy background of displacements of the retinal image against which real target movement would have to be discriminated in darkness. Since these movements produce correlated shifts of the retinal image of test target and visible background, they should be of less significance when a visible background is employed.

It has been noted that during pursuit of a moving target against a textured background the latter tends to move very much more slowly in a direction opposite to the target (FILHENE, 1922; GREGORY, 1958). It has not yet been determined how this relates to functioning of the extraretinal signal, to background conditions, or to differential sensitivities of the central and peripheral retinas to movement.

3. Variation of Visual Direction during Pursuit Eye Movements

STOPER (1968) has carried out psychophysical experiments which provide measures of relative visual direction during pursuit movements. Although the method employed was based on the one described above for saccades, direct

[19] The small values of target velocity required for nulling and producing reversal of the autokinetic motion in these extreme viewing positions provide some interesting questions when juxtaposed with subjective estimates of autokinetic velocity. Values as large as 60°/sec are frequently reported.

determinations of eye position were not made. Instead, two types of controls were employed; in one case the control gave some assurance that deviations of the eye from the moving fixation target were not greater than ± 2°, and in a second case that ocular velocity was between 6°/sec and 12°/sec when tracking a target moving at 9°/sec. In one experiment, STOPER's subjects tracked a small fixation target moving (rightward) horizontally in darkness over a 27° distance at a velocity of either 0°/sec, 9°/sec, 13.5°/sec or 27°/sec. When this target reached the midpoint of its traverse a vertical line was flashed 0.36° to the right of the fixation target's momentary location. At some later time (102, 204, or 306 msec) a second vertical line was flashed at a location that varied from trial to trial. The subject reported whether the second target appeared to the left or right of the first target. In a second experiment interflash intervals ranged from 306 to 1734 msec with the fixation target traveling at 9°/sec and the first flash presented 7° to the left of the moving fixation target at the moment that the latter crossed the midline of the field. PSEs for two subjects in the second experiment are shown in Fig. 14.

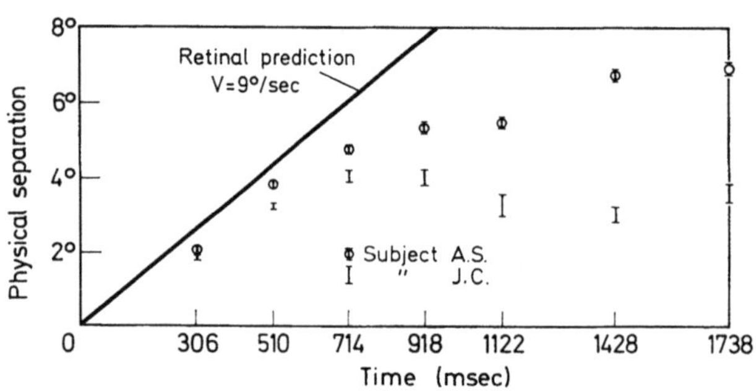

Fig. 14. Physical separation of two flashed lines reported to lie in the same visual direction, whose presentations were separated by the time interval shown on the abscissa. The eye pursued a fixation target at the velocity indicated. The diagonal line in the figure is the locus of points for which the two lines would strike the same horizontal retinal locus if ocular pursuit was accurate. Data would fall along abscissa if report was accurate with regard to physical location. Data for first experiment (not shown) lie close to diagonal. (Data from second experiment by STOPER, 1968)

If we assume accurate tracking by STOPER's subjects we must conclude that up to interflash intervals of 300–700 msec there is only a slight indication of extraretinal signal involvement in the discrimination. Up to then the judgments do not depart substantially from those that would be made were the subjects to have required that the two targets strike the same vertical retinal meridian; whatever apparent deviation does occur from such a requirement might be due to failure of the eye to keep up with the target. However, for interflash intervals beyond 700 msec deviations from a "retinal identity" basis cannot reasonably be attributed to such failure; the deviations here are too large. Since the target (and presumably the eye also) had already traveled 13.5° when the first flash occurred (for the 9°/sec velocity, the moving fixation target and eye had then been traveling for 1.5 sec), we may infer from STOPER's data that departure from a discrimination based on identity of horizontal retinal locus during pursuit (i.e., where a shift of retinal local sign is first manifested) does not depend on time from onset of the target movement or ocular movement, but simply on the delay between presentations of the first and second flashes. This result is similar to the one described above in relation to saccades, and suggests some common aspects between the mechanisms for judgments of visual direction in the presence of voluntary saccades and pursuit eye movements. There are not yet enough data for the two types of situations, however, to permit any evaluation of the degree of commonality.

It has generally been assumed that stability of visual direction in the presence of voluntary saccades and the appearance of visual movement of the moving fixation target during ocular pursuit are manifestations of the same mechanism. For the former it has been presumed that the extraretinal signal regarding ocular movement "compensates" visual direction for the shift in location of the retinal images of stationary objects; for the latter it has been presumed that the extraretinal signal operates in a similar fashion but is "unopposed" by a shift in location of the retinal image. No direct evidence exists on this question, however.

C. Involuntary Eye Movements

1. Visual Direction during Fixation of a Visible Target

During fixation of a visible target (see Fig. 3) the probability that an involuntary saccade will return the eye toward a mean or "optimum" position increases monotonically and approaches 1.0 as the deviation of the eye from this position approaches 7′ (Cornsweet, 1956). Some correction of ocular position is also carried out by means of slow drifts (Nachmias, 1959). Since there is a considerable increase in amplitude and rate of the involuntary eye movements when the fixation target is removed and the subject attempts to maintain a steady eye position in the dark (Ditchburn, 1955; Cornsweet, 1956; Nachmias, 1960; Matin *et al.*, 1966; Matin, Matin, and Pearce, 1970; Skavenski and Steinman, 1970), it is clear that this correction is controlled mainly by information arising from the displacement of the image on the retina from some preferred position[20] and at most in only a minor way by information regarding deviation of the eye itself from a preferred position. Furthermore, since subjects do not "perceive the retinal locus stimulated," but rather perceive targets in particular visual directions, it is clear that the retinal displacement of the image of the fixation target could provide an effective signal regarding error in eye position only if the involuntary ocular displacement is not perfectly compensated by an extraretinal signal involved in the stabilization of visual direction. A similar conclusion follows if we assume that the useful information in eye position correction is direction of retinal image travel rather than a specific retinal offset (or set of offsets). The conclusions drawn in an earlier section regarding failure of the extraretinal signal to maintain stability of visual direction for successive stimulations separated by short durations, along with data regarding typical drift durations (0.5 sec) during attempts

[20] It has on occasion been suggested that the central 15′ or so in the "fovea" constitutes a "dead zone" within which detection of target displacement is not possible. Clearly this is not so. Cornsweet's (1956) results and also those of Beeler (1967) quite conclusively rule out the possibility of such a dead zone.

at steady fixation, and the values of thresholds for detection of direction of real target movement, all have a sufficient correspondence to support the conclusion drawn here that visual direction of a stationary target is not stabilized by an extraretinal signal at least during movement away from the optimum position.

Further evidence on this point stems from some binocular observations. With continuous binocular central fixation on a stereoscopically-presented target adjusted for zero fixation disparity, small brief flashes to eccentrically-located corresponding points of the two eyes will sometimes appear spatially separate ("binocular flash diplopia"). The frequency of this report increases with increase in delay between flashes to the two eyes and with decrease in the area of the flashed targets (MATIN, 1962). If accurate compensation of visual direction were associated with the involuntary eye movements, spatial doubling ought not to increase with delay.

Standard deviations of fluctuation in convergence between the two eyes are about 2′—3′ during attempts at steady fixation (KRAUSKOPF *et al.*, 1960). The sizeable correlation between the positions of the two eyes is almost wholly due to the synchrony and correlation in magnitude and direction of the involuntary saccades; drift components show no significant relationship. Although the relative size of synchronous saccades in the two eyes tend to correct for vergence errors, KRAUSKOPF *et al* (1960) have provided evidence that monocular errors in fixation rather than vergence errors provide the stimulus for saccades. The eye that is further from its optimum position generally triggers the saccade and its saccade magnitude is generally larger.

The magnitude of these fluctuations in convergence are roughly the same as PALMER (1961) finds in subjects' reports regarding whether the upper of two 1.5′ targets is to the left or right of the lower when the targets are presented simultaneously for 10 msec, one to each eye. The extent of PANUM's area measured with a similar pair of targets with no vertical disparity was about 15′ in the central fovea (PALMER, 1961). PALMER determined this from reports of "singleness" or "doubleness." The ability to report on spatial doubling is thus in part limited by processes of summation and fusion between stimulations to the two eyes. OGLE (1963) has found that reliable reports of depth in response to flashes presented successively to regions of the two eyes which vary in disparity from 0 to 2.5′ extend up to interstimulus intervals between 60 and 100 msec.

2. Visual Direction in Darkness

As indicated above, the increase in magnitude of the involuntary eye movements which occur in total darkness implies that accuracy of fixation of a visible target is controlled mainly, or perhaps wholly, by the displacement of the image on the retina from some preferred position. Typically, these movements contain very many fewer involuntary saccades than do movements in the presence of a visible target (Fig. 15). Available data indicate that the mean (unsigned) deviation of the eye from the prior fixation position increases with time in the dark, reaching about 25′ in 3 seconds (MATIN, MATIN and PEARCE, 1970) and 2° in 2 minutes (SKAVENSKI and STEINMAN, 1970). In addition, the eye irregularly changes mean position with time in the dark although the eye movement pattern deviates from a random walk (MATIN, MATIN, and PEARCE, 1970).

The increase in variablity in control of ocular position is accompanied by sizeable errors in the report of visual direction of a brief flash presented after fixation target removal to that of the previously-viewed fixation target (MATIN and KIBLER, 1966; MATIN, PEARCE, MATIN, and KIBLER, 1966). With a three second dark interval the proportion of correct reports increased monotonically with physical separation of the flash and fixation target with standard deviations of the response distributions that ranged from 17.4′ to 46.3′ with viewing in primary position; these increased systematically in secondary viewing positions. PSEs systematically shifted leftward and upward as viewing position was moved rightward and downward respectively, changing within a single subject by as much as 1°11′ in the horizontal dimension for a 69° change in viewing position, and 42′ in the vertical dimension for a 67–1/2° change in viewing position (Matin and Kibler, 1966).

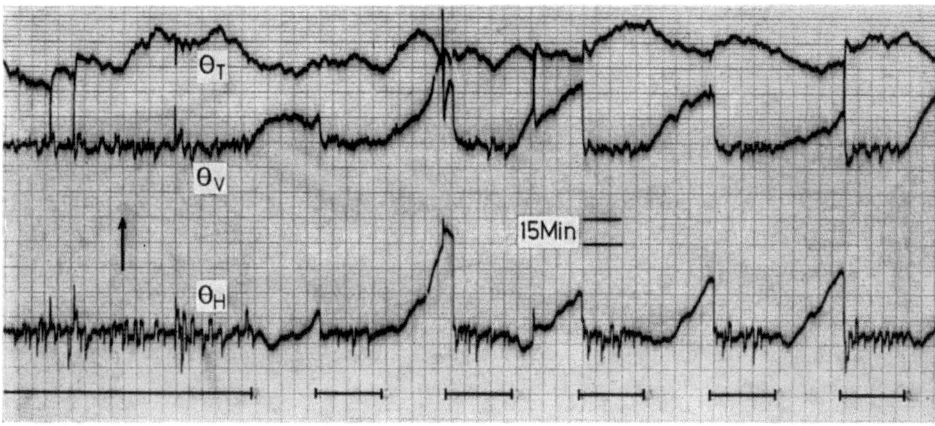

Fig. 15. Involuntary horizontal (Θ_H), vertical (Θ_V), and torsional (Θ_T) eye movements of left eye during periods in which fixation target was alternately visible and extinguished in an otherwise dark environment. The dark horizontal line at the bottom indicates periods during which target was visible; gaps indicate periods of total darkness. Subject attempted to maintain a steady fixation position. The 15′ calibration applies to all three traces. Arrow indicates ocular rotation to right in Θ_H, downward in Θ_V, and top of eye nasalward in Θ_T. Time lines separated by 1 sec. (From Matin and Pearce, 1964)

Between 2/3 and 3/4 of the variance of the response distribution for the horizontal discrimination in primary position was accounted for by making use of simultaneous measurements of eye position (Matin, Pearce, Matin, and Kibler, 1966). Independently of where the eye was located at the moment of flash presentation, the proportion of reports that the flash was to the right of the fixation target increased monotonically as the retinal location of the test flash lay further to the right. Since the psychophysical report for any particular retinal locus of flash stimulation was independent of eye position it was concluded that systematic participation of extraretinal signals containing accurate information regarding eye position was not involved in the report of flash direction relative to the previously-viewed fixation target. Offset of PSE at the retina of as much as 12′ from the central fovea (the mean retinal locus that had been occupied by the image of the fixation target), however, indicated that systematic distortions in local sign had taken place. Similar conclusions were reached by Fiorentini and Ercoles (1968) for similar kinds of experiments employing stabilized images.

In further experiments (Matin, Matin, and Pola, 1968), two vertical lines, one above and the other below a fixation target, were sequentially flashed in darkness each for 2 msec 400 msec after the removal of the fixation target and a report of horizontal vernier offset was obtained. Trial-to-trial variability of the response distribution increased with the interstimulus temporal interval through 800 msec along a negatively accelerated curve (Fig. 16). As in the experiments described above in which the visual direction of a subsequently-presented flash was compared to that of a previously-viewed fixation target, a portion of the response variability was predictable simply from the offset at the retina of the two flashes.

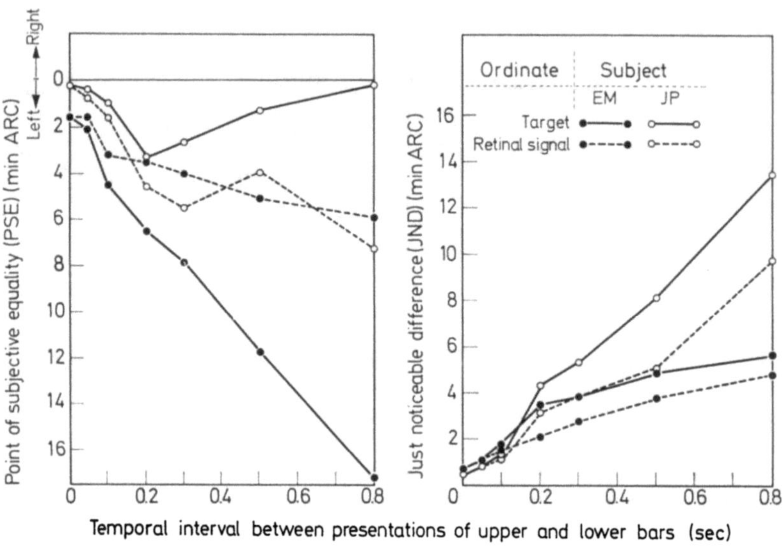

Fig. 16. Points of subjective equality (PSEs) and just noticeable differences (JNDs) for detection of horizontal vernier offset as a function of time between flashed presentations of two vertical lines. "Target" values refer to visual angle distances at the stimulus array. "Retinal Signal" values refer to visual distances at the retina; these were calculated from horizontal offset of the two flashed targets and eye positions at the moments that the two targets were flashed. (From MATIN, MATIN, and POLA, 1968)

Thus, for example Fig. 17 shows the response distribution over trials for one subject when the two lines had a fixed spatial relation to each other on all trials and were sequentially presented with a 100 msec interflash interval. The horizontal retinal offset (abscissa) between the two lines is thus a result of the 21" of target offset fixed over all trials represented in Fig. 17 *plus* the offset resulting from the eye movement between the flashed presentation of the two lines (variable from trial). Not only did response variability increase with interflash interval when target offset at the stimulus array was considered without considerations of eye movement, but an increase also was obtained with horizontal *retinal* offset treated as the stimulus (as in Fig. 17); this is also shown in Fig. 16. By employing distributions such as Fig. 17 for different target offsets at any given interstimulus interval, it was possible to compare the response to a given retinal offset under conditions in which the eye had moved different distances in the interflash interval. Since no systematic differences in response were obtained it was possible to conclude that systematic participation of extraretinal signals containing accurate information about the eye movement that had occurred in the interflash interval was not involved in the report of relative visual direction. The latter conclusion held at all interflash intervals and was in agreement with the conclusions reached in the experiments described above in which the previously-viewed fixation target was compared to a subsequent flash.

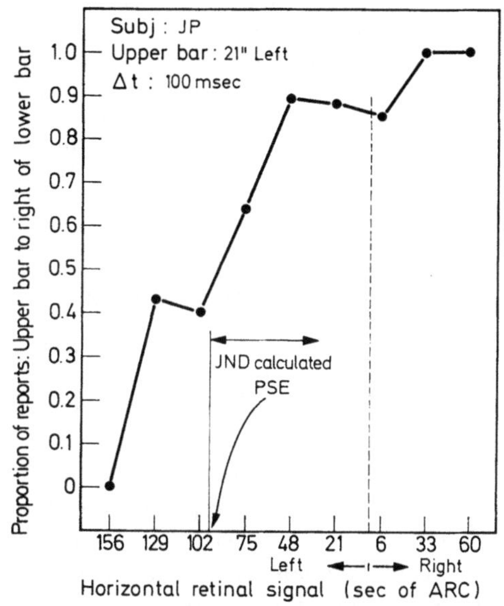

Fig. 17. Proportion of trials in which subject JP reported that the upper vertical bar appeared to the right of the lower vertical bar when one was flashed 100 msec after the other. At the target array the upper bar was 21″ to the left of the lower bar. The abscissa is the horizontal offset between the retinal loci of the two flashes; trial-to-trial variation in this retinal distance is wholly due to trial-to-trial variation in the eye movement between the two flashes. (From MATIN, MATIN, and POLA, 1968)

However, as in the previous experiments, the PSEs showed substantial offsets from physical colinearity of the targets (Fig. 16). Considered in terms of *retinal* offset, PSEs increased monotonically from values of 20″ when the lines were simultaneously presented through interflash intervals of 800 msec at which point values of about 6′ were obtained (Fig. 16).

It was suggested that the increase in variability of retinal offset for the discrimination of visual direction as well as the systematically increased mean "error" as time elapses between viewing of the two targets whose visual directions are being compared are both indications of a "gradual loss of memory" for the location of the target viewed first (MATIN, PEARCE, MATIN, and KIBLER, 1966; MATIN, MATIN, and POLA, 1968). It was also suggested that the lack of a systematic influence of eye position in these experiments (apart from its effect on the retinal locus stimulated by a flash from a target at a particular location) might be a consequence of a stochastic accumulation of errors in the relation between magnitudes of actual eye position change and the associated extraretinal signals, and that such "noise" might in part underlie the loss of memory (MATIN, PEARCE, MATIN, and KIBLER, 1966).

This "loss of memory" would not be easy to reconcile with KOFFKA's (1935) related view that no stable localization is possible without a stable visual framework. For KOFFKA the apparent vertical and horizontal are determined by the main lines of organization of the visual field, and localization is made relative to them. Since no visual field is present during the experimental session, KOFFKA's formulation predicts that memory loss should progress throughout a session in spite of periodic presentation of the fixation target-test flash sequence. Such a progressive increase in errors was not found.

A deeper analysis than we can provide here would consider the question of whether a memory loss involves a change in remembered direction (e.g. a target striking a retinal locus which originally signaled "straight ahead" is remembered as lying "to the left" when recall or recognition is tested X seconds later) or such remembered directions remain stable and subsequent inputs to the same retinal locus are seen in different directions than previous ones. Similar questions need to be raised regarding the shifts in local signs related to saccades and pursuit movements.

3. Ocular Torsion in Relation to Visual Direction and Orientation

When a subject assumes a particular direction of gaze, rotation of the eye about the visual axis relative to the orbit may be defined as a torsional rotation. Production of torsional movement is not under voluntary control. However, it has been suggested that torsional responses are stimulated by (a) viewing several different kinds of visual stimuli, and (b) rotation of the head in the frontal plane. In both cases the existence and quantitative properties of such movements need to be considered, and if they exist the question arises as to whether or not they are accompanied by extraretinal signals which influence visual direction. Torsion also accompanies rotations of the globe to tertiary positions of gaze (this has often been called "false torsion"). The discussion below will be limited to (a).

a) Tilt Adaptation. If a line tilted from the vertical within a frontal plane is viewed monocularly for a period of time it appears less tilted. Immediately after viewing the tilted line, the subject reports that a vertical line appears tilted from the vertical (GIBSON and RADNER, 1937; GIBSON, 1937). The change is of the order of 1.5° after viewing a line tilted by 5° for 20 seconds. GIBSON (1937) considered the effect in the context of successive contrast and adaptation to norms. KÖHLER and WALLACH (1944) suggested that it could be treated simply as a figural aftereffect whose general characteristic was an apparent displacement of the test figure away from the location of the inspection figure. The existence of a factor other than or in addition to figural aftereffect displacement is indicated by the fact that after viewing a line tilted from the vertical, a horizontal line appears tilted in the same direction as does a vertical line. The horizontal line appears tilted toward the previously-viewed line which is contrary to the displacement principle of figural aftereffects. In fact, tilt aftereffects of several kinds have been distinguished (MIKELIAN and HELD, 1964; MORANT and BELLER, 1965; EBENHOLTZ, 1968; MORANT and MISTOVICH, 1970).

The apparent tilts of both vertical and horizontal lines are compatible with the occurrence of a torsional eye movement in the same direction as the tilt of the line turned from vertical. Nevertheless, although HOWARD and TEMPLETON's (1964) subjects displayed a 2° tilt aftereffect to viewing a line tilted 10° from vertical for 10 seconds, they were unable to measure any mean change of torsional eye position by means of a technique capable of 0.2° resolution.

b) Cyclofusion and Torsion. HOFMANN and BIELSCHOWSKY (1900) used cards of identical print on the two sides of a haploscope. A horizontal line was above center on one card and below center on the other. The fused view is of a single card of print with two horizontal parallel lines. When the two cards are slowly rotated in opposite directions about their centers, fusion is maintained and the lines continue to appear parallel until rotations of 5° to 8° are reached at which point the lines gradually begin to deviate from parallelism and with further rotation fusion breaks. From this it has been concluded that as long as the lines remain parallel, in both eyes ocular torsion has occurred of a magnitude equal to the card rotation (OGLE, 1946).

A sizeable number of other phenomena suggest a similar conclusion. For example: When a binocularly fixated vertical line is tilted around its center in the median plane it no longer can strike the same retinal meridians on the two retinas that it did when it was vertical unless torsional movements occur in opposite directions in the two eyes. Yet such a tilted line has been reported to continue to appear vertical without the onset of diplopia (OGLE, 1946).

By means of meridional afocal magnification lenses, OGLE and ELLERBROCK (1946) simultaneously introduced binocular retinal disparities of equal magnitudes in a vertical and horizontal line, but in directions such that, if the binocular disparity for the vertical line were to be eliminated by ocular torsion, the disparity for the horizontal line would be simultaneously doubled, and vice versa (Fig. 18).

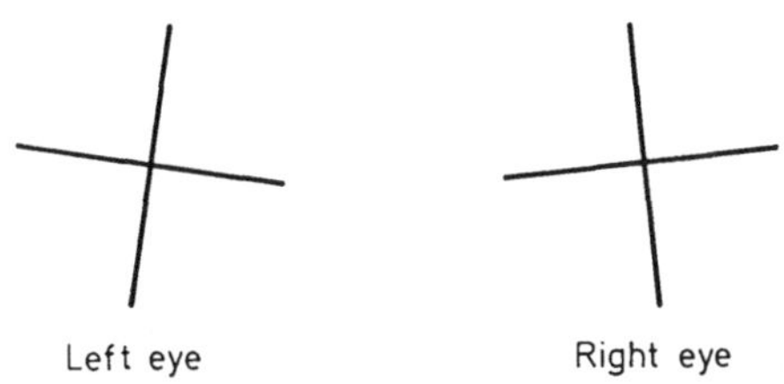

Fig. 18. Stimuli presented to the left and right eyes by OGLE and ELLERBROOK (1946). The fused image of the lines nearer the vertical appears like a line in the median plane with the top tilted toward the observer. By rotating the near-vertical lines alone (in effect, this rotation was by equal angles to the two eyes, but in opposite directions in the frontal plane) a setting was determined at which the line no longer appeared tilted

If such targets produce stimuli for torsion, then the stimuli from the two lines were for torsion in opposite directions. Under these conditions the vertical line does appear tilted out of the frontal plane in the direction of the physical tilt predictable from its disparity. OGLE and ELLERBROCK then had their subjects adjust the line tilted from vertical until it appeared vertical. This was done over an 80° range of induced tilts and yielded settings which suggested that torsion of a magnitude sufficient to remove the binocular disparity for the horizontal line had occurred (see Fig. 19).

A substantial number of related phenomena have been subsumed under the name "binocular depth contrast" (WERNER, 1937; OGLE, 1946). WERNER (1937) suggested that these phenomena involved a change in retinal correspondence between the two eyes. OGLE (1946) later suggested that these phenomena and the ones described above indicate that torsion takes place in the interest of maintaining fusion. However, he also reports that when one or more vertical lines are placed on each side of a line tilted within the median plane, the tilted line appears tilted in the direction appropriate to the physical tilt within the median plane and the vertical lines appear tilted in the opposite direction. In this case, while torsion can succeed in placing the retinal images of either the vertical or tilted lines on corresponding meridians, it cannot accomplish both simultaneously. Yet all lines continue to appear single, which indicates, like the examples described above, that torsion is not necessary for fusion to take place.

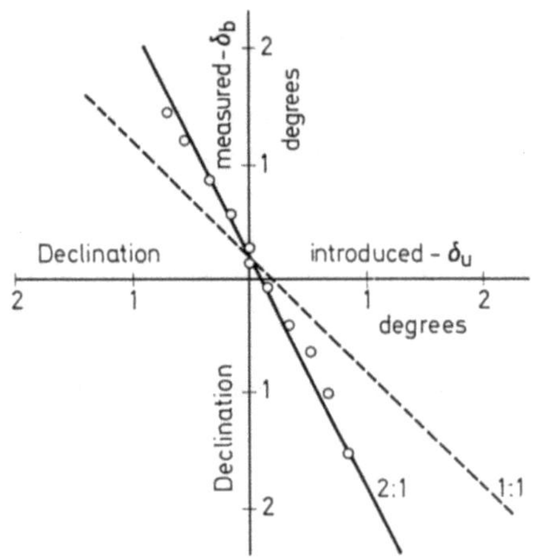

Fig. 19. Data for the configuration in Fig. 18. Declination introduced — δ_u (abscissa) is the deviation of the near-horizontal lines from horizontal. Declination measured — δ_b (ordinate) is the deviation of each of the retinal images of the near-vertical lines from the physical vertical when the fused image appears vertical. (A value of about 1.9° for δ_b would be produced under normal conditions when both eyes view a line tilted in the median plane by 50° at 2 meter viewing distance). That the data follow the 2 : 1 ratio is ascribed by OGLE and ELLERBROOK (1946) to the eyes' torting so as to eliminate declination at the retinas for the near-horizontal lines; the subject's setting eliminates declination at the retinas for the near vertical lines

Some of the binocular depth contrast phenomena were later independently treated in the context of three dimensional figural aftereffects (KÖHLER and EMERY, 1947). That something other than figural aftereffect displacement is probably involved, however, is indicated by the fact that such aftereffects are not predicted when the same single tilted line serves both as inspection and test figure; but as indicated above, the latter is an important case in point.

In 1936 BEASLEY and PECKHAM looked at the eye through a telescope and reported in a brief note that they could observe no torsion under conditions in which vertical stimuli were rotated by $\pm 10°$ (or horizontal stimuli rotated by $\pm 3°$) in stereoviewing while fusion was maintained. Recently, KERTESZ and JONES (1970) have reported the maintenance of fusion for rotations by $\pm 5°$ in each eye of stereoscopically-presented horizontal lines (as in Fig. 18). But measurement of torsion by a contact-lens technique and by observation of a radial conjunctival blood vessel did not reveal any change in torsional position of the eye while fusion was so maintained. (They report a resolution of 0.5 and 0.25° for the two methods respectively). Further, by comparing the magnitude of binocular vertical retinal disparity introduced by the rotation of the horizontal lines to MITCHELL'S (1966) values for the sizes of Panum's area, KERTESZ and JONES (1970) conclude that fusion could have been maintained within Panum's area entirely without the occurrence of torsion.

Although the fact that fusion does not require torsion in the situations described above was clear in the older data, KERTESZ and JONES' failure to find torsion suggests the possibility of local sign flexibility in some of the phenomena described above and the need for new explanations. Thus, the facts that a line tilted in the median plane appears vertical when viewed alone, and appears appropriately tilted when viewed along with a fused horizontal line with equal sized but "oppositely-directed" disparity (Fig. 18) are left unexplained. The former may be a manifestation of simultaneous tilt adaptation in the two eyes. The latter phenomenon and some of the binocular depth contrast phenomena can be similarly interpreted.

A simplified statement of one such interpretation is: Simultaneous viewing of the two lines in Fig. 18 by each eye alone would induce opposite tendencies for tilt adaptation; hence no net adaptation would occur in each eye. Thus when the targets in Fig. 18 are viewed, the fused image arising from the lines tilted from vertical in the frontal plane should continue to yield the appearance of a line tilted in the median plane. However, the basis of tilt adaptation itself is not understood. In addition, in the original demonstration by HOFMANN and BIELSCHOWSKY, the two horizontal lines (one to each eye) would have changed their relative retinal orientations by 10° to 16° if no torsion had taken place. More work is needed on these problems.

D. Convergence

Within some limits objects do not normally appear to undergo substantial changes in size when viewing distance is changed despite size changes in the retinal image. When fixation is shifted from a distant point to a near point the triple response of convergence, accommodation, and pupillary contraction occurs. Whether extraretinal signals associated with any of these oculomotor adjustments are involved in the mechanisms underlying size constancy is a question that has proved difficult to analyze. No clear information is presently available with regard to either accommodation or pupillary size changes. However, HEINEMANN, TULVING, and NACHMIAS (1959) have quite convincingly shown that variation in convergence does result in changes of apparent size in a direction appropriate to assist in the production of size constancy.

In their experiments subjects were required to compare the sizes of two discs sequentially presented at different distances under conditions in which contextual cues were eliminated. Use of 0.5 mm artificial pupils eliminated changes in accommodative adjustment in response to a change in viewing distance, and under one condition variations of accommodation were eliminated with drugs. When the subjects carried out a monocular comparison of a variable disc presented at a distance of 400 cm with a 1° standard disc presented at 25, 33.3, 50, 100, or 300 cm, the size equation (with the artificial pupil in place) resulted in settings that were essentially retinal size matches. However, when a binocularly-viewed fixation point was fused under different degrees of convergence (with artificial pupils) the size comparison of the discs (again monocularly-viewed) changed with viewing distance in a way that did not result in an equation of the retinal images of the two discs. The retinal image of the more distant disc (at 400 cm, viewed monocularly with convergence appropriate to the distance) had to be made smaller than that of the nearer disc (at variable distance but always subtending 1°, and viewed monocularly with convergence appropriate to its distance) in order to appear equal to it. This decrease in size changed systematically with viewing distance of the nearer disc (in the direction of a tendency towards size constancy). The total effect of convergence itself, however, is only a small part of size constancy. Identical effects were obtained with and without paralysis of accommodation. The latter condition eliminated changes in accommodation consequent to changed convergence and the resultant possibility of an extraretinal involvement due to accommodative change itself. Essentially similar results have been obtained by BIERSDORF, OHWAKI, and KOZIL (1963).

E. Basis for Extraretinal Signals Related to Eye Movements

HELMHOLTZ (1866) concluded from the appearance of visual movement consequent on attempts at turning the paralyzed eye and consequent to passive ocular movement that an extraretinal signal derived from the "effort of will" was responsible for maintaining the normal appearance of stability when the direction of gaze was changed ("outflow theory"). Unopposed by the normal displacement of the image at the retina in the paralyzed eye, this signal was presumed to give rise to the visual appearance of movement. Unopposed by the "effort of will", the retinal image displacement caused by passive eye movement was also presumed to give rise to visual movement. On the other hand, JAMES (1906) and SHERRINGTON (1918) argued that muscle spindles in the extraocular musculature provided the source for the extraretinal signal resulting in perceptual stability when eye movements occur ("inflow theory"). The evidence presented in earlier sections above makes it clear that the extraretinal signal, regardless of its source, is not sufficient to account for the normal stability of perception of stationary objects. Nevertheless, the basis for the extraretinal signal remains a problem.

The results with the immobilized (MACH, 1906) or paralyzed eye have weighed most heavily in the considerable number of subsequent evaluations of the problem, and KORNMULLER's (1930) work, in which the subject reported visual apparent movement when he attempted to turn his eyes following novacaine injection into his extraocular muscles, is generally considered to provide the clearest support for the older observations. This is also generally considered decisive in favor of outflow theory. Since the paralyzed eye does not move it has been presumed that change in muscle spindle discharge could not be involved when an attempt is made to turn the eye. Furthermore, the observation that an afterimage viewed in darkness does not appear to move as a consequence of passive eye movement (HELMHOLTZ, 1866) has also been cited in support of outflow theory, as has the finding that involuntary movements during attempts at steady fixation in darkness do not systematically influence fluctuations in local sign (MATIN *et al.*, 1966. See above).

These results are less than critical, however, and further considerations are in order. (These considerations are taken here not to affirm the validity of the hybrid mechanism described below, but to point out that the "paralyzed-eye" experiments cannot, without further kinds of manipulations, rule out the utility of an inflow signal in determining visual perception of direction.) KORNMÜLLER (1930) did not believe that the novacaine which he injected into the extraocular muscles in the region of the insertion in the globe produced paralysis, but that instead the large mass of injected fluid produced an exophthalmic condition which in effect immobilized the eye. Further, if muscle spindles continue to be active in such immobilization, or in experimental or clinical paralysis, apparent movement on attempts to turn the eye does not at all rule on whether the extraretinal signal is inflowing or outflowing. It is now well-known that two sources can modify the afferent signal from muscle spindles: (1) Modification occurs when the extrafusal muscle is stretched or contracted. (2) Modification occurs when motor innervation to the intrafusal muscle fiber that is part of the spindle is changed (GRANIT, 1955). The latter innervation is via the gamma efferent motor fibers, some of whose sources of control are central and do not appear to lie within direct reflex paths such as might be expected to produce stretch reflexes. It is thus possible that when the extrafusal muscle of extraocular musculature was paralyzed, intrafusal fibers remained active. Certainly this would be so in experiments which involve immobilization without paralysis. One possible consequence of a subject attempting to turn his eye then is a centrally-arising increase in excitation of the gamma-efferents leading to spindles in the agonist muscle and a reduction of excitation or an inhibition of the gamma efferents leading to spindles in the antagonist. These changes would result in an increase in tension in the associated intrafusal muscle of the spindles in the agonist and a decrease in tension in the associated intrafusal muscle of spindles in the antagonist. Such a consequence would produce oppositely-directed modifications in the afferent signals from muscle spindles in the two muscles and thus could give rise to a directionally-biased extraretinal signal which produces a change in the relation between perceived visual direction and retinal locus when the subject attempts to change his direction of gaze. Such a result does not depend at all then on whether the eye position, and so muscle length, actually changes or not. If the attempt does not yield an eye movement, as in the paralyzed or immobilized eye, the extraretinal signal would produce an appearance of visual movement; if the attempt yields an eye movement, as in the normal eye, visual movement would not result (MATIN and MATIN, in preparation).

Since the location of most spindles is at the other end of the muscle from the site of KORNMÜLLER's novacaine injection, and since the anesthetic did not appear to diffuse rapidly, continued spindle activity is not unlikely. Whether spindles remain active in fresh cases of clinical paralysis, when visual apparent movement occurs with attempts to turn the eye by the paralyzed muscle(s), is also unclear. Still further, SIEBECK (1954) reports that curare injections into extraocular muscle resulted in apparent movement only during the prodromal period when attempts were made to turn the eye. He reports that when paralysis was complete such attempts did not result in apparent movement, and ascribes this to the subject's awareness of his limitation of change of the direction of gaze. Since transmission in extrafusal neuromuscular junctions is more sensitive to curare than transmission at intrafusal myoneural junctions (MATTHEWS, 1964) it would also be expected that the gamma control of spindle afference would be eliminated later during the developing paralysis. SIEBECK's results are thus easily interpretable in terms of the hybrid mechanism pointed to in the previous paragraph. This hybrid mechanism could also serve to explain some aspects of the information presented above. For one thing the sizeable shifts in local sign for stimulation presented as early as 240 msec before the saccade (MATIN, MATIN, and POLA, 1970; see also Fig. 10) are not reasonably treated in terms of SHERRINGTON's inflow theory which requires the occurrence of the eye movement before extraretinal signal generation can occur. In addition, the influence of either eye position or saccade length on the shift of local sign for test flashes following the saccade (Fig. 10) requires that outflow theory become somewhat more complicated. It can be handled directly, however, by the hybrid mechanism. A more detailed analysis of the psychophysical and pharmacological aspects of the "paralyzed eye" could do much to clarify the mechanism. Among other things, it would be worth knowing whether the elimination of apparent movement after the prodromal period in SIEBECK's experiments could be caused by the effects of learning during that period.

Although the dual control of spindle output, and the consequent possibility of a hybrid mechanism, make the available "paralyzed eye" data less crucial for support of the outflow theory (indeed SIEBECK's report provides negative evidence), a variety of related considerations have led a number of workers to conclude that muscle spindles play no role in our sense of position — for the eye or for limbs — or in determining perceived visual direction (IRVINE and LUDVIGH, 1936; LUDVIGH, 1952a, b; ROSE and MOUNTCASTLE, 1959; BRINDLEY and MERTON, 1960; MERTON, 1961, 1964). Noting that afferent signals from muscle spindles are not uniquely related to muscle length (and so, in limbs, to joint angle and limb position), due to modulation of these signals by the gamma efferent fibers which control the tension of the intrafusal muscle fibers of the spindle, ROSE and MOUNTCASTLE (1959) conclude that signals from the spindles cannot reliably inform on limb position. In addition, they question previous reports that spindle signals arrive at somatosensory cortex, considering such arrival necessary if spindles are to subserve a sense of limb position. The necessity for such arrival if spindles are to mediate a position sense may be questioned. In any case, the presence of spindle signals from forelimb muscle arriving at the cortex has been established in cat (OSCARSSON and ROSEN, 1966), and the possibility of further instances cannot be ruled out.

Perhaps most damaging to the possibility that signals from muscle spindles inform on position sense or influence visual direction is the attractiveness of the interpretation which treats them as "misalignment detectors" (MERTON, 1951, 1964; ELDRED, GRANIT, and MERTON, 1953). This interpretation assumes (a) that such detectors serve to maintain muscle length constant under varying load, and (b) that voluntary attempts at movement result in gamma barrage which produces an increased spindle output preceding the contraction of extrafusal muscle, and that extrafusal muscle contracts only so far as is necessary in order to return the signals from spindles back to the level they had before the command to move was given. If this is the case, then spindle signals could hardly serve to signal muscle length. Too little is known about single units during voluntary movements to consider it as more than an interesting hypothesis at the moment. MATTHEWS (1964) states "the idea that movements are ever normally initiated solely by means of the γ route is not yet established." Although GRANIT (1966) contests this, his argument does not refer to voluntary movements in the intact preparation. In fact the results of TAUB *et al.* (1966) on monkeys with spinal deafferentation raise serious questions for the misalignment hypothesis as fundamental in voluntary movement.

For jointed limbs it is clear that position sense for passive movements is subserved in a major way by receptors in the joints since anesthetization of a joint either considerably reduces or completely eliminates the ability of a subject to report on passive movement of the attached limb (see ROSE and MOUNTCASTLE, 1959, and MERTON, 1964 for summaries). Further, MERTON reports that when a pneumatic tourniquet is placed on the wrist, making the joint and skin of the thumb anesthetic without any effect on the muscles, the subject becomes insensitive to passive movements of the top joint of the thumb. Active movements (without visual stimulation) are made with the same accuracy as without ischemia, and if movement is restrained by holding the thumb while the subject attempts to move it he believes that he has succeeded in moving it. In MERTON's subject stretch reflexes remained, as indicated by increased electromyographically recorded discharge from the flexor when the upper joint of the thumb was forcibly extended while the subject was attempting to maintain steady flexion. MERTON reports that the subject could generally detect the forced extension but attributes it to slight consequent movements of the forearm causing slight changes in pressure to the skin rather than to changes in spindle output.

In jointed limbs a given limb position may be associated with a large range of loads on the associated muscle. It is not known for the case of voluntary movement whether such variations in muscle tonus at fixed limb positions are associated with variation of afferent signals from muscle spindles, although this appears to be likely. If this is so, the likelihood of spindle signals as useful sources for informing on limb position is reduced. However, for the extraocular muscles under normal conditions, muscle load and length (and thus eye position) are in an essentially invariant relation. Nor do the muscles serve an antigravity function. Stretch reflexes do not seem to be present. Something approaching an invariant steady state relation between gamma input, spindle output, and muscle length is thus a more likely possibility for extraocular muscle.

In experiments partially analogous to those MERTON (1964) reports for the anesthetized thumb, BRINDLEY and MERTON (1960) have found that when the eyes of subjects in total darkness are passively rotated (by pulling with forceps on the anesthetized conjunctiva), the subject is not able to report a change in eye position even for rotations as large as 30°. Since the muscle spindles present in human extraocular muscle (COOPER and DANIEL, 1949) must have been stimulated, it was concluded that whatever information is available for verbal communication regarding eye position or change in eye position does not arise from spindles. On the other hand, when the eyes were prevented from rotating (again in total darkness) while the subjects attempted to turn them, they reported that the eyes did turn (BRINDLEY and MERTON, 1960). The authors interpret these results as supporting an outflow mechanism for the position sense, as does MERTON (1964) for the experiments on the thumb. However, the latter result could be a consequence of a hybrid mechanism at work with gamma motor input changing during the attempt at turning the eyes and producing a change in spindle output which is treated as change in eye position by the subject. In addition, SKAVENSKI (1970) has recently reported that when a subject's eye is pulled from a resting position in darkness while he attempts to maintain a prior fixation position during maintained application of the force, his subsequent movements return the eye toward the prior position. The subject is able to correctly report the direction of pull when a force of at least 10 gm is imposed (1.25 gm/deg. is the normal relation between applied force and ocular rotation: ROBINSON, 1964; SKAVENSKI, 1970). The basis for the disagreement between the results of BRINDLEY and MERTON (1960) and of SKAVENSKI (1970) is as yet unclear. Although it is not altogether likely in view of the large rotations to which BRINDLEY and MERTON subjected the eyes of their subjects, the possibility exists that the passivity of their subjects (they were not attempting to hold their eyes in a given position) played some role in their inability to report that their eyes were turned by unloading the spindles via the gamma motor fibers. Some support for this possibility, and for this version of a hybrid approach to the ocular position sense, can be found in WHITTERIDGE'S (1959) report that increased input to the gamma motor fibers subserving spindles in the extraocular muscle of the goat resulted in an increased sensitivity of the spindle to stretch (i.e., an increased slope of the function relating spindle firing rate to applied stretch). If this were the case in humans it would provide a basis for interpretation by the hybrid mechanism for both of BRINDLEY and MERTON'S key observations and for both of SKAVENSKI'S.

Selective elimination of spindle output from extraocular muscle has not yet been feasible although it would clearly be a desirable means of separating inflow and outflow signals. Monkeys with complete spinal deafferentation can reach accurately for seen objects without viewing the hand (TAUB *et al.*, 1966; TAUB and BERMAN, 1968), thus demonstrating the presence of an outflow signal involved in position sense for the arm and the lack of necessity for signals from muscle spindles. The possibility of inflow involvement, however, is indicated by the finding that adaptation to horizontal displacement of the visual field induced by wearing wedge prisms, normal monkeys showed only a 39 % initial aftereffect on prism removal, whereas for deafferented animals the initial aftereffect was 100 % (TAUB *et al.*, 1966; TAUB and BERMAN, 1968). Whether the inflow involvement is spindle-mediated, or mediated by cutaneous and joint receptors cannot yet be decided, however, since spinal deafferentation was complete.

In effect, then, for the visual system we are left with no clear picture as yet whether an inflowing signal (via a hybrid mechanism) or an outflowing signal, or both, are involved in the ocular position sense or in the visual perception of direction. This ambiguity of outcome is perhaps mirrored in uncertainty about the neural locus of such an extraretinal signal. Although not entirely ruled out, the primary visual projection system through striate cortex is unlikely. The frontal eye fields have sometimes been considered as a prime possibility for such a locus. However, this possibility has not yet been sufficiently explored. BIZZI (1968) and BIZZI and SCHILLER (1970) report two types of cells related to eye movements in the frontal eye fields. Units of Type 1 discharged during (but not before) saccades in a given direction and during the fast phase of optokinetic or vestibularly-induced nystagmus, but were silent during slow eye movements and during steady fixation. Units of Type II responded during steady fixation, during slow movements, and during the slow phase of nystagmus with discharge frequency monotonically related to eye position. These show quiescence during saccades. Neither type appears to be influenced by visual stimulation. The authors mention some indirect evidence against the relation of their results to an inflowing mechanism, but the interpretation is by no means certain as yet. Some single cells in the superior colliculus have visual receptive fields (SCHAEFER, 1966; McILWAIN and BUSER, 1968; STERLING and WICKELGREN, 1969), others receive vestibular (SCHAEFER, 1967) or proprioceptive inputs (COOPER *et al.*, 1953), while others without apparent direct sensory control fire before eye movements (WURTZ and GOLDBERG, 1971). This has suggested the superior colliculus as a focus at which extraretinal signals may influence the perception of space. Of course, it is entirely possible that transformations of local signs by extraretinal inputs involves activity at more than one central neural locus.

It is reasonable to think that a subject's difficulty or inability to verbally report eye position and to control eye position in darkness, and his ability to counteract and report the direction of an imposed rotational force applied to the eye bear on the question of the basis of the extraretinal signal involved in visual direction. In this discussion, these effects have been considered separately as well as together. The connection, however, is not a necessary one. Although it is frequently presumed that the extraretinal signal involved in visual direction should be identical to the one used for reporting on eye position and for controlling it, it has not been conclusively shown that information on eye position influences the perception of direction of visual stimuli. There are, however, a number of studies in which subjects were required to report on the direction of visually-presented targets and the data are interpreted as measures of an ocular position sense. Clearly the question of where a subject feels his eye to be and where he sees a visual target are separable questions. How the two are related is an additional question. Although some basis for a relation is evident in experiments involving modification by experience, this issue takes us beyond the scope of the present chapter. (See HELD and FREEDMAN, 1963; HARRIS, 1965; ROCK, 1966; HOWARD and TEMPLETON, 1966, for related considerations.)

Acknowledgement. The writing of this chapter was supported by research grant NSF GB-5947 from the National Science Foundation and by PHS Grant R01-5-EY00375 from the National Eye Institute, National Institutes of Health.

References

ADAMS, H. F.: Autokinetic sensations. Psychol. Monogr. **14**, 1—45 (1912).

ALPERN, M.: Metacontract. J. opt. Soc. Amer. **43**, 648—657 (1953).

ANDERSEN, E. E., WEYMOUTH, F. W.: Visual perception and the retinal mosaic. 1. Retinal mean local sign — an explanation of the fineness of binocular perception of distance. Amer. J. Physiol. **64**, 591—594 (1923).

ANDREWS, D. P.: Perception of contours in the central fovea. Nature (Lond.) **205**, 1218—1220 (1965).

— Perception of contour orientation in the central fovea, part 1. Short lines. Vision Res. **7**, 975—997 (1967a).

— Perception of contour orientation in the central fovea, part II. Spatial integration. Vision Res. **7**, 999—1013 (1967b).

ARNULF, A., DUPUY, O.: La transmission des contrastes par le système optique de l'oeil et les seuils des contrastes rétiniens. C. R. Acad. Sci. (Paris) **250**, 2757—2759 (1960).

Aubert, H.: Eine scheinbare bedeutende Drehung von Objekten bei Neigung des Kopfes nach rechts oder links. Arch. path. Anat. **20**, 381—393 (1861).
— Die Bewegungsempfindung. Arch. ges. Physiol. **39**, 347—370 (1886).
Averill, H. L., Weymouth, F. W.: Visual perception and the retinal mosaic. II. The influence of eye-movements on the displacement threshold. J. comp. Psychol. **5**, 147—176 (1925).
Baker, K. E.: Some variables influencing vernier acuity. 1. Illumination and exposure time. 2. Wave-length of illumination. J. opt. Soc. Amer. **39**, 567—575 (1949).
Barmack, N.: Dynamic visual acuity as an index of eye movement control. Vision Res. **10**, 1431—1441 (1970).
Bauermeister, M.: Effect of body tilt on apparent verticality, apparent body position, and their relation. J. exp. Psychol. **67**, 142—147 (1964).
Beasley, W. C., Peckham, R. H.: An objective study of cyclotorsion. Psychol. Bull. **33**, 741—742 (abstract) (1936).
Beck, J.: Accommodative astigmatism and pattern acuity. Presented at Eastern Psychological Association 1965.
Becker, W., Fuchs, A. F.: Further properties of the human saccadic system: eye movements and correction saccades with and without visual fixation points. Vision Res. **9**, 1247—1258 (1969).
Beeler, G. W.: Visual threshold changes resulting from spontaneous saccadic eye movements. Vision Res. **7**, 769—775 (1967).
Békésy, G. von: Neural volleys and the similarity between some sensations produced by tones and by skin vibrations. J. acoust. Soc. Amer. **29**, 1059—1069 (1957).
— Experiments in Hearing. New York: McGraw-Hill 1960.
— Sensory Inhibition. Princeton: Princeton Univ. 1967.
Berry, R. N.: Quantitative relations among vernier, real depth, and stereoscopic depth acuities. J. exp. Psychol. **40**, 708—801 (1948).
— Riggs, L. A., Duncan, C. P.: The relation of vernier and depth discriminations to field brightness. J. exp. Psychol. **40**, 349—354 (1950).
Biersdorf, W. R., Ohwaki, S., Kozil, D.: The effect of instructions and oculomotor adjustments on apparent size. Amer. J. Psychol. **76**, 1—17 (1963).
Bizzi, E.: Discharge of frontal eye field neurons during saccadic and following eye movements in unanesthetized monkeys. Exp. Brain Res. **6**, 69—80 (1968).
— Schiller, P.: Single unit activity in the frontal eye fields of unanesthetized monkeys during eye and head movement. Exp. Brain Res. **10**, 151—158 (1970).
Bouma, H., Andriessen, J. J.: Perceived orientation of isolated line segments. Vision Res. **8**, 493—607 (1968).
— — Induced changes in the perceived orientation of line segments. Vision Res. **10**, 333—349 (1970).
Bourdon, B.: La perception visuelle de l'espace. Paris: Librairie C. Reinwald 1902.
Brindley, G. S., Merton, P. A.: The absence of position sense in the human eye. J. Physiol. (Lond.) **153**, 127—130 (1960).
Campbell, F. W., Kulikowski, J. J.: Orientational selectivity of the human visual system. J. Physiol. (Lond.) **187**, 437—445 (1966).
— — Levinson, J.: The effect of orientation on the visual resolution of gratings. J. Physiol. (Lond.) **187**, 427—436 (1966).
Carr, H. A.: The autokinetic sensation. Psychol. Rev. **17**, 42—75 (1910).
Cooper, S., Daniel, P. M.: Muscle spindles in human extrinsic eye muscles. Brain **72**, 1—24 (1949).
— — Whitteridge, D.: Nerve impulses in the brainstem of the goat. Responses with long latencies obtained by stretching the extrinsic eye muscles. J. Physiol. (Lond.) **120**, 491—513 (1953).
Cornsweet, T. N.: Determination of the stimuli for involuntary drifts and saccadic eye movements. J. opt. Soc. Amer. **46**, 987—993 (1956).
Crone, R., Lunel, H.: Autokinesis and the perception of movement: the physiology of eccentric fixation. Vision Res. **9**, 89—102 (1969).
Deckert, G. H.: Pursuit eye movements in the absence of a moving stimulus. Science **143**, 1192—1193 (1964).

Ditchburn, R. W.: Eye-movements in relation to retinal action. Optica Acta **1**, 171—176 (1955).
— Ginsborg, B. L.: Vision with a stabilized retinal image. Nature **170**, 36—37 (1952).
Dodge, R.: Visual perception during eye movement. Psychol. Rev. **7**, 454—465 (1900).
— The illusion of clear vision during eye movement. Psychol. Bull. **2**, 193—199 (1905).
— Travis, R. C., Fox, J. C.: Optic nystagmus III. Characteristics of the slow phase. Arch. Neurol. **24**, 21—34 (1930).
Ebenholtz, S.: Some evidence for a comparator in adaptation to optical tilt. J. exp. Psychol. **77**, 94—100 (1968).
Eldred, E., Granit, R., Merton, P.: Supraspinal control of the muscle spindles and its significance. J. Physiol. (Lond.) **122**, 498—523 (1953).
Fender, D. H., Nye, P. W.: An investigation of the mechanisms of eye movement control. Kybernetik **1**, 81—88 (1961).
— — The effects of retinal image motion in a simple pattern recognition task. Kybernetik **2**, 192—199 (1962).
Filhene, W.: Über das optische Wahrnehmen von Bewegungen. Z. Sinnesphysiol. **53**, 134—145 (1922).
Fiorentini, A., Ercoles, A. M.: Visual direction of a point source in the dark. Atti Fond. G. Ronchi **23**, 405—428 (1968).
Ganz, L.: Mechanism of the figural aftereffects. Psychol. Rev. **73**, 128—150 (1966).
Gertz, H.: Über die gleitende (langsame) Augenbewegung. Zeitschrift für Psychologie und Physiologie der Sinnesorgane. Abteilung 2: Z. Sinnesphysiol. **49**, 29—58 (1916).
Gibson, J. J.: Adaptation with negative aftereffect. Psychol. Rev. **44**, 222—243 (1937).
— Radner, M.: Adaptation, after-effect and contrast in the perception of tilted lines. 1. Quantitative studies. J. exp. Psychol. **20**, 453—457 (1937).
Gilbert, D. S.: Monocular estimates on distance and direction with stabilized and non-stabilized retinal images. Vision Res. **9**, 103—115 (1969).
Graham, C. H.: Depth and movement. Amer. Psychologist **23**, 18—26 (1968).
Granit, R.: Receptors and Sensory Perception. New Haven: Yale University Press 1955.
— Effects of stretch and contraction on the membrane of motor neurons. In: Granit, R. (Ed.) Muscular Afferents and Motor Control. Nobel Symp. **1**, 37—50 (1966).
Gregory, R. L.: Eye movements and the stability of the visual world. Nature (Lond.) **182**, 1214—1216 (1958).
Hamblin, J. E., Winsor, T. H.: On the resolution of gratings by the astigmatic eye. Opt. Soc. (Lond.) **29**, 28—42 (1927—1928).
Harris, C. S.: Perceptual adaptation to inverted, reversed, and displaced vision. Psychol. Rev. **72**, 419—444 (1965).
Heinemann, E. R., Tulving, E., Nachmias, J.: The effect of oculomotor adjustments on apparent size. Amer. J. Psychol. **72**, 32—45 (1959).
Held, R., Freedman, S. J.: Plasticity in human sensorimotor control. Science **142**, 455—462 (1963).
Helmholtz, H. von: Handbuch der Physiologischen Optik. Leipzig: Voss 1866. English translation from Edit. 3, 1925. Southall, J. P. C. (Ed.): A Treatise on Physiological Optics, 1963, Vol. 3. New York: Dover 1963.
Henderson, D.: Movement perception and the displacement threshold. Perc. Psychophys. **10**, 313—320 (1971).
Hering, E.: Der Raumsinn und die Bewegungen des Auges. In: Hermann, L.: Handbuch der Physiologie 3 (Part 1), 1879. English translation, Radde, C. A. (Ed.): Spatial Sense and Movement of the Eye. Amer. J. Optom. 1942.
— Über die Grenzen der Sehschärfe. Ber. Königl. Sächs. ges. Wiss. math.-phys. Kl. Leipzig **20**, 16—24 (1899).
Higgins, G. C., Stultz, K. V.: Variation of visual acuity with various test object orientations and viewing conditions. J. opt. Soc. Amer. **40**, 135—137 (1950).
Hofmann, F. B., Bielschowsky, A.: Über die der Willkür entzogenen Fusionsbewegungen der Augen. Plügers Arch. ges. Physiol. **80**, 20—28 (1900) (quoted in Ogle, 1950).
Holt, E. B.: Eye movement and central anesthesia. Harv. Psychol. Stud. **1**, 3—45 (1903).

HOWARD, I. P., TEMPLETON, W. B.: Visually-induced eye torsion and tilt adaptation. Vision Res. **4**, 433—437 (1964).

— — Human Spatial Orientation. New York: Wiley, 1966.

HUBEL, D. H., WIESEL, T. N.: Receptive fields, binocular interaction and functional architecture in the cat's visual cortex. J. Physiol. (Lond.) **160**, 106—154 (1962).

— — Receptive fields and functional architecture of monkey striate cortex. J. Physiol. (Lond.) **195**, 215—243 (1968).

IRVINE, S., LUDVIGH, E.: Is ocular proprioceptive sense concerned in vision. Arch. Ophthal. **15**, 1037—1049 (1936).

JAMES, W.: The Principles of Psychology. Vol. II. Holt, 1890. Reprinted New York: Dover 1950.

KAHNEMAN, D.: Method, findings, and theory in studies of visual masking. Psychol. Bull. **70**, 404—425 (1968).

KEESEY, U. T.: Effects of involuntary eye movements on visual acuity. J. opt. Soc. Amer. **50**, 769—774 (1960).

KERTESZ, A. E., JONES, R. W.: Human cyclofusional response. Vision Res. **10**, 891—896 (1970).

KOFFKA, K.: Principles of Gestalt Psychology. New York: Harcourt 1935.

KÖHLER, W., EMERY, D. A.: Figural aftereffects in the third dimension of visual space. Amer. J. Psychol. **60**, 159—201 (1947).

— WALLACH, H.: Figural aftereffects: an investigation of visual processes. Proc. Amer. Phil. Soc. 88, 269—357 (1944).

KOLERS, P. A.: Intensity and contour effects in visual masking. Vision Res. **2**, 277—294 (1962).

— ROSNER, B. S.: On visual masking (metacontrast): dichoptic observation. Amer. J. Psychol. **73**, 2—21 (1960).

KORNMÜLLER, A. E.: Eine experimentelle Anaesthesie der äußeren Augenmuskeln am Menschen und ihre Auswirkungen. J. Psychol. Neurol. **41**, 354—366 (1930).

KRAUSKOPF, J., CORNSWEET, T. N., RIGGS, L. A.: Analysis of eye movements during monocular and binocular fixation. J. opt. Soc. Amer. **50**, 572—578 (1960).

LATOUR, P. L.: Visual threshold during eye movements. Vision Res. **2**, 261—262 (1962).

LEIBOWITZ, H.: Some observations and theory on the variation of visual acuity with the orientation of the test object. J. opt. Soc. Amer. **43**, 902—905 (1953).

LOTZE, H.: Outline of Psychology. Translated and edited by Ladd, G. T. Boston: Ginn 1886.

LUDVIGH, E.: Possible role of proprioception in the extraocular muscles. Arch. Ophthal. **48**, 436—441 (1952a).

— Control of ocular movements and visual interpretation of the environment. Arch. Ophthal. **48**, 442—448 (1952b).

— Direction sense of the eye. Amer. J. Ophthal. **36**, 139—143 (1953).

MACH, E.: Analysis of Sensations. Trans. from first Germ. Ed. (1885) by WILLIAMS, C. M., Rev. and Suppl. from fifth Germ. Ed. New York: Dover 1959.

MACKAY, D. M.: Elevation of visual threshold by displacement of retinal image. Nature (Lond.) **225**, 90—92 (1970).

MARSHALL, W. H., TALBOT, S. A.: Recent evidence for neural mechanisms in vision leading to a general theory of sensory acuity. Biol. Symp. **7**, 117—164 (1942).

MATIN, E., CLYMER, A., MATIN, L.: Metacontrast and saccadic suppression. In preparation.

— MATIN, L., POLA, J., KOWAL, K.: The intermittent light illusion and constancy of visual direction during voluntary saccades. Presented at Psychonomic Society 1969.

MATIN, L.: Binocular summation at the absolute threshold of peripheral vision. J. opt. Soc. Amer. **52**, 1276—1286 (1962).

— Measurement of eye movements by contact-lens techniques: Analysis of measuring systems and some new methodology for three dimensional recording. J. opt. Soc. Amer. **54**, 1008—1018 (1964).

— Eye movements and visual direction. Symposium: Problems of sensorimotor control in the C. N. S.: The role of feedback, feedforward and the corollary motor discharge. Amer. Psychol. Assoc. 1968.

— KIBLER, G.: Acuity of visual direction in the dark for various positions of the eye in the orbit. Perc. Mot. Sk. **22**, 407—420 (1966).

MATIN, L., MACKINNON, E.: Autokinetic movement: selective manipulation of directional components by image stabilization. Science **143**, 147—148 (1964).
— MATIN, E.: A possible hybrid mechanism for modification of visual direction associated with eye movements — The paralyzed eye experiment reconsidered. In preparation.
— — PEARCE, D. G.: Visual perception of direction when voluntary saccades occur: 1. Relation of visual direction of a fixation target extinguished before a saccade to a flash presented during the saccade. Perc. Psychophys. **5**, 65—80 (1969).
— — — Eye movements in the dark during the attempt to maintain a prior fixation position. Vision Res. **10**, 837—857 (1970).
— — POLA, J.: Detection of vernier offset, eye movements, and autokinetic movement. Presented at Eastern Psychological Association 1968.
— — — Visual perception of direction when voluntary saccades occur: II. Relation of visual direction of a fixation target extinguished before a saccade to a subsequent test flash presented before the saccade. Perc. Psychophys. **8**, 9—14 (1970).
— — — Visual perception of direction when voluntary saccades occur: III. Relation af visual direction of a fixation target extinguished before a saccade to a test flash after the saccade. In preparation.
— — — BOWEN, R.: Relative visual direction of two flashes presented at different times or intensities during a voluntary saccade — retinal constraints in the operation of extra-retinal signals. Presented at Eastern Psychological Association 1971.
— — — PEARCE, D. G.: Visual perception of direction for stimuli flashed before, during, and after voluntary saccadic eye movements. Presented at Psychonomic Society 1968.
— PEARCE, D. G.: Three-dimensional recording of rotational eye movements by a new contact-lens technique. MURRY, W. E., SALISBURY, P. F. (Ed.): Biomedical Sciences Instrumentation, pp. 79—95. New York: Plenum Press 1964.
— — Visual perception of direction for stimuli flashed during voluntary saccadic eye movements. Science **148**, 1485—1488 (1965).
— — MACKINNON, G. E.: Variation in directional components of autokinetic movement as a function of the position of the eye in the orbit. J. opt. Soc. Amer. **53**, 521 (abs.) (1963).
— — MATIN, E., KIBLER, G.: Visual perception of direction in the dark: roles of local sign, eye movements, and ocular proprioception. Vision Res. **6**, 453—469 (1966).
MATTHEWS, P. B. C.: Muscle spindles and their motor control. Physiol. Rev. **44**, 219—288 (1964).
MCCOLLOUGH, C.: Color adaptation of edge-detectors in the human visual system. Science **149**, 1115—1116 (1965).
MCILWAIN, J. T., BUSER, P.: Receptive fields of single cells in the cat's superior colliculus. Exp. Brain Res., **5**, 314—325 (1968).
MCLAUGHLIN, S. C.: Parametric adjustment in saccadic eye movements. Perc. Psychophys. **2**, 359—362 (1967).
MERTON, P. A.: The silent period in a muscle of the human hand. J. Physiol. (Lond.) **114**, 183—198 (1951).
— The accuracy of directing the eyes and the hand in the dark. J. Physiol. (Lond.) **156**, 555—577 (1961).
— Human position sense and sense of effort. Symp. Soc. exp. Biol. **18**, 387—400 (1964).
MIKELIAN, H., HELD, R.: Two types of adaptation to an optically-rotated visual field. Amer. J. Psychol. **77**, 257—263 (1964).
MILLER, E. F., II.: Counterrolling of the human eyes produced by head tilt with respect to gravity. Acta Oto-Laryng. **54**, 479—501 (1962).
MITCHELL, D. E.: A review of the concept of Panum's fusional areas. Amer. J. Ophthal. **43**, 387—401 (1966).
MORANT, R. B., BELLER, H. K.: Adaptation to prismatically rotated visual fields. Science **148**, 530—531 (1965).
— MISTOVICH, M.: Tilt after-effects between the vertical and horizontal axes. Perc. Mot. Sk. **10**, 75—81 (1970).
MÜLLER, G. E.: Über das Aubertsche Phänomen. Z. Sinnesphysiol. **49**, 109—244 (1916).
NACHMIAS, J.: Two-dimensional motion of the retinal image during monocular fixation. J. opt. Soc. Amer. **49**, 901—908 (1959).

Nachmias, J.: Meridional variations in visual acuity and eye movements during fixation. J. opt. Soc. Amer. **50**, 569—571 (1960).

Ogilvie, J. C., Taylor, M. M.: Effect of orientation on the visibility of fine wire. J. opt. Soc. Amer. **48**, 628—629 (1958).

Ogle, K. N.: The binocular depth contrast phenomenon. Amer. J. Psychol. **59**, 111—126 (1946).

— Researches in Binocular Vision. Philadelphia: W.B. Saunders 1950.

— Stereoscopic depth perception and exposure delay between images to the two eyes. J. opt. Soc. Amer. **53**, 1296—1304 (1963).

— Ellerbrock, V. J.: Cyclofusional movements. Arch. Ophthal. **36**, 700—735 (1946).

— Weil, M. P.: Stereoscopic vision and the duration of the stimulus. Arch. Ophthal. **59**, 4—17 (1958).

Onley, J. W., Volkmann, J.: The visual perception of perpendicularity. Amer. J. Psychol. **71**, 504—516 (1958).

Oscarsson, O., Rosen, I.: Short-latency projections to the cat's cerebral cortex from skin and muscle afferents in the contralateral forelimb. J. Physiol. (Lond.) **182**, 164—184 (1966).

Osgood, C. E., Heyer, A. W., Jr.: A new interpretation of figural after-effects. Psychol. Rev. **59**, 98—118 (1952).

Oyster, C. W., Barlow, H. B.: Direction-selective units in rabbit retina: distribution of preferred directions. Science **155**, 841—842 (1967).

Palmer, D. A.: Measurement of the horizontal extent of Panum's area by a method of constant stimuli. Optica Acta 8, 151—159 (1961).

Pearce, D.: Consistency of individual patterns of autokinetic direction. Perc. Mot. Sk. **23**, 1119—1123 (1966).

— Matin, L.: The measurement of autokinetic speed. Can. J. Psychol. **20**, 160—172 (1966).

— — Variation of the magnitude of the horizontal-vertical illusion with retinal eccentricity. Perc. Psychophys. **6**, 241—243 (1969).

— Porter, E.: Changes in visual sensitivity associated with voluntary saccades. Psychon. Sci. **19**, 225—227 (1970).

Pettigrew, J. D., Nikara, T., Bishop, P. O.: Responses to moving slits by single units in cat striate cortex. Exp. Brain Res. **6**, 373—390 (1968).

Pola, J.: Visual direction of a flash presented during or following saccades of variable length to an 8° peripheral target. Presented at Eastern Psychologial Association 1971.

Puckett, J. D., Steinman, R. M.: Tracking eye movements with and without saccadic correction. Vision Res. **9**, 695—703 (1969).

Raab, D. H.: Backward Masking. Psychol. Bull. **60**, 118—129 (1963).

Rashbass, C.: The relationship between saccadic and smooth tracking eye movements. J. Physiol. (Lond.) **159**, 326—338 (1961).

Ratliff, F.: Mach Bands: Quantitative Studies on Neural Networks in the Retina. San Francisco: Holden-Day 1965.

Richards, W.: Saccadic suppression. J. opt. Soc. Amer. **59**, 617—623 (1969).

Riggs, L. A., Armington, J. C., Ratliff, F.: Motions of the retinal image during fixation. J. opt. Soc. Amer. **44**, 315—321 (1954).

— Ratliff, F., Cornsweet, J., Cornsweet, T. N.: The disappearance of steadily fixated visual test objects. J. opt. Soc. Amer. **43**, 495—501 (1953).

Robinson, D. A.: The mechanics of human saccadic eye movement. J. Physiol. (Lond.) **174**, 245—264 (1964).

— The mechanics of human smooth pursuit eye movement. J. Physiol. (Lond.) **180**, 569—591 (1965).

Rochlin, A. M.: The effect of tilt on the visual perception of parallelness. Amer. J. Psychol. **68**, 223—236 (1955).

Rock, I.: The Nature of Perceptual Adaptation. New York: Basic Books 1966.

Rose, J. R., Mountcastle, V. B.: Touch and Kinesthesis. In: Handbook of Physiology: Sect. 1. Neurophysiology, Vol. 1. Field, J., Magoun, H., Hall, V. E. (Eds.) Amer. Physiol. Soc., Wash., D. C. Ch. **17**, 409—415 (1959).

SCHAEFER, K.-P.: Mikroableitungen im Tectum opticum des frei beweglichen Kaninchens: Ein experimenteller Beitrag zum Problem des Bewegungssehens. Arch. Psychiat. Nerv. **208**, 120—146 (1966).

— Neuronale Entladungsmuster im Tectum opticum des Kaninchens bei passiven und aktiven Eigenbewegungen. Arch. Psychiat. Nerv. **209**, 101—125 (1967).

SCHÖNE, H.: Über den Einfluß der Schwerkraft auf die Augenrollung und auf die Wahrnehmung der Lage im Raum. Z. vergl. Physiol. **46**, 57—87 (1962).

SEKULER, R. W., RUBIN, E. L., CUSHMAN, W. H.: Selectivities of human visual mechanisms for direction of movement and contour orientation. J. opt. Soc. Amer. **58**. 1146—1150 (1968).

SHERRINGTON, C. S.: Observations on the sensual role of the proprioceptive nerve supply of the extrinsic ocular muscles. Brain **41**, 332—343 (1918).

SHORTESS, G. K., KRAUSKOPF, J.: Role of involuntary eye movements in stereoscopic acuity. J. opt. Soc. Amer. **51**, 555—559 (1961).

SIEBECK, R.: Wahrnehmungsstörung und Störungswahrnehmung bei Augenmuskellähmungen. Graefes Arch. Ophthal. **155**, 26—34 (1954).

SKAVENSKI, A.: Mechanisms underlying control of eye position in the dark. Ph. D. Dissertation, University of Maryland, 1970.

— STEINMAN, R. M.: Control of eye position in the dark. Vision Res. **10**, 193—203 (1970).

SMITH, V. C.: Scotopic and photopic functions for visual band movement. Vision Res. **9**, 293—304 (1969a).

— Temporal and spatial interactions involved in the band movement phenomenon. Vision Res. **9**, 665—676 (1969b).

STARK, L., VOSSIUS, G., YOUNG, L. R.: Predictive control of eye tracking movements. Institute of Radio Engineers. Transactions on Human Factors in Electronics HFE-3, 52—57, 1962.

ST-CYR, G. J., FENDER, D. H.: Nonlinearities of the human oculomotor system: time delays. Vision Res. **9**, 1491—1503 (1969).

STERLING, P., WICKELGREN, B. G.: Visual receptive fields in the superior colliculus of the cat. J. Neurophysiol., **32**, 1—15 (1969).

STIGLER, R.: Chronothotische Studien über den Umgebungskontrast. Pflügers Arch. ges. Physiol. **134**, 365—435 (1910).

STOPER, A. E.: Vision during pursuit movement: the role of oculomotor information. Ph. D. Dissertation. Brandeis University, 1968.

SULZER, R. L.: A determination of several functions relating sensitivity of perception of parallelness to stimulus dimensions. Ph. D. dissertation, Duke University, 1954.

— ZENER, K.: A quantitative analysis of relations between stimulus determinants and sensitivity of the visual perception of parallelness. Amer. Psychologist **8**, 444 (1953).

TAUB, E., BERMAN, A.: Movement and learning in the absence of sensory feedback. In: The Neuropsychology of Spatially Oriented Behavior. FREEDMAN, S. (Ed.), Ch. 11, pp. 173—192. Homewood: Dorsey 1968.

— ELLMAN, S., BERMAN, A.: Deafferentation in monkeys: effect on conditioned grasp response. Science **151**, 593—594 (1966).

VENIAR, F.: Difference thresholds for shape distortion of geometrical squares. J. Psychol. **26**, 461—476 (1948).

VOLKMANN, F.: Vision during voluntary saccadic eye movements. J. opt. Soc. Amer. **52**, 571—578 (1962).

— SCHICK, A. M. L., RIGGS, L. A.: Time course of visual inhibition during voluntary saccades. J. opt. Soc. Amer. **58**, 562—569 (1968).

WALLS, G. L.: Factors in human visual resolution. J. opt. Soc. Amer. **33**, 487—505 (1943).

WEISSTEIN, N.: What the frog's eye tells the human brain: single cell analyzers in the human visual system. Psychol. Bull. **72**, 157—176 (1969).

WERNER, H.: Studies on contour: 1. Qualitative analyses. Amer. J. Psychol. **47**, 40—64 (1935).

— Dynamics in depth perception. Psychol. Monogr. **49**, 1—127 (1937).

WESTHEIMER, G.: Eye movement responses to a horizontally moving visual stimulus. Arch. Ophthal. **52**, 932—941 (1954).

Westheimer, G., Conover, D. W.: Smooth eye movements in the absence of a moving visual stimulus. J. exp. Psychol. **47**, 283—284 (1954).
Weymouth, F. W.: Visual sensory units and the minimal angle of resolution. Amer. J. Ophthal. **46**, 102—113 (1958).
— Stimulus orientation and threshold: an optical analysis. Amer. J. Ophthal. **48**, 6—10 (1959).
— Andersen, E. E., Averill, H. H.: Retinal mean local sign: a new view of the relation of the retinal mosaic to visual perception. Amer. J. Physiol. **63**, 410—411 (1923).
Whitteridge, R.: The effect of stimulation of intrafusal muscle fibres on sensitivity to stretch of extraocular muscle spindles. Quart. J. exp. Physiol. **44**, 385—393 (1959).
Witkin, H. A., Asch, S. E.: Studies in space orientation: III. Perception of the upright in the absence of a visual field. J. exp. Psychol. **38**, 603—614 (1948).
Woellner, R. C., Graybiel, A.: Reflex ocular torsion in healthy males. Proj. NM. 17.01.11 Subtask 1, Rep. No. 47. U. S. Nav. Sch. aviat. Med., Pensacola, Fla., 1958.
Wurtz, R. H., Goldberg, M. E.: Superior colliculus cell responses related to eye movements in awake monkey. Science **171**, 82—84 (1971).
Zuber, B. L., Stark, L.: Saccadic suppression: Elevation of visual threshold associated with saccadic eye movements. Exp. Neurol. **16**, 65—79 (1966).

Chapter 14

Theoretical Issues of Color Vision

By

DOROTHEA JAMESON, Philadelphia, Pennsylvania (USA)

With 9 Figures

Contents

I. Introduction

The scope and purpose of color theory are differently defined by different investigators (LE GRAND, 1968, Ch. 19). For some, the overriding problem is to account for trivariance and trichromasy. For some, also the only valid scientific "givens" are those numerical data that can be obtained by using the eye as a "null detector". These are the results of what BRINDLEY (1960) calls "Class A" experiments. One can, of course, describe the data of perceived color identity without ever making any reference to hue names and without specifying the qualities that are presumably generated by means of spectrally selective mechanisms of physiological response to light stimulation. It is, however, more common for experimenters *qua* interpreters to tag the mechanisms they discuss with hue names that imply a specific quality code.

A broader view of the objective of color theory is that it constitutes an attempt to explain, by hypothesis, the mechanisms whereby (a) we see the particular colors that we see and (b) make, or fail to make, the visual discriminations that we do on the basis of perceived color differences. In this chapter, the broader definition is assumed, and it is from this point of view that we shall review the current status of color theory with respect to a series of issues, some of which seem near resolution, others that are still far from resolution at the present time.

The problem of trivariance and the psychophysical data of color identity or just-detectable non-identity bring us directly to grips with the theoretical concentration on receptor pigment distributions as the physiological substrate which seems, for many, to be of exclusive or nearly exclusive interest. Such restricted concentration on visual cone pigments would, of course, be justified if it seemed likely, on theoretical, anatomical, or physiological grounds, that the retinal mechanisms basic to the "quality code" for color vision were simply the cone receptors together with an uncomplicated reflection of their properties in the subsequent substrates of neural transmission. The picture we now have of the fine structure of the retina and its synaptic connections is, however, not consistent with such a simplistic view.

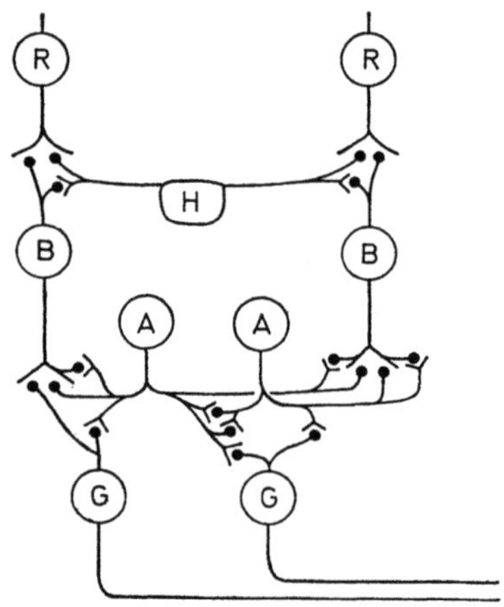

Fig. 1. Diagrammatic representation of the various retinal structures and their synaptic interrelations, based on the work of Dowling and Werblin (1969) on the vertebrate retina. Receptors (*R*) drive both bipolar (*B*) and horizontal (*H*) cells; horizontals synapse laterally on adjacent bipolars; bipolar terminals to both ganglion (*G*) and amacrine (*A*) cells. Amacrines make feedback synapses on *B* terminals, feed-forward synapses on *G* cells, feed-forward and lateral, serial synapses on other A cell processes

Fig. 1 is a diagrammatic representation of the various retinal structures and their synaptic interrelations, based on the work on the vertebrate retina of Dowling and his associates (Dowling and Boycott, 1966; Dowling and Werblin, 1969; Dowling, 1970). The retinal organization is seen to be one in which the receptor cells form synaptic contacts with both bipolar and horizontal cells, and bipolars are synaptically related to both horizontal[1] and amacrine cells as well as serving in the "transmission line" between receptors and retinal ganglion cells. Electrophysiological recordings show only sustained hyperpolarizing responses to light stimulation in the receptors and in the horizontal cells, hyperpolarizing and depolarizing responses in the bipolars and amacrine cells, and both

[1] A recent report by Kolb (1970) based on electron microscopy gives a somewhat different representation of horizontal cell contacts, showing dendritic contact with 7 to 12 cones, and axonal contact to numerous rod spherules, with an overlap of 4 to 6 horizontal cells onto a single cone pedicule.

"on-" and "off-" type spike discharges in the ganglion cells (WERBLIN and DOWLING, 1969; DOWLING, 1970).

Evidence from a variety of species has now accumulated, since the early demonstration by SVAETICHIN (1956), which shows that responses from individual units are spectrally selective, and that those units that show both hyperpolarizing and depolarizing responses, or both on- and off-spike discharges, may reverse the response made for different regions of the spectrum. The precise ways in which the spectral selective responses are altered between the receptors and ganglion cells cannot yet be specified on the basis of individually identified units, although recent technical improvements in both recording (TOMITA *et al.*, 1967) and dye-marking (MILLER and DOWLING, 1970) make such knowledge predictably immanent.

As we shall see in the following sections of this chapter, many issues crucial to a detailed specification of the functional basis of normal color vision remain unresolved in terms of the physiological evidence, hence hypotheses deduced from perceptual experiments on intact organisms continue to have a decisive influence on our interpretations of the mechanisms involved.

Some of the issues that will be discussed in this context include the precise specification of cone receptor sensitivities as they relate to cone photopigment absorptions on the one hand and spectral color-mixture and luminosity data on the other; problems of linear and non-linear transducer mechanisms as they relate to both changes in color appearance with change in luminance and related measures of color discrimination; and issues concerned with short- and long-term characteristics of physiological responses and interactions as they enter in the complex spatio-temporal dependences of color perceptions and discriminations.

II. Color Mixture and Spectral Luminosity

The primary data that imply the existence of three cone types with different spectral selectivities, or three different cone pigments, are the data of three-stimulus color mixture. (See WRIGHT, chapter 16, this volume.) The basic assumption is very simply that different spectral energy distributions produce identical visual effects if and only if the different lights are equally absorbed in each of the spectrally selective receptor photopigments. Since only three independent stimulus manipulations are required for complete color matches, only three independent visual pigment absorptions are needed to satisfy the matching requirement. Furthermore, for lights restricted to the fovea, at least, the rhodopsin pigment of the rods is assumed to play no part in photopic vision, hence three cone photopigments must be present in the retina in addition to the rhodopsin of the scotopic rod receptor system.

Although photochemical studies of retinal extracts have been successful in revealing the absorption characteristics, photoproducts of bleaching, structural and functional properties of vitamin A_1 based rhodopsin and the parallel, Vitamin A_2 based, rod pigments, the cone pigments have not yielded so easily to such analysis. Hence the search has continued for many decades for psychophysical techniques that might lead, through analysis and inference, to a specification of the receptor sensitivities, and thus the photopigment absorptions, of the human cones. (For a discussion of spectrally selective wave-guide properties of receptors, see CRAWFORD, chapter 18, this volume.) A fundamental, and universally accepted restriction on any such hypothetical set of derived receptor functions is that they must be linearly related to the three-variable color-mixture data.

That this restriction alone still leaves a wide latitude in the choice of potential candidates for the "true" spectral distributions sought is illustrated in Fig. 2. Here we show the transformation of average color-mixture data to the $\bar{x}_\lambda$, $\bar{y}_\lambda$, $\bar{z}_\lambda$,

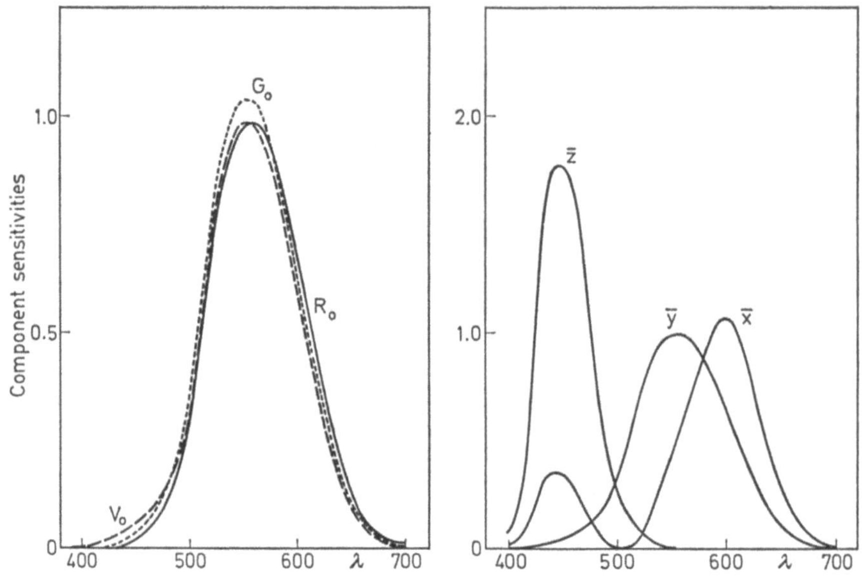

Fig. 2. HECHT's (1934) V_0, G_0, R_0 curves (left) and CIE tristimulus curves (right). Both sets are linear transformations of average experimental color-mixture data. $\bar{x}_\lambda$, $\bar{y}_\lambda$, $\bar{z}_\lambda$ plotted from WYSZECKI and STILES (1967) Table 3.2; V_0, G_0, R_0 plotted from transformation equations given by GRAHAM (1965), Eq. 15.36

curves of the CIE 1931 standard for colorimetry (Fig. 2, right) together with V_0, G_0, R_0, curves (Fig. 2, left) derived by HECHT (1934) in his own formulation of the Young theory. (For transformation equations, see GRAHAM, 1965.) Both sets of curves are equally satisfactory representations of the experimental color-matching data, but neither set now seems at all plausible to represent the cone photopigment distributions. The CIE curves have been taken to represent cone responses in one form of "zone theory" (see discussion by JUDD, 1966). It should be pointed out, however, that the CIE tristimulus values were not originally intended to describe receptor functions directly, but rather, this particular transformation was chosen largely on grounds of computational convenience for the colorimetrist and photometrist in that the $\bar{y}_\lambda$ curve also duplicates the standard photopic luminosity function, V_λ. (See LE GRAND chapter 15, this volume.) The Hecht curves, on the other hand, were intended to represent the spectral sensitivities of three cone types whose activities were presumably correlated in simple one-to-one fashion with three "fundamental" hue sensations. A similar set of distributions was suggested by HURVICH and JAMESON to represent the sensitivities of a set of cones which we labeled simply α, β, γ, since they were derived in the context of a very different theoretical model that does not locate the physiological hue-coding responses in the receptor mechanisms per se (HURVICH and JAMESON, 1955, 1957). A revised model of this same theory describes the receptor functions, α, β and γ approximately as shown in Fig. 3 (JAMESON and HURVICH, 1968). The issue of the cone photopigments as they relate to color-mixture data is, unfortunately, not yet resolved however, as we shall see below.

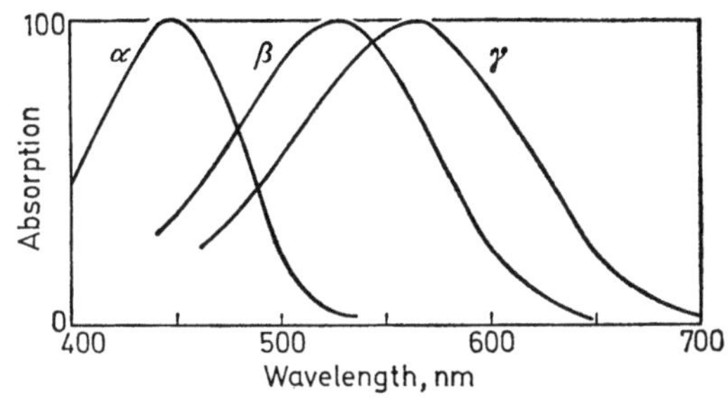

Fig. 3. Receptor distribution functions suggested by microspectrophotometric measures of individual human cones. (From JAMESON and HURVICH, 1968)

During the last decade, technical advances have made possible the measurement of visual pigments in the intact receptors, rather than in retinal extracts, and these measures have both confirmed the existence of three cone photopigments and have located, at least approximately, their wavelengths of maximal absorption (BROWN and WALD, 1963; 1964; MARKS *et al.*, 1964). The measures are not yet sufficiently extensive or precise to specify in detail the complete absorption spectra of the three cone pigments for the human eye. Presumably these absorptions will have the characteristic form described by the Dartnall nomogram (DARTNALL, 1953), and the data obtained by microspectrodensitometry of single cones from monkey and human retinas do seem to be consistent with the Dartnall rule. The curves of Fig. 3 are Dartnall-type absorption spectra with maxima at 448 nm, 528 nm, and 567 nm. These are average estimates of the measures of the human cone absorptions available at this time. The curves are uncertain in two respects: first, the total sample of human cones is very small and hence estimates of the average maxima for the different types are far from definitive; and second, neither the actual measures nor the nomogram representation extends throughout the visible spectrum and there is no firm basis for extrapolation. For comparison with the psychophysical color-mixture data, the latter difficulty is the more important one since three-valued absorption data are needed throughout the spectrum to derive three-variable color-mixture functions. One can, however, reverse the procedure, to see to what extent theoretically derived transforms of color-mixture data can be taken as consistent with the approximate maxima and spectrally limited forms of photopigment absorptions. As WYSZECKI and

Stiles (1967) have observed, when psychophysical results are analyzed and interpreted as representations of cone sensitivities, it is useful to compare the spectral distributions so interpreted with the form of the Dartnall visual pigment nomogram.

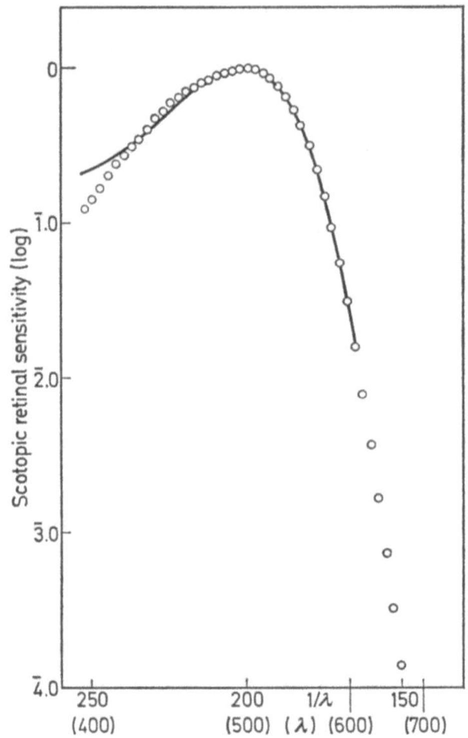

Fig. 4. Corrected scotopic luminosity function compared with absorption spectrum of rod rhodopsin. Plotted from Wyszecki and Stiles (1967) Table 7.9

Fig. 4 shows the extent to which we are justified in assuming that psychophysical measures of any sort can be expected to coincide with pigment distributions of the Dartnall type. This figure shows log rhodopsin absorption drawn as the solid line, and compared with it the standard scotopic luminosity function (V'_λ) after correction for the selective transmission of the ocular media and for quantum absorption. The agreement is clearly excellent.

Fig. 5a shows a linear transformation of the CIE 1931 color-mixture data to a set of curves with maxima at 450 nm, 540 nm and 560 nm. The transformed data points are represented by the symbols, and the curves are nomogram functions with appropriately located peak absorptions. The points are based on numerical results tabulated by Wyszecki and Stiles (1967, Table 5.5) shown here after correction for pre-retinal light losses and quantal absorption, and they are consistent with presumed receptor sensitivities that satisfy various theoretical postulates put forward by König. Although the 560 nm maximum distribution follows quite well a visual pigment form throughout most of its spectral extent, the fit to the 540 nm max distribution is somewhat less satisfactory, and the curve with the short-wave maximum at 450 nm is clearly too narrow in its band width to be represented acceptably by the pigment nomogram. The derivation of this particular set of functions depends on assumptions about photopic luminosity, the

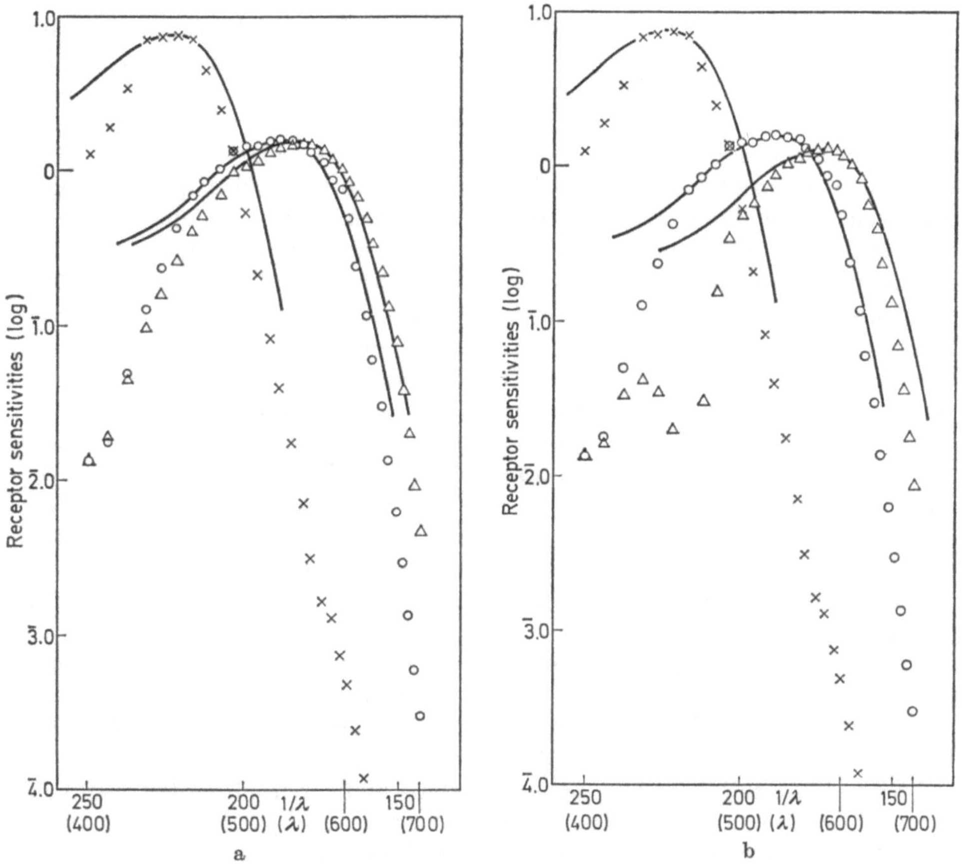

Fig. 5. a) Receptor distributions consistent with König theory and with color-mixture data. b) Receptor distributions consistent with Fick hypothesis and with color-mixture data. In both *a* and *b* curves are expected forms of pigment absorption functions

V_λ curve, for both normal trichromatic and dichromatic vision. The normal spectral luminosity function is assumed to reflect a simple linear combination of the component sensitivities (appropriately weighted) with maxima at 450 nm, 540 nm, and 560 nm, respectively. Protanopic dichromats, whose luminosity function is depressed in the long-wave spectral region, are assumed to have only the functions with maxima at 450 nm and 540 nm, and deuteranopic dichromats, whose spectral luminosity functions differ only slightly from the normal V_λ, and in the opposite direction from the protanopic deviation, are assumed to retain only the receptor components with maximal absorptions at 450 nm and 560 nm. (See Hurvich, chapter 23, this volume.) If the König assumption about deuteranopia is substituted by an alternative hypothesis, namely, that the three-variable information is degraded to a two-variable system by a collapse or fusion of two "channels" into one, rather than by the loss of one of the receptor pigments, then the curves of Fig. 5B result as the hypothetical receptor distributions for normal color vision. The 450 and 540 nm max curves are unchanged, but the third function is shifted to longer wavelengths with maximum at 580 nm. Again the data are based on the transformed results tabulated by Wyszecki and Stiles (1967, Table 5.5) for Fick's hypothesis, and in Fig. 5b they have been corrected for pre-retinal light losses and quantal absorption for comparison with the pigment nomogram (solid line). The 580 nm data show a small secondary maximum in the short-wave region of the spectrum. The existence, in the visible spectral range, of a secondary band of increased absorption in photolabile visual pigments cannot be definitively ruled out on the basis of cone pigment absorptions reported so far because of both the scarcity and noisiness of the available data. (For the latter, see Marks' 1965, results on Vitamin A_2 pigments for a large sample of goldfish cones.) Such a secondary maximum is not an infrequent result in transformations intended to account for both color-mixture data and various other psychophysical measures. Helmholtz, in fact, derived three "double-humped" curves by his line-element technique to account for some of the early data on both color mixture and wavelength discrimination (Helmholtz, 1896; Hurvich *et al.*, 1965). The study of visual pigments by difference spectra, involving as they do the formation of short-wave photoproducts, leaves the form of the absorption curve at the shortwave spectral extreme in considerable doubt until both the cone photopigments and their bleaching photoproducts have been chemically analyzed (Dartnall, 1962).

It is somewhat disappointing to the visual theorist that the studies of human cones by microspectrodensitometry have not been pressed forward to accumulate more definitive data after the initial very promising reports. Wald (1964; 1965; 1966; 1967; Wald and Brown, 1965) in fact, has taken the alternative approach and has pursued the cone photopigment analysis by inference from the results of psychophysical experiments. His procedure is the same as the Stiles (1959) two-color increment threshold technique (see Enoch, chapter 21, this volume), except that Wald limits his experimental conditions to a single, very high luminance background level of each of a few chromaticities selected to yield the narrowest possible spectral distribution of increment threshold sensitivities. The functions resulting from Stiles' analysis of his own more extensive two-color increment threshold data are plotted in Fig. 6 (from Wyszecki and Stiles, 1967, Table 7.6) where they are also compared with nomogram curves of the standard form for visual pigments. These functions appear rather frequently as instruments of data analysis in the current visual literature, and they are often treated as if they represented human cone absorptions, even though Stiles (1959) does not interpret them in this fashion, nor does he assume that they reflect only the activities of the receptor cells of the retina. Stiles has pointed out, moreover, that these functions cannot be derived by any simply linear transformation of the color-mixture data.

In summary, then, the present status of color theory with respect to cone receptor function seems to be as follows. The assumption that light is selectively absorbed by three cone photopigments with maximal absorptions, respectively, near 440–450 nm, 530–540 nm, and 560–580 nm seems consistent with all the data that can legitimately be brought to bear on this question. The assumption that the data of three-variable color mixture (correctly expressed in terms of retinal stimulus values) and the absorption spectra of the three cone photopigments are related to each other by a linear transformation has yet to be

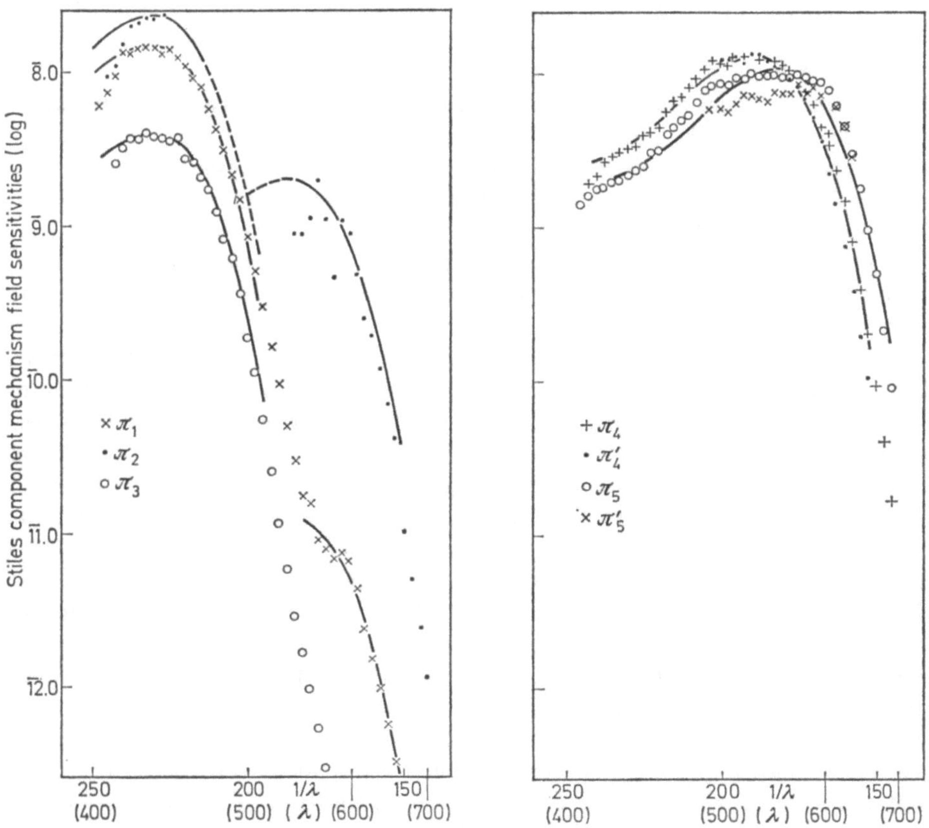

Fig. 6. Stiles π mechanism distributions (at retina) compared with expected forms of pigment absorption functions

validated[2]. We have discussed above the uncertainties in the specification of receptor pigments that make precise quantitative comparisons difficult. We have not yet touched upon the uncertainties inherent in the color-mixture data themselves. The fact that the CIE color-mixture data have been standardized by international agreement and that their values can be found tabulated exactly to many decimal places does not mean that they have been purged of the usual errors and uncertainties inherent in the original experimental measures on which they are

[2] Le Grand (1969) has suggested that the cone photopigments may have absorption spectra narrower than the rhodopsin form and that they therefore may not be based on retinal.

based (NIMEROFF, 1967). Unquestionably, the errors are sufficiently small so that the functions can serve as a useful standard for the color-equivalents of normal color vision. This is not true of the 1931 V_λ curve which is represented in the tristimulus values by the $\bar{y}_\lambda$ function (see LE GRAND, chapter 15, this volume) and which specifies short-wave luminosity values that are much too low to yield acceptable luminance specifications for light stimuli whose energies are concentrated in the short-wave region of the spectrum.

The inaccuracy of this function has served to becloud another issue of color theory that also remains unresolved at this time, and this issue concerns the concept and basis of photopic luminance.

The conventional analysis of the photopic luminosity curve has been that it results from a linearly additive combination of the activities engendered in the three types of cone receptors. In accordance with this analysis, luminances are arithmetically additive, and strictly so. The luminance additivity postulate is, furthermore, at the foundation of photometry, since it makes possible the conversion from physical units of radiant energy with wavelength specified to photometric light units by cross-multiplying the spectral energy distribution with the photopic luminosity function and then summing the products for all wavelengths to obtain a single-valued specification of the integrated luminance of the light. The usefulness of the photometric units further depends on the corollary assumption that two lights will appear equally bright when their photometric luminances are equal. Failure to verify the "equal-luminance, equal-brightness" prediction has often been reported for luminances specified by the CIE 1931 V_λ function (e.g., CHAPANIS and HALSEY, 1955), but the significance of such reports was difficult to evaluate, given the known inadequacy of the V_λ curve itself. More recently, however, the question has been intensively explored by methods that circumvent this particular function. Conclusions vary from one that luminances are far from additive (GUTH, 1967) to one that the luminance additivity assumption is strictly correct but that the corollary assumption of "equal-luminance, equal-brightness" is demonstrably false (BOYNTON and KAISER, 1968). The latter conclusion is consistent with, although not identical to, the opinions of earlier investigators that brightness judgments in heterochromatic comparisons are often contaminated by the observer's inability to maintain a clear distinction between brightness, on the one hand, and saturation, on the other. If it is the distinction between matched heterochromatic brightness and equality of luminance that underlies the apparent additivity failures, then the issue is not relevant for the relation of receptor absorptions activities to photopic luminosity and luminance specification, and the linearly additive combination of receptor activities can continue to stand as one of the fundamental propositions of color theory that relate to events at the receptor level of the retina.

The entire preceding discussion concerning the relation of receptor function to photopic luminosity and three-variable color mixture is necessarily restricted to the foveal region of the retina. Beyond this region, rod density increases, cone density decreases, and color vision deteriorates progressively and rapidly with increasing eccentricity. With this deterioration, the so-called laws of color mixture cease to hold (see MORELAND, chapter 20, this volume), and small non-linearities enter in the psychophysical data even for centrally viewed stimulus fields when the field diameter is increased to as much as 10 degrees (STILES and BURCH, 1959). These behaviors of the extra-foveal regions of the retina are related to receptor populations and populations of post-receptoral neural units, and it is likely that they also involve receptive field organizations that differ from the situation in the central, so-called photopic (WALD, 1967) area. We shall return to these matters in a later section.

III. Receptor Sensitivities, Neural Organization, and Physiological Color-code

For most of its history, the central focus of disagreement in color theory has been the relation between receptor events and the hues seen by human observers with normal color vision. In the Young-Helmholtz tradition, the hue coding was presumably represented in a one-to-one correspondence between receptor activities and three fundamental hue qualities (usually specified as red, green, and blue), but with non-fundamental, emergent qualities (yellow and white) generated in the visual centers (presumably visual cortex) (HECHT, 1928). In the rival Hering tradition, hue coding was presumably associated with opponent modes of response in the neural elements of the retina and related visual neural system, and not correlated in one-to-one fashion with receptor absorptions. In the current literature, there is evidence of much conceptual, or at least, semantic confusion in that the cone absorptions are often labelled with hue names that imply the simple correspondence notion of coding, even when no such hypothetical mechanism is explicitly intended (WALRAVEN, 1962, Fig. 20). To avoid such confusion, we have preferred to use the Greek letters α, β, and γ to identify the three types of cones that contain, respectively, the three photopigments with maximal absorptions near 450 nm, 530 nm, and 570 nm.

As pointed out in the preceding section, activities initiated by light absorption in all three types of cones are presumably combined at some level of the neural system in an additive fashion, and, to the extent that luminances are arithmetically additive, the combination must occur at a level prior to any non-linear transformation between the radiant energy incident at the retina and the physiological response[3]. The combination can be supposed, then, to occur quite early in the chain of physiological events, i.e., at a level not far removed from the most peripheral of the responding elements. This requirement has led to the suggestion that there might be a special class of cone that contains all three of the differently selective photopigments (PIÉRON, 1945), but what little evidence is available on the spectral absorptions of isolated cones (MARKS, 1965; MARKS, *et al.*, 1964; BROWN and WALD, 1964), and on the spectral distributions of electrical responses recorded from single cones (TOMITA *et al.*, 1967; BAYLOR and FUORTES, 1970) fails to support the idea of such a specialized "luminosity" type cone. If the receptor responses are linear, however, then there is no need

[3] It should be noted that derivation of a spectral equality-of-brightness function by a line-element procedure (SCHROEDINGER, 1920; STILES, 1946) leads to non-linear predictions, but these non-linearities would produce effects opposite to the deviations found in experiments (WYSZECKI and STILES, 1967, pp. 516–518).

for such a specialized receptor that combines all three selective photopigments, but there is need for a neural element (bipolar cell ?) that receives input directly from all three types of cone receptor. There is physiological evidence for ganglion cell responses that reflect inputs that must originate in more than one receptor type (GRANIT, 1947; WAGNER *et al.*, 1960; MICHAEL, 1968; DAW, 1968) and some evidence, though not so clear, that graded potentials recorded from some horizontal cells also may reflect multiple types of receptor activation (MACNICHOL and SVAETICHIN, 1958; NAKA and RUSHTON, 1966). The records of graded, S-potentials come mostly from fish retinas, in which the synaptic and functional organization need not, of course, match in detail the properties of the human retina. In fact, NAKA and RUSHTON (1966a) interpret their studies of S-potentials in the tench to mean that this retina functions with a fourth cone-pigment, in addition to the three identified in direct pigment studies. If confirmed, this four pigment system would represent a radical departure from the human, trivariant situation.

The ganglion cell responses are not, of course, linearly related to stimulus energy, and it seems not unlikely that the linearity of the system is already lost at the bipolar level. This is a question that cannot be decided by psychophysical experiment, but must await more evidence from unit recordings in the different retinal layers. At issue is the response criterion in the electrical recordings. Receptor potentials, for example, show amplitude changes over only restricted stimulus ranges, but response latencies and time to peak continue to decrease at stimulus levels well beyond the amplitude ceiling (WERBLIN and DOWLING, 1969). In any event, the psychophysical evidence points to an additive combination of excitatory inputs that are linearly related to the incident energy as one of the three variables of the color coding system. Thus,

$$V_1 = f_1 \left[\Sigma_\lambda \left(a_{11}\, e_\lambda\, \alpha_\lambda + a_{12}\, e_\lambda\, \beta_\lambda + a_{13}\, e_\lambda\, \gamma_\lambda\right)\right] \qquad (1)$$

where α, β, and γ represent the three cone sensitivities and are assumed to be both linear transforms of the color-mixture data and approximations to the photopigment distributions shown in Fig. 3. In this expression, the linear product sum has the spectral distribution of V_λ, the photopic luminosity curve, and a_{11}, a_{12} ,a_{13} are appropriate weighting constants for the three cone spectral sensitivities. Typically, the weighting factor a_{11} that is applied to the cone distribution with maximum in the short-wave spectral region has a value considerably less than a_{12} or a_{13}, consistent with a relatively small contribution of this kind of receptor activity to spectral luminosity. In WALD's (1967) analysis of luminosity functions measured by threshold determinations for the dark-adapted fovea, individual differences in the form of this function are attributed to the assumption that different individuals are relatively "rich" in one or another of the three different cone types. BAKER and RUSHTON (1963; 1965; RUSHTON and BAKER, 1964) similarly refer to their normal observers as having retinas that are "rich" in *erythrolabe* or in *chlorolabe* relative to one another, using RUSHTON's terms for the cone pigments with maxima in the 560–580 nm and 530–540 nm regions, respectively. Thus, as expressed here, the factors a_{11}, a_{12}, and a_{13} would presumably show individual variations that would depend on the relative numbers of the three cone types in the foveal regions of different retinas. WALD (1967) also asserts that the relative numbers of the short-wave, (α-type) cones are considerably reduced in the very central, "fixation" region (8′) of the nearly rod-free "photopic" fovea (1−2°). Interpretation of changes in population density of different cone elements in the foveal region is complicated, however, by variations in optical density of macular pigment within the same region (HURVICH, 1970). To the extent that sensitivity changes due to retinal factors can be clearly distinguished from the purely optical effects of the selective filtering action of the macula (see RUDDOCK, chapter 17, this volume), the factors a_{11}, a_{12}, and a_{13} must also be assumed to take on different values depending on precisely which retinal region is stimulated.

The term f in Eq. (1) symbolizes the transducer function that operates on the linear product sum, and this function is, by all the evidence, non-linear. It may be logarithmic, pseudo-logarithmic, or a power function. Such a transform certainly has occurred by the time responses are measured from the retinal ganglion cells, and quite possibly prior to this level. The non-linear transform need not, and does not, as conceptualized here, distort the linear relations of luminance to energy or the additivity of luminance units, but it does render non-linear the relation between luminance and perceived brightness, or whiteness, if that is the way in which the V_1 coded response is to be perceptually interpreted. Presumably the coding for the intensitive dimension of this variable is spike frequency at either on- or off-. The overlay on the all-positive combination of inputs from different cone types of excitatory and inhibitory influences from neighboring spatial areas of the receptive field will, of course, further modify the V_1 magnitudes, but we leave these spatial interaction effects aside at this point in the discussion and shall return to them in a later section.

Representations of inputs from more than one cone type are also found in physiological records of unit responses that show a reversal in mode of response from one region of the spectrum to another. Such reversals in response mode may be from depolarization to hyperpolarization in the case of graded potential responses, or from on- to off- in the case of spike discharges. Examples of both types, in different species, and in different parts of the visual tract (retina, optic nerve, lateral geniculate, optic tectum, visual cortex) may be found in the work of SVAETICHIN (1956), SVAETICHIN *et al.* (1965), WAGNER *et al.* (1960), DE VALOIS (1965a and b), MICHAEL (1968), JACOBSON (1964), WIESEL and HUBEL (1966), and GOURAS (1970). In terms of the psychophysical data, the relations of the receptor activities to the variables showing opposite modes of response in different parts of the spectrum may be expressed as follows:

$$V_2 = f_2\,[\Sigma\,(a_{21}\,e_\lambda\,\alpha_\lambda + a_{23}\,e_\lambda\,\gamma_\lambda - a_{22}\,e_\lambda\,\beta_\lambda)] \qquad (2)$$

$$V_3 = f_3\,[\Sigma\,(a_{32}\,e_\lambda\,\beta_\lambda + a_{33}\,e_\lambda\,\gamma_\lambda - a_{31}\,e_\lambda\,\alpha_\lambda)]\,.$$

The plus/minus convention used in these equations expresses the opposite modes of response, or, in perceptual terms, the mutually exclusive hue responses of the two separate variables. Whether the resultant of the algebraic sums takes on negative or positive values has no absolute significance beyond the convention. The spectral distributions of responsiveness for the three variables, V_1, V_2, and V_3 are shown in Fig. 7, where V_1 is interpreted as whiteness or brightness, V_2 is interpreted as redness for positive values and greenness for negative ones, and V_3 is interpreted as yellowness for positive values and blueness for negative ones. The

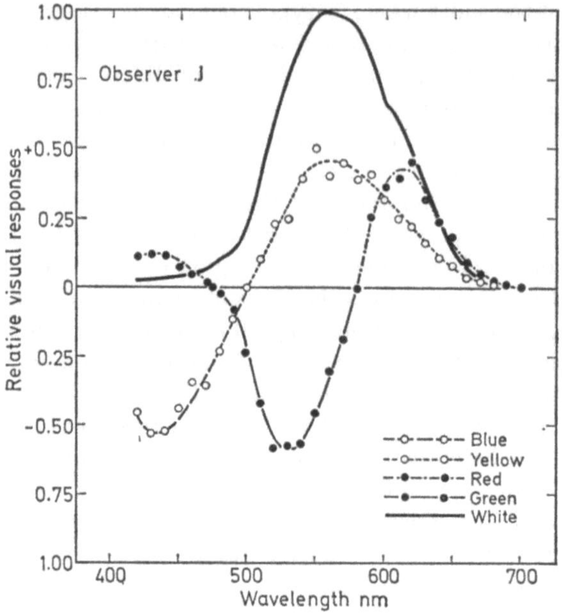

a

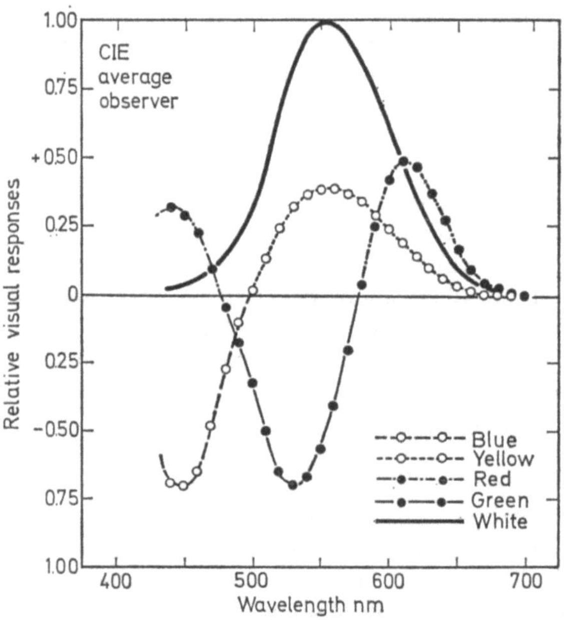

b

Fig. 7. a) Experimental curves for three quality coded variables of normal foveal color vision. b) Curves calculated for CIE Standard Observer for three quality coded variables of normal foveal color vision

data of Fig. 7a are experimental results for a single observer, for which the achromatic function was measured by foveal threshold, with the eye bright-adapted and in the presence of an illuminated surround of 5500° K, which appeared neutral white to this observer (HURVICH and JAMESON, 1953). The data for the hue variables were obtained for the same observer and same viewing conditions, but by a hue-cancellation technique, in which pairs of wavelengths that elicited opposite hue responses (blue and yellow, respectively, in one case, red and green in the other), were superimposed and their relative energies varied until the criterion ratio was determined at which neither of the opposite hues could be detected in the mixture (JAMESON and HURVICH, 1955). The relative energies required for the hue cancellation served as a measure of the amplitude of the relevant function at each wavelength. For comparison, Fig. 7b shows curves for the same three variables that are linear transformations of the 1931 CIE color-mixture data (tristimulus values) of Fig. 2 (JUDD, 1951, HURVICH and JAMESON, 1955).

The weighting factors a_{ij} of Eqs. (1), (2), and (3) depend on the precise set of functions chosen as most representative of the α, β, and γ cone distributions. For the incomplete visual pigment nomogram functions of Fig. 3, the most suitable values for V_1 were found to be

$$0.45\,\alpha + 0.85\,\beta + 1.30\,\gamma$$

for V_2

$$0.55\,\alpha + 0.55\,\gamma - 1.00\,\beta$$

and for V_3

$$0.15\,\beta + 0.15\,\gamma - 1.00\,\alpha$$ (JAMESON and HURVICH, 1968).

If the König distributions of Fig. 5a represent the receptor sensitivities, then the values a_{ij} become
for V_1

$$0.00\,\alpha + 0.15\,\beta + 0.85\,\gamma$$

for V_2

$$0.37\,\alpha + 1.66\,\gamma - 2.23\,\beta$$

and for V_3

$$0.06\,\beta + 0.34\,\gamma - 0.71\,\alpha.$$

It should be noted that the zero weighting of the König distributions for the short-wave, α contribution to the achromatic brightness variable is more likely to reflect the erroneously small CIE values for the short-wave region of the luminosity function than a plausible failure of the short-wave absorbing cone activities to channel any input whatsoever into the system that codes luminosity or brightness. (Compare the curves in Figs. 7a and 7b.) It should also be noted that although this variable can be interpreted as representing both whiteness and brightness, it is not necessarily the only interpretation. BOYNTON and KAISER (1968), for example, have suggested that this variable codes whiteness, but that brightness involves a further interaction between this variable and the other two systems that presumably are responsible for the hue coding of the visual system. Specifically, they suggest that brightness may be related to the sum of all elements, whether of the whiteness or the hue-coding type. They further suggest that it is this distinction between whiteness and brightness that can explain the failure of luminance additivity in experiments that involve brightness matches between fields in which the individual components of mixed lights have "brightnesses" that depend on both whiteness and hue-coding elements, whereas mixtures of these components, particularly in the case of complementaries, may have "brightnesses" determined only by the linear additions that activate the "whitness-coding" elements. The distinction made by BOYNTON and KAISER is a matter of perceptual criterion or judgment. Other investigators (GUTH *et al.*, 1969; WASSERMAN, 1968) have suggested that there is a physiological interaction among the chromatic and achromatic variables, and that it may involve both summative and subtractive (inhibitory) contributions of the chromatic mechanisms to the physiological response that ultimately codes perceived brightness. These recent suggestions are reminiscent of the notions of "inherent brightening and darkening" of different hues suggested in the older literature (HILLEBRAND, 1889; MÜLLER, 1930), and the notion that blue and green hue responses are associated with an "inherent darkening", whereas yellow and red responses are associated with an "inherent brightening", has been shown to account for the slight Purkinje shift found in the 1° central fovea if one wishes to reject the possibility that this area is not, in fact, totally rod-free (HURVICH and JAMESON, 1953). The idea remains, however, now as well as when originally proposed, without convincing supporting evidence.

With respect to Eqs. (2) and (3) that represent the contributions of the three cone types to the oppositely coded hue variables (HERING, 1964) the need for inputs from α, β, and γ to each paired hue response function arises from the human psychophysical data, and in particular, to accord with the hues seen throughout the spectrum by the human observer with normal color vision. In his recordings from opponent cells in the LGN of the macaque, DE VALOIS (1965) has noted that there is no evidence of any contribution from α-type cone activity to the responses of cells that he labels $+R - G$ and $-R + G$, and he also remarks that the "very good agreement between the recording and the psychophysical data breaks down at the short wavelengths" (p. 575). His recordings show no evidence of the short-wave "red" lobe of the sort plotted in Fig. 7 for the hue responses of the intact human. Moreover, his analysis of the combined effects of the opponent RG cells together with those that he codes $+Y - B$ and $-Y + B$ would suggest that in the short-wave spectral region where the human sees reddish-blue or violet hues, the monkey would "see" mostly greens with a secondary blue hue component. If the geniculate picture is maintained at the visual cortex (DE VALOIS suggests only that there may be some further amplification of the "blue"-coded responses at that level), then the color vision of the macaque might more closely resemble that of a human with a tritan defect than the normal human trichromat (see HURVICH, chapter 23, this volume). A recent report by GOURAS (1970), however, indicates influences of all three cone receptor types on spectrally opponent units in the monkey cortex, and this result seems more consistent with what is to be expected for normal human trichromats.

Most of the unit recordings from opponent cells in monkey LGN are responses to diffuse light stimulation of the retina. When patterned stimulation (e.g., center-spot and annulus, or small spot vs large spot) is used to explore the receptive field characteristics of the neural units, spatial non-homogeneities of receptor contributions are detected in some classes of cells, and, although one might anticipate that the receptive field organization would show a clear analogy to perceived color contrast effects, this does not seem to be the case for the relatively small sample of cells thus far investigated in this manner (WIESEL and HUBEL, 1966). We shall see below, moreover, that there are additional difficulties encountered in trying to decipher the "quality code" from unit responses in the monkey LGN or cortex.

In the experimental curves of Fig. 7a, the function representing the spectral distribution of red and green hues shows null values at about 475 nm and near 580 nm, and the corresponding wavelengths are closely similar in the theoretical curves of Fig. 7b. These wavelengths represent, respectively, the unique blue and yellow hues for a neutral condition of adaptation. The null point of the experimentally determined function representing the spectral distribution of blue and yellow hues occurs near 500 nm, and similarly in the corresponding theoretical function. This wavelength region corresponds to the locus of unique green for the neutral adaptation condition (HURVICH and JAMESON, 1951). One might expect that if the retinas of different individuals are indeed differently "rich" in cones that contain one or another of the three cone pigments, such differences would give rise to a dispersion of these unique hue loci for a population of normal observers. Thus, unless there were a compensatory change in synaptic connections, relative "richness" in α-type cones would shift both the unique blue and green toward longer wavelengths, richness in β-type (Rushton's chlorolabe) cones would shift the unique blue and green toward shorter wavelengths and the yellow toward longer ones, and richness in γ-type (Rushton's erythrolabe) would shift both the unique green and yellow toward shorter wavelengths. And these wavelength loci would presumably show predictable correlations with the form of the photopic luminosity function for the different individuals. A flurry of reports in recent years has focused on the distribution of unique green loci, with claims and counterclaims concerning the normality or bimodality of this distribution in a normal population (RUBIN, 1961; RICHARDS, 1967; HURVICH *et al.*, 1968). Correlational analyses of the sort described here in the context of cone inputs to both luminosity and hue functions would be of interest, but the evidence is not yet at hand. The unique hue loci are known to be highly sensitive to the state of chromatic adaptation of the visual system (JAMESON and HURVICH, 1951; HURVICH *et al.*, 1968), hence any such studies require the utmost care to guarantee that the state of adaptation is the same, and neutral, for all individuals in the population.

IV. Postulated Mechanisms of Appearance Changes with Changes in Luminance

The linearities of the color vision system that apply to the color-mixture data and their transformations (see WRIGHT, chapter 16, this volume) clearly do not extend to the transducer functions that intervene between the amount of radiant energy incident at the retina and the intensitive variables of perceived color, i.e., brightness and color strength of the individual hues. With respect to brightness, the Fechnerian psychophysical function, that is, a logarithmic relation between energy (or luminance) and perceived brightness was long considered to be the leading candidate for the non-linear intensitive transform. Stevens (1960; 1961), marshalling his evidence from direct "magnitude-scaling" experiments in many sense domains and buttressing it with cross-modality matching data that are predictable from the scaling results, has made an impressively documented case for the "repeal of Fechner's law" and the ratification of a power law in its stead. The specific power varies for different senses and for different sensory attributes within a given modality, but for brightness the exponent seems often to be quoted as equal to 1/3. Thus, in the various formulas that have been proposed, $B = kL^n$, $B = k(L - L_0)^n$, $B = kL^n - c$, and so on, and that are suggested to fit specific experimental data, the exponent n, is usually close to or equal to 1/3. (For a more detailed discussion of the scaling problem, see Krantz, chapter 26, this volume.) There seems to be no significant variation in the form of the psychophysical brightness versus luminance function that is specifically dependent on wavelength (Wilson, 1964; Ekman, 1961; Jameson, 1970) for conditions of neutral adaptation. For evidence concerning the physiological substrate of this relationship, we would probably want to look to the stimulus-response relations in the records of the so-called "non-opponent" cells. The "non-opponent" tag refers, of course, only to the non-opponent characteristic of such cells with respect to variations in wavelength. Cells of this sort do, indeed, show opponent response characteristics with respect to spatial variables of stimulation within their receptive fields. One would want to know, also, to what extent the unit response characteristics are altered going from the ganglion cells of the retina to units in the LGN and ultimately to those in the visual cortex.

For many of the phenomena of perceived color, it is not so much the individual transducer functions per se that are of primary influence, but the differences in these functions that may exist among the three differently coded variables as represented in Eqs. (1), (2), (3). Thus, for example, the Bezold-Brücke phenomenon, the variation in hue with variation in luminance for a fixed wavelength or wavelength distribution, implies that blueness and yellowness responses increase with luminance more rapidly than do redness and greenness responses. Such a difference in the gradients of the response functions is consistent with the observed phenomenon that both reddish-blue and greenish-blue hues look more blue and less red or green at high luminances than at lower ones, and that reddish-yellow and greenish-yellow hues look more yellow and less reddish or greenish at high luminances than at lower ones. It has been shown (Hurvich and Jameson, 1955) that quantitative measures of these hue shifts can be described quite well by specific assumptions about the differences in gradients in the two variables, that is, by specific differences between the functions f_2 and f_3.

Quantitative measures of the hue shifts of spectral colors with changes in luminance were obtained by Purdy (1937) who determined the difference in wavelength required to match spectral lights in hue when they differ in luminance by different amounts. Purdy's results, which span more than 2 log units, have been confirmed both by a replication of his matching procedure and by a "color-naming" method of hue scaling (Boynton and Gordon, 1965). They can be accounted for by assuming that, with a log unit increase in luminance, there is a differential increase for yellow and blue coded responses of about 20% relative to the increase in red and green hue magnitudes (HURVICH and JAMESON, 1955). We have attributed the relative increase to a differential amplification function in the two opponent hue systems, whereas JUDD (1951) suggested that it might be attributable to a difference in rate of adaptation between the two neural opponent-hue systems. When the eye is continuously exposed to a chromatic stimulus and its appearance is followed over time by a percentage hue-scaling method (JAMESON and HURVICH, 1959), with continued exposure for as long as 2 minutes steady viewing, perceived red or green hue components fade more rapidly than do yellow and blue ones (EICHENGREEN, 1971). In an experimental study recently carried out in our laboratory, however, the wavelength differences measured for hue matches between 2 mL and 20 mL stimuli are very nearly identical when exposure duration is varied in a series of steps from 150 msec to 2000 msec (COHEN, 1971). Hence, although there is evidence that red and green fading does occur more rapidly than yellow and blue for continued steady stimulation at a given luminance level, there seems to be no support for the idea that this difference alone is responsible for the hue shift with luminance change that is perceived in stimuli viewed for relatively short times. It has been shown, however, that luminance change, per se, is not the crucial factor in the perceived hue dependence. If the brightness reduction associated with a given decrease in luminance is brought about, rather, by presenting the higher luminance stimulus within a brightly illuminated surround, the perceived hues are identical to those of the lower luminance stimulus in a dark surround (COREN and KEITH, 1970). This result suggests that the intense surround stimulation, which depresses the brightness response in the test area, also depresses the magnitudes of the physiological activating events at the level of the *input* to the opponent hue response mechanisms, without affecting the operating characteristics of those mechanisms. It should be noted that this equivalence of contrast darkening and luminance reduction in its effect upon apparent hue is limited, of course, to illuminated surrounds that are achromatic or perceptually neutral in appearance. Strongly chromatic surrounds that might produce the same amount of darkening would, of course, drastically alter the perceived hues in the test area, (JAMESON and HURVICH, 1959) and in the extreme case convert a spectral stimulus to a complementary hue appearance (HELSON, 1938; HELSON and JEFFERS, 1940).

The COREN and KEITH result would be expected if, for example, the spatial interactions were mediated by the horizontal cells acting as controller elements through feedback synaptic loops to the cone receptors, or as a feed-forward controller system through synaptic connections at the inputs of the bipolar cells (see Fig. 1). In either event, the effect would be to reduce the magnitude of the receptor light response as a stimulus to the bipolar cells. These cells might then respond to the reduced input precisely in the same way that they would respond to an input reduced by reduction of the light energy incident on the receptor elements.

It has also long been known (HELMHOLTZ, 1866) that the perceived saturations of all colors vary with level of luminance; very dim colors are relatively desaturated, maximum saturations are perceived at intermediate levels, and all colors become relatively desaturated again at extremely high luminances. These variations in saturation with variation in luminance are related in part to differences in chromatic and achromatic thresholds, but also to differences in response function slopes for the achromatic relative to the two chromatic variables of the color vision system.

Consistent with these systematic variations in perceived color with changes in luminance, the various discrimination functions (purity discrimination, wavelength discrimination) also vary systematically with luminance level. Again, the quantitative data that are available on these discrimination measures can be shown to be satisfactorily represented by theoretical functions based on specific differences in the transducer functions for the three primary variables. The assumed relations are, of course, the same as those used to account for the hue shift and perceived color data (HURVICH and JAMESON, 1955).

There is an interesting relation that emerges from these effects and from their theoretical treatment. There appears to be a direct relation between the slopes of the functions and the levels of the specific thresholds in the case of the two hue variables. Thus, although yellow and blue hues predominate at high luminance levels, discriminations based on these hues are strongly degraded at very low levels, particularly when both low luminances and small field sizes are used. FARNSWORTH (1955), because of the latter effect, referred to the small field discrimination losses as near-threshold tritanopia type phenomena. We, too, have treated the small field, low luminance, tritanopia effects as near-threshold phenomena, and as consistent with relatively high specific threshold levels for blueness and yellowness as opposed to those for perceptions of and discriminations between greenness and redness (HURVICH and JAMESON, 1958). Evidence for similar relations between threshold and magnitude gradients can be found in other sense domains such as touch and hearing (BÉKÉSY, 1960). In the auditory sense, when the phenomenona occur in a particular type of deafness it is referred to as "recruitment". It shows up again when threshold and brightness magnitude scales are measured in foveal and peripheral parts of the retina (JAMESON, 1966).

One would, of course, like to know more about the physiological substrate for all three of the magnitude functions for the three color variables, and again it would be of interest to follow all of these functions from the retinal level to the visual cortex. This is not to imply, of course, that a strict parallelism is to be sought between the perceptual and physiological domains at the level of individual neural unit responses. Although impulse frequency at stimulus on- or off- is ordinarily taken to code the intensitive aspect of sensory response, temporal response patterning, latency, and synchrony of discharge in many units may all enter in the complex relations between stimulus energies and perceived sensory magnitudes (MOUNTCASTLE, 1968). It is likely, moreover, that relations established for electrophysiological responses to diffuse light stimulation of the retina may have little significance for ordinary vision of patterned light stimuli, where receptive field organization can be expected to play a more determinative role.

V. Postulated Mechanisms of Appearance Changes with Changes in Spatial Extent and Retinal Locus

Most of the theorizing about mechanisms of color vision and most theoretical analyses of the relevant psychophysical data restrict consideration to events related to the 2° fovea. Since it is this region of the retina that affords us not only our best visual acuity but also the fineness of our color discriminations, this restricted concern is perhaps as it should be. It is, nevertheless, true that the visual field is an extended one and that much of our appreciation of color in everyday life is related to the extended visual field. The fact that the retinal mechanisms are decidedly non-homogeneous in their characteristics throughout the visual field is therefore of some significance for the postulated mechanisms whereby color appearances are generated.

To begin with, of course, we must remember that the effective light distribution across the retinal surface cannot be uniform even for a perfectly uniform extended source of external illumination because of the spectrally selective macular pigment that is distributed in varying thickness over the foveal and immediately surrounding parafoveal retina. (See RUDDOCK, chapter 17, this volume.) Although the macula must alter the quantity and quality of retinal illumination in a localized area of the visual field, the fact that it does not make itself visible under ordinary viewing conditions can be attributed to the circumstance that the localized non-homogeneities in the retinal light pattern that it produces are fixed and independent of eye-movements. Like any other fixed image, the "image" of the macula fades and disappears completely, and, also like any other fixed image, the color of the surrounding area seems to "fill in" the faded image area to produce a uniform appearance (HERING, 1964). Thus the selective absorption of the macular filter fails to "interfere" with perception of uniform extended surfaces under ordinary circumstances, and it can be brought into view only by the use of techniques specifically designed to break up momentarily the fixed-image adaptation.

Apart from the macular filter, the distribution of receptor elements of different types across the retina is a still more important basis for physiological non-homogeneity of color responses across the visual field. The central fovea, about 2°, where cones are most densely packed, is relatively rod-free; beyond the fovea the rod-cone proportions are reversed, both rods and cones become more sparse in the far periphery, but the cones more so, so that the far periphery can be described as relatively cone-free. Given the progressive reduction in the cone receptor population with increasing eccentricity, the progressive deterioration in color discrimination that is known to characterize the retinal periphery is only to be expected. The reduction in capacity for color discrimination and in the colors perceived is not uniform for all hues, however. Red and green hues, and discriminations based on them, are lost at a retinal eccentricity at which yellows and blues are still seen and discriminated.

The red-green blind dichromasy of the mid-periphery of the normal retina is attested to both by the older work on color zones (BAIRD, 1905; DIMMICK, 1948), and by more recent quantitative data of color matching in the periphery (CLARKE, 1960, 1962) and of color equations between a matching field presented at the fovea and test stimuli imaged at various retinal eccentricities (MORELAND and CRUZ, 1958; see also MORELAND, chapter 20, this volume). Only at still more peripheral locations do yellows and blues also drop out to yield a condition of monochromasy.

If we accept, for example, DE VALOIS' classification of spectrally opponent cells into classes that are coded either "red/green" or "yellow/blue", then the obvious theoretical assumption to account for the characteristics of the different color zones of the retina would be a relative reduction in the number of cells of both populations related to retinal positions of increasing eccentricity, but with a more rapid reduction in the spectrally opponent "red/green" type than in the "yellow/blue" class.

This assumed change in opponent-cell distributions, although likely enough, is most probably not the whole story. We have no evidence, for example, on the way in which the reduction in overall cone population density is distributed among the three cone sub-populations, whether proportionately or otherwise. Measures of spectral luminosity show relatively increased short-wave sensitivity in the periphery as compared with the fovea (WEALE, 1951; 1953), and it is not clear that this can be accounted for entirely by the absence of macular pigment as opposed to a change in proportion of receptor types in favor of the α-type cones. Nor is the role of rod receptors in photopic, peripheral vision in any sense agreed upon. Theoretical interpretations vary from the conclusion that rod responses are "saturated" and play no role at all at photopic levels of illumination to analyses that suggest an inhibitory interaction of rod activities on mechanisms related to the cone receptor system (see MORELAND, chapter 20, this volume). The hypothesis that there is a relatively more rapid reduction in neural red/green response processes than in yellow/blue ones with increasing eccentricity in no way excludes the simultaneous role of other receptoral and neural factors that may also contribute to the particular manifestations of red-green blind dichromasy in the normal periphery.

The fact that the characteristics of the perceived visual field do not reflect either the gradient of retinal stimulation, in the case of the macula, or the gradient of retinal color sensitivity or responsiveness, might be taken as support for a view that the visual system responds only to abrupt changes in gradients, both spatial and temporal. The physiological organization that gives rise to on- and off-discharges would seem to be well suited to such a functional design, as is the receptive field organization in which adjacent retinal areas are related in a mutually opponent, excitatory-inhibitory interdependence in their influences on a single neural unit. We know, particularly from the work of HUBEL and WIESEL (1960; 1962; 1965), that there is a progressive increase in specialization of patterning of receptive field organization from retina through geniculate to visual cortex in both cat and primate. We can also infer, from psychophysical results with human observers, that such specialized patterning of receptive field organization is probably responsible for specialized adaptation effects that cannot be attributed simply to desensitization, through exposure, of particular regions of the retina. Thus, for example, an observer can be desensitized, through continued exposure with the moving eye, to an alternating light-dark spatial bar pattern or grating of a particular spatial frequency (BLAKEMORE and CAMPBELL, 1969; BLAKEMORE and SUTTON, 1969). Moreover, the receptive field organization seems also to retain relative independence of hue coding associated with particular spatial configurations. There is no evidence, to our knowledge, yet available from electrophysiological studies on the wavelength dependence of cortical units with so-called "complex" receptive fields. The evidence for specialized color effects again rests on psychophysical adaptation experiments with humans, and, in this instance, on the phenomenon that has come to be known as the McCollough effect. McCollough (1965) first demonstrated that exposure of the retina alternately for a few seconds at a time to a vertical, light-dark, square-or-rectangular-wave grating pattern of one color (say, red), followed by the same pattern in a horizontal orientation and a different color (say, green), could result in after-image colors appropriate to the exposure color-plus-orientation linkages on subsequent presentation of achromatic patterns in either the vertical or horizontal orientations. There have since been many confirmations and extensions of her study. We have, moreover, observed the chromatic exposure after-effect specificities as frequency-dependent for spatial grating patterns of the same orientations.

All of these effects would seem to suggest that hue is coded neurally in terms of a particular mode of discharge (either on- or off-) in a particular cell that carries the opponent hue label (e.g., red-on/green-off) and that is further specialized to respond maximally to a particular spatial configuration of stimulation at the retina. But such a conclusion, as we have pointed out elsewhere (Hurvich and Jameson, 1970), is not only a gross oversimplification, it is demonstrably false. A given cell, for one size of stimulus field and one state of adaptation, can indeed seem to signal, say, "red-on/green-off". But if the eye is then dark-adapted, the same cell can respond in non-opponent fashion with on responses to stimuli at all wavelengths, and in this state its spectral sensitivity mimics that of the scotopic, rod rhodopsin system (Wiesel and Hubel, 1966). De Valois (1965) has expressed concern about similar findings in his own electrophysiological work on the lateral geniculate units in the macaque. It is not surprising to find that there is a Purkinje shift in the non-opponent cells when one goes from a light-adapted to a dark-adapted preparation; "a rod-cone shift can be demonstrated not only in non-opponent cells, however, but also in many opponent cells which may, under scotopic conditions, act like scotopic non-opponent cells. How the same response of such a cell can have completely different significance to the organism under conditions of light and dark adaptation is a puzzling question." (De Valois, 1965b, p. 570).

If it is true, as it seems to be in terms of the physiological evidence thus far available, that we do not yet have our feet securely planted on the ground in specifying the quality code for the color vision system, it should not be surprising that we have even less to go on in terms of physiological evidence for the intensitive relations within given qualitative variables, for the specificity of quality and patterning variables or, as we shall see in the next section, for the temporal relations that also play a decisive role in perceived color effects.

VI. Postulated Mechanisms of Appearance Changes that Depend on Temporal Parameters of Stimulation

Some of the most intriguing perceived color effects are those that arise as a consequence of manipulating the temporal pattern of successive brief stimuli that vary only in luminance. Among the many devices for producing such patterned stimulation, perhaps the best known is the so-called Benham disk, shown in Fig. 8a. The disk is made up of areas that differ only in total reflectance with no difference in spectral selectivity, and it appears as a black and white pattern when the disk is at rest and viewed under ordinary illumination (i.e., daylight or incandescent indoor illumination). When the disk is set into rotation so that the same part of the retina is stimulated in rapid succession by the different levels of reflected light, a pattern of rings of different hues is perceived, the so-called "subjective colors".

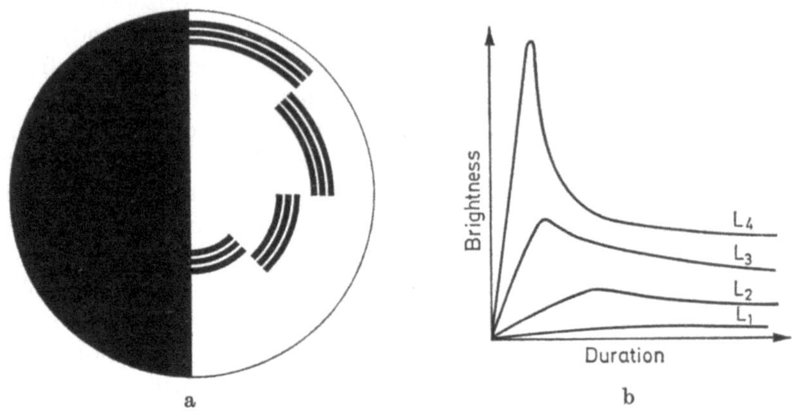

Fig. 8. a) Typical Benham disk pattern for producing "subjective colors". b) Illustration of time course of development of brightness sensation. $L_1 \ldots L_4$ indicate increasing levels of stimulus luminance

A wide variety of explanations has been brought forward to account for the subjective colors, and many of them refer to the possibility of different sensation rise times for the different hues. Fig. 8b is an illustration of the well-known time course of the development of the brightness sensation (BROCA and SULZER, 1902; 1903). At low levels of stimulation, the sensation rises gradually to a maximum within (say) 100 msec after stimulus onset, and at higher levels not only is the maximum reached earlier, but for strong stimulation there is also an "overshoot", as illustrated in the graph.

Among the earliest proposals to explain the subjective color phenomena from black and white patterns was the suggestion that the variation in time course of development of a visual sensation (or the time course of excitation) depended not only on the stimulus luminance but also on the particular hue mechanism involved. The particular temporal pattern of luminance variation provided by the different sets of arcs in the Benham disk presumably favors the development of one or another of these specific hue responses, hence the rings are perceived in different hues (PIÉRON, 1931).

A detailed critical examination of some of the earlier thinking about the mechanisms responsible for the subjective colors can be found in FRÖHLICH (1929), and a brief synopsis of the various theoretical suggestions put forth over the years is given by CAMPENHAUSEN (1969).

CAMPENHAUSEN summarizes the theoretical views in five groups. The oldest view and the one endorsed by FECHNER (1838), was the one mentioned above, namely that the different color sensations rise and fall at different rates and that periodic light stimulation has the effect of separating the different hue components and also their momentary after-effects. Many investigators, including BENHAM (1894; 1895), BIDWELL (1896; 1897; 1901), EBBECKE (1920) related the subjective colors to after-images. A number of investigators, including FRY (1933a and b), SEGAL (1940), ROELOFS and ZEEMAN (1957; 1958), thought the phenomena could be interpreted in terms of TROLAND's (1921) modulation theory of color vision, which assumed a frequency-modulation pattern of nerve impulses as the physiological code for color hue. Duplication of the pattern by an appropriate temporal pattern of achromatic flickering light stimulation would then, presumably, give rise to the associated hue response. Some investigators have sought to relate the colors to lateral interactions of specific sorts (BIDWELL, 1897; PIÉRON, 1922; 1923), and a number of studies have explored the spatial characteristics of the luminance pattern (ROELOFS and ZEEMAN, 1958; FRY, 1933a and b) as well as patterns that vary in both luminance and chromaticity. The possible role played by the chromatic aberration of the eye in its effect on subjective colors has also been examined.

It is likely that there is some validity to all of the hypotheses that have been advanced, and that the subjective colors of the Benham disk, like our everyday color experiences, can be shown to depend to some extent on all the factors cited.

FRÖHLICH (1929), for example, agrees with EBBECKE's idea that, for most conditions of illumination, the eye is not in a chromatically neutral state of adaptation, but tends to be desensitized to long-wave light. It is primarily to this state of long-wave adaptation that EBBECKE attributed the frequently observed red coloration that occurs when the "red-desensitized" state is momentarily interrupted by the period of greatly reduced illumination while the black portion of the sectored disk is imaged on a part of the retina. Re-illumination after this "release" from red adaptation then permits the momentary re-arousal of the red hue sensation. This view is consistent with the report of VERRIEST and SEKI (1964) on the colors seen on the Benham disk when it is illuminated by CIE Source A (color temperature about 2800° K, energy distribution weighted in long-wave spectral region) as compared with when it is illuminated by CIE Source C (artificial daylight, energy distribution more closely approximating equal energy). Under the latter illumination, the subjective colors are greatly desaturated, and there is very little red to be seen in the rings.

VERRIEST and SEKI consider their result to confirm PIÉRON's (1928) report that the subjective colors depend on the spectral distribution of the illuminant, rather than on its colorimetric properties, probably because both Source A and Source C are commonly referred to, albeit erroneously, as "white light". The results are irrelevant to PIÉRON's report, however, since these two illuminants are not metamers in the colorimetric sense. The two different distributions would not match when viewed side-by-side in a bi-partite stimulus field. Each illuminant viewed alone might be said to "look white" under the appropriate viewing conditions, but then only because of the compensatory nature of chromatic adaptation which has the effect of shifting toward a neutral appearance most chromatic stimuli to which the eye is continuously exposed. If it were, in fact, the case that subjective colors differ depending on the actual spectral distribution of the broad-band light stimulation, even when the broad-band lights used are identical in their colorimetric properties, it would undermine one of the basic tenets of color theory. However many points color theorists may find to disagree on, they do agree on the principle of color reception that metameric light stimuli are identical in color appearance when projected on the same or equivalent parts of the retina if and only if the different spectral light distributions are equally absorbed in each of the three different cone receptor pigments. There is no basis for different response latencies in a given receptor when it absorbs the same number of light quanta, whether of the same or different wavelengths. Because of the fundamental contradiction implied by the reported difference in subjective colors for metameric light stimuli, CAMPENHAUSEN (1969) recently reexamined this possibility in a systematic experimental study in which he used nine different pairs of metamers. His results show no differences, and he suggests that the successive comparison method used in the earlier studies may have been inadequate to insure precise color matches between the lights that were presumably identical in appearance for steady viewing conditions.

As a model for the physiological basis of the subjective colors CAMPENHAUSEN (1968) proposes a schema of the sort illustrated in Fig. 9. Excitatory activities engendered in three differently selective cone types are assumed to be modified in their temporal characteristics by units acting as "kinetic filters", each specific

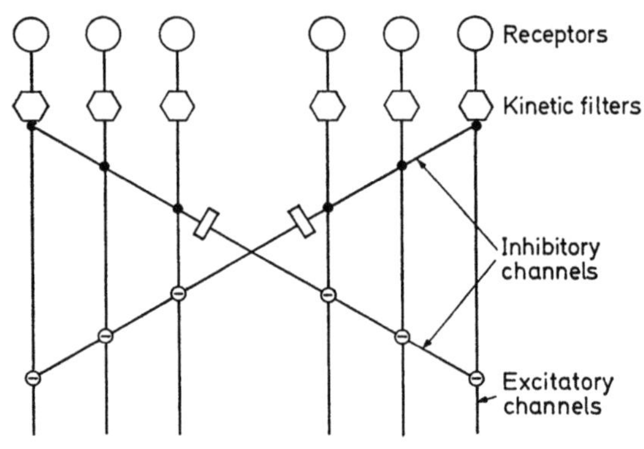

Fig. 9. Diagrammatic representation of phase-dependent lateral inhibition concept to account for "subjective colors" (based on CAMPENHAUSEN, 1968)

for its own channel. Lateral inhibitory connections to and from neighboring excitatory channels serve to depress the excitatory flow. When both the excitatory flow and the lateral inhibitory influences are modulated by particular temporal patterns of stimulation, the phase relations of the two types of activities become determinative for the net excitatory outflow, and because the temporal characteristics of the different spectrally selective channels are not identical, the inhibitory modulation is such as to selectively supress or favor one or another channel of different spectral selectivity. Since the crux of the model is the concept of phase-dependent lateral inhibition, subjective hue effects are predicted only for intermediate frequencies of temporally varying stimulation for which phase relations become important. CAMPENHAUSEN conceives of the horizontal cells as the inhibitory links in the mechanism, and he points out that the spatial characteristics of the Benham type patterns that give rise to color effects in the fovea and in the more peripheral retina are consistent with the different lateral spreads of horizontal cells in different parts of the retina. This model does not take into account the spectrally opponent processes that seem to be related to the physiological mechanisms of hue coding. If, however, the phase-dependent lateral inhibitory effects are assumed to operate at the level of the opponent processes, then its explanatory power is also extended to the red-yellow and blue-green hues that are seen when a simple half-black/half-white disk is rotated, or a strobe light is flashed repeatedly at an intermediate frequency.

A postulate of different temporal characteristics for neural events that are excitatory (say, depolarizing *S*-potentials or spike discharges) versus inhibitory (say, hyperpolarizing *S*-potentials or inhibition of nerve impulses) is a highly likely one in terms of what is known of neurophysiology. Further analysis of the "tonic" and "phasic" retinal cells described by GOURAS (1968) may provide information relating to the temporal aspects of hue-coded response mechanisms. So far, however, specific differences in temporal characteristics between different (r/g vs. y/b) hue processes lack convincing physiological documentation, and the psychophysical evidence is also uncertain. (See, for example, the discussion of some of the earlier evidence on this question by FRÖHLICH, 1929, and see also GUTH, 1968, for negative findings on specific hue latencies or rise times as measured by a "displacement" effect.)

Specific wavelength dependent phase differences have been revealed in studies of visual flicker (DE LANGE, 1958a and b; KELLY, 1962) and further psychophysical evidence on the temporal characteristics of specific hue processes is likely to be forthcoming from this method of experimental analysis.

Acknowledgement. Preparation of this chapter was supported in part by NIH Grant EY-00249. The development and analyses reported here are based heavily on research carried out jointly by the author and LEO M. HURVICH.

References

BAIRD, J. W.: The color sensitivity of the peripheral retina. Publication No. 29, Carnegie Institution: Washington 1905.

BAKER, H. D., RUSHTON, W. A. H.: Erythrolabe in the normal eye. J. Physiol. (Lond.) **161**, 91–92 (1963).

— — The red-sensitive pigment in normal cones. J. Physiol. (Lond.) **176**, 56—72 (1965).

BÉKÉSY, G. VON: Experiments in Hearing (Translated by WEVER, E. G.). New York: Wiley 1960.

BENHAM, C. E.: Notes. Nature (Lond.) **51**, 113—114 (1894a).

— Letters to the Editor. Nature (Lond.) **51**, 200 (1894b).

— Letters to the Editor. Nature (Lond.) **51**, 321 (1895).

BIDWELL, S.: On subjective colour phenomena attending sudden changes of illumination. Proc. roy. Soc. (Lond.) B **60**, 368—377 (1896).

— On the negative after-images following brief retinal excitation. Proc. roy. Soc. (Lond.) B **61**, 268—271 (1897).

BIDWELL, S.: On negative after-images and their relation to certain other visual phenomena. Proc. roy. Soc. (Lond.) B **68**, 262—285. (1901).

BLAKEMORE, C., CAMPBELL, F. W.: On the existence of neurones in the human visual system selectively sensitive to the orientation and size of retinal images. J. Physiol. (Lond.) **203**, 237—260 (1969).

— SUTTON, P.: Size-adaptation: A new after-effect. Science **166**, 245—247 (1969).

BOYNTON, R. M., GORDON, J.: Bezold-Brücke hue shift measured by color-naming technique. J. opt. Soc. Amer. **55**, 78—86 (1965).

— KAISER, P. K.: Vision: The additivity law made to work for heterochromatic photometry with bipartite fields. Science **161**, 366—368 (1968).

BRINDLEY, G. S.: Physiology of the Retina and the Visual Pathway. London: Arnold 1960.

BROCA, A., SULZER, D.: La sensation lumineuse en fonction du temps. J. Physiol. Path. gén. **4**, 632—640 (1902).

— — La sensation lumineuse en fonction du temps pour les lumières colorées; discussion des résultats. C. R. Acad. Sci. (Paris) **137**, 1046—1049 (1903).

BROWN, P. K., WALD, G.: Visual pigments in human and monkey retinas. Nature (Lond.) **200**, 37—43 (1963).

— — Visual pigments in single rods and cones of the human retina. Science **144**, 45—52 (1964).

CAMPENHAUSEN, C. VON: Über die Farben der Benhamschen Scheibe. Z. vergl. Physiol. **60**, 351—374 (1968).

— The colors of Benham's top under metameric illuminations. Vision Res. **9**, 677—682 (1969).

CHAPANIS, A., HALSEY, R. M.: Luminance of equally bright colors. J. opt. Soc. Amer. **45**, 1—6 (1955).

CLARKE, F. J. J.: Extra-foveal colour metrics. Optica Acta **7**, 355—384 (1960).

— Further studies of extra-foveal colour metrics. Optica Acta **10**, 257—284 (1962).

COHEN, J. D.: Temporal independence of the Bezold-Brücke hue shift. Ph. D. Thesis, University of Pennsylvania (1971).

COREN, S., KEITH, B.: Bezold-Brücke effect: Pigment or neural locus? J. opt. Soc. Amer. **60**, 559—562 (1970).

DARTNALL, H. J. A.: The interpretation of spectral sensitivity curves. Brit. med. Bull. **9**, 24—30 (1953).

— The identity and distribution of visual pigments in the animal kingdom. In: The Eye. Vol. 2, pp. 367—426. DAVSON, H. (Ed.). New York: Academic Press 1962.

DAW, N. W.: Colour-coded ganglion cells in the goldfish retina: Extension of their receptive fields by means of new stimuli. J. Physiol. (Lond.) **197**, 567—592 (1968).

DELANGE, H.: Research into the dynamic nature of the human fovea-cortex systems with intermittent and modulated light. I. Attenuation characteristics with white and colored light. J. opt. Soc. Amer. **48**, 777—784 (1958a).

— Research into the dynamic nature of the human fovea-cortex systems with intermittent and modulated light. II. Phase shift in brightness and delay in color perception. J. opt. Soc. Amer. **48**, 784—789 (1958b).

DE VALOIS, R. L.: Behavioral and electro-physiological studies of primate vision. In: Contributions to Sensory Physiology. Vol. 1, pp. 137—178. NEFF, W. D. (Ed.). New York: Academic Press 1965a.

— Analysis and coding of color vision in the primate visual system. Cold. Spr. Harb. Symp. quant. Biol. **30**, 567—579 (1965b).

DIMMICK, F. L.: Color. In: Foundations of Psychology. BORING, E. G., LANGFELD, H. S., WELD, H. P. (Eds.) pp. 269—296. New York: Wiley 1948.

DOWLING, J. E.: Organization of vertebrate retinas. Invest. Ophthal. **9**, 655—680 (1970).

— BOYCOTT, B. B.: Organization of the primate retina: Electron microscopy. Proc. roy. Soc. (Lond.) B **166**, 80—111 (1966).

— WERBLIN, F. S.: Organization of the retina of the mudpuppy. *Necturus maculosus*. I. Synaptic structure. J. Neurophysiol. **32**, 315—338 (1969).

EBBECKE, U.: Über das Sehen im Flimmerlicht. Pflügers Arch. ges. Physiol. **185**, 196—223 (1920).

EICHENGREEN, J.: Time-dependent chromatic adaptation. Ph. D. Thesis, University of Pennsylvania (1971).
EKMAN, G.: Some aspects of psychophysical research. In: Sensory Communication. ROSENBLITH, W. (Ed.) pp. 35—47, New York: Wiley 1961.
FARNSWORTH, D.: Tritanomalous vision as a threshold function. Farbe **4**, 185—196 (1955).
FECHNER, G. T.: Über eine Scheibe zur Erzeugung subjektiver Farben. Ann. Phys. Chem. **45**, 227—332 (1838).
FRÖHLICH, F. W.: Die Empfindungszeit. Jena: Gustav Fischer 1929.
FRY, G. A.: Modulation of nerve current as basis for color vision. Amer. J. Psychol. **45**, 488—492 (1933a).
— Color phenomena from adjacent retinal areas for different temporal patterns of intermittent white light. Amer. J. Psychol. **45**, 714—721 (1933b).
GOURAS, P.: Identification of cone mechanisms in monkey ganglion cells. J. Physiol. (Lond.) **199**, 533—547 (1968).
— Trichromatic mechanisms in single cortical neurons. Science **168**, 489—491 (1970).
GRAHAM, C. H.: Color: Data and theories. In: Vision and Visual Perception, GRAHAM, C. H. (Ed.), pp. 414—452. New York: Wiley 1965.
GRANIT, R.: Sensory Mechanisms of the Retina. London: Oxford University Press 1947.
GUTH, S. L.: The effect of wavelength on visual perceptual latency. Vision Res. **4**, 567—578 (1964).
— Nonadditivity and inhibition among chromatic luminances at threshold. Vision Res. **7**, 319—328 (1967).
— DONLEY, N. J., MARROCCO, R. T.: On luminance additivity and related topics. Vision Res. **9**, 537—575 (1969).
HECHT, S.: The binocular fusion of colors and its relation to theories of color vision. Proc. nat. Acad. Sci. (Wash.) **14**, 237—241 (1928).
— Vision: II. The nature of the photoreceptor process. In: Handbook of General Experimental Psychology. MURCHISON, C. (Ed.), pp. 704—828. Worcester, Mass.: Clark University Press 1934.
HELMHOLTZ, H. L. F. VON: Handbuch der Physiologischen Optik (1st ed.) Hamburg: Voss 1866.
— Handbuch der Physiologischen Optik (2nd ed.) Hamburg: Voss 1896.
HELSON, H.: Fundamental problems in color vision. I. The principle governing changes in hue, saturation, and lightness of nonselective samples in chromatic illumination. J. exp. Psychol. **23**, 429—476 (1938).
— JEFFERS, V. B.: Fundamental problems in color vision. II. Hue, lightness, and saturation of selective samples in chromatic illumination. J. exp. Psychol. **26**, 1—27 (1940).
HERING, E.: Grundzüge der Lehre vom Lichtsinn. [Outlines of a Theory of the Light Sense.] Berlin: Springer 1920 (Translated by HURVICH, L. M., JAMESON, D.). Cambridge: Harvard University Press 1964.
HILLEBRAND, F.: Über die spezifische Helligkeit der Farben. (Intro. by E. HERING) S.-B. Akad. Wiss. Wien, math.-nat. Kl. , Abt. III, **98**, 70—120 (1889).
HUBEL, D. H., WIESEL, T. N.: Receptive fields of optic nerve fibres in the spider monkey. J. Physiol. (Lond.) **154**, 572—580 (1960).
— — Receptive fields, binocular interaction and functional architecture in the cat's visual cortex. J. Physiol. (Lond.) **160**, 106—154 (1962).
— — Receptive fields and functional architecture in two nonstriate visual areas (18 and 19) of the cat. J. Neurophysiol. **28**, 229—289 (1965).
HURVICH, L. M.: Is the central fixation area of the fovea blue-blind? In: International Colour Meeting Stockholm 1969, pp. 49—57. Göttingen: Musterschmidt-Verlag 1970.
— JAMESON, D.: The binocular fusion of yellow in relation to color theories. Science **114**, 199—202 (1951).
— — Spectral sensitivity of the fovea. I. Neutral adaptation. J. opt. Soc. Amer. **43**, 485—494 (1953).
— — Some quantitative aspects of an opponent-colors theory. II. Brightness, saturation, and hue in normal and dichromatic vision. J. opt. Soc. Amer. **45**, 602—616 (1955).
— — An opponent-process theory of color vision. Psychol. Rev. **64**, 384—404 (1957).

HURVICH, L. M., JAMESON, D.: Further development of a quantified opponent-colours theory. In: Visual Problems of Colour, Vol. II, pp. 691—723. London: H. M. Stationery Office 1958.
— — Color vision and color coding. In: Perception and its Disorders. HAMBURG, D. A., PRIBRAM, K. H., STUNKARD, A. J. (Eds.) pp. 12—25. Baltimore: Williams and Wilkins 1970.
— — COHEN, J. D.: The experimental determination of unique green in the spectrum. Perc. Psychophys. **4** (2), 65—68 (1968).
— — KRANTZ, D. H.: Theoretical treatments of selected visual problems. In: Handbook of Mathematical Psychology, Vol. 3, pp. 99—159. LUCE, R. D., BUSH, R. R., GALANTER, E. (Eds.) New York: Wiley 1965.
JACOBSON, M.: Spectral sensitivity of single units in the optic tectum of the goldfish. Quart. J. exp. Physiol. **49**, 384—393 (1964).
JAMESON, D.: Threshold and supra-threshold relations in vision. Internationale Farbtagung Luzern 1965, pp. 128—136. Göttingen: Musterschmidt-Verlag 1966.
— Brightness scales and their interpretation. In: International Colour Meeting Stockholm 1969. pp. 377—385. Göttingen: Musterschmidt-Verlag 1970.
— HURVICH, L. M.: Use of spectral hue-invariant-loci for the specification of white stimuli. J. exp. Psychol. **41**, 455—463 (1951).
— — Some quantitative aspects of an opponent-colors theory. I. Chromatic responses and spectral saturation. J. opt. Soc. Amer. **45**, 546—552 (1955).
— — Perceived color and its dependence on focal, surrounding, and preceding stimulus variables. J. opt. Soc. Amer. **49**, 890—898 (1959).
— — Opponent-response functions related to measured cone photopigments. J. opt. Soc. Amer. **58**, 429—430 (1968).
JUDD, D. B.: Basic correlates of the visual stimulus. In: Handbook of Experimental Psychology. STEVENS, S. S. (Ed.) pp. 811—867. New York: Wiley 1951.
— Fundamental studies of color vision from 1860 to 1960. Proc. nat. Acad. Sci. (Wash.) **55**, 1313—1330 (1966).
KELLY, D. H.: Visual responses to time dependent stimuli. IV. Effects of chromatic adaptation. J. opt. Soc. Amer. **52**, 940—947 (1962).
KOLB, H.: Organization of outer plexiform layer of the primate retina: Electron microscopy of Golgi-impregnated cells. Phil. Trans. (Lond.) B **258**, 261—283 (1970).
LE GRAND, Y.: Light, Colour and Vision (2nd ed., HUNT, R. W. G., HUNT, F. R. W., Translators). London: Chapman and Hall, 1968.
— Photopigments des cônes humains. Documenta ophthal., **26**, 257—263 (1969).
MACNICHOL, E. F., SVAETICHIN, G.: Electrical responses from the isolated retinas of fishes. Amer. J. Ophthal. **46**, 26—34 (1958).
MARKS, W. B.: Visual pigments of single goldfish cones. J. Physiol. (Lond.) **178**, 14—32 (1965).
— DOBELLE, W. H., MACNICHOL, E. F.: Visual pigments of single primate cones. Science **143**, 1181—1183 (1964).
MCCOLLOUGH, C.: Color adaptation of edge-detectors in the human visual system. Science, **149**, 1115—1116 (1965).
MICHAEL, C. R.: Receptive fields of single optic nerve fibers in a mammal with an all-cone retina. III. Opponent color units. J. Neurophysiol. **31**, 268—282 (1968).
MILLER, R. F., DOWLING, J. E.: Intracellular responses of the Müller (Glial) cells of mudpuppy retina: Their relation to b- wave of the electroretinogram. J. Neurophysiol. **33**, 323—341 (1970).
MORELAND, J. D., CRUZ, A. C.: Colour perception with the peripheral retina. Optica Acta **6**, 117—151 (1958).
MOUNTCASTLE, V. B.: The problem of sensing and the neural coding of sensory events. In: The Neurosciences. QUARTON, G. C., MELNECHUCK, T., SCHMITT, F. O. (Eds.) pp. 393—408. New York: Rockefeller University Press 1967.
MÜLLER, G. E.: Über die Farbenempfindungen. II. Leipzig: Barth 1930.
NAKA, K. I., RUSHTON, W. A. H.: S-potential from colour units in the retina of fish (Cyprinidae). J. Physiol. (Lond.) **185**, 536—555 (1966a).

NAKA, K. I., RUSHTON, W. A. H.: An attempt to analyse colour reception by electrophysiology. J. Physiol. (Lond.) **185**, 556—586 (1966b).

— — S-potentials from luminosity units in the retina of fish (Cyprinidae) J. Physiol. (Lond.) **185**, 587—599 (1966c).

NIMEROFF, I.: The variability of color measurement. Color Eng. **5**, 24—29 (1967).

PIÉRON, H.: Loi de la vitesse d'établissement des processus chromatiques fondamentaux en fonction de l'intensité de l'excitation lumineuse. C. R. Acad. Sci. (Paris) **174**, 1294—1296 (1922a).

— Des lois déséquilibre chromatique initial et de la préponderance de la diffusion chromatique dans l'excitation lumineuse de la rétine. C. R. Soc. Biol. (Paris) **86**, 922—925 (1922b).

— Le méchanisme d'apparition des couleurs subjectives de Fechner-Benham. Ann. psychol. **23**, 1—48 (1923).

— Influence de la composition de la lumière sur la nature des couleurs subjectives de Fechner-Benham. Ann. psychol. **29**, 229—233 (1928).

— La sensation chromatique. Données sur la latence propre et l'établissement des sensations de couleur. Ann. psychol. **32**, 1—29 (1931).

— La Sensation, Guide de Vie. Paris: Gallimard 1945.

PURDY, D. M.: The Bezold-Brücke phenomenon and contours for constant hue. Amer. J. Psychol. **49**, 313—315 (1937).

RICHARDS, W.: Differences among color normals: Classes I and II. J. opt. Soc. Amer. **57**, 1047—1055 (1967).

ROELOFS, C. O., ZEEMAN, W. P. C.: Colour phenomena associated with increases and decreases in physical brightness. Acta psychol. (Amst.) **13**, 173—196 (1957).

— — Benham's top and the colour phenomena resulting from interaction with intermittent light stimuli. Acta psychol. (Amst.) **13**, 334—356 (1958).

RUBIN, M. L.: Spectral hue loci of normal and anomalous trichromats. Amer. J. Ophthal. **52**, 166—172 (1961).

SCHROEDINGER, E.: Grundlinien einer Theorie der Farbenmetrik im Tagessehen. Ann. Physik (IV), **63**, 481—520 (1920).

SEGAL, J.: Une nouvelle manifestation de couleurs subjectives. C. R. Soc. Biol. (Paris) **133**, 259—261 (1940).

STEVENS, S. S.: The psychophysics of sensory function. Amer. Scientist **48**, 226—253 (1960).

— To honor Fechner and repeal his law. Science **133**, 80—86 (1961).

STILES, W. S.: A modified Helmholtz line-element in brightness-colour space. Proc. phys. Soc. (Lond.) **58**, 41—65 (1946).

— Color vision: The approach through increment threshold sensitivity. Proc. nat. Acad. Sci. (Wash.) **45**, 100—114 (1959).

— BURCH, J. M.: N.P.L. colour-matching investigation: Final report (1958). Optica Acta **6**, 1—26 (1959).

SVAETICHIN, G.: Spectral response curves from single cones. Acta physiol. scand. **39**, Supp. 134, 17—46 (1956).

— NEGISHI, K., FATEHCHAND, R.: Cellular mechanisms of a Young-Hering visual system. In: Colour Vision, Physiology and Experimental Psychology (Ciba Found. Symp.), DE REUCK, A. V. S., KNIGHT, M. (Eds.), pp. 178—203. Boston: Little, Brown 1965.

TOMITA, T., KANEKO, A., MURAKAMI, M., PAUTLER, E. L.: Spectral response curves of single cones in the carp. Vision Res. **7**, 519—531 (1967).

TROLAND, L. T.: The enigma of color vision. Amer. J. physiol. Optics **2**, 23—48 (1921).

VERRIEST, G., SEKI, R.: Les chromaticités des couleurs subjectives suscitées par la rotation du disque de Fechner-Benham. Rev. Opt. (Paris) **43**, 53—63 (1964).

WAGNER, H. G., MACNICHOL, E. G., WOLBARSHT, M. L.: The response properties of single ganglion cells in the goldfish retina. J. gen. Physiol. **43** (Suppl.) 45—62 (1960).

WALD, G.: The receptors of human color vision. Science **145**, 1007—1017 (1964).

— Receptor mechanisms in human vision. Proc. 13th Int. Physiol. Congr., Tokyo, 1965, Lectures and Symposia, pp. 69—79. Amsterdam: Excerpta Medica Foundation 1965.

— Defective color vision and its inheritance. Proc. nat. Acad. Sci. (Wash.) **55**, 1347—1363 (1966).

— Blue-blindness in the normal fovea. J. opt. Soc. Amer. **57**, 1289—1301 (1967).

WALD, G., BROWN, P. K.: Human color vision and color blindness. Cold Spr. Harb. Symp. quant. Biol. **30**, 345—361 (1965).
WALRAVEN, P. L.: On the mechanisms of colour vision. Soesterberg: Institute for Perception RVO-TNO 1962.
WASSERMAN, G. D.: Heterochromatic additivity failure. Psychol. Rev. **76**, 221—222 (1969).
WEALE, R. A.: The foveal and para-central spectral sensitivities in man. J. Physiol. (Lond.) **114**, 435—446 (1951).
— Spectral sensitivity and wavelength discrimination of the peripheral retina. J. Physiol. (Lond.) **119**, 170—190 (1953).
WERBLIN, F. S., DOWLING, J. E.: Organization of the retina of the mudpuppy, *Necturus maculosus*. II. Intracellular recording. J. Neurophysiol. **32**, 339—355 (1969).
WIESEL, T. N., HUBEL, D. H.: Spatial and chromatic interactions in the lateral geniculate body of the rhesus monkey. J. Neurophysiol. **29**, 1115—1156 (1966).
WILSON, B. C.: An experimental examination of the spectral luminosity construct. PhD thesis, New York University. Ann Arbor: University Microfilms (1964).
WYSZECKI, G., STILES, W. S.: Color Science: Concepts and Methods, Quantitative Data and Formulas. New York: Wiley 1967.

Chapter 15

Spectral Luminosity

By

Yves Le Grand, Paris (France)

With 8 Figures

Contents

Introduction

The human retina is sensitive to a large variety of radiations: X-rays (see Schober, 1964), perhaps cosmic rays (d'Arcy and Porter, 1962), ultraviolet (as far as 300 nm for aphakic subjects without crystalline lens; normally ultraviolet absorption by the lens limits the blurring of the retinal image due to chromatic aberration) and, on the other hand, infrared up to more than 1000 nm (Griffin *et al.*, 1947). But only a limited range of wavelengths is actually effective in human vision, the so-called visible spectrum which lies roughly between 400 and 700 nm. This chapter deals with measurements of the efficiency of different wavelengths to produce vision. In technical terms, this problem is referred to as *luminous efficiency of monochromatic radiations* or more briefly *spectral luminosity*.

A precise definition of this concept may be obtained as follows. Let us consider two monochromatic radiations of wavelengths λ_1 and λ_2, and an experimental device enabling these radiations to fall upon the retina, either simultaneously or successively. Geometrical specifications are identical for both beams of light: in simultaneous comparison, for instance, the radiations fill (uniformly or with the same pattern of spatial distribution) the two halves of a bipartite test field; in successive comparison, they fill the same test field one after the other with the same exposure time. In the device a control knob allows a continuous change in the ratio of the energies W_1 and W_2 of the two beams during a given time (duration of a flash, or one second in case of steady exposure). The energy W_1 remains at a fixed setting while W_2 may vary between two limiting values. It is essential also to adopt an *equivalence criterion* between the two radiations with respect to their visual effect. As will be seen later, this criterion is more or less arbitrary, but it must give the observer the possibility of determining without ambiguity the value of W_2 which fulfills the equivalence condition. When equivalence is reached, there is no reason for W_1 and W_2 to be equal, and actually this happens only by chance. But it is always possible to write

$$V_1 W_1 = V_2 W_2 \tag{1}$$

V_1 and V_2 being positive weighting factors. The choice of the symbol V is due to the historical fact that these quantities were called "visibility factors" by NUTTING some sixty years ago. This terminology is now obsolete, but the symbol remains.

If the argument is continued in the same way, it is possible to assign to each wavelength λ a factor V_λ. As these factors have so far been defined only by their ratios, it is possible arbitrarily to fix the value of V_λ for a certain wavelength λ_m as unity, which yields values less than unity for all other wavelengths, and thus to define the *relative luminous efficiency* of any monochromatic radiation.

It is essential to remember that the V_λ values are relative to a given observer whose retina is in a given state of adaptation, and also to a conventional equivalence criterion for well-defined conditions of observation. It is well known that cone vision can be isolated by confining the stimulus to the rod free center of the fovea; the diameter of the test field must then be less than 1°. When the test field is fixated centrally and the light level is high enough (luminance of at least a few cd/m^2), the cones still predominate and these conditions are said to be *photopic*. On the other hand, with a retina fully dark-adapted, at a low luminance level (less than 10^{-3} cd/m^2) and a large peripheral test field, vision is mediated by rods only and the conditions are said to be *scotopic*. The intermediate range, when both cones and rods are active, is called *mesopic*.

It is less important, although interesting, to note that the equality $V_2 W_2 = V_3 W_3$ combined with Eq. (1) does not necessarily mean that $V_1 W_1 = V_3 W_3$ with a fixed set of V_i and W_i values, unless the mathematical condition of *transitivity* is obeyed. Experimentally it seems to be true to a reasonable approximation, so that we may speak of a single-valued function V_λ for specified conditions without giving the sequence $\lambda_1 \lambda_2 \ldots \lambda_n$ used in the actual measurements.

The usual graphical representation of this function is a plot of the *relative luminous efficiency curve* with V_λ as ordinate and λ as abscissa. The bell-shaped curves thus obtained are asymptotically tangent to the abscissa axis at the ends of the visible spectrum, so that graphical precision is poor except in the middle of the spectrum; thus it is better, and we shall adopt this procedure, to plot $\log_{10} V_\lambda$ as ordinate. For the abscissae we shall also depart from the classical linear wavelength scale; graduation linear in *frequency* is better for reasons which will appear later, but the numbers will be given in wavelengths (nm) because they are more familiar to the average reader than frequencies or wave-numbers.

Since vision is primarily a photochemical process, it is related more directly to numbers of light quanta (photons) absorbed in the retinal photopigments than to energies. Accordingly Eq. (1) which defines luminous efficiencies should more logically be written with numbers N_1 and N_2 of quanta than with the total energies W_1 and W_2 carried by them. The well-known Planck relation tells us that the energy of one quantum of light is proportional to its frequency, hence inversely proportional to the wavelength; the new luminous efficiency should then be proportional to V_λ/λ. Although these new factors should be more convenient, because directly comparable to absorption spectra of photopigments, we shall not use them – a little reluctantly – but rather we shall still adhere to the traditional definition (1).

Photopic Luminous Efficiency

For the history of relative luminous efficiency functions, reference should be made to accounts by SLOAN (1928) and LE GRAND (1968).

The first equivalence criterion to be used for a statistical determination of the photopic efficiency was that of the *flicker* method. A source constantly emitting the same white light at a fixed luminance alternated, at a rate of 10 to 20 times per second, with monochromatic light λ_1 of energy W_1. The circular field of about 3° diameter, was uniformly and successively filled with the white and monochromatic lights without dark interruption. The value of W_1 was adjusted by the observer until flicker was at a minimum. The minimum would have been reduced to nothing and the appearance perfectly steady if the frequency of alternation had been high enough, but to get the best precision it is useful to retain a slight flicker since the condition of minimum can be determined more precisely than complete disappearance. The operation is repeated with another wavelength λ_2 and the energy W_2 adjusted until the flicker is again at a minimum, and so on.

A second equivalence criterion was that of *direct comparison*: a bipartite photometric field (for example a 2° circular test area divided along a vertical diameter) was uniformly filled on one side with light λ_1 and on the other with light λ_2. When λ_1 and λ_2 are well apart in the spectrum, for instance if one half of the field is red and the other green, this problem of *heterochromatic photometry* is difficult to solve because, due to the difference in colour, the equivalence criterion is highly unstable: it is different from one observer to another and even from day to day for the same subject. This difficulty diminishes as λ_1 and λ_2 become more nearly the same and vanishes when the difference between λ_1 and λ_2 falls below the differential threshold of chromaticity. But since there are as many as 250 discernible hues in the spectrum, a complete determination of luminous efficiency by direct comparison would be very laborious and has never been done. A simplified variation of it, *the step-by-step method*, is used instead: at, say, 20 points in the spectrum a direct comparison is made between wavelengths λ_1 and λ_2, the difference varying between 2 to 5 nm in order that the difference in hue remain very slight. In fact it is the derivative $dV_\lambda/d\lambda$ which is obtained by this method for 20 values of λ and the V_λ curve is deduced by integration.

There is a systematic deviation between results obtained from flicker and step-by-step methods, as can be seen from the classical results obtained by the U.S.A. Bureau of Standards between 1917 and 1923 (Fig. 1). But this difference is much smaller than the spread between different subjects using the same method, so that a mean curve based on both techniques was adapted in 1924 by the Commission Internationale de l'Éclairage (C.I.E.) and is universally used under the name of

C.I.E. Photopic Standard Observer. This fictitious entity is based on more than 200 adult white observers looking centrally at a 2° test field. In order to assist the retina to adapt itself to the light level of this test field, it is generally surrounded by a large peripheral field of the same luminance. In the flicker measurements referred to above, this luminance was constant and was equivalent to about 1.5 cd/m² seen with the natural pupil; in the step-by-step method, it varied between about 3 cd/m² in the middle of the spectrum to less than 0.5 cd/m² at the ends. These levels are mesopic rather than photopic.

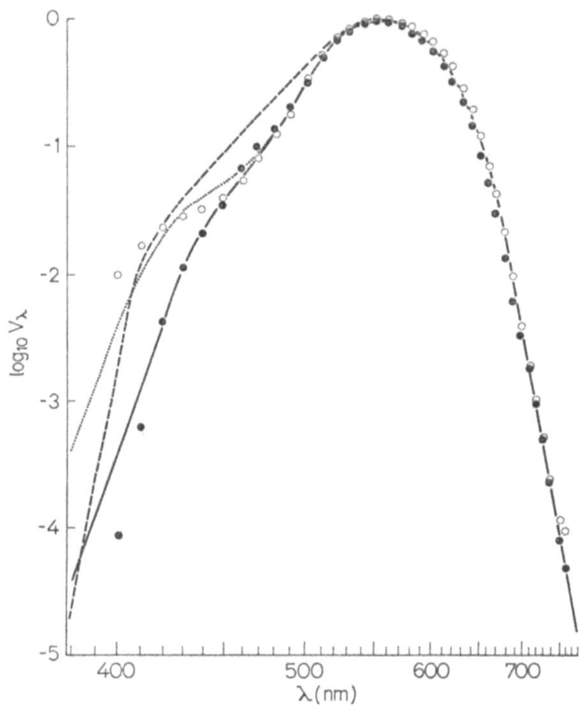

Fig. 1. Photopic luminosity curves: ○ flicker, ● step-by-step. C.I.E. standard observer (——), modifications proposed by Judd (1949) (······), C.I.E. supplementary observer (-----)

The C.I.E. standard observer is constantly used in photometry and has much practical value though its physiological definition seems far from perfect. As can be seen in Fig. 1, the choice of the C.I.E. photopic efficiency curve was somewhat arbitrary, especially at the blue end of the spectrum. Values of V_λ may be found in Table 1. The maximum ($V_\lambda = 1$) is for $\lambda_m = 555$ nm.

Real subjects, even with normal colour vision, may differ considerably from the C.I.E. observer. For example, for the 125 subjects studied by flicker, the individual maximum varied between 549 and 570 nm, and the average was at 557.6 nm. For 52 subjects in one step-by-step study, the following limits were obtained at the extremities of the spectrum

$$\lambda = 430 \text{ nm}, \quad 0.014 < V_\lambda < 0.064,$$

$$\lambda = 700 \text{ nm}, \quad 0.0028 < V_\lambda < 0.0069.$$

Table 1. *C.I.E. Standard observers: a, photopic; b, supplementary; c, scotopic*

λ(nm)	*a*	*b*	*c*
380	0.00004	0.00002	0.0006
390	0.00012	0.00025	0.0022
400	0.0004	0.0020	0.0093
410	0.0012	0.0088	0.0348
420	0.0040	0.0214	0.0966
430	0.0116	0.0387	0.1998
440	0.023	0.0621	0.3281
450	0.038	0.0895	0.455
460	0.060	0.1282	0.567
470	0.091	0.1852	0.676
480	0.139	0.2536	0.793
490	0.208	0.3391	0.904
500	0.323	0.4608	0.982
510	0.503	0.6067	0.997
520	0.710	0.7618	0.935
530	0.862	0.8752	0.811
540	0.954	0.9620	0.650
550	0.995	0.9918	0.481
560	0.995	0.9973	0.3288
570	0.952	0.9556	0.2076
580	0.870	0.8689	0.1212
590	0.757	0.7774	0.0655
600	0.631	0.6583	0.0332
610	0.503	0.5280	0.0159
620	0.381	0.3981	0.0074
630	0.265	0.2835	0.0033
640	0.175	0.1798	0.0015
650	0.107	0.1076	0.00068
660	0.061	0.0603	0.00031
670	0.032	0.0318	0.00015
680	0.017	0.0159	0.000072
690	0.0082	0.0077	0.000035
700	0.0041	0.0037	0.000018
710	0.0021	0.0018	0.000009
720	0.00105	0.00085	0.000005
730	0.00052	0.00041	0.000003
740	0.00025	0.00020	0.000001
750	0.00012	0.00010	0.000001
760	0.00006	0.00005	
770	0.00003	0.00003	
780	0.000015	0.000013	

In cases of abnormal colour vision, discrepancies are much higher, especially for protans whose spectrum is shortened in the long wave region.

Investigations of Japanese and Egyptian subjects seem to show that ethnological differences do not affect V_λ, except perhaps through racial differences in macular pigmentation (see below). For a given observer, variations related to astronomical periodicities or other causes have sometimes been described, but the only certain dependence is a progressive change with age. A thorough study of this problem was done by RUDDOCK (1965) on some 400 observers from 16 to 70 years of age. Flicker and direct comparison methods were used with a 1°20′ square field and a light level (equivalent luminance with natural pupil) from 5 to 10 cd/m² except for 420 nm (about 0.2 cd/m²). The mean V_λ values obtained for each age group, relative to unity at 560 nm, show a slight increase with age for 600 nm, a slight decrease at 515 and a very large decrease at 420 (Fig. 2). It seems that the retina does not change with age and that the effect is due to a gradual yellowing of the crystalline lens, a phenomenon known for a long time (see Ruddock, chapter 17, this volume).

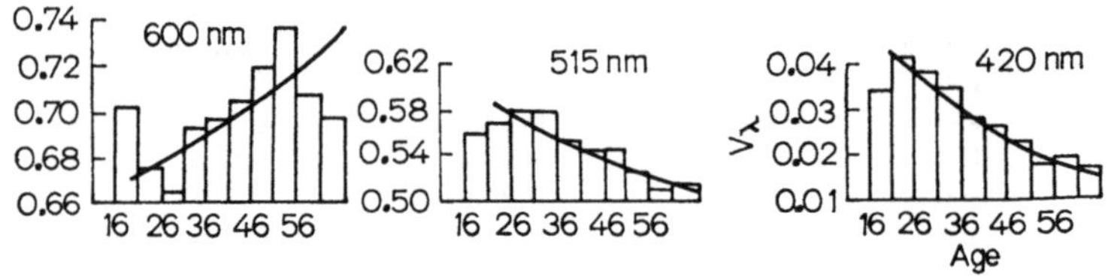

Fig. 2. Mean V_λ values for different age groups ($V_\lambda = 1$ at 560 nm). The curves have been drawn on the assumption of a continuous change with age (after Ruddock, 1965)

Colorimetric Method

Another equivalence criterion for photopic luminous efficiency makes use of a *colour match* between a monochromatic radiation filling one half of a photometric field, and the superposition on the other half of three monochromatic radiations, called *primaries* (usually wavelengths that appear mostly red, green and blue). When the match is obtained, there is a perfect visual identity, both in colour and brightness, between both halves of the field, and consequently the equality of luminances is far more precise than for heterochromatic photometry. Flicker or direct comparison methods are restricted to the determination of the luminous units of the primaries themselves and all other measurements are purely physical (energy determinations). It is important, however, to note that the validity of this method rests upon a postulated additivity of luminances in the additive mixture of primaries, which is far from being evident and to which we shall return later. For a complete discussion of this method, see Wyszecki and Stiles (1967).

Briefly the first step is to choose monochromatic primaries, for instance $\boldsymbol{R}$ (645.2 nm), $\boldsymbol{G}$ (526.3 nm) and $\boldsymbol{B}$ (444.4 nm) and to measure the energies W_R, W_G and W_B of the primaries which by addition give a colour match to a standard white light. Then (by flicker, for instance) the relative luminous efficiencies of the primaries, V_R, V_G and V_B are measured. These heterochromatic determinations are the only ones required in the process. The luminous units of the primaries are then defined as

$$L_R = V_R W_R, \quad L_G = V_G W_G, \quad L_B = V_B W_B.$$

Then a colour match is realized between the unit energy of any given monochromatic radiation λ and three energies $\bar{r}_\lambda$, $\bar{g}_\lambda$ and $\bar{b}_\lambda$ of the primaries; these quantities are the colour-matching functions and their determination involves only energy determinations when the match is obtained. Finally the luminous efficiency of the radiation is given by

$$V_\lambda = L_R \bar{r}_\lambda + L_G \bar{g}_\lambda + L_B \bar{b}_\lambda. \tag{2}$$

Actually for all wavelengths (except the primaries) one of the values of $\bar{r}_\lambda$ $\bar{g}_\lambda$ and $\bar{b}_\lambda$ is negative when (as assumed) the primaries are monochromatic radiations. That means that it is necessary to add (in one half of the photometric field) one of the primaries to the radiation λ in order to desaturate it and permit a match to the other two primaries (added in the second half of the field) (see WRIGHT, chapter 16, this volume).

Instead of calculating V_λ from Eq. (2), it is mathematically equivalent to change the primaries and define three new reference stimuli $\boldsymbol{X}\ \boldsymbol{Y}\ \boldsymbol{Z}$ deduced from $\boldsymbol{R}\ \boldsymbol{G}\ \boldsymbol{B}$ by three linear equations; if the stimuli $\boldsymbol{X}$ and $\boldsymbol{Z}$ are located on the *alychne* (straight line of zero luminosity), then V_λ is given simply by the colour matching function $\bar{y}_\lambda$.

The most important work based on the colorimetric method was done in the British National Physical Laboratory by STILES and BURCH (1959) on 49 subjects with a circular, horizontally divided, bipartite field of 10° diameter with a narrow surround extending the illuminated field to a total diameter of 14°. The light level was high: the equivalent luminance for a natural pupil was maintained between 10 and 180 cd/m² except at the shortwave end of the spectrum where it fell to about 2 cd/m². The observers were instructed, in making colour matches, not to stare fixedly at the centre of the field while approaching the colour match, but on the other hand, to base their final judgment on the field appearance with the gaze directed to the centre and then to disregard in their judgment the central region (1° to 2° diameter) where the well known Maxwell spot due to macular yellow pigmentation of the retina makes it impossible to obtain an identity of the half-fields over their whole area for any setting of the primaries. All the observers also made direct-comparison heterochromatic brightness matches between the primaries and a white field, and 26 of them made a flicker match for the same purpose of measuring the luminous units of the primaries. Wide variations (up to a ratio of 30 to 1) were found for colour-matching functions in the short wavelengths. They are due to individual differences in the yellow pigmentation of the macula, and also in spectral absorption of the crystalline lens. For a discussion of the respective importance of these two absorptions, the reader may consult the original paper. (See also RUDDOCK, chapter 17.)

In 1964, the C.I.E. adopted a *supplementary standard observer* for a 10° field, based mostly on STILES and BURCH's results and to a lesser extent on SPERANSKAYA's (1959) experiments in the Soviet Union. The values are listed in Table 1, the maximum being at $\lambda_m = 557$ nm. The main differences from the standard 2° observer occur in the short wavelengths, partly because the old values are somewhat uncertain in that region and also because of macular absorption (see Fig. 1). Since the light level is much higher for the supplementary observer than for the classical one, it might be thought that the true photopic luminosity function is closer to the supplementary observer than to his elder brother[1]. But the large field might cause some rod intrusion: a correction for it was applied to arrive at the final mean data, but the correction is small. In fact, C.I.E. experts think that both observers may be used for photopic conditions, depending on the field dimensions.

Threshold and other Methods

In the past, a very different method was often used for the purpose of obtaining photopic spectral efficiencies; the *absolute threshold* within the fovea was measured,

[1] Flicker determinations of V_λ for 10 subjects, a 10° field and a luminance of about 50 cd/m² by KANZOW (1964) give a curve closer to the standard photopic than to the supplementary C.I.E. observer.

that is the smallest energy of a monochromatic flash which is still perceived. The light source must be small enough to be imaged on the rod-free area, and the fixation controlled so that no rods may come into action. In principle the source is seen as coloured as soon as it is perceived, whereas with rod vision it is seen as colourless. The reader may consult Pirenne (1962) for an excellent review of such experiments. These threshold studies are very interesting but they do *not* measure spectral luminosity and it is easy to understand why. In connexion with Thomas Young's theory of colour vision, it was thought without proof during a century and a half that there existed in the human retina three different types of cones, all anatomically identical but with different photosensitive pigments. In recent years this hypothesis has been experimentally demonstrated for the goldfish retina by microspectrophotometry of individual cones, and for the carp retina by electrical recordings from individual cones (see Jameson, chapter 14, this volume). It is highly probable that it is also true for man. Luminous efficiency is based on cooperative work done by the three types of cones. (It has sometimes been postulated that a fourth type of cone might contain a mixture of the three pigments; were this the case, luminous efficiency would depend on these "luminosity" cones, whilst colour vision would depend on the three other types. This hypothesis is wrong, as proved by experiments on the goldfish and the carp referred to above.) At threshold there is no summation because one only of the cone mechanisms is active, i.e., the most sensitive for the stimulus which is used. As Pirenne (1962) writes, the foveal sensitivity curve based on absolute threshold measurements is not the sum of the sensitivities of the individual cone mechanisms, but rather an "envelope" of the sensitivity curves of the various mechanisms acted upon by the stimulus. In fact, the so-called "luminous efficiency curves" measured at threshold in the fovea by numerous authors exhibit various humps which may be used to define transition points among the three types of cones. This is very useful to elucidate mechanisms of colour vision, but of no assistance in the true problem of luminosity.

Numerous other equivalence criteria have been proposed, but all are actually measurements of other functions with no direct relation to luminosity. For example, the idea of using pupil diameter as an index of sensitivity to various wavelengths has often been tried, but there is no reason why it should give the same results as the classical methods and Bouma (1965), for instance, has clearly shown that short wavelengths are much more efficient in the pupillary reflex than in photopic vision. Ultraviolet has an effect on the pupil even when it is not seen.

The opposite conclusion may be reached for another criterion, the equal acuity method. Even if the chromatic aberration of the eye is corrected, acuity is worse at the short wave end of the spectrum at constant luminance; this is probably related to a smaller density of population of "blue" cones than of the others, as demonstrated by Brindley (1960)[2].

The only equivalence criterion that gives results in good agreement with the direct-comparison, flicker and colorimetric methods, is based on electrophysiology and will be dealt with in another section of this book (see Riggs and Wooten, chapter 27, this volume).

---

[2] With the acuity criterion, and also for an equal contrast criterion, Khazanov (1967) finds a curve with several maxima, but the maxima differ in these two cases.

Photopic Peripheral Luminosity

All experiments hitherto described refer to central vision, the subject being instructed to fixate the center of the field. It is also important to study the peripheral retina and two different methods may be used.

In the first a peripheral test field is compared to a central one, both being presented simultaneously for a short time because properties of extra-foveal vision change very quickly. Equivalence criteria of direct comparison or colorimetry may be used, but not flicker, which disappears in a few seconds in the peripheral retina. As an example of such a study, we may cite MORELAND and CRUZ's (1959) measurements by colorimetry: a foveal trichromatic mixture in a rectangular test field of $40' \times 80'$ was matched with a monochromatic stimulus of the same dimensions seen peripherally. The luminance was equivalent to about 2 cd/m² seen with the natural pupil. Luminous units of the primaries were measured by purely foveal matches. The V_λ curves for two observers were determined between 10° and 50° of excentricity (angular distance between the fields). In these experiments matches are difficult and of low precision, but the general features are quite clear: the maximum λ_m shifts toward short wavelengths and is below 500 nm for great excentricities. But if the entire retina is in darkness except for the two test fields, the usual form of the V_λ curve does not change significantly.

In the second method, both fields to be matched are peripheral and near one another. When a large conditioning field of high luminance surrounds the test fields, the shape of the curve is considerably distorted and a prominent hump appears in the blue near 440 nm. This fact has been reported frequently but the most interesting results are those of WEALE (1953) for direct comparison, and of MORELAND (1955) for colorimetry (Fig. 3). At 10° excentricity the blue hump is very apparent and at 25° the short wave sensitivity is further enhanced and becomes higher than anywhere else in the spectrum.

It is sometimes said that these results are characteristic of the "light-adapted" peripheral retina. This terminology is confusing because the word adaptation may have different meanings. The older meaning (AUBERT, 1865) refers to *temporal adaptation*: a long-lasting stay in bright sunshine, or in very dim light, results in a state of the retina that persists for some minutes even if the illumination conditions change. This light or dark adaptation is mainly a photochemical phenomenon, due to bleaching or regeneration of pigments in the outer segments of cones and rods. It is also due in part to changes in retinal nervous connections, especially for rods: scotopic vision is mediated by groups of rods whose excitations converge, and rod superiority is caused by the fact that they work in parallel with greater facility than do cones. But there is also a second meaning of the word adaptation, the *spatial adaptation* which is really a neural inhibition, as in contrast or glare effects, and which is better named *masking*. Clearly in the experiments summarized here (Fig. 3), the so-called "adapting" field of high luminance which surrounds the test fields depresses the sensitivities of retinal mechanisms, but less for the "blue" cones than for the others. It is striking that the "blue fundamental" behaves in a special way, characterized by the smallness of its contribution to luminance in the central retina, by laws of adaptation to colour peculiar to itself, and by its primitive type, shown by the rarity of anomalies affecting this "fundamental" which seems oldest in evolutionary history. On account of their robustness, "blue" cones are more resistant to the masking effect of a high conditioning surround; in central vision, lateral inhibition is much less than in excentric vision, and the apparent enhancement of luminosity at short wavelengths (due to masking of "green" and "red" fundamentals) is scarcely apparent; it increases with excentricity and becomes enormous in the retinal periphery.

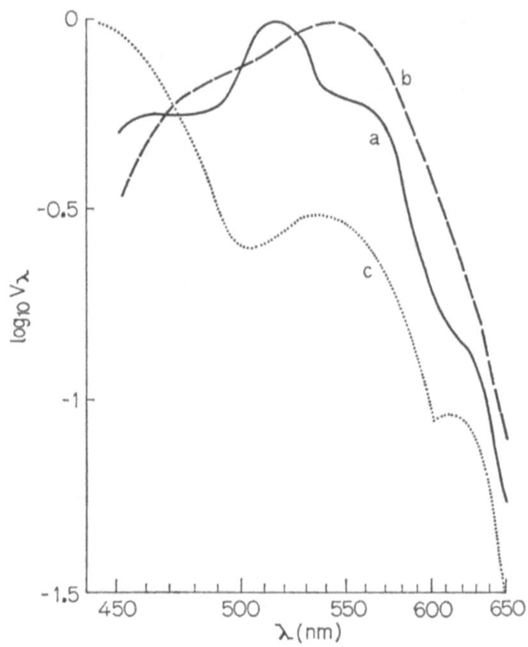

Fig. 3. Photopic luminosity in peripheral retina with a conditioning surround: *a* MORELAND, 10°; *b* WEALE, 10°, *c* WEALE, 25°

Scotopic Luminous Efficiency

This problem is much easier to solve than the photopic one. The retina is now fully dark-adapted by at least 20 minutes of total darkness, luminous levels are kept very low during the measuring in order not to destroy dark adaptation, test fields are large so that cooperative properties of rods may function freely, and they are presented peripherally at about 10° excentricity where the rod population is most dense. As for the equivalence criterion to be used, flicker is impossible because fusion is reached very quickly in lateral vision. Direct comparison is much easier than for cone vision since colour differences disappear in scotopic vision. The threshold method is also usable and gives results in good agreement with direct comparison: there is only one kind of rod (at least for man) and therefore no difficulties arise from a multiplicity of receptors at threshold.

The best scotopic luminosity determinations are those of CRAWFORD (1949) made by direct comparison between a white and a monochromatic light in a 20° field with vertical separation. Fixation was on the upper end of the dividing line.

The luminance was about 3.10^{-5} cd/m^2 viewed with a natural pupil. Fifty observers under 30 years of age took part in the measurements after spending an hour in darkness. The threshold method was used by WALD (1945) with 22 observers averaging 20 years of age. At a meeting in 1951, the C.I.E. decided to recommend a *scotopic standard observer* based on CRAWFORD's and WALD's results and considered to represent the average scotopic luminosity for dark-adapted subjects under

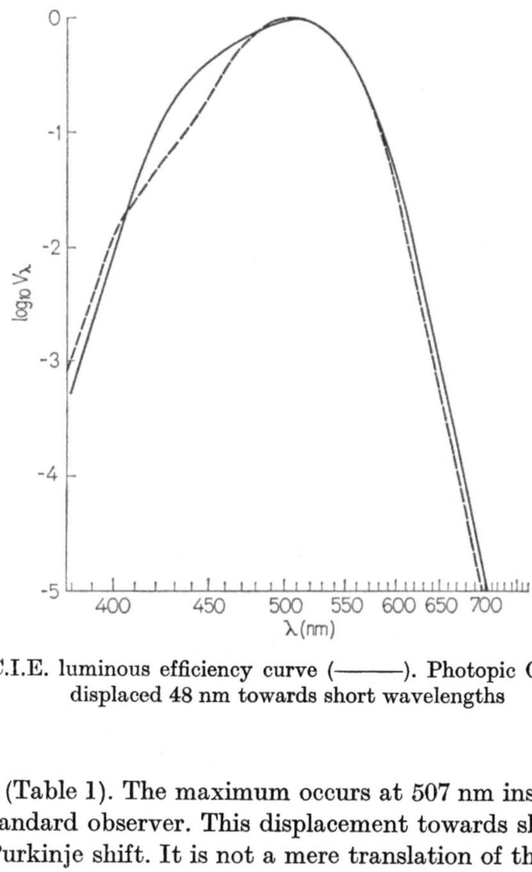

Fig. 4. Scotopic C.I.E. luminous efficiency curve (———). Photopic C.I.E. curve (- - - - - -) displaced 48 nm towards short wavelengths

30 years of age (Table 1). The maximum occurs at 507 nm instead of 555 nm for the photopic standard observer. This displacement towards short wavelengths is known as the Purkinje shift. It is not a mere translation of the curves, as can be seen in Fig. 4 where the photopic curve has been displaced toward the short wave end to make both maxima coincide. In fact, the scotopic curve V_λ, when corrected for the absorption in the crystalline lens (macular absorption does not play any role in peripheral vision), or better, the V_λ/λ curve for reasons given above, is closely related to the action spectrum of *rhodopsin*, the rod photosensitive pigment (see chapter 14). All the action spectra of known photopigments are identical, given a translation parallel to the abscissa axis, if this axis is scaled in frequency, which is one of the advantages of using frequency scaling and not wavelength. This generality, known as DARTNALL's (1957) rule, evidently cannot be extended to describe the relation between photopic and scotopic V_λ which indicates that cones contain more than one photopigment.

It is clearly apparent in Fig. 4 that in the long wavelengths the photopic and scotopic curves are straight lines that run parallel and may be represented by the formula

$$\log_{10} V_\lambda = a + b/\lambda$$

the factor b being about 14,000 nm for both curves.

The explanation of this fact has been given independently by STILES (1948) and DE VRIES (1948): if the decomposition of a molecule of photosensitive pigment requires energy W, the quantum of light $h\nu$ must in principle convey at least this amount if none comes from the molecule. At long wavelengths, $h\nu$ becomes less than W and the thermal energy of the molecule may provide the necessary supplement $E = W - h\nu$. If it is assumed that the fraction of molecules having at least this amount of thermal energy E follows Boltzmann's law in exp $(-E/kT)$, it is possible to calculate the long wave absorption curves of any photosensitive pigments; on a logarithmic scale they will be parallel straight lines to a first approximation if the abscissa scale is frequency, whatever the chemical constitution of the substance. A second approximation (LEWIS, 1955) predicts slight departures from straight lines, which gives a theoretical explanation of BRINDLEY's (1955) observations of minor changes in hue in the deep red for cone vision. Another consequence of STILES' and DE VRIES' theory is that increase in temperature T increases the sensitivity to deep red, which has been experimentally verified.

A last question about scotopic luminosity efficiency is what happens when the age exceeds 30 years, since the values in Table 1 apply only to younger subjects. According to CRAWFORD, for wavelengths λ below 500 nm, there is a decrease in V_λ depending on age A which can be represented by

$$\Delta(\log_{10} V_\lambda) = 10^{-4}(500 - \lambda)(A - 30).$$

As already said, this phenomenon must be due to the progressive yellowing of the lens. With aphakic subjects, scotopic efficiency increases considerably in the short-wave violet and ultraviolet: DODT and WALTHER'S (1958) electroretinogram measurements give values of V_λ of about 0.1 at 350 nm.

Mesopic Vision

It is generally agreed that scotopic vision extends to about 10^{-3} cd/m^2 and that above that luminance cones are activated and vision becomes mesopic. The upper limit of mesopic vision, that is the saturation of rods, is not so well defined and varies with the dimensions of the field. According to JOHNSON (1937) the necessary luminance is about 5 cd/m^2 with a 3° diameter field (seen centrally, of course), and at least 15 cd/m^2 for a 25° diameter field.

Much work has been done on mesopic luminosity curves (for the history see LE GRAND, 1968) and it was early evident that intermediate luminosity functions cannot be simulated by linear combinations of photopic and scotopic functions. The problem is much more complicated and depends upon various parameters. We shall not try to examine this question in detail and shall give only the most important results concerning rod and cone interactions.

Experimental evidence for rod-cone interaction in the mesopic range has been produced by many authors. For example, BROWN (1968) has confirmed the suggestion, already proposed by several investigators, that red light may have a sensitizing effect on rods: exposure to red light at a low luminance seems to hasten dark adaptation, the absolute threshold falling more quickly than in total darkness. It is not impossible for this effect to be a pure photochemical rod phenomenon, as *photorestoration* by long wavelengths is classical in photobiology, but it seems more probable that it is a neural facilitation of rods by "red" cones. BROWN has also tried to test the opposite interaction, that is an inhibition of one receptor process on the function of the other. He concludes that there is no evidence that cones may be inhibited by the emergence of the scotopic process; actually the equivalence criterion used by BROWN was an acuity one, which has little to do with luminosity problems.

Interesting results were obtained by HOUGH (1968) when measuring the flicker luminosity function of his own parafovea at 7° from the fixation point, in the temporal part of the retina. The field was a circular one of 55′ diameter, the spectral range extended from 400 to 570 nm, and 3 levels of retinal illumination were used, corresponding to about 0.5, 0.1 and 0.02 cd/m² seen by the natural pupil. The foveal luminosity function was also measured for the same conditions. At the highest level, the difference is entirely due to macular pigmentation, since this difference agrees closely with the spectral absorption found by RUDDOCK (1963). A change with excentricity in the relative populations of "red" and "green" cones, suggested by WEALE (1968), would also affect the V_λ function although not the colour matching functions; it does not appear in HOUGH's results.

At the two other levels, the mesopic V_λ curve is displaced towards short wavelengths. It was not possible to use a level lower than 0.02 cd/m² due to poor fixation and difficulties in making flicker judgments. If the V_λ change was caused only by increasing rod intrusion, the difference in the V_λ functions between the highest and one of the lower levels would give the scotopic V_λ function with a maximum near 500 nm, whereas the actual maximum is at about 450 nm and thus seems related to the "blue" cones. HOUGH thinks that the Purkinje shift in the mesopic range is effected both by rods and "blue" cones, perhaps because at low levels there arises a facilitation of the "blue" mechanisms by rods.

A confirmation of this idea was obtained by HOUGH and RUDDOCK (1969) from measurements of the Purkinje shift on a tritanope whose "blue" cones are lacking. The foveal V_λ curve of this subject is quite normal, which is not surprising because "blue" cones make only a small contribution to foveal luminosity. But at a 7° extrafoveal location, the tritanope has a classical V_λ scotopic luminosity curve even at relatively high luminances; it is only above 20 cd/m² that his Purkinje shift is complete, due to the saturation of the rods. Therefore the Purkinje shift in a normal observer is facilitated by the functioning of the "blue" cone mechanism. It is interesting to note that some relationship between rods and "blue" cones had already been postulated by various authors, for example BLACKWELL and BLACKWELL (1961).

In conclusion, it seems certain that a simple mixing of photopic and scotopic vision in the mesopic range is not correct from the point of view of physiology. However, for technical purposes, we shall see later how this intricate problem may be solved in an approximate way.

Luminance Additivity

Up to now we have dealt only with monochromatic luminosities. But this is an artificial case, and in practical applications light sources emit in the visible range either a line spectrum or a continuous one or sometimes both simultaneously, as in fluorescent tubes where the mercury line spectrum is superimposed on the continuous spectrum of the coating.

In the case of a line spectrum containing discrete monochromatic radiations $\lambda_1 \lambda_2 \ldots \lambda_n$, the simplest assumption about the total luminance L is Abney's law of additivity

$$L = L_1 + L_2 + \cdots + L_n \tag{3}$$

where L_i represented the component luminance of the radiation λ_i. It has long been known that this law holds very well in scotopic vision, whereas in photopic vision it holds only as an approximation which is generally sufficient for practical purposes. Departures from Abney's law are dependent on the choice of the equivalence criterion. There is little to be said about the colorimetric method because additivity of the three primary luminances is implicitly assumed as the basis of this technique, and therefore the only way of testing Abney's law is to compare V_λ values obtained through colorimetry with those obtained by other methods. This procedure is far too indirect to be precise, but SPERLING (1958) and RICHARDS and LURIA (1964) concluded that additivity failures were not severe enough to warrant abandoning Abney's law. In flicker photometry, departures from additivity are small, as shown by IVES as early as 1912 and later by SHIPLEY (1961). On the other hand, with direct brightness comparison, discrepancies are sometimes very large (see TESSIER and BLOTTIAU, 1951).

A thorough study of this problem has been done anew by GUTH *et al.* (1969), using two equivalence criteria, threshold and direct comparison. In the threshold method, the general approach was to establish a subliminal field of wavelength λ, and to determine the added luminance of a variety of wavelengths including λ, in order to bring the field to threshold. In these conditions, Abney's law does not hold at all, which is not surprising. We know that the threshold criterion seems valid for rods to determine V_λ, but does not apply to V_λ for cones. SWETS (1960) has suggested a *vector model* as an alternative to Abney's law. Any monochromatic stimulus is represented by a vector whose length and direction indicate its luminance and wavelength, respectively; the resultant luminance of several lights is represented by the vectorial sum. It is possible to calculate a vectorial space so that the experimental facts can be approximately predicted, but it is a symbolic way of expressing interactions and inhibitions among the three types of cones, and its physiological meaning is not clear. The same conclusion holds for the *incremental threshold* method of STILES. He measures the threshold for a small test stimulus, for example, a circular patch of 1° diameter, appearing in flashes and foveally fixated, superimposed at the center of a 10° adapting field seen continuously. The test and adapting lights are monochromatic radiations of different wavelengths. The reader may find in MARRIOTT'S review (1962) a summary of the main results obtained by this technique (see also ENOCH, chapter 21, this volume). Here too uncertainties about interactions do not permit any firm conclusion about additivity.

In GUTH's direct brightness matching method, a circular bipartite field of 1.5° diameter was presented in Maxwellian view with a dark surround. In one half of this photometric field, white light from an iodine lamp was presented at a constant luminance. In the other half, a first monochromatic light λ_1 (for instance, 521 nm) was adjusted in intensity until the observer thought it matched the white in brightness; the same adjustment was made with a second monochromatic light

λ_2 (647 nm, for instance); the energy of 521 nm was then halved exactly, and 647 nm was added until a new match to the white was obtained. If Abney's law were valid, the energy of 647 nm would then have been half of its former value. Nine subjects, ten wavelengths and three photopic levels were used; factorial analysis of variance yielded a non-significant effect of level. As an example, Fig. 5 shows the mean results for $\lambda_1 = 521$ nm as a function of λ_2. In the long wavelengths there is a large loss of luminance, in accordance with the classical results that

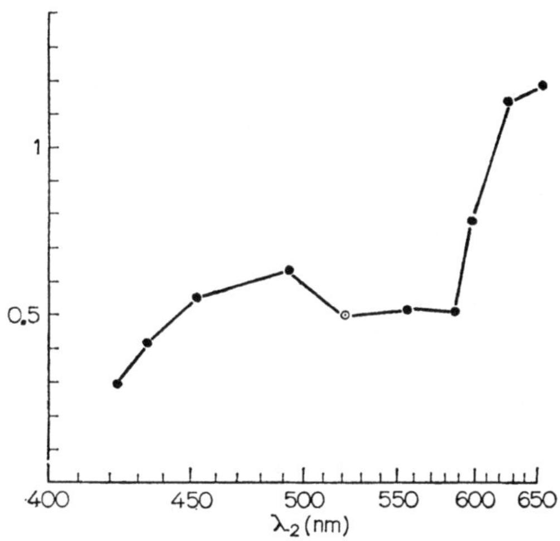

Fig. 5. Mean luminance of λ_2 added to $\lambda_1 = 521$ nm in order to bring the mixture to unit luminance, after GUTH *et al.* (1969)

showed, in particular, that superposition of lights that are complementary results in a clear cancellation of brightness as well as of chromaticness (PIÉRON, 1942). But a curious *enhancement* effect appears when λ_2 is in the short-wave violet, the whole being greater than the sum of the parts: on the average about 0.3 unit of 422 nm plus 0.5 unit of 521 nm matches a unit luminance of white. In the case of such enhancement, it is impossible to use a real vector space to represent failures of Abney's law.

Until recently it was difficult to find a physiological basis for luminance additivity, even if it were only a crude approximation. It is well known that, except near threshold, where apparent brightness may be linearly related to luminance (EKMAN and GUSTAFSSON, 1968), this relation is represented for higher levels either by Fechner's logarithmic law or by Plateau's power function. It is thus highly probably that luminosity signals in the optic nerve fibers, coming from the three cone mechanisms, are not linear functions of luminance, and this lack of linearity is confirmed by electrophysiological records. A possible way of escaping this contradiction was to postulate in the retina a fourth type of cone containing a mixture of pigments: but such a "luminosity cone" is not found in goldfish or carp retinas, as seen above. Another possibility was the hypothesis (HURVICH and JAMESON, 1957) of a linear combination of "brightness" signals before the non-linear physiological encoding. Happily the discovery of the ERP (Early Receptor Potential) clarifies the physiology. One of the ERP components is linearly related to the amount of pigment bleached by light in the photoreceptor during a unit of time. If the first stage of the luminosity signal is the resultant of the 3 ERP's converging on the same bipolar, Abney's law will hold whatever may be the subsequent changes in brightness coding at later stages in neural transmission.

Now the difficulty is reversed, and we must explain departures from additivity. GUTH *et al.* discuss their results within the framework of an opponent-colours theory in which direct brightness matching judgments are mediated by the combined effects of an opponent-type chromatic system and a non-opponent achromatic system, whereas flicker judgments are mediated only by the non-opponent system. In simpler words, it means that in heterochromatic photometry, colour and brightness are mixed in such a way that brightness matching becomes very difficult (actually there are very large variations from one observer to another in individual curves such as those in Fig. 5). It is possible also that the so-called Helmholtz-Kohlrausch effect (see LE GRAND, 1968), that is, a V_λ change through adaptation by coloured lights, may explain some features of these experiments, and especially the curious enhancement in the short wave region. As an argument in favour of this interpretation, we may cite a paper by BOYNTON and KAISER (1968) where it is shown that additivity holds in direct comparison photometry if, instead of the subjective criterion of equal brightness, the observer uses a criterion of minimally distinct border between two precisely juxtaposed fields. Small eye movements prevent different adaptation on the two sides of this separation line, and apparent failures of Abney's law disappear because they are mainly consequences of the Helmholtz-Kohlrausch adaptation effect.

Photometric Consequences

If Abney's law is assumed to hold, at least as a practical approximation, we may apply it to a source emitting a continuous spectrum light, and extending Eq. (3) write

$$L = K \int V_\lambda N_\lambda \, d\lambda \,, \tag{4}$$

where K is a constant factor depending on the choice of units and N_λ the *spectral radiance* of the source. In principle, the limits of the integral are zero and infinity, but as $V_\lambda = 0$ outside the visible spectrum, we may take the limits as those of the visible spectrum.

The K value has been fixed by the C.I.E. using a black body at the absolute temperature T of the solidification of platinum under normal pressure. By convention the value of L is then exactly 60 cd/m^2, this rounded value being chosen so that the new candela should not differ too much from the ancient "international candle". Since N_λ is known by Planck's formula, it is then possible to calculate K for any given V_λ function. Classical K values are 1746 for the scotopic standard observer if radiance is measured in watts per cm^2 and steradian (LE GRAND, 1968), and 683 or 645 for the photopic or supplementary observer, respectively (Comité E-1.4.1, 1968).

I have recalculated K values from the tables giving V_λ at 1 nm intervals by WYSZECKI and STILES (1967). Planck's formula is

$$N_\lambda = 2c^2h\,\lambda^{-5}(\exp(c_2/\lambda T) - 1)^{-1}. \quad (5)$$

For the velocity of light in vacuum c and Planck's constant h, I adopted the values $c = 2.997925 \cdot 10^8$ m/sec and $h = 6.62517 \cdot 10^{-34}$ joules sec. For the ratio c_2/T we take 7.04212, which is the value recommended by the Bureau International des Poids et Mesures ($c_2 = 14380$ and $T = 2042$). The values of K obtained by an electronic computer are 680.23, 654.45 and 1746.70 for the C.I.E. photopic, supplementary and scotopic observers, respectively.

In order to take into account departures from Abney's law and the Helmholtz-Kohlrausch effect, the photometric concept of *equivalent luminance* has recently gained much favour among Russian workers (VOLKENSHTEIN, 1965). This notion is defined as follows by the Comité E-1.4.1 of the C.I.E. (1968): "The equivalent luminance of the field of an arbitrary spectral composition of the radiation is the luminance (standard, photopic) of another field which has the relative composition of black body radiation with 2042°K and which under certain specified visual photometry conditions appears to be in photometric equality with the first field." The shape and dimensions of the stimulus field, state of adaptation of the subject and other technical points, are specified. It is also recommended that for mesopic vision intermediate V_λ values given for 6 luminances be adopted.

In my opinion, the "equivalent" luminance concept is unwise: it is already disturbing enough to have 3 different luminances defined by Eq. (4) and the 3 sets of standard K and V_λ values. These true luminances obey Abney's law. The so-called "equivalent luminance" is actually a subjective brightness concept founded on direct comparison heterochromatic matching, a method which is known to vary widely with the observer.

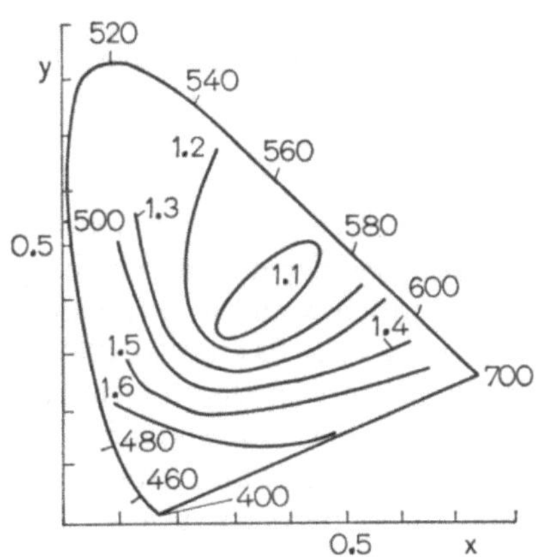

Fig. 6. C.I.E. chromaticity chart with loci of the Helmholtz-Kohlrausch factor, after SANDERS and WYSZECKI (1963)

Another possibility to make allowance for the Helmholtz-Kohlrausch effect is to multiply the classical luminance by a correction factor which depends on the chromaticity coordinates of the light, and which was determined for 20 observers by SANDERS and WYSZECKI (1963) (Fig. 6). But the practical utility of such refinements is not obvious. For instance, every lighting engineer knows that a given moderate luminance obtained from "daylight" fluorescent tubes seems sad and dull if compared with incandescence, but the correction factor in Fig. 6 is quite small in this case. Psychological effects preclude a general mathematical formula for such situations.

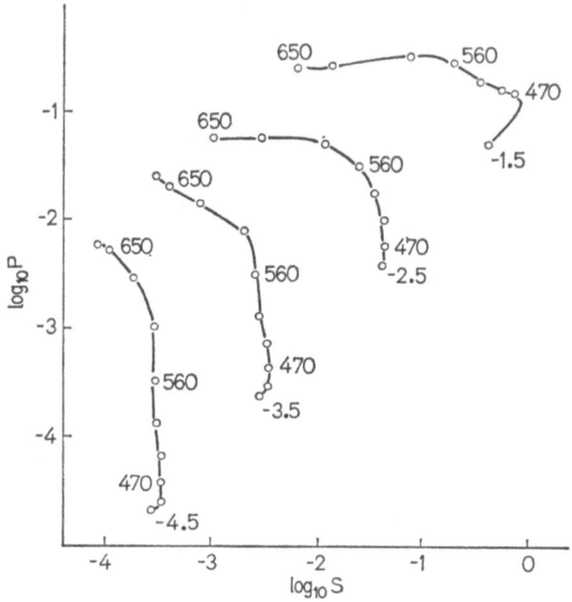

Fig. 7. Logarithmic plot of photopic luminance P against scotopic luminance S for monochromatic tests lights (in nm) that match the white standard in a 15° field for 4 levels L ($\log_{10} L$ is given near each curve). Mean of 18 subjects. All luminances in cd/m² (after Palmer, 1967)

About the mesopic range, we have already stated that interactions between cones and rods are so complicated and depend on so many parameters that it seems hopeless to speak of a V_λ curve which would be a function of the mean luminance in the visual field. A much better way is Palmer's (1967) suggestion. Let P and S be the photopic and scotopic luminances deduced from Eq. (4); then using a given equivalence criterion, the observer matches a standard "white", for example, a black body at 2042° K, with the test light, and determines for this light the function $L(S, P)$ for the experimental conditions in use. As examples, Fig. 7 represents for a 15° field the mean results obtained on 18 subjects by direct brightness matching with nearly monochromatic lights as test stimuli (interference filters of 30 nm half-width transmission and maxima at 410, 440, 470, 500, 530, 560, 590, 620, 650 and 680 nm) at 4 levels of mesopic vision. Ideally the $S-P$ loci should be straight lines parallel to the P axis at low levels and to the S axis at high levels, but actually they are never straight lines. Fig. 8 shows similar results for one observer with 5° and 45° fields, at 5 levels. It is seen that the long wave end rises progressively with increasing level, while the short wave end swings up abruptly at a moderately high level.

In conclusion, we may say that scotopic luminosity is a rather simple affair, photopic is already more intricate, and mesopic so difficult that experiments of the sort indicated by PALMER are necessary in each experimental situation to represent what is happening. Happily, for practical purposes, scotopic vision is of interest only in wartime, and mesopic photometry of little use in engineering problems. But for the physiologist, the entire problem is fascinating because it reveals the complexity of the human retina, even in so apparently simple a question as spectral luminosity.

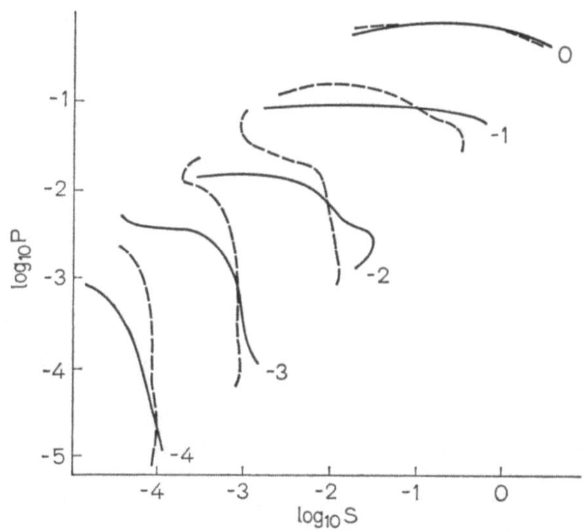

Fig. 8. Same as Fig. 7, but for one observer only viewing a 5° (———) and a 45° field (- - - - - -) at 5 luminance levels (after PALMER, 1967)

References

D'ARCY, F. J., PORTER, N. A.: Detection of cosmic ray μ-mesons by the human eye. Nature (Lond.) **196**, 1013—1014 (1962).

AUBERT, H.: Physiologie der Netzhaut. Breslau: Morgenstern 1865.

BLACKWELL, H. R., BLACKWELL, O. M.: Rod and cone receptor mechanisms in typical and atypical congenital achromatopsia. Vision Res. **1**, 62—107 (1961).

BOUMA, H.: Receptive systems mediating certain reactions on the pupil of the human eye. Thesis, Eindhoven, 1965.

BOYNTON, R. M., KAISER, P. K.: Vision: the additivity law made to work for heterochromatic photometry with bipartite fields. Science **161**, 366—368 (1968).

BRINDLEY, G. S.: The colour of light of very long wavelength. J. Physiol. (Lond.) **130**, 34—44 (1955).

— Physiology of the Retina and Visual Pathway. London: Arnold 1960.

BROWN, J. L.: Problems in the specification of luminous efficiency. Techn. Rep. 5, Department of Psychology, Kansas State Univ., 1968.

Comite E-**1.4.1**: Vision photopique, mésopique et scotopique. Compte-Rendu 16e Session C.I.E., 152—162 (1968).

CRAWFORD, B. H.: The scotopic visibility function. Proc. phys. Soc. (Lond.) B **62**, 321—334 (1949).

Dartnall, H. J. A.: The Visual Pigments. London: Methuen 1957.
Dodt, E., Walther, J. B.: Fluorescence of the crystalline lens and electroretinographic sensitivity determination. Nature (Lond.) **181**, 286—287 (1958).
Ekman, G., Gustafsson, V.: Threshold values and the psychophysical function in brightness vision. Vision Res. 8, 747—758 (1968).
Griffin, D. R., Hubbard, R., Wald, G.: Sensitivity of the human eye to infra-red radiation. J. opt. Soc. Amer. **37**, 546—554 (1947).
Guth, S. L., Donley, N. J., Marrocco, R. T.: On luminance additivity and related topics. Vision Res. **9**, 537—575 (1969).
Hough, E. A.: The spectral sensitivity function for parafoveal vision. Vision Res. 8, 1423—1430 (1968).
— Ruddock, K. H.: The Purkinje shift. Vision Res. **9**, 313—315 (1969).
Hurvich, L. M., Jameson, D.: An opponent-process theory of color vision. Psychol. Rev. **64**, 384—404 (1957).
Ives, H. E.: On heterochromatic photometry. Phil. Mag. **24**, 845—853 (1912).
Johnson, L. B.: Upper limit of mesopic vision. Trans. Ill. Eng. Soc. **32**, 646—650 (1937).
Kanzow, J.: Bestimmung der relativen spektralen Hellempfindlichkeit für das 10°-Gesichtsfeld. Farbe **13**, 143—155 (1964).
Khazanov, V. S.: Visual task effect in spectral eye sensitivity. Vision Res. **7**, 329—339 (1967).
Le Grand, Y.: Light, Colour and Vision. 2nd Ed. London: Chapman & Hall 1968.
Lewis, P. R.: A theoretical interpretation of spectral sensitivity curves at long wavelengths. J. Physiol. (Lond.) **130**, 45—52 (1955).
Marriott, F. C. H.: Colour vision. In: Davson, H. (Ed.): The Eye, Vol. 2, pp. 219—320. New York: Academic Press 1962.
Moreland, J. D.: Modifications of the Wright trichromatic colorimeter for extrafoveal and peripheral observations. Optica Acta **2**, 101—104 (1955).
— Cruz, A.: Colour perception with the peripheral retina. Optica Acta **6**, 117—151 (1959).
Palmer, D. A.: The definition of a standard observer for mesopic vision. Vision Res. **7**, 619—628 (1967).
Piéron, H.: Recherches sur la validité de la loi d'Abney. Ann. Psychol. **40**, 52—83 (1942).
Pirenne, M. H.: Spectral luminous efficiency of radiation. In: Davson, H. (Ed.): The Eye, Vol. 2, pp. 65—91. New York: Academic Press 1962.
Richards, W., Luria, S. M.: Color mixture functions at low luminance levels. Vision Res. **4**, 281—313 (1964).
Ruddock, K. H.: Evidence for macular pigmentation from colour matching data. Vision Res. **3**, 417—429 (1963).
— The effect of age upon colour vision. Vision Res. **5**, 37—58 (1965).
Sanders, C., Wyszecki, G.: Correlate for brightness in terms of C.I.E. colour-matching data. Compte-Rendu 15e Session C.I.E., 221—230 (1963).
Shipley, T.: The veiling function and non-additivity in flicker fusion. Vision Res. **1**, 301—309 (1961).
Schober, H.: Die Direktwahrnehmung von Röntgenstrahlen durch den menschlichen Gesichtsinn. Vision Res. **4**, 251—269 (1964).
Sloan, L. L.: The effect of intensity of light, state of adaptation of the eye, and size of photometric field on the visibility curve. Psychol. Monogr. **28**, No. 173 (1938).
Speranskaya, N. I.: Determination of spectrum color coordinates for twenty-seven normal observers. Optics and Spectroscopy **7**, 424—428 (1959).
Sperling, H. G.: An experimental investigation on the relationship between colour mixture and luminous efficiency. In: Visual Problems of Colour, Vol. 1, pp. 249—277. London: H. M. Stationery Office 1958.
Stiles, W. S.: The physical interpretation of the spectral sensitivity curve of the eye. In: Trans. Opt. Conv. of the Worshipful Co. of Spectacle Makers, pp. 97—107. London: Spectacle Makers Co. 1948.
— Burch, J. M.: N.P.L. colour-matching investigation, final report. Optica Acta **6**, 1—26 (1959).
Swets, J. A.: Color vision. Quarterly progress rep., Res. Lab. of Electronics. Cambridge, Mass.: Mass. Inst. of Technology 1960.

TESSIER, M., BLOTTIAU, M.: Variations des caractéristiques photométriques de l'oeil aux luminances photopiques. Rev. Opt. **30**, 309—322 (1951).
VOLKENSHTEIN, A. A.: Vizualnaya photometriya malih yarkostey. Moscou: Izd. Energiya 1965.
DE VRIES, H.: Der Einfluß der Temperatur des Auges auf die spektrale Empfindlichkeitskurve. Experientia (Basel) **4**, 357—358 (1948).
WALD, H.: Human vision and the spectrum. Science **101**, 653—658 (1945).
WEALE, R. A.: Spectral sensitivity curves and the absorption of light by the ocular media. Brit. J. Ophthal. **37**, 148—156 (1953).
— Photochemistry of the human central fovea. Nature (Lond.) **218**, 238—240 (1968).
WYSZECKI, G., STILES, W. S.: Color Science. New York: Wiley 1967.

Chapter 16

Colour Mixture

By

W. D. Wright, London (Great Britain)

With 10 Figures

Contents

The Mixing of Colours

Since colour mixture is a somewhat ambiguous term it is necessary at the outset of this chapter to make clear the sense in which the term is being used here. In colour technology a distinction is made between additive and subtractive mixture. By additive mixture is meant the adding together of beams of light from different parts of the spectrum or of different spectral compositions. Sometimes this addition is achieved by means of quite complex optical instruments known as additive colorimeters. Sometimes it is achieved by means of projectors which throw beams of coloured light on to the same area of a screen or a stage. It occurs when we look at a colour television picture in which the light from the minute red, green and blue phosphor dots of which the picture is composed merge in the eye because the dot pattern is too fine to be resolved by the mosaic of retinal receptors.

Additive mixture also, in fact, occurs whenever we look at a uniformly coloured surface, since although the average dye or pigment absorbs fairly broad bands of the spectrum it also allows a quite extensive range of wavelengths to be reflected. Hence when an image of the surface is formed on the retina, the retinal receptors are bombarded with a continuous stream of light quanta made up of an intimate mixture of all the frequencies represented in the spectral composition of the light reflected from the surface. Thus when a yellow surface is being viewed (Fig. 1), the spectral composition of the light extends from the far red (700 nm) end of the spectrum to the green (near 500 nm) (Fig. 1) so that the retina is illuminated by a highly heterogeneous additive mixture of quanta with frequencies ranging from about 4×10^{14} to 6×10^{14} cycles per second.

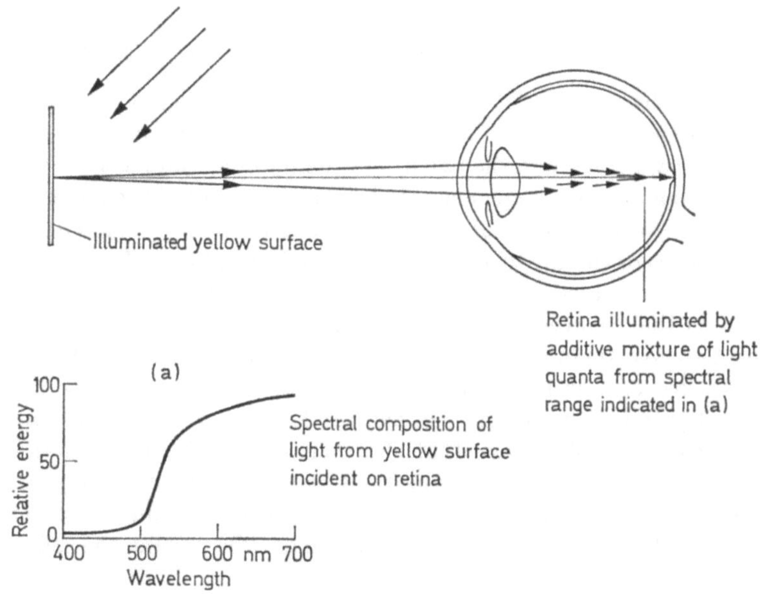

Fig. 1. Diagram to illustrate additive mixture of light quanta of wide range of frequencies when retina is illuminated by light from a yellow surface

Subtractive mixture occurs when we mix dyes or pigments together, or when we place two or more colour filters in series. It is called subtractive mixture because when a beam of white light passes through a succession of filters or a mixture of dyes, the spectral composition of the light which finally emerges is determined by the parts of the spectrum which are absorbed or subtracted from the incident light by each of the component dyes or filters. Thus if a yellow dye which absorbs primarily in the blue and violet is mixed with a blue dye which absorbs mainly in the yellow and orange and red, the colour of the light which emerges is green, as is well known. In this case, one dye has subtracted the short-wave end of the spectrum and the other has subtracted the long-wave end, leaving the residual wavelengths which are transmitted by both dyes to come from the middle, or green, band of wavelengths.

Even in the case of subtractive mixture, however, we have to note that the emergent light still consists of quite a broad band of wavelengths, so that when the light is focused on the retina, we have, for this waveband, an additive mixture of quanta of a range of frequencies striking the receptors. In fact, in virtually every visual situation the light that is ultimately focused on the retina is an additive mixture of a number, and generally a large number, of different frequencies, and it is for this reason that the study of additive colour mixture is so important to our understanding of the process of colour perception. It is, then, this additive combination of lights of different frequencies with which we are concerned in this chapter on colour mixture.

Spectral Composition and Colour Appearance

It might have happened that additive colour mixture did not take place in the visual system, in which case there would have been no mixture phenomena worthy of study. In the case of the ear, the particular quality of a sound has to be analysed in terms of its component frequencies and harmonics, but the manner in which the eye responds to a mixture of light vibrations is entirely different from the analytical response of the ear to a mixture of sound vibrations. We can appreciate this already from the case illustrated in Fig. 1, since when we look at a yellow surface such as that represented in this diagram, we are conscious of a unitary yellow sensation. We are quite unaware, from the visual appearance of the surface, that there are red and orange and green radiations as well as yellow radiations being reflected from the surface into our eyes. In fact, the yellowness of the surface is hardly to be distinguished from that of a monochromatic radiation at a wavelength of 580 or 590 nm. One of the questions we therefore have to try to answer is what has happened to the redness and greenness that we might expect to see in a beam of light that contains radiations in the 620–700 nm and the 550–500 nm wavebands.

In some respects an even more striking situation exists in the case of a white surface. Here the whole of the spectrum is reflected yet we are conscious simply of the unitary sensation of whiteness. At least in the case of the yellow surface there is a yellow band of wavelengths in the reflected light, but there is no band of "white" wavelengths in the white light spectrum. White is a unique sensation not to be found among the spectral colours.

We might, then, reasonably begin our study of colour mixture phenomena by relating the colours of different surfaces with their spectral reflection characteristics and with the colours in the spectrum. In Fig. 2, for example, we show the curves of spectral luminance factor against wavelength for typical red, yellow, green, blue and white surfaces; for comparison, a black and white representation of the spectrum is included, with the hues associated with particular wavebands printed in. We would have little difficulty in deducing the hues of the red, green and blue surfaces since their reflection maxima occur in these parts of the spectrum. It is the yellow and the white surfaces that pose the real problem, which can only be answered when we know more about how the eye responds to a mixed radiation.

Coloured surfaces may differ in appearance not only in respect of their hue but also in respect of their lightness and the vividness or depth of the coloration. Lightness presents no great problem, since if all the reflection curves of Fig. 2 were reduced to a half or a quarter of their heights, we should clearly expect the surfaces to be darker. How light or how dark a surface may appear is, however, not only a function of the height of its reflection curve but also of the background against which it is seen. A dark background enhances the lightness, a light background induces some greyness into the colour appearance. This aspect of colour appearance, which involves the phenomenon of contrast and of related colours, lies outside the subject of colour mixture and will not be considered further in this chapter.

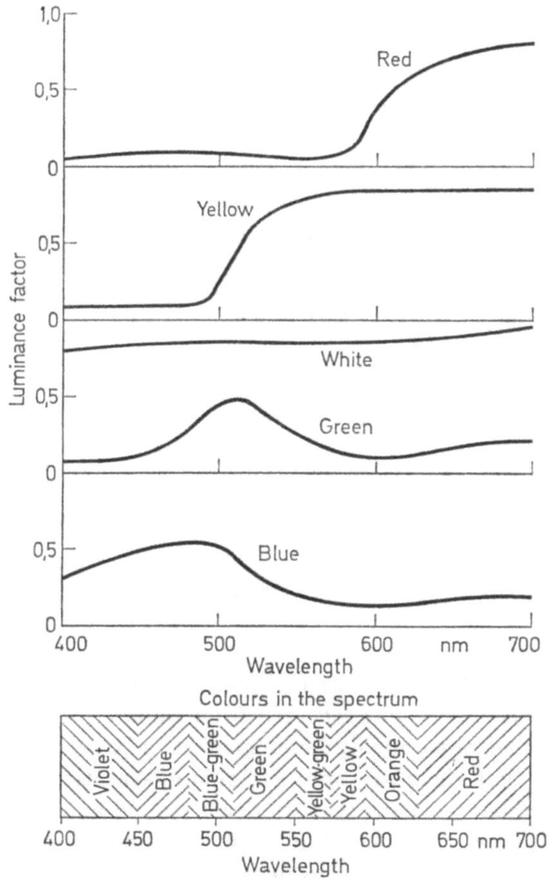

Fig. 2. Curves of luminance factor against wavelength to show spectral reflection curves for typical red, yellow, green, blue and white surfaces. Below: Division of the spectrum into its main hues

It had, nevertheless, to be mentioned if only to make it clear that colour appearance is not merely a function of spectral composition (see HEINEMANN, chapter 6 and JAMESON and HURVICH, chapter 22, this volume).

The vividness or depth of coloration of a surface is often described as the colour saturation. A pastel colour, for example, would be a desaturated colour, while a bright, vivid colour would be highly saturated. In the Munsell system this attribute is known as Chroma and Fig. 3 shows the spectral reflection curves of a series of Munsell red chips of increasing chroma. Here the spectral composition is changing in the sense of an increase in the reflection of the main long wave red band of wavelengths and a decrease in the reflection of the remainder of the spectrum. If we consider the spectral composition as made up of two parts, a main band in the long wave red and a white component represented by a roughly uniform reflection through the whole spectrum, we see that an increase in chroma or saturation corresponds to an increase in the proportion of the "red" component relative to the "white" component.

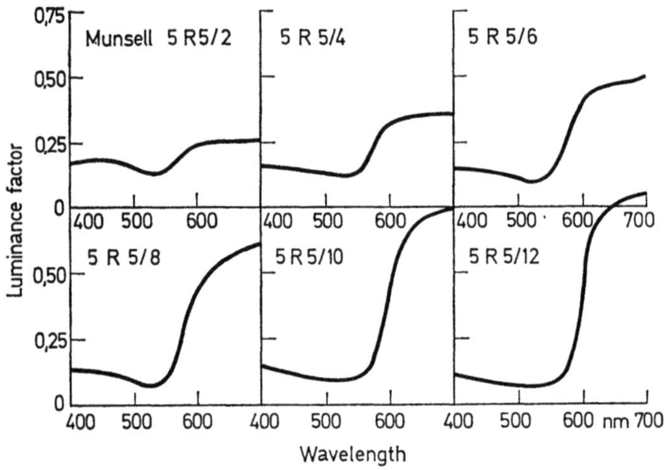

Fig. 3. Spectral reflection curves of Munsell red chips of increasing chroma (Munsell Hue 5R, Value 5, Chroma 2—12)

These, then, are the kind of relations which we can deduce from a study of the spectral composition of the light reflected from coloured surfaces and the visual response created when these highly heterogeneous mixtures stimulate the retina. We can recognise that there are only six unique sensations, white, black, red, yellow, green and blue; we learn that we never see red and green simultaneously in a colour, nor yellow and blue. But from this type of spectral analysis and synthesis alone, we are still unable to deduce just how the retina responds to a mixed radiation. For this, we have to undertake more sophisticated colour mixture experiments in which, first, we observe the colour appearances obtained when we mix coloured lights in different proportions, and, second, undertake quantitative studies of colour mixture and colour matching.

Two-Colour and Three-Colour Mixture

In this section we will describe in qualitative terms the more important effects which can be observed when two or three selected radiations are mixed additively. It will be convenient to assume that the radiations to be mixed are either monochromatic radiations, so that they can be readily specified by their wavelengths, or a broad-band of radiations which, for simplicity, we will consider as an "equal-energy" white.

Suppose, first, we consider the result of mixing the equal-energy white with a red of wavelength 650 nm. The colours that result as the proportion of white to red is varied, are very much as expected, namely a steady desaturation of the red as more and more white is added and, as the amount of red is reduced, so the whiteness predominates until it becomes only slightly tinged with red. In other words, there is a continuous variation in colour appearance between the two terminal colours, red and white.

There is no need to describe the essentially similar changes that occur as we mix white with monochromatic yellow of, say, wavelength 580 nm, or with green

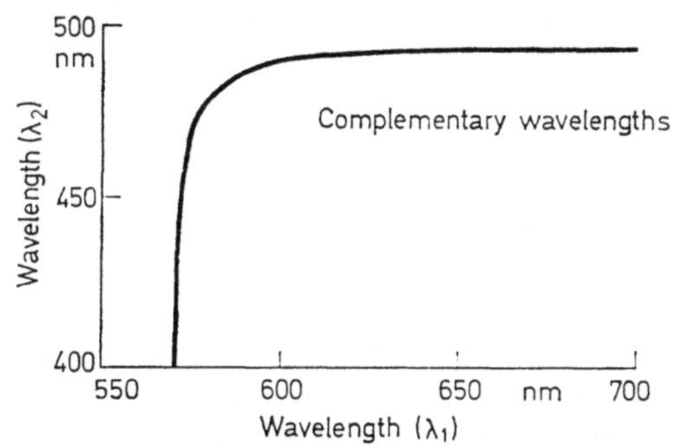

Fig. 4. Curve relating complementary pairs of wavelengths, λ_1 and λ_2. When λ_1 is mixed additively with λ_2 in the correct proportions, the mixture will match the equal-energy white

of wavelength 530 nm, or blue of wavelength 460 nm. The same desaturation occurs in a continuing series between the terminal colours, yellow and white, green and white, and blue and white respectively.

Suppose, now, we mix two monochromatic wavelengths, say a yellow of 580 nm and a blue of wavelength 480 nm. As the blue is added to the yellow, the yellow becomes desaturated until, when the appropriate proportions of the two wavelengths are reached, the mixture is neither yellow, nor blue, but white. Then as the amount of blue increases and yellow decreases, the colour changes from white to a blue of increasing saturation. A very similar sequence of colour changes will occur between other pairs of complementary wavelengths, Fig. 4, in which, at a certain point in the mixture, the mixed beam, as it becomes white, loses all trace of the hues of the two terminal wavelengths. At no point, in fact, in the mixture of 580 nm and 480 nm does the mixture possess the attributes of both yellowness and blueness simultaneously, but only of yellowness and whiteness or whiteness and blueness.

It is unfortunate that sheer familiarity with the result of mixing complementary wavelengths has tended to dull our appreciation of the remarkable nature of the phenomenon. Equally remarkable is the result of mixing monochromatic light from the long-wave, red, end of the spectrum, say of wavelength 650 nm, with monochromatic light from the middle, green, region, say of wavelength 530 nm. As 530 nm is added to 650 nm, so the colour loses some of its redness to become more orange and then, at a certain point in the mixture, the colour changes to a yellow which is almost indistinguishable from a monochromatic yellow. As in the case of the white produced by the mixture of complementary wavelengths, so the yellow possesses none of the attributes of redness or greenness possessed by the two terminal colours. The redness and the greenness have been replaced by a saturated yellowness. As the proportion of 530 nm increases and 650 nm decreases, the colour appearance changes progressively from yellow towards green through yellow-green. Again, as in the case of the complementaries, at no point in the mixture of 650 nm and 530 nm does the resultant colour possess the attributes of both redness and greenness simultaneously, but only of redness and yellowness, or yellowness and greenness.

These subjective, descriptive effects are probably among the most important phenomena that have to be explained by any acceptable theory of the visual process even though they have not been expressed in quantitative terms. The extension of the mixture relations from two-colour mixture to three-colour mixture does not really introduce any new subjective element although the quantitative colour-matching functions derived from three-colour mixture experiments are, of course, of key importance.

Experiments on three-colour mixture are generally carried out with a red, a green and a blue light, and typical radiations that have been used are 650 nm, 530 nm and 460 nm. From the description just given of the results of two-colour mixture, it is easy to see that a wide range of colours can be produced by combining three such radiations in various proportions. Thus the orange, yellow and yellow-green hues can be reproduced by various mixtures of 650 and 530 nm. The addition of 460 nm to these mixtures will then introduce varying degrees of desaturation towards and including white. Similarly, the blue-green hues can be reproduced by various mixtures of 530 and 460 nm, and be desaturated by the addition of 650 nm, while the mixture of 460 and 650 nm will produce the purples which can be desaturated by the addition of 530 nm. The use of three stimuli in colour mixture experiments are thus necessary and sufficient to reproduce all hues with their varying degrees of desaturation. This still holds in principle even though a mixture of 530 and 460 nm yields blue-green colours which appear desaturated by comparison with pure spectral colours in the wavelength range 480–510 nm, so that these cannot be reproduced by a positive mixture of 650, 530, and 460 nm radiations. However, a match can be made by adding 650 nm to the pure blue-green spectral colour, which is equivalent to saying that the spectral colour can be reproduced by a mixture of a positive amount of 530 and 460 nm with a negative amount of 650 nm. It then only remains for some awkward person to ask whether this is additive or subtractive mixture!

This section has reviewed the colours that are seen for various two-colour and three-colour mixtures, as an introduction to an account of the more detailed colour matching experiments which form the foundation of the whole subject of trichromatic colorimetry. We are not concerned in this chapter with colorimetry as such, but we do have to take note of the relation of the colour-matching functions to the probable spectral sensitivity curves of the retinal receptors, and also the implications which phenomena such as the stability of colour matches and the additivity of colour-matching equations have for our understanding of the visual process. These topics will be dealt with in the following sections.

The Determination of the Spectral Mixture Curves

The spectral mixture curves, or colour matching functions as they are now frequently called, record the amounts of defined red, green and blue stimuli which, when mixed additively, give a colour match to each wavelength in turn in the equal-energy spectrum. These curves are fundamental data for colour matching because with them it is possible to work out whether any two stimuli defined by their spectral compositions are a colour match or whether they are a mis-match. The curves are also basic visual data because,as mentioned above, they must be directly related to the spectral sensitivities of the receptors in the retina.

The first attempt to derive spectral colour mixture curves was made by MAXWELL (1860). His colour box was a relatively crude prism spectroscope system in which three entrance slits produced three overlapping spectra. A single exit-slit selected three different wavelengths from these spectra so that when the observer placed his eye behind the exit-slit, he saw the prism face illuminated by the mixture of these wavelengths. The proportions in which they were mixed could be varied by adjusting the widts of the three entrance slits. The curves obtained with this apparatus were of interest in demonstrating the validity of the principle underlying the curves but were too limited in accuracy to be of much scientific importance.

A more elaborate apparatus was developed by HELMHOLTZ (1924) in which a prism spectroscope was equipped with two collimator systems. Each collimator contained a double-image prism which again produced two overlapping spectra in the focal plane of the viewing telescope. The relative energies of each pair of spectra could be varied by the rotation of two polarising prisms mounted behind the collimator entrance slits. The observer placed his eye behind the exit-slit of the telescope and saw two half-fields illuminated by a mixture of two pairs of monochromatic lights. Colour matches could then be made between the two fields, and in the hands of KONIG and DIETERICI (1892), this apparatus provided the first set of colour mixture curves with any claim to reliability.

At about the same time, ABNEY also recorded a set of mixture curves using his colour-patch apparatus (see ABNEY, 1913). In this prism instrument, wavebands in the red, green and blue were selected by locating three slits in the appropriate parts of the spectrum and were mixed additively by focussing the three beams on to the same area of a white diffusing screen. The proportions in which the three beams were mixed were controlled by adjusting the widths of the three slits.

Until the 1920's the data obtained by KONIG and DIETERICI, and by ABNEY, represented the most reliable information available on the colour mixing properties of the eye. Then studies by GUILD (1931) and the author (WRIGHT, 1928, 1929) provided a more modern set of data for a field of view subtending 2° and observed by foveal vision. In these investigations GUILD (1925) used a trichromatic colorimeter in which the red, green and blue stimuli were obtained with colour filters and the three beams were mixed by means of a rotating prism which passed successively in front of the three filters. The proportions in which the three colours were mixed were controlled by three sector apertures over the filters.

In the author's colorimeter (WRIGHT, 1927, 1946), Fig. 5, a spectrum was formed with a prism dispersing system, and roof reflecting prisms were located in the spectrum at 650 nm, 530 nm, and 460 nm; these prisms reflected red, green and blue wavebands back through the dispersing prisms to produce an additive mixture of the wavebands. The mixture could be varied with photometer wedges mounted in front of the roof prisms.

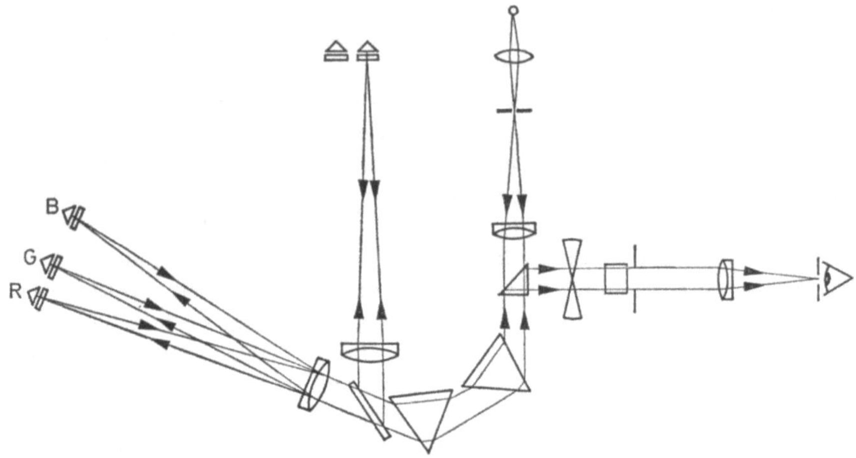

Fig. 5. Optical system of WRIGHT trichromatic colorimeter (WRIGHT, 1927, 1946)

The most recent and sophisticated colour mixing equipment of this type is the Stiles trichromator (STILES, 1955), Fig. 6. Here again a spectrum was formed with a prism dispersing system, wavebands at 645 nm, 526.3 nm, and 444.4 nm were selected by means of three slits located in the spectrum, and a field lens focused the three beams into a second dispersing system to produce an additive mixture. Photometer wedges in front of the three slits were used to control the red-green-blue mixture. With this equipment, STILES obtained colour mixture data for a field size of 2° angular subtense viewed foveally and for a field subtending 10° in which the central 2 or 3 degrees was ignored. In effect, therefore, the 10° data

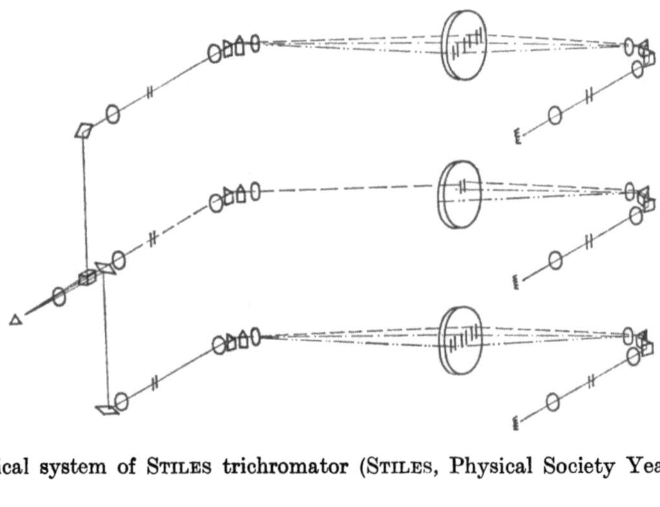

Fig. 6. Optical system of STILES trichromator (STILES, Physical Society Year Book, 1955)

referred to a field that was annular in shape (see LE GRAND, chapter 15, this volume).

There is no occasion here to elaborate on the experimental details of the investigations undertaken by GUILD, STILES and the author since they have been described at length elsewhere and are fully documented in the literature. We need only recognise that they were full-scale scientific investigations undertaken with all the optical and photometric resources available at the time. The authority of the work was acknowledged by the Commission Internationale de l'Éclairage (C.I.E.) when the Guild-Wright data were used to define the colour matching characteristics of the standard observer in the 1931 C.I.E. system of colorimetry, and in 1964 a supplementary system of colorimetry for large-field conditions was established by the C.I.E. based largely on the Stiles data, and to a lesser extent on SPERANSKAYA's (1959) data for the same field size. No doubt future investigations will add refinements to these studies but it can now be claimed that the essential facts of colour mixture and matching for photopic vision are known.

The form in which the 1931 standard observer was defined is shown in Fig. 7. The matching stimuli used in this definition were three monochromatic radiations of wavelength 700 nm (red), 546.1 nm (green) and 435.8 nm (blue) and their units were adjusted to be equal in a colour match on an equal-energy white. The curves then give the relative amounts of the three radiations required to match each wavelength in the equal-energy spectrum. They are described in colorimetric terms as the equal-energy distribution curves, and the proportions of the red, green and blue radiations are described on this unit basis as distribution coefficients, with the symbols $\bar{r}_\lambda$, $\bar{g}_\lambda$, $\bar{b}_\lambda$ (they are also often known as spectral tristimulus values). It will be seen that there is a deep negative lobe to the $\bar{r}_\lambda$ curve between the wavelengths of the green and blue matching stimuli, 546.1 nm and 435.8 nm, but this merely arises from the need to desaturate the monochromatic blue-green wavelengths, as described in the previous section, when attempting to match

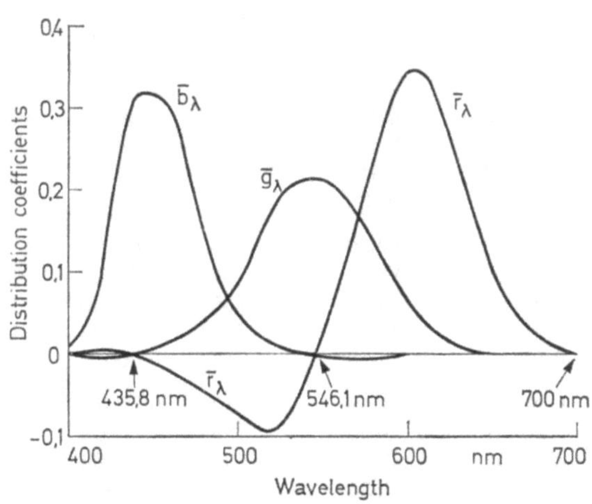

Fig. 7. The colour-matching characteristics of the 1931 C. I. E. standard observer, expressed in terms of the matching stimuli 700 nm, 546.1 nm and 435.8 nm required to match each wavelength in the equal-energy spectrum and with their units adjusted to be equal in a colour match on an equal-energy white

Table 1. *The spectral tristimulus values (or distribution coefficients) $\bar{r}(\lambda)$, $\bar{g}(\lambda)$, $\bar{b}(\lambda)$ defining the colour matching characteristics of the 1931 standard observer using radiations of wavelengths 700 nm, 546.1 nm, 435.8 nm as matching stimuli with their units adjustrd to be equal in a match on an equal-energy white. The relative luminances of unit quantities of the matchung stimuli on this system of units are 1.00:4.5907:0.0601 for the red:green:blue stimuli*

λ	Spectral tristimulus values			λ	Spectral tristimulus values		
(nm)	$\bar{r}(\lambda)$	$\bar{g}(\lambda)$	$\bar{b}(\lambda)$	(nm)	$\bar{r}(\lambda)$	$\bar{g}(\lambda)$	$\bar{b}(\lambda)$
380	0.00003	—0.00001	0.00117	580	0.24526	0.13610	—0.00108
385	0.00005	—0.00002	0.00189	585	0.27989	0.11686	—0.00093
390	0.00010	—0.00004	0.00359	590	0.30928	0.09754	—0.00079
395	0.00017	—0.00007	0.00647	595	0.33184	0.07909	—0.00063
400	0.00030	—0.00014	0.01214	600	0.34429	0.06246	—0.00049
405	0.00047	—0.00022	0.01969	605	0.34756	0.04776	—0.00038
410	0.00084	—0.00041	0.03707	610	0.33971	0.03557	—0.00030
415	0.00139	—0.00070	0.06637	615	0.32265	0.02583	—0.00022
420	0.00211	—0.00110	0.11541	620	0.29708	0.01828	—0.00015
425	0.00266	—0.00143	0.18575	625	0.26348	0.01253	—0.00011
430	0.00218	—0.00119	0.24769	630	0.22677	0.00833	—0.00008
435	0.00036	—0.00021	0.29012	635	0.19233	0.00537	—0.00005
440	—0.00261	0.00149	0.31228	640	0.15968	0.00334	—0.00003
445	—0.00673	0.00379	0.31860	645	0.12905	0.00199	—0.00002
450	—0.01213	0.00678	0.31670	650	0.10167	0.00116	—0.00001
455	—0.01874	0.01046	0.31166	655	0.07857	0.00066	—0.00001
460	—0.02608	0.01485	0.29821	660	0.05932	0.00037	0.00000
465	—0.03324	0.01977	0.27295	665	0.04366	0.00021	0.00000
470	—0.03933	0.02538	0.22991	670	0.03149	0.00011	0.00000
475	—0.04471	0.03183	0.18592	675	0.02294	0.00006	0.00000
480	—0.04939	0.03914	0.14494	680	0.01687	0.00003	0.00000
485	—0.05364	0.04713	0.10968	685	0.01187	0.00001	0.00000
490	—0.05814	0.05689	0.08257	690	0.00819	0.00000	0.00000
495	—0.06414	0.06948	0.06246	695	0.00572	0.00000	0.00000
500	—0.07173	0.08536	0.04776	700	0.00410	0.00000	0.00000
505	—0.08120	0.10593	0.03688	705	0.00291	0.00000	0.00000
510	—0.08901	0.12860	0.02698	710	0.00210	0.00000	0.00000
515	—0.09356	0.15262	0.01842	715	0.00148	0.00000	0.00000
520	—0.09264	0.17468	0.01221	720	0.00105	0.00000	0.00000
525	—0.08473	0.19113	0.00830	725	0.00074	0.00000	0.00000
530	—0.07101	0.20317	0.00549	730	0.00052	0.00000	0.00000
535	—0.05316	0.21083	0.00320	735	0.00036	0.00000	0.00000
540	—0.03152	0.21466	0.00146	740	0.00025	0.00000	0.00000
545	—0.00613	0.21487	0.00023	745	0.00017	0.00000	0.00000
550	0.02279	0.21178	—0.00058	750	0.00012	0.00000	0.00000
555	0.05514	0.20588	—0.00105	755	0.00008	0.00000	0.00000
560	0.09060	0.19702	—0.00130	760	0.00006	0.00000	0.00000
565	0.12840	0.18522	—0.00138	765	0.00004	0.00000	0.00000
570	0.16768	0.17087	—0.00135	770	0.00003	0.00000	0.00000
575	0.20715	0.15429	—0.00123	775	0.00001	0.00000	0.00000
580	0.24526	0.13610	—0.00108	780	0.00000	0.00000	0.00000

them with an additive, all-positive, red-green-blue mixture of radiations. As we shall see later, it is possible to make linear transformations of these curves and to produce a set of all-positive curves. It is these transformed curves that we shall discuss in due course in relation to the sensitivity curves of the retinal receptors.

Table 1 gives the data from which the curves in Fig. 7 were drawn and Table 2 gives the corresponding data used to define the 1964 standard observer for matches made with a 10° field.

Table 2. *The spectral tristimulus values (or distribution coefficients) $\bar{r}_{10}(\bar{v})$, $\bar{g}_{10}(\bar{v})$, $\bar{b}_{10}(\bar{v})$ defining the colour matching characteristics of the 1964 standard observer for large-field (10°) conditions. In this table the standard observer is defined in terms of matching stimuli of wavenumbers 15500, 19000 and 22500 (corresponding to wavelengths of 645.2 nm, 526.3 nm and 444.4 nm). The tristimulus values are given in power units adjusted to unity at the wavenumbers of the three matching stimuli*

Wave-length λ (nm)	Wave-number $\bar{v}$ (cm^{-1})	Spectral tristimulus values $\bar{r}_{10}(\bar{v})$	$\bar{g}_{10}(\bar{v})$	$\bar{b}_{10}(\bar{v})$
360.4	27750	0.000000079100	—0.000000021447	0.000000307299
363.6	27500	0.00000029891	—0.00000008125	0.00000116475
367.0	27250	0.00000108348	—0.00000029533	0.00000423733
370.4	27000	0.0000037522	—0.0000010271	0.0000147506
373.8	26750	0.0000123776	—0.0000034057	0.0000489822
377.4	26500	0.000038728	—0.000010728	0.000154553
381.0	26250	0.000114541	—0.000032004	0.000462055
384.6	26000	0.00031905	—0.00009006	0.00130350
388.3	25750	0.00083216	—0.00023807	0.00345702
392.2	25500	0.00201685	—0.00058813	0.00857776
396.0	25250	0.0045233	—0.0013519	0.0198315
400.0	25000	0.0093283	—0.0028770	0.0425057
404.0	24750	0.0176116	—0.0056200	0.0840402
408.2	24500	0.030120	—0.010015	0.152451
412.4	24250	0.045571	—0.016044	0.251453
416.7	24000	0.060154	—0.022951	0.374271
421.1	23750	0.071261	—0.029362	0.514950
425.5	23500	0.074212	—0.032793	0.648306
430.1	23250	0.068535	—0.032357	0.770262
434.8	23000	0.055848	—0.027996	0.883628
439.6	22750	0.033049	—0.017332	0.965742
444.4	22500	0.000000	0.000000	1.000000
449.4	22250	—0.041570	0.024936	0.987224
454.5	22000	—0.088073	0.057100	0.942474
459.8	21750	—0.143959	0.099886	0.863537
465.1	21500	—0.207995	0.150955	0.762081
470.6	21250	—0.285499	0.218942	0.630116
476.2	21000	—0.346240	0.287846	0.469818
481.9	20750	—0.388289	0.357723	0.333077
487.8	20500	—0.426587	0.435138	0.227060
493.8	20250	—0.435789	0.513218	0.151027
500.0	20000	—0.438549	0.614637	0.095840

Table 2 (continued)

Wave-length λ (nm)	Wave-number $\bar{v}$ (cm^{-1})	Spectral tristimulus values		
		$\bar{r}_{10}(\bar{v})$	$\bar{g}_{10}(\bar{v})$	$\bar{b}_{10}(\bar{v})$
506.3	19750	—0.404927	0.720251	0.057654
512.8	19500	—0.333995	0.830003	0.029877
519.5	19250	—0.201889	0.933227	0.012874
526.3	19000	0.000000	1.000000	0.000000
533.3	18750	0.255754	1.042957	—0.008854
540.5	18500	0.556022	1.061343	—0.014341
547.9	18250	0.904637	1.031339	—0.017422
555.6	18000	1.314803	0.976838	—0.018644
563.4	17750	1.770322	0.887915	—0.017338
571.4	17500	2.236809	0.758780	—0.014812
579.7	17250	2.641981	0.603012	—0.011771
588.2	17000	3.002291	0.452300	—0.008829
597.0	16750	3.159249	0.306869	—0.005990
606.1	16500	3.064234	0.184057	—0.003593
615.4	16250	2.717232	0.094471	—0.001844
625.0	16000	2.191156	0.041693	—0.000815
634.9	15750	1.566864	0.013407	—0.000262
645.2	15500	1.000000	0.000000	0.000000
655.7	15250	0.575756	—0.002747	0.000054
666.7	15000	0.296964	—0.002029	0.000040
678.0	14750	0.138738	—0.001116	0.000022
689.7	14500	0.0602209	—0.0005130	0.0000100
701.8	14250	0.0247724	—0.0002152	0.0000042
714.3	14000	0.00976319	—0.00008277	0.00000162
727.3	13750	0.00375328	—0.00003012	0.00000059
740.7	13500	0.00141908	—0.00001051	0.00000021
754.7	13250	0.000533169	—0.000003543	0.000000069
769.2	13000	0.000199730	—0.000001144	0.000000022
784.3	12750	0.0000743522	—0.0000003472	0.0000000068
800.0	12500	0.0000276506	—0.0000000961	0.0000000019
816.3	12250	0.0000102123	—0.0000000220	0.0000000004

The Additivity of Trichromatic Colour Matches

When a colour match has been made using a trichromatic colorimeter such as one of the instruments illustrated in Figs. 5 or 6, the viewing situation can be represented by a diagram such as Fig. 8. We can suppose that the upper half of the square field of view of the instrument is illuminated by the colour C which is to be matched, while the lower half of the field is illuminated by the red, green and blue waveband mixture required to match C. Suppose the number of lumens of C in the upper field is F, and the lumens of the red, green and blue matching stimuli in the lower half of the field are F_R, F_G and F_B respectively.

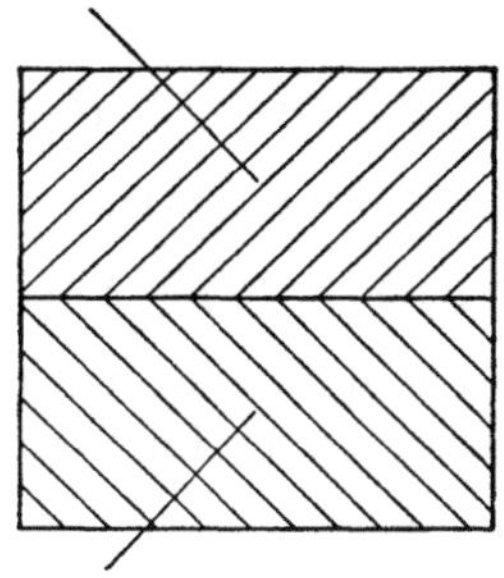

Fig. 8. The viewing situation when making a match of a colour C with a mixture of the red, green and blue matching stimuli in a trichromatic colorimeter

The colour match of Fig. 8 can then be expressed algebraically by the equation

$$F(C) \equiv F_R(R) + F_G(G) + F_B(B)\,, \tag{1}$$

where the bracketed symbols (C), (R), (G), and (B) are merely descriptive symbols to identify the particular spectral radiations in the two halves of the field and have no quantitative significance. The $\equiv$ sign is to be read "is matched by" to show that the equation is really a shorthand way of describing the colour match and is not a normal algebraic equation (see LE GRANT, chapter 15, colorimetric method).

Suppose, having made the match in the instrument, that we had some way of, say, doubling or halving the light flux in both halves of the field. This might be done, for example, by means of a rotating sector which could be introduced into or removed from the two beams in the instrument. Would the colour match still remain a match? Experiments show that it would, at least when observations are made with a 2° foveal field in which only cone vision is effectively involved and provided also that the illumination does not reach extremely high or very low levels. For a middle range of illuminations and for cone vision, it has been shown that colour matches do remain a match over a considerable range of illuminations (WRIGHT, 1946).

We will consider the visual significance of this conclusion later. For the moment we are concerned to establish the additivity of colour matches, and this experiment of doubling the light flux in both halves of the field is one aspect of additivity, since it is equivalent to adding two similar colour matches together. We now have to examine what happens when we add two different colour matches together. Thus suppose a second colour C' is matched in the instrument and that this match is represented by the equation

$$F'(C') \equiv F'_R(R) + F'_G(G) + F'_B(B)\,. \tag{2}$$

We now bring the original colour C back into the instrument and add it to C'. This gives a new colour to which we will give the symbol C'' and we proceed to make a fresh match in the instrument. We can express this third match by the equation

$$F''(C'') \equiv F''_R(R) + F''_G(G) + F''_B(B)\,. \tag{3}$$

Since $F''(C'')$ is made up of $F(C) + F'(C')$, we can write

$$F(C) + F'(C') \equiv F''_R(R) + F''_G(G) + F''_B(B)\,. \tag{4}$$

To determine whether colorimetric additivity holds, we have to examine how closely the following equations are confirmed experimentally:

$$\begin{aligned} F''_R &= F_R + F'_R\,, \\ F''_G &= F_G + F'_G\,, \\ F''_B &= F_B + F'_B\,. \end{aligned} \tag{5}$$

The algebra is extremely simple but it does not necessarily follow that the visual process functions in such a simple way. C'' is likely to be an entirely different hue from C and C'; for example, if C were a red and C' a green, then C'' might be a yellow, or if C were a yellow and C' a blue, then C'' might be a white. This radical change in colour appearance might very possibly involve some non-linear function in the visual system and this could upset the additivity.

In fact, additivity is found to hold quite closely for the red and green stimulus combinations and virtually within a discrimination step for the yellow and blue ones, provided the observations are made with a 2° field viewed foveally. Additivity is an essential assumption for trichromatic colorimetry (WRIGHT, 1969) and the wide use of the 1931 C.I.E. system of colour measurement in many different applications of colour technology is itself evidence that any departures from additivity must be quite small.

The importance of establishing the additivity principle in colour mixture and colour matching phenomena is that it justifies the treatment of colour matching equations as if they were normal linear algebraic equations. Addition, subtraction, multiplication and division can be applied and also the substitution of an amount of one colour stimulus by any other colour combination that matches it. This in turn implies freedom to transform colour matching data expressed in terms of one set of red, green and blue matching stimuli (R), (G), (B) into terms of another set (R'), (G'), (B'), provided the colour equations of (R), (G) and (B) are known in terms of (R'), (G') and (B'). This is very important in practical colour matching as it enables colour matches made with one type of colorimeter to be compared with matches made with a different type of instrument. It also enables colour mixture curves such as those shown in Fig. 7 to be transformed to curves expressed in terms of a different set of matching or reference stimuli. This enables the colour matching data to be related to the spectral sensitivity curves of the retinal receptors, as we shall see in the next section.

The discussion of additivity has been confined so far to experiments carried out with matching fields subtending 2° and viewed foveally. The situation with larger fields is more complicated, partly because of the intrusion of the rod receptors into the matching situation and partly because the yellow macular pigment introduces a non-homogeneity into the field (see RUDDOCK, chapter 17, this volume). These difficulties were experienced, for example, in the colour matching experiments undertaken by Stiles and Burch (1959), and by Speranskaya (1959) which led to the 1964 C.I.E. Supplementary Standard Observer for large-field conditions. (For an extensive account and tabulation of these and other colour matching data, see Wyszecki and Stiles, 1967. A shorter account is given by Wright, 1969.)

The most recent discussion of departures from additivity with large fields is that of Lozano and Palmer (1968) and the most likely cause of non-additivity is the changing contributions of the rod and cone processes to the visual response as both the spectral composition and the illumination level of the colours under examination are altered. Since we are restricting our discussion in this chapter to photopic levels of illumination and to the cone receptors, we need not be concerned with the complexities that emerge under large-field conditions. Nevertheless, the additivity and colour-match stability which is found in foveal, cone vision, as discussed in the next two Sections, acquires heightened significance because of the non-additivity of the extra-foveal retina.

Colour Mixture Curves and Receptor Sensitivities

The colour mixture curves of Fig. 7 had the embarrassing feature that the "red" curve had a pronounced negative lobe and in fact the "green" and "blue" curves also become slightly negative although their negative lobes are too small to be visible in Fig. 7. We saw that these negative quantities merely arose from the need to desaturate the spectral colours to enable an all-positive match to be made and were therefore little more than an algebraic contrivance. Nevertheless, if we are to interpret colour mixture data in terms of three types of receptor in the retina, we need to transform the colour mixture curves into an all-positive system. The additivity principle established in the previous section enables us to do this, but many alternative positive transformations are possible. The algebra of the transformation process need not concern us here as it is well known and described in text-books on colorimetry. The question does arise, however, as to which particular all-positive transformation is most likely to represent the actual colour processes in the retina.

The theory that there were only three types of colour receptor in the cones dates back to a suggestion of Thomas Young which he made as long ago as 1802. In spite of many vicissitudes and contrary arguments over the years, there does now seem to be a growing concensus of opinion that there really are three types of cone. This part, at least, of the Young-Helmholtz theory can be accepted, the most direct objective evidence in support coming from absorption measurements of individual cones using a micro-spectrophotometer (Marks, Dobelle, and MacNichol, 1964; Brown and Wald, 1964).

It is impossible to be dogmatic as yet as to which set of mixture curves correspond to the actual receptor sensitivities. Supplementary data on defective colour vision, adaptation, colour discrimination and the like are called in to support one set of curves in preference to another. To some extent this must be speculation, because we are still ignorant of the underlying physiological processes which produce colour defects, control adaptation and determine discrimination sensitivity.

One possible set of curves that have been proposed are shown in Fig. 9, but all we should claim for these is that they are typical of the mixture curves that could represent the receptor sensitivities. What we must emphasise, however, is that any receptor sensitivity curves which are eventually put forward as definitive, must be capable of being linearly related to the experimentally determined colour matching data of Fig. 7.

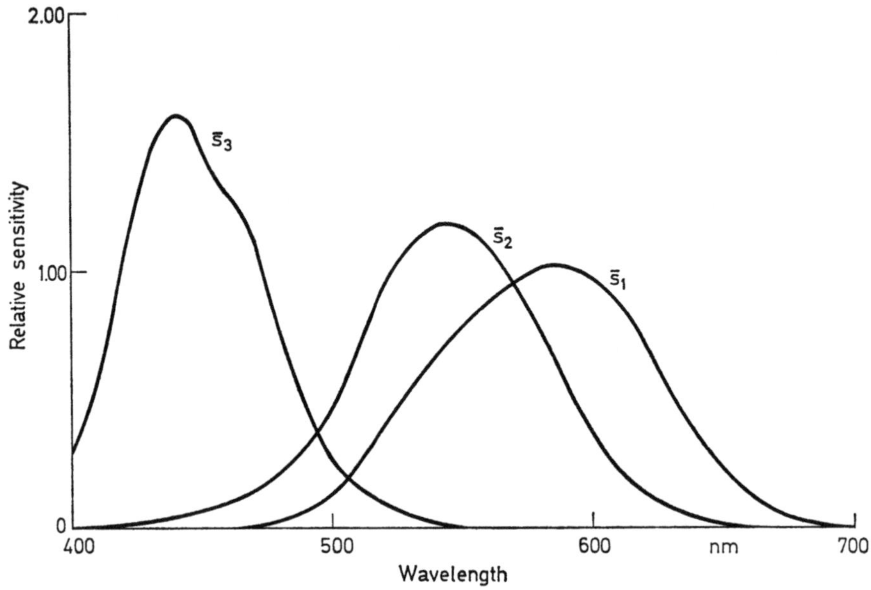

Fig. 9. Possible set of sensitivity curves of the retinal receptors responsible for the first stage of the colour perception process, as derived by Thomson and Wright (1953)

The Stability of Trichromatic Colour Matches

Trichromatic colour matching is a very surprising phenomenon. It can, however, be explained on the theory of three receptor processes with sensitivity curves similar to those in Fig. 9, since two stimuli will match in colour provided they produce similar activities in these three processes even though they have very different spectral compositions. Additivity of colour matches is a further surprising feature of the colour perception process for it implies a linear absorption of the light in the receptors over a considerable range of stimulation of the receptors. Perhaps the most surprising feature of all is the stability of trichromatic colour matches under a wide range of adaptation conditions of the eye.

When a colour match is made in a trichromatic colorimeter, the observer will tend to be partially dark-adapted if the surround to the matching field is dark, but he will also be partially adapted to the matching field itself. After a match has been made under those conditions, the observer can arrange to look away from the instrument and to adapt himself to a quite different field. He might even go outdoors and become adapted to daylight, or he might adapt to some light box illuminated by white or coloured light. If, having adapted himself in this way, he looks back into the colorimeter he will find, unless the adaptation level is very high (WRIGHT, 1946), that the two halves of the field still match, although they may have changed quite considerably in colour appearance.

The explanation of this stability of colour matching in terms of receptor sensitivity curves such as those in Fig. 9 is that the effect of adaptation is to depress the sensitivity of the receptors without altering the shapes of the sensitivity curves. If the adaptation light is coloured, one set of receptors is likely to be depressed in sensitivity more than the others, but still the shapes of the curves will remain unchanged. It is easy to show, for example, that if the height of one of the curves in Fig. 9 were reduced, say, to $^1/_{10}$th of its value at all wavelengths, then two stimuli of different spectral compositions which gave a matched response in that receptor before adaptation would still give a matched, though much smaller, response after adaptation.

Colour-match stability is an important experimental fact whose visual significance has not always been fully appreciated. It provides, for example, convincing evidence against the existence of an independent, fourth receptor in addition to the other three receptors. This is so important that it is worth while studying the argument in some detail.

Fig. 10 illustrates the matching situation when a monochromatic light of wavelength 585 nm is matched by a mixture of monochromatic light of wavelength 650 nm and a monochromatic light of wavelength 530 nm. (For our present purpose we can ignore the need to add a small amount of desaturating blue light to the monochromatic yellow to secure a perfect match.) Under normal conditions of adaptation, the two halves of this matched field will look yellow. Suppose, now, the observer adapts his eye to a moderately bright long wave red light for a minute or two and then looks back at the matched field of Fig. 10. What does he

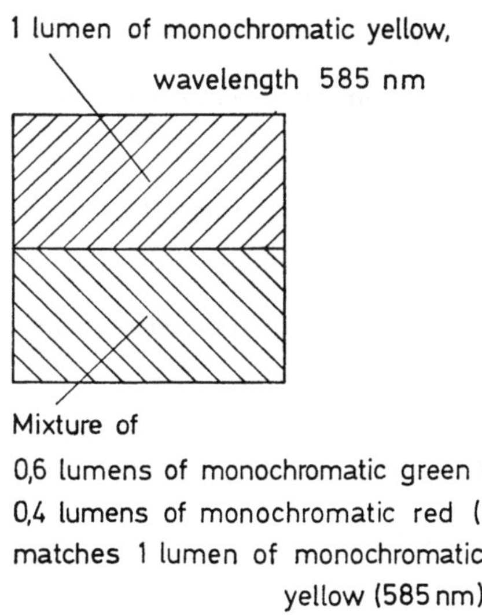

Fig. 10. The matching situation in a colorimeter field when 1 lumen of a monochromatic yellow, wavelength 585 nm, is matched by an additive mixture of 0.6 lumens of monochromatic green (530 nm) and 0.4 lumens of monochromatic red (650 nm)

see ? He again sees a matched field but both halves of the field will now look green. As he continues to look at the field, the two halves will gradually but simultaneously regain their original yellow appearance as the eye recovers from the red adaptation. If the experiment is repeated using a mid-spectral green adapting light instead of a long wave red one, a similar situation will be observed except that this time the two halves will look orange or red immediately after the green adaptation. The extent of the change in colour appearance is, of course, a function of the luminance of the adapting light, the spectral purity of the adapting light, and the duration of the adaptation.

The explanation of this experiment in terms of a set of sensitivity curves such as those of Fig. 9 is then as follows: When a colour match is made, the amounts of the 650–530 nm mixture have to be adjusted to satisfy the equations

$$(P\,\bar{s}_1)_{650} + (P\,\bar{s}_1)_{530} = (P\,\bar{s}_1)_{585}$$

and

$$(P\,\bar{s}_2)_{650} + (P\,\bar{s}_2)_{530} = (P\,\bar{s}_2)_{585} \tag{6}$$

where P is the radiant flux at the wavelengths indicated by the suffix outside the brackets and $\bar{s}_1$ and $\bar{s}_2$ are the sensitivities of the two receptor processes at the same wavelengths. In effect, these equations specify the stimulus relations of the two halves of the matching field of Fig. 10 to ensure that identical reactions are produced in the s_1 and s_2 receptor processes and hence that the two halves of the field are an exact colour match under normal conditions of adaptation.

If, now, the eye is adapted to long wave light the sensitivity of the s_1 process is reduced to a greater extent than the s_2. (The precise biological process through which this adaptation occurs is irrelevant to our argument.) By way of numerical example, we might suppose that the s_1 sensitivity is reduced to $^1/_{10}$th of its previous value and the s_2 to $\frac{1}{2}$. The response of the s_1 receptors to the 650–530 nm mixture will then be

$$\left(P\,\frac{\bar{s}_1}{10}\right)_{650} + \left(P\,\frac{\bar{s}_1}{10}\right)_{530}$$

and their response to the monochromatic 585 nm stimulus will be

$$\left(P\,\frac{\bar{s}_1}{10}\right)_{585}.$$

Similarly, the response of the s_2 receptors to the 650–530 nm mixture will be

$$\left(P\,\frac{\bar{s}_2}{2}\right)_{650} + \left(P\,\frac{\bar{s}_2}{2}\right)_{530}$$

and their response to the monochromatic 585 nm stimulus will be

$$\left(P\,\frac{\bar{s}_2}{2}\right)_{585}.$$

But from the Eqs. (6) given above for the matching situation before adaptation, it is evident that the following equations will also hold,

$$\frac{1}{10}\,(P\,\bar{s}_1)_{650} + \frac{1}{10}\,(P\,\bar{s}_1)_{530} = \frac{1}{10}\,(P\,\bar{s}_1)_{585}$$

and

$$\frac{1}{2}\,(P\,\bar{s}_2)_{650} + \frac{1}{2}\,(P\,\bar{s}_2)_{530} = \frac{1}{2}\,(P\,\bar{s}_2)_{585}\,. \tag{7}$$

Hence it follows that the match will still hold after adaptation.

But suppose there had been a fourth receptor with, we will assume, a rather narrow sensitivity curve with its maximum at 585 nm. A colour match will still be possible, only now the amounts of P_{650} and P_{530} in the mixture will have to be such that they stimulate the s_1 and s_2 receptors so as to give a yellow of the same hue and brightness as the radiation P_{585} will give due to its combined stimulation of the 585 nm receptor and the s_1 and s_2 receptors. We can, however, no longer represent this match situation in useful algebraic form because we are no longer dealing with an equation involving the s_1 and s_2 receptors alone.

To understand the situation after adaptation we can suppose that the s_1 sensitivity would again be reduced to $^1/_{10}$th of its pre-adaptation value and the s_2 to $\frac{1}{2}$, but the sensitivity of the 585 nm receptor would be hardly affected because of its narrow sensitivity curve and therefore its insensitivity to the long wave red adaptation. This necessarily means that the adaptation would have a different effect on the response to the mixture of 650 and 530 nm than it would on the response to the single wavelength 585 nm. In other words the match would break down. In colour appearance terms, while the red adaptation would cause the red-green mixture to change from yellow to green, it would merely cause a slight drop in intensity of the monochromatic yellow with no change in its yellow appearance. This is not what is observed so there cannot be a fourth receptor of the sort described here.

The Limited Visual Significance of Three-Colour Mixture Data

The two previous Sections of this paper have discussed the relation of the colour mixture curves to the retinal receptors. There can be little room for doubt that the quantitative facts of colour matching are determined entirely by the spectral sensitivity curves of the retinal receptors and presumably, therefore, by the spectral absorption curves of the light-sensitive substances in the receptors. Hence we can expect the colour mixture curves to give us very direct information about these absorption curves.

This is, however, the limit of their visual significance. It is, of course, very important indeed to know as much as we can about this first stage in the visual process, but it is, after all, only the first stage. The mixture curves tell us nothing about how the colour information is coded in the retina for transmission to the visual cortex nor how the qualities of redness, greenness, blueness, yellowness and whiteness are generated.

This chapter is not concerned with theories of colour vision but it is perhaps appropriate to emphasise in conclusion that the colour mixture curves in themselves tell us nothing about the colour sensations. When we make a colour match the only visual judgment required is whether the two halves of the field are identical in appearance, but not what that appearance happens to be. Yet the changes in colour that occur when we mix different stimuli are of the greatest possible interest to our understanding of the visual process and it was for that reason that special attention was given in an earlier Section of this chapter to a descriptive account of the effects of two-colour and three-colour mixture.

References

ABNEY, W. DE W.: Researches in Colour Vision. London: Longmans Green 1913.

BROWN, P. K., WALD, G.: Visual pigments in single rods and cones of the human retina. Science **144**, 45—52 (1964).

GUILD, J.: A trichromatic colorimeter suitable for standardisation work. Trans. opt. Soc. (Lond.) **27**, 106—128 (1925—26).

— The colorimetric properties of the spectrum. Phil. Trans. roy. Soc. (Lond.) A, **230**, 149—187 (1931).

HELMHOLTZ, H. von: Physiological Optics. Trans. of 3rd Ed., Rochester: Optical Society of America 1924.

KÖNIG, A., DIETERICI, C.: Die Grundempfindungen in normalen und anomalen Farbensystemen und ihre Intensitätsverteilung im Spektrum. Z. Psychol. Physiol. Sinnesorg. **4**, 241—397 (1892).

LOZANO, R. D., PALMER, D. A.: Large-field color matching and adaptation. J. opt. Soc. Amer. **58**, 1653—1656 (1968).

MARKS, W. B., DOBELLE, W. H., MACNICHOL, E. F.: Visual pigments of single primate cones. Science **143**, 1181—1183 (1964).

MAXWELL, J. C.: On the theory of compound colours, and the relations of the colours of the spectrum. Phil. Trans. roy. Soc. (Lond.), **150**, 57—84 (1860).

SPERANSKAYA, N. I.: Determination of spectrum color coordinates for twenty-seven normal observers. Optics and Spectroscopy **7**, 424—428 (1959).

STILES, W. S., BURCH, J. M.: N. P. L. colour-matching investigation: Final report (1958). Optica Acta **6**, 1—26 (1959).

— The basic data of colour-matching. Year Book, Phys. Soc. (Lond.), pp. 44—65 (1955).

THOMSON, L. C., WRIGHT, W. D.: The convergence of the tritanopic confusion loci and the derivation of the fundamental response functions. J. opt. Soc. Am. **43**, 890—894 (1953).

WRIGHT, W. D.: A trichromatic colorimeter with spectral primaries. Trans. opt. Soc. (Lond.) **29**, 225—241 (1927—28).

— A re-determination of the trichromatic coefficients of the spectral colours. Trans. opt. Soc. (Lond.) **30**, 141—159 (1928—29).

— A re-determination of the mixture curves of the spectrum. Trans. opt. Soc. (Lond.) **31**, 201—211 (1929—30).

— Researches on Normal and Defective Colour Vision. London: Kimpton 1946.

— The Measurement of Colour, 4th Ed. London: Hilger 1969.

WYSZECKI, G., STILES, W. S.: Color Science. New York: Wiley 1967.

Chapter 17

Light Transmission through the Ocular Media and Macular Pigment and its Significance for Psychophysical Investigation

By

K. H. Ruddock, London (Great Britain)

With 6 Figures

Contents

1. Introduction

The light which is detected by photochemical absorption in the receptoral pigments must firstly traverse the ocular media and the retina. The refractive powers of the ocular media enable the eye to form a retinal image, but in addition, these media have significant attenuating properties. Attenuation of the incident light beam on its passage through the eye arises from two sources, namely, absorption and scatter. Both forms of light loss may be wavelength dependent, and may therefore influence the spectral composition of "white" light absorbed by the photopigments. Scattering of light from an incident beam also degrades the visual image (see Westheimer, chapter 7, this volume).

2. The Ocular Media

a) The Ocular Media (Fig. 1) comprise the cornea, aqueous and vitreous humours, and the crystalline lens. The spectral transmission properties of the pre-retinal ocular media taken as a whole were determined by LUDVIGH and MCCARTHY (1938), working with freshly enucleated eyes. A small area of the foveal retina and pigment epithelium was removed from the region around an aperture cut in the sclera and choroid. The fraction of light transmitted through the eye and out through this small area was then determined as a function of wavelength. The

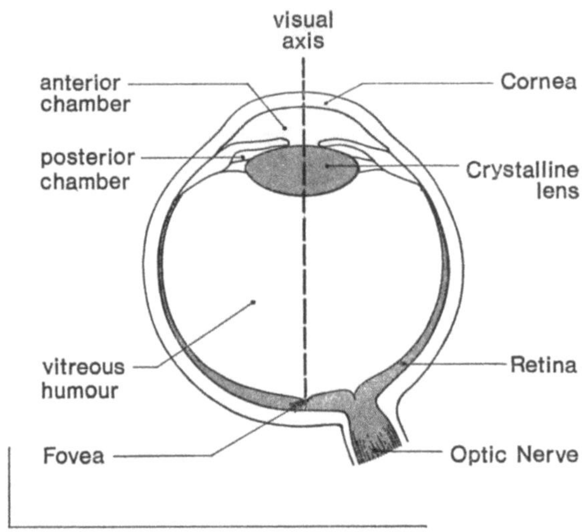

Fig. 1. Schematic cross-section through the eye, showing the ocular media and retina

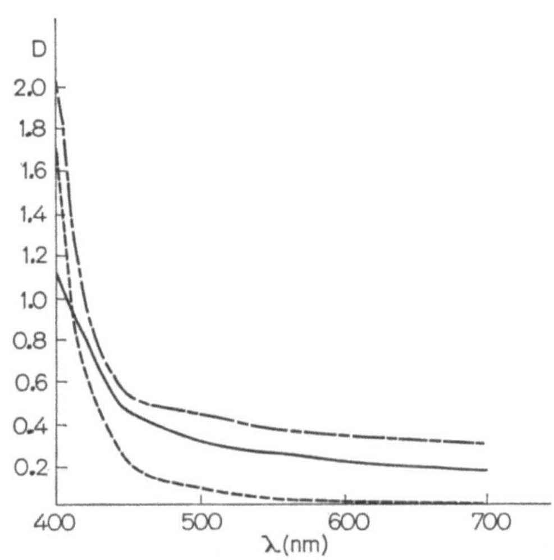

Fig. 2. The optical density, D, of the ocular media as determined by LUDVIGH and MCCARTHY (1938) — continuous curve; by GEERAETS *et al.* (1960) — broken curve; and by BOETTNER and WOLTER (1962) semi-broken curve

data were obtained from old eyes (average age 62 years), but were "corrected" for age changes so as to yield data applicable to young eyes (Fig. 2). This correction was made by taking into account age changes in lens absorption, determined by separate measurements on extirpated lenses. The correction data were not, however, published with the transmission values for the ocular media.

Also shown in Fig. 2 are transmission data for the ocular media published by GEERAETS *et al.* (1960) and BOETTNER and WOLTER (1962). The former give average data for the two eyes of a 28 year old subject, measurements being made 4 hours post mortem. BOETTNER and WOLTER (1962) measured the spectral transmission properties of each component of the ocular media. Nine eyes taken from subjects aged between 4 weeks and 75 years were studied, and thus age dependence of the transmission factors was also investigated. Their data will be discussed further in the following sections 2.2 to 2.5, which deal with transmission measurements for the individual elements of the ocular media. From their experimental results, BOETTNER and WOLTER computed a transmission curve for passage through the whole eye of a young observer, and it is this which is presented in Fig. 2.

It can be seen that all three sets of data shown in Fig. 2 have the same general characteristics, with the results of LUDVIGH and MCCARTHY (1938) intermediate between the others.

b) The Cornea is of average thickness 0.54 mm and mean refractive index 1.377. It is responsible for most of the refractive power of the optical system of the eye. Incident light suffers about 4 % reflection at the air-corneal interface, but otherwise the cornea is of high transmissivity for visible radiation. Thus, BOETTNER and WOLTER (1963) measured corneal transmission values of 80 % to 95 %, although the values for the non-scattered component dropped to 70 % at 700 nm and 40 % at 400 nm. This light scatter apparently arises in the stroma (MAURICE, 1957) which constitute some 90 % of the corneal thickness. MAURICE found that *in vivo* back scatter from the cornea was greater for short-wave than long-wave light, suggesting a Rayleigh-type spectral dependence.

Scatter and absorption in the cornea are the most significant sources of light loss in the ocular media, next to that occurring in the lens. Thus, both VOS and BOOGAARD (1963) and BOYNTON and CLARKE (1964) conclude that 25–30 % of the total light scatter in the eye arises at the cornea. VOS (1963) states that the overall light scatter in the eye is not wavelength dependent, but this conclusion is at variance with the careful studies of LE GRAND (1937a, b) who found evidence that the eye scatters short-wave light to a greater extent than long-wave light.

c) The Anterior Chamber is clear under slit lamp examination and light losses in the aqueous humour are almost certainly negligible, as can be seen from BOETTNER and WOLTER'S (1962) data.

d) The Crystalline Lens, which is largely responsible for the accommodation capacity of the eye, is of variable refractive index, the value of the refractive index increasing from 1.39 at the periphery to 1.42 at the centre of the lens (DUKE-ELDER, 1938). Studies indicate that the lens is an important source of both absorption and scatter of light from an incident beam.

The extirpated lens appears yellow, an appearance which is confirmed by the spectral absorption data for human lenses recorded "*in vivo*" by SAID and WEALE

(1959). Their published data are shown in Fig. 3, and the marked age dependence of the absorption values will be discussed in Section 3, p. 460. These results were obtained by densitometric analysis of photographic records of the Purkinje reflex images of an incident light beam, formed by reflection at the front and back surfaces of the lens. BOETTNER and WOLTER (1962) measured light transmission factors for a number of extirpated lenses, and their results were largely in agreement with the "*in vivo*" lens absorption factors determined by SAID and WEALE

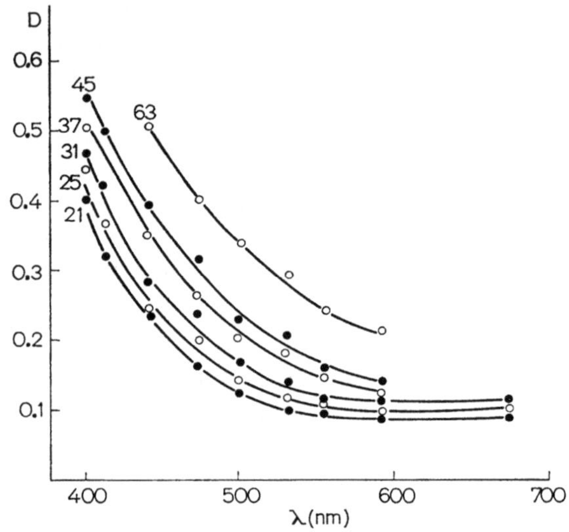

Fig. 3. The optical density, D, of living human crystalline lenses plotted as a function of wavelength, λ. Numbers refer to the ages of the observer (taken from SAID and WEALE, 1959)

(1959). WALD (1949) gives a spectral absorption curve for the extirpated lens of a 68 year old observer, which has a relative wavelength distribution similar to the curves of Fig. 3, but is of greater absolute density. WEALE (1961 b) has criticized WALD'S data on the grounds that the extirpated lens probably suffered post-mortem clouding, resulting in increased optical density. The lens pigment has been variously identified as melanin (FISCHER, 1948) or as some urochrome related pigment (not melanin) (MCEWEN, 1959). COOPER and ROBSON (1969) have published U.V. and visible absorption spectra for the lens pigment, which they found to be water soluble, but which they did not identify chemically. WOLF and GARDINER (1965) investigated the scattering properties of the lens "*in vivo*" using slit lamp illumination, and found that significant scatter occurred. VOS and BOOGAARD (1963) have published photographic evidence of light scatter arising in the lens (and cornea) under slit lamp examination.

Psychophysical determinations of lens absorption have depended largely on the study of aphakic observer response. GAYDON (1938) showed that the visual sensitivity of an aphakic observer extends into the near U-V, with little reduction in sensitivity between 400 and 320 nm. This demonstrates clearly that the lens effectively acts as a shortwave cut off filter for the eye. WALD (1949) deduced the spectral characteristics of lens absorption from threshold studies with an aphakic observer and RUDDOCK (1964) showed that the colour matches established by an aphakic observer were consistent with the removal of a yellow filter from the visual system. STILES and BURCH (1959) analysed observer variations in colour matching data and found clear indications of differences between observers in the amount of light absorption in the lens. In general, SAID and WEALE'S values for the optical density of the lens (Fig. 3) are lower than those derived by psychophysical methods. The experiments of BOYNTON and CLARKE (1964) and VOS (1963) indicate that light scatter in the lens is significant, but in neither case was the question of wavelength dependence examined.

e) The Vitreal Chamber contains the vitreous humour, which apparently gives rise to some light scatter (WOLF and GARDINER, 1965). BOETTNER and WOLTER (1962) found that less than 10% of the incident light is absorbed on its passage through the vitreous humour.

f) The Retina contains the photosensitive receptoral elements of the visual system, the early stages of the nervous channels leading to the cortex, and the capillary blood vessels. The most important source of light absorption in the retina is the macular pigmentation, which is discussed in detail in the next section. KISHTO (1968) has produced evidence of variations in visual thresholds associated with screening by blood vessels and VOS and BOUMAN (1964) have estimated that light scatter in the retina constitutes some 30% of the total light scatter in the eye.

g) Macular Pigmentation. Under ophthalmoscopic examination it can be seen that the central region of the retina absorbs blue-green and blue light. This absorption, apparent up to some 5° from the fovea centralis, is ascribed to a yellow pigment, called the macular pigment. The pigment responsible for the light absorption has been identified as a carotinoid pigment, xanthophyll, by both GULLSTRAND (1905) and WALD (1949). The former believed the pigment to be a result of post-mortem changes in the retina, although the effect of such a pigment upon psychophysical data is clearly demonstrable, in addition to its being visible ophthalmoscopically. Using an ophthalmoscopic arrangement, ISHAK *et al.* (1962) have photographed the fundus in monochromatic light and densitometric analysis of the results enabled them to determine spectral absorption characteristics for the macular region. Their data agree quite closely with the psychophysical results obtained by RUDDOCK (1963), but the difficulty of interpreting ophthalmoscopic data noted in the last paragraph of this section must be borne in mind.

In an early paper HERING (1893) discussed the influence of macular pigment on colour matches and WRIGHT (1928–1929) showed that spectral colour matches involving blue-green stimuli are extremely variable between different observers. This he ascribed to light absorption by macular pigmentation, the optical density of which varies greatly from observer to observer. RUDDOCK (1963) derived data for the spectral absorption and retinal distribution of the macular pigment from an analysis of colour mixture data (Fig. 4). The spectral absorption curve so obtained deviated somewhat from the xanthophyll absorption spectrum (also shown in Fig. 4), especially at the longer wavelengths. WALD (1949) published psychophysical data for macular absorption which agree closely with the spectrum derived by RUDDOCK. STILES (1953) also deduced the spectral absorption characteristics of the macular pigment from colour matching data and his results are consistent with the identification of the pigment as xanthophyll.

The absorption losses in the macular pigment are polarization sensitive (NAYLOR and STANWORTH, 1954; RUDDOCK, 1965c), and the entoptic phenomena known as Maxwell's spot and Haidinger's brushes (HELMHOLTZ, 1924) are manifestations of the same absorption process. Observers who fail to see one also

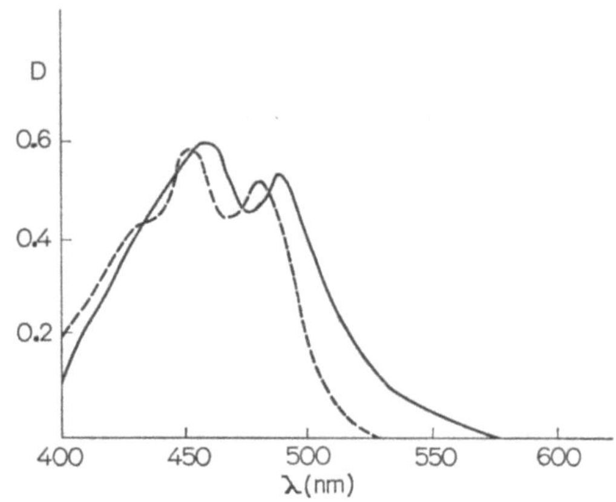

Fig. 4. Continuous line — optical density of the macular pigment, D, as a function of wavelength, λ, (after RUDDOCK, 1963). Broken line — absorption spectrum of xanthophyll

fail to see the other. ISHAK (1952a, b) demonstrated that the optical density of the macular pigment for a group of Egyptian observers was greater than that of the average white English observer (taken as the 1931 C.I.E. 2° standard observer). Thus, it is possible that the density of the macular pigment is subject to racial variation. It is interesting to note that some classes of colour defective observers may fail to detect Maxwell's spot in some illuminations but not in others (WALLS and MATHEWS, 1952; KALMUS, 1965; WALLS and HEATH, 1956; MURRAY, 1954; see also HURVICH, chapter 23, this volume).

In spite of the close similarity in their retinal distribution and spectral transmission characteristics, there is no conclusive proof that the macular absorption detected by ophthalmoscopic examination gives rise to the various psychophysical phenomena described above. One puzzling fact is that macular absorption of blue and blue-green light is detected by ophthalmoscopic examination of retinae which, on the basis of psychophysical data, would be judged as being free from macular pigment (e.g. the case of observer J.A.S. of RUDDOCK's 1963 investigation).

3. Observer Age

An important feature of the published data regarding light losses in the ocular media is their dependence upon the age of the observer. The general properties of the ageing eye have been discussed at length by WEALE (1963). The cornea appears yellower in the older eye and an associated increase in corneal scatter may also occur (WEALE, 1961a). BOETTNER and WOLTER (1962) found a small but significant increase in corneal light losses with increasing age.

The major age changes in light transmission through the ocular media seem to arise in the lens. SAID and WEALE (1959) demonstrated that the optical density of the crystalline lens increases with age, particularly for short wavelength stimuli (Fig. 3). Their results show a systematic increase in density with increasing observer age, although WALD (1949) and STILES and BURCH (1959) have suggested that lens absorption is variable even amongst observers of the same age. BOETTNER and WOLTER (1963) found age changes in transmission through their extirpated lenses which were consistent with the data of SAID and WEALE, but they too are of the opinion that the age increases in absorption are less systematic than was suggested by SAID and WEALE. HESS (1911) studied lens absorption by measuring threshold sensitivities for a group of unilaterally aphakic observers of different ages, and WEALE (1963) has shown that HESS's results are consistent with those of SAID and WEALE (1959).

The lens continues to grow throughout its life-span, causing compression of the fibres already present towards its centre. This growth is accompanied by a decrease in the water content of the lens, with a resulting accumulation of non-soluble protein (WEALE, 1963). Thus, it is to be expected that non-uniformities of refractive index within the lens volume will be associated with ageing. This is partly borne out by the data of WOLF and GARDINER (1965) who demonstrated that lens scattering increased linearly with age beyond 40 years, but was constant up to that age. Further, COOPER and ROBSON (1969) were not able to extract more pigment from old than from young lenses, despite the greater optical density of the former. This suggests that Rayleigh-type scattering may be at least partly responsible for the increased "yellowness" of the older lens, although COOPER and ROBSON (1969) deduce that a second, U.V. absorbing pigment, probably occurs in older lenses.

In a psychophysical investigation of colour vision, RUDDOCK (1965a, b) showed that age changes in the photopic V_λ curve and in the colour matching data of some 500 observers could be closely correlated with the age changes in lens absorption as determined by SAID and WEALE (1959). No correlation with increase in macular pigment absorption was found (see WRIGHT, 1946). It was demonstrated that the spectral distribution of the age dependent light losses in the ocular media are consistent with Rayleigh's law, indicating that scatter may be an important factor in causing these losses. STILES and BURCH (1959) analysed observer variations in the results of their 10° colour matching investigation. They found a small but significant correlation with age, and showed that this resulted from a systematic increase in lens absorption. Further, age changes in the colour matching functions were not consistent with light absorption by a single pigment and it was therefore suggested that both macular pigment and lens absorption vary with observer age.

A number of workers have carried out surveys of observer response to the Farnsworth-Munsell 100-hue test (FARNSWORTH, 1943) and other colour vision tests (see e.g. BIRCH, 1964; LAKOWSKI, 1958; KELLY 1958; VERRIEST *et al.*, 1962). The results of these surveys undoubtedly depend on the transmission properties of the ocular media, as is discussed later (Section 4c, p. 463), but their analysis is more difficult than that of colorimetric investigations with spectral matching stimuli.

4. Effects of Light Loss in the Ocular Media and the Macular Pigment

a) General Considerations. The work surveyed in the previous sections shows that light passing through the eye from the cornea to the retinal receptors suffers significant absorption in traversing the lens and the macular pigment. Absorption losses in the other optical media and losses by scatter can be neglected with little error. (It should be noted, however, that "absorption" losses measured in the lens may in part arise from wavelength dependent scattering, particularly in the case of older observers). The light losses in the lens and macula modify the results of psychophysical measurements, and in order to take account of this, it is necessary to adopt values for the spectral transmission factors of the lens and macular pigment. We are generally concerned only with the relative values of the transmission coefficients as a function of wavelength, but occasionally absolute transmission values are required (see Section 4b, p. 463).

The most reliable values for the spectral transmission factors of the lens seem to be those of SAID and WEALE (1959) given in Fig. 3. Although these values do not agree in all respects with psychophysical data (see Sections 2f and 3), there are good reasons for choosing them in preference to other data. Firstly, they were obtained "*in vivo*" by means of an objective technique and secondly, they show clearly the dependence of the lens transmission upon observer age. Alternatively, the data of Fig. 2 (e.g. those of LUDVIGH and MCCARTHY, 1938), for transmission through the total pre-retinal ocular media may be used. Unfortunately, LUDVIGH and MCCARTHY published no information regarding the age dependence of their data, which they claim apply to a young (20–30 year old) eye, and BOETTNER and WOLTER (1963) do not give sufficiently detailed values for the effect of age.

The relative absorption spectrum of the macular pigment is given by Fig. 4, either by the psychophysical curve or, alternatively, by the xanthophyll absorption curve (WALD, 1949). Average optical densities for the macular pigment present in the eye are tabulated by WYSZECKI and STILES (1967). However, it has been shown by WRIGHT (1928/29) and RUDDOCK (1963) that the optical density of the macular pigment is very variable from observer to observer. Thus, it is not possible to make even an approximate calculation to allow for macular absorption in an individual eye, unless some estimate has been made of the optical density of the pigment. Such an estimate is most readily obtained by differential measurements between the fovea and a parafoveal region preferably some 5° to 8° away. This is the general method applied by WALD (1949) and RUDDOCK (1963), the former deriving the transmission of the macular pigment from the differences between the foveal and parafoveal spectral sensitivity functions and the latter from the differences between foveal and parafoveal colour matching characteristics. A simpler, but much less accurate, estimate of the density of the macular pigment can be obtained from the appearance of Maxwell's spot (MILES, 1949) or Haidinger's brushes. Observers who fail to see either of these phenomena also show no influence of macular absorption in their colour matching or their spectral sensitivity functions (RUDDOCK, 1965c).

b) Spectral Sensitivity Functions. Visual spectral sensitivity functions (e.g., the photopic function, V_λ) are defined in terms of the radiant energy flux, E_λ, of wavelength λ, which is required to produce a given visual response. The response criterion may be threshold detection or brightness equality as determined by a flicker technique or by heterochromatic matching (compare LE GRAND, chapter 15, this volume). The visual spectral sensitivity at wavelength λ is defined as:

$$V_\lambda = \frac{K}{E_\lambda} \tag{1}$$

where K is a normalizing constant and E_λ is the energy flux at the cornea.

If we wish to find the spectral sensitivity S_λ of the photoresponse mechanism, we must evaluate:

$$S_\lambda = \frac{K'}{t_\lambda E_\lambda} = \frac{K'' V_\lambda}{t_\lambda} \tag{2}$$

where t_λ is the transmission factor for the eye prior to the absorption of the light in the photopigment, and K' and K'' are normalizing constants. (Note: if t_λ arises from a number of successive absorption processes, the transmission factors for these successive absorptions are multiplied together to give t_λ.) We can consider that the function S_λ represents the function V_λ "corrected" for light losses in the ocular media.

Both the lens and the macular pigment absorb more heavily at short wavelengths than at long wavelengths (Figs. 3 and 4). Thus, from Eq. (2), we can see that correction for light loss in either the lens or the macular pigment yields a function S_λ which is of higher sensitivity at shorter wavelengths than is V_λ. STILES (1959) corrected the spectral sensitivity functions of the inferred colour mechanisms in this way and compared the corrected functions with the standard visual pigment absorption spectrum proposed by DARTNALL (1953).

We can look at Eq. (2) in another way. If S_λ were constant, a change in t_λ would cause a change in V_λ. For example, t_λ could represent the age changes in the spectral transmission curve of the lens. If we assume that the absorption spectra, S_λ, of the photopigments do not change with age, then from Eq. 2 we can compute the changes in the V_λ function. In this way, WEALE (1963) and RUDDOCK (1965b) showed that variations with observer age in both absolute threshold sensitivity and the photopic V_λ function are consistent with the age changes in lens transmission.

In theory, the number of photons which must be absorbed in the photopigment(s) for threshold detection, S_λ, could be calculated from the corresponding photon flux, V_λ, measured at the cornea. However, it is necessary to include a figure for the quantum efficiency of the photopigment(s) in the value of t_λ, and t_λ must also account for non-wavelength dependent light losses due e.g. to back reflection at the cornea and white light scatter. Thus in practice, it should be much easier to determine the threshold photon requirement from statistical considerations, although there is a remarkable discrepancy between different estimates made in this way (see e.g., HECHT *et al.*, 1942; VAN DER VELDEN, 1944; BRINDLEY, 1960).

c) Colour Specification and Screening Tests. A filter of transmission characteristic t_λ interposed between the eye and a light beam of spectral radiant flux distribution E_λ changes the colour specification of the incident beam. The C.I.E.

specification of the flux received by the eye is given by

$$\begin{aligned} X &= \int_\lambda E_\lambda t_\lambda \bar{x}_\lambda d\lambda , \\ Y &= \int_\lambda E_\lambda t_\lambda \bar{y}_\lambda d\lambda , \\ Z &= \int_\lambda E_\lambda t_\lambda \bar{z}_\lambda d\lambda , \end{aligned} \tag{3}$$

where X, Y, Z, are the tristimulus values of the light and $\bar{x}_\lambda$, $\bar{y}_\lambda$ and $\bar{z}_\lambda$, are the equal energy distribution coefficients of the C.I.E. standard observer (Compte Rendu of the C.I.E. 1931, 1963). In practice, integration over λ is replaced by a summation over a finite number of discrete spectral values (usually 31 equally spaced λ-values in wavelength range 400–700 nm).

The corresponding chromaticity co-ordinates which specify the colour quality, but not the flux, are given by:

$$x = \frac{X}{X+Y+Z}\,; \quad y = \frac{Y}{X+Y+Z}\,; \quad z = \frac{Z}{X+Y+Z} \tag{4}$$

so that $x + y + z = 1$.

Now the C.I.E. standard observer corresponds to a 25–30 year old observer and age changes in the ocular media must modify the overall visual response of an older observer. For example, if we let t_λ represent the *change* in transmission for the older observer relative to the standard young observer, then the C.I.E. specification of a colour for the older observer is given by Eqs. (3) and (4).

RUDDOCK (1964) has computed the colour specification of the Farnsworth-Munsell 100 hue test for young and old observers, making use of the spectral transmission curves of Fig. 2 to take account of the age changes in transmission through the ocular media. Applying Eqs. (3) and (4), the chromaticity co-ordinates of the 100 hue test samples were computed for a 25 year old observer (equivalent to the 1931 C.I.E. 2° standard observer) and a 65 year old observer. Values of t_λ corresponded to the differences in lens transmission between these two ages (Fig. 3). The results of the calculation are shown in Fig. 5, expressed both in the C.I.E. x–y diagram and in the BRECKENRIDGE and SCHAUB (1939) uniform chromaticity scale. Examination of the latter shows that for certain regions of the hue circle, consecutive hue samples are significantly more closely grouped for the older than for the younger observer. Thus, the older observer should be less able to discriminate between these groups of hues (specifically, the blue-green hue samples numbered 45–55 and the red hue samples numbered 80–85 and 1–5).

This conclusion, which is confirmed by results of the experimental investigations of VERRIEST *et al.* (1962) and BIRCH (1964), demonstrates that the transmission properties of the eye influence the results of visual screening tests. In consequence, the results of such tests require careful interpretation. For example, it would be quite incorrect to conclude that the changes with age in ability to discriminate the 100-hue test samples arise from an age-change in post-retinal discrimination capacity.

Unfortunately, calculations based on Eqs. (3) and (4) take no account of visual adaptation to the illuminant. It has been clearly shown (BURNHAM *et al.*, 1952; JAMESON and HURVICH, 1951; 1959; WASSEF, 1958; 1959), that the visual system may partially compensate for changes in colour appearance associated with a change of illuminant. Since all light detected by the receptors is transmitted through the lens etc., it is conceivable that the eye may partially compensate for changes in pigmentation by adaptation. What is not all clear, however, is the extent to which the shift in apparent colour associated with such adaptation modifies the ability of the eye to discriminate colours.

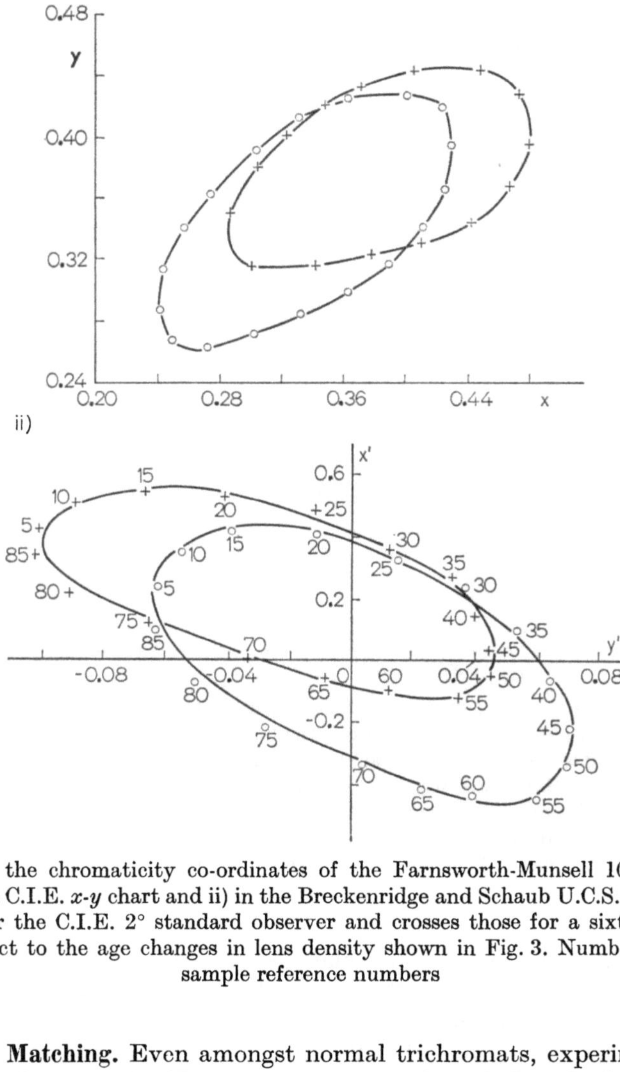

Fig. 5. Loci of the chromaticity co-ordinates of the Farnsworth-Munsell 100 hue samples plotted i) in the C.I.E. x-y chart and ii) in the Breckenridge and Schaub U.C.S. Circles give the co-ordinates for the C.I.E. 2° standard observer and crosses those for a sixty-five year old observer, subject to the age changes in lens density shown in Fig. 3. Numbers are the test sample reference numbers

d) Colour Matching. Even amongst normal trichromats, experimental colour matches are subject to significant observer variation. Although these variations may result from differences in the absorption spectra of the visual photopigments, they are more usually associated with observer differences in transmission characteristics of the ocular media and retina. Thus, we frequently wish to calculate the effect on a colour match of variation in lens or macular pigment absorption, assuming constant photopigment absorption and receptor response. For this purpose, it is necessary to use a system of colour measurement based entirely upon spectral stimuli, such as the W.D.W. system (WRIGHT, 1928/29). We cannot apply directly the results of computation based on the C.I.E. system, but we can transform such results into the W.D.W. system (ISHAK, 1952b; WARBURTON, 1954). We may still use Eqs. (3) und (4) of the previous section to compute the effect of the filter t_λ, but we must transform Eq. (4) into a W.D.W. type system in order to make useful comparisons with experimental colour matching data. The reason for using the W.D.W. or some other similar colorimetric system is that changes in pigment absorption do not alter the chromaticity co-ordinates of

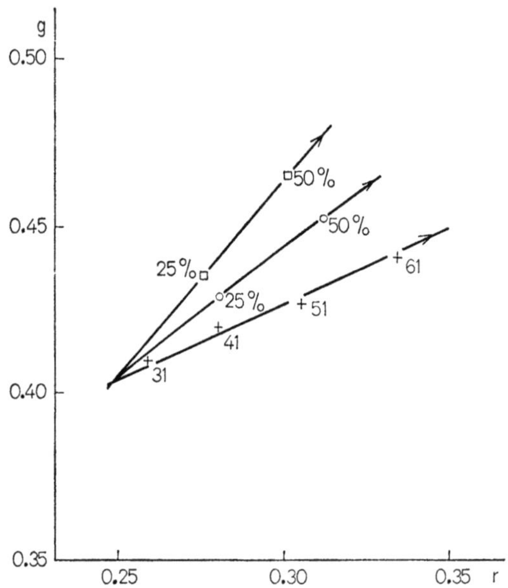

Fig. 6. Loci of chromaticity co-ordinates of the C.I.E. 2° standard source S_B, plotted in the W.D.W. *r-g* system. *Crosses* — co-ordinates calculated for the C.I.E. 2° standard observer, subject to yellowing of the lens with age, as shown in Fig. 3. The numbers refer to observer age. *Circles* — co-ordinates calculated for the C.I.E. 2° standard observer, modified by increases in density of the macular pigment. Figures refer to the percentage increase in the density values shown in Fig. 4 required to produce the corresponding co-ordinates. *Squares* — as above, but calculated on the basis of the spectral transmission function of xanthophyll (Fig. 4)

spectral stimuli. If, however, colour matches are made with test stimuli having continuous energy distribution E_λ, the resulting chromaticity co-ordinates are dependent upon pre-receptoral light absorption in the eye. A detailed mathematical discussion of this point is given by WYSZECKI and STILES (1967).

RUDDOCK (1965b) has computed the changes in the W.D.W. chromaticity co-ordinates of the C.I.E. source S_B which result from age changes in lens transmission (Fig. 3) or from changes in the optical density of the macular pigment. The results of these computations are shown in Fig. 6, and it can be seen that both variables produce similar effects, although the dominant wavelength for lens ageing (581 nm) is somewhat greater than that for macular pigment changes (574 nm to 578 nm). Experimental data show that age changes in colour matching correspond closely to the calculated changes arising from increased lens absorption (RUDDOCK,

1965b). Similarly, ISHAK (1952b) correlated colour matching differences between English and Egyptian observers with differences in the optical density of the macular pigment.

The optical density of the macular pigment decreases away from the fovea and so colour matches established in the parafovea and extra-fovea are subject to little or no absorption by this pigment. Thus, changes in colour matching between foveal and non-foveal retinal locations must, at least in part, reflect the differences in the macular pigment absorption at the two field locations. It is interesting to note, however, that the differences between the C.I.E. 2° and 10° colour matching functions cannot be caused solely by macular pigment absorption and must therefore also represent differences in receptoral response.

e) The Stiles-Crawford Effect. WEALE (1961b) has discussed at length the photometric significance of the human crystalline lens, on the assumption that light losses in the lens are caused by a uniformly distributed pigment. If this assumption were true, a pencil of light passing through the periphery of the lens would be subject to less absorption than an axial pencil, due to its shorter path through the lens body (FINCHAM, 1937). Thus, a reverse Stiles-Crawford type effect should be introduced and, as WEALE points out, this must be accounted for in any analysis of the Stiles-Crawford effect proper. (See CRAWFORD, chapter 18, this volume.) It seems that light scattering centres are non-uniformly distributed through the lens volume (VOS and BOOGAARD, 1963) and thus scatter losses cannot be accurately accounted for by WEALE's approach. Nonetheless, the shorter optical path through the lens of eccentric light pencils must significantly modify their absorption in the lens.

References

BIRCH, J.: Private communication. Report on Colour Vision and Age to the Medical Research Council 1964.

BOETTNER, E. A., WOLTER, J. R.: Transmission of the ocular media. Invest. Ophthal. **1**, 776—783 (1962).

BOYNTON, R. M., CLARKE, F. J. J.: Sources of entoptic scatter in the human eye. J. opt. Soc. Amer. **54**, 110—119; 1170—1171 (1964).

BRECKENRIDGE, F. C., SCHAUB, W. R.: Rectangular uniform chromaticity scale coordinates. J. opt. Soc. Amer. **29**, 370—380 (1939).

BRINDLEY, G. S.: Physiology of the Retina and Visual Pathway. Ch. 6. London: Arnold 1960.

BURNHAM, R. W., EVANS, R. M., NEWHALL, S. M.: Influence on color perception of adaptation to illumination. J. opt. Soc. Amer. **42**, 597—605 (1952).

Commission Internationale de l'Éclairage (C.I.E.) Compte rendu des séances. Cambridge: The University Press 1931.

— Compte rendu of 15th session. Volume A (Paris) 1963.

COOPER, G. F., ROBSON, J. G.: The yellow colour of the lens of man and other primates. J. Physiol. (Lond.) **203**, 411—417 (1969).

DARTNALL, H. J. A.: The interpretation of spectral sensitivity curves. Brit. Med. Bull. **9**, 24—30 (1953).

DUKE-ELDER, W. S.: Textbook of Ophthalmology, Vol. 1, p. 746. London: Kimpton 1938.

FARNSWORTH, D.: The Farnsworth-Munsell 100-hue test for colour blindness. J. opt. Soc. Amer. **33**, 568—578 (1943).

FINCHAM, E. F.: The Mechanism of Accommodation. London: Pulman 1937.

FISCHER, F. P.: The senescence of the eye. In: SORSBY, A. (Ed.). Modern Trends in Ophthalmology, Vol. 2. London: Butterworth 1948.

Gaydon, A. G.: Colour sensations produced by ultra-violet light. Proc. Phys. Soc. (Lond.) **50**, 714—720 (1938).

Geeraets, W. J., Williams, R. C., Chan, G., Ham, W. T., Guerry, D., Schmidt, F. H.: The loss of light energy in retina and choroid. Arch. Ophthal. **64**, 606—615 (1960).

Gullstrand, A.: Zur Maculafrage. Graefes Arch. Ophthal. **66**, 141—188 (1907).

Hecht, S., Shlaer, S., Pirenne, M. H.: Energy, quanta and vision. J. gen. Physiol. **25**, 819—840 (1942).

Helmholtz, H. von: Physiological Optics, Vol. 2, Ch. 25. Southall, J. P. C., (Transl.) Rochester: Optical Society of America 1924.

Hering, E.: Über den Einfluß der Macula lutea auf spectrale Farbengleichungen. Pflügers Arch. ges. Physiol. **54**, 277—312 (1893).

Hess, C.: Gr. Saemisch Handbuch Augenheilk. 3rd. Ed., part 2, Ch. 9. Leipzig: Engelmann 1911.

Hurvich, L. M., Jameson, D.: A psychophysical study of white. III. Adaptation as variant. J. opt. Soc. Amer. **41**, 787—801 (1951).

Ishak, I. G. H.: The photopic luminosity curve for a group of fifteen Egyptian trichromats. J. opt. Soc. Amer. **42**, 529—534 (1952a).

— The spectral chromaticity co-ordinates for one British and eight Egyptian trichromats. J. opt. Soc. Amer. **42**, 534—539 (1952b).

— Housni, F. A., Said, F. S., Abd El-Sayed, S. Z.: Measurements of absorption spectrum curve of the yellow macular pigmentation in the living eye. Excerpta medica international congress series No. 146, pp. 1101—1106. Proc. of the XXth International Congress of Ophthalmology, Munich 1966.

Jameson, D., Hurvich, L. M.: Perceived color and its dependence on focal, surrounding and preceding stimulus variables. J. opt. Soc. Amer. **49**, 890—898 (1959).

Kalmus, H.: Diagnosis and Genetics of Defective Colour Vision, Ch. 6. London: Pergamon Press 1965.

Kelly, K. L.: Observer differences in colour-mixture functions studied by means of a pair of metameric grays. J. Res. Nat. Bur. Stand. (Wash.) **60**, 97—103 (1958).

Kishto, B. N.: The photometric evaluation of flashing light sources in relation to their conspicuity. Ph. D. Thesis. University of London 1968.

Lakowski, R.: Age and colour vision. Advan. Sci. **59**, 231—236 (1958).

Le Grand, Y.: Recherches sur la diffusion de la lumière dans l'oeil humain. Rev. Opt. (Paris) **16**, 201—214 (1937a).

— Recherches sur la diffusion de la lumière dans l'oeil humain. Rev. Opt. (Paris) **16**, 241—266 (1937b).

Ludvigh, E., McCarthy, E. F.: Absorption of visible light by the refractive media of the human eye. Arch. Ophthal. **20**, 37—51 (1938).

Maurice, D. M.: The structure and transparency of the cornea. J. Physiol. (Lond.) **136**, 263—286 (1957).

McEwen, W. K.: The yellow pigment of human lenses. Amer. J. Opthal. **47**, pt. II, 144—146 (1959).

Miles, W. R.: On the central zone of the human fovea. Science **109**, 441—442 (1949).

Murray, E.: Book review: G. L. Walls, R. W. Mathews' New Means of Studying Color Blindness and Normal Foveal Color Vision. Amer. J. Psychol. **67**, 182—188 (1954).

Naylor, E. J., Stanworth, A.: Retinal pigment and the Haidinger effect. J. Physiol. (Lond.) **124**, 543—552 (1954).

Ruddock, K. H.: Evidence for macular pigmentation from colour matching data. Vision Res. **3**, 417—429 (1963).

— The effect of age upon colour matching and colour discrimination. Ph. D. Thesis. University of London, 1964.

— The effect of age upon colour vision-I. Response in the receptoral system of the human eye. Vision Res. **5**, 37—45 (1965a).

— The effect of age upon color vision-II. Changes with age in light transmission of the ocular media. Vision Res. **5**, 47—58 (1965b).

— Foveal and parafoveal color vision. J. opt. Soc. Amer. **55**, 1180 (1965c).

SAID, F. S., WEALE, R. A.: The variation with age of the spectral transmissivity of the living crystalline lens. Gerontologia (Basel) **3**, 213—231 (1959).

STILES, W. S.: Further studies of visual mechanisms by the two colour threshold technique. Coloquio sobre problemas opticas de la vision. (Madrid) Union Internationale de Physique pure et appliquée **1**, 65—103 (1953).

— Color vision: The approach through increment threshold sensitivity. Proc. nat. Acad. Sci. (Wash.) **45**, 100—114 (1959).

— BURCH, J. M.: N.P.L. colour-matching investigation: Final report (1958). Optica Acta **6**, 1—26 (1959).

VAN DER VELDEN, H. A.: Over het aantal lichtquanta dat nodig is voor een lichtprikkel bij het menselijk oog. Physica **11**, 179—189 (1944).

VERRIEST, G., VALDEVYVERE, R., VANDERDONCK, R.: Variations de la discrimination chromatique. Rev. Opt. (Paris) **41**, 499—509 (1962).

VOS, J. J.: On the mechanisms of glare PhD. thesis. University of Utrecht 1963.

— BOOGAARD, J.: Contribution of the cornea to entoptic scatter. J. opt. Soc. Amer. **53**, 869—873 (1963).

— BOUMAN, M. A.: Contribution of the retina to entoptic scatter. J. opt. Soc. Amer. **54**, 95—100 (1964).

WALD, G.: The photochemistry of vision. Documenta Ophthal. **3**, 94—137 (1949).

WALLS, G. L., HEATH, G. G.: Neutral points in 138 protanopes and deuteranopes. J. opt. Soc. Amer. **46**, 640—649 (1956).

— MATHEWS, R. W.: New Means of Studying Color Blindness and Normal Foveal Color Vision. Berkeley: University of California Press 1952.

WARBURTON, F. L.: Variations in normal colour vision. Proc. Phys. Soc. (Lond.) B **67**, 477—484 (1954).

WASSEF, E. G. T.: Investigation into the theory of prediction of the appearance of colours and its bearing on theory of colour vision. Optica Acta **5**, 101—108 (1958).

— Linearity of the relationship between the tristimulus values of corresponding colours seen under different conditions of chromatic adaptation. Optica Acta **6**, 378—386 (1959).

WEALE, R. A.: Retinal illumination and age. Trans. Illum. Soc. (Lond.) **26**, 95—100 (1961a).

— Notes on the photometric significance of the human crystalline lens. Vision Res. **1**, 183—191 (1961b).

— The Aging Eye. London: Lewis 1963.

WOLF, E., GARDINER, J. S.: Studies on the scatter of light in the dioptric media of the eye as a basis of visual glare. Arch. Ophthal. **74**, 338—345 (1965).

WRIGHT, W. D.: A re-determination of the trichromatic coefficients of the spectral colours. Trans. opt. Soc. (Lond.) **30**, 141—158 (1928—1929).

— Researches on Normal and Defective Colour Vision, Ch. 12. London: Kimpton 1946.

WYSZECKI, G., STILES, W. S.: Color Science, Ch. 2 and 5. New York: Wiley 1967.

Chapter 18

The Stiles-Crawford Effects and their Significance in Vision

By

B. H. CRAWFORD, London (Great Britain)

With 9 Figures

The Stiles-Crawford effect (of the first kind) was discovered in about 1932 as a photometric discrepancy (STILES and CRAWFORD, 1933). Following an idea of STILES', a small piece of apparatus was made in which the brightness of one half of a photometric field, seen through the whole aperture of the eye pupil, was compared with the brightness of the other half, seen through a small central area of the pupil only. The apparatus is sketched in Fig. 1. The brightness of the first half of the field (reflected from P_2) would depend upon size of pupil, while that of the second half would be independent of it. Assuming that the retinal illuminance is proportional to pupil area (as with exposure in a camera), changes in pupil size with change in general illumination could be deduced from the corresponding

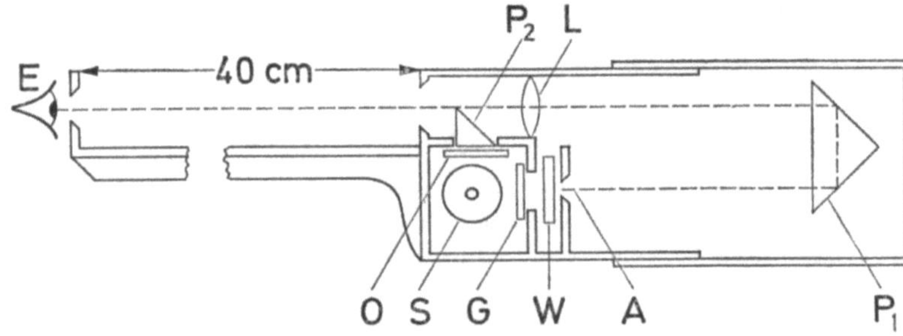

Fig. 1. Photometric pupillometer (after STILES and CRAWFORD, 1933). S lamp; G ground glass; W neutral wedge; A aperture imaged at E by L; P_1, P_2 reflecting prisms; L lens; O opal glass; E eye

changes in photometric balance as measured on a suitably calibrated neutral wedge. It would be necessary to make one determination of pupil size, most easily at a high level of illumination, by direct mensuration against a scale or by photography: other pupil sizes could then be related to this one. It may be mentioned that the photometric method was not intended to replace the direct methods, but only to provide a rapid and convenient check on pupil size during measurements of various visual capacities.

In fact, things did not turn out this way at all: the pupil sizes deduced for lower levels of illumination were much too small to be correct when compared with the various data available from direct measurement (e.g., REEVES, 1920; LYTHGOE, 1932).

The most obvious implication of this photometric discrepancy was that light entering the eye through the outer parts of the expanded pupil was for some reason less effective in eliciting the sensation of brightness than that entering through the central parts. The most obvious experiment to carry out was to compare the brightness of a field produced by a fixed beam passing through the geometric centre of the pupil aperture with the brightness from a beam which could be traversed across the pupil aperture. The results of this experiment are exemplified in Fig. 2. Closely similar results were obtained for several other observers with slight variations in the position of the maximum relative to the geometric centre of the eye pupil.

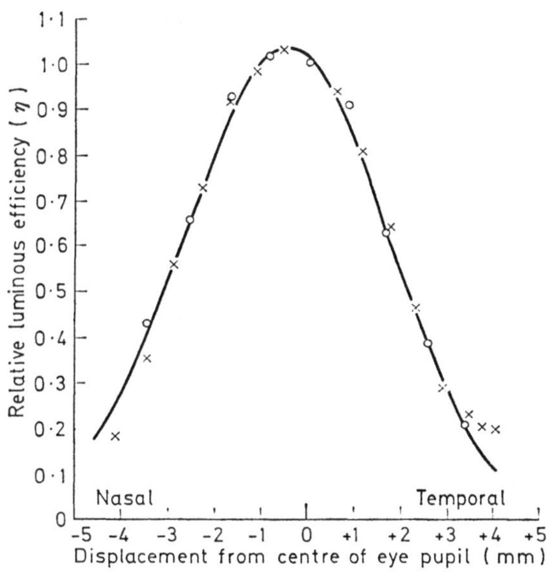

Fig. 2. Relative luminous efficiency (η) of light entering the eye pupil at different points for foveal vision. ×, measurements by photometric matching method (STILES and CRAWFORD, 1933); ⊙, measurements by brightness threshold method (CRAWFORD, 1937); curve $\eta = 1.04\, e^{-0.108\,(r+0.47)^2}$

It was natural for the discoverers of this unexpected effect to search at once for a reasonable hypothesis of its origin and it seemed more than likely that it was associated with the long, thin shape of the foveal cones and necessity for light to pass axially down them if it was to elicit the maximum response. Before this likelihood could be taken as a certainty, however, additional evidence was necessary. As the years passed, this was forthcoming in a variety of forms. The experiment of GOLDMANN (1942) is particularly important because of its directness. When one observer matched in apparent brightness the fields from beams with peripheral and central entry through the pupil, another observer, looking at the first observer's retina through an ophthalmoscope, could see an easily distinguishable difference between the two fields. That is, different light intensities incident on the retina from different directions could produce the same sensation of brightness: this can only happen if the seat of the effect is within the retinal layers.

Evidence of a different kind, but still fairly direct and unambiguous, comes from measurements of the Stiles-Crawford effect by observers with certain retinal abnormalities (FANKHAUSER, ENOCH, and CIBIS, 1961; DUNNEWOLD, 1964). The former authors describe, for instance, a case of retinoschisis. On one and the same apparatus they determined the Stiles-Crawford efficiency curve for a normal subject as well as for the pathological subject before and after operation by photocoagulation on the peripheral retina. The contrast-threshold curve for the normal subject (Fig. 3), if plotted in reciprocal form is closely similar to the early examples shown in Fig. 2. The curve for the pathological subject (Fig. 4) is much flatter than the normal, though still symmetrical with respect to the pupil. After photocoagulation, however, the curve (Fig. 5) is notably distorted in shape and in

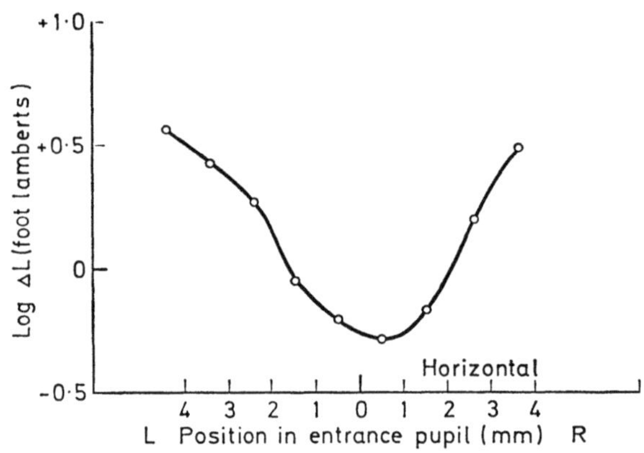

Fig. 3. Normal subject (J. E.) (from FANKHAUSER, ENOCH and CIBIS, 1961)

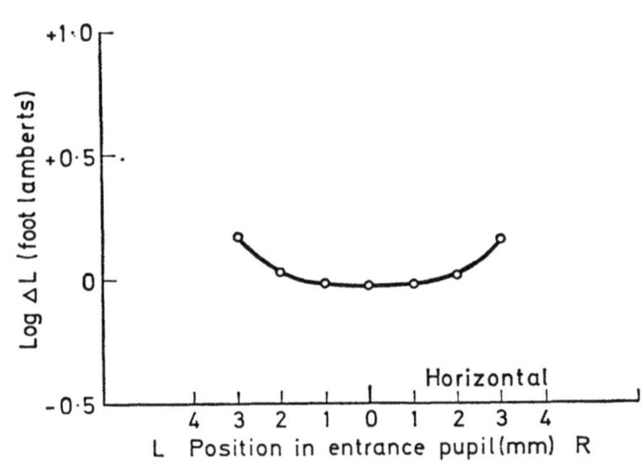

Fig. 4. Case I (C. R.) retinoschisis (prior to photocoagulation) (from FANKHAUSER, ENOCH and CIBIS, 1961)

position of minimum. Since photocoagulation produces stressed in the retina, pulling it transversely, the distortion shown in Fig. 5 is precisely what might be expected to result from such a state of stress, the proximal surface moving sideways, the distal surface, stuck to the choroid, remaining fixed: the cones in consequence shear over and so lead to a displacement of the axis of symmetry of the Stiles-Crawford curve. Putting the matter briefly, the retina is moved, the Stiles-Crawford effect is modified, *ergo*, the effect is in the retina.

The work of DUNNEWOLD provides evidence which is also of pathological origin, but slightly different in character. In one of his clinical cases, of prepapillar toxoplastic inflammation in the right eye, the left eye was normal and showed a normal Stiles-Crawford effect. In the right eye, however, the foveal polar sensitivity curve was flat (Fig. 6) and there was an appearance of fine retinal traction-folds covering the macular region (the macular region in the left eye appeared normal). The association of the shape of the Stiles-Crawford curve with retinal disorientation and normality respectively is again clear evidence of the location of the effect in the retina.

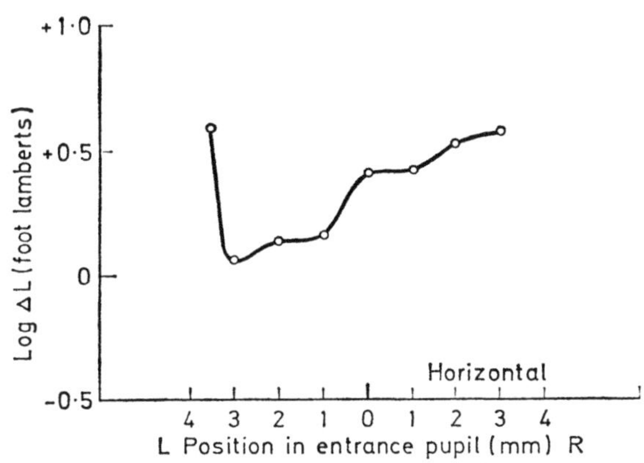

Fig. 5. Case I (C. R.) retinoschisis (post photocoagulation) (from FANKHAUSER, ENOCH and CIBIS, 1961)

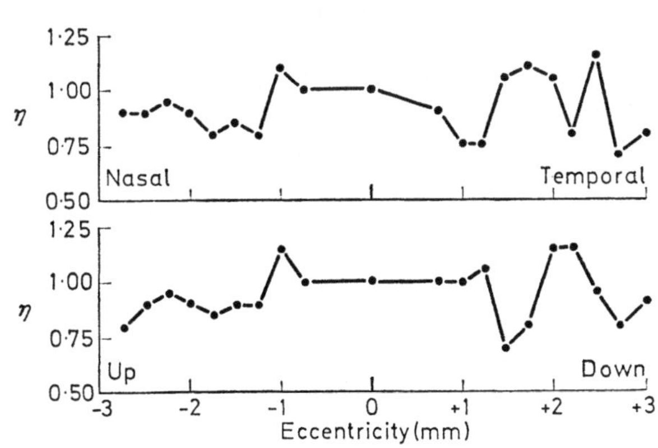

Fig. 6. After DUNNEWOLD (1964): patient C. v. d. W.; the Stiles-Crawford effect in the diseased eye with traction-folds over the macular area

Finally, a very significant experiment of quite a different character was carried out by RIPPS and WEALE (1964). For two observers and two colours of light, they were able to compare the Stiles-Crawford effect determined in the classical subjective manner with a corresponding effect measured in terms of bleaching by the objective technique of retinal reflex photometry (see Volume VII/1, this Handbook). The results are shown in Fig. 7 and the high degree of correlation between subjective and objective measurements again leaves little doubt of the location of the effect in the retina; it is, of course, assumed that the pigments which are bleached are the ones which mediate vision.

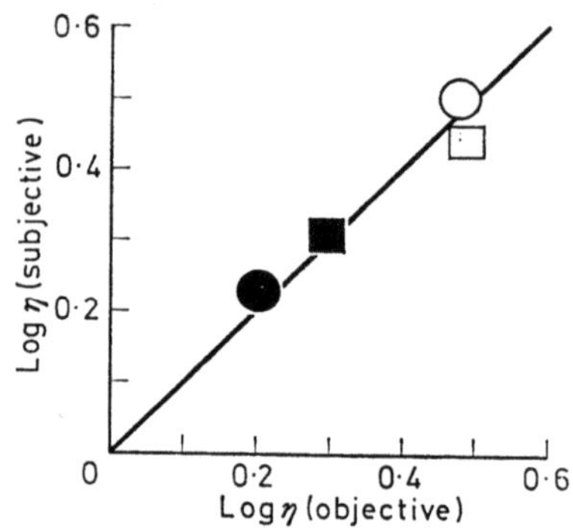

Fig. 7. Correlation between the directional effects of the fovea measured by objective bleaching and by visual, i. e., subjective, comparison for two observes (circles and squares). The black symbols refer to blue, the open symbols to orange light (RIPPS and WEALE, 1964)

Having described the evidence that the Stiles-Crawford effect is located in the retinal cones of the fovea, some further manifestations of the effect must be described. CRAWFORD (1937) investigated it in the parafoveal retina, using a threshold technique. In the fovea this technique gave results identical with those from the brightness matching technique – see Fig. 2 – and so it could be considered a reliable method in general. When applied in the parafovea at a series of background luminance levels from high to zero, it was found that the Stiles-Crawford effect virtually disappeared at zero field luminance, the change being progressive rather than sudden, as shown in Fig. 8. The clear implication is that the effect is shown by the cones, in fovea and in parafovea, but not by the rods which, in the parafovea, take over the function of visual perception at low luminance levels. (Note that all these experiments relate to white light.) The explanation of this difference between rods and cones will be discussed later, but it may be said at once that it still remains something of an enigma.

We now turn to the Stiles-Crawford effect of the second kind (STILES, 1937, 1939). STILES found that when the fixed and traversing beams of the usual apparatus for measuring the effect were fed by independent monochromators, the traversing beam changed in hue relative to the fixed, centrally entering beam. The hue change could be matched by a change in wavelength of one or other of the beams and the change was by no means small. Further investigations are

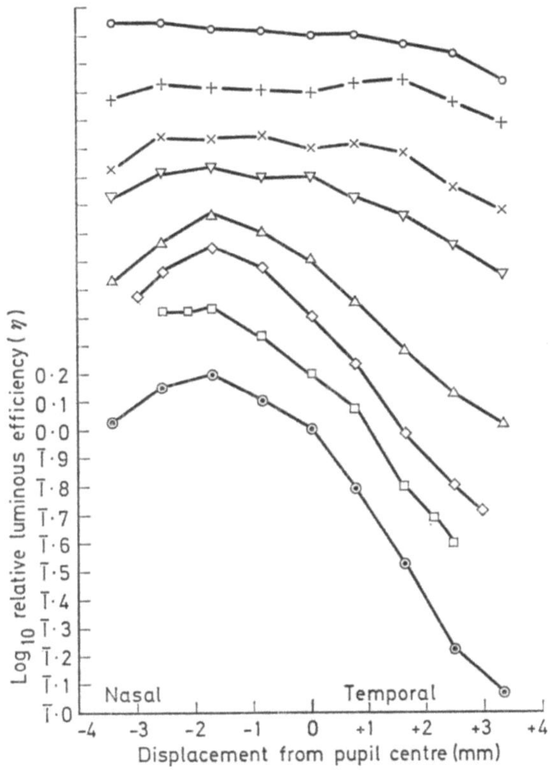

Fig. 8. Polar efficiency curves at various field luminances for retinal area 5° from the fovea (Crawford, 1937). Each curve shifted by 0.2 units for clarity of presentation. ○, $L = 0$, △, $L = 0.096$ c/ft², +, $L = 0.000060$ c/ft², ◇, $L = 1.29$ c/ft², ×, $L = 0.0107$ c/ft², □, $L = 8.9$ c/ft², ▽, $L = 0.0102$ c/ft², ⊙, $L = 22$ c/ft²

reported by Enoch and Stiles (1961) and by Walraven and Bouman (1960). Fig. 9 gives a summary of the various workers' results, also the theoretical curve discussed later.

Now that the location of the Stiles-Crawford effect and manifestations of some of its variables are known, the next logical step is to try to explain it. Historically, of course, the assumption that the effect is retinal and attempts at explanation were made almost immediately after the initial discovery in 1932, but history is seldom logical: if it were, the world would be a dull and unprogressive place. One can come very close to a satisfactory theory of the effect of the first kind by considering the cone outer limb as an isotropic dielectric rod. This line of thought has several variants. The first possibility, explored by Stiles and Crawford (1933), is that the cones, or at least their outer extremities, are embedded in the choroidal pigment: this would produce a screening effect for light incident at an angle to the cone axis, a smaller volume of cone substance would be traversed and stimulated by the light and so the cone would appear to be less sensitive. Unfortunately, there is no anatomical evidence for pigment sheathing of any part of the cones of the human retina and the theory was therefore early discarded.

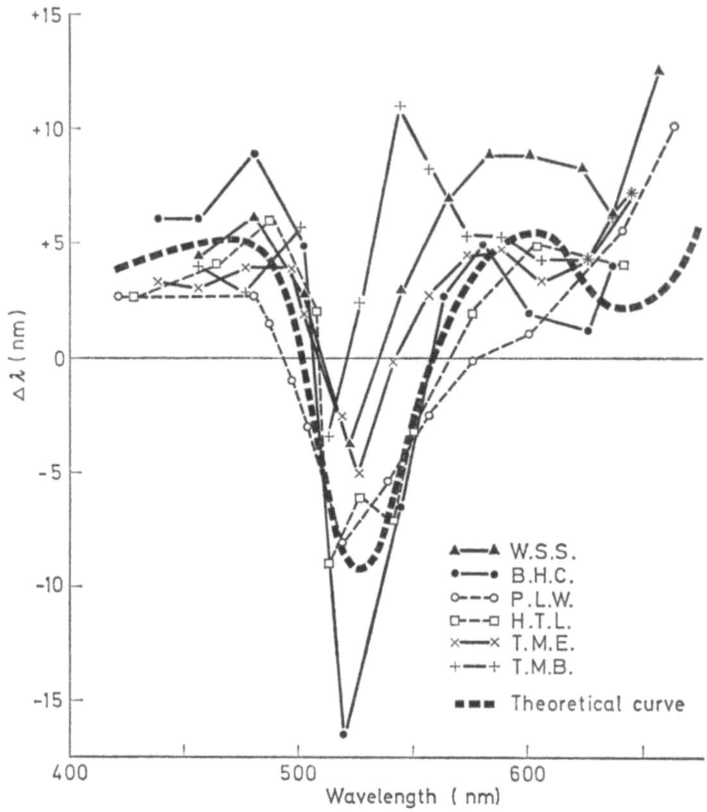

Fig. 9. Stiles-Crawford effect of the second kind: shift of apparent hue as a function of wavelength for six subjects at an excentricity of 3.5 mm (after Vos, 1960)

The next alternative rests upon the fairly well established fact that the substance of the cones has a slightly higher refractive index than the surrounding tissues (Barer, 1957; Sidman, 1957; Toraldo di Francia, 1948a, b; Wright and Nelson, 1936). Even a simple consideration of the problem in terms of rays of light contained by total internal reflection for small angles of incidence, but lost at larger angles, yields reasonable agreement with experiment. In addition, the theory has been tested by an analogue experiment using radio microwaves and a cone model made of polystyrene foam of appropriate size and effective refractive index (Jean and O'Brien, 1949). Agreement between experiment and analogue is quite good for the foveal cones, but no very convincing explanation follows for the striking difference between rods and cones, although it has been suggested that small differences in size and refractive index may be sufficient to make the optical acceptance angle of the rod broad enough for no Stiles-Crawford effect to be apparent within the range of angles of incidence upon the retina allowed by the pupil when fully expanded. This theory of the effect is still not very precise. It has been extended by Walraven and Bouman (1960), however, in an interesting way to explain the Stiles-Crawford effect of the second kind. The escape of light from a cone to an increasing degree with increasing angle of incidence would lead to a decreasing path through the substance of the cone and hence through the contained pigment. Combined with the known phenomenon of change in pigment absorption characteristics with concentration and thickness of solution, a theoretical curve for the effect of the second kind has been worked out by WALRAVEN and BOUMAN and is shown in Fig. 9. The agreement appears good, but unfortunately the concentrations of pigment necessary for this quantitative fit of theory to experiment are at variance with concentrations deduced in other ways. This and other theories are fully discussed by STILES (1962) but, as he says, none are entirely satisfactory and we await further developments before a really acceptable theory can be formulated.

A deal of consideration has been given to the receptor outer limb as a waveguide and to the waveguide modes which should occur in it. Some of these modes have been demonstrated for actual retinal cones by ENOCH (1960, 1961). Their significance in the response to light by visual rods and cones has been discussed theoretically by MYERS (1962) and his deductions are revolutionary as well as interesting. Briefly, he links spectral sensitivity with cone size (diameter), not with a number of different photopigments. So long as a single photopigment is present and has a maximum of absorption somewhere in the central part of the visible spectrum, variation of cone size over a small range will produce cone selectivities which could account for colour discrimination. The Rushton-Weale results from reflexion densitometry would also follow, the apparent presence of erythrolabe, chlorolabe and cyanolabe being the result of one pigment, rhodopsin, in three classes of cone outer limbs, large, medium and small respectively. It is interesting to note that the results reported by IVES (1918) indicating polychromatic rather than trichromatic colour vision find now on Myers' theory a ready explanation. It appears probable that Myers' theory might also explain the Stiles-Crawford effect of the second kind, but a detailed treatment has not yet been worked out. The explanation of the effect of the second kind may be regarded as a critical test of any general theory of the effect of the first kind[1].

Another early theory (WRIGHT and NELSON, 1936; CRAWFORD, 1937) has recently been revised by SAFIR and HYAMS (1969) and leads us to yet another realm of speculation regarding the origin of the Stiles-Crawford effect. WRIGHT and NELSON pointed out that the shape of the polar efficency curve was closely similar to a Gaussian probability distribution curve and put forward the suggestion that this might be due to an appropriate random distribution of orientation of receptors which, individually, have very narrow polar curves of acceptance. An example of the fit of such a curve to experimental points is shown in Fig. 2. SAFIR and HYAMS have produced more evidence of the strictly Gaussian shape of the polar efficiency curve, especially for extreme displacements from the pupil centre. Much more experimental evidence is needed before this idea can be effectively developed, but it is pertinent to reflect that the detailed structure of the outer limb of a cone or rod as

[1] It should be noted in connection with Myers' theory that experimental evidence of three different cone pigments has been obtained for a number of vertebrates, including man, in the well-known work of BROWN and WALD (1964), MARKS, DOBELLE, and MACNICHOL (1964) and MARKS (1965). Whether or not this evidence is at variance with Myers' theory is still a matter for discussion.

revealed by electron microscopy (SJÖSTRAND, 1948, 1953) is of great complexity and precision. The structure suggests, indeed, that the outer limb may be a multiple aerial array rather than a dielectric rod aerial. If appropriate transfer phasing existed between successive elements, the result could be either very highly directional or almost non-directional. Transistor-type amplification between successive elements is also a possibility and would provide a mechanism for transforming the small signal energy which can be visually detected, a few quanta, into the substantial signal which is transmitted to the brain via the optic nerve. A further possibility is that the inter-loop coupling, or the intra-loop circuit, may include a photosensitive element of solid state type: this would directly lead to a time-coded response as the mechanism of spectral differentiation first suggested, rather vaguely, by SMIRNOV and BONGARD (1958). Such a time-coded transmission of signal along the cone would almost certainly be somewhat variable with angle of reception, giving a qualitative explanation of the Stiles-Crawford effect of the second kind. This, perhaps, is as far as speculation should be taken in the present context, but it is plain to see that investigation of the Stiles-Crawford effects and their modi operandi is still a stimulating and profitable approach to the heart of the study of vision.

Finally, a word about the list of references: this is very long and only a fraction has been referred to in this chapter, but it should all be read, or at least glanced at, by anyone desiring to carry out further experiments or devise better theories.

References

AGUILAR, M., PLAZA, A.: Effecto Stiles-Crawford en vision fotopica extra-foveal. Coloquios sobre problemas ópticos de la visión, (Madrid), Union Internationale de Physique pure et appliqué. **1**, 232 (1953).

— — Ann. real. soc. Espan. fis. y quim. **50**, 119 (1954).

— STILES, W. S.: Saturation of the rod mechanism of the retina at high levels of stimulation. Optica Acta **1**, 59—65 (1954).

ALPERN, M., BENSON, D.: Directional sensitivity of the pupillomotor photoreceptors. Amer. J. Optom. **30**, 569—580 (1953).

ARNULF, A.: Influence of the pupillary diameter and the Stiles-Crawford effect on the luminance of images in visual instruments. Comm. Lab. Inst. d'Opt., (Paris) **1**, 23 (1944).

BAHR, G. VON: On the effect of peripheral rays in testing of light sense. Acta Ophthal. (Kbh.) **19**, 114 (1941).

BARANY, E.: The Stiles-Crawford effect in polarised light. Acta Ophthal. (Kbh.) **24**, 93 (1946).

BARER, R.: Refractometry and interferometry of living cells. J. opt. Soc. Amer. **47**, 545—556 (1957).

BEST, F.: The decrease in brightness when light enters through the peripheral area of the pupil. Z. Ophthal. Opt. **31**, 65 (1943).

BOCCHINO, G.: Studio della variazione della luminosità di un cannocchiale al variare della pupilla d'uscita. Ottica **1**, 136—142 (1936).

— Relazione tra l'ingrandimento e la luminosità di un cannocchiale. Ottica **1**, 213—224 (1936).

— Influenza delle pupille di entrata e di uscita sulla luminosità delle immagini dei cannocchiali. Ottica **2**, 39—44 (1937).

BRINDLEY, G.: The effects on colour vision of adaptation to very bright lights. J. Physiol. (Lond.) **122**, 332—350 (1953).

— RUSHTON, W. A. H.: The colour of monochromatic light when passed into the human retina from behind. J. Physiol. (Lond.) **147**, 204—208 (1959).

BRINK, G. VAN DEN: Measurements of the geometrical aberrations of the eye. Vision Res. **2**, 233—244 (1962).

Brown, P. K., Wald, G.: Visual pigments in single rods and cones of the human retina. Science **144**, 45—51 (1964).

Brücke, E.: Über die physiologische Bedeutung der stabförmigen Körper und der Zwillingszapfen in den Augen der Wirbeltiere. Arch. Anat. Physiol. **11**, 444—451 (1843).

Burns, J. R.: The Stiles-Crawford effect: a modified clinical instrument and some preliminary applications. B. Sc. Dissertation, University of Edinburgh 1967.

— The Stiles-Crawford effect and the yellow-blue equation. Comm. Vis. Lab., Psychol. Dept., University of Edinburgh 1968.

Campbell, F. W.: A retinal acuity direction effect. J. Physiol. (Lond.) **144**, 25P—26P (1958).

— Effect of oblique incidence of light on the spatial resolving power of the human retina. J. opt. Soc. Amer. **50**, 515 (1960).

— Gregory, A. H.: The spatial resolving power of the human retina with oblique incidence. J. opt. Soc. Amer. **50**, 831 (1960).

Collier, L. J., Taylor, W. G. A.: A telephotometer employing the Maxwellian view principle and its use in measuring atmospheric transmission. J. sci. Instrum. **15**, 5—17 (1938).

Commoner, B.: On the interpretation of the absorption of ultra-violet light by cellular nucleic acids. Science **110**, 31—40 (1949).

— Lipkin, D.: The application of the Beer-Lambert law to optically anisotropic systems. Science **110**, 41—43 (1949).

Craik, K. W. J.: Transmission of light by the eye media. J. Physiol. (Lond.) **98**, 179—184 (1940).

Crawford, B. H.: The luminous efficiency of light entering the eye pupil at different points and its relation to brightness threshold measurements. Proc. roy. Soc. (Lond.) B **124**, 81—96 (1937).

Denton, E. J.: On the orientation of molecules in the visual rods of *Salamandra maculosa*. J. Physiol. (Lond.) **124**, 17P—18P (1954).

— The contributions of the orientated photosensitive and other molecules to the absorption of whole retina. Proc. roy. Soc. (Lond.) B **150**, 78—94 (1959).

Donner, K. O., Rushton, W. A. H.: The Stiles-Crawford effect in the frog's retina. J. Physiol. (Lond.) **132**, 37P (1956).

— — Rod-cone interaction in the frog's retina analysed by the Stiles-Crawford effect and by dark adaptation. J. Physiol. (Lond.) **149**, 303—317 (1959).

Dunnewold, C. J. W.: On the Campbell and Stiles-Crawford effects and their clinical importance. Soesterberg: Institute for Perception. RVO-TNO 1964.

Dziobek, W.: Der Stiles-Crawford-Effekt und seine Bedeutung für die Photometrie. Licht **4**, 150—152 (1934).

Enoch, J. M.: Amblyopia and the Stiles-Crawford effect. Amer. J. Optom. **34**, 298—309 (1957).

— Summated response of the retina to light entering different parts of the pupil. J. opt. Soc. Amer. **48**, 392—405 (1958).

— Further studies on the relationship between amblyopia and the Stiles-Crawford effect. Amer. J. Optom. **36**, 111—128 (1959).

— Receptor amblyopia. Amer. J. Ophthal. **48**, 262—274 (1959).

— Optical interaction effects in models of parts of the visual receptors. Arch. Ophthal. **63**, 548—558 (1960a).

— Response of a model retinal receptor as a function of wavelength. J. opt. Soc. Amer. **50**, 315—320 (1960b).

— Waveguide modes in retinal receptors. Rep. Dept. Ophthal., Washington School of Medicine and Oscar Johnson Inst., St. Louis, Mo., U.S.A. (1961).

— Waveguide modes in retinal receptors. Science **133**, 1353—1354 (1961).

— Nature of the transmission of energy in the retinal receptors. J. opt. Soc. Amer. **51**, 1122—1126 (1961).

— Visualisation of waveguide modes in retinal receptors. Amer. J. Ophthal. **51**, 1107—1118 (1961).

— Optical properties of the retinal receptors. J. opt. Soc. Amer. **53**, 71—85 (1963).

— Physical properties of the retinal receptors and response of the retinal receptors. Psychol. Bull. **61**, 242—251 (1964).

Enoch, J. M.: An approach towards the study of retinal receptor optics. Amer. J. Optom. **42**, 63—70 (1965).
— The retina as a fiber optics bundle. In: Fiber Optics, Principles and Applications. Kapany, N. S., (Ed.) New York: Academic Press 1967.
— Fry, G. A.: Characteristics of a model retinal receptor studied at microwave frequencies. J. opt. Soc. Amer. **48**, 899—911 (1958).
— Stiles, W. S.: The colour change of monochromatic light with retinal angle of incidence. Optica Acta **8**, 329—358 (1961).
Ercoles, A. M., Ronchi, L., Toraldo di Francia, G.: The relation between pupil efficiencies for small and extended pupils of entry. Optica Acta **3**, 84—89 (1956).
Fankhauser, F., Enoch, J. M.: The effects of blur upon perimetric thresholds. Arch. Ophthal. **68**, 240—251 (1962).
— — Cibis, P.: Receptor orientation in retinal pathology. Amer. J. Ophthal. **52**, 767—783 (1961).
Fine, B. S.: Limiting membranes of the sensory retina and pigment epithelium. Arch. Ophthal. **66**, 846—860 (1961).
Fiorentini, A.: Sulla non additivita degli stimoli coerenti provenienti da punti diversi della pupilla. Atti Fond. G. Ronchi **7**, 294 (1952).
— Toraldo di Francia, G.: La vision des franges d'interférence formées directement sur la rétine. Coloquio sobre problemas ópticos de la visión, (Madrid) Union Internationale de Physique pure et appliqué **2**, 72—76 (1953).
Flamant, F.: Contribution à l'étude du phénomène Stiles-Crawford. Comm. Lab. Inst. d'Opt. (Paris) **2**, 47 (1946).
— Contribution à l'étude du phénomène Stiles-Crawford. Rev. Opt. **28**, 44 (1949).
— Contribution à l'étude de l'effet Stiles-Crawford. Coloquio sobre problemas ópticos de la visión, (Madrid) Union Internationale de Physique pure et appliqué. **2**, 184 (1953).
— Etude de la répartition de lumière dans l'image d'une fente. Rev. Opt. **34**, 433—459 (1955).
— Stiles, W. S.: The directional and spectral sensitivities of the retinal rods to adapting fields of different wavelengths. J. Physiol. (Lond.) **107**, 187—202 (1948).
Fuortes, M., Gunkel, R., Rushton, W. A. H.: Increment thresholds in a subject deficient in cone vision. J. Physiol. (Lond.) **156**, 179—192 (1961).
Goldmann, H.: Stiles-Crawford Effekt. Ophthalmologica **103**, 225 (1942).
Goodeve, C. F.: Relative luminosity in the extreme red. Proc. roy. Soc. (Lond.) A **155**, 664—683 (1936).
Hansen, G.: Zur Kenntnis des physiologischen Apertur-Farbeffektes (Stiles-Crawford-Effekt zweiter Art). Naturwissenschaften **35/36**, 416 (1943).
— The influence of the Stiles-Crawford effect on measurements with the Pulfrich photometer. J. opt. Soc. Amer. **36**, 321—325 (1946).
— Abhängigkeit des Farb-Aperturеffektes (Stiles-Crawford-Effekt zweiter Art) von der Adaptation. Coloquio sobre problemas ópticos de la visión, (Madrid) Union Internationale de Physique pure etappliqué **2**, 192 (1953).
Ives, H. E.: The resolution of mixed colours by differential visual diffusivity. Phil. Mag. **35**, 413—421 (1918).
Jean, J. N., O'Brien, B.: Microwave test of a theory of the Stiles-Crawford effect. J. opt. Soc. Amer. (Abstr.) **39**, 1057 (1949).
Kapany, N. S.: Appendix. In: Concepts of Classical Optics. Strong, J.: San Francisco: Freeman 1958.
— Fibre optics. V. Light leakage due to frustrated total reflection. J. opt. Soc. Amer. **49**, 770—778 (1959).
— Fibre optics. VI. Image quality and optical insulation. J. opt. Soc. Amer. **49**, 779—787 (1959).
— Burke, J. J.: Fiber optics. IX. Waveguide effects. J. opt. Soc. Amer. **51**, 1067—1078 (1961).
— — Light conduction along absorbing fiber by evanescent boundary wave. J. opt. Soc. Amer. (Abstr.) **51**, 1474 (1961).

le Grand, Y.: Recherches sur la diffusion de la lumière dans l'oeil humain. Rev. Opt. **16**, 241—257 (1937).
— Recherches sur l'effet Stiles-Crawford. Rev. Opt. **27**, 759 (1948).
Loever-Sieger, D. H.: Amblyopie, een studie over de kenmerken en de behandeling. Thesis, Amsterdam G.U. (1962).
Lythgoe, R. J.: The measurement of visual acuity. Spec. Rep. Ser., No. 173. Med. Res. Council. London: H. M. Stationery Office 1932.
Marks, W. B.: Visual pigments of single goldfish cones. J. Physiol. (Lond.) **178**, 14—32 (1965).
— Dobelle, W. H., MacNichol, E. F.: Visual pigments of single primate cones. Science **143**, 1181—1183 (1964).
Martinelli, L.: Sulla luminosità delle immagini viste con un cannochiale. Ottica **2**, 45—53 (1937).
Metcalf, H.: Stiles-Crawford apodization. J. opt. Soc. Amer. **55**, 72—74 (1965).
Miller, N. D.: The changes in the Stiles-Crawford effect with high luminance adapting fields. Amer. J. Optom. **41**, 599—608 (1964).
Moon, P., Spencer, D. E.: On the Stiles-Crawford effect. J. opt. Soc. Amer. **34**, 319—329 (1944).
— — The transient Stilcs-Crawford effect. J. opt. Soc. Amer. **34**, 744—750 (1944).
Myers, O.: Spectral sensitivity of visual receptor cells. Nature (Lond.) **193**, 449—451 (1962).
O'Brien, B.: A theory of the Stiles-Crawford effect. J. opt. Soc. Amer. **36**, 506—509 (1946).
— The Stiles and Crawford effect in polarised light. J. opt. Soc. Amer. **37**, 275—278 (1947).
— Comment on the note entitled "Retinal cones as dielectric antennas". J. opt. Soc. Amer. **39**, 324 (1949).
— Local variation of the Stiles-Crawford effect. J. opt. Soc. Amer. (Abstr.) **40**, 796 (1950).
— Vision and resolution in the central retina. J. opt. Soc. Amer. **41**, 882—894 (1951).
Østerberg, G.: Topography of the layer of rods and cones in the human retina. Acta Ophthal. **13**, Suppl. 6, 1—103 (1935).
Osterberg, F., Snitzer, E., Polanyi, M., Hilberg, R.: Optical waveguide modes in small glass fibers. II. Experimental (see also Snitzer and Hicks). J. opt. Soc. Amer. (Abstr.) **49**, 1128 (1959).
Platt, J. R.: On the Wright-Nelson explanation of the Stiles-Crawford effect. J. opt. Soc. Amer. **37**, 669—670 (1947).
— Further remarks on the Stiles-Crawford effect. J. opt. Soc. Amer. **39**, 614 (1949).
Pugh, M.: Visual distortions in amblyopia. Brit. J. Ophthal. **42**, 449—460 (1958).
Raab, O.: Troland und Stiles-Crawford-Effekt. Farbe **3**, 73 (1957).
Reeves, P.: The response of the average pupil to various intensities of light. J. opt. Soc. Amer. **4**, 35—43 (1920).
Ripps, H., Weale, R. A.: Photolabile changes and the directional sensitivity of the human fovea. J. Physiol. (Lond.) **173**, 57—64 (1964).
— — Directional properties of cone pigments. J. opt. Soc. Amer. **55**, 205—206 (1965).
Ronchi, L.: On the influence of mydriatics and miotics on visual functions. Atti Fond. G. Ronchi **10**, 285 (1955).
— Influence d'un mydriatique sur l'effet Stiles-Crawford. Optica Acta **2**, 47—49 (1955).
— Toraldo di Francia, G.: Ricerche sulla diretivita dei ricettori retinici. Atti Fond. G. Ronchi **7**, 197—203 (1952).
— — Ulteriori misure sulla diffusione direzionale della retina. Atti Fond. G. Ronchi **8**, 109—113 (1953).
Rushton, W. A. H.: Physical measurement of cone pigment in the living human eye. Nature (Lond.) **179**, 571—573 (1957).
Safir, A., Hyams, L.: Distribution of cone orientations as an explanation of the Stiles-Crawford effect. J. opt. Soc. Amer. **59**, 757—765 (1969).
Said, F. S., Weale, R. A.: The variation with age of the spectral transmissivity of the living human crystalline lens. Gerontologia **3**, 213—231 (1959).
Schroeder, A.: Theory on the receptor mechanism in color vision. J. opt. Soc. Amer. **50**, 945—949 (1960).
Sidman, R. L.: The structure and concentration of solids in photoreceptor cells studied by refractometry and interference microscopy. J. Biophys. Biochem. Cytol. **3**, 15—30 (1957).
— Histochemical studies on photoreceptor cells. N. Y. Acad. Sci. **74**, 182—195 (1958).

Sjöstrand, F. S.: The ultrastructure of the retinal rods of the guinea pig eye. J. appl. Phys. **19**, 1188 (1948).

— The ultrastructure of the outer segments of rods and cones of the eye as revealed by electron microscopy. J. cell. comp. Physiol. **42**, 15—44 (1953).

Sloan, L. L.: Size of pupil as a variable factor in measurements of the threshold. An experimental study of the Stiles-Crawford phenomenon. J. opt. Soc. Amer. **30**, (Abstr.) 271 (1940).

— Size of pupil as a variable factor in the determination of the light minimum. Arch. Ophthal. **24**, 258—275 (1940).

Smirnov, M. S., Bongard, M. M.: Hypothesis concerning the mechanism of photoreception in the retina (analogy between retinal receptors and semiconductor photocells). (In Russian.) Biophysica **4**, 181—186 (1959).

Snitzer, E.: Cylindrical dielectric waveguide modes. J. opt. Soc. Amer. **51**, 491—498 (1961).

— Glass fibers acting as receiving dielectric endfire antennas in the visible spectrum. J. opt. Soc. Amer. (Abstr.) **51**, 1463 (1961).

— Hicks, J.: Optical waveguide modes in small glass fibers. I. Theoretical. J. opt. Soc. Amer. (Abstr.) **49**, 1128 (1959).

— Osterberg, H.: Observed dielectric waveguide modes in the visible spectrum. J. opt. Soc. Amer. **51**, 499—501 (1961).

— Polanyi, M.: Possible waveguide mode effects in retinal receptors. J. opt. Soc. Amer. (Abstr.) **51**, 476 (1961).

Snyder, A. W.: Excitation of waveguide modes in retinal receptors. J. opt. Soc. Amer. **56**, 705—706 (1966).

Spring, K. H., Stiles, W. S.: Variation of pupil size with change in the angle at which the light stimulus strikes the retina. Brit. J. Ophthal. **32**, 340—346 (1948).

Stanworth, A., Naylor, E. J.: Haidinger's brushes and the retinal receptors with a note on the Stiles-Crawford effect. Brit. J. Ophthal. **34**, 282—291 (1950).

Stenius, S.: Dark adaptation and the platinum chloride method of staining visual purple. Acta physiol. scand. **1**, 380—382 (1941).

Stiles, W. S.: The luminous efficiency of monochromatic rays entering the eye pupil at different points and a new colour effect. Proc. roy. Soc. (Lond.) B **123**, 90—118 (1937).

— The directional sensitivity of the retina and the spectral sensitivities of the rods and cones. Proc. roy. Soc. (Lond.) B **127**, 64—105 (1939a).

— The directional sensitivity of the retina. Science Progress **33**, 676—689 (1939b).

— The directional sensitivity of the retina. Ann. roy. Coll. Surgeons **30**, 73—101 (1962).

— Crawford, B. H.: The luminous efficiency of rays entering the eye pupil at different points. Proc. roy. Soc. (Lond.) B **112**, 428—450 (1933).

— — Luminous efficiency of rays entering the eye pupil at different points. Nature (Lond.) **139**, 246 (1937).

Tansley, K., Johnson, B. K.: The cones of the grass snake's eye. Nature (Lond.) **178**, 1285—1286 (1956).

Toraldo di Francia, G.: Ricettori retinici e microonde. Atti Fond. G. Ronchi **3**, 137—144 (1948).

— Per una teoria dell'effetto Stiles-Crawford. Nuovo Cimento **5**, 589—590 (1948).

— Retinal cones as dielectric antennas. J. opt. Soc. Amer. (Letter) **39**, 324 (1949).

— The radiation pattern of retinal receptors. Proc. phys. Soc. (Lond.) B, **62**, 461—462 (1949).

— Ronchi, L.: Directional scattering of light by the human retina. J. opt. Soc. Amer. **42**, 782—783 (1952).

— — Scattering of light by the retina. Coloquio sobre problemas ópticos de la visión, (Madrid) Union Internationale de Physique pure et appliqué. **2**, 138—142 (1953).

— Sbrolli, W.: Sulla legge integrale dell'effetto Stiles-Crawford. Atti Fond. G. Ronchi **2**, 100—104 (1947).

Vos, J. J.: A new apparatus to measure the Stiles-Crawford effect all over the pupil. Rep. No. IZF1959-14 and annex. Soesterberg: Institute for Perception. RVO-TNO 1960.

— Some new aspects of colour stereoscopy. J. opt. Soc. Amer. **50**, 785—790 (1960).

— 25 years of the Stiles-Crawford effect. Advan. Ophthal. **10**, 32—48 (1960).

Vos, J. J.: On the mechanisms of glare (Thesis, Univ. Utrecht). Rep. No. IZF 1963-16. Soesterberg: Institute for Perception. RVO-TNO 1963.
— Huigen, A.: A clinical Stiles-Crawford apparatus. Amer. J. Optom. **39**, 68—76 (1962).
— Walraven, P. L.: The Stiles-Crawford effect, a survey. Pub. dell'Ist. Naz. di Ottica, Serie IV, No. 380, Firenze 1962.
de Vries, H., Kuiper, J. W.: Optics of the insect eye. Ann. N. Y. Acad. Sci. **74**, 196—203 (1958).
Walraven, P. L.: On the mechanisms of colour vision. (Thesis, Univ. Utrecht) Rep. No. IZF 1962-16. Soesterberg: Institute for Perception. RVO-TNO 1962.
— Recovery from the increase of the Stiles-Crawford effect after bleaching. Nature (Lond.) **210**, 311—312 (1966).
— Bouman, M. A.: Relation between directional sensitivity and spectral response curves in human cone vision. J. opt. Soc. Amer. **50**, 780—784 (1960).
— Leebeek, H. J.: Handflickerphotometer. Rev. Sci. Instrum. **29**, 320—321 (1958).
— — The chromatic Stiles-Crawford effect of anomalous trichromats. Rep. No. IZF 1962-5. Soesterberg: Institute for Perception. RVO-TNO 1962.
— — The chromatic Stiles-Crawford effect of anomalous trichromats. J. opt. Soc. Amer. **52**, 836—837 (1962).
— Vos, J. J., Dunnewold, J. W.: The Stiles-Crawford effect as an instrument of research. Studies in Perception. pp. 145—158. Soesterberg: Institute for Perception. RVO-TNO 1966.
Weale, R. A.: Note on the photometric significance of the human crystalline lens. Vision Res. **1**, 183—191 (1961).
White, W. J.: Experimental studies of the effects of accelerative stress on visual performance. Diss. Ohio State Univ., Columbus, Ohio 1958.
— Jarve, W. R.: The effects of gravitional stress upon visual acuity. WADC Tech. Rep. No. 56-247 (Wright-Patterson Air Force Base, Ohio) (1956).
Wolken, J. J.: Studies of photoreceptor structures. Ann. N. Y. Acad. Sci. **74**, 164—181 (1958).
Wright, W. D., Nelson, J. H.: The relation between the apparent intensity of a beam of light and the angle at which the beam strikes the retina. Proc. phys. Soc. (Lond.) **48**, 401—405 (1936).
Zimmerman, L. E.: Applications of histochemical methods for the demonstration of acid mucopolysaccharides to ophthalmic pathology. Trans. Amer. Acad. Ophthal. Otolaryngol. **62**, 697—703 (1958).
Zoli, M. T.: Influenza dell'effetto Stiles-Crawford sulla luminosità dea cannochiali. Atti Fond. G. Ronchi **5**, 245—250 (1950).

Chapter 19

Color Discrimination Data

By

M. A. Bouman, Utrecht and P. L. Walraven, Soesterberg (Netherlands)

With 27 Figures

Contents

I. Introduction

The sense of sight provides us with information on how the radiance of the environment is distributed in time and space. Such information pertains to both the energy and the spectral distribution of the radiance. Researchers in the field of color vision generally assume that, as attributes of visual perception, brightness and color stem from mechanisms which respond specifically to the physical variables of energy and spectral distribution of the stimulus. This assumption has led to the hypothesis that the eye's capability of distinguishing differences in energy level of a stimulus relies only on the properties of a brightness mechanism. The color mechanisms are then supposed to be separately tested by changing the spectral energy distribution of a stimulus while its brightness is kept constant by weighting the energy of any wavelength according to a spectral sensitivity curve of the luminosity channel of the visual system. The requirement that such a curve be independently determined, however, cannot be met. The basic problem is not satisfactorily solved by canonization of procedures for such a determination by flicker (or step-by-step) photometry. Studies of color discrimination are often based on the rather reckless assumption that flicker photometry is a methodological panacea. In each of them the author has compromised in some way with this essential methodological difficulty. An extensive discussion on this point was presented recently by GUTH *et al.* (1969). Nevertheless, much useful information has become available from this line of research, and representative studies will be reviewed briefly below. However, for the preservation of an appropriate open-mindedness in the scientist, and as a prelude to recent new views mentioned in later sections, we shall dwell here briefly upon the retina's duplicity and its implications for our topic.

The two essential pillars of evidence for this duplicity are first, the two phases in the retina's time-dependent sensitivity during dark adaptation, and second, the incidence of chromatic vision at high luminances with a light-adapted eye and the incidence of achromatic vision at low luminances with the dark-adapted eye. The rigorous attribution of visual processes during light-adapted periods to cone activity and those during dark-adapted periods to the activity of rods is the keystone of the generally accepted hypothesis regarding processing of brightness and color signals in the retina. Such attribution obviates explanations as to how one group of receptors can produce such essentially different perceptions as chromatic and achromatic ones when only the energy of the stimulus is changed.

The question of the rods' contribution to perception at higher luminances is then usually waved aside by vaguely specified inhibitory actions of the cones on the rods' discrimination function. Furthermore, changes of apparent color with luminance at high illumination levels, as demonstrated in the Bezold-Brücke phenomenon, are then supposed to be due to second-order saturation effects (WALRAVEN, 1961). However, at low luminances the rod-free fovea produces achromatic perceptions which are exactly those arising from peripheral rod stimulation. Although one can say that a more intensive stimulus is needed for identification than for mere detection, such a statement explains next to nothing and does not help an understanding of the mechanistic basis of the difference. We may also say that cones as well as rods can participate in achromatic perception and that rods might positively contribute to the eye's performance not only at scotopic, but also at photopic luminance levels.

In this introduction we have tried to make the reader aware of some problems connected with measurements of "pure" color discrimination functions. To have some order in the treatment of these functions, this chapter is subdivided into a number of sections; first, color discrimination, measured in the usual way by comparison of two fields of different color will be discussed. The recent developments concerning modulation transfer functions are included. A separate section will deal with a special technique, namely, color naming. The chapter is concluded by a short survey of the description of color discrimination by the so-called line element.

II. Color Discrimination

A. General Properties

Most investigations of just noticeable color differences employ a bipartite field as shown in Fig. 1.

A difference in chromaticness can be adjusted by the observer and set at a level such that the difference is just perceptible. A prerequisite for a proper measurement is that there be no brightness difference between the fields. As mentioned in the introduction this is one of the difficulties encountered in this kind of experiment.

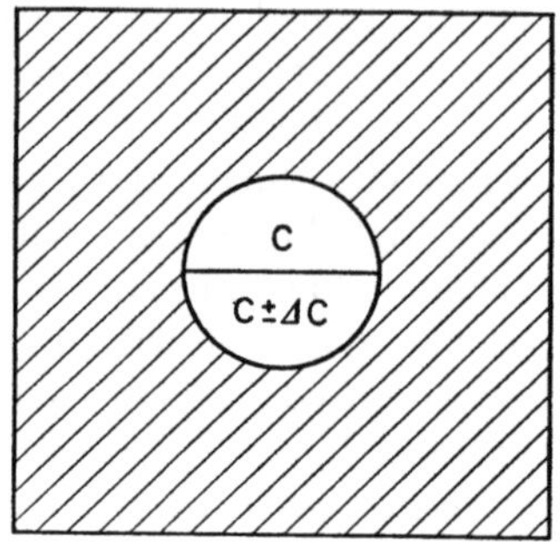

Fig. 1. A bipartite field often used in color discrimination experiments. Hatched area indicates surrounding field

Most data on color discrimination are obtained with 2° fields, the CIE standard field size, assuming the foveal 2° area as rod-free. Examples of data for normal subjects are shown in Fig. 2 in the form of a wavelength discrimination curve, and in Fig. 3 in the form of discrimination ellipses in the color diagram.

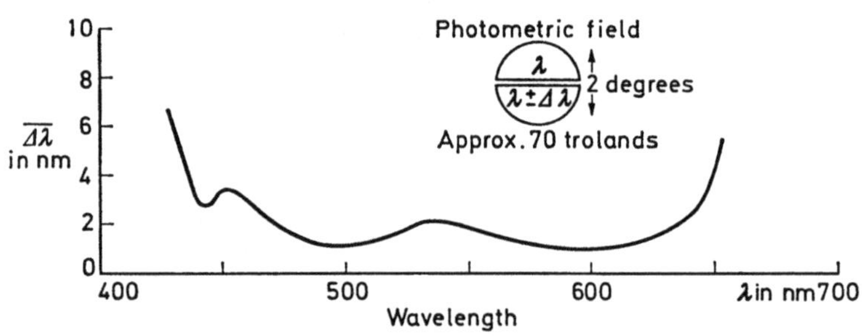

Fig. 2. Wavelength discrimination curve based on observations made by Wright and Pitt (1934)

These data were obtained for relatively high luminance levels. Details will be discussed in the following sections. Essential characteristics of wavelength discrimination curves are two main minima, and a minor third in the short-wave part of the spectrum. A typical example is the curve shown in Fig. 2, as measured by Wright and Pitt (1934). Investigations in which the whole area of the chromaticity chart has been tested are those by MacAdam (1942) and Wright (1943), resp., shown in Figs. 3 and 4. Along the 440–645 nm line additional data in the purple region of the chromaticity diagram are reported by Connors and Siegel (1964). The MacAdam ellipses in the chromaticity diagram are based on standard deviations of color matches. The Wright-Pitt curve and the MacAdam ellipses are generally considered as representative for color discrimination. However, a number of circumstances influence the size of the just noticeable difference. The extensive literature on color discrimination shows this clearly.

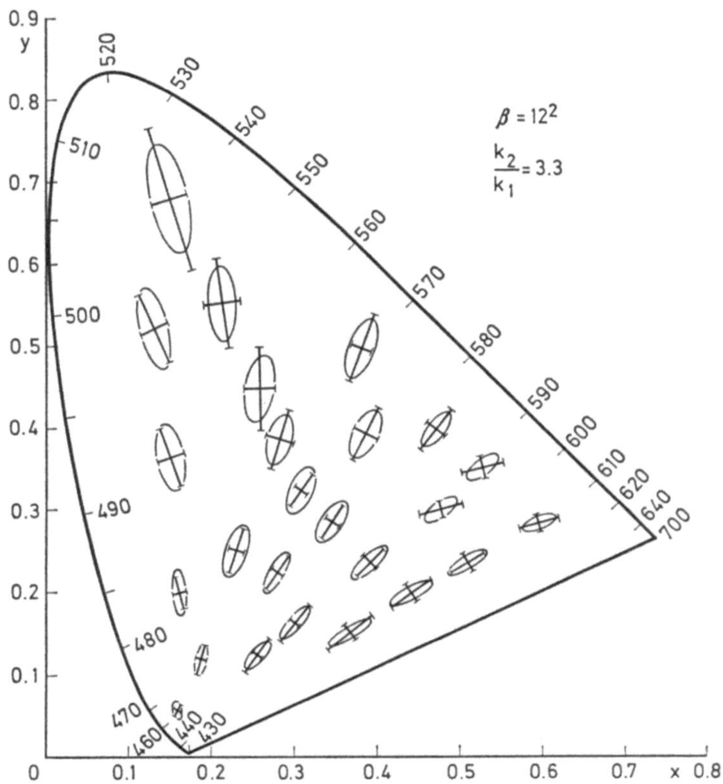

Fig. 3. The CIE color-mixture diagram with the experimental and theoretical MacAdam ellipses (MacAdam, 1942). The axes drawn belong to the experimental ellipses, the solid ellipses are theoretical and conform to Eqs. 8 and 9 (Section 4). The ellipses are 10 × the size of the threshold ellipses

In order to describe the many experimental data systematically, this section is subdivided according to two experimental conditions: field size and luminance. Other experimental conditions are, for example, the technique of observation, viz., fixation or scanning, the surround of the test field, etc. For insight into the physiological mechanisms, however, field size and luminance are more important parameters, and the other conditions will be considered at appropriate places in the text. In the subsections reference will also be made to the properties of color defective observers. This chapter is not meant to describe the nervous mechanisms for color discrimination which extract the requisite information from the receptors. A separate chapter on electrophysiology will deal with this. (This Handbook, volume VII/3.) However one single reference might be useful. This concerns the study by DeValois (1965) who did electrophysiological work on the lateral geniculate nucleus of the macaque and recorded also some psychophysical data on wavelength discrimination in these primates. DeValois found by behavioral studies that the wavelength discrimination function of the macaque

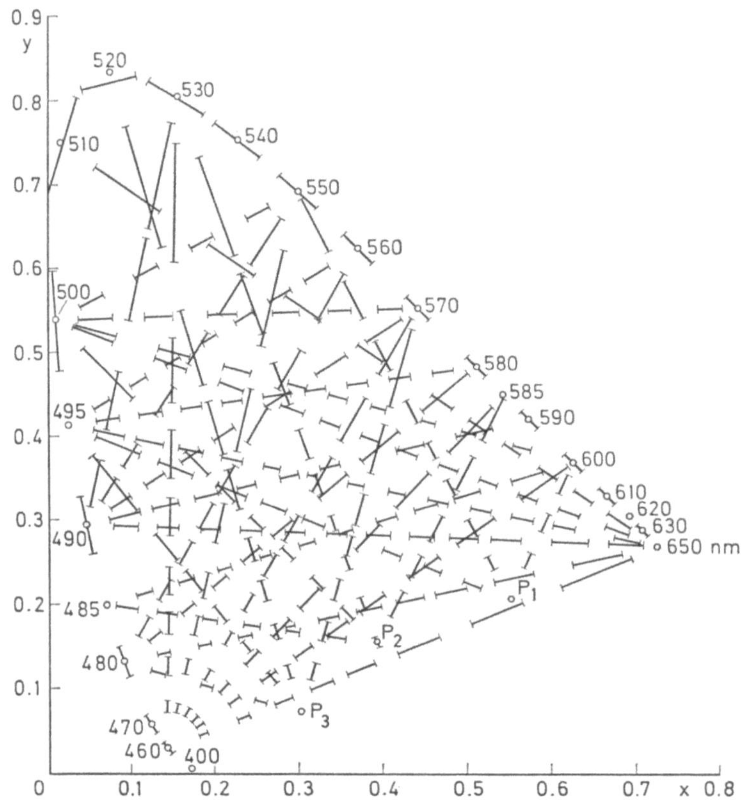

Fig. 4. Subjectively equal color steps plotted in the CIE chromaticity chart. The lines represent a color difference about three times greater than the just noticeable difference for a 2° field (Wright, 1946)

monkeys is very similar that of the human. By recording the changes in firing rate of the opponent cell types (red-green and yellow-blue cells) one is able to relate a high change in firing rate with good discrimination. It seems from this comparison that the short wavelength discrimination is governed in particular by the yellow-blue cells and the long wavelength discrimination by the red-green cells. One recognizes this also in the next sections in the theoretical analysis of color discrimination data.

B. Just Noticeable Color Differences as a Function of Field Size

Typical examples of measurements of wavelength discrimination as a function of field size are those by McCree (1960). Fig. 5 illustrates this dependence.

The observations were made on the Wright colorimeter (WRIGHT, 1946). They were begun with a divided field in which the two halves had been set to the same wavelength. The observer then altered the wavelength of the lower half a little, adjusted its brightness to match that of the upper half, and looked for any possible difference in color, scanning the field all the time in order to avoid any fixation effects. No attempt was made to keep the field within the central foveal part of the retina.

The adjustable wavelength was changed in steps until there was a definite difference in color, and then moved back until this difference just disappeared. Readings were taken on both sides of the fixed wavelength and averaged. The data obtained by McCREE are plotted in this graph on a logarithmic scale. This

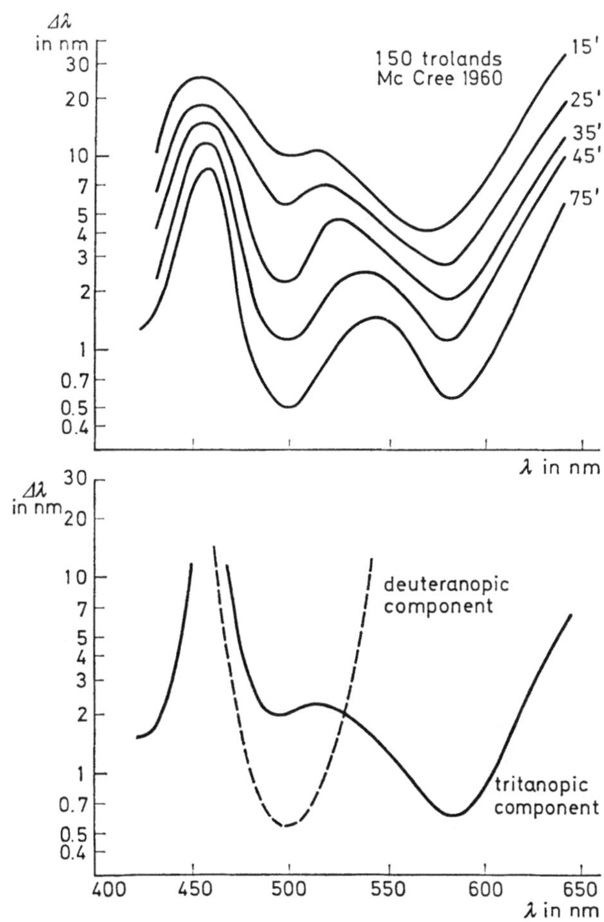

Fig. 5. The upper graph shows discrimination curves measured by McCREE (1960) at high luminance with different field sizes. Experimental points are not plotted in order to avoid confusion in reading the graph. The lower graph shows the two components into which these curves can be split. The effect of so-called small-field tritanopia is due to a decrease of the influence of the deuteranopic component with decreasing field size, according to the analysis by WALRAVEN and BOUMAN (1966)

scale is used to show that there is a change in shape of the curves in addition to deterioration of $\Delta\lambda$ with reduction in angular subtense; a non-proportional variation is hard to recognize on a linear scale. The luminance of the test field was 150 trolands. As the field size decreases, a tendency toward tritanopic wavelength discrimination appears. This was confirmed by Ruddock (1966) who found that at 490 nm $\Delta\lambda$ showed a sharper increase with decreasing field size

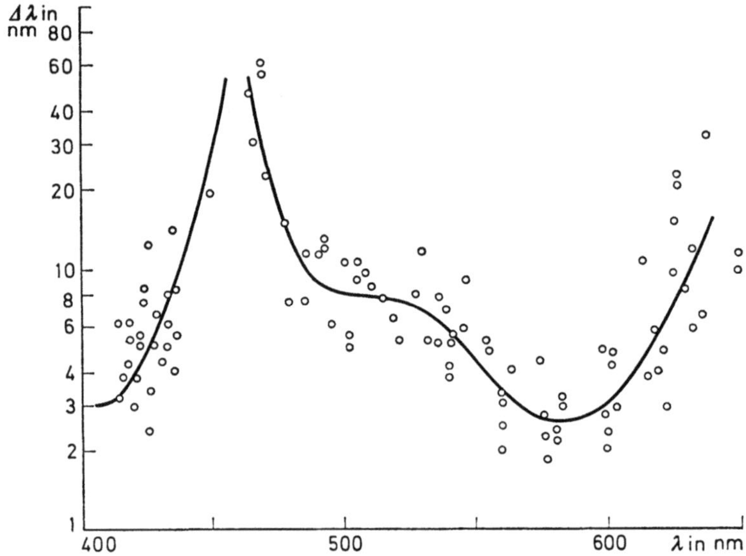

Fig. 6. Wavelength discrimination in tritanopia. Measured points according to Wright (1952) and Fischer *et al.* (1951)

than at 590 nm. In order to make this comparison, wavelength discrimination in tritanopia is shown in Fig. 6. The points in this graph include the measurements of a number of tritanopes from different studies (Fischer *et al.*, 1951; Wright, 1952).

With a small field, wavelength discrimination seems to have the properties one has in tritanopia. This is usually called small-field tritanopia. However, McCree points out that complete tritanopia, that is, dichromatic vision, did not occur, but color vision remained trichromatic. It is therefore better to speak of a small-field tritan effect. This small-field tritan effect is also apparent in measures obtained at a lower luminance. There is, moreover, a remarkable difference between the shapes of the curves at high and at low luminance. Fig. 7 gives the data at a luminance of 0.85 troland. One sees that the minimum in the blue-green region of the spectrum is located at 470 nm rather than at 500 nm. Again, however, with decreasing field size discrimination in the blue-green region deteriorates faster than in the yellow-red region. Again the small-field tritan effect with decreasing field size exists.

Recognizing this fact, one can analyze the discrimination into two components (see Fig. 5). Consider the $\Delta\lambda$-curve at 150 trolands. If the $\Delta\lambda$-curve of the tritanope is taken as one component, another component with a minimum at

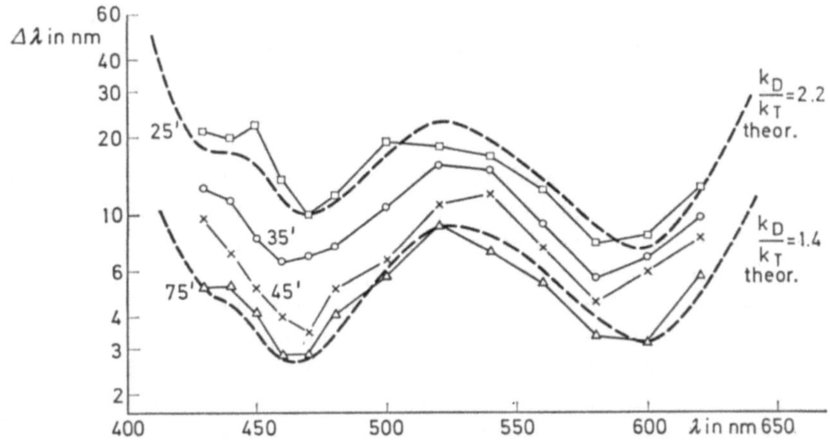

Fig. 7. Wavelength discrimination at a luminance of 0.85 trolands as a function of visual angle (McCREE, 1960). Dotted curves represent theoretical curves according to Eqs. 8 and 9 in Section 4

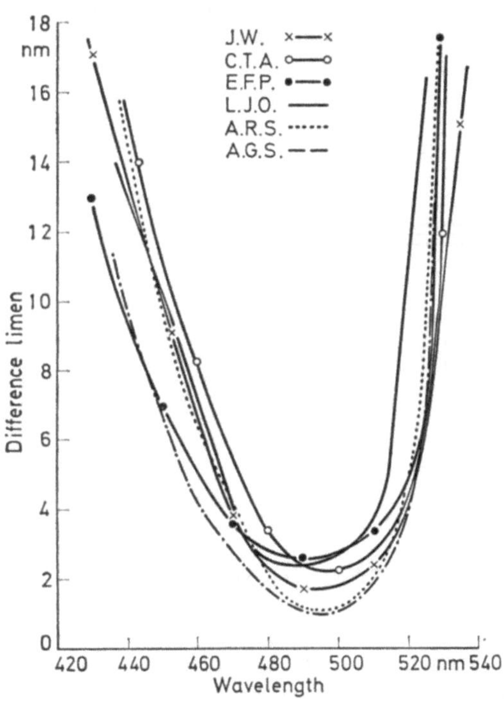

Fig. 8

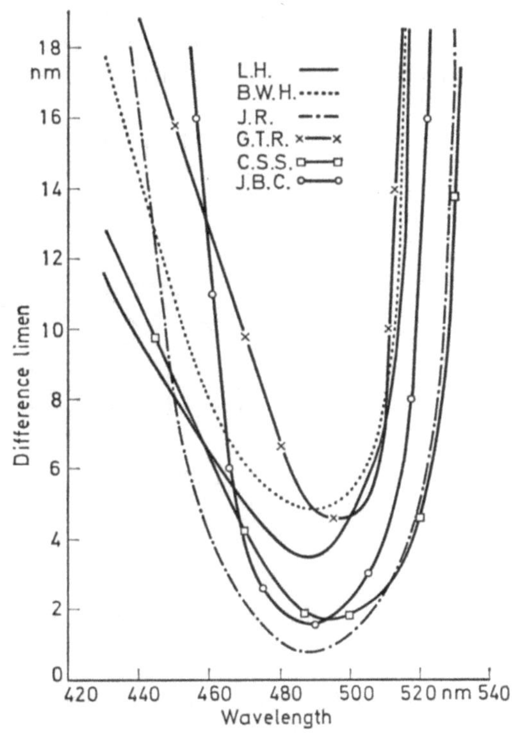

Fig. 9

Fig. 8. Wavelength discrimination curves for 6 deuteranopes (WRIGHT, 1946)

Fig. 9. Wavelength discrimination curves for 6 protanopes (WRIGHT, 1946)

500 nm completes the picture. The latter component can be described as the deuteranopic component (Walraven and Bouman, 1966), because the curve has the typical shape found for the deuteranope (Fig. 8). This is not called the protanopic component (Fig. 9), because a normal observer does not have reduced light sensitivity at the long-wave end of the spectrum, as the protanope has. Although it seems from the wavelength discrimination curves in Figs. 8 and 9 that these observers are complete dichromats, colour-naming experiments reveal that most of the subjects classified as dichromats still have some residual red-green discrimination (Scheibner and Boynton, 1968).

However, Judd and Yonemura (1970) consider this indeed as a protanopic component by considering normal vision as a combination of protanopia and tritanopia, as suggested by the second stage of the Müller theory of color vision. The same analysis of the discrimination curve can also be made at low luminance. The deuteranopic component is in this case shifted towards shorter wavelengths, a luminance dependence which is also found in deuteranopia (see Fig. 17).

In order to understand, the color discrimination of normal trichromats, it is useful to consider normal color vision as a combination of tritanopic and deuteranopic vision. The relative contributions of these two kinds of vision are dependent upon the visual angle of the test field.

In view of the evidence presented by microspectroscopy of single receptors the existence of three different cone types with sensitivities peaked in the short, middle and long-wave part of the spectrum is generally accepted (Brown and

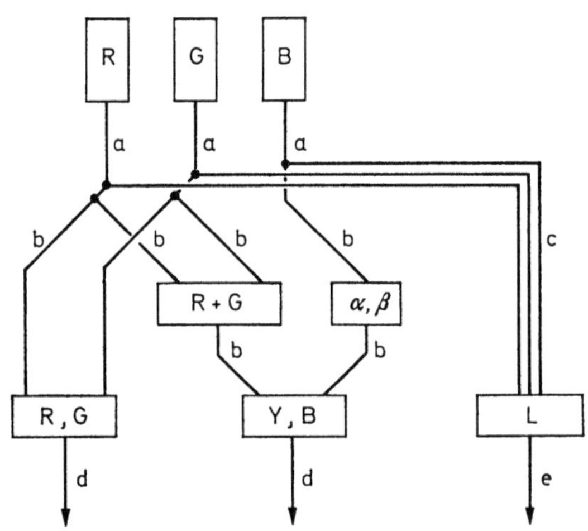

Fig. 10. Scheme of a zone theory of color vision (Walraven, 1962)

Wald, 1963; Marks and MacNichol, 1963). That there are also neural discrimination mechanisms present was recognized as early as 1880 by Hering, and later emphasized by Hurvich and Jameson (1955). The combination is accounted for in a zone theory, as for instance described by Walraven (1962, 1966).

The scheme proposed in Fig. 10 tries to combine the two features. There are three kinds of cones, which we call "red", "green", and "blue" cones, in a ratio of roughly 10:10:1. It is suggested that the absorption curves of the visual pigments in these cones are a revision of the Wright-Thomson curves (Walraven and Bouman, 1966) corrected for absorption in the eye media. The brightness signal L is the sum of the brightness contributions of the three different cone systems after going through the channels a and c, and it is transmitted through channel e. The chromaticness information is transmitted through the channels b. The information from the "red" and "green" cone systems goes to a "red-green" centre, from which the R, G signal is transmitted along a channel d to higher centres. A yellow (Y) signal is assumed to result from the addition of the red and green signals $R + G = Y$. It arrives in a "yellow-blue" centre, from which the Y, B signal is transmitted to the higher centres. The "blue" system contributes little to brightness, but as far as chromaticness is concerned, it is of as much value as the "red" and "green" systems. The chromaticness valence factor $\alpha = 10$ in channel b of the "blue" system accomplishes that. The weighting factor β is a luminance-dependent variable necessary to describe the behavior of color discrimination as a function of luminance (see Section 4).

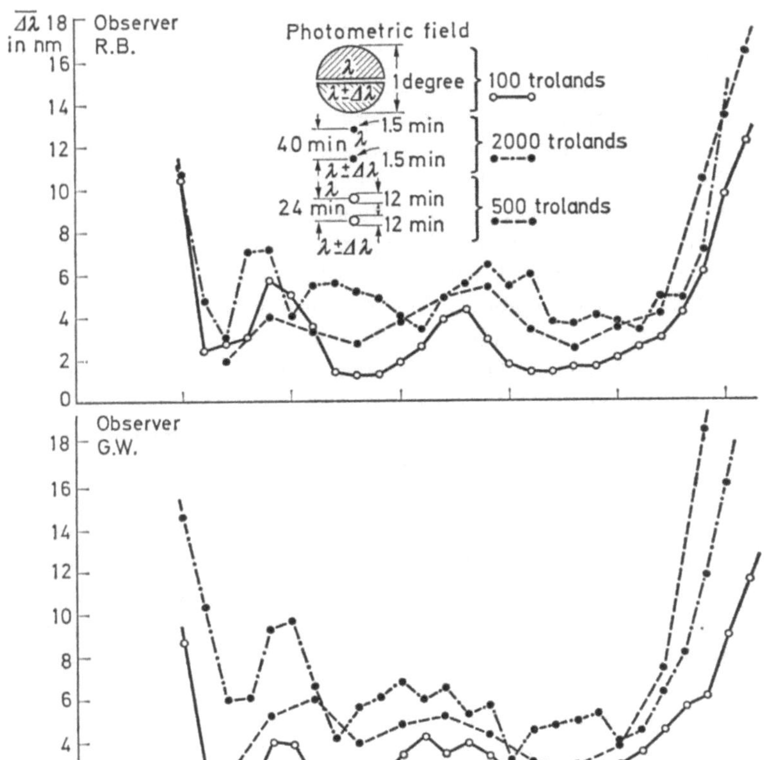

Fig. 11. Wavelength discrimination curves based on observations made by Bedford and Wyszecki (1958) for different field sizes and retinal illuminances (trolands)

Other investigators have also studied the effect of field size. A change in diameter from 2° to 12° improves color discrimination, but the magnitude of the improvement is independent of the position of the colors in the color diagram and of the direction of the lines in the color diagram along which the color differences are measured (BROWN, 1951). Fig. 11 shows the measurements of BEDFORD and WYSZECKI (1958), who used very small test patches. The small-field tritan effect apparently did not occur. One has to bear in mind that the measurements for different field sizes were not done at the same luminance and furthermore, that due to ever-present eye movements, the part of the retina stimulated was not the same, so that the observations were effectively over an area larger than the 1.5 arc min stimulus field. But even when this effect is eliminated by presenting brief stimuli, and even when the luminance is just above threshold (see Fig. 23 in section "Color naming"), it is clear that small-field color vision is trichromatic, since responses such as "red", "green" and "violet" occur.

One still cannot say therefore that small-field tritanopia does exist in its ultimate form of dichromatic vision when the test patch is as small as possible, but a change in the relative prominence of the tritanopic and the deuteranopic components with change in field size remains apparent. This is clear not only for wavelength discrimination, but also in non-spectral color discrimination measurements represented in the color diagram. The measurements of MACADAM (1959) are an example. Here two test patches of 3′ diameter separated from each other by 6′ were compared. The background, completely surrounding the test patches, was a not further specified fluorescent "white". The average value of the decrease of the deuteranopic component with respect to the tritanopic component was 2.6, compared with the well-known MACADAM data (Fig. 3), irrespective of the general deterioration in discrimination. Another experiment has been done by WALRAVEN (1962) in which a color difference existed between a test patch and its surround. This color difference was a difference in saturation produced by adding some monochromatic light to the test patch, and subtracting some of the white light from it in order to have equal brightness of test patch and surround. The saturation degree is then defined as the ratio (in %) of the luminance of monochromatic light to the total luminance. (Saturation degree is the same as colorimetric purity.) The color difference threshold was measured as a function of the diameter of the test patch. The results are given in Fig. 12 for a "white" surround (2824° K) for different wavelengths which correspond to different directions in the chromaticity diagram. But rather than plotting saturation degree, the saturation degree × area is plotted as a function of the diameter. This way of plotting gives the relation between the "amount of energy of the spectral light" in the test patch, and the diameter. This has the advantage that one easily can see in the graph that, up to about 3′ to 4′, the total amount of spectral light in the test patch is the determining factor for discrimination (Riccò's law).

In Fig. 12b, the curves for $\lambda = 590$ nm (more or less in the direction of a tritanopic confusion line), show an inflexion, indicating the existence of the small field tritan effect very clearly. The dependence of color discrimination on field size is therefore a complex function, depending upon the color combinations used, and also dependent upon the observation conditions.

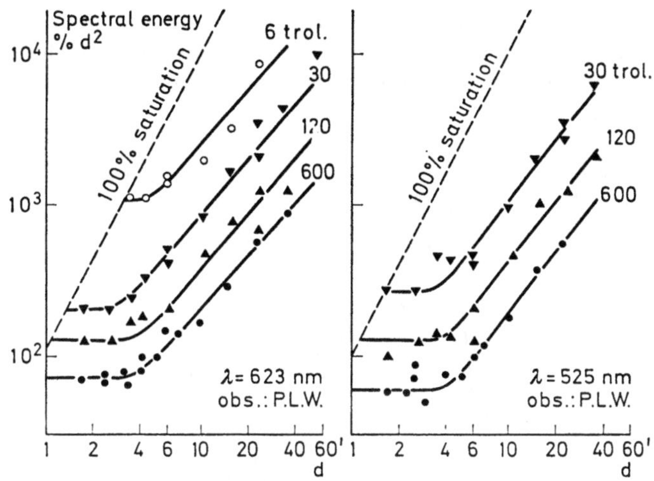

Fig. 12 a. Dependence of amount of spectral energy in test patch needed in order for it to be seen as a function of diameter at the wavelengths indicated for a few luminance levels (WALRAVEN, 1962)

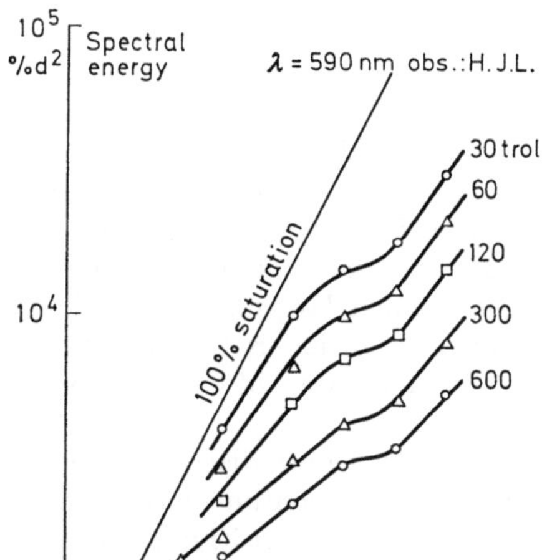

Fig. 12 b. Note the inflections at about 25′ representing the small field tritan effect (WALRAVEN, 1962)

Shown in Fig. 13 is another example of the influence of observation conditions. Rather than scanning the field, strict fixation of the test patch was maintained. It now turns out that blue-green discriminations become extremely poor. Thus the fixation method apparently plays a role in the determination of the relative contributions of tritanopic and deuteranopic vision to normal color vision.

BALL and FRY (1959) have shown that this tritanopic behavior can also be recognized inside the chromaticity diagram. The "blue" corner of the color mixture diagram is in fact nearly dichromatic, and the poor discrimination around 470 nm is just one aspect of this. They showed that the isochromatic lines in this dichromatic zone of the normal observer correspond to the confusion lines of a tritanope.

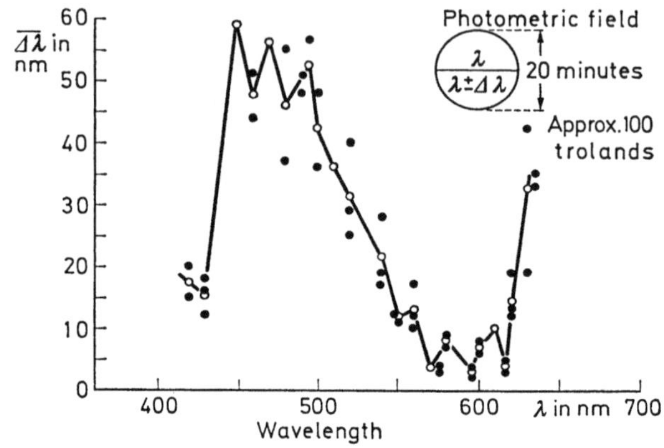

Fig. 13. Wavelength discrimination curve based on observations made by Willmer and Wright (1945), using a small field and strict foveal fixation (from Bedford and Wyszecki, 1958)

The influence of the position on the retina of the test fields is also very important. Weale (1953), in a review of color vision in the peripheral retina, mentions that wavelength discrimination is at its best in the blue. Measurements at perimetric angles of 25° and 45° show that the just noticeable wavelength steps are, except at short wavelengths, much larger in the periphery than in the fovea. At 45° considerable red-green confusion is taking place. The farther periphery tends therefore to exhibit characteristics of dichromatic vision. (See Moreland, chapter 20, this volume.)

Siegel (1965) showed that wavelength discrimination improves with exposure time. Sensitivity to color differences continued to increase even at 5 sec exposure time, although the differences in sensitivity for exposure times of 0.2 sec and longer are only slight.

The influence of the surround on discrimination cannot be neglected. Connors (1964) studied the effect of the luminance ratio of surround and test field. Averaged for a range of luminances from 0.06–2 ftL of the test field, the $\Delta\lambda$ for 550 nm is plotted in Fig. 14. Siegel (1969) used a more extended range of luminances of the test field from 0.1–100 ftL. His data, measured around 570 nm, are averaged for all these luminances and also plotted in Fig. 14. From this graph one easily can see that there is an optimum ratio of stimulus to surround luminance, and that, starting from a ratio 10:1 of surround and test stimulus, color discrimination deteriorates rapidly when this ratio is increased.

The influence of the surround is, however, more complex than a proportional change in the wavelength step all across the spectrum. Hurvich and Jameson (1961) have shown that the form of the wavelength discrimination function

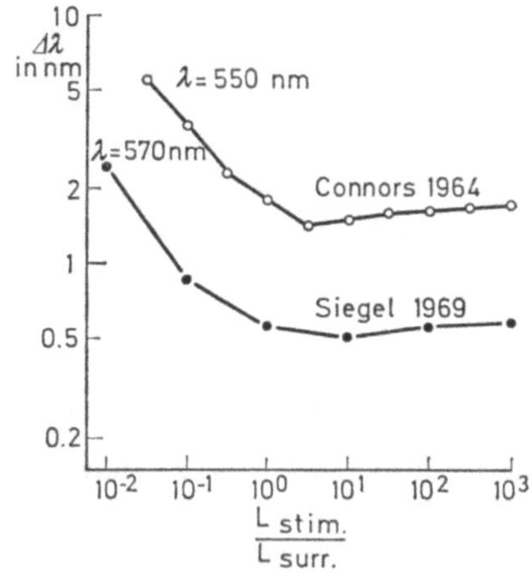

Fig. 14. Just noticeable wavelength step as a function of the ratio of luminance of test field and luminance of surround, according to CONNORS (1964) and SIEGEL (1969)

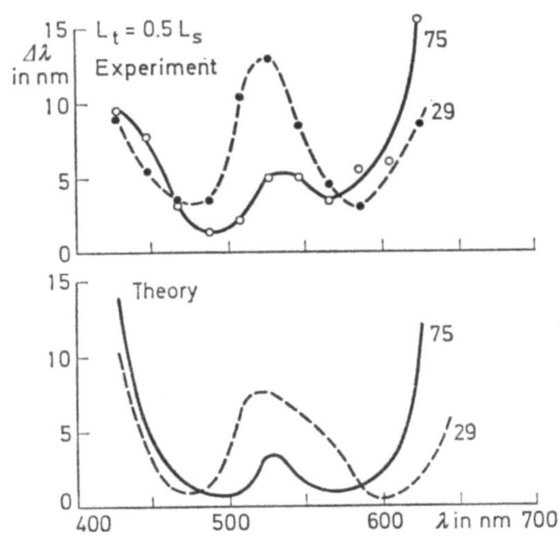

Fig. 15. Wavelength discrimination as influenced by color of the surround (75 = green 29 = yellow-red). Luminance of test field 5 mL, surround 10 mL. Theoretical curves according to the analysis by HURVICH and JAMESON (1961)

varies with a chromatic surround. Fig. 15 shows this for one observer for a "yellowish-red" and for a "green" surround of 10 mL luminance and test field of 5 mL ($L_t = 0.5\,L_s$). These data show that, with "yellow-red" adaptation, discrimination among long wavelengths is not worse but rather better than for "green" adaptation. The long-wave minimum in the $\Delta\lambda$-curve shifts towards longer wavelengths. The reverse is the case for "green" adaptation. HURVICH and JAMESON analysed this dependence on chromatic surround in terms of an opponent-colors mechanism. A yellowish-red surround increases the green response in the test-field. In the mid-spectral wavelengths, with a high percentage of greenness, this added green response will make the rate of change in hue from one wavelength to the next relatively slow. The wavelengths with the fastest rate of change will therefore be shifted towards longer wavelengths. Also in the traditional trichromatic theory such a shift is to be expected on the same reasoning. The activity of the red in the test-field will be decreased by a yellowish-red surround. If treated mathematically in the same way as the induced greenness in the opponent colors theory, the conclusions in terms of wavelength-discrimination are the same.

C. Modulation Transfer Functions in Time and Space

In the use of photometric fields such as that shown in Fig. 1 and in studies of color discrimination and dependence on the dimensions of such fields, homogeneity of the retinal test area is often assumed. An effective tool for research on retinal detection and discrimination mechanisms in which the test area dimensions are of less importance, is the use of sinusoidal variation of luminance in space and in time. (See Kelly, chapter 11, and Westheimer, chapter 7, this volume). In this chapter our concern is especially with the application of the sinusoidal modulation technique when test stimulus and reference are heterochromatic.

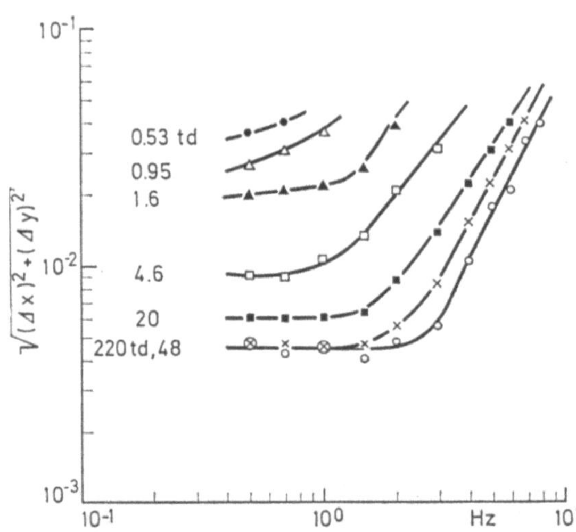

Fig. 16. Chromatic threshold contrast modulation of flicker frequency. Reference stimulus $x = 0.38$, $y = 0.52$. Average illuminances 220, 48, 20, 4.6, 1.6, 0.95 and 0.53 trolands (van der Horst, 1969)

In Fig. 16 typical temporal frequency characteristics for several luminances are represented. Such data provide information about the limited accuracy of color flicker photometry. They were obtained (van der Horst, 1969) for a centrally fixated test area, 5.3° wide $\times$ 2.8° high, that was sinusoidally modulated in color in a red-green direction around an average yellow, $x = 0.38$, $y = 0.52$. For larger modulation amplitudes critical fusion frequency approximates the Ferry-Porter law, $CFF = a \log B + b$.

Analogous to temporal frequency dependence of discrimination, spatial frequency has been studied by the use of grid patterns as visual stimuli (van der Horst, de Weert, Bouman, 1967; Schober and Munker, 1967). The mutual influence of spatial and temporal characteristics on thresholds is considered next.

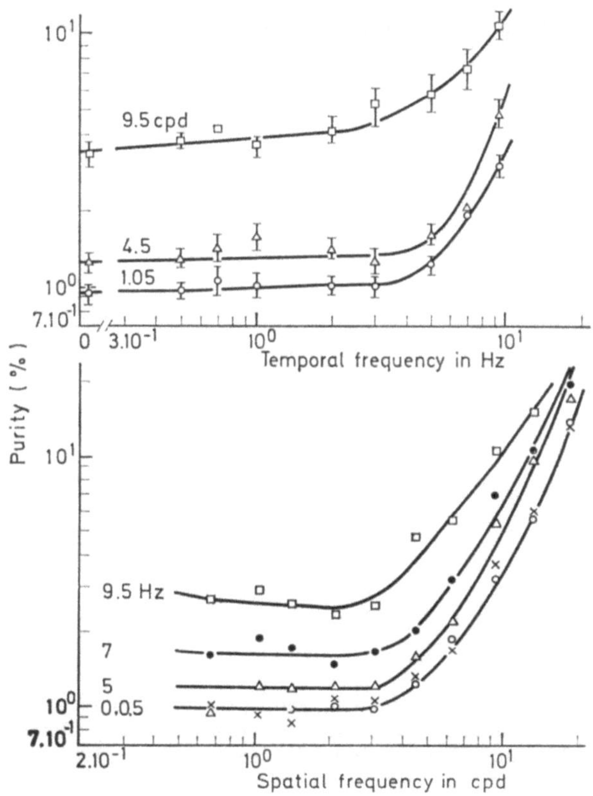

Fig. 17. Chromatic threshold contrast for travelling sine waves. *Lower part:* contrast modulations at 5 temporal frequencies 0 (0), 0.5 (×), 5, 7 and 9.5 Hz. *Upper part:* threshold contrast dependence on temporal frequency for gratings of 1.05, 4.5 and 9.5 cycles per degree. Retinal illuminance 160 trolands, reference color standard "white" E, with "red-green" chromaticity modulation. Purity is expressed in percent with respect to a dominant wavelength of 492 nm (van der Horst and Bouman, 1969)

Relevant data for spatially sinusoidal grids are illustrated in Fig. 17 (van der Horst and Bouman, 1969). In this figure detection thresholds are represented for regularly moving grids that were obtained by combination of a temporal with a spatial frequency modulation in the same test area. They show a typical size and time dependence of transmission that is readily described by the actions of spatial and temporal low pass filters. The general shapes of both spatial and temporal transfer functions seem to a large degree to be mutually independent as well as resistant to changes in average luminance level. Such behavior points to linear functioning of the relevant transmission channel, at least around threshold levels. This supposed linearity is tested by comparison of thresholds for sinusoidal modulation with thresholds for other types of modulation such as triangular and square-wave forms. For modulation in time as well as in space, the fundamental Fourier component in the stimulus was expected to be the only significant frequency for the modulation detection. Although significant deviations from this picture occur, especially for square waves, they are small enough, so that calculation of the Fourier transform function is probably justified.

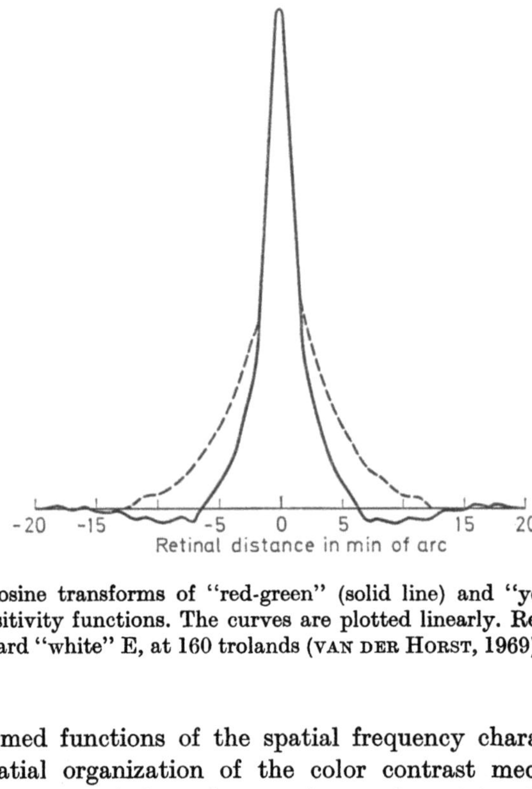

Fig. 18. Fourier cosine transforms of "red-green" (solid line) and "yellow-blue" (dashed line) chromatic sensitivity functions. The curves are plotted linearly. Reference color, standard "white" E, at 160 trolands (van der Horst, 1969)

Such transformed functions of the spatial frequency characteristics clearly illustrate the spatial organization of the color contrast mechanisms. Fig. 18 shows a summation area of the red-green chromatic activity that is about half the size of the area of the yellow-blue channel (van der Horst, 1969). This, of course, again affirms the small-field tritan effect. The differences in spatial characteristics between the visual channels will have repercussions in the time domain as well. Different latencies and different phase characteristics then complicate the interpretation of color flicker data (Walraven, Leebeek, and Bouman, 1957–58; Walraven and Leebeek, 1964).

The curves in Fig. 18 exhibit little or no negative region and thus little or no inhibition. This is in sharp contrast to what is found for the brightness channel, where a greater spatial sensitivity at higher luminances goes with obvious inhibitory qualities. Brightness is consequently transmitted far from linearly.

Frequency characteristics for this transmittance are of the band pass type, particularly at high luminances, and they are strongly dependent on average luminance level. Moreover the transmissions in the domains of time and space are not independent, which explains the familiar experience that a regularly moving, luminance modulated grid is seen more readily than a steady one (VAN NES, 1969). Such enhancement by motion does not exist for color modulated targets. VAN DER HORST (1969) has suggested that spatial resolution for differences in luminance as well as in chromaticness is limited by the diffraction of light by the pupil.

D. Just Noticeable Color Differences as a Function of Luminance

Two aspects of color discrimination as a function of luminance have to be distinguished. The first is the general deterioration of discrimination with decreasing luminance. The second is the shift in the location of the minimum of the wavelength discrimination curve in the blue-green part of the spectrum. The latter effect has already been mentioned in the foregoing section (compare Figs. 5 and 7). In view of the fact that this effect is only associated with the deuteranopic component in color discrimination, one would expect that this would also occur in deuteranopic vision. This is indeed the case, as is shown in Fig. 19 (WALRAVEN and BOUMAN, 1966). Here a bipartite 1° field was used,

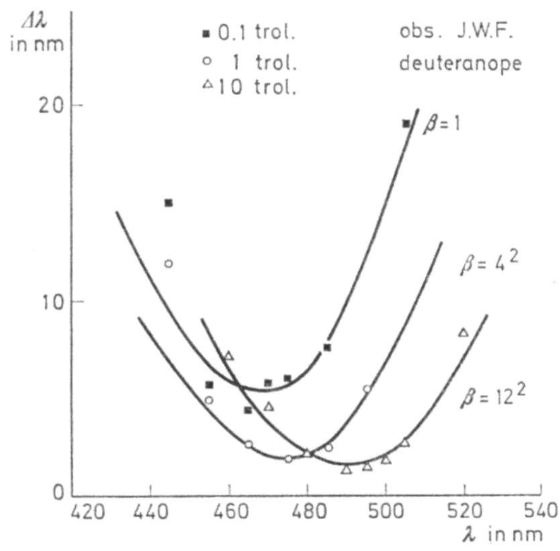

Fig. 19. Wavelength discrimination of a deuteranope at different luminances. The shift of the position of the minimum is very clearly shown. The solid curves are the best-fitting theoretical curves (WALRAVEN and BOUMAN, 1966)

viewed foveally. Much care was taken to use the centre of the pupil to avoid disturbance by the Stiles-Crawford luminance and color effects. (See CRAWFORD, chapter 18, this volume.) These can be very large in color-defective vision (WALRAVEN and LEEBEEK, 1962). The shift in the minimum interacts with the general deterioration of wavelength discrimination, so that at certain wavelengths an increase in discrimination with decreasing luminance can even be obtained. This is also apparent in the McCREE data on normal color vision mentioned earlier.

The same shift of the short-wave minimum was also found for protanomalous vision by Thomson and Trezona (1951), as constructed from their data by Bouman and Walraven (1962). The theoretical curve for the lowest luminance has been derived from the quantum theory of color discrimination. (Fig. 20). The kind of curves given in Fig. 20 are typical for protanomalous and deuteranomalous vision (Wright, 1964). A reduction in sensitivity to wavelength diffe-

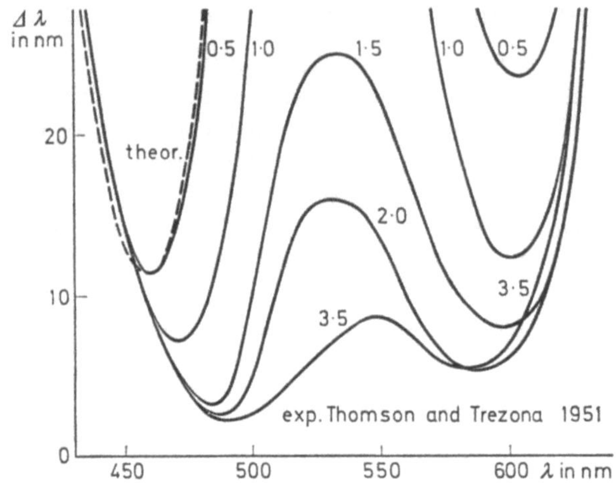

Fig. 20. Wavelength discrimination of a protanomalous observer at a number of luminances (parameter is log relative luminance)

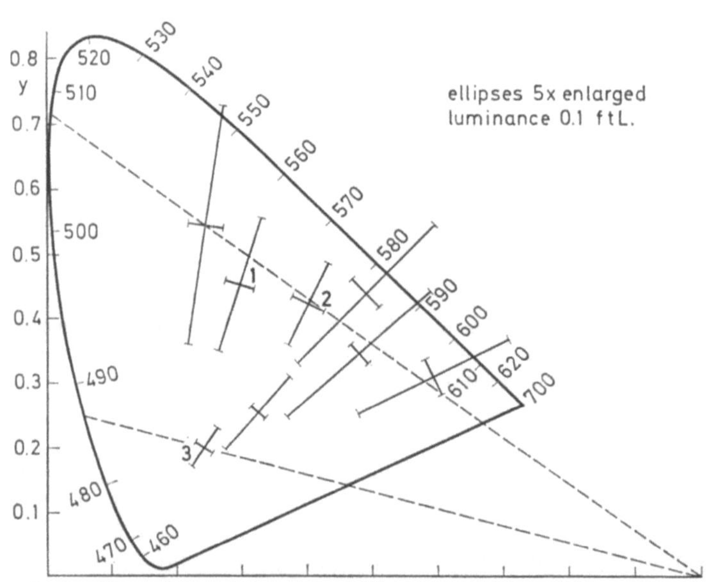

Fig. 21. Discrimination ellipses, indicated by their axes, average of two subjects (Brown, 1951). A case of pseudo-tritan effect

rences is largely confined to the "red-yellow-green"-part of the spectrum. The size of the reduction is dependent upon the degree of the defect. In the ultimate case of dichromatism this reduction is complete, as is apparent from Figs.8 and 9.

WEALE (1951) found the shift of the shortwave minimum not only in the fovea, but also in the periphery, using a 50′ field. In the latter case one might suppose that rod intrusion plays a role in the effect. In view of the fact that, in the measurements for the deuteranope, a 1° foveal field was used in order to avoid rod-intrusion, the shift seems to be a genuine cone effect. This has to be mentioned explicitly, because MCCREE (1960) chose deliberately not to fixate centrally.

The same effect can be recognized in the work of BROWN (1951), who measured discrimination ellipses in CIE chromaticity space as a function of luminance. Fig. 21 shows the axes of discrimination ellipses averaged for two observers at a luminance level of approximately 0.1 ftL. Two points must be considered: all ellipses except no. 3 are markedly elongated at low luminance. BROWN's data indicate, for example, that ellipses 1 and 2 undergo an average elongation of nearly 3-fold from 5 ftL to 0.1 ftL. The elongation can also be seen by comparing these ellipses with the ellipses of MACADAM (1942) which were measured at a high luminance level under the same viewing conditions, i. e., a 2° field in a dark surround. However, ellipse 3 does not change in shape! The conclusion by BROWN (1951), that at a low luminance a normal observer appears to become tritanomalous, is not fully correct. Such a conclusion would be valid only if the deterioration in discrimination occurred to the same degree along the complete length of a tritanopic confusion locus. This is apparently not the case, because the elongation does not occur for ellipse 3. Rather than calling the elongation for the other ellipses tritanomaly, this is better described as a pseudo-tritan effect. CORNU and HARLEY (1969), by studying color discrimination as a function of luminance with the 100-hue Farnsworth-test, also found a tritan effect with low luminances. Their viewing conditions are more natural than looking into a colorimeter. One wonders, in view of the foregoing discussion, whether their finding of a tritan effect is also a pseudo-tritan effect. This would need further analysis of their data.

In order to compare the data with the deuteranopic component of wavelength discrimination, deuteranopic confusion loci are drawn through the upper ellipses and ellipse 3. The intersections with the spectrum locus are at 508 and 487 nm. When one considers these wavelengths in Fig. 19, one can indeed see that at 508 nm wavelength discrimination deteriorates more rapidly than at 487 nm. The shift of the minimum in the wavelength curve of the deuteranope and the pseudo-tritan effect in BROWN's data are in fact the same phenomenon.

Fig. 22 gives a typical example of measurements of color discrimination as a function of retinal illuminance, in this case wavelength is parameter. These measurements are of the same type as those described in Fig. 12. A test patch of the indicated diameter is seen against a large "white" background. For comparison with luminance discrimination, measurements for equivalent conditions were made with a darker field in the white surround. In the color discrimination graphs, the just noticeable saturation degree for a number of wavelengths has been plotted. Saturation degree is defined as the ratio (in %) of the luminance of the monochromatic light to the total luminance. In the range of 1 to 10^3 trolands a square-root relation holds, thus saturation degree is inversely proportional to the square root of the retinal illuminance. This is the de Vries-Rose law, (DE VRIES, 1943; ROSE, 1942) on which the treatment in section 4 is based.

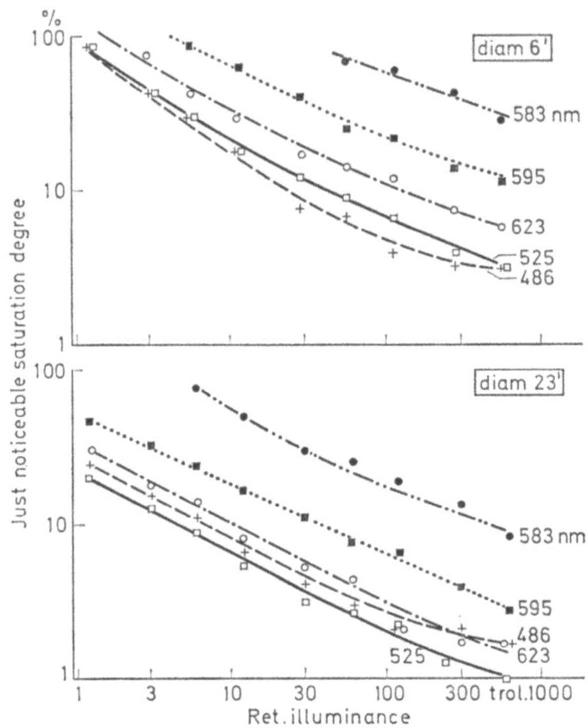

Fig. 22. Graphs represent just noticeable saturation degree as a function of retinal illuminance for the wavelengths and diameters indicated (WALRAVEN, 1962)

It is well known that for values higher than 1 000 trolands the Weber-law is valid, thus color contrast is independent of illuminance. The recent study by VAN DER HORST and BOUMAN (1969), presents more extended material on the validity of these laws for color discrimination.

Before we move to luminances where the square-root behavior of discrimination thresholds no longer holds, a recently suggested mechanism (BOUMAN, 1959, 1964, 1969) is worth mentioning. Although each absorbed quantum of light sets up a signal in the retina, not all these quantum signals are individually transmitted to the brain. The retina applies a data-processing action upon these signals by a scaling procedure. Each last quantum of a package of k quanta in a sample period produces a discrete potential for the next neuron layer. This scaling factor k varies in proportion to the square-root of the luminance to which the eye is adapted. Thus, the inevitable but irrelevant (for the eye) statistical variations in quantum numbers are excluded from further penetration into the visual pathways.

The retina evidently performs this job without an elaborate statistical analysis. The only possible way in which this optimal situation can then be reached was shown by BOUMAN and AMPT (1965) to be arithmetical adaptation. In its simplest form it means that, for each next ongoing action potential within the integration period of the adapting scaler, a fixed number of ϱ more input pulses are needed than were required for the last output pulse. Where n output pulses were registered in this period, they were produced by $\frac{1}{2} \varrho\, n\,(n+1)$ input pulses. When $\varrho = 2$, output frequency $F_0 \sim F_i^{1/2}$, where F_i is input frequency. For two just significantly different stimuli, the numbers of output pulses of such a coincidence centre differ by one. Consequently, this adapting scaler mechanism produces the square-root threshold behavior. Electrophysiological evidence for such a scaler, including arithmetical adaptation processes, is to hand (BOUMAN, 1969; BOUMAN and TEN DOESSCHATE, 1969). Such a square-root "de Vries-Rose" scaler is essentially a coincidence centre that is fed by the single quantum signals in the receptors of the centre's receptive field. In the de Vries-Rose adapting scalers, a feedback inhibition process is assumed. In case an arithmetical adaptation acts in feed-forward manner, a scaler results whose scale factor increases by one for each successive package of ϱ input pulses. For such a scaler, the scale factor in the steady state is proportional to the input, and consequently becomes its output independent of input level (VAN DE GRIND and BOUMAN, 1969). Just one extra output pulse is produced for a fast transient that is proportional to the steady input level: Weber's law.

Such a feed-forward arithmetically adapting scaler can only be located in the receptors. Quantal absorption probability is proportional to the available amount of photopigment. However, the receptor's coincidence requirement k for these quantal absorptions is proportional to the number of pigment molecules recently decomposed by preceding absorption. Evidently this "Weber" adaptation of the receptors becomes operational when 2 or more quantum-hits occur within the summation time. Although only a rough estimate can be made of the average quantum-absorption rate, on the basis of absolute threshold measurements, foveal cones should enter their Weber luminance region at about 300 trolands and peripheral rod vision at about 30 trolands. This is because maximum absorption rate for rods is about ten times as high as for cones (BOUMAN, 1950). The summation time for the faster Weber scaling is taken to be three times shorter than for the de Vries-Rose scaling.

The Weber fraction at which the receptors of a particular recipient unit operate at higher luminances is determined by the scale value of de Vries-Rose scaler of the unit concerned. This value is $[\Sigma\, n_p\,(1 - e^{-P}/_3)]^{+1/2}$ where n_p is the number of receptors of type p, P is the average number of quantum hits per p-receptor per summation time of the square-root scaler, and $(1 - e^{-P}/_3)$ the fraction of the p-receptors that is hit at least once per Weber integration period (BOUMAN, 1969). Data presented in this chapter do not conflict significantly with such a picture. Answers to the question as to which receptors feed the square-root scalers and which signal the luminosity and chromaticity channels, are deduced by BOUMAN (1969) from color-naming experiments at very low luminances (BOUMAN and WALRAVEN, 1957; WALRAVEN, 1962).

III. Color Naming

Color naming is recognized as a good tool for studying color discrimination. (See KRANTZ, chapter 26, this volume, for a more general discussion of scaling). It is possible to obtain reliable and consistent results (BOYNTON and GORDON, 1965). Applied to color defective subjects, significant information about defective color recognition and discrimination can be obtained (SCHEIBNER and BOYNTON, 1968). The discussion here will be limited to color naming by normal subjects.

At very low luminances the performance of the color vision mechanism becomes very poor. This can most obviously be seen in the color naming of weak, small and short light flashes. In such circumstances, light of wavelengths normally called yellow may be called green, occasionally blue may be called red, and very close to the absolute threshold, color vision gives way completely. We then perceive light without any chromatic impression, not even a white one. This instability in the appearance of test stimuli makes direct hue-discrimination

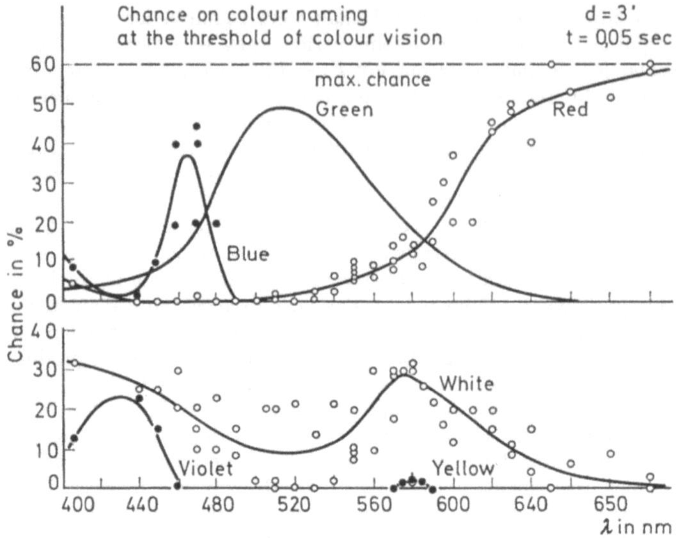

Fig. 23 a. The frequencies of seeing particular colors as indicated, at the threshold of color as a function of wavelength (Walraven, 1962; Bouman and Walraven, 1957)

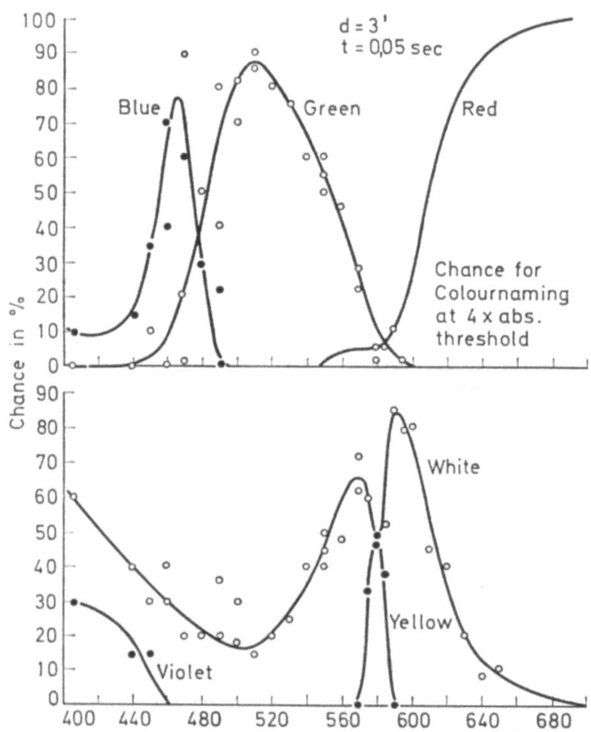

Fig. 23 b. The frequencies of seeing particular colors as indicated at 4 × absolute threshold, as a function of wavelength (Walraven, 1962; Bouman and Walraven, 1957)

measurements or direct matching of colors almost impossible. Qualitative reasoning indicates that this can happen only if the number of quanta involved is extremely small. The smaller this number, the greater the influence of chance effects becomes; for instance, a long-wave receptor may be hit solely by 500 nm quanta. A representative set of results is given in Figs. 23, 24, and 25. KRAUSKOPF (1965) has attempted to derive the receptor sensitivity curves from color naming at threshold levels.

Key roles in the further analysis of such color-naming experiments were played by the results for 580 and for 700 nm (Fig. 23 a, b). The latter is in the wavelength region where "wrong" hue reports are never given. Subjects report either red or achromatic, but never yellow, green, white or any other color. This is understandable because at these wavelengths the absorption of the "green system" (540 nm peak receptor absorption) is negligible when compared to that of the "red system" (590 nm peak receptor absorption). The ratio between chromatic and achromatic thresholds, the achromatic zone, is 1.3—1.4 at 700 nm and is independent of test flash size. It was consequently concluded that

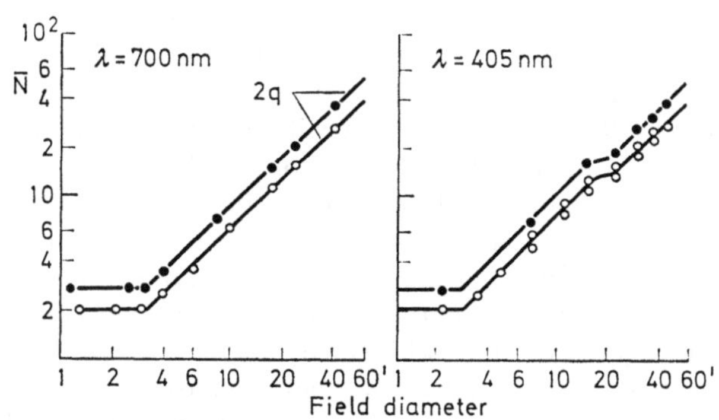

Fig. 24. Achromatic (lower curves) and chromatic (upper curves) threshold energies $\bar{N}$ as a function of field diameter for 700 and 405 nm, in the dark-adapted fovea. The slopes of the curves indicate a two-quanta coincidence mechanism. The inflection in the 405 nm-curve is due to inhomogeneity in sensitivity of the fovea at that wavelength (BOUMAN and WALRAVEN, 1957; WALRAVEN, 1962)

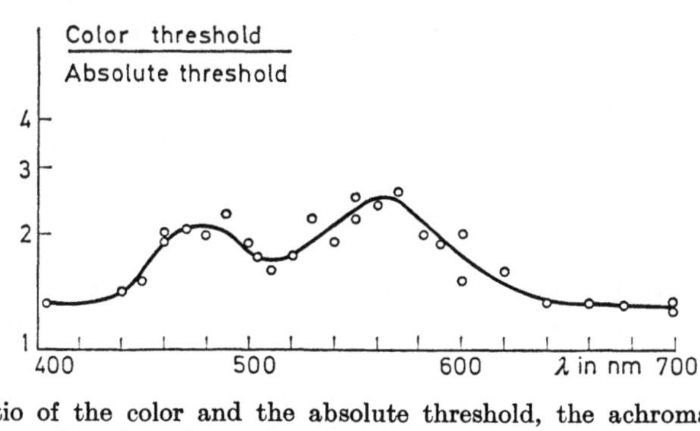

Fig. 25. The ratio of the color and the absolute threshold, the achromatic zone at large diameter (60′) as a function of wavelength (WALRAVEN, 1962; BOUMAN and WALRAVEN, 1958)

a 700 nm flash is seen uncolored before it is seen as red because of a greater summation area for achromatic than for chromatic vision. In the fovea this difference does not show up in the area-threshold relation, Riccò's law, because optical blur intervenes. It was found that the summation area for the achromatic signals is about twice (1.4^2) the area required for the chromatic signal. (Fig. 24). Because under appropriate circumstances Piper's law in the area-threshold relation ($I_{\text{threshold}}$ is proportional to diameter) means a twofold quantum coincidence requirement for threshold (van der Velden, 1944, 1946; Bouman, 1950), Bouman concluded that single hits in each of discrete groups of two or three "red cones" lead to an achromatic response, but double hits of one "red cone" are needed to give a red response. Similarly, if two single hits occur in receptors not belonging to a single "red cone" group, no light is perceived, no matter how closely these cones are located to each other.

This concept was extended for results at other wavelengths. At 580 nm the achromatic zone is larger than at any other spectral locus (Fig. 25). In the 500–700 nm region, the sum of red and green response percentages is smallest around 580 nm, and white perceptions occur more frequently here than anywhere else in the spectrum. Yellow evidently occurs at the cost of these white signals, but is still seen very rarely around the color threshold and only between 570–590 nm. Recognition of equal sensitivity of "red and green receptors" as the basis for these peculiar results for 580 nm naturally led to extending the assumed group of "red cones" to include two "green cones". In these postulated groups of four receptors, two or more single hits result in achromatic perception. Corresponding to what was assumed for "red cones", "green signals" are produced by multiple hits of individual "green cones". The name "human ommatidia" was suggested for such discrete receptor groups. A more complex picture, harder to analyse, is met for "yellow" and "white signals".

Bouman suggested as most probable that "yellow signals" are produced when "red" and "green" multiple color hits are balanced in any single "ommatidium". When this $R - G = 0$ balance is achieved by the simultaneous color excitations of several "ommatidia", pure white is perceived if the "ommatidia" involved are sufficiently close together. When they are not, distinct reddish and greenish spots are seen. Such groups of interacting "ommatidia" represent the next level of retinal organization where mutually overlapping receptive units are operating, each consisting of 5–7 "ommatidia", and each "ommatidium" belonging to 5 to 7 of such units depending on squareness or hexagonality of the retinal mosaic. If quanta are absorbed in the "blue cones" of a unit, "blue signals" are added to the perception. One such "blue signal" turns one "yellow signal" of any of the receptive unit's "ommatidia" into a "white" one. These specific suggestions were deduced from a rough quantitative analysis of percentages, of hue naming at threshold level, as represented in Figs. 21, 22 and 23. The assumptions about "blue-cone" excitation stem mainly from the fact that in the short-wave part of the spectrum color naming responses are variable for short, small flashes, whereas for more extended stimulus areas, colored appearances are always blue even at the color threshold. According to the hypothetical scheme, the luminosity channel of a unit is represented by its $R + G$ input, its tritanopic channel by its $R - G$ value, and the deuteranopic channel by its

$(R + G) - B$ input. The receptor's Weber adaptation, because of its multiple-hits basis, operates only in chromatic signal production; the achromatic pathways carry the "ommatidium's" quantum-concidence requirements that must be fulfilled by the test stimulus in order to pass the threshold for its visibility. The "ommatidium's" square-root scaler determines these threshold conditions, and derives them from the quantum flux $(R + G)$ of the whole unit in which the "ommatidium" concerned is the central element.

The foveal achromatic "cone perceptions" look exactly like those mediated exclusively by rods. This again naturally led to the suggestion that "scotopic vision by cones" is mechanistically equivalent to that of rods (BOUMAN, 1969). Consequently rods also could show a distinction between multiple coincidences by single and by multiple hits on each rod, the first leading to achromatic and the second to chromatic, probably white, perception (BOUMAN and TEN DOESSCHATE, 1969). The achromatic luminance range, being proportional to the square-root of the number of receptors in a unit, should then depend on eccentricity. The range throughout which apparent color depends on luminance should then be of the same size as the achromatic zone. Both ranges together constitute the luminance range in which threshold shows a square-root dependence on luminance. Consequently this total range is proportional to the number of receptors per receptive unit at the eccentricity concerned.

In this view, small field and short time tritanopia is a consequence of the absence of achromatic excitations from "blue-receptors" because coincidence of single quantum absorptions produces "blue-signals" in the receptive unit concerned. This implies less strict temporal and spatial coincidence requirements for the arousal of "blue-signals". It means that the tritanopic channel benefits more than the deuteranopic channel from increase in the test – stimulus duration or area. "Blue-blindness" of the fovea evidently does not exist: weak, small and short 450 nm flashes do produce blue color-naming responses in the fovea. It has to be recognized, that the sensitivity for short wavelengths is diminished in the central part of the fovea (Fig. 24). However, lack of interference by "rod-white signals" gives the fovea red-green discrimination that is far superior to that in peripheral parts of the retina. Defective color vision in the periphery is presumably due to flooding of the chromaticity channels by the "rod-white signals". Thus the retina is a far better brightness discriminator in the periphery than in the fovea. Spatially, detection abilities for color and for luminance differences are distributed over the retina in a complementary fashion.

IV. Description of Color Discrimination as a Line Element

Many attempts have been made to describe empirical color discrimination data in terms of the so-called line element. The following definition of the line element

$$(ds)^2 = \sum_{i,k} g_{ik}\, dx_i\, dx_k \tag{1}$$

is based upon the assumption that the subjective difference between two closely similar colors can be described by an infinitesimal expression which is quadratic in the differences in color coordinates. This is the Riemannian form for the line element, which is generally used in color theory, although some have questioned its validity. Le Grand (1957, 1970) for instance, doubts whether the MacAdam ellipses are really ellipses; Parra (1969) has measured a number of "MacAdam ellipses" and, according to him, these ellipses show humps and bumps. Moreover, Crawford (1970) shows that the ellipses are essentially not symmetric, which would indicate non-linearities in the color discrimination system.

Let it be assumed that the MacAdam ellipses are really ellipses to a first approximation. Then the problem is to determine the metric coefficients g_{ik}. A detailed analysis of several proposals for line elements can be found in Wyszecki and Stiles (1967).

Helmholtz (1896) was the first to propose a line element. He suggested a scheme in which the amounts of light absorbed in the three receptor systems are represented by R, G and B.

Thus $R = \int P_\lambda \bar{r}_\lambda d\lambda$, $G = \int P_\lambda \bar{g}_\lambda d\lambda$, and $B = \int P_\lambda \bar{b}_\lambda d\lambda$ where P_λ is the spectral energy distribution and $\bar{r}_\lambda$, $\bar{g}_\lambda$ and $\bar{b}_\lambda$ are the spectral response functions of the three independent response mechanisms.

The line element is then given by

$$(ds)^2 = \left(\frac{dR}{R}\right)^2 + \left(\frac{dG}{G}\right)^2 + \left(\frac{dB}{B}\right)^2 \tag{2}$$

Eq. (2) clearly reflects Helmholtz's ideas about a three-receptor color-mediating system. A fractional increase in intensity, $\frac{dR}{R} = \frac{dG}{G} = \frac{dB}{B} = f$, results in $(ds)^2 = f^2$. Since constancy of the line element means subjective equality, this means that the relative difference threshold is independent of intensity: Weber's law. Helmholtz, of course, formulated his line element in such a way that it would produce Weber-like threshold behaviour. The prediction of the wavelength-discrimination curve from Eq. (2), turns out to be rather bad, which makes the Helmholtz line element mainly of historical interest.

Schrödinger (1920) proposed another line element:

$$(ds)^2 = \frac{1}{R+G+B}\left[\frac{(dR)^2}{R} + \frac{(dG)^2}{G} + \frac{(dB)^2}{B}\right] \tag{3}$$

Here too, the line element complies with Weber's law when $\frac{dR}{R} = \frac{dG}{G} = \frac{dB}{B} = f$, then $(ds)^2 = f^2$.

Schrödinger's point in proposing this line element was that in his system brightness and wavelength are orthogonal. One can show this as follows.

Suppose the three-dimensional color space is plotted with transformed coordinates $\sqrt{R}$, $\sqrt{G}$ and $\sqrt{B}$, then the Schrödinger line element takes the form

$$(ds)^2 = \frac{1}{R+G+B}\left[(d\sqrt{R})^2 + (d\sqrt{G})^2 + (d\sqrt{B})^2\right] \tag{4}$$

which means that the $(\sqrt{R}, \sqrt{G}, \sqrt{B})$ space is Euclidean at any point. In this space radius vectors, characterized by $\sqrt{R}:\sqrt{G}:\sqrt{B} =$ constant, and thus by $R:G:B =$ constant, are lines of constant spectral composition, and spheres around the origin $(\sqrt{R})^2 + (\sqrt{G})^2 + (\sqrt{B})^2 = R + G + B =$ constant, are surfaces of constant luminance. Apparently, in the Schrödinger space, luminance and wavelength are perpendicular to each other. It can easily be shown that this is not the case in the Helmholtz space. Comparison with experimental data, however, proved unsatisfactory.

STILES (1946) proposed a modification of the Helmholtz line element by introducing different weights for the color-mediating systems.

$$(ds)^2 = \frac{(dR)^2}{(0.78\,R)^2} + \frac{(dG)^2}{(1.00\,G)^2} + \frac{(dB)^2}{(4.46\,B)^2}\,. \tag{5}$$

STILES has shown that this modified line element accords more closely with the experimental data. The use of a significantly different weighting factor for the 'blue' system reflects the consistently different behaviour of this system from that of the 'red' and 'green' ones. (For a discussion of STILES' later work, see ENOCH, chapter 21, this volume.)

Objections have been raised against analyses in which three receptor systems play the only role. In particular, HURVICH and JAMESON (1957) have stressed the point that two color discriminating mechanisms, a "yellow-blue" and a "red-green" system as well as a "white-black" one, must be working in the retina. This is in line with Hering's opponent-color theory. With this opponent scheme in mind, several attempts have been made to express a line element. SHKLOVER (1958) may be mentioned in this connection. FRIELE (1961, 1966) has made a very elaborate attempt, in which a brightness mechanism and two chromatic differencing mechanisms are postulated. This formulation fits in with the Müller type of opponent-color theory, but is modified in an empirical way in order to adapt the formulation to the experimental data.

So far a mechanistic basis for discriminability has not been used. BOUMAN and WALRAVEN (1962, 1966) proposed that the noise of the incident light in the three receptor systems is the limiting factor for discrimination. WALRAVEN added to it the opponent scheme. The formulation of the subsequent line element is given by VOS and WALRAVEN (1970). This formulation resembles Schrödinger's line element, but differs from it mainly in that SCHRÖDINGER tried to make his formula agree with Weber's law, whereas here the validity of the de Vries-Rose law is assumed. As shown in section 3 (in particular Fig. 22), color discrimination obeys the de Vries-Rose law: contrast is inversely proportional to the square root of the luminance over a large range of luminances.

The statistical uncertainty in the number of quanta absorbed is given by the square root of the number of incident quanta. In the physical (R, G, B) space, the surface of equally R, G, B discernable points is given by

$$(ds)^2 = \frac{(dR)^2}{R} + \frac{(dG)^2}{G} + \frac{(dB)^2}{B}\,. \tag{6}$$

The quadratic summation reflects the mutual independence of the three receptor processes. Here, R, G and B represent numbers of quanta, and are designated in Fig. 26 by $\bar{n}_r$, $\bar{n}_g$ and $\bar{n}_b$. (In the text this designation will not be used further.) Now the opponent scheme has to be taken into account. According to the scheme of Fig. 10, $R + G + B = L$ (Brightness) and $R + G = Y$ (Yellow), and it is assumed that there are separate R, G and Y, B-channels. The influence on the

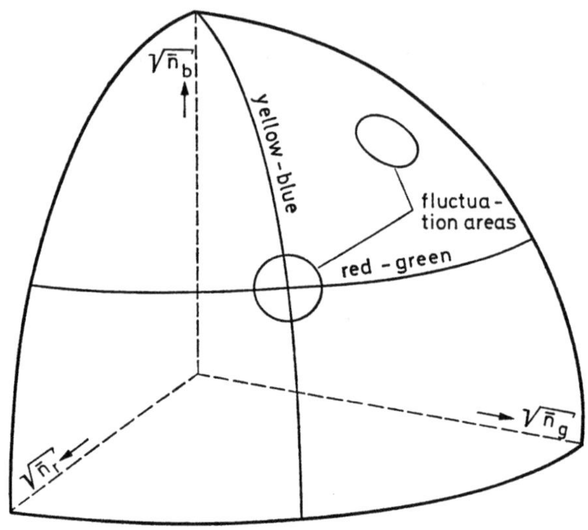

Fig. 26. The three-dimensional square-root diagram. The fluctuations cover spheres in this space, and circles on the surface of equal luminance $\bar{n}_r + \bar{n}_y + \bar{n}_b$ = constant. According to the model of Fig. 10, discrimination along the meridians is yellow-blue discrimination (deuteranopic vision) and along the parallels of latitude, red-green discrimination (tritanopic vision)

formulation of the line element is that, because data transmission is not equally accurate in the (R, G)-, (Y, B)- and L-channels, the ellipsoid of Eq. (6) is considerably changed in size, shape and orientation. In order to deal with this, it is useful to plot, as in the Schrödinger case (Eq. 4), $\sqrt{R}$, $\sqrt{G}$ and $\sqrt{B}$ as coordinates. The physical line element then becomes

$$(ds)^2 = (d\sqrt{R})^2 + (d\sqrt{G})^2 + (d\sqrt{B})^2 \tag{7}$$

which means that the space is uniformly Euclidean on a square-root basis. Spheres about the origin represent surfaces of equal luminance, $R + G + B = L$ = constant (Fig. 26). The infinitesimal spheres representing $(ds)^2$ according to (Eq. 7) are transformed into ellipsoids with the axes:

along the radius	(L-component),
along the parallels of latitude	(R, G-component),
along the meridians	(Y, B-component).

Introducing k_L as the accuracy factor for the L-component, k_D for the deuteranopic component and k_T for the tritanopic component, then Eq. (7) changes into:

$$\begin{aligned}(ds)^2 = \frac{1}{L}\Bigg[&\left(k_L + k_T \cdot \frac{G\cdot L}{R\cdot Y} + k_D \cdot \frac{B}{Y}\right)(dR)^2 + \left(k_L + k_T \cdot \frac{R\cdot L}{G\cdot Y} + k_D \cdot \frac{B}{Y}\right)(dG)^2 \\ &+ \left(k_L + k_D \cdot \frac{Y}{B}\right)(dB)^2 + 2\left(k_L - k_T \cdot \frac{L}{Y} + k_D \cdot \frac{B}{Y}\right) dR dG \\ &+ 2\,(k_L - k_D)\, dR dB + 2\,(k_L - k_D)\, dG dB\Bigg]\,. \end{aligned} \tag{8}$$

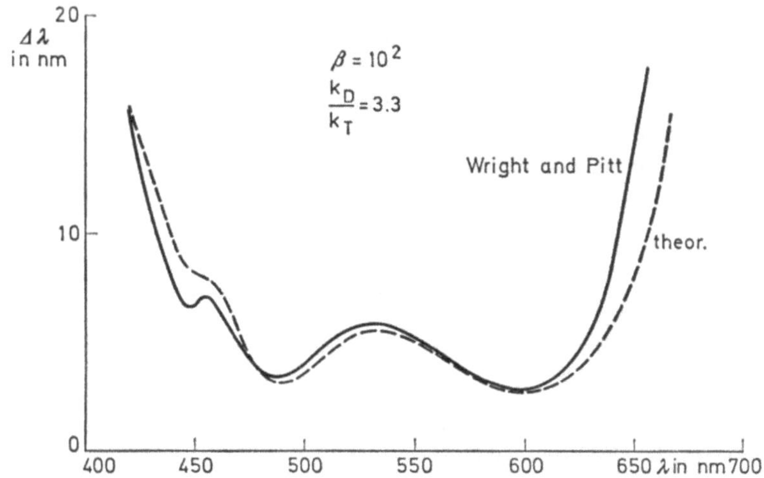

Fig. 27. Experimental wavelength discrimination curve measured by WRIGHT and PITT (1934), compared with the theoretical one (WALRAVEN and BOUMAN, 1966)

In the case of color discrimination at constant luminance, $k_L = 0$, which means that discrimination is *not* made on the basis of luminance differences. In the case of deuteranopia, $k_T = 0$, and in the case of tritanopia, $k_D = 0$.

It is obvious that the resulting line element is more complex than those of HELMHOLTZ, SCHRÖDINGER, or even STILES. This is because of the cross-products, which indicate that the ellipsoid is no longer oriented along the R-, G- and B-axes. This is due to the zone-processing introduced. This line element satisfactorily describes color discrimination at low luminances, using as fundamental response curves the revised Thomson-Wright curves (WALRAVEN and BOUMAN, 1966).

Two distinct minima at 460 nm and a little below 600 nm occur in the wavelength discrimination curve. A modification, an extra parameter, has to be introduced to deal with the shift of the minimum from 460 to 490 nm with increasing luminance. Following STILES (Eq. 5), a weighting factor β for the 'blue' system has to be introduced. This modification means that, rather than taking the discrimination step on the surface $R + G + B =$ constant, it is taken on the surface $R + G + \beta B =$ constant, giving the B an extra weighting factor β.

This changes Eq. (8) in that k_D has to be replaced by k_D^* in which

$$k_D^* = k_D \cdot \frac{(Y + B) \cdot (Y + \beta^2 B)}{(Y + \beta B)^3} \,. \tag{9}$$

In the case of constant luminance, only two parameters have to be specified to fit the experimental data. In Fig. 3 the values $\beta = 12^2$ and $k_D/k_T = 3.3$ are chosen. They describe the MacAdam ellipses very well. The wavelength discrimination curve of WRIGHT and PITT is best approximated with $\beta = 10^2$ and the same k_D/k_T value (Fig. 27) (WALRAVEN and BOUMAN, 1966).

Bouman's "ommatidium-scaler" model and a corresponding slightly modified opponent scheme lead to a mathematical specification of just noticeable differences that deviates in some respects from Eq. (8) (BOUMAN, 1969). He incorporated the supposition that change of luminance implies changes of input to the chromaticity channels. This is because these inputs are treated as difference signals like $R - G$, and $(R + G) - B$. He suggested that photopic signal elicitation is responsible for the transition from de Vries-Rose into Weber threshold behavior, as shown in the previous section. Thus it seems that there are many ways in which further research might reveal new perspectives on the field of color vision.

References

Ball, R. J., Fry, G.: Lines of constant hue in the blue corner of the color mixture diagram. Amer. J. Optom. **36**, 200—212 (1959).

Bedford, R. E., Wyszecki, G.: Wavelength discrimination for point sources. J. opt. Soc. Amer. **48**, 129—135 (1958).

Bouman, M. A.: Quanta explanation of vision. Documenta ophthal. **4**, 23—115 (1950).

— History and present status of quantum theory in vision. In: Sensory Communication Rosenblith, W. (Ed.) New York: Wiley 1959.

— Efficiency and economy in impulse transmission in the visual system. Acta psychol. (Amst.) **23**, 239—241 (1964).

— My image of the retina. Quart. Rev. Biophys. **2**, 25—64 (1969).

— Ampt, G. G. F.: Fluctuation theory in vision and its mechanistic model. In: Performance of the eye at low luminances. Amsterdam: Exc. Med. Congr. Ser. 1965.

— Ten Doesschate, J.: Adaptation and the electrical excitability of the eye. Documenta ophthal. **26**, 240—247 (1969).

— Walraven, P. L.: Some color-naming experiments for red and green monochromatic lights. J. opt. Soc. Amer. **47**, 834—649 (1957).

— — A study of defective and normal colour vision. In: Visual Problems of Colour, Vol. 2, p. 463. London: H. M. Stationery Office 1958.

— — Quantum theory of color discrimination of dichromats. Vision Res. **2**, 177—187 (1962).

Boynton, M. B., Gordon, J.: Bezold-Brücke hue shift measured by color naming technique. J. opt. Soc. Amer. **55**, 78—86, 1965.

Brown, P. K., Wald, G.: Visual pigments in human and monkey retinas. Nature (Lond.) **200**, 37—43 (1963).

Brown, W. R. J.: The influence of luminance level on visual sensitivities to colour differences. J. opt. Soc. Amer. **41**, 684—688 (1951).

Connors, M. M.: Effect of surround and stimulus luminance on the discrimination of hue. J. opt. Soc. Amer. **54**, 693—695 (1964).

— Siegel, M. H.: Differential color sensitivity in the purple region. J. opt. Soc. Amer. **54**, 1374—1377 (1964).

Cornu, L., Harlay, F.: Modifications de la discrimination chromatique en fonction de l'éclairement. Vision Res. **9**, 1273—1287 (1969).

Crawford, B. H.: Lop-sided ellipses of colour sensitivity. In: International Colour Meeting Stockholm 1969, Vol. 1, 302—311. Göttingen: Musterschmidt 1970.

DeValois, R.: Analysis and coding of color vision in the primate visual system. Cold Spr. Harb. Symp. quant. Biol. **30**, 567—579 (1965).

Fischer, F. P., Bouman, M. A., Ten Doesschate, J.: A case of tritanopy. Documenta ophthal. **5**, 55—67 (1951).

Friele, L. F. C.: Analysis of the Brown-MacAdam colour-discrimination data. Farbe **10**, 193 (1961).

— Further analysis of colour-discrimination data. Proc. Int. Colour Meeting (Lucerne). Göttingen: Musterschmidt 1966.

Grind, W. A. van de, Koenderink, J. J., Bouman, M. A.: Models of the processing of quantum signals by the human peripheral retina. Kybernetik **6**, 213—227 (1970).

Guth, S. L., Donley, N. J., Marrocco, R. T.: On luminance additivity and related topics. Vision Res. **9**, 537—576 (1969).

HELMHOLTZ, H. von: Handbuch der Physiologischen Optik, 2. Aufl. Hamburg: Voss 1896.

VAN DER HORST, G. J. C.: Chromatic flicker. J. opt. Soc. Amer. **59**, 1213—1217 (1969).

— Fourier analysis and color discrimination. J. opt. Soc. Amer. **59**, 1670—1676 (1969).

— BOUMAN, M. A.: Spatiotemporal chromaticity discrimination. J. opt. Soc. Amer. **59**, 1482—1488 (1969).

— DE WEERT, C. M. M., BOUMAN, M. A.: Transfer of spatial chromaticity contrast at threshold in the human eye. J. opt. Soc. Amer. **57**, 1260—1267 (1967).

HURVICH, L. M., JAMESON, D.: Some quantitative aspects of an opponent-color theory. II. Brightness, saturation and hue in normal and dichromatic vision. J. opt. Soc. Amer. **45**, 602—616 (1955).

— — An opponent-process theory of color vision. Psychol. Rev. **64**, 384—404 (1957).

— — Opponent chromatic induction and wavelength discrimination. In: The Visual System: Neurophysiology and Psychophysics. JUNG, R., KORNHUBER, H. (Eds.). Berlin-Göttingen-Heidelberg: Springer 1961.

JUDD, D. B., YONEMURA, G. R.: CIE 1960 UCS diagram and the Müller theory of color vision. J. Res. nat. Bur. Standards A **74**, 23—30 (1970).

KRAUSKOPF, J., SREBRO, R.: Spectral sensitivity of color mechanisms: Derivation from fluctuations of color appearance near threshold. Science **150**, 1477—1479 (1965).

LE GRAND, Y.: Light, Colour and Vision. New York: Wiley 1957.

— Théories sur la métrique de l'espace des couleurs. In: International Colour Meeting Stockholm 1969. Göttingen: Musterschmidt 1970.

MACADAM, D. L.: Visual sensitivities to color difference in daylight. J. opt. Soc. Amer. **32**, 247—274 (1942).

— Small field chromaticity discrimination. J. opt. Soc. Amer. **49**, 1143—1146 (1959).

MCCREE, K. J.: Small field tritanopia and the effects of voluntary fixation. Optica Acta **7**, 317—323 (1960).

MARKS, W. B., MACNICHOL, E. F.: Difference spectra of single goldfish cones. Fed. Proc. **42**, Abstr. 2143 (1963).

VAN NES, F. L.: Enhanced visibility by regular motion of retinal images. Amer. J. Psychol. **81**, 367—374 (1969).

PARRA, F.: Recherches sur le seuil différentiel de couleur. Thèse de l'Université de Paris 1966.

ROSE, A.: The relative sensitivities of television pick-up tubes, photographic film and the human eye. Proc. Inst. Radio Engrs. **30**, 295—308 (1942).

RUDDOCK, K. H.: Integration processes in colour vision. Farbe **15**, 63—72 (1966).

SCHEIBNER, H. M. O., BOYNTON, R. M.: Residual red-green discrimination in dichromats. J. opt. Soc. Amer. **58**, 1151—1158 (1968).

SCHOBER, H., MUNKER, H.: Untersuchungen zu den Übertragungseigenschaften des Gesichtsinns für die Farbinformation. Vision Res. **7**, 1015—1027 (1967).

SCHRÖDINGER, E.: Grundlinien einer Theorie der Farbenmetrik im Tagessehen. Ann. Physik **63**, 481 (1920).

SHKLOVER, D. A.: The equicontrast colorimetric system. In: Visual Problems of Colour, Vol. 2, London: H. M. Stationery Office 1958.

SIEGEL, M. H.: Colour discrimination as a function of exposure time. J. opt. Soc. Amer. **55**, 566—568 (1965).

— Color discrimination and luminance. Perc. Psychophys. **66**, 163—166 (1969).

STILES, W. S.: A modified Helmholtz line element in brightness-colour space. Proc. phys. Soc. (Lond.) **58**, 41—65 (1946).

THOMSON, L. C., TREZONA, W. P.: The variation of hue discrimination with change of luminance level. J. Physiol. (Lond.) **114**, 98—106 (1951).

VAN DER VELDEN, H. A.: Over het aantal lichtquanta, dat nodig is voor een lichtprikkel bij het menselijk oog. Physica **11**, 179—189 (1944).

— The number of quanta necessary for perception of light of the human eye. Ophthalmologica (Basel) **111**, 321—331 (1946) [Translation].

VOS, J. J., WALRAVEN, P. L.: An analytical description of the line-element in the zone fluctuation model of colour vision. Report No. IZF 1970-5. Soesterberg: Institute for Perception RVO-TNO 1970.

de Vries, Hl.: The quantum character of light and its bearing upon threshold of vision, the differential sensitivity and visual acuity of the eye. Physica **10**, 553—564 (1943).

Walraven, P. L.: On the Bezold-Brücke phenomenon. J. opt. Soc. Amer. **51**, 113—1116 (1961).

— On the mechanisms of colour vision. University Thesis, Utrecht 1962.

— A zone theory of colour vision. Farbe **15**, 17—20 (1966).

— Bouman, M. A.: Fluctuation theory of color discrimination of normal trichromats. Vision Res. **6**, 567—586 (1966).

— Leebeek, H. J.: Chromatic Stiles-Crawford effect of anomalous trichromats. J. opt. Soc. Amer. **52**, 836—837 (1962).

— — Phase shift of sinusoidally alternating colored stimuli. J. opt. Soc. Amer. **54**, 78—82 (1964).

— — Bouman, M. A.: Some measurements about the fusion frequency of colors. Acta Electronica **2**, 50—55 (1957/1958); Optica Acta **5** (1958) special number.

Weale, R. A.: Hue discrimination in para-central parts of the human retina measured at different luminance levels. J. Physiol. (Lond.) **113**, 115—121 (1951).

— Colour vision in the peripheral retina. Brit. med. Bull. **9**, 55—60 (1953).

Willmer, E. N., Wright, W. D.: Colour sensitivity of the fovea centralis. Nature (Lond.) **156**, 119—121 (1945).

Wright, W. D.: The graphical representation of small color differences. J. opt. Soc. Amer. **33**, 632—636 (1943).

— Researches on Normal and Defective Colour Vision. London: Kimpton 1946.

— The characteristics of tritanopia. J. opt. Soc. Amer. **42**, 509—521 (1952).

— Pitt, F. H. G.: Hue discrimination in normal color vision. Proc. phys. Soc. (Lond.) **46**, 459 (1934).

Wyszecki, G., Stiles, W. S.: Color Science. New York: Wiley 1967.

Chapter 20

Peripheral Colour Vision

By

J. D. MORELAND, Waterloo, Ontario (Canada)

With 7 Figures

Contents

There is a sense in which a transit out from the fovea is like a journey back in evolutionary time: a descent from the acme of form and colour vision to more rudimentary perceptions. If the changes met with in that descent were merely quantitative the periphery would present only a limited field for research but that is not so. Indeed peripheral vision differs qualitatively as well as quantitatively from that in the fovea and those differences are fundamental to an understanding of the physiology of vision.

Anatomy

There are considerable regional variations in neuronal topography, both in the retina and in the visual pathways, that underly the differing characteristics of foveal and peripheral vision. Classical studies of photoreceptor population distributions in flat retinal preparations have been reported by POLYAK (1941) for cones and in a meticulous work by ØSTERBERG (1935) on a single human retina for both rods and cones. VILTER (1949) has published distributions for rods, cones (outer segments and pedicles separately), bipolars and ganglions, but these were derived from sagittal sections which are susceptible to not inconsiderable counting errors. Quantitative data for regional variations in the sizes or domains of the dendritic trees of retinal neurones are very sparse (MORELAND, 1969b, 1970) as indeed they are for other sites in the visual pathway.

The topographical relationship between photoreceptoral counts and visual acuity has been noted by POLYAK (1941), HARRISON (1953), DOESSCHATE (1946a, b) and WRIGHT (1949) and similar comparisons have been made for light sensitivity by DOESSCHATE (1949), RUSHTON *et al.* (1955) and WEALE (1956). The correlations obtained by these workers, though not perfect, may be considered satisfactory in view of such factors as differences between individual retinas and experimental conditions, and unknowns such as the degree of lateral convergence of receptors and dioptric aberrations.

The organisation of the higher centres of the visual pathway emphasizes the overiding importance of the central region of the retina. This region (diameter 20 degrees in the visual field) occupies only about 1.7 % of the visual field, but the retino-cortical projection constructed by HOLMES and LISTER (1916) and HOLMES (1945) from scotoma resulting from gunshot wounds of the brain shows that about 22 % of the cortex is devoted to that part of the retina. That is, the central region receives about 16 times its "fair share" of the cortex and it might be supposed that a greater factor would apply to the foveal region itself. FULTON'S (1949) work on the lateral geniculate of the chimpanzee shows that a similar disproportionate share of that body is appropriated by the central retina. It is of interest to note, in this connection, that LAKOWSKI and ASPINALL (1969), using the method of static perimetry, have reported that young children (about 6 years) have such low peripheral sensitivities compared with their elders that only events in a central region of ± 15 degrees are of "interest". The authors surmise that there may be a cortical suppression of peripheral information while perceptual development takes place foveally, or that peripheral "learning" has yet to occur.

Problems Peculiar to the Periphery

These factors and others make necessary the use of special techniques and precautions to ensure precise work on peripheral vision.

Refraction. Curiously the correction of peripheral refractive defects, which may be as much as 3 dioptres, has been found to be of little benefit in so far as visual acuity is concerned (WEALE, 1956; CLARKE and BELCHER, 1962) although such defects must play an important role in any observations of thresholds for small fields. WEYMOUTH (1958) has shown, however, that extrafoveal refractive defects are insignificant compared with the resolving power of the retina itself.

Fixation. To study a specific extrafoveal retinal location a fixation target is necessary for foveal viewing while the test field itself is projected at the required angle from it. The head should be immobilised. Various methods of head location are used from a mere chin and forehead rest (as in clinical perimetry) to full dental bites for precise work especially when Maxwellian view is employed. Of course the normal small involuntary eye movements that occur during fixation will alter the region of retina under test. Over observation periods of some 2 minutes or so meridional movements of about 1/4 degree might be expected to occur which would produce equal displacements of the test field whatever its position in the field of view. Tortional movements, however, would increase in importance proportionately with increasing distance of the test from the fovea. In fact all these movements would reduce the effects of local adaptation but to a limited extent depending upon the size of test field employed.

The double requirement of foveal fixation and of extrafoveal perception can be mastered with some practice but it does present to the naive subject a task of divided attention that he may well find difficult. Indeed the temptation to "look" at the test field is very strong in such cases.

Local Adaptation (Troxler's Effect). The price paid for good fixation is local adaptation. It has long been known that a small test field seen peripherally at one retinal location fades rapidly (TROXLER, 1804). The effect may be observed foveally too but the changes are much reduced (CLARKE, 1957). On the other hand MCCREE (1960a, b) has reported a dramatic reduction in colour discrimination for some subjects who could maintain good fixation for extended periods, and KANEKO (1965) also has found short term (< 1 sec) changes mostly in saturation. Such large changes in foveal vision may be due to a reduction in size and frequency of the flick component of involuntary eye movements during the act of fixation. (See ALPERN, chapter 12, this volume.)

Faced with the problem of local adaptation and the appearance of after-images, some investigators (e.g., THOMSON and WRIGHT, 1947; WEALE, 1951; RICHARDS and LURIA, 1964) employ a "glance" technique of viewing, in which the eye is averted or closed to allow time for recovery. One criticism of this technique is that neither the exposure nor the recovery time is known and since changes in sensitivity in different mechanisms may occur at different rates accurate work would require a defined time control. The degree of control necessary to achieve the desired level of precision will depend upon the experimental conditions: for example, when two fields that are being compared are projected onto parts of the retina with very diverse characteristics, the need for control is more acute (MORELAND, 1955a) than when those characteristics are similar (as is usually assumed for a bipartite field).

MORELAND (1955a, b) introduced a flash and recovery cycle (see below) to reduce and control local adaptation. Flash presentations had been used much earlier, of course, by STILES and CRAWFORD (1933) but for the different purpose of defining a threshold criterion.

Visual Acuity. Poor visual acuity in the periphery militates against the use of juxtaposed bipartite fields either in matching or in discrimination experiments. Small bipartite fields (about 2 degrees diameter) have been used by WRIGHT (1946), GILBERT (1947, 1950) and RICHARDS and LURIA (1964) but only at small eccentricities. Larger (10 degree) bipartite fields have been used by STILES (1955), and his co-workers, SPERANSKAYA (1958, 1959), LOZANO and PALMER (1967) and NIMEROFF (1964), but these were centrally fixated. CLARKE (1962) has used such a field at an eccentricity of 10 degrees. The use of a gap between two small fields to provide clear resolution at eccentricities of 10 degrees or more was introduced by WEALE (1951a) and adopted by MORELAND (1955a) and CLARKE (1960).

Experimental Methods

One of the most striking aspects of peripheral colour vision is the change in appearance of a coloured stimulus as it is moved out across the field of view. Early descriptions of these changes usually involved qualitative techniques, frequently undefined stimuli and scantily described experimental conditions and are, consequently, of mainly historic interest. An interesting review of such early work is given by BAIRD (1905). More recent reviews have been given by WEALE (1953b, 1956).

Colour Naming. Colour naming criteria have been used to describe hue and saturation changes or to establish stimuli of "unique" or invariant hue but only the most stringent precautions in method (see below) yield results of worthwhile precision. Although HESS (1889) employed spectral lights, in place of the bits of coloured paper used in earlier work, for his work on invariant hues, the use of broadband heterochromatic stimuli still persists (see, for example, BÄUML and ENGELHARDT, 1951; and VERRIEST and ISRAEL, 1965), Following HESS, increasing attention was given to the dependance of peripheral judgements on experimental

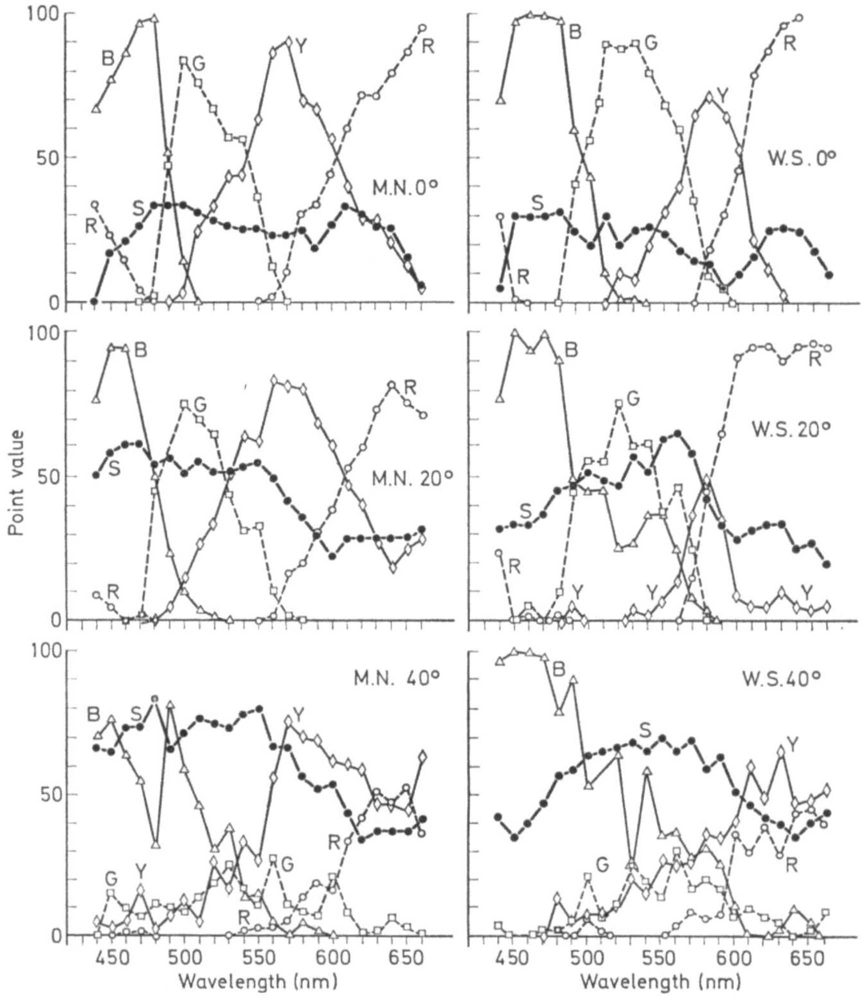

Fig. 1. Proportion of judgements named blue *B*, green *G*, yellow *Y*, red *R* and white *S*. The test field, diameter 3 degrees, retinal illuminance 1000 trolands, is presented 0.3 sec every 6 sec on a dark background at eccentricities 0, 20 and 40 degrees in the nasal visual field. Subjects M.N. and W.S. From BOYNTON *et al.* (1964)

conditions. ABNEY (1913) reported the dependance of the size of colour fields on wavelength (see also RINDE, 1932), luminance and angular subtense of the stimulus. LYTHGOE (1931) found that colour naming at various retinal locations differed when the eye was light- or dark-adapted. YAKOVLEV (1938) reported an influence of sound on the size of certain colour fields and it is of interest to note in this connection similar findings by KRAVKOV (1941) for quantitatively determined sensitivity changes at the fovea as a function of wavelength using either sound or instilled adrenalin. More recently JAMESON and HURVICH (1967) have noted that the colour of fixation targets may have a pronounced effect on the hue-naming of test lights.

These are a few examples of the wide range of physical parameters influencing the perception of colour in the peripheral retina: the technique of colour naming becomes a reliable tool only when they are controlled and achieves acceptable precision when the "end-point" is decided by a forced choice naming procedure.

Such a method was devised by THOMSON (1954) in his determination of the "unique" hues for foveal vision. Its essential feature is the severe restriction of the number of responses allowed to the subject, (e.g. the "yellow" point in the spectrum was defined as that wavelength for which the subject responded "red and green" with equal frequency: no intermediate colour name was allowed). A less restricted method has, with other desirable precautions, been applied to the fovea and periphery by BOYNTON *et al.* (1964). Hue and desaturation responses for spectral lights were reported for two subjects at three retinal locations for a 3 degree field at 1000 trolands. The colour categories were restricted to red, yellow, green, blue and white but three kinds of hue response were allowed for each: "Unique hue", "mixed hue", "White-no hue"; in addition three responses were allowed for desaturation magnitudes. An arbitrary set of weights was assigned to the responses from which the functions of Fig. 1 were calculated.

These functions give a reasonable description of the hue changes through the spectrum for foveal vision and reveal significant differences between the two subjects. Foveal "saturation[1]" curves are less satisfactory and do not show the minimum at 590 nm found in the classical work of PRIEST and BRICKWEDDE (1938), MARTIN *et al.* (1933), and WRIGHT and PITT (1937) for normal trichromats. This suggests that "saturation" is a far more elusive attribute than hue to "name" and indeed this is borne out by the analysis of correlation coefficients by BOYNTON and his co-workers. In moving from the fovea out to 20 and 40 degrees there is a marked reduction in the saturation of all wavelengths shorter than 600 nm and in addition there is a dramatic collapse of hue-naming discrimination particularly at 40 degrees suggesting a dichromatic system with blue and yellow to red responses predominating. Similar results have been obtained by WEITZMANN and KINNEY (1969) who employed the same colour-naming procedure for small test fields (11 and 21 min of arc) and two durations (200 and 20 msec) at the fovea and at 5 and 10 degrees extrafoveally. These authors used a white surround field of 0.17 mL viewed through the natural pupil (probable retinal illuminance: 12 trolands) and obtained a foveal "white" response curve more in accord with classical work (see above). There is no fundamentally satisfactory way of relating these arbitrarily

[1] There is an unfortunate confusion in this paper: the terms saturation and desaturation appear to be used synonymously.

weighted data to quantitative colour matching functions but see BOYNTON and SCHEIBNER (1967) for an approach to this problem that uses a multidimensional scaling procedure.

Asymmetric Colour Matching. The quantitative correlate of "colour naming" is the technique of asymmetric matching whereby a peripherally viewed test field is matched for one or all of its attributes by a foveal comparison field. In this way the semantic pitfalls inherent in colour designation may be avoided and peripheral equivalents can be expressed in terms of the matching foveal stimuli.

One of the earliest descriptions of such a technique is given by DREHER (1911) who employed monochromatic spectral lights and projected one to the fovea and the other to the periphery. The wavelength of the *peripheral* test light was adjusted until it matched the foveal comparison field in hue. Hue changes at 14 degrees in the visual field of view were estimated using a 4.25 degree field and their dependance on the state of adaptation was observed. DREHER'S apparatus, which was a diffraction grating single monochromator would have suffered from stray light. NEWHALL (1936) was probably the first to describe a complete photometric and colour match between foveal and peripheral responses. Using a three filter colorimeter that provided a 2 degree square foveal comparison field he matched this to the "blue arcs of the retina". (These were induced by a rectangular light patch projected nasally.) Paradoxically the "blue arcs", a transient effect appearing in the space between the rectangular stimulus and the blind spot, although luminous are not real lights (see MORELAND 1968, 1969a, b). NEWHALL was able to show that their blue colour was constant and independant of the colour of the initiating stimulus. His results were expressed in the CIE x, y, z coordinate system with the units based on a white match. This is unsatisfactory because of the large dependance of such a match on the yellow pigmentation of the human lens and possibly of the macula lutea.

A fragmentary account is given by VOLK and FRY (1947) of matches made between a red-green mixture at the fovea and nonspectral red, yellow and green test lights in the periphery. Hue shifts of red and green toward yellow were reported as the test was moved out from the fovea to 7.5 degrees.

GILBERT (1950) briefly recorded an experiment in which the test and comparison fields of WRIGHT'S (1946) colorimeter were separated by 3 degrees; foveal colour mixtures in the comparison field were used to match the parafoveal test at various wavelengths. The technique was marred, however, by the matches used as the basis of the units. Although WRIGHT'S (1946) stratagem was employed to nullify the effect on the test stimulus of non-photosensitive ocular pigments, the unit matches were made asymmetrically, i.e., foveal mixture *versus* parafoveal test. Such a match places an arbitrary restriction on any peripheral hue changes in the unit stimuli (in this case 494 nm and 582.5 nm) and, of course, influences the calculation of coefficients for all other spectral stimuli.

MORELAND (1955a, b) modified the Wright trichromatic colorimeter to facilitate separation of the test and comparison beams for the purpose of asymmetric matching. All matches were made using the instrumental primaries 650, 530 and 460 nm (R, G and B respectively) and normalised by means of foveal (i.e., symmetric) matches on 494 nm and 582.5 nm such that $B = G$ for the former and $R = G$ for the latter. In this way all asymmetric matches could be expressed in terms of foveal colour space. CRUZ and MORELAND (1955) and MORELAND and CRUZ (1958) reported a comprehensive series of measurements for test field positions ranging from 10 to 30 degrees on the lower vertical meridian and from 15 to 50 degrees on the nasal horizontal meridian. Both test and comparison fields (each 80×40 min of arc) were presented simultaneously for 0.5 sec every 2 sec to reduce and control local adaptation. Matches were made while viewing a sequence of some 20 to 30 exposures. The fields, Fig. 2, were viewed on a dark background by the dark-adapted eye. The extrafoveal field was kept approximately at constant luminosity for all locations and most wavelengths: the corresponding retinal illuminance for the foveal field was about 30 trolands.

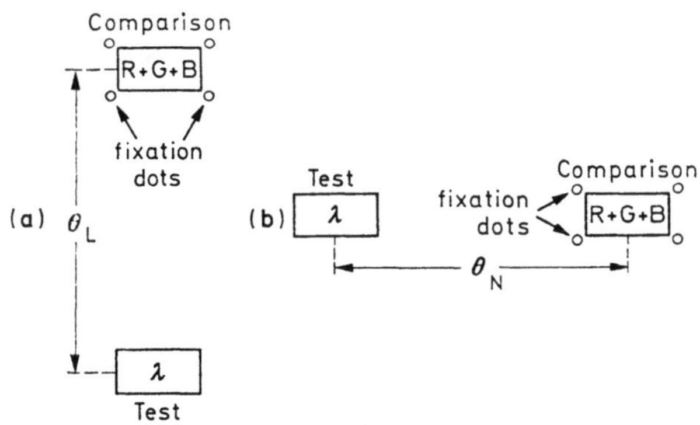

Fig. 2. Fields used in asymmetric colour matching. The extrafoveal test of wavelength λ is matched by a 30 troland mixture of 650, 530 and 460 nm ($R + G + B$) in the foveal comparison field. The fields, size 80×40 min of arc, are presented 0.5 sec every 2 sec on a dark background at eccentricities $(a)\,\theta_L$ in the lower vertical meridian $(b)\,\theta_N$ in the nasal horizontal meridian. From MORELAND and CRUZ (1958)

The main findings showed a progressive reduction in size and shape of the spectrum locus with increasing distance from the fovea (Figs. 3 and 4). The most dramatic effects were found at 25 to 30 degrees where the locus was almost straight (Fig. 4) and by 40 to 50 degrees the collapse was almost complete. A straight line would imply dichromatic colour vision (assuming additivity) but the 25 to 30 degree loci show a residual curvature that might result (see below) from rod intrusion. The contraction of the spectrum locus found for increasing eccentricity is remarkably similar to the change of perceived colour of small and of large centrally fixated fields of fixed chromaticity seen under different surround luminances found by HUNT (1950, 1953). He assumes that the rod mechanism is inoperative and explains his results in terms of postulated neural links (HUNT, 1950) between the three cone mechanisms which are formed in dark adaptation and break down in light adaptation. It is quite feasable that the contraction of peripheral spectrum loci could be explained by increasing neural links with distance from the fovea, but rod intrusion cannot be discounted (MORELAND, 1955b; MORELAND and CRUZ, 1958).

The results gave no support to the concept of invariant hues: a careful analysis showed that those wavelengths with zero hue change depended not only on the

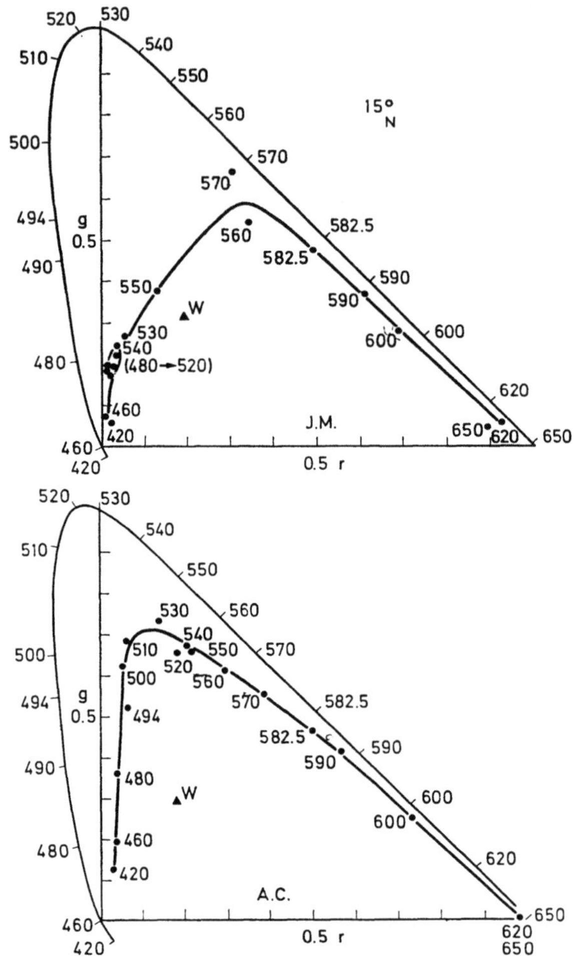

Fig. 3. Asymmetric colour matches of extrafoveal test stimuli, at 15 degrees nasally, expressed in the WDW chromaticity diagram for subjects A.C. and J.M. The bold line drawn through the points is the extrafoveal spectrum locus. The foveal spectrum locus and the white point (triangle: standard illuminant *C*) provide individual frames of reference for each subject. Wavelengths are marked in nm. Matches are normalised for $B = G$ at 494 nm and $R = G$ at 582.5 nm. From Moreland and Cruz (1958)

subject but on the retinal location under test. This finding has since been confirmed by Boynton *et al.* (1964) and Weitzman and Kinney (1969) using colour-naming techniques. These authors also report the occurrence of dichromacy with increasing retinal eccentricity, but at different eccentricities due presumably to the different test field sizes, luminances and exposure times employed.

In the above asymmetric colour matching experiments there is a progressive reduction of discrimination in the region of 530 nm with increasing eccentricity and at 25 degrees it involved the whole range 480–550 nm. This can be thought of as resulting from (a) increasing participation in vision by rod-cone groups or (b) the

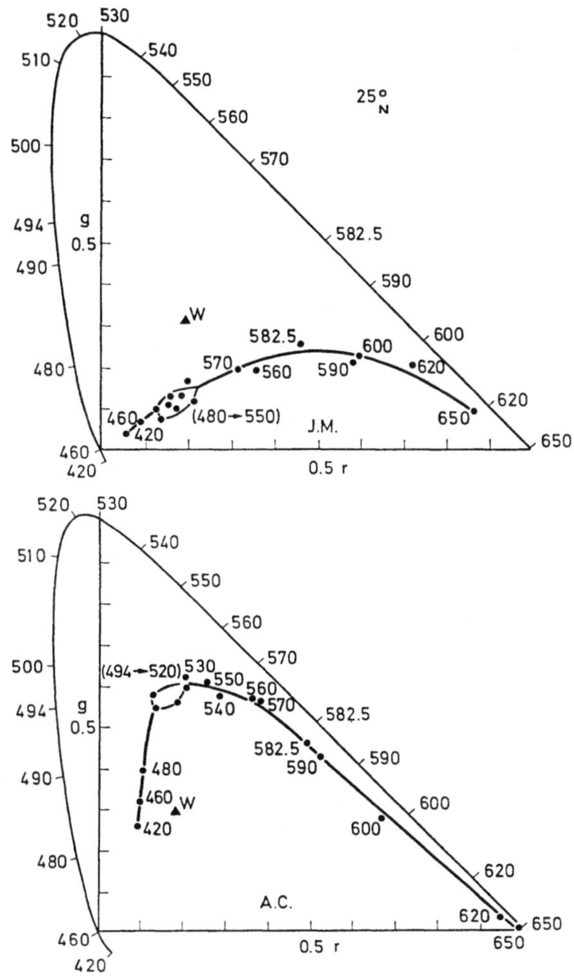

Fig. 4. Same as Fig. 3 but with extrafoveal test stimuli at 25 degrees nasally. From MORELAND and CRUZ (1958)

reduction in cone population covered by the test field by analogy with "small field" tritanomaly. CRUZ and MORELAND (1955) did indeed suggest a similarity to small field[2] data but the spectrum loci found do not support this notion. The work of WILMER and WRIGHT (1945) and of WRIGHT (1952) shows that both congenital and "small field" tritanopia should be characterised by a straight spectrum locus that folds back on itself at 460 nm. The MORELAND and CRUZ asymmetric colour matching data do not behave in this way (Fig. 4).

[2] It was stated in this paper that the test field, measuring 80 × 40 min of arc and placed at 15, 30 and 40 degrees was equivalent (on a cone population basis) to circular fields of 1.6, 1.2 and 1.0 min of arc diameter respectively at the fovea. The decimal was wrongly placed: the correct values being 16, 12 and 10 min, i.e., comparable to the foveal field sizes for which tritanopic characteristics are reported.

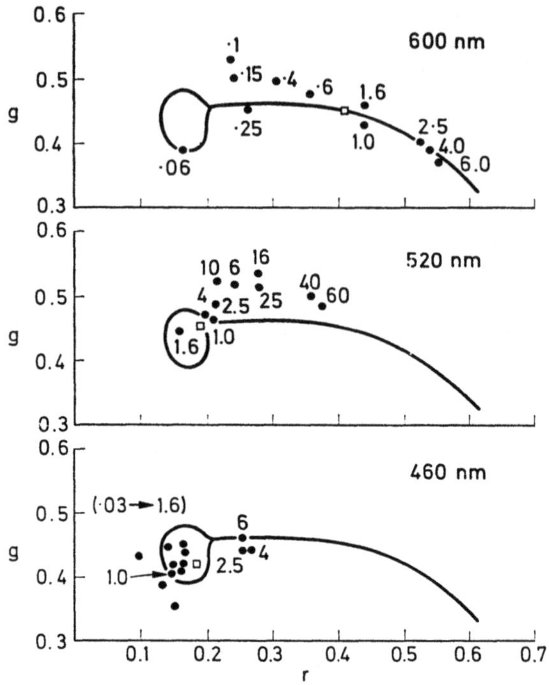

Fig. 5. The change in asymmetric colour matches with illuminance for extrafoveal test stimuli, 600, 520 and 460 nm, at 30 degrees in the lower vertical meridian. The continuous curve is the spectrum locus for this location: the end loop contains matches for the range 420 to 590 nm which are all confused. Unfilled squares are the original matches (for 600, 520, or 460 nm) on the locus. Filled circles are matches made at the relative test illuminances indicated. From Moreland and Cruz (1958)

The ubiquitous effect of local adaptation may also play a significant part in these findings for although measures (see above) were taken for its reduction and control it is doubtful whether it was absent entirely. The effect of exposure time was found to be quite marked for long wavelengths (Moreland, 1955b), and Clarke (1960) has demonstrated significant changes depending on the number of exposures of the test observed prior to a match.

The need for stringent control of luminance in such experiments cannot be over emphasized. In one exploratory experiment at 30 degrees Moreland and Cruz (1958) found (Fig. 5) that the matches for a 600 nm stimulus changed, with a 100 fold change in luminance, over the whole gamut of the spectrum locus established for the 30 troland condition. Matches made on 520 and 460 nm changed in a *similar* sense suggesting that the "dichromatic" condition was maintained in the presence of changing colour responses.

Symmetric Colour Matching[3]. Trichromatic mixture coefficients of the spectrum at 4 degrees extrafoveally were reported by Wright (1946) for a 2 degree bipartite

[3] A generalized description of the conditions governing symmetry and asymmetry in colour matching is given by Wyszecki and Stiles (1967).

field. Compared to normal foveal data he found a reduced negative 650 nm lobe between 460 and 530 nm and an increased negative 460 nm lobe between 530 and 650 nm. GILBERT (1950), using the same apparatus, found that the 4 degree extrafovea became dichromatic at luminances lower than 2 trolands. Using only the blue (460 nm) and red (650 nm) mixture stimuli, she found colour mixture functions which resemble those found later by WRIGHT (1952) in his classic investigation of tritanopia. MORELAND (1955b) repeated these experiments at 10 degrees at a luminance of 30 trolands, separated the test and comparison fields with a gap of 40 min of arc to obtain good resolution, and confirmed the above mentioned trends found by WRIGHT. Colour discrimination at this location was poor however and impeded the ready choice of desaturation stimulus luminances. In changing from excessive to liminal desaturants the calculated chromaticity coordinates changed significantly demonstrating additivity failure. NIMEROFF (1964b) compared MORELAND'S matches on the standard sources A, B and C with those predicted from the colour matching functions obtained with liminal desaturants and found further evidence of additivity failure. CLARKE (1960, 1962) has made an extensive study of additivity failures for extrafoveal vision at 10 degrees under a variety of mesopic conditions for mixtures of paired spectral stimuli. CLARKE separated his test and comparison fields by a space of 80 min of arc when they were small (80×40 min each) but kept them juxtaposed when they were large (10 degree diameter bipartite field). He adopted precautions necessary to reduce and control local adaptation and refined the MORELAND and CRUZ (1958) 20–30-flash match criterion yet further by adopting a match reached between the 27th and 33rd flash. Measurements were made under both dark-adapted and light-adapted conditions. The loci of mixtures of the pairs 430 + 530 nm and of 480 + 650 nm were markedly curved for small fields but not for large fields (Fig. 6) under dark adapted conditions. CLARKE (1960) postulated cone-rod inhibition to account for this curvature. Under light adapted conditions Clarke employed the pairs 440 + 560 nm and 494 + 650 nm whose mixture loci were found to be straight but, as in the case of the large-field dark adapted condition, departures from additivity were still recorded *along* the locus (Fig. 6b). Large fields showed somewhat smaller departures from additivity than did small fields.

An interesting feature of the 494 + 650 nm mixture loci for both large and small fields is the apparent failure to satisfy the condition of retinal symmetry since they do not pass through the chromaticity point (1,0) corresponding to the 650 nm instrumental primary (Fig. 6b). Although anatomical and psychophysical evidence suggests that retinal asymmetry is largely radial, it is not possible to assume that radial division (or separation) of two fields is sufficient to eliminate the effects of asymmetry. Indeed CLARKE concludes that a significant tangential asymmetry is present. It is not known why the effect is manifest in the light- but not dark-adapted condition. It is not found in any of the other above mentioned researches in which the division or separation of the fields is radial. Nor is the effect reported in a determination of colour matching functions by RICHARDS and LURIA (1964) who used a 2 degree field divided *tangentially* at 3.33 degrees extrafoveally (i.e. involving a high degree of asymmetry) and a white surround at mesopic levels. This experiment lacked precision however, due perhaps to inadequate control of local adaptation which may have masked the expected asymmetry. An interesting

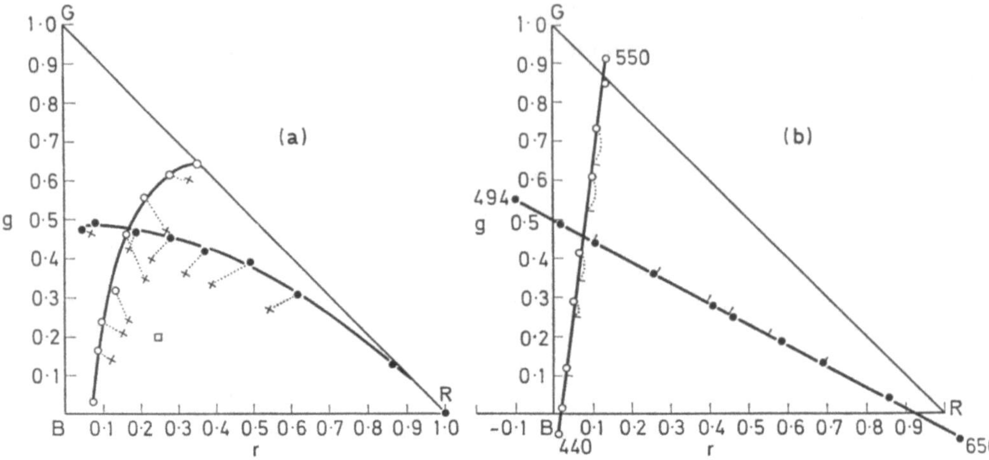

Fig. 6 (*a*) and (*b*). Additivity failure in extrafoveal symmetric colour matching at 10 degree nasally. (*a*) Small fields (80 × 40 min of arc), dark adapted. Mixtures of 430 + 530 nm (unfilled circles) and of 480 + 650 nm (filled circles). Crosses are additive mixtures predicted from the most saturated "all positive" extrafoveal matches. The unfilled square is a possible chromaticity for "rod colour". The primaries *R*, *G* and *B* are 650, 500 and 450 nm respectively and matches are normalised for *B* = *G* at 480 nm and *R* = *G* at 570 nm. (*b*) Large fields (10 degrees diameter), light adapted. Mixtures of 440 + 550 nm (unfilled circles) and of 494 + 650 nm (filled circles). The bars on the straight lines indicate the additive mixtures predicted from the most saturated "all positive" extrafoveal matches. The primaries *R*, *G* and *B* are 650, 530 and 460 nm respectively and matches are normalized on *B* = *G* at 494 nm and *R* = *G* at 582.5 nm. From CLARKE (1962)

result of this experiment is the breakdown of additivity at mesopic levels (0.1 troland) both for the extrafovea and for the fovea. GRIGOROVICI and ARICESCU-SAVOPOL (1958) had made colour matches under similar conditions for 1.6 degree and 9 degree foveally fixated fields and found that matches became effectively dichromatic at about 0.1 troland. These authors found *no differences* between the small- and large-field matches. It seems probable that these results were obtained due to poor fixation at low luminances.

BONGARD *et al.* (1958) claim that, by using four mixing primaries in place of the usual three, large field extrafoveal colour matching functions could be obtained that were stable with changes in luminance and undisturbed therefore by rod intrusion. They do not describe how a *unique* set of matches was obtained from the infinitude possible with four primaries, but TREZONA (1970) has proposed a method of systematically iterating between matches made at two mesopic luminances in such a way that a unique match is finally achieved when rod and cone contributions remain unchanged on changing luminance.

Intensive experiments have been carried out in recent years to define a standard colorimetric observer for large centrally fixated fields. While the prime aim of such work lies outside the scope of this chapter (see WRIGHT, chapter 16, this volume) several important problems are encountered concerning retinal asymmetry, rod intrusion and non-additivity which are of particular interest. Thus it is found that, when a colorimeter field of 10 degrees subtense is centrally fixated,

Maxwell's spot is usually observed and that a match obtained for peripheral regions of the field does not hold near the centre. To overcome this difficulty, STILES' (1955) subjects were instructed to ignore the Maxwell spot while making a match, but SPERANSKAYA (1958, 1959) simply removed a 2 degree diameter area from the centre of the field. NIMEROFF (1964a), on the other hand, made a best-compromise match over the whole field claiming that it was more representative of normal matching practices.

STILES' and SPERANSKAYA'S data were combined and adopted by the CIE (1964) to define a 10 degree standard observer. The colour matching functions of that observer are supposed to be free from the effects of rod intrusion and several devices had to be employed to ensure it. Since the rod mechanism saturates at about 1000 scotopic trolands (AGUILAR and STILES, 1954) it is necessary to use high luminances for a constant scotopic effect. STILES (1955, 1958) used retinal illuminances in the range 20 to 3,000 trolands, and he found it necessary to employ large band widths at the extremes of the spectrum, to substitute a "yellow" mixing primary in place of the "green," to change the "blue" mixing primary from 445 to 471 nm and to add equal amounts of "green" to both sides of the field as occasion demanded to achieve the required illuminance. SPERANSKAYA'S data were obtained at lower levels (1 to 40 trolands) and were corrected for rod intrusion (see STILES and BURCH, 1959) before combination with STILES' results.

When field trials are carried out at the lower levels of luminance typical of every day matching experience, KELLY (1958), STILES and WYSZECKI (1962), and WRIGHT and WYSZECKI (1960) find small but significant discrepancies when actual colour matches made on samples are compared with the predictions of the standard observer. These discrepancies may be due to rod intrusion, non-additivity, population differences, residual errors in the rod-corrected standard observer or other but non-physiological factors.

Specific tests of the additivity principle for individual subjects by CRAWFORD (1965), LOZANO and PALMER (1967, 1968), NIMEROFF (1964b) and STILES (1963) also show significant departures from the law. These tests eliminate population differences, the standard observer and non-physiological factors from the above mentioned list of possible causes of non-additivity in centrally fixated 10 degree fields. (See also LE GRAND, chapter 15, this volume.)

Spectral Sensitivity and Wavelength Discrimination. If fields of 2 degrees or more are viewed extrafoveally under dark adapted conditions spectral sensitivity is found to conform very closely to the scotopic V'_λ function. When fields smaller than 1 degree or an adapting field or surround is used then spectral sensitivity curves with more or less marked secondary peaks are found. Such reports have been made by CLARKE (1960, 1962), KINNEY (1955), MORELAND and CRUZ (1958), SPERLING and HSIA (1957), STILES and CRAWFORD (1933), WEALE (1951b, 1953a) and WRIGHT (1946) who employed a wide variety of techniques. (A detailed discussion of these experiments is beyond the scope of this chapter.)

In all of these studies with one notable exception[4] short wavelengths show enhanced sensitivity with increasing retinal eccentricity or with higher stimulus or

[4] SPERLING and HSIA (1957) used very short duration (0.005 sec) exposures and these are known to depress sensitivity especially at short wavelengths (see IKEDA and BOYNTON, 1962; MORELAND, 1955b).

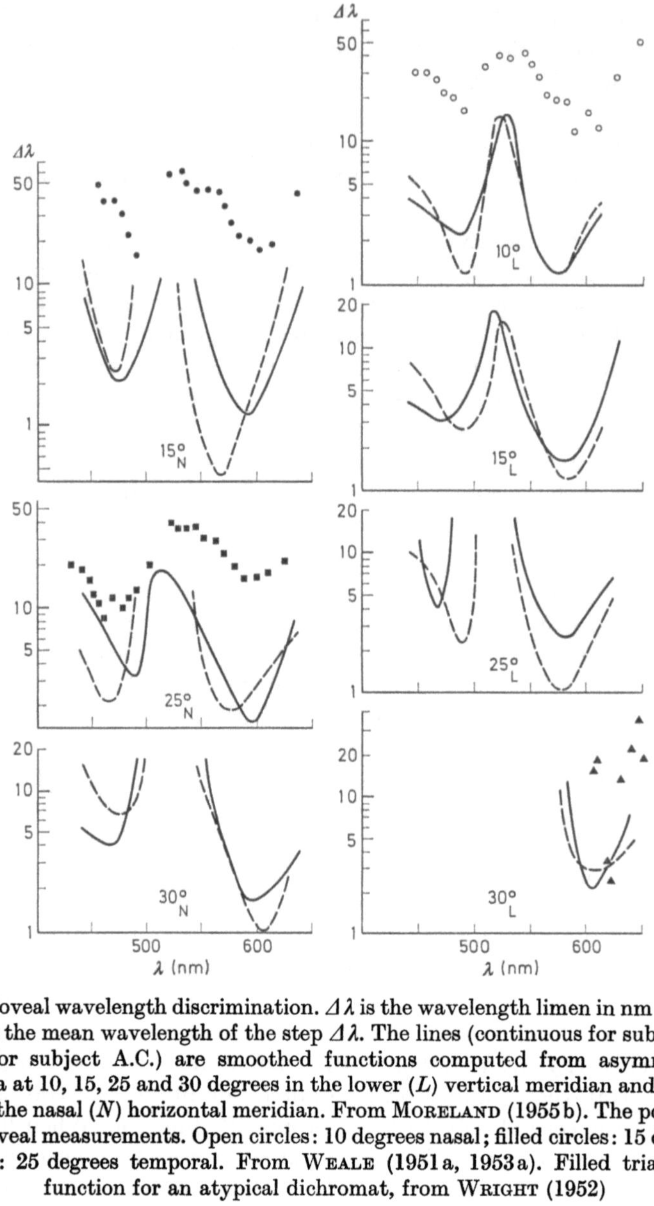

Fig. 7. Extrafoveal wavelength discrimination. $\Delta\lambda$ is the wavelength limen in nm on a logarithmic scale. λ is the mean wavelength of the step $\Delta\lambda$. The lines (continuous for subject J.M. and interrupted for subject A.C.) are smoothed functions computed from asymmetric colour matching data at 10, 15, 25 and 30 degrees in the lower (*L*) vertical meridian and at 15, 25 and 30 degrees in the nasal (*N*) horizontal meridian. From MORELAND (1955b). The points are from direct extrafoveal measurements. Open circles: 10 degrees nasal; filled circles: 15 degrees nasal; filled squares: 25 degrees temporal. From WEALE (1951a, 1953a). Filled triangles: foveal function for an atypical dichromat, from WRIGHT (1952)

adaptation luminances. In particular WEALE (1953b) has reported an enhancement dependant on adaptation for eccentricities greater than 25 degrees thus precluding explanations in terms of macular pigmentation.

HOUGH (1968) investigated the changes in shape of extrafoveal spectral sensitivity at 7 degrees as a function of retinal illuminance and found, at the lower mesopic levels, that the difference curves (between succesive spectral sensitivity curves) approximated the Stiles' π_1 mechanism. (See ENOCH chapter 21, this volume.) An analysis of WALTERS and WRIGHT's (1943) extrafoveal data showed a similar trend and HOUGH concludes that the Purkinje shift is caused partly by rods interacting with the 'blue' cone mechanism.

Extrafoveal wavelength discrimination has been measured by GILBERT (1947, 1950) using a bipartite field at 2 and at 4 degrees and by WEALE (1951 a, 1953 a) using separated fields (for good resolution) at 10, 15, 25 and 45 degrees from the fovea. MORELAND (1955 b) calculated wavelength discrimination functions for 10, 15, 25 and 30 degrees from his two subjects' asymmetric colour matching data by transformation to the so-called uniform chromaticity chart of BRECKENRIDGE and SCHAUB (1939). These functions are shown (after correction for the residual non-uniformity of the chart determined from WRIGHT'S (1943) chromaticity discrimination data) in Fig. 7 together with some of WEALE'S results obtained under similar luminance conditions. In common with GILBERT, these authors found that wavelength discrimination is worst in the region of 520 nm and interpreted it as tritanopia caused by rod intrusion. MORELAND and CRUZ (1958) later withdrew the description "tritanopia" on the grounds that the tritanopic pessimum (see WRIGHT, 1952) was at 460 nm and that their "dichromatic" spectrum locus did not conform to that of tritanopia. At higher luminances where rod intrusion would be less marked, WEALE'S (1953 b) wavelength discrimination maximum at 25 and 45 degrees shows a shift towards longer wavelengths and the whole function conforms closely to extreme protanomaly. He suggests that this is in accord with LE GROS CLARK'S and CHACKO'S (1947) conception of the fusion of the "peripheral" layers of the geniculate nucleus. MORELAND'S calculated wavelength discrimination function do not show protanomaly at such eccentricities and only one of his two subjects (see MORELAND and CRUZ, 1958) shows hue shifts predicted by the fusion hypothesis.

Peripheral Colour Vision of Colour Defectives

In the preceding sections we have been concerned with peripheral colour vision in normals, i.e., foveal trichromats. It is to be hoped that this review will help dispel the (sometimes taught) notion that colour vision resides only in the fovea.

Although NAGEL (1907) discovered that he was a deuteranope on his anomaloscope using a central field of about 3 degrees but a trichromat when this field was increased to more than 10 degrees, this finding is not widely known. The phenomenon was investigated further by JAEGER and KROKER (1952) who, using centrally fixated fields of diameters 1.25 and 22 degrees under daylight conditions, studied a small group of congenital foveal dichromats and found that 2 out of 7 deuteranopes and 3 out of 9 protanopes were trichromatic with the larger field. WALD (1967) has made the interesting commentary that some forms of colour deficiency might result therefore from the invasion of the central retinal zone by the *normally* colour deficient outer peripheral regions. It is also possible that NAGEL'S and perhaps to a lesser extent, JAEGER and KROKER'S finding could have been due to rod intrusion acting as an independant "colour" mechanism.

It is usually assumed that congenital foveal dichromats obey the laws of additivity and their acceptance of trichromatic matches is a point in favour. However GRAHAM and HSIA (1958 a, b) found that the mixture coefficients for a unilateral dichromat depended to a marked degree on the amount of desaturant mixed with short wavelength test lights. This indicates a breakdown of additivity and merits further investigation. In more recent work on acquired unilateral tritanopia Graham *et al.* (1967), using their binocular hue-matching technique wherein the unaffected normal eye is used for comparison, find that matches change with test luminance. In this instance the presumptive test area was within a retinal lesion some 18 degrees across and about 5 degrees out from the presumptive fovea. Under these conditions changes of colour with luminance are to be expected. Especial care is required to determine whether fixation is indeed foveal for eyes in which the cone function is residual and rod activity invades the presumptive fovea (Blackwell and Blackwell, 1961; Sloan, 1954).

In one case of so-called incomplete rod monochromacy, Fuortes *et al.* (1961) and Siegel *et al.* (1966) have shown that, for low test luminances under dark adapted conditions, fixation was consistently 4 degrees on the nasal side of the fovea, but at photopic luminances fixation was precisely foveal (i.e., coincident with the foveal reflex). Rushton (1961) could not detect any pigment in this monochromat's fovea, but rhodopsin in the periphery was normal in amount and in rate of regeneration. Fuortes *et al.* (1961) measured the increment threshold at 7 degrees and found that it coincided with that for normal rods (Aguilar and Stiles, 1954). At 1,000 trolands, the monochromat's rod mechanism saturated as for the normal but all perception of contrast was lost. They concluded that, since the spectral sensitivity of the background that just saturates was that of rhodopsin, the abolition of rod function in both monochromats and normals by bright backgrounds is *not* due to inhibition of rods by cones. Siegel *et al.* (1966) measured the extrafoveal spectral sensitivity function of this monochromat by the increment threshold on a white field at 7 degrees. It showed no change in shape on changing the field from zero to 0.55 mL whereas the same functions for a normal subject showed marked changes and especially an enhanced relative sensitivity at short wavelengths. This finding differs from the results obtained by Blackwell and Blackwell (1961) for a "blue-cone" monochromat.

Hough and Ruddock (1969a, b) measured the spectral sensitivity functions of a tritanope by the method of flicker photometry at 7 degrees from the fovea, and colour matching data were obtained for the fovea (symmetric technique) and also for the extrafovea at 6 degrees (asymmetric technique with foveal comparison). The Purkinje shift for the tritanope became manifest only at 200 photopic trolands, lagging considerably behind that for the normal. Since at absolute threshold there is no difference between the normal and the tritanope for test wavelengths shorter than 510 nm, Hough and Ruddock deduce that below the "blue cone" threshold the tritanopic rod response is normal but above it inhibition of rods by the "blue" mechanism occurs. A simple additive theory of rod intrusion at mesopic levels successfully described the differences between foveal and extrafoveal colour matches made by the tritanope.

Blackwell and Blackwell (1961) have suggested that inhibition of rods by "blue cones" occurs in their "blue-cone" monochromats and Trezona (1970), in a review of rod participation in the "blue" mechanism claims that all the evidence, for and against the idea that rods elicit a blue sensation under photopic conditions, can be reconciled if rods and "blue" cones were discrete receptors sharing one neural pathway.

References

ABNEY, W. DE W.: Researches in Colour Vision. London: Longmans, Green 1913.

AGUILAR, M., STILES, W. S.: Saturation of the rod mechanism of the retina at high levels of stimulation. Optica Acta **1**, 59—65 (1954).

BÄUML, J., ENGELHARDT, A.: Das Sehen von Buntfarben in der Netzhautperipherie. Z. Biol. **104**, 307—334 (1950).

BAIRD, J. W.: Colour sensitivity of the peripheral retina. Publication No. 29, Washington: Carnegie Institution (1905).

BLACKWELL, H. R., BLACKWELL, O. M.: Rod and cone receptor mechanisms in typical and atypical congenital achromatopsia. Vision Res. **1**, 62—107 (1961).

BONGARD, M. M., SMIRNOV, M. S., FRIEDRICK, L.: The four-dimensional colour space of the extrafoveal retinal area of the human eye. In: Visual Problems of Colour, Vol. 1, pp. 325—330. London: H. M. Stationery Office 1958.

BOYNTON, R. M., SCHAFER, W., NEUN, M. A.: Hue-wavelength relation measured by color-naming method for three retinal locations. Science **146**, 666—668 (1964).

— SCHEIBNER, H.: On the perception of red by "red-blind" observers. Acta Chromatica **1**, 205—220 (1967).

BRECKENRIDGE, F. C., SCHAUB, W. R.: Rectangular uniform-chromaticity scale co-ordinates. J. opt. Soc. Amer. **29**, 370—380 (1939).

CIE Proc. (1963) Vienna: Paris Bureau Central CIE 1964.

CLARKE, F. J. J.: Rapid light adaptation of localized areas of the extrafoveal retina. Optica Acta **4**, 69—77 (1957).

— Extra-foveal colour metrics. Optica Acta **7**, 355—384 (1960).

— Further studies of extra-foveal colour metrics. Optica Acta **10**, 257—284 (1962).

— BELCHER, S. J.: On the localisation of Troxler's effect in the visual pathway. Vision Res. **2**, 53—68 (1962).

CRAWFORD, B. H.: Colour matching and adaptation. Vision Res. **5**, 71—78 (1965).

CRUZ, A. C., MORELAND, J. D.: Small field tritanomaly in peripheral vision. Farbe **4**, 241—245 (1955).

DOESSCHATE, J. TEN: Visual acuity and distribution of percipient elements on the retina. Ophthalmologica (Basel) **112**, 1—18 (1946a).

— Acuity of vision in connection with the distribution of the percipient elements over the retina. Ophthalmologica (Basel) **112**, 159 (1946b).

— Extra-foveal scotopic absolute threshold and the distribution of retinal rods. Ophthalmologica (Basel) **117**, 110—115 (1949).

DREHER, E.: Methodische Untersuchung der Farbentonänderungen homogener Lichter bei zunehmender Intensität. Z. Sinnesphysiol. **46**, 1—82 (1911).

FULTON, J. F.: Physiology of the Nervous System. New York: Oxford University Press 1949.

FUORTES, M. G. F., GUNKEL, R. D., RUSHTON, W. A. H.: Increment thresholds in a subject deficient in cone vision. J. Physiol. (Lond.) **156**, 179—192 (1961).

GILBERT, M.: Colour perception in extra-foveal vision. Ph. D. Thesis, University of London, 1947.

— Colour perception in parafoveal vision. Proc. phys. Soc. (Lond.) B **63**, 83—89 (1950).

GRAHAM, C. H., HSIA, Y.: Some visual functions of a unilaterally dichromatic subject. In: Visual Problems of Colour Vol. 1, pp. 279—295. London: H. M. Stationery Office 1958a.

— — Color defect and color theory. Science **127**, 675—682 (1958b).

— — STEPHAN, F. F.: Visual discriminations of a subject with acquired unilateral tritanopia. Vision Res. **6**, 469—479 (1967).

GRIGOROVICI, R., ARICESCU-SAVOPOL, I.: Luminosity and chromaticity in the mesopic range. J. opt. Soc. Amer. **48**, 891—898 (1958).

HARRISON, E. R.: Visual acuity and the cone cell distribution of the retina. Brit. J. Ophthal. **37**, No. 9, 538—542 (1953).

HESS, C. VON: Über den Farbensinn bei indirektem Sehen. Graefes Arch. Ophthal. **35**, 1—42 (1889).

HOLMES, G.: The organization of the visual cortex in man. Proc. roy. Soc. (Lond.) B **132**, 348—361 (1945).

HOLMES, G., LISTER, W. T.: Disturbances of vision from cerebral lesions with special reference to the cortical representation of the macula. Brain **39**, 34—73 (1916).
HOUGH, E. A.: The spectral sensitivity functions for parafoveal vision. Vision Res. 8, 1423—1430 (1968).
— RUDDOCK, K. H.: The Purkinje shift. Vision Res. **9**, 313—315 (1969a).
— — The parafoveal visual response of a tritanope and an interpretation of the V_λ sensitivity functions of mesopic vision. Vision Res. **9**, 935—946 (1969b).
HUNT, R. W. G.: The effects of daylight and tungsten light adaptation on color perception. J. opt. Soc. Amer. **40**, 362—370 (1950).
— The perception of color in 1° fields for different states of adaptation. J. opt. Soc. Amer. **43**, 479—484 (1953).
IKEDA, M., BOYNTON, R. M.: Effect of test-flash duration upon the spectral sensitivity of the eye. J. opt. Soc. Amer. **52**, 697—699 (1962).
JAEGER, W., KROKER, K.: Über das Verhalten der Protanopen und Deuteranopen bei großen Reizflächen. Klin. Mbl. Augenheilk. **121**, 445—449 (1952).
JAMESON, D., HURVICH, L. M.: Fixation-light bias: an unwanted by-product of fixation control. Vision Res. **7**, 805—809 (1967).
KANEKO, T.: A study of rapid declining processes of color sensation. Acta Chromatica **1**, 156—163 (1965).
KELLY, K. L.: Observer differences in colour-mixture functions studied by means of metameric grays. J. Res. nat. Bur. Stand. (Wash.) **60**, 97—103 (1958).
KINNEY, J. A. S.: Sensitivity of the eye to spectral radiation at scotopic and mesopic intensity levels. J. opt. Soc. Amer. **45**, 507—514 (1955).
KRAVKOV, S. V.: Colour vision and the autonomous nervous system. J. opt. Soc. Amer. **31**, 335—337 (1941).
LAKOWSKI, R., ASPINALL, P. A.: Static perimetry in young children. Vision Res. **9**, 305—312 (1969).
LE GROS CLARK, W. E., CHACKO, L.: A possible central mechanism for colour vision. Nature (Lond.) **160**, 123—124 (1947).
LOZANO, R. D., PALMER, D. A.: The additivity of large field colour matching functions. Vision Res. **7**, 929—937 (1967).
— — Large-field colour matching and adaptation. J. opt. Soc. Amer. **58**, 1653—1656 (1968).
LYTHGOE, R. J.: Dark adaptation and the peripheral colour sensations of normal subjects. Brit. J. Ophthal. **15**, 193—210 (1931).
MCCREE, K. J.: Colour confusion produced by voluntary fixation. Optica Acta **7**, 281—290 (1960a).
— Small field tritanopia and the effects of voluntary fixation. Optica Acta **7**, 317—323 (1960b).
MARTIN, L. C., WARBURTON, F. L., MORGAN, W. J.: The determination of the sensitiveness of the eye to differences in the saturation of colours. Spec. Rep. Ser. No. 188, pp. 1—42. Med. Res. Coun. (Lond.) 1933.
MORELAND, J. D.: Modifications of the Wright trichromatic colorimeter for extrafoveal and peripheral observations. Optica Acta **2**, 101—104 (1955a).
— The perception of colour by extrafoveal and peripheral vision. Ph. D. Thesis. University of London, 1955b.
— Threshold measurements of the blue arcs phenomenon. Vision Res. 8, 1093—1106 (1968).
— Possible mechanisms of the blue arcs of the retina. J. Physiol. (Lond.) **201**, 60—61P. (1969a).
— The distribution of dendritic domains of retinal neurones. Vision Res. **9**, 529—535 (1969b).
— Retinal topography and the blue arcs phenomenon. Vision Res. **9**, 965—976 (1969c).
— Selectivity in two retinal staining techniques. Vision Res. **10**, 205—206 (1970).
— CRUZ, A. C.: Colour perception with the peripheral retina. Optica Acta **6**, 117—151 (1958).
NAGEL, W. A.: Neue Erfahrungen über das Farbensehen der Dichromaten auf großem Felde. Z. Sinnesphysiol. **41**, 319—337 (1907).
NEWHALL, S. M.: The constancy of the blue arc phenomenon. J. opt. Soc. Amer. **27**, 165—176 (1937).
NIMEROFF, I.: Colorimetry in parafoveal fields. I. Color-matching functions. J. opt. Soc. Amer. **54**, 824—832 (1964a).

Nimeroff, I.: Colorimetry in parafoveal fields. II. Additivity failure. J. opt. Soc. Amer. **54**, 833—838 (1964b).

Østerberg, G.: Topography of the layer of rods and cones in the human retina. Acta Ophthal. (Kbh.) Suppl. **6**, 76—102 (1935).

Polyak, S. L.: The Retina. Chicago: Chicago University Press 1941.

Priest, I. G., Brickwedde, F. G.: The minimum perceptible colorimetric purity as a function of dominant wavelength. J. opt. Soc. Amer. **28**, 133—139 (1938).

Richards, W., Luria, S. M.: Color-mixture functions at low luminance levels. Vision Res. **4**, 281—313 (1964).

Rinde, C. A.: Retinal chromatic fields as a function of wavelength. J. opt. Soc. Amer. **22**, 333—356 (1932).

Rushton, W. A. H.: Rhodopsin measurement and dark adaptation in a subject deficient in cone vision. J. Physiol. (Lond.) **156**, 193—205 (1961).

— Campbell, F. W., Hagins, W. A., Brindley, G. S.: The bleaching and regeneration of rhodopsin in the living eye of the albino rabbit and of man. Optica Acta **1**, 183—190 (1955).

Siegel, I. M., Graham, C. H., Ripps, H., Hsia, Y.: Analysis of photopic and scotopic function in an incomplete achromat. J. opt. Soc. Amer. **56**, 699—704 (1966).

Sloan, L. L.: Congenital achromatopsia: A report of 19 cases. J. opt. Soc. Amer. **44**, 117—128 (1954).

Speranskaya, N. I.: Methods of determination of the co-ordinates of spectrum colours. In: In: Visual Problems of Colour, Vol. I, pp. 317—323. London: H. M. Stationery Office 1958.

— Determination of spectrum color co-ordinates for 27 normal observers (translation). Optics and Spectroscopy **7**, 424—428 (1959).

Sperling, H. G., Hsia, Y.: Some comparisons among spectral sensitivity data obtained in different retinal locations and with two sizes of foveal stimulus. J. opt. Soc. Amer. **47**, 707—713 (1957).

Stiles, W. S.: The basic data of colour-matching. Phys. Soc. Year Book (Lond.), pp. 44—65 (1955).

— The average colour matching functions for a large matching field. In: Visual Problems of Colour, Vol. 1, pp. 211—247. London: H.M. Stationery Office 1958.

— NPL colour-matching investigation: addendum on additivity. Optica Acta **10**, 229—232 (1963).

— Burch, J. M.: NPL colour-matching investigation, final report. Optica Acta **6**, 1—26 (1959).

— Crawford, B. H.: The liminal brightness increment as a function of wavelength for different conditions of the foveal and parafoveal retina. Proc. roy. Soc. (Lond.) B **113**, 496—530 (1933).

— Wyszecki, G.: Field trials of color-mixture functions. J. opt. Soc. Amer. **52**, 58—75 (1962).

Thomson, L. C.: Sensations aroused by monochromatic stimuli and their prediction. Optica Acta **1**, 93—102 (1954).

— Wright, W. D.: The colour sensitivity of the retina within the central fovea of man. J. Physiol. (Lond.) **105**, 316—331 (1947).

Trezona, P. W.: Rod participation in the 'blue' mechanism and its effect on colour matching. Vision Res. **10**, 317—332 (1970).

Troxler, D.: Über das Verschwinden gegebener Gegenstände innerhalb unseres Gesichtskreises. In: Ophthalm. Bibliothek. II. pp. 51—53. Himly and Schmidt. (Eds.) Jena: 1804.

Verriest, G., Israel, A.: Application du perimetre statique de Goldmann au relève topographique des seuils differentiels de luminance pour de petits objets colorés projetés sur un fond blanc. Vision Res. **5**, 151—174 (1965).

Vilter, V.: Récherches biométriques sur l'organisation synaptique de la rétine humaine. C.R. Soc. Biol. (Paris) **143**, 830—832 (1949).

Volk, D., Fry, G. A.: Effect of quality of illumination and distance of observations upon performance in the Ishihara test. Amer. J. Optom. **24**, 99—122 (1947).

Wald, G.: Blue-blindness in the normal fovea. J. opt. Soc. Amer. **57**, 1289—1301 (1967).

Walters, H. V., Wright, W. D.: The spectral sensitivity of the fovea and extra-fovea in the Purkinje range. Proc. roy. Soc. (Lond.) B **131**, 340—361 (1943).

Weale, R. A.: Hue-discrimination in para-central parts of the human retina measured at different luminance levels. J. Physiol. (Lond.) **113**, 115—122 (1951a).
— The foveal and para-central spectral sensitivities in man. J. Physiol. (Lond.) **114**, 435—446 (1951b).
— Spectral sensitivity and wavelength discrimination of the peripheral retina. J. Physiol. (Lond.) **119**, 170—190 (1953a).
— Colour vision in the peripheral retina. Brit. med. Bull. **9**, 55—60 (1953b).
— Problems of peripheral vision. Brit. J. Ophthal. **40**, 392—415 (1956).
Weitzman, D. O., Kinney, J. A. S.: Effect of stimulus size, duration, and retinal location upon the appearance of color. J. opt. Soc. Amer. **59**, 640—643 (1969).
Weymouth, F.: Visual sensory units and the minimum angle of resolution. Amer. J. Ophthal. **46**, 102—113 (1958).
Wilmer, E. N., Wright, W. D.: Colour sensitivity of the fovea centralis. Nature (Lond.) **156**, 119—121 (1945).
Wright, H., Wyszecki, G.: Field trials of 10° color-mixture functions. J. opt. Soc. Amer. **50**, 647—650 (1960).
Wright, W. D.: The graphical representation of small color differences. J. opt. Soc. Amer. **33**, 632—636 (1943).
— Researches on Normal and Defective Colour Vision. London: Kimpton 1946.
— Photometry and the Eye. London: Hatton Press 1949.
— The characteristics of tripanopia. J. opt. Soc. Amer. **42**, 509—521 (1952).
— Pitt, F. H. G.: The saturation-discrimination of two trichromats. Proc. phys. Soc. (Lond.) **49**, 329—331 (1937).
Wyszecki, G.: Reanalysis of the NRC field trials of color-matching functions. J. opt. Soc. Amer. **54**, 710—714 (1964).
— Stiles, W. S.: Color Science. New York: Wiley 1967.
Yakovlev, P. A.: The influence of acoustic stimuli upon the limits of visual fields for different colours. J. opt. Soc. Amer. **28**, 286—289 (1938).

Chapter 21

The Two-Color Threshold Technique of Stiles and Derived Component Color Mechanisms

By

JAY M. ENOCH, St. Louis, Missouri (USA)

With 10 Figures

Contents

Introduction

In order to understand color vision mechanisms, it is necessary to learn how visual stimuli are coded for neural transmission and the nature of data processing at different points along the visual pathway. In quest of a solution to at least part of this difficult problem, STILES has experimentally and theoretically defined a set of color response functions (π functions) through the application of a classical psychophysical technique. Here, an attempt will be made to describe these functions as well as to bring together what is known about their characteristics.

The systematic nature of the approach, the elegance of the analysis, the diversity of questions asked, and the broad application of these studies to a whole range of visual problems make the study of these properties important as an experimental model. In this context, the student will find Chapter IV in BRINDLEY'S book, "Physiology of the Retina and the Visual Pathway" (1960) a stimulating discussion.

In Chapter 4, BLACKWELL discusses the general topic of brightness discrimination. In such studies one determines the just perceptible energy increment of a small test stimulus which is generally superimposed on a larger background field.

This experimental design appears in visual psychophysics under many names, e.g., intensity discrimination, increment threshold, contrast threshold, just noticeable difference threshold, static perimetric threshold, (and plotted in a somewhat different manner) the Weber fraction, etc. In such experiments the observer indicates whether he has or has not *detected* the test stimulus. The subject need not report the subjectively appreciated characteristics of the stimulus. Rather, he merely has to use a consistent response criterion. This technique is of great value in many experiments, because a threshold level stimulus minimally disturbs the response characteristic which is being studied. The response to the test flash largely reflects the properties of the retinal area investigated (and its subsequent elaborations along the visual pathways) as conditioned or adapted by the background field.

The experimental criterion of "mere detection" on the part of the observer can be extended from the classical discrimination experiment to include the use of background and incremental stimuli[1] of different spectral compositions or colors. This is the essential innovation of the two-color threshold technique. *Assuming the presence of more than one color vision mechanism,* STILES *sought to isolate or reveal the individual color components by selectively reducing the sensitivity (or influence) of competing mechanisms.* He used one wavelength for the background or adapting field, and a different wavelength for the threshold test flash. As will be shown, the validity of inferences from the results depends in the acceptance of certain assumptions and the development of interesting experimental and analytical strategies. While the key analysis appeared in STILES' (1939) paper, measurements by a two-color technique were reported earlier in papers by ROAF (1932), and STILES and CRAWFORD (1933a).

The stimulus pattern used by STILES (1939) is shown in Fig. 1. A small 1° square test field was superimposed on a larger (10° diameter) conditioning, background or adapting field.

λ = wavelength of the test field.

μ = wavelength of the conditioning or adapting field.

N_λ = threshold radiance measurement[2] of the test field at wavelength λ expressed in quanta/sec deg².

M_μ = radiance[2] of the background, conditioning, or adapting field set at wavelength μ and expressed in quanta/sec deg².

The principle is demonstrated in Fig. 2a. For the sake of the argument, the reader is asked to accept the notion that more than one color response process or mechanism may be defined. STILES designated derived processes with „pi" numbers (p for process, π for p). If the observer was first dark adapted, central fixation established, and the background field not exposed ($M_\mu = 0$, the "zero field" condition), the foveal threshold may be determined for different wavelength stimuli (N_λ). The filled dots at the bottom of Fig. 2a represent such a set of data obtained on one of STILES' observers. Superimposed on these data points are drawn three of

[1] STILES prefers the term increment threshold when describing his work because the test and background fields he used were usually of different wavelengths and more than just a brightness change was at issue.

[2] In early studies radiance was expressed in terms of ergs/sec deg².

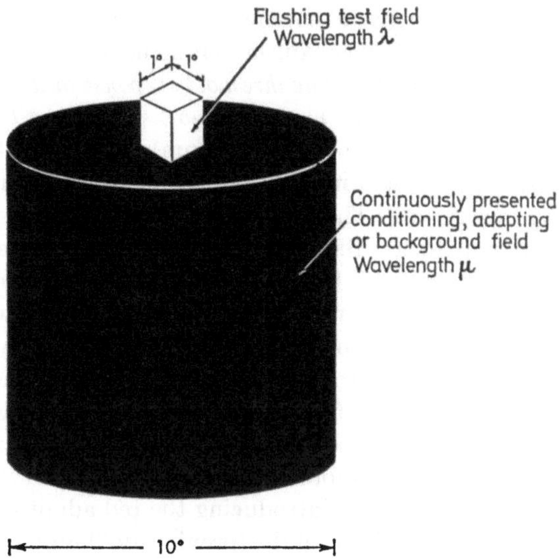

Fig. 1. The stimulus display employed in studies of the two-color threshold technique is shown in this figure. The radiance of the large background adapting field is designated as M_{μ}, and the threshold radiance of the smaller test field is indicated by the symbol N_{λ}

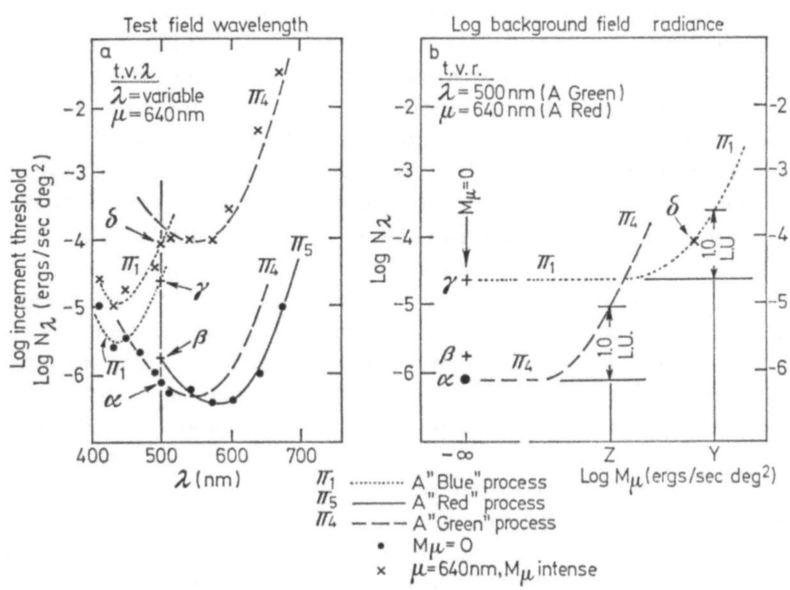

Fig. 2. a. This figure includes two sets of *t.v.λ.* data taken from STILES (1949). Superimposed on the data points are separately derived component color (π) functions. $\alpha = N_{500\,\mathrm{nm}}$ when $M_{640\,\mathrm{nm}} = 0$. $\delta = N_{500\,\mathrm{nm}}$ when $M_{640\,\mathrm{nm}}$ was intense. β and γ represent the spectral sensitivities of π_5 and π_1 at $\lambda = 500$ nm when $M_{640\,\mathrm{nm}} = 0$. These latter two values are not revealed in the data presented in Fig. 2a. b. This part of the figure is a hypothetical *t.v.r.* plot paralleling data obtained in part a of this figure. Points α and δ are the same values as are seen in part a. α, β, and γ represent absolute threshold values of π_4, π_5, and π_1 respectively at $\lambda = 500$ nm. Points Y and Z are values of log M_{μ} derived for plotting on a *f.v.μ.* data format.

Stiles' derived color response functions, π_1, a "blue" mechanism; π_4, a "green" mechanism; and π_5, a "red" mechanism. These have been defined on the basis of many experimental procedures. *The threshold response at any given wavelength λ is determined by whichever response process is most sensitive at that wavelength.*

If an intense red stimulus (e.g., $\mu = 640$ nm) is used for the large conditioning or adapting field, it may be assumed that it will substantially reduce the sensitivity of the "red" π_5 mechanism. The individual mechanisms respond to stimulation over a broad spectral band. Because of considerable overlap of π_4 and π_5, the "green" π_4 mechanism will also be affected to a considerable degree by adaptation to a red background field. However, this adapting field should only reduce "blue" sensitivity (π_1) slightly. This is precisely what happened. The increment-threshold data obtained on this subject for the intense red background stimulus condition are shown by the x symbols. After adaptation to this background, the "red" π_5 mechanism can no longer be detected, the threshold measurements defining the "green" π_4 mechanism rose by more than two log units, and the "blue" π_1 function was only minimally affected. By introducing the red adapting field more information was obtained about the shape of the (previously "hidden") π_1 and π_4 functions. Hence, by selectively chromatically adapting a retinal area, a great deal of information regarding the contributing response functions was elicited. Obviously, many combinations of background and test wavelengths were needed in order to define the individual mechanisms. It was necessary to learn how and under what conditions the individual processes were translated, and techniques had to be developed to further reveal the individual characteristics of the π mechanisms. Effects of stimulus level, test flash area, summation properties of the mechanisms, the stability of these properties in different retinal areas, interactions between mechanisms, and so forth, had to be explored. In turn, attempts had to be made to locate the derived relationships in the visual system, and to consider response anomalies. Many questions regarding these properties remain as yet unresolved.

Before proceeding with the analysis, let us more completely define the experiment. In this chapter only "steady state" conditions are considered, that is, following initial dark adaptation, the observer was adapted fully to the background field. By this means, transient effects were minimized and the system allowed to achieve a state of equilibrium. This is not a minor consideration. In the experiment from which Fig. 2a was derived (Stiles, 1949), data were also obtained from measurements of the increment threshold, N_λ, two seconds after the intense red adapting field was turned off. At that time the π_5 "red" mechanism exhibited rapid recovery, the π_4 "green" showed some recovery of sensitivity, but the π_1 "blue" dramatically lost sensitivity and could not be discerned in the resultant data (Stiles, 1949, 1953a). Boynton and his co-workers (1956, 1959) have studied transients of these mechanisms which occur at the onset of a stimulus.

Stiles flashed the test field for 63 msec every 3.6 seconds; the background was continuously exposed, and the observer responded to each presentation. In most experiments the test and background stimuli were centered on the fovea, and the 1° test flash therefore fell in the rod-free area. In later experiments 0.2 sec test flash was employed.

The test field size exceeded the small central foveal "fixation" area; the latter is known to be relatively insensitive to short wavelengths and it is necessary to avoid this bias. Outside of the test field area a pattern of small dim lights helped to direct fixation centrally or eccentrically (as desired). Test flashes were separated sufficiently in time to prevent one threshold level test flash stimulus from significantly influencing the following presentation. The use of a large conditioning or background field (10°) reduced the effect of border interactions, and small eye movements did not alter retinal adaptation in the test area.

Refractive correction, accommodation, and pupil size were controlled. A Maxwellian field was used and careful control of point of entry of the beams in the entrance pupil was maintained. In selected experiments the effect of varying the point of entry in the pupil was determined. (STILES and CRAWFORD, 1933b; STILES, 1939.)

Data Formats

In the experiment as defined there are three independent variables and one dependent variable, the test field increment threshold, N_λ.

$$N_\lambda = f(M_\mu, \mu, \lambda) .$$

The following three different data formats have been used in exploring these relations:

1. Log N_λ has been determined as a function of λ for a fixed value of μ and M_μ. This is the *threshold versus wavelength curve* = *t.v.λ.*

2. Log N_λ has been measured as a function of log M_μ for fixed values of λ and μ. The resultant relation is known as a *threshold versus radiance curve* = *t.v.r.* (In earlier publications this was called a *t.v.i.* curve where i stood for *intensity*.)

3. Log M_μ has been varied with μ. In these studies λ was fixed at a given wavelength and M_μ was the experimentally determined value of the background (known as the *field radiance*) needed to raise the increment threshold (log N_λ) to some fixed multiple of its value when $M_\mu = 0$. This technique provides functions known as *field radiance versus field wavelength curves* = *f.v.μ.*

The first of these three data formats, the *t.v.λ.*, as sampled in Fig. 2a, is quite straightforward. One merely sets the background at a wavelength μ, and its radiance at M_μ, and determines the threshold log N_λ at various wavelength settings (λ) of the test field. Of course, when $M_\mu = 0$, log N_λ depends only on λ and the parameters defining the test stimulus.

The other two forms of data presentation require some consideration. Fig. 2b shows a hypothetical set of data derived from the same observer. It is plotted as a *t.v.r.* curve. Here the wavelengths of the test field (500 nm) and the background (640 nm) were fixed, and the radiance of the background or adapting field was increased from zero to an intense level in successive steps. Two points, α and δ on the *t.v.r.* curve as drawn in Fig. 2b can be taken from the two corresponding points which appear in Fig. 2a at $\lambda = 500$ nm (see arrows). In Fig. 2a the effect of the background set at $\mu = 640$ nm was sampled across the spectrum, in Fig. 2b the same background was used, only here the effect of varying its radiance was determined. The resultant effect on test flash threshold (log N_λ) was measured. When considering this type of format, it is useful for the reader to pause and mentally reconstruct the stimulus array. That is, given mechanisms π_a, π_b, π_c, given test flash wavelength 500 nm, a green, and a background wavelength of 640 nm, a red, one asks which mechanism will be most sensitive when the background is zero or insignificant, which mechanisms will most probably be affected as $M_{640\,\mathrm{nm}}$ is increased, etc.? Because $M_{640\,\mathrm{nm}}$ is plotted as the logarithm, there is a break at the foot of the function (Fig. 2b) and along the abscissa for the log $M_\mu = -\infty$ or

$M_\mu = 0$ case, which is merely the absolute threshold value of log N_λ. When M_μ is set at low level, the adapting field has little effect, and measured values of log N_λ tend to asymptote towards the absolute threshold.

The curves in Fig. 2b are similar to those obtained in any number of experiments designed to establish the duplicity theory of vision, i.e., a break occurs in the measured function as a second response mechanism supercedes a first as the most sensitive when background radiance is increased. In duplicity theory, photopic mechanisms (cones) take over from the scotopic system (rods). Here a similar transition occurs, one color response mechanism takes over from another with increasing background radiance. This can be predicted from the description of Fig. 2a. When the test field wavelength $\lambda = 500$ nm, in the dark adapted state (when $M_{640\,\text{nm}} = 0$) π_4, a "green" mechanism, is most sensitive. The red adapting field acts most effectively on the "red" π_5 mechanism, but also substantially on the "green" π_4 mechanism. As $M_{640\,\text{nm}}$ is increased, it reduces the sensitivity of the "green" π_4 mechanism more rapidly than the "blue" π_1 component, and at some point on the log $M_{640\,\text{nm}}$ scale, π_1 becomes the most sensitive mechanism. This gives rise to the break in the function (Fig. 2b). If this stimulus display were displaced into the parafoveal region, a third "rod" component would appear at the *lower end* of the function in Fig. 2b. For certain combinations of blackground and test field wavelengths, it is also possible to show a third cone component in a *t.v.r.* plot.

The individual curves comprising the *t.v.r.* functions are the same as those found in studies of the just detectable increment threshold determined as a function of background luminance or radiance when $\lambda = \mu$. Such curves may have three basic parts as seen in Fig. 3, left ordinate scale. This relation was taken from a paper by AGUILAR and STILES (1954), and represents rod or scotopic data. STILES refers to the scotopic mechanism as π_0.

As indicated, the "foot" of this function asymptotes towards the absolute threshold, as the adapting field exerts less and less influence on the measurement of N_λ. The middle or rising portion of the curve has been classically fitted by the Weber fraction[3], as defined in the works of the pioneering psychophysicists, WEBER and FECHNER. In this part of the curve,

$$\frac{N_\lambda}{M_\mu} = \text{constant.}^4$$

(In Fig. 3 the ordinate and abscissa are expressed in terms of retinal illuminance rather than radiance.[5]) Cross multiplying and rewriting this simple relation in logarithmic terms, one obtains a simple straight line on a log-log plot. To conform with classical studies of the Weber function, the reference constant for each π function is determined for the test situation where $\lambda = \mu$ (see Table 1).

The justification for applying this same concept in a situation where $\lambda \neq \mu$ must be based on the notion that one mechanism is being considered at a time, and

[3] Several authors, including STILES, term this the Fechner fraction. It has its origin in the work of WEBER.

[4] Or at least these values approximate a constant.

[5] This would alter the resultant constant somewhat because of the unequal multiplicative factors which would enter the numerator and the denominator in the radiometric to photometric conversion (in this instance based on the V'_λ curve) when $\lambda \neq \mu$. (See LE GRAND, chapter 15, this volume.) However, since these in turn are constants (for given values of λ and μ), there is no need to complicate the discussion.

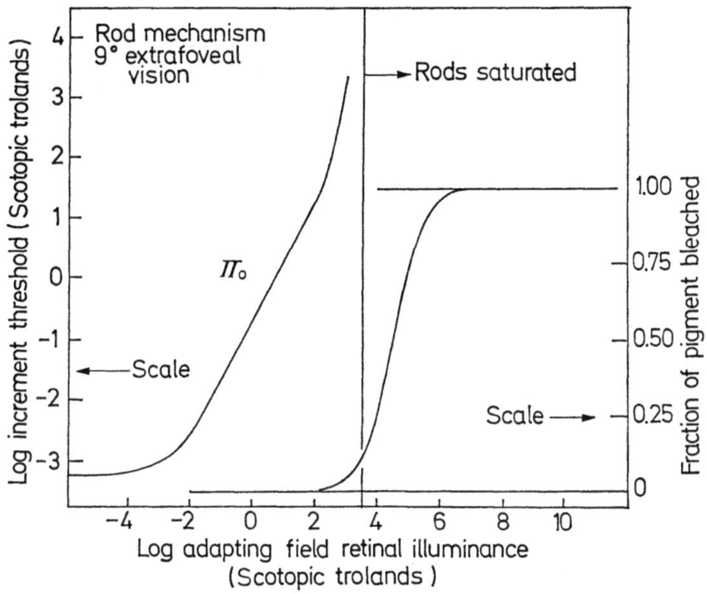

Fig. 3. This illustration is adapted from a paper by AGUILAR and STILES (1954). The increment threshold of the scotopic visual system is measured (at a point 9° from the fovea) as a function of background field retinal illuminance. The background field ranged from 0 to 1000 scotopic trolands. The curve to the left clearly has three separate portions, a "foot" where the threshold approaches a constant (the absolute threshold), a linear rising portion where the ratio of threshold/background approximates a constant, and finally a more sharply rising component where the threshold approaches infinity. The reader is referred to the original paper for details of the technique used to obtain this function. — To the right, RUSHTON's rhodopsin bleaching data are expressed as a function of retinal illuminance (1956, 1958a, 1959). The curve is based on the assumption that rhodopsin obeys the laws of a first order photochemical reaction. When the increment threshold approaches infinity (left hand curve), this means the response system is saturating, that is, it is losing the ability to make additional discriminations. This occurs in the scotopic system when only a small fraction of the available rhodopsin pigment has been bleached. The effective response of the scotopic system ranges from reaction to single molecules being bleached in a few rods scattered in a finite area, to a state where approximately 100,000 molecules or a bit more are bleached in each rod.

that varying either λ or μ only results in translation or displacement of the curve on a log-log plot rather than an alteration in its shape. That is, the slope of the linear mid-section of the curve in Fig. 3, left, is a property of the mechanism, and the position of the curve on the graph is a property of the stimulus conditions (see section on displacement rules below).

Each of the π mechanisms has a series of identifying properties, e.g., its spectral sensitivity, and its Weber fraction. In addition, the retinal directional sensitivities of the respective π mechanisms may differ (Stiles-Crawford effect, STILES and CRAWFORD, 1933b; STILES, 1939; see also CRAWFORD, chapter 18, this volume.) These properties aid in the identification of individual color processes.

At the upper part of the function (Fig. 3, left), even a small increase in background energy causes a very marked increase in the energy needed to detect an

Table 1

Mechanism	Symbol	Remarks		Weber fraction (percent), $\lambda = \mu$ (1°; 0.2 sec test stimulus) (Stiles)	Wavelength of maximal sensitivity (nm) Stiles $\pi_\mu.v.\mu.$	Wald[a] $t.v.\lambda.$
Rod	π_0	Absent at the fovea		(30)	503	
"Blue" cone	π_1	Ratio of blue to yellow sensitivity (440/590)	approx. 2.6 log units	8.7	440	"Blue" 440
	π_2	Ratio of blue to yellow sensitivity (440/590)	order of 1 log unit	? (Probably as for π_1 and π_3)	? (Between 440 and 480)	
	π_3	Ratio of blue to yellow sensitivity (440/590)	approx. 4.0 log units	8.7	440	
"Green" cone	π_4			1.9	540	"Green"
	π'_4	Modified high-intensity state		...	540	548
"Red" cone	π_5			1.8	575 (very flat max.)	"Red" 580
	π'_5	Modified high-intensity state		...	587	

[a] When Wald's data are corrected for absorption due to ocular media and macula pigment, the maximum of the "red" action spectrum is 575 nm, the "green", 540 nm, and the "blue", 430 nm (Wald, 1964).

added increment of light. This indicates that the system is saturating or reaching its limit in terms of response capability. Interestingly, as seen from the curve to the right of Fig. 3, this occurs in the scotopic system when only a small part of the available rhodopsin has been bleached. It is not clear whether comparable saturation effects occur in cone response (Stiles, 1961). Certainly saturation of this function does not occur at low bleaching levels in cones (see below), although other psychophysical relations tend to break down. For example, color matches made at moderate luminance levels are significantly altered at 10,000 photopic trolands.

In order to evaluate the contribution of the background in the two-color threshold method, Stiles developed a third data format, the $f.v.\mu.$ This is not displayed in Fig. 2, but the technique used in deriving it is shown. From the above, it is obvious that an assessment of the contribution of the background, adapting or conditioning field is the more meaningful the greater the range of the individual two-color threshold curve which is measured in the experiment. But the entire curve need not be available in each case if the foot and a reasonable part of the ascending portion can be observed.

In the *field radiance versus field wavelength curves*, at each wavelength μ, the value of log M_μ is determined which raises the increment threshold N_λ ten times (value arbitrarily chosen) above its absolute threshold. Raising the threshold N_λ one log unit locates a reference measurement point on the upward sloping portion of the *t.v.r.* curve. In addition, the absolute threshold determination of N_λ, or the backward extension of the *t.v.r.* curve to the asymptote locates the "foot" of the function. In essence, a common "template" or curve can be fit to these data. In earlier studies, STILES believed that the curve varies some with the π mechanism. In WYSZECKI and STILES (1967), he indicates that these differences are probably slight.

Two hypothetical determinations are shown in Fig. 2b. The derived values of $\log M_\mu$ for μ fall at Z for π_4, and Y for π_1. From several such values a $f.v.\mu.$ function may be derived (see Fig. 5 and 6). A wide separation of the different mechanisms is not needed in order to obtain an adequate estimate of the positions of the components making up the curve, provided one can assume a stable shape for the reference template. Within reason, it is possible to extend the curve for any given mechanism somewhat beyond that revealed in the data profile. Obviously, in order to do this and to make such statements, it is necessary to obtain a vast amount of data under many test conditions. In such situations, independence of the component processes is assumed. Derived $f.v.\mu.$ curves for the several π mechanisms are seen in Fig. 4. These are based on mean data obtained from four subjects.

The curves of Fig. 4 are expressed in the form $1/f.v.\mu.$ This is a sensitivity rather than threshold display, and sensitivity is the inverse of threshold. These curves are often referred to a $\pi_\mu.v.\mu.$ where $\pi_\mu = 1/M_\mu$ with M_μ set at the value which raises the increment threshold to $10 \times$ the absolute threshold value for the mechanism (WYSZECKI and STILES, 1967).

STILES prefers to specify his stimuli in terms of wavenumber. The wavenumber of a stimulus is the inverse of the wavelength. The unit is cm^{-1}. A brief table of comparative values follows:

$1/\lambda$ Wavenumber (cm^{-1})	λ Wavelength (nm or mμ)
25,000	400
22,222	450
20,000	500
18,182	550
16,667	600
15,385	650

DARTNALL (1953) and WALD (1965) also favor using wavenumber designations. (See also LEGRAND, chapter 15, this volume.) While the advantages are many, traditional usage has inhibited this development. The wavenumber, $1/\lambda$ is related to the frequency of electromagnetic radiation.

$$\nu = \frac{c}{\lambda} = \frac{v}{\lambda_m}.$$

Here ν = frequency (cycles/sec), c = velocity of light in vacuum or air (cm/sec), $1/\lambda$ = wavenumber in air or vacuum in cm^{-1}, v = velocity of light in any specified medium and λ_m is the wavelength of light in that medium. From this simple relation, one of the advantages of the wavenumber designation becomes immediately evident. Frequency is invariant, the wavelength varies with the medium. λ in psychophysical experiments is always specified in terms of the measured value in vacuum or air. Hence, this value of λ does not apply to retinal receptors, glass, or the vitreous humor, etc. From the simple expression above, $\lambda_m = \lambda/n$, or $n\lambda_m = \lambda$, where $n = c/v$. If $\lambda = 590$ nm in air, in a retinal receptor outer segment, if index of refraction

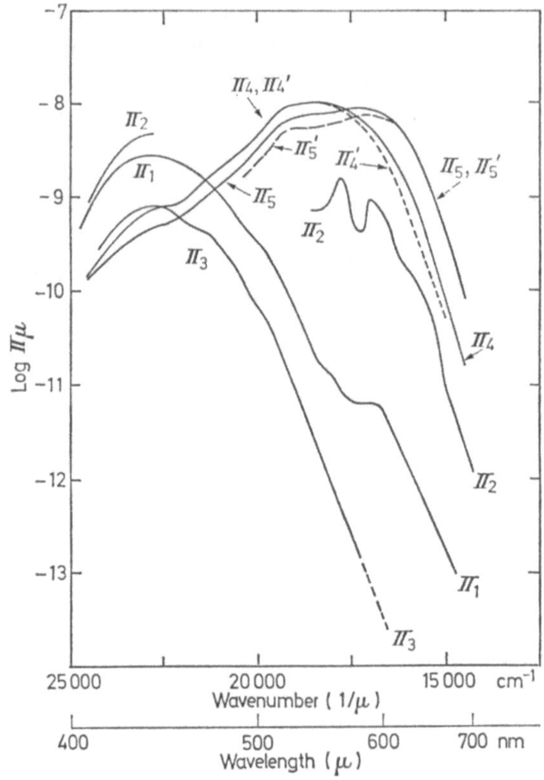

Fig. 4. These are Stiles' derived field radiance versus field wavelength curves (*f.v.μ.*). Actually the individual curves are plotted as sensitivity (rather than threshold) distributions, $\pi_\mu = 1/M_\mu$ (see discussion in text). There are three "blue" mechanisms, π_1, with a long wave sub-peak, π_3, a higher intensity form which lacks the long wave sub-peak, and π_2, which has been only partially defined. Note π_2 is plotted in two sections. There are two "green" mechanisms, π_4 and a high intensity state, π'_4. π'_4 differs from π_4 mainly at longer wavelengths. Similarly, two "red" processes have been defined, π_5 and π'_5. π'_5 again is the higher intensity form of π_5. In this case, differences in spectral sensitivity between the two forms occur at the shorter wavelengths. — The numerical mean data may be found in Table 7.6 in Wyszecki and Stiles (1967). Notice the extended range over which measurements may be made using these techniques

$= 1.4$, $\lambda_m = 421$ nm[6]. However, frequency would not change. Since λ is measured in air and since c is a constant, it is not necessary to compute ν. Hence the wavenumber, $1/\lambda$, is sufficient. Several added physical and physical chemical arguments are cited in Wald (1965). Wyszecki and Stiles (1967) discuss problems involved when quantum and wavenumber units are integrated, e.g., when integrating an absolute spectral energy distribution (p. 576).

The *f.v.μ.* format (Fig. 4) has greater "power" than the *t.v.λ.* (Fig. 2a) approach, in part, because each derived *f.v.μ.* point obtained from a *t.v.r.* distribution (Fig. 2b) is based on a sum of determinations contributing to the individual *t.v.r.* curve for the mechanism. In turn, these data may be fit and tested against a

[6] Actually, the problem becomes even more complicated in an absorbing medium, because the index of refraction takes on an imaginary factor.

common *t.v.r.* curve ot template (for values, see Table 7. 5 in WYSZECKI and STILES, 1967). In addition, and probably more important, the *f.v.μ.* approach allows broader separation of the π mechanisms across the spectrum. For example, this approach is particularly meaningful in terms of defining π_5.

Displacement Rules

Displacement rules, in general, refer to *t.v.r.* (Fig. 2b) curves. They describe the characteristic changes of the component mechanisms as λ and μ are varied. They may be used in part to test the independence of the mechanisms and they aid in the identification of the individual components. These rules were largely worked out by STILES in 1939. The author will first state the rules, then try to describe the changes which occur in some detail.

1. A change in λ, keeping μ constant, should merely displace a component *t.v.r.* curve (without change in shape on a log-log plot) parallel to the axis of ordinates by an amount determined by the relative spectral sensitivity of the mechanism being studied.

2. A change in μ, keeping λ constant, should, on the other hand, displace the individual *t.v.r.* curve along the axis of abscissas by an amount also fixed by the mechanism's relative spectral sensitivity.

As noted above, the data plotted as black dots in Fig. 2a were obtained by varying λ and determining N_λ when $M_\mu = 0$. Depending on λ, parts of π_1, π_4, and π_5 could be detected. One might ask how the remainder of each of these superimposed curves might be determined at absolute threshold level. Here, *t.v.r.* curves prove valuable. Regardless of the setting of μ, when $M_\mu = 0$, the individual π mechanisms asymptote at their absolute threshold for wavelength λ. That is, if one extends the π_1 curve back to its asymptote at γ (Fig. 2b), one may deduce the absolute spectral sensitivity of π_1 (a "blue" mechanism) at $\lambda = 500$ nm. This derived point has been plotted at γ on Fig. 2a. Other wavelength backgrounds, μ, may be chosen to more completely expose the π_1 function, at different test field wavelengths λ. β is the threshold of π_5 (a "red" mechanism) at λ, but since at $\lambda = 500$ nm (a green), π_5 is less sensitive than π_4 (a "green" mechanism), and since a red background (M_μ) more rapidly reduces the sensitivity of π_5, this point is not revealed by this combination of λ and μ. In short, α, β, and γ are independent of μ, but varying μ allows the experimenter to determine these values over an extended range of λ.

If one varies λ, and holds μ constant, the individual functions shift on the ordinate of the *t.v.r.* curve. The amount of shift is related to the sensitivity of the individual mechanisms at the *new* test field wavelength, λ'. For example, holding $\mu = 640$ nm, and selecting $\lambda' = 470$ nm, π_4 would shift upward on the *t.v.r.* curve to about the position of β (Fig. 2b) and π_1 would shift downward to a point about halfway between γ and β. These displacements can be deduced from Fig. 2a, lower set of data and curves. The effects described are shown in Fig. 5a. Here $\mu = 600$ nm (an orange) and λ was variable. The individual curves have been displaced vertically somewhat to provide more equal spacing. When $\lambda = 410$ nm and 430 nm, at lower values of $M_{600\,\mathrm{nm}}$, only the "blue" π_1 is seen; as λ increases, the "green" π_4 becomes

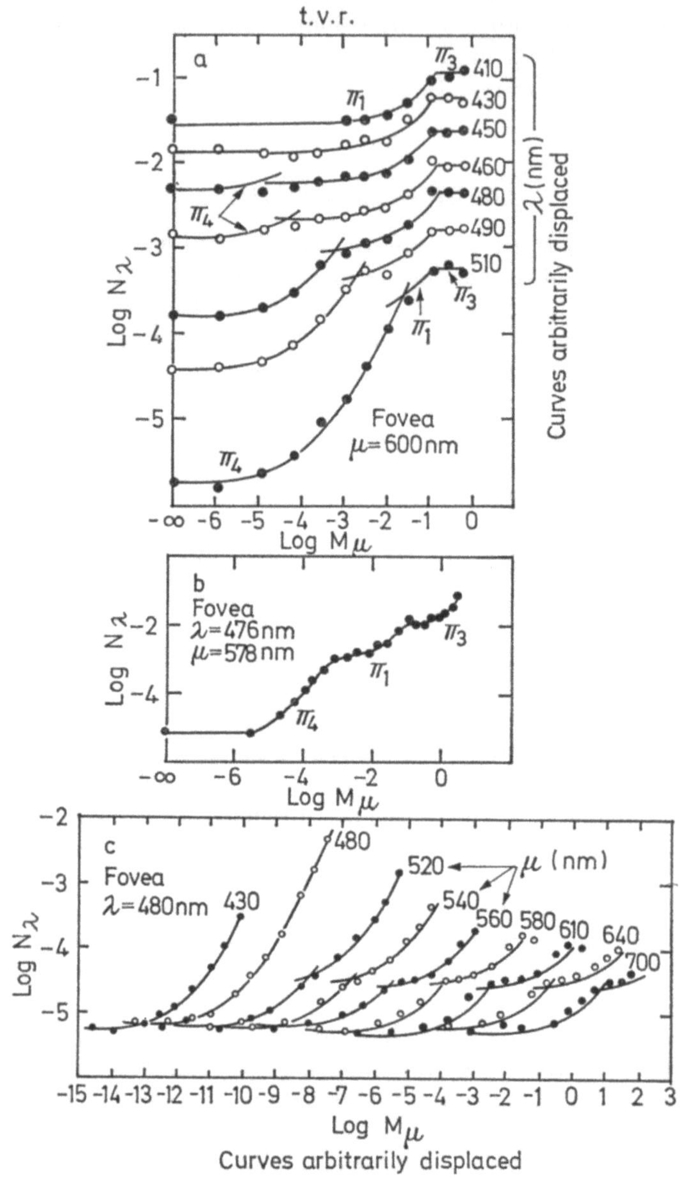

Fig. 5. a. The effect of varying λ and holding μ constant is shown in this figure. The individual curves have been displaced vertically to minimize overlap. Values of λ are shown to the right. Filled and non-filled data points differentiate data sets (Stiles, 1939). b. This three section foveal *t.v.r.* curve reveals the presence of three separate component color mechanisms. π_4 is a "green" mechanism, and π_1 and π_3 are "blue" mechanisms (Stiles, 1959). c. The effect of varying μ while λ is held constant is revealed in this figure. The individual curves and data points have been translated laterally to minimize overlap. Regardless of the choice of μ, when $M_\mu = 0$, N_λ must equal a constant, its absolute threshold at λ. Keeping this point in mind, the reader can judge the magnitude of the individual displacements. These data have been reproduced in several of Stiles' papers (1939, etc.)

increasingly visible (for lower values of $M_{600\,\mathrm{nm}}$). At $\lambda = 510$ nm (a green) only a small part of π_1 remains.

At higher values of $M_{600\,\mathrm{nm}}$ in Fig. 5a, there is a flattening of the π_1 function about 0.6 L.U. above the π_1 threshold. This flattening occurs at backgrounds of about 30,000 photopic trolands for $\mu > 570$ nm. In earlier publications, STILES termed this the "limiting conditioning effect on the blue mechanism." It was thought to be associated with the long wave hump on the π_1 function seen in Fig. 4. More recent studies identify this as the π_3 function, *another* "blue" mechanism which lacks the long wave hump of the π_1 function. π_3 (Fig. 4, 5b) has essentially the same wavelength peak as π_1 (Table 1).

Thus, varying λ and holding μ constant alters the *t.v.r.* curves by causing vertical translation of the individual functions, the amount of which is related to the spectral sensitivities of the individual π mechanisms.

If λ is held constant and μ is varied (Fig. 5c), the curves shift laterally, not vertically. As in Fig. 5a, the several sets of data have been spread out to minimize overlap. Again, the vertical position of each mechanism on the *t.v.r.* curve is set by the absolute threshold of the most sensitive mechanism. All of these curves must have a common data point at this value.

At $\lambda = 480$ nm, when $M_\mu = 0$, π_4 is most sensitive (Fig. 2a). The background field, $\mu = 430$ nm (Fig. 5c), acts most effectively to reduce the sensitivity of the "blue" mechanism π_1. At $\mu = 480$ nm, where $\lambda = \mu$, the π_1 mechanism is less sensitive than π_4 for all values of M_μ, and multi-branched curves are not seen. Where $\mu > 520$ nm, as M_μ increases, π_4 is superceded by the now more sensitive π_1, and at $\mu = 580$ nm and 610 nm, the beginning of the π_3 component is again visible. Lateral translation of the functions occurs because the different background field wavelengths are more or less effective in altering the sensitivity of the several π functions. The rise of the curve from the value of the absolute threshold will occur sooner or later depending on the sensitivity of the mechanism most sensitive at wavelength λ to the chromatic adapting stimulus of wavelength μ.

The derivation of an individual *f.v.μ.* function is seen in Fig. 6. Here λ is again fixed, and μ is variable (the curves have not been translated). Measured log unit values of N_λ above absolute threshold are transferred below on to the Log M_μ scale. Only one mechanism is pictured. These values are associated with the specific background field wavelength employed. The combination yields a spectral sensitivity curve of the component color mechanism, in this case, π_4. If more than one component is present in the *t.v.r.* curve, as in Fig. 2b or 5, contributions to more than one π function may be recorded from a single set of *t.v.r.* data.

In special cases it is useful to add a second wavelength to the background or adapting field. This has been termed the "auxiliary field method" and has been used in particular to further reveal part of the "blue" π_1 function (STILES, 1953b). WALD (1964) uses a variant of this technique to help reveal his "green" mechanism (see below).

When discussing the effects of varying λ or μ, it has been assumed that the individual mechanisms behave in the manner indicated. This is a test of the validity of the argument. In fact, this is only partially true. π_1, and π_3 do act in the manner described (i.e., they obey the displacement rules). A third "blue" mechanism π_2, with a maximum of sensitivity at a somewhat longer wavelength (not completely defined in Fig. 4) and an odd long wavelength perturbation is poorly defined. This mechanism is best revealed when $\lambda < 460$ nm and $\mu > 600$ nm. It reveals itself as a breakdown in the displacement rules for π_4. π_2 has not been recorded for all test subjects.

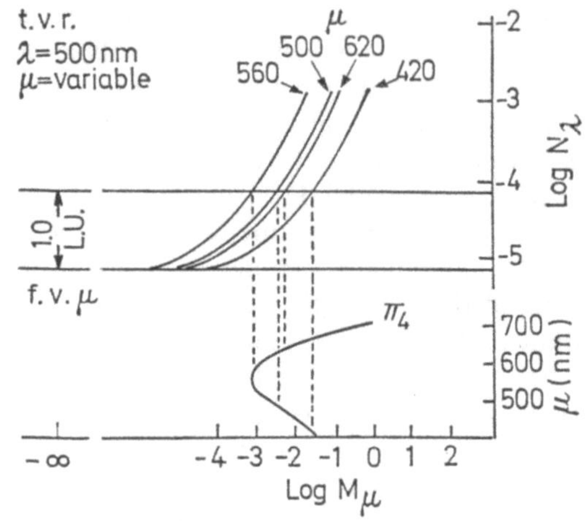

Fig. 6. In this figure, the same manoeuver was carried out as was shown in Fig. 5c. That is, λ was held constant and μ varied. To simplify the problem only one mechanism is shown. This graph shows how a $f.v.\mu$. function may be derived. In each instance, the value of M_μ was determined which raised the threshold, N_λ, 1.0 log unit above the absolute threshold. The derived M_μ values were then translated downward to a second curve. On the ordinate to the right there are two separate sections, the top is log N_λ and the bottom μ. This figure was taken from Marriott's chapter in Volume 2 of Davson's, The Eye (1962)

π_4 and π_5 only partially obey the defined displacement characteristics. They conform satisfactorily to the basic rules of the analysis for backgrounds of 150 trolands or less. There is a breakdown when more intense background fields are employed. This has made it necessary to define high intensity forms of these mechanisms known as π'_4 and π'_5 which have some what different spectral sensitivities from π_4 and π_5. The mean foveal spectral sensitivity curves of the several π functions defined by Stiles (1953a, b, 1959) appear in Fig. 4. A summary of the characteristics of the several mechanisms appears in Table 1. Note, in the remarks section of Table 1, that the sensitivities of the three "blue" π mechanisms at 440 nm are compared to their sensitivities at 590 nm. All three functions can be measured at 440 nm, but 440 nm may not represent peak sensitivity for π_2.

In summary, three forms of "blue" mechanism, and two forms each of "red" and "green" mechanisms have been defined. In addition, a π_0 designation has been given to the scotopic function similarly obtained in non-foveal testing.

Assumptions

At first glance the presentation given here seems a rather backwards approach to the problem. That is, the presence of a set of underlying color mechanisms has been assumed, and some of their properties have been described before all the underlying assumptions defining the experiments have been considered. However, the author has found this approach valuable in order to clarify the need for several of the assumptions inherent in the theoretical development, and to explain some of the experimental manoeuvers which were required in the establishment of the relations.

The following list of assumptions has been taken or paraphrased from WYSZECKI and STILES (1967). Some have been mentioned above.

1. In the retinal area where the test stimulus is imaged, there are several component color mechanisms, any one of which may trigger off a response "seen" when the test flash is applied.

2. Each component mechanism is believed to be an association of a selected proportion of end organs (rods and cones) in the area, the association being effected somewhere in the neural system through which the nervous activity, which was initiated by light absorption in the end organs, is transmitted to the brain.

3. It is assumed that the end organs of a component mechanism need not necessarily be all of the same kind or contain just one pigment, nor that end organs need belong exclusively to one component mechanism.

4. The color response mechanisms are assumed to have sufficient independence for the idea of a particular component mechanism acting alone to have meaning. In effect, this assumes that the response of all but one component mechanism may be blocked (at least ideally), leaving the remaining mechanism to respond in its normal way. This may not be totally achievable in practice.

5. For a given test stimulus and given background conditioning stimulus, the observed increment threshold in the retinal area tested is assumed to depend only on the respective increment thresholds of the component mechanisms that would be observed under the same conditions if they were acting alone.

6. It is assumed that the observed increment threshold will not exceed any of the component increment thresholds and will generally approximate the smallest of these.

7. Each component mechanism is assumed to have a characteristic relative spectral sensitivity function. The effect on the mechanism of an irradiance E_1 of λ_1, forming the whole or part of a test or background stimulus, is just the same as that of an irradiance E_2 of λ_2 that may be substituted for it, provided that E_1 and E_2 are in the inverse ratio of their relative spectral sensitivity values at these wavelengths (STILES, 1959).

Given these assumptions and the experimental approach described above, the intent of the research was to determine whether the observed quantities could arise in the manner proposed, and if so, to describe the relative spectral sensitivities and other properties of the assumed component color mechanisms.

Certain of these assumptions have been questioned. For example, WALD (1964) believes the functions he has derived using intense adapting fields and the *t.v.λ.* technique are action spectra of cone "red," "green," and "blue" photosensitive pigments. HURVICH *et al.* (1965) have pointed out that STILES' displacement rules are based on what is, in principle a von Kries type coefficient analysis to account for the effects of colored adaptations. Since the simple coefficient analysis has been shown to be inadequate for other data of chromatic adaptation, e.g., haploscopic color matches (HURVICH and JAMESON, 1958, 1960), they have suggested that the analysis of increment threshold data may also require an arithmetic displacement component in addition to the logarithmic one of STILES' displacement rules. Work by BOYNTON, IKEDA, and STILES (1964) and related studies raise questions regarding the independence of, and the interaction of the individual mechanisms, particularly near points of crossings of the *t.v.r.* functions. These issues and additional ones will be considered when STILES' π functions are compared with other available data.

Comparison of STILES' and Other Steady State Two-Color Threshold Data

Contributions to the two-color increment threshold technique made before STILES' 1939 paper were not extensive enough to allow definition of color mechanisms; a broad systematic treatment was required. DEVRIES (1946) presented a set of three functions based on this technique.[7] Actually, his equivalent of π_1 matched STILES' function well within the limits of wavelengths tested. The peak of his "green" mechanism was similar to that of STILES, but his function was considerably narrower than π_4 on the short wavelength side. The "red" function had a rather short wavelength peak when compared with π_5. STILES plots his 1939 data with those of DEVRIES in a brief note (1946a).

A set of comparable functions obtained using the *t.v.λ.* format has recently been presented by WALD (1964, 1966, 1967). He used broad band filters (rather than narrow spectral bands) for the background illumination, and these conditioning stimuli were very intense. He tested subjects with normal and abnormal color vision, he evaluated the effect of macular pigment, and measured responses at various retinal loci.

WALD (1964) employed a continuously presented background field 3.5° in diameter, and a 1.0° circular test field, the flash duration of which was 45 msec. A Maxwellian view was employed with a 3.5 mm entrance pupil. A zirconium arc source was used in conjunction with a series of filters for the adapting field, and monochromatic spectral lights for the test stimuli.

A yellow filter (Corning Glass number 3482) was used to selectively reduce the sensitivity of the "red" and "green" mechanisms, and to reveal the "blue" mechanism. Background adapting retinal illuminance was measured and a figure of 7.0 log photopic trolands was quoted. To isolate the "red" mechanism he used one of two blue filters for the background field (Kodak, Wratten number 47B, 4.3 log photopic trolands, or Kodak, Wratten number 47, 6.2 log photopic trolands). The "green" mechanism was defined by using a purple filter containing both a red and blue band (Kodak, Wratten number 35, 5.4 log photopic trolands). The latter approach is similar in concept to STILES' auxiliary field device, and to a technique employed by BRINDLEY (1953). WALD used other filter combinations for specific purposes. It has been questioned whether WALD's estimates of adapting illuminance, particularly for the yellow field, are not too high (STILES, private communication).

WALD's functions show surprisingly small difference from either STILES' *t.v.λ.* (1953b, 1964) curves or STILES' $\pi_\mu.v.\mu.$ (or $1/f.v.\mu.$) functions (Fig. 4) except in the case of π_5 (slightly less difference for π'_5, see Fig. 7 and 8). In Fig. 7, WALD's "blue" mechanism is graphed with two of STILES' *t.v.λ.* functions (STILES, 1953b). STILES' functions were obtained at somewhat lower background stimulus levels. Differences

[7] He was not aware of STILES' 1939 paper.

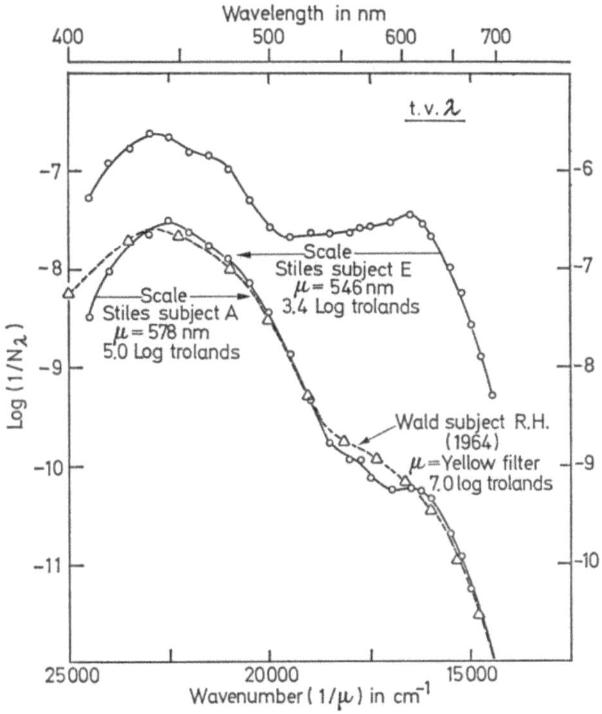

Fig. 7. This *t.v.λ.* plot matches two sets of STILES' data (1953) with a determination of WALD's "blue" mechanism (1964). WALD used a broad band yellow filter to selectively adapt the "red" and "green" mechanisms. His background field was 7.0 log photopic trolands. STILES used narrow spectral bands. Subject *E* was adapted to a yellow-green $M_{546\,\mathrm{nm}} = 3.4$ log photopic trolands. Subject A was adapted to an intense yellow stimulus $M_{578\,\mathrm{nm}} = 5.0$ log photopic trolands. The ordinates refer to STILES' two sets of data. WALD's curve, same scale, has been arbitrarily located coincident with data of STILES' subject A. Obviously there has been vertical translation of these sets of data. The significant point is that differences between these functions are not great

in the measured "blue" mechanisms seem limited. In Fig. 8, STILES' π_4 and π'_4 ($\pi_\mu .v.\mu$) are plotted with WALD's "green" mechanism, and π_5 and π'_5 with WALD's "red" function. The two sets of "green" mechanisms are not markedly different, but the "red" π_5 mechanisms are poorly matched. In the case of the "green" and "red" mechanisms, the higher intensity π'_4 and π'_5 curves more closely approximate WALD's data.

In a later report (1966) WALD changed from a zirconium arc to a tungsten filament lamp (for purposes of stability) as the light source for his adapting field. In addition, he added a Jena heat filter KGl to the Corning glass filter 3482, and a Jena BG18 to the Wratten 47. With this new arrangement he used much less intense adapting fields. Ignoring the Stiles-Crawford effect (1933b), his white light source before passing through the yellow Corning filter (plus KGl) was 15,300 photopic trolands (as compared with 7.0 log photopic trolands in the earlier study); it was 48,600 photopic trolands before passing through the Wratten 47 (plus BG18); and it provided 64,700 photopic trolands before transmission through the

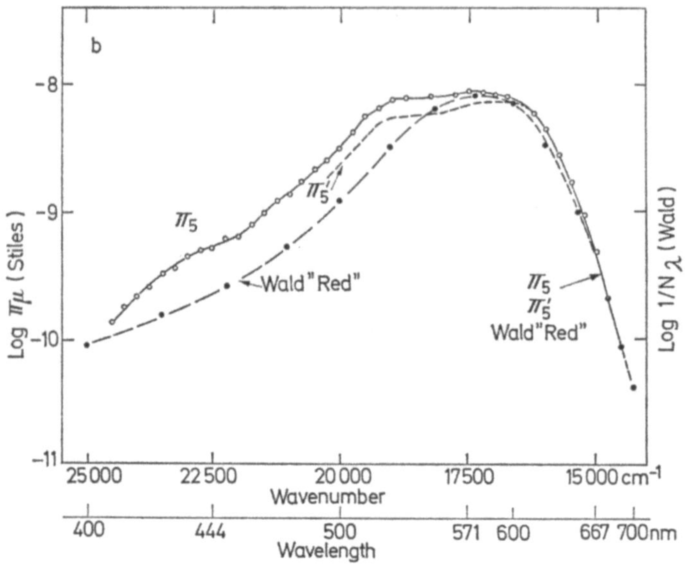

Fig. 8a

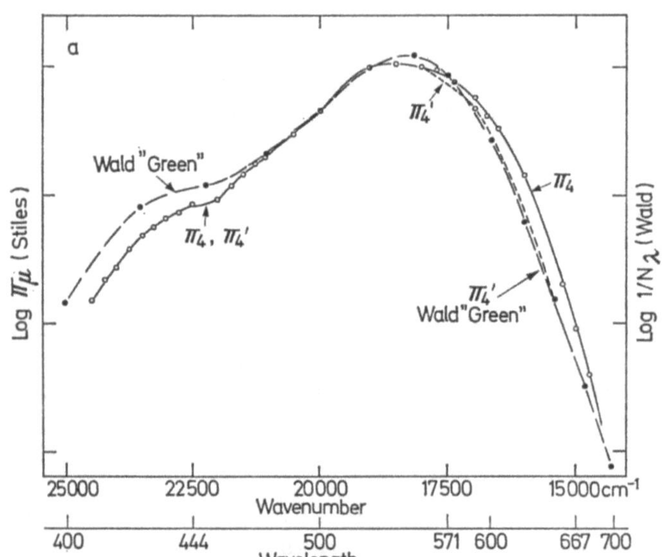

Fig. 8b

Fig. 8. a. Wald's "green" function ($t.v.\lambda.$) is compared with Stiles' mean π_4 and π'_4 ($\pi_\mu.v.\mu.$) relations. The functions have been translated vertically on the log scale for purposes of comparison. b. Wald's "red" function ($t.v.\lambda.$) is compared in this figure to Stiles' π_5 and π'_5 ($\pi_\mu.v.\mu.$)

purple Wratten 35 filter. Obviously each of these filters significantly reduced the retinal illuminance of the background stimulus. With these less intense adapting stimuli, WALD recorded results which were essentially comparable with his earlier data (1964). He does not report significant differences in the shape of his three spectral curves in the two sets of data (1964 and 1966). Rather, he notes that normal subjects tend to differ in terms of measured proportions of the three different color mechanisms. This author therefore assumes the curves in the two studies to be similar in nature.

INGLING (1969) recently published a π_5 function which matches STILES' mean data quite well except for a small perturbation around wavenumber 17,000 cm^{-1}.

Are the π Functions Measurements of Action Spectra of Cone Pigments?

Assumptions 2 and 3 listed above deal with the general questions, what is being measured, and how do these experimentally determined mechanisms relate to photoreceptor pigment absorption characteristics? These are extremely important questions. Obviously, STILES has carefully not committed himself on these issues. WALD (1964) has stated that the functions he derived using an essentially identical technique provide cone photosensitive pigment action spectra. His arguments (paraphrased by this author) are as follows:

1. If there is only one pigment present, selective chromatic adaptation should not alter resultant spectral sensitivity whether that spectral sensitivity is measured in the absolute sense ($N_\lambda = f(\lambda)$ with $M_\mu = 0$) or if it is determined against any chromatic background (N_λ for $M_\mu \neq 0$). This statement assumes limited pigment density.

2. If more than one pigment is present, carefully chosen chromatic adapting stimuli will effectively reduce response (or more completely deplete chosen pigments), leaving a resultant spectral response representing the pigment moiety being studied. This is best achieved using intense adapting fields. In fact, WALD sees his technique as the limiting case of STILES' experiment.

3. Resultant functions tend to be remarkably invariant (of course, recognizing individual differences in pigment concentration, pre-receptor absorption media, etc.). This invariance is an essentially photochemical criterion characterizing the operation of single visual pigments. However, the invariance is that belonging to a pigment, and not necessarily to a class of receptors.

4. In measured cases of color vision anomalies, the individual color mechanisms (pigments) are shown to be deficient, and the effect is similar to that found in chromatic adaptation experiments.

5. The narrower the spectral peak obtained using the two-color technique, the more closely the resultant curve conforms to the action spectrum of the visual pigment.

6. Conformity to the displacement rules may be regarded as a means of isolating the action spectrum of a single visual pigment. A mechanism which does not obey the displacement rules (e.g., π_4 and π_5 when going from low to higher background

stimulus levels) represents the resultant mixture of more than one pigment action spectrum.

It is important to note that WALD accepts STILES' third assumption, i.e., that the two-color threshold technique provides no information regarding the distribution of the photopigments in and among end-organs (receptors). STILES' discussion of the general question is found in his 1953 and 1959 papers and in Chapter 7 of WYSZECKI and STILES (1967).

A number of comparisons may be made between STILES' data, similar data, e.g., WALD'S, and data representative of pigment absorption curves or other functions that are highly influenced by the spectral absorption curves of cone pigments. In several instances there is rather good agreement between the π functions and these data. For example, π_4 is fit well by a rhodopsinlike pigment distribution when plotted using a wavenumber abscissa (i.e., it is well matched by the Dartnall nomogram, DARTNALL, 1953);[8] the "green" function of the Thomson-Wright color fundamentals based on color-mixture data provides a good fit (STILES, 1959; THOMSON and WRIGHT, 1953);[9] it is quite well matched by the pigment chlorolabe (RUSHTON, 1963) determined by fundus reflectometry (π'_4 provides a slightly better match); and it is fit by BRINDLEY'S (1953) "artificial monochromacy" function (revealed by an intense red-blue bleach) as well as by WALD'S two-color threshold "green" mechanism. This suggests that π_4 or π'_4 reflects the spectral absorption characteristics of a cone pigment. If this is the case, STILES asks why the spectral sensitivity of π_4 changes at increased radiance levels to π'_4? Further, HSIA and GRAHAM'S (1957) protanopic spectral sensitivity curve is somewhat narrower than π_4 (see below).

π_1 and π_3 compare favorably with other available data, if one overlooks the long-wave sub-peak on π_1. In "blue cone monochromacy," (BLACKWELL and BLACKWELL, 1959; RUSHTON, 1964; ALPERN *et al.*, 1965) reasonable agreement of spectral sensitivity with π_1 has been found. However, what is π_2, and why are there three "blue" mechanisms?

π_5 and π'_5 provide the poorest comparisons with other established data. The Thomson-Wright "red" color-mixture function does not match π_5. The Dartnall nomogram does not fit either STILES' π_5 distribution nor WALD'S "red" mechanism,

[8] DARTNALL (1953) found that "rhodopsin" and other "rhodopsin-like" pigments could be fit by a common nomogram when plotted on a wavenumber axis. More recently DARTNALL noted small differences between pigments having origins in Vitamin A_1 and Vitamin A_2 (WYSZECKI and STILES, 1967, Table 7.9). If the nomogram is applied to a distribution, and a reasonably acceptable fit is achieved, it may be argued that the distribution is related to this class of pigments. Of course, psychophysical functions are altered by the transmission properties of intervening ocular media. This partially limits interpretation. Also, the failure of a function to match the nomogram only means that the distribution does not have properties similar to rhodopsinlike pigments, i.e., it is possible that another pigment form is present.

[9] Foveal color matching functions (excluding very intense stimuli) are almost certainly based on linear combinations of the spectral photosensitivities of three visual pigments (STILES, 1959). Quoting from p. 109 in the latter reference. "Thus, if the spectral sensitivity of a component mechanism could be represented as a linear combination of the color matching functions, it would also be a linear combination of the pigment photosensitivities. This would indicate that the end-organs of the mechanisms contained the pigments represented in linear combination (i.e., those having non-zero coefficients) and that the effects of light absorption in these different pigments add up linearly." Thus, it is valuable to compare such data with the derived functions.

nor does a linear combination of two such distributions fit π_5. Initially, the long-wave absorbing pigment erythrolabe (RUSHTON, 1958b), was found to fit π_5 poorly. This pigment has been studied by fundus reflectometry by RUSHTON and WEALE and their co-workers. More recently, BAKER and RUSHTON (1965), with improvements in technique, found a far better match. π'_5 provides a slightly better match. Since the fundus reflectometry technique requires substantial pigment bleaching for measurement, it is logical that data be compared to π'_5.

HSIA and GRAHAM'S (1957) deuteranopes have spectral sensitivity functions with narrower distributions than π_5 and a broader distribution than WALD'S "red" mechanism. RUSHTON'S erythrolabe falls roughly between STILES' π_5 and HSIA and GRAHAM'S function (RUSHTON, 1966). One must ask if π_5 and/or π'_5 represent end-organs containing more than one pigment? If so, why is the π'_5 function seemingly so stable at high luminances where red-green anomaloscope matches break down?

WALD'S "red" function measured in color normals and color deficients is on the whole different from STILES' π_5. However, individual curves show wide variation from one observer to the next. WALD shows similar data for very intense bleaches (1964), and later for lower luminance adapting fields (1966). If he is defining the limiting case — why does the curve not change when the adaptation level is lowered?

Many additional points need to be considered. What happens physically in the retina as steady state retinal illuminance is increased? First, if pigment density is high enough, and appreciable pigment bleaching is produced, *self-screening* may be altered. Self-screening is a characteristic of an absorbing medium.

Given a spectrally selective filter of some density and a finite thickness, the initial or front part of the filter will be most effective at its absorption peak. As the remaining radiant energy proceeds through the filter, there is proportionately less energy in the energy distribution at the absorption maximum. Hence, the spectral composition of the incident distribution is measureably different as the residual energy reaches the rear of the filter. This alters the absorption probability. For these same reasons, with bleaching, the front of the filter (or receptor) is bleached first, and the spectral absorption of the filter as a whole changes.

Second, WEALE (1964) has shown the retina to "grey" during fundus reflectometry at high luminances, and BUSACCA (1947) has recorded the clouding of the retina in normals during steady slit-lamp observations. In addition, there is evidence for change in receptor dimensions and optical properties. KÜHNE (1877) quotes a medical student, VON HORNBOSTEL, who reported swelling of frog receptors following bleaching! More recently KUWABARA (personal communication) has shown swelling, and disturbances in lamellar disc spacing and membrane irregularities in primate receptor outer segments following intense bleaching. His standard and scanning electron micrographs are striking. Some of his earlier work has been published in a paper by FRIEDMAN and KUWABARA (1968). On the basis of data obtained from infrared interference microscopic examination of single photoreceptors in the frog before and after bleaching, this author found measureable photoreceptor outer segment swelling coupled with a decrease of index of refraction. One implication of these changes is that previously described waveguide properties may be altered at high bleaching levels and the non-uniform distributions of energy (modes) in these cells (which vary as a function of wavelength) may change. Similarly, efficiency of transmission as a function of wavelength of the guide may be altered if the parameters defining its properties change with bleaching.

In his 1939 paper, STILES showed that in most instances a change from one mechanism to another was accompanied by an alteration in retinal directional sensitivity, (the Stiles-Crawford effect of the first kind, 1933b). It is generally accepted that the Stiles-Crawford effect is largely mediated by the optical properties of receptors. (See CRAWFORD, chapter 18.) Thus, a change in mechanisms may be accompanied either by a change in optical properties of the same cells, or by a change in the set of cells contributing to the response. Presumably in the latter case, the cells pooling their excitations would have measureably different directional sensitivity. The author can find no descriptive data concerning this question for the high intensity transitions of π_4 to π'_4, π_5 to π'_5, and π_1 to π_3. Such a study would provide insight as to whether optical or cell selective processes were active in these transfers. Further complicating the issue, recent studies (discussed at length below) have shown that the π mechanisms are not as independent as hoped, particularly at or near overlap of *t.v.r.* curves.

Spectral response curves obtained from the two-color threshold method are action rather than difference spectra. Most efficient comparison of psychophysical with photochemical data is made after first converting energy determinations into quantal units. WYSZECKI and STILES (1967) note that corrections for absorption in intervening ocular media must be made – generally on a mean basis, although significant individual variance does exist, e.g., in the concentration of macular pigment. (See RUDDOCK, chapter 17, this volume.) They note that oriented pigment in the retinal photoreceptor has a higher absorption coefficient than pigment studied in solution. This becomes a problem only if more than one absorption axis exists in the pigment molecule. Problems also arise when comparing an action spectrum with a difference spectrum. For example, at the isobestic point these data cannot be compared. The isobestic point occurs where the difference spectrum goes to zero and then turns negative. Interestingly, studies of primate and human cone difference spectra measured in single cells (reported to date) have not revealed any products of bleaching! This is only one of many problems one encounters in these difficult studies.

The two-color threshold technique provides reliable data extending over many log units (Fig. 4). Available cone pigment absorption curves rarely provide accurate data beyond a 1.0 log unit range. Further, the absorption data are most accurate near their maxima, with reliability falling off as signal approaches the noise or background level.

Data currently available from microspectrophotometry or even from fundus reflectometry are less reliable and less well defined than those reported in two-color threshold measurements. The new pigment measurement techniques represent *tours de force* by the scientists contributing to this field. This author feels that all of these studies are conducted at the limits of current technology. It is important that solutions to outstanding problems be found and test techniques be further refined. RIGGS presents the argument cogently in his Friedenwald lecture (1967) when he simply plots the various sets of data obtained from microspectrophotometry and fundus reflectometry on a single graph. Virtually a continuous set of overlapping functions is presented (with a slight break in the short-wave region).

Obviously, multiple pigments are present, and most probably there are three. At this stage fundus reflectometry (except for the short-wave absorbing or cyanolabe pigment) provides a better estimate than microspectrophotometry.

One last argument relative to this question, does cone receptor response saturate when truly intense adapting fields are used? STILES in an interesting experiment (1961) finds that within the extensive range he tested, the Weber fraction remained constant up to a level approaching a total bleach (Fig. 9).

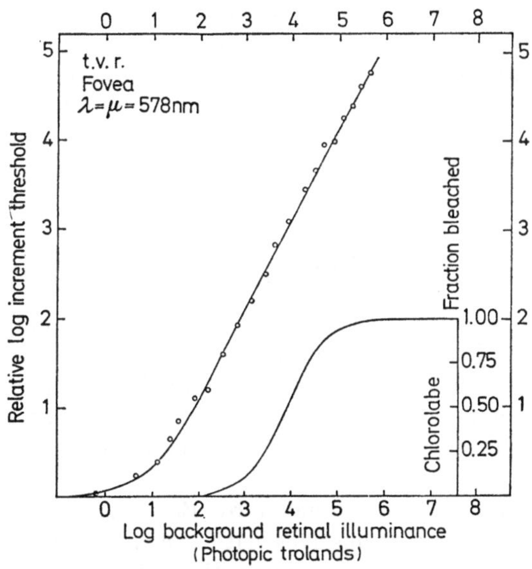

Fig. 9. This is a foveal increment threshold distribution measured as a function of background field retinal illuminance (STILES, 1961). It is interesting to compare these data with Fig. 3. At 578 nm both π_4 and π_5 are almost equally affected (Fig. 4). At the levels of retinal illuminance tested, no evidence of saturation was found. The chlorolabe bleaching curve to the right was taken from RUSHTON (1963). At this wavelength one assumes approximately equivalent bleaching of chlorolabe and erythrolabe

At 578 nm (a yellow) π_4 and π_5 are nearly equally active. Thus, if $\lambda = \mu = 578$ nm, both mechanisms should be bleached in approximately the same proportion, and on a *t.v.r.* curve one might expect no break. In Fig. 9, STILES has plotted such data. To the right of this figure he has added RUSHTON's data (1963) that show the fraction of chlorolabe bleached by the background. This function follows a first order photochemical reaction. Presumably erythrolabe follows a rather similar bleaching course. The format is similar to that employed in Fig. 3 which applied to scotopic vision. In Fig. 9, however, even when bleaching is marked, the *t.v.r.* curve shows no saturation. This author wishes such studies would be extended. It is hard to believe that at levels where color matches break down, odd after-image effects occur, receptor and retinal changes may be taking place, etc., that some alteration (saturation or otherwise) in the photopic *t.v.r.* curve does not occur.

In summary, the two-color increment threshold method provides curves which certainly are ***substantially influenced*** by cone pigments, but a large number of intervening physical, chemical, and neural interactive events probably limit conclusive interpretations. Wald's data, with the possible exception of the "red" mechanism, are not sufficiently "limiting" to suggest a unique relation. His "red" mechanism is different and this difference should be investigated further. To state that a function acts as if it were a pigment is not proof that it is a pigment *per se*, and that the measured function is not influenced by intervening processes. This author finds Stiles' more conservative position on this issue more acceptable at this time. That is, he assumes the measured mechanisms represent an association of a selected proportion of end organs (cones only in the fovea) in the area, and that this association is effected somewhere in the nervous system through which the neural activity, initiated by light absorption in the end organs, is transmitted to the brain. This point will become more obvious as the analysis continues into questions of interaction between mechanisms.

Are the π Mechanisms Independent?

Several of Stiles' assumptions refer to the question of independence of the mechanisms, and their displacement properties. Stiles obviously has been concerned with interactions between mechanisms and their stability under different test conditions. He made preliminary determinations of interactions between mechanisms using a threshold method which leads to what he calls a summation index (Stiles, 1967).

The work was modified and extended by Boynton, Ikeda, and their co-workers who have concerned themselves with the interactive properties of the retina and visual pathways and the characteristics of the psychophysical functions being measured. In essence, the questions they raise are the opposite of those introduced by Wald, although they too seek to define basic color mechanisms. Wald accepts the independence of the functions — in fact, he tries to get at pigment characteristics and to bypass intermediary processes by intense adaptation. Boynton questions the validity of some the principles upon which Stiles' model is based. Boynton, Ikeda, and Stiles (1964) agree that Stiles' assumptions hold in certain situations, and tend to break down at other times. Boynton's arguments are perhaps best summarized in a paper published early in 1963. Boynton argues as follows:

1. In the 1° test flash area there are several thousand receptors whose state of adaptation is controlled by the much larger adapting field. The latter stimulates these receptors as well as many more in the surrounding area.

2. The rate of quantum absorption of these end organs is probably very high, especially at higher levels of adaptation. Bleaching of pigment is believed to be only one factor in the direct elevation of the increment threshold as background radiance is increased.

3. Subjectively, that which is perceived at threshold is quite variable. Boynton surmises that hundreds of receptors operating in a highly organized state influence the individual judgement, "seen or not seen." This is based on border characteristics, etc., reported by observers.

4. STILES' results suggest that the hundreds of receptors and their neural interconnections which make up a mechanism (in the test field area) have a stable collective spectral sensitivity, and some degree of independence from other mechanisms all of which are located in the same general retinal region. BOYNTON questions whether all of the receptors of a single mechanism can have exactly the same spectral sensitivity (and total independence from other neural retinal elements). STILES would ask the same question.

5. Mechanisms differ in ways other than spectral sensitivity, e.g., the *t.v.r.* curve need not be assumed to be the same for all mechanisms; the Weber fraction of the different π functions varies (Table 1); the manner in which the Weber fraction varies as a function of test field area, test flash duration, and retinal position, may differ between mechanisms; different mechanisms have different adaptation characteristics; etc.

6. The spectral sensitivity of a given mechanism may be examined only under conditions where the sensitivity of that mechanism, over a fairly wide range of values of λ and μ, is distinct from and lower than that of all other mechanisms. This tends to restrict the experimental possibilities.

7. There is a degree of human judgement involved in deciding how to fit a *t.v.r.* curve. This problem becomes rather acute when notches in (separations of) these functions are small, e.g., as often occurs when "red" and "green" mechanisms are studied.

8. There is an unknown degree of interaction between the various mechanisms for conditions which cause them to have nearly equal sensitivities.

9. The technique requires unusual precision and stability of optical alignment and radiometric measurement, since relative measures will not suffice, and absolute values recorded over a single session must be comparable with those obtained during other sessions often quite separated in time.

10. The data obtained by STILES' methods generally do not fit spectral sensitivity curves obtained in color deficient individuals (HSIA and GRAHAM, 1957; BOYNTON *et al.*, 1959). These data are fit by narrower spectral curves particularly in comparison with π_4 and π_5. This argument assumes that these individuals have a "reduced" form of otherwise normal color vision.

STILES' own assumptions are designed to deal with some of these problems and he discusseds these questions in some detail in his Newton lecture (1967).

Specific forms of neural interactive mechanisms are shown in Fig. 10. Two overlapping spectral sensitivity curves (assume a $1/t.v.\lambda.$ data format) are presented in Fig. 10a, left. At λ_0 the two mechanisms π_a and π_b are equally sensitive. Three possible relations are shown in Fig. 10a. The curve to the left in Fig. 10a demonstrates the case of no summation. The curve at the top of Fig. 10a, right, indicates complete summation, and the curve below that bridging the two mechanisms corresponds to probability summation. Complete summation assumes that response is determined by total quanta absorbed, whichever mechanism absorbs the quanta. Thus, the top curve Fig. 10a, right, represents the linear sum of the two underlying π functions. Such a result might be expected in a linearly acting part of the visual pathway.

Probability summation is a bit more complex. Basically the argument is that two observers, or two eyes, or two mechanisms, if equally, or nearly equally sensitive

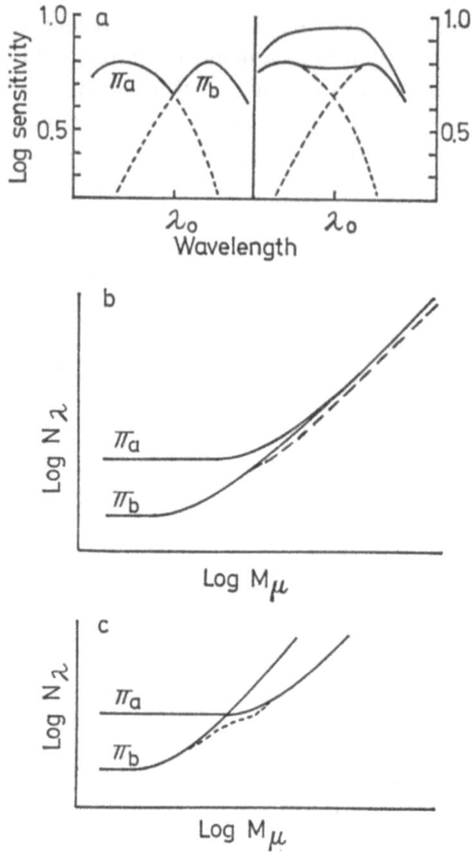

Fig. 10. a. Spectral sensitivity functions of two hypothetical component color mechanisms π_a and π_b are shown on the left hand side of this figure. They do not interact. The top curve on the right hand side of the figure represents the linear summation of $\pi_a + \pi_b$. Probability summation is indicated on the curve bridging the dashed π_a and π_b curves. b. When component mechanisms π_a and π_b have an overlapping or near overlapping rising section (not uncommon in distributions where π_4 and π_5 are being studied) error may be introduced by summation (dashed line). c. Summation often occurs at transitions from one mechanism to a second, where near equivalence in sensitivity exists. These three figures have been adapted from Boynton (1963)

and operating independently, have a greater probability of detecting a signal than one acting alone.[10] Obviously, if the sensitivity of one mechanism is greater than that of the second, probability summation will change in relation to the disparity between the sensitivities of the two "observers". Boynton argues that the third possibility, no summation at all, probably requires an active inhibitory process. In fact, he suggests that opponent processes might give rise to such phenomena.

[10] The threshold case (when either mechanism acting alone has a 50% chance of responding to the flash) at λ_0 is equivalent to asking the probability of at least one head turning up on two independent tosses of a coin. The answer is a 75% chance of seeing, or at least one head turning up.

STILES, in his Newton lecture (1967), talks of the need for a color differencing system to bring about this result.

For specific experimental conditions, BOYNTON, IKEDA, and STILES (1964), and IKEDA (1963) have reported each of these forms of interaction. These experiments were complex in nature and required a double-flash arrangement with each of the two flashes presented simultaneously and usually of a different wavelength. Adaptation level and flash duration proved to be key variables, since the result obtained depended in large measure on these test conditions. They found that when the two flashes influenced the same π mechanism, complete summation was achieved. In fact, this is predicted in STILES' assumption number 7 above. Where more than one mechanism was involved, there was sometimes probability summation, and in many cases more or less summation was found. The data actually revealed a series of complex relations. Effects that might be created by summative properties (which are most significant near transitions between mechanisms) are shown in Fig. 10b and c, taken from BOYNTON (1963). These effects raise questions regarding the independence of mechanisms in these test situations. One can only conclude that transitions must be regarded as less reliable for purposes of data interpretation.

In another set of important but complex experiments, ALPERN and RUSHTON (1965) (see also ALPERN, 1965), claim independence of action of the π functions in the after-flash effect. BOYNTON, DAS, and GARDINER (1966) question the validity of ALPERN and RUSHTON'S models and feel that their results conflict with those of BOYNTON, IKEDA, and STILES (1964). In the 1966 paper BOYNTON *et al.* extend the earlier studies of π mechanism interactions. They point out that *t.v.r.* functions used to distinguish π_5 are often of the type seen in Fig. 10b. The rather small lateral separation of the π_4 and π_5 mechanisms, and the resultant interactions between these functions tend to make the interpretation difficult. They conclude that π_4 and π_5 are not unitary functions, rather they seem to be made up of underlying mechanisms whose spectral sensitivities remain reasonably well fixed with respect to one another. They further conclude that for the specific test conditions described, thresholds are not wholly determined by the most sensitive mechanism acting alone. This conclusion contradicts some of STILES' basic assumptions. However, as noted, STILES has never claimed that his model is all inclusive and has repeatedly indicated where the functions fail to act in the anticipated manner. The issue has not yet been fully resolved. Interestingly, BOYNTON (1963), IKEDA (1963) and more recently INGLING (1969) suggest that four narrower band mechanisms or pigments are needed to account for the measured effects. They would include a "yellow" function. BOYNTON'S student, INGLING, argues that a four pigment stage which immediately converges to a three channel stage fits available data.

In summary, BOYNTON and his co-workers have raised some valid points concerning STILES' experimental model. Working together, BOYNTON, IKEDA, and STILES (1964) have investigated the problem of π mechanism interaction. Whereas the results of those studies create problems, they do not destroy the rationale of the technique. Rather, the questions raised are important if the mechanisms subserving adaptation and color vision are to be understood. In a sense, these studies open a new and important phase in the analysis of the component color processes.

Other Related Studies

A growing number of studies are appearing in the literature which are directly related studies of the π mechanisms using STILES' two-color threshold technique. They fall into certain logical categories. There are experiments which are concerned with transient effects such as those conducted by BOYNTON (mentioned above). Other investigations are concerned with detecting the presence of the π functions by other psychophysical or electrophysiological procedures, e.g., DU CROZ and RUSHTON (1966). These authors identified π_1, π_4, and π_5 by selective chromatic light adaptation and the measurement of subsequent dark adaptation functions using test flashes of different wavelengths. Essential independence of these mechanisms was found for these test conditions, although evidence for limited interactions was presented. AUERBACH and WALD (1954) using a similar technique had previously defined what they called a "violet detector".

BOYNTON and WAGNER (1961) first sought to use the two color threshold technique as a clinical tool, and studies by BAKER (1966), WALD (1966), and ALPERN *et al.* (1965, 1968) have contributed additional data for color deficient individuals. The technique, as used so far, fails to discriminate between anomalous trichromats and related dichromats, e.g., between protanopes and protanomalous.

Other investigators use the Stiles technique to isolate a π mechanism, and then study the response characteristics of that component color process, e.g., GREEN (1968) has evaluated the resolution characteristics of several π components. In particular, GREEN found (as had STILES, 1949, and BRINDLEY, 1960, p. 235) that the "blue" mechanism had rather reduced resolution capability. The "blue" mechanism is something of an enigma. It has a rather different retinal distribution from the other mechanisms (e.g., WALD, 1967), and a much higher Weber fraction (Table 1). It would seem valuable to examine additional properties of this mechanism, as well as the characteristics of the others.

This chapter has concentrated on defining the basic procedure and its current status. For a review of several of the developments touched on above, the reader is referred to an extensive discussion by ALPERN (1968), and to RIPPS and WEALE (1969) for many pertinent references.

Conclusions

The two-color increment threshold method of STILES represents an important development in the effort to understand mechanisms subserving color vision. One must be impressed by the number of studies which have been stimulated by this theoretical and experimental development culminating in the definition of component color processes known as π functions. These mechanisms are not simple representations of cone pigment action spectra, but are clearly highly influenced by the photosensitive pigments. The π mechanisms are not as free of interactive processes as STILES had obviously hoped, but they are not so compromised by these phenomena that their value is lost. In short, the π functions most probably represent a relatively stable, early, reproduceable stage in the biological processing of color vision "data". As such, they serve as a criterion or reference in our efforts to further define color vision processes. As is so often the case, many questions remain unresolved.

Acknowledgements. The author wishes to thank W. S. STILES for critically reading this manuscript and for his many constructive suggestions.

The illustrations contained in this chapter have been taken largely from earlier studies by STILES. Dr. STILES has been kind enough to update and correct data. He prepared Figs. 7, 8 and 9 for inclusion in this manuscript. Fig. 6 was obtained from F. H. C. MARRIOTT'S excellent chapter dealing with STILES' two-color threshold technique which appeared in H. DAVSON (Editor). The Eye, *II. The Visual Process*, Academic Press, N. Y. 1962, p. 253. Fig. 10 was taken from BOYNTON, 1963. The data attributed to WALD in Figs. 7 and 8 are based on subject R.H. in his 1964 paper. The origin of other figures has been identified in the text. The author wishes to thank the publishers and authors for their permission to reproduce these illustrations.

This work has been supported in part by Research Grant Number NBO-2168-11, and Career Development Award Number NB-K3-15, 138-08 of the National Institute of Neurological Diseases and Blindness (now National Eye Institute), National Institutes of Health Bethesda, Maryland, U.S.A.

References

AGUILAR, M., STILES, W. S.: Saturation of the rod mechanism of the retina at high levels of stimulation. Optica Acta **1**, 59—65 (1954).

ALPERN, M.: Rod-cone independence in the after-flash effect. J. Physiol. (Lond.) **176**, 462—472 (1965).

— Distal mechanisms of vertebrate color vision. Ann. Rev. Physiol. **30**, 279—318 (1968).

— LEE, G. B., SPIVEY, B. E.: π_1 Cone monochromatism. Arch. Ophthal. **74**, 334—337 (1965).

— MINDEL, J., TORII: Are there two types of deuteranopes? J. Physiol. (Lond.) **199**, 443—456 (1968).

— RUSHTON, W. A. H.: The specificity of the cone interaction in the after-flash effect. J. Physiol. (Lond.) **176**, 473—482 (1965).

— TORII, S.: Prereceptor colour vision distortions in protanomalous trichromacy. J. Physiol. (Lond.) **198**, 549—560 (1968).

AUERBACH, E., WALD, G.: Identification of a violet receptor in human volor vision. Science **120**, 401—405 (1954).

BAKER, H. D.: Single-variable anomaloscope matches during recovery from artificial red blindness. J. opt. Soc. Amer. **56**, 686—689 (1966).

— RUSHTON, W. A. H.: The red-sensitive pigment in normal cones. J. Physiol. (Lond.) **176**, 56—72 (1965).

BLACKWELL, H. R., BLACKWELL, O. M.: Identification of rod and cone receptor mechanisms in atypical congenital achromatopsia. Arch. Soc. Amer. Oftal. Optom. (Bogata) **2**, 73—94 (1959). See also Vision Res. **1**, 62—107 (1961).

BOYNTON, R. M.: Rapid chromatic adaptation and the sensitivity functions of human color vision. J. opt. Soc. Amer. **46**, 172—179 (1956).

— Contributions of threshold measurements to color discrimination theory. J. opt. Soc. Amer. **53**, 165—178 (1963).

— DAS, S., GARDINER, J.: Interaction between photopic visual mechanisms revealed by mixing conditioning fields. J. opt. Soc. Amer. **56**, 1775—1780 (1966).

— IKEDA, M., STILES, W. S.: Interactions among chromatic mechanisms as inferred from positive and negative increment thresholds. Vision Res. **4**, 87—117 (1964).

— KANDEL, G., ONLEY, J.: Rapid chromatic adaptation of normal and dichromatic observers. J. opt. Soc. Amer. **49**, 654—666 (1959).

— WAGNER, M.: Two-color threshold as test of color vision. J. opt. Soc. Amer. **51**, 429—440 (1961).

BRINDLEY, G. S.: The effects on color vision of adaptation to very bright lights. J. Physiol. (Lond.) **122**, 332—350 (1953).

— Physiology of the Retina and the Visual Pathway. London: Arnold 1960.

BUSACCA, A.: Les aspects du fond de l'oeil normal étudié par la stéréoophthalmoscopie. Arch. Ophthal. (Paris) **7**, 361 (1947).

COLE, B. L., WATKINS, R.: Increment thresholds in tritanopia. Vision Res. **7**, 939—947 (1967).

DARTNALL, H. J. A.: The interpretation of spectral sensitivity curves. Brit. med. Bull. **9**, 24—30 (1953).

DAS, S. R.: Foveal sensitivity for a protanope in relation to Stiles' "blue" and "green" mechanisms. J. opt. Soc. Amer. **54**, 839—841 (1964).

DEVRIES, HL.: On the basic sensation curves of the three-color theory. J. opt. Soc. Amer. **36**, 121—127 (1946).

DUCROZ, J. J., RUSHTON, W. A. H.: The separation of cone mechanisms in dark adaptation. J. Physiol. (Lond.) **183**, 481—496 (1966).

FRIEDMAN, E., KUWABARA, T.: The retinal pigment epithelium: IV. The damaging effects of radiant energy. Arch. Ophthal. **80**, 265—279 (1968).

GREEN, D. G.: The contrast sensitivity of the colour mechanisms of the human eye. J. Physiol. (Lond.) **196**, 415—429 (1968).

HSIA, Y., GRAHAM, C. H.: Spectral luminosity curves for protanopic, deuteranopic, and normal observers. Proc. nat. Acad. Sci. (Wash.) **43**, 1011—1019 (1957).

HURVICH, L. M., JAMESON, D.: Further development of a quantified opponent-colors theory. In: Visual Problems of Colour, Vol. II, pp. 691—773, London: H. M. Stationery Office 1952.

— — Color vision. Ann. Rev. Psychol. **11**, 99—130 (1960).

— — KRANTZ, D. H.: Theoretical treatments of selected visual problems. In: Handbook of Mathematical Psychology, Vol. 3, pp. 100—159. LUCE, R. D., BUSH, R. R., GALANTER, E. (Eds.) New York: Wiley 1965.

IKEDA, M.: Study of interrelations between mechanisms at threshold. J. opt. Soc. Amer. **53**, 1305—1313 (1963).

— Further use of the summation index for the study of color vision. J. opt. Soc. Amer. **54**, 89—94 (1964).

— Temporal summation of positive and negative flashes in the visual system. J. opt. Soc. Amer. **55**, 1527—1534 (1965).

— BOYNTON, R. M.: Effect of test-flash duration upon the spectral sensitivity of the eye. J. opt. Soc. Amer. **52**, 697—699 (1962).

— — Negative flashes, positive flashes, and flicker examined by increment threshold technique. J. opt. Soc. Amer. **55**, 560—566 (1965).

INGLING, C. R., JR.: A tetrachromatic hypothesis for human color vision. Vision Res. **9**, 1131—1148 (1969).

KÜHNE, W.: Untersuchungen über den Sehpurpur. Untersuchungen aus dem Physiol. Inst. Heidelberg, Bd. 1, S. 409—411. (1877).

MARRIOTT, F. H. C.: Color vision: The two color threshold technique of Stiles. In: The Eye, Vol. 2, Ch. 14, pp. 251—272. DAVSON, H. (Ed.) New York: Academic Press 1962.

RIGGS, L.: Electrical evidence on the trichromatic theory. Invest. Ophthal. **6**, 6—17 (1967).

RIPPS, H., WEALE, R. A.: Color vision. Ann. Rev. Psychol. **20**, 193—216 (1969).

ROAF, H. E.: The influence of coloured surrounds and coloured backgrounds on visual thresholds. Proc. roy. Soc. (Lond.,) B **111**, 448—482 (1932).

RUSHTON, W. A. H.: The difference spectrum and photo-sensitivity of rhodopsin in the living human eye. J. Physiol. (Lond.) **134**, 11—29 (1956).

— Kinetics of cone pigments measured objectively in the living human fovea. Ann. N. Y. Acad. Sci. **74**, 291—304 (1958a).

— The cone pigments of the human fovea in colour blind and normal. In: Visual Problems of Colour; Vol. 1, pp. 71—105. London: H. M. Stationery Office 1958b.

— Visual pigments in man and animals and their relation to seeing. Prog. Biophys. **9**, 239—283 (1959).

— Cone pigment kinetics in the protanope. J. Physiol. (Lond.) **168**, 374—388 (1963).

— Colour blindness and cone pigments. Amer. J. Optom. **41**, 265—282 (1964).

— Chemical basis of colour vision and colour blindness. Nature (Lond.) **206**, 1087—1091 (1965).

— Densitometry of pigments in rods and cones of normal and color defective subjects. Invest. Ophthal. **5**, 233—241 (1966).

RUSHTON, W. A. H., HENRY, G. H.: Bleaching and regeneration of cone pigments in man. Vision Res. **8**, 617—631 (1968).

STILES, W. S.: The directional sensitivity of the retina and the spectral sensitivity of the rods and cones. Proc. roy. Soc. (Lond.) B **127**, 64—105 (1939).

— The basic sensation curves of the three-color theory. J. opt. Soc. Amer. **36**, 491—492 (1946a).

— Separation of the "blue" and "green" mechanisms of foveal vision by measurements of increment thresholds. Proc. roy. Soc. (Lond.) B **133**, 418—434 (1946b).

— Increment thresholds and the mechanisms of colour vision. Documenta Ophthal. **3**, 138—165 (1949).

— Visual properties studied by subjective measurements on the colour-adapted eye. Brit. med. Bull. **9**, 41—49 (1953a).

— Further studies of visual mechanisms by the two-colour threshold method. Coloquio sobre problemas opticos de la vision (Madrid), Union Internationale de Physique pure et appliquée, **1**, 65—103 (1953b).

— Color vision: The approach through increment-threshold sensitivity. Proc. nat. Acad. Sci. (Wash.) **45**, 100—114 (1959).

— Adaptation, chromatic adaptation, colour transformation. An. real Soc. Esp. Fisica Quimica. A, **57**, 149—175 (1961).

— Foveal threshold sensitivity on fields of different colors. Science **145**, 1016—1017 (1964).

— Newton Lecture, Mechanism concepts in colour theory, J. Colour Group (Lond.), No. 11, 105—123, November (1967).

— CRAWFORD, B. H.: The liminal brightness increment as a function of wave-length for different conditions of the foveal and parafoveal retina. Proc. roy. Soc. (Lond.) B **113**, 496—530 (1933a).

— — The luminous efficiency of rays entering the eye pupil at different points. Proc. roy. Soc. (Lond.) B **112**, 428—450 (1933b).

THOMSON, L. C., WRIGHT, W. D.: The convergence of the tritanopic confusion loci and the derivation of the fundamental response functions. J. opt. Soc. Amer. **43**, 890—894 (1953).

WALD, G.: The receptors of human color vision. Science **145**, 1007—1016 (1964).

— Frequency or wavelength. Science **150**, 1239—1240 (1965).

— Defective color vision and its inheritance. Proc. nat. Acad. Sci. (Wash.) **55**, 1347—1363 (1966).

— Blue-blindness in the normal fovea. J. opt. Soc. Amer. **57**, 1289—1301 (1967).

— Molecular basis of visual excitation. Science **162**, 230—239 (1968).

WEALE, R. A.: Comparison of reactions of human and rabbit fundi to photic exposures. J. opt. Soc. Amer. **54**, 120 (1964).

WYSZECKI, G., STILES, W. S.: Color Science: Concepts and methods, quantitative data and formulas. New York: Wiley 1967. Items of main interest appear in Chapter 7.

Chapter 22

Color Adaptation: Sensitivity, Contrast, After-Images

By

DOROTHEA JAMESON and LEO M. HURVICH, Philadelphia, Pennsylvania (USA)

With 3 Figures

Contents

I. Introduction

This chapter deals with the problems of chromatic adaptation and its mechanisms. In our analysis of chromatic adaptation and its use to reveal specific properties of the mechanism of color vision, we shall discuss sensitivity changes, contrast effects and after-images. Despite the intrinsic interest of each of these topics, we are not here concerned with a detailed and comprehensive description of the multiplicity of visual effects conventionally grouped under the separate rubrics, contrast, after-images, etc.

For an early annotated bibliography of contrast phenomena that summarizes and comments on several hundred reports that date from ancient times through the year 1877, the reader is referred to Sections V and VI of PLATEAU's comprehensive review (1878). Section 24 of KÖNIG's bibliography in the second edition of HELMHOLTZ's Physiological Optics carries the bibliographic material through the year 1894, and the best review article through the end of the last century that treats the facts, laws, and theories of contrast and irradiation is probably TSCHERMAK's paper (1903). Later accounts can be found in PARSONS (1924) and GRAHAM and BROWN (1965). Excellent comprehensive reviews of the early work on adaptation and after-images can also be found in other sections of PLATEAU's review, in HELMHOLTZ, and in PARSONS' classic work on color vision. A good inclusive contemporary review of the work on after-images is available in BROWN's chapter in Vision and Visual Perception (1965).

II. Coefficient Law

Chromatic adaptation phenomena have long been used to try to analyze the physiological properties of the visual mechanism (VON KRIES, 1878; WRIGHT, 1934; MACADAM, 1956). In addition, many psychophysical studies of chromatic adaptation have been concerned with elucidating the lawful relations that hold between phenomena of color appearance when the eye is exposed to illuminated scenes of different illuminant qualities, i.e., illuminants of different spectral compositions (HELSON *et al.*, 1952; BURNHAM *et al.*, 1952). In the latter context, it is of first importance to note that metameric color equations, that is, equations between lights of different spectral distributions, continue to hold when the state of chromatic adaptation is changed at normal photopic levels. This metamer invariance does break down with a change from photopic to scotopic adaptation for stimuli not confined to the nearly rod-frce center of the fovea, or upon exposure to extremely high energy levels of chromatic light (WRIGHT, 1936; BRINDLEY, 1953). The cause of the former breakdown is obvious, since the rod system enters into the light reception process at low levels of illumination and adaptation as a fourth, mathematically independent variable. At higher light levels, however, the rod system is presumably saturated and thus not capable of variations in response; vision is accomplished primarily by variations in cone response (AGUILAR and STILES, 1954). The breakdown of metameric matches at extremely high levels of light exposure is a strong indication that the forms of the spectral distributions of the three types of cone receptor have been altered, whereas chromatic adaptation at normal (i.e., useful) levels of exposure seems to produce changes in the balance of sensitivities of the three kinds of cone photoreceptor with no change in the form of the spectral distribution of each but only a variation of its amplitude. Thus, if α_λ, β_λ, γ_λ represent the spectral distributions of the cone-receptor elements for one state of adaptation, and α'_λ, β'_λ, γ'_λ represent the altered sensitivities of these elements brought about by exposure to chromatic illumination, then

$$\begin{aligned} \alpha'_\lambda &= k_1 \alpha_\lambda \\ \beta'_\lambda &= k_2 \beta_\lambda \\ \gamma'_\lambda &= k_3 \gamma_\lambda . \end{aligned} \tag{1}$$

The relations expressed in Eqs. (1) comprise what has come to be known as the von Kries Coefficient Law (VON KRIES, 1905), when the magnitudes of k_1, k_2, k_3 are interpreted as inversely related to the relative strengths of activation of α, β, γ by the particular energy distribution of the chromatic adapting light in question.

This conceptualization is a fairly simple one, and it would seem to provide not only a ready analytical concept for visual scientists to systematize and describe the perceptual effects of chromatic adaptation, but also a tool by which the underlying distributions, α_λ, β_λ, γ_λ might be precisely specified on the basis of carefully measured psychophysical data for chromatic adaptation to various lights of known spectral energy distributions. The von Kries coefficient logic has been basic to a great deal of experimental psychophysical research and it continues to be so, either implicitly or explicitly, both in current psychophysical work (TAKASAKI, 1969; JUDD, 1960; PEARSON *et al.*, 1969) and in electrophysiological experiments concerned with unit cellular responses thought to be part of the mechanism of color vision (De Valois, 1965; Naka and Rushton, 1966a, b; Gouras, 1970).

The psychophysical measures that have been used extensively in studies of chromatic adaptation are threshold measures, on the one hand, and matching data, on the other. For the threshold measures, the basic idea is simply to selectively suppress one of the basic cone mechanisms by spectrally selective light exposure and thus to reveal the sensitivities of the other mechanisms without contamination by the adapted one, or better still, to selectively suppress two of the three cone responses and reveal the third in isolation. The essential feature of this approach is that, within the logic of the conceptual analysis, the isolated sensitivity distribution that can be measured by the spectral distribution of the threshold data is precisely the same for all physiological states of the system, with variations possible in amplitude only. It is, of course, essential to the logic that the mechanisms act completely independently insofar as the determination of the threshold measures is concerned, since any interdependence would clearly contaminate the spectral distribution revealed by the threshold measures.

The particular psychophysical technique most commonly used in recent years for this kind of experiment is that of increment thresholds. For these measures, the spectrally selective adapting light remains visible throughout the experiment, and detectibility of threshold flashes is determined for test lights superimposed on the adapting light as background. This is the technique used by Wald (1964) in recent years in his attempt to supplement the direct spectrophotometric measures of cone absorption (Brown and Wald, 1964; Marks *et al.*, 1964) by psychophysical measures of the same absorption characteristics. Wald's application of the increment threshold technique has involved the use of very high energy background adapting lights exclusively. Thus, to reveal the spectral characteristics of the mechanism with maximal sensitivity in the region of 440—450 nm, he measures thresholds throughout the spectrum for test lights superimposed on a very intense yellow background, i.e., a background light that consists of energy from the mid- and long-wave regions but with relatively little energy from the short-wave spectral region (less than about 500 nm). To reveal the function with maximum at 530 to 540 nm, the background light is one that contains both short- and long-wave radiation of high energy content and relatively little in the mid-spectral region. The function with maximum at 550—570 nm is measured against a high energy background of radiation concentrated in the short-wave spectral region. Wald's psychophysical threshold experiments are designed on a logical basis that is a direct parallel to that of his selective bleach experiments to measure photopigment difference spectra. The selective bleach technique is used to reveal separate photopigments in a mixture of photosensitive materials that contains more than a single visual pigment. The technique was first used successfully by him to reveal the cone pigment *iodopsin* as a difference spectrum in an extract from chicken retina that was measured after a long-wave bleaching light irradiated a solution of mixed rod and cone pigments (Wald, 1937; Wald *et al.*, 1955). The long-wave bleaching light was, of course, relatively ineffective with respect to the rod pigment *rhodopsin* which absorbs relatively little long-wave light and has its maximum around 500 nm.

It is important to note that Wald's increment-threshold, selective-bleach experiments, and his interpretation of the psychophysical results as revealing the absorption (action) spectra of the three selective cone photopigments, in no sense either test or confirm the validity of the von Kries Coefficient Law for chromatic adaptation. This law can be considered valid only under conditions for which it can be demonstrated that the three underlying mechanisms act independently, for which there is persistence of metameric color matches, and for which the "proportionality rule" can be shown to hold. We shall discuss the proportionality rule and the question of its validity in a later context. The very high intensity background bleaching lights used in the WALD increment-threshold technique are precisely the kinds of energy levels that have been shown to produce a breakdown in the persistence of metameric matches (WRIGHT, 1936; BRINDLEY, 1953). If the color-match breakdowns can be attributed exclusively to a change in the form of the effective spectral distribution of that mechanism that is selectively desensitized by the adapting light, then this departure from von Kries' requirements need have no contaminating effect on the sensitivities revealed by the threshold technique for that particular adapting light, since the measured sensitivities refer to mechanisms that have *not* been strongly depressed by the adapting or bleaching stimulus. If the mechanisms do not act independently, however, that is, if the measured sensitivity that is primarily determined by one of the three is altered by interaction with another mechanism, then the force of this interaction on the threshold data can be assumed to differ for different levels of activation of the interacting mechanism, and the precise meaning of the different measured functions becomes a more complex matter than is its parallel meaning in the selective bleach experiments of the photochemist dealing with extracted photosensitive materials in solutions. Unfortunately for the simplicity of the analysis of experiments of this sort, the independence postulate, when tested in the more extensive increment-threshold experiments of the STILES type (1949, 1959), has been shown to be invalid under some circumstances (BOYNTON *et al.*, 1964). STILES' experiments, which are described and analyzed in detail by ENOCH in Chapter 21 of this volume, provide a more rigorous test of the properties of the systems that determine threshold sensitivities: complete functions are determined for given test lights against given background lights over a wide range of energy values. Under these more rigorous conditions, it has been demonstrated by STILES (1959) that the increment thresholds must be related, not simply to three differently selective spectral mechanisms, but rather to five, or perhaps seven such mechanisms. For this reason, STILES does not describe the mechanisms revealed by increment threshold in his hands as cone absorption functions, but rather as π mechanisms whose precise physiological interpretation is left unspecified. It is also under the more rigorous testing conditions of the Stiles type increment-threshold analyses that the independence postulate is shown not to be universally valid. In summary, therefore, it can be said that the logic of the von Kries formulation of chromatic adaptation leads to threshold experiments that anticipate the separate revelation and specification of three different spectrally selective mechanisms of color vision, but that the experiments carried out so far do not entirely confirm the basic premises of the von Kries analysis.

The third requirement for the validity of the von Kries interpretation of chromatic adaptation is, as VON KRIES himself explicitly recognized in his original formulation (1905), that the proportionality rule must be shown to hold under any conditions in which the coefficient analysis is applied. If the relations of Eqs. (1) (p. 569) correctly describe the differences in component sensitivities between one state of chromatic adaptation and another, then the following relations describe the state of affairs for metameric matches that hold for both states of adaptation. For one state of adaptation,

$$\begin{aligned} e_{\lambda(A)}\,\alpha_\lambda &= e_{\lambda(B)}\,\alpha_\lambda \\ e_{\lambda(A)}\,\beta_\lambda &= e_{\lambda(B)}\,\beta_\lambda \\ e_{\lambda(A)}\,\gamma_\lambda &= e_{\lambda(B)}\,\gamma_\lambda \end{aligned} \tag{2}$$

when

$$e_{\lambda(A)} \equiv e_{\lambda(B)}\,,$$

which is the metamer rule.

For a different state of chromatic adaptation, α, β, γ become α', β', γ', but since Eqs. (1) is assumed to hold, then

$$\begin{aligned} e_{\lambda(A)}\,k_1\alpha_\lambda &= e_{\lambda(B)}\,k_1\alpha_\lambda \\ e_{\lambda(A)}\,k_2\beta_\lambda &= e_{\lambda(B)}\,k_2\beta_\lambda \\ e_{\lambda(A)}\,k_3\gamma_\lambda &= e_{\lambda(B)}\,k_3\gamma_\lambda\,, \end{aligned} \tag{3}$$

the persistence rule.

By the rules of "color arithmetic", or Grassman's Laws (see WRIGHT, Chapter 16, this volume), we can also write:

$$a_1 e_{\lambda(A)} \equiv a_1 e_{\lambda(B)}\,,$$

and thus,

$$\begin{aligned} a_1 e_{\lambda(A)}\,\alpha_\lambda &= a_1 e_{\lambda(B)}\,\alpha_\lambda \\ a_1 e_{\lambda(A)}\,\beta_\lambda &= a_1 e_{\lambda(B)}\,\beta_\lambda \\ a_1 e_{\lambda(A)}\,\gamma_\lambda &= a_1 e_{\lambda(B)}\,\gamma_\lambda\,, \end{aligned} \tag{4}$$

the proportionality rule. The rule applies equally, of course, whether the mechanism sensitivities for both sides of Eqs. (4) are α_λ, β_λ, γ_λ for one state of adaptation, or $k_1\alpha_\lambda$, $k_2\beta_\lambda$, $k_3\gamma_\lambda$ for a different adaptive state. If the adaptive state differs on the two sides of the equation, then the original metameric match between $e_{\lambda(A)}$ and $e_{\lambda(B)}$ will no longer hold, and a new match

$$e_{\lambda(A)} \equiv e_{\lambda(C)}$$

must be established. If the coefficient rule for chromatic adaptation correctly describes the new match situation, then,

$$\begin{aligned} e_{\lambda(A)}\,\alpha_\lambda &= e_{\lambda(C)}\,k_1\,\alpha_\lambda \\ e_{\lambda(A)}\,\beta_\lambda &= e_{\lambda(C)}\,k_2\beta_\lambda \\ e_{\lambda(A)}\,\gamma_\lambda &= e_{\lambda(C)}\,k_3\gamma_\lambda\,. \end{aligned} \tag{5}$$

When the proportionality rule is applied in this, asymmetrical adaptation situation, it must also be true that

$$\begin{aligned} a_1 e_{\lambda(A)}\,\alpha_\lambda &= a_1 e_{\lambda(C)}\,k_1\,\alpha_\lambda \\ a_1 e_{\lambda(A)}\,\beta_\lambda &= a_1 e_{\lambda(C)}\,k_2\beta_\lambda \\ a_1 e_{\lambda(A)}\,\gamma_\lambda &= a_1 e_{\lambda(C)}\,k_3\gamma_\lambda\,, \end{aligned} \tag{6}$$

the proportionality rule for asymmetrical chromatic adaptation that is consistent with the von Kries Coefficient Law.

III. Non-Validity of Proportionality Rule

If the von Kries formulation is valid, then the proportionality rule of Eqs. (6) must be shown to be valid. The conditions under which it is reasonable to test this rule should not, of course, include those under which persistence breaks down. The test would necessarily fail for test lights of such low luminance values that they can legitimately be considered scotopic and thus involve the rod receptor system. It would also be predicted to fail for adapting lights so intense that they can reasonably be expected to bleach a large fraction of a given cone pigment and give rise to a new screening pigment or otherwise cause an alteration in the effective spectral distribution function of any one of the cone receptors. For moderate photopic levels of adapting and test lights, however, for which the persistence rule [Eqs. (3)] holds, the proportionality rule can also be expected to hold if the adaptation mechanism has been correctly described by the coefficient formulation.

Although there has always been good reason to assume that the proportionality rule could not be completely valid, its validity or approximate validity has been implicitly assumed over the years in many studies of chromatic adaptation that involve the determination of color matches for two different states of adaptation (e.g., MacAdam, 1956).

Suppose conditions such that $e_{\lambda(A)} \equiv e_{\lambda(B)}$ when the eye is adapted at a photopic level to a neutral or white light. Suppose also that the same metameric match holds when the eye is adapted at a moderate photopic level to a strongly chromatic, say, deep red, light. The matched fields, $e_{\lambda(A)}$ and $e_{\lambda(B)}$, although identical to each other for both conditions of adaptation, will appear very different in color to the chromatically adapted eye as contrasted with the neutrally adapted one. To determine the way in which the matching light distributions must be changed in order to produce the same color appearance for the two different states of adaptation, it is necessary to compare matches made in a bipartite field when the eye is adapted to, say, neutral light for the left hand side of the color match and to the deep red chromatic light for the other side of the color match. This can be done (1) by pre-exposing the eye to juxtaposed neutral and red adapting lights each of which is incident on the respective part of the retina that is to be tested subsequently by the test lights $e_{(A)}$ and $e_{(C)}$ that are to be matched; (2) by presenting the test stimuli for the matching equation separately to the two separate eyes of a single observer, for example, $e_{(A)}$ to the left eye and $e_{(C)}$ to the right. The distributions required for the color equation are then compared, first when both eyes had been pre-exposed to the neutral light, and second when one eye is pre-exposed to the neutral light and the other eye to the colored adapting stimulus. The latter situation has been used frequently in studies of color adaptation that employ a matching measurement procedure, and it is variously called binocular, dichoptic, or haploscopic color matching. We prefer the latter term, viz., haploscopic, for those situations in which both eyes are involved but the stimuli presented to the two separate retinas are not the same and are independently controlled. We avoid the term "binocular" for this situation since binocular vision implies the normal everyday manner of viewing lights in which the same external source is imaged at corresponding points on the two retinas and is not controlled independently for the two eyes.

The importance of the haploscopic matching paradigm is that, if the von Kries formulation is valid, then asymmetrical color matches of this sort for different conditions of adaptation and for a variety of test lights of different wavelengths or spectral compositions can yield the information necessary to derive, by analysis, the underlying spectral distributions, α_λ, β_λ, γ_λ.

Metameric color-match data for any given uniform state of adaptation can be satisfied by any set of three spectral distributions that are linear transformations of the "true" physiological distributions. The data for equivalent color appearance for different states of adaptation can, however, within the paradigm, be accounted for by only a single such set, presumably the "true" physiological ones. Disappointingly, the many carefully carried out experiments of this sort over the years have failed to yield this important and simple result (WRIGHT, 1947; BREWER, 1954; MACADAM, 1956; BURNHAM *et al.*, 1957). When subjected to a least-squares mathematical analysis to solve for the underlying distributions, either the data yield complex roots or, if the number of variables is not limited *a priori* to the assumed three, a number greater than three is found. When, as an alternative, the matching data are subjected to mathematical analysis in order to derive generalized empirical relations between stimuli that yield equivalent color appear-

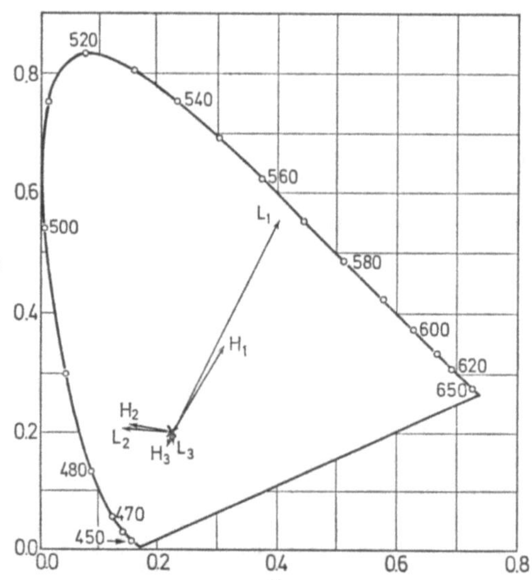

Fig. 1. Chromaticity shifts for a single test color at two luminance levels (10 mL and 1 mL) for three pairs of haploscopic conditions. The large X in the diagram at $x = 0.23$, $y = 0.20$ represents the CIE chromaticity of the small variable matching stimulus in the left eye for both a high and low luminance level of the test field of fixed spectral distribution in the right eye when no surround is present in either eye. When the left eye is adapted to a heterogeneous near-neutral distribution (10 mL) and the right eye to a 450 nm stimulus of the same luminance, the match for the high luminance test stimulus is the chromaticity indicated by the arrow head at H_1 on the chart, and for the same adapting and surround conditions, the match to the low luminance stimulus is at the point labelled L_1. For the right eye adapted to 650 nm, and all other conditions the same, the comparable matches for the two test levels are at H_2 and L_2, respectively. For right eye adaptation to 580 nm, the matches are located at the points H_3 and L_3, respectively

ance for different conditions of adaptation without attempting to use such data to solve for the three fundamental physiological variables, the generalized empirical relations that emerge are more complex than the simple linear relations described above.

Our own analysis of the chromatic adaptation situation responsible for this unfortunately complex state of affairs suggested that the difficulty lay in the failure of the proportionality rule, even within the restricted range of conditions for which it should hold (HURVICH and JAMESON, 1958; JAMESON and HURVICH, 1959). Fig. 1 reproduces results published in 1958 that show, on a standard CIE chromaticity diagram, the haploscopic color matches for different states of adaptation in the two eyes when test stimuli were presented at each of two different energy levels, both within the photopic range. The figure shows the way in which a matching stimulus must be varied in chromaticity when the nature of the chromatic adapting light is varied, and it also shows the different chromaticity shifts that are measured when the same test stimulus is presented at either a high or a low level of luminance. If the proportionality rule of Eq. 6 were valid, the chromaticity shifts for both levels of test luminance would be identical within the error of measurement. Clearly, this is far from the case. Data such as those shown in Fig. 1 demonstrate that when $e_{\lambda(A)} \equiv e_{\lambda(C)}$ for the asymmetrical adaptation case,

$$a_1 e_{\lambda(A)} \not\equiv a_1 e_{\lambda(C)}\,.$$

The logic of the simple linear von Kries coefficient law is inadequate to handle the chromatic adaptation phenomena.

IV. "Two-Process" Interpretation

Our analysis (JAMESON and HURVICH, 1959) of chromatic adaptation data such as those shown in Fig. 1, as well as those of many other adaptation studies for which the coefficient rule proved less than adequate (e.g., HELSON, 1938; HELSON and JEFFERS, 1940; JUDD, 1940; WALTERS, 1942; WRIGHT, 1947; MACADAM, 1956; BURNHAM *et al.*, 1957), suggested that the phenomena require a "two-process" interpretation, namely, an incremental process in addition to the multiplicative process of the coefficient rule. The way in which we have interpreted the two different processes attributes the multiplicative sensitivity change to the cone receptor level, and the incremental shift to the post-receptoral neural units or systems in which the opponent, presumably color-coded, neural responses are detected.

Figs. 2 and 3 illustrate the differences in the component functions of a normal trivariant color vision system at these two different levels. In Fig. 2a, the three curves are assumed to represent a system balanced for a chromatically neutral state of adaptation. These three all positive functions are linear transformations of the standard color-mixture data of the CIE 1931 Standard Observer (see WRIGHT, Chapter 16, this volume). The spectral peaks of the three functions are not inconsistent with the most recent data on human cone absorptions, although the forms of the functions are not precisely those to be anticipated for visual photopigments. (See JAMESON, Chapter 14, this volume, where these functions are appropriately corrected to represent their "absorption" characteristics at the retinal level;

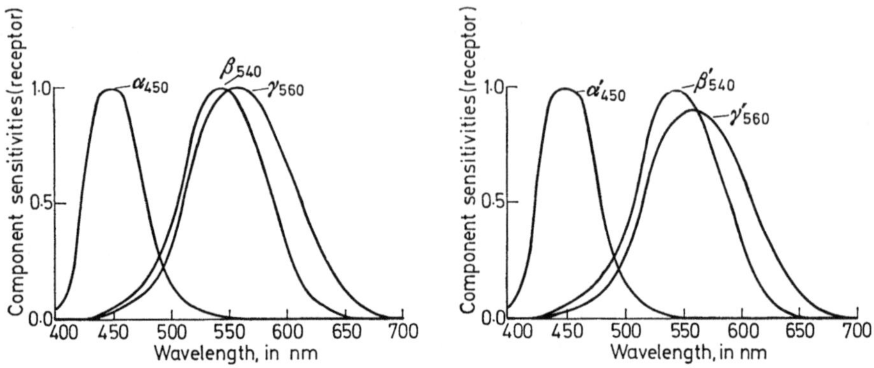

Fig. 2. Component sensitivities (receptor level). For equal energy level at cornea. Not corrected for ocular transmission or quantal absorption. *a* Neutral balance of sensitivities. *b* Balance of sensitivities altered for adaptation to 650 nm

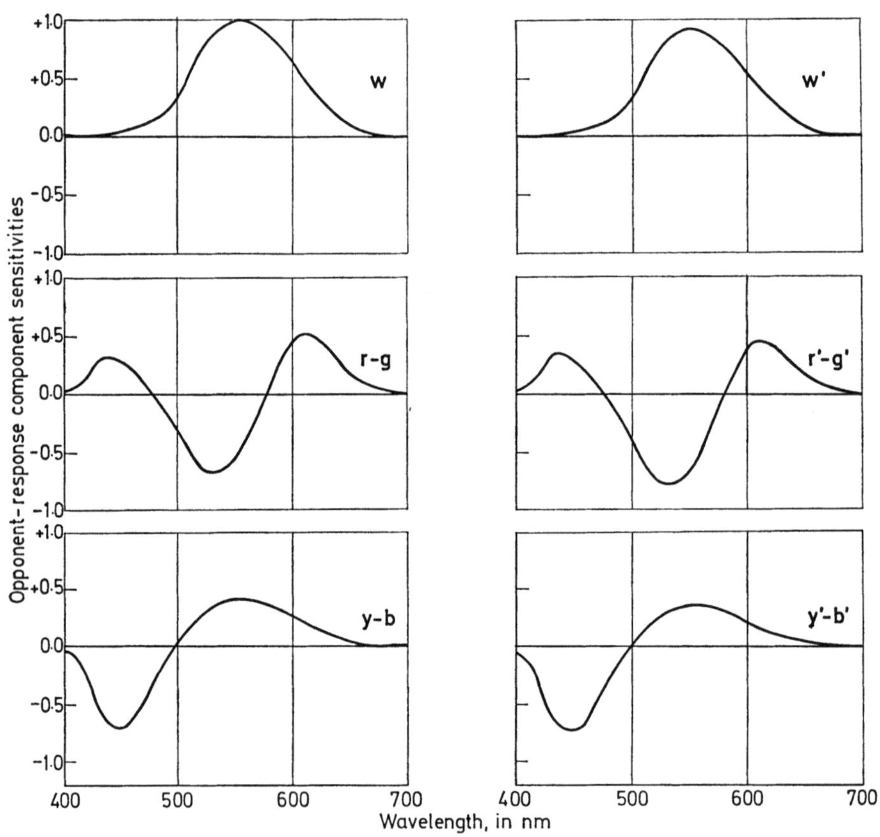

Fig. 3. Opponent-response component sensitivities. *a* Neutral balance of sensitivities. *b* Balance of sensitivities altered for adaptation to 650 nm. Note that the only changes represented here are those controlled by changes at receptoral level

Fig. 5a of Chapter 14.) The curves may serve, nevertheless, as useful illustrations in the context of the general principles of chromatic adaptation that are under consideration here. If we now imagine an eye presumably endowed with the three-variable system of Fig. 2a subjected to continued stimulation by light of 650 nm at a moderate level of luminance, the curves of Fig. 2b can be taken to represent the new balance of component sensitivities. Since a 650 nm light has a ten-fold greater effectiveness for the γ_{560} component than for the β_{540} one, its continued action is assumed to have a ten-fold greater desensitizing effect on the γ_{560} component than on the β_{540} one, and the new balance of sensitivities as plotted in Fig. 2b reflects just this change. The changes illustrated between the curves of Figs. 2a and 2b follow precisely the von Kries coefficient rule.

Figs. 3a and 3b show the corresponding differences, controlled by these receptoral changes, but at the level of the post-receptoral antagonistic neural processes. These three functions are related to the all-positive receptoral stage by the following linear transformation equations:

$$\begin{aligned} w &= 0.8524\,\gamma_{560} + 0.1538\,\beta_{540} \\ r - g &= 1.6643\,\gamma_{560} - 2.2299\,\beta_{540} + 0.3676\,\alpha_{450} \\ y - b &= 0.3410\,\gamma_{560} + 0.0615\,\beta_{540} - 0.7130\,\alpha_{450} \end{aligned} \tag{7}$$

Note that the antagonistic aspect of the "w" component, namely, "black" (bk) is not represented in these relations, since it enters only when the incremental process mentioned above is also taken into account. Note also that there is no representation of α_{450} in the "w" variable. This is a defect of this particular transformation and derives from incorrect short-wave luminosity values in the CIE standardization. (See discussion in WYSZECKI and STILES, 1967; also JAMESON, Chapter 14, this volume.) Measures of spectral luminosity following short-wave adaptation make it quite clear that differential desensitization of a short-wave sensitive receptor system brings about a selective luminosity loss in the short-wave spectral region (HURVICH and JAMESON, 1954; JAMESON and HURVICH, 1953; AUERBACH and WALD, 1955; BRENNEMAN, 1958).

The main effects of the multiplicative sensitivity changes on the opponent response functions of Fig. 3 occur in the $r - g$ distribution, where after adaptation the long-wave "r" amplitude is decreased, the mid-spectral "g" amplitude is increased, and the r/g transition wavelength at which unique yellow is predicted to occur is shifted by about 6 nm toward longer wavelengths. Changes in the curves for the other two variables are very small: a slight depression in the "y" amplitude of the $y - b$ function, and a slight shift in the maximum of the "w" function toward shorter wavelengths. It should be remembered that all the changes illustrated here are consistent with only moderate energy levels of the chromatic adapting stimulus, since very strong adapting lights that are capable of bleaching selectively large fractions of the cone photopigments give rise to very different effects (see above, Section II), and they yield visual states that might better be considered as temporarily pathological.

As stated above, the changes illustrated in Figs. 2 and 3, which are controlled by multiplicative changes in sensitivities, would predict that the proportionality rule would hold, i.e., color matches once achieved between states A and B would continue to be matches at increased or decreased test stimulus luminances. Suppose, however, that the adapting field that causes a reduction in the amplitude of the "r" lobe of the $r - g$ function of Fig. 3b also induces a fixed amount of greenness activity in the test area. Perceptually, this statement is equivalent to a simultaneous contrast effect; physiologically, it may be conceptualized as an effect of lateral inhibition between surround and center of the effective receptive field. Mathematically, it is equivalent to a shift in the baseline in the positive direction in the $r - g$ function of Fig. 3b, thereby incrementing all values measured in the negative direction by a constant amount. Interestingly, it can also be thought of as equivalent to having a constant background light, which, in the case of our 650 nm adapting stimulus, would produce a constant upward deflection in the baseline (redness response direction), with the responses to the spectral test lights all measured relative to this biassed base-line[1]. The concept of the incremental process thus serves as a convergence point for mechanisms that have been in the forefront of analyses of achromatic contrast on the one hand (lateral inhibition), and light and dark-adaptation on the other (equivalent background light). For detailed discussions of these topics, see BARLOW, Chapter 1, HEINEMANN, Chapter 6, FIORENTINI, Chapter 8, and WEISSTEIN, Chapter 10, this volume[2]. Comparable incremental processes are assumed to occur also, of course, in the $y - b$ and $w - bk$ variables. Such a process is thought to be wholly responsible for the blackness, or darkening response in the achromatic system (the spectrally non-opponent cells of the neurophysiologist).

The generalized expressions for the perceptually correlated responses at the opponent-process neural level thus become:

$$\begin{aligned} w_\lambda - bk_\lambda &= f_1\ [e_\lambda(a_{11}\alpha_\lambda + a_{12}\beta_\lambda + a_{13}\gamma_\lambda)] + i_{w-bk} \\ r_\lambda - g_\lambda &= f_2\ [e_\lambda(a_{21}\alpha_\lambda + a_{22}\beta_\lambda + a_{23}\gamma_\lambda)] + i_{r-g} \\ y_\lambda - b_\lambda &= f_3\ [e_\lambda(a_{31}\alpha_\lambda + a_{32}\beta_\lambda + a_{33}\gamma_\lambda)] + i_{y-b} \end{aligned} \tag{8}$$

A change in chromatic adaptation that alters α, β, γ to α', β', γ' by a coefficient rule also alters i_{w-bk}, i_{r-g}, i_{y-b} to i'_{w-bk}, i'_{r-g}, i'_{y-b}. In general, the induction increment, i, can be considered as a shift in the equilibrium base-line of each variable in the same direction as the response of that system to the adapting light. For after-images seen in total darkness, the base-line shifts seem to undergo an oscillatory return to the original equilibrium value, with a consequent fluctuation in after-image appearance. These oscillations, moreover, are not synchronous for all three variables, so that after-image hues may fluctuate from, say, blue-red to blue-green to yellow-red, etc., when viewed in the dark. The presence of a field of secondary light stimulation on which the after-image is "projected" seems to have a strong damping effect, so that, unless the primary adapting stimulus has been very

[1] The notion described as "discounting the illuminant" is also mathematically equivalent to this same process, although workers in the area since the time of HELMHOLTZ have given this notion a cognitive interpretation rather than a physiological one. (See, for example HELMHOLTZ, 1896; JUDD, 1960; RICHARDS and PARKS, 1971.)

[2] For discussions and evaluations of various mathematical models that incorporate incremental variables for brightness contrast (*not* color), see BLISS and MACURDY (1961), RATLIFF (1965), MARSDEN (1969), GIGER and FANKHAUSER (1969), and WÄSSLE and HEINRICH (1970).

intense, the after-image fading process undergoes a much more steady course. For extremely intense adapting stimuli, rapid hue oscillations may be seen even while the primary stimulus is still present. These intense light effects may well be related to rapid (flash) bleaching at the receptoral level as well as to "overdrive-instability" in the postreceptoral antagonistic neural systems (EICHENGREEN, 1971).

The importance of the chromatic adaptation analysis lies primarily, however, in understanding and accounting for color perceptions within the moderate stimulus levels encountered in normal viewing situations. The quantitative outcomes of incremental processes of the sort described here for perceptual scaling data, spectral discrimination functions, and experiments concerned with approximate brightness and color constancy are given in detail in JAMESON and HURVICH (1959, 1961, 1964), HURVICH and JAMESON (1960, 1961, 1966), HURVICH (1965), JAMESON (1970). Here we wish simply to point out that the two-process description of chromatic adaptation accounts both for the validity (within the limits discussed above) of the persistence rule and for the failure of the proportionality rule. A constant increment of, say, greenness that must be matched by a green appearing stimulus at one level of luminance will not be proportionately amplified when the test stimulus on the adapted retina is increased in luminance, but the green-appearing stimulus on the neutrally adapted retina will be so amplified with an equivalent increase in luminance, and the original color match will perforce be destroyed.

It should also be made clear here that an incremental process alone can account for chromatic adaptation phenomena no better than a coefficient sensitivity change alone. This is a difficulty in attempting to conceptualize degrees of light and dark-adaptation exclusively in terms of "equivalent background light", "dark light" or "after-image light". It is, in fact, of interest that von Kries, who was responsible for the formalization of the coefficient analysis, came to the coefficient rule only after testing and rejecting the likelihood that color adaptation effects could be explained exclusively by assuming that a given amount of "after-image light" is added to the real light of a test stimulus. He was able to demonstrate very easily that a fixed amount of real light complementary to the after-image hue could neutralize a test field appearance at one level of luminance, but was inadequate to neutralize it at a higher level of luminance. He thus concluded, and correctly, that sensitivity changes must be involved. Unfortunately, his coefficient analysis was formalized without also including the incremental, or what he thought of as after-image, component. Had the more complex formulation been stated originally, much experimental effort might have been saved in the many frustrated attempts to arrive at the "true" component sensitivities of the color vision mechanism on the incorrect assumption that proportional sensitivity changes alone were involved in the process of chromatic adaptation.

Acknowledgement. Preparation of this chapter was supported in part by NIH Grant EY-00249.

References

AGUILAR, M., STILES, W. S.: Saturation of the rod mechanism of the retina at high levels of stimulation. Optica Acta **1**, 59—65 (1954).

AUERBACH, E., WALD, G.: The participation of different types of cones in human light and dark adaptation. Amer. J. Ophthal. **39**, 24—40 (1955).

Bliss, J. C., Macurdy, W. B.: Linear models for contrast phenomena. J. opt. Soc. Amer. **51**, 1373—1379 (1961).

Boynton, R. M., Ikeda, M., Stiles, W. S.: Interactions among chromatic mechanisms as inferred from positive and negative increment thresholds. Vision Res. **4**, 87—117 (1964).

Brenneman, E. J.: Dependence of luminance required for constant brightness upon chromaticity and chromatic adaptation. J. opt. Soc. Amer. **48**, 228—232 (1958).

Brewer, W. L.: Fundamental response functions and binocular color matching. J. opt. Soc. Amer. **44**, 207—212 (1954).

Brindley, G. S.: The effects on colour vision of adaptation to very bright lights. J. Physiol. (Lond.) **122**, 332—350 (1953).

Brown, J. L.: Afterimages. In: Vision and Visual Perception, Ch. 17. Graham, C. H. (Ed.). New York: Wiley 1965.

Brown, P. K., Wald, G.: Visual pigments in single rods and cones of the human retina. Science **144**, 45—52 (1964).

Burnham, R. W., Evans, R. M., Newhall, S. M.: Influences on color perception of adaptation to illumination. J. opt. Soc. Amer. **42**, 597—605 (1952).

— — — Prediction of color appearance with different adaptation illuminants. J. opt. Soc. Amer. **47**, 35—42 (1957).

De Valois, R. L.: Behavioral and electrophysiological studies of primate vision. In: Contributions to Sensory Physiology. Neff, W. D. (Ed.). New York: Academic Press 1965.

Eichengreen, J.: Time dependent chromatic adaptation. Ph. D. thesis, University of Pennsylvania (1971).

Giger, H., Fankhauser, F.: Die linearen Modelle des Helligkeitssehen. Vision Res. **9**, 785—801 (1969).

Gouras, P.: Trichromatic mechanisms in single cortical neurons. Science **168**, 489—491 (1970).

Graham, C. H., Brown, J. L.: Color Contrast and Color Appearances: Brightness Constancy and color constancy. In: Vision and Visual Perception, Ch. 16. Graham, C. H. (Ed.). New York: Wiley 1965.

Helmholtz, H. L. F. von: Handbuch der Physiologischen Optik, (2nd Edit.). Hamburg-Leipzig: Voss 1896.

Helson, H.: Fundamental problems in color vision. I. The principle governing changes in hue, saturation, and lightness of non-selective samples in chromatic illumination. J. exp. Psychol. **23**, 439—476 (1938).

— Jeffers, V. B.: Fundamental problems in color vision. II. Hue, lightness, and saturation of selective samples in chromatic illumination. J. exp. Psychol. **26**, 1—27 (1940).

— Judd, D. B., Warren, M.: Object-color changes from daylight to incandescent filament illumination. Illum. Eng. **47**, 221—233 (1952).

Hurvich, L. M.: The indispensibility of a bimodal black-white color vision process. In: Internationale Farbtagung Luzern 1965, pp. 167—172. Göttingen: Musterschmidt 1966.

— Jameson, D.: Spectral sensitivity of the fovea. III. Heterochromatic brightness and chromatic adaptation. J. opt. Soc. Amer. **44**, 213—222 (1954).

— — Further development of a quantified opponent-colours theory. In: Visual Problems of Colour. Vol. 2, pp. 691—723. London: H. M. Stationery Office 1958.

— — Perceived color, induction effects, and opponent-response mechanisms. J. gen. Physiol. **43** (Suppl.), 63—80 (1960).

— — Opponent chromatic induction and wavelength discrimination. In: The Visual System: Neurophysiology and Psychophysics, pp. 144—152. Jung, R., Kornhuber, H. (Eds.). Berlin: Springer 1961.

— — Introductory Lecture. In: Recent Progress in Photobiology. Bowen, E. J. (Ed.). Oxford: Blackwell 1965.

Jameson, D.: Brightness scales and their interpretation. In: International Color Meeting Stockholm 1969, pp. 377—385. Göttingen: Musterschmidt 1970.

— Hurvich, L. M.: Spectral sensitivity of the fovea. II. Dependence on chromatic adaptation. J. opt. Soc. Amer. **43**, 552—559 (1953).

— — Perceived color and its dependence on focal, surrounding, and preceding stimulus variables. J. opt. Soc. Amer. **49**, 890—898 (1959).

JAMESON. D., HURVICH, L. M.: Opponent chromatic induction: Experimental evaluation and theoretical account. J. opt. Soc. Amer. **51**, 46—53 (1961).
— — Theory of brightness and color contrast in human vision. Vision Res. **4**, 135—154 (1964).
JUDD, D. B.: Hue, saturation and lightness of surface colors with chromatic illumination. J. opt. Soc. Amer. **30**, 2—32 (1940).
— Appraisal of Land's work on two-primary color projections. J. opt. Soc. Amer. **50**, 254—268 (1960).
KRIES, J. VON: Beitrag zur Physiologie der Gesichtsempfindungen. Arch. Anat. Physiol. **2**, 505—524 (1878).
— Die Gesichtsempfindungen. In: Handbuch der Physiologie des Menschen, Vol. 3, pp. 109—282. NAGEL, W. (Ed.). Braunschweig: Vieweg 1905.
MACADAM, D. L.: Chromatic adaptation. J. opt. Soc. Amer. **46**, 500—513 (1956).
MARKS, W. B., DOBELLE, W. H., MACNICHOL, E. F., JR.: Visual pigments of single primate cones. Science **143**, 1181—1183 (1964).
MARSDEN, A. M.: An elemental theory of induction. Vision Res. **9**, 653—663 (1969).
NAKA, K. I., RUSHTON, W. A. H.: S-potentials from colour units in the retina of fish *(Cyprinidae)*. J. Physiol. (Lond.) **185**, 536—555 (1966a).
— — An attempt to analyze colour reception by electrophysiology. J. Physiol. (Lond.) **185**, 556—586 (1966b).
PARSONS, J. H.: An Introduction to the Study of Colour Vision. (2nd Edit.) Cambridge: Cambridge University Press 1924.
PEARSON, D. E., RUBINSTEIN, C. B., SPIVACK, G. J.: Comparison of perceived color in two-primary computer-generated artificial images with predictions based on the Helson-Judd formulation. J. opt. Soc. Amer. **59**, 644—658 (1969).
PLATEAU, J.: Bibliographie analytique des principaux phénomènes subjectifs de la vision Cinquième section. Phénomènes ordinaires de contraste. Sixième section. Ombres colorées. Mém. Acad. roy. Belg. **42** (5), 1—35; (6), 1—38 (1878).
RATLIFF, F.: Mach Bands: Quantitative Studies on Neural Networks in the Retina. San Francisco: Holden-Day 1965.
RICHARDS, W., PARKS, E. A.: Model for color conversion. J. opt. Soc. Amer. **61**, 971—976 (1971).
STILES, W. S.: Increment thresholds and the mechanisms of colour vision. Documenta Ophthal. **3**, 138—163 (1949).
— Colour vision: the approach through increment-threshold sensitivity. Proc. nat. Acad. Sci. (Wash.) **45**, 100—114 (1959).
TAKASAKI, H.: von Kries coefficient law applied to subjective color change induced by background color. J. opt. Soc. Amer. **59**, 1370—1376 (1969).
TSCHERMAK, A.: Über Kontrast und Irradiation. Ergeb. Physiol. **2**, 726—798 (1903).
WALD, G.: Photo-labile pigments in the chicken retina. Nature (Lond.) **140**, 545—546 (1937).
— The receptors of human color vision. Science **145**, 1007—1017 (1964).
— BROWN, P. K., SMITH, P. H.: Iodopsin. J. gen. Physiol. **38**, 623—681 (1955).
WÄSSLE, H., HEINRICH, F.: Untersuchungen zum Helligkeitskontrast. Vision Res. **10**, 361—373 (1970).
WALTERS, H. V.: Some experiments on the trichromatic theory of vision. Proc. roy. Soc. (Lond.) B **131**, 27—49 (1942).
WIESEL, T. N., HUBEL, D. H.: Spatial and chromatic interactions in the lateral geniculate body of the rhesus monkey. J. Neurophysiol. **29**, 1115—1156 (1966).
WRIGHT, W. D.: The measurement and analysis of colour adaptation phenomena. Proc. roy. Soc. (Lond.) B **115**, 49—87 (1934).
— The breakdown of a colour match with high intensities of adaptation. J. Physiol. (Lond.) **87**, 23—33 (1936).
— Researches on Normal and Defective Colour Vision. St. Louis: Mosby 1947.
WYSZECKI, G., STILES, W. S.: Color Science. New York: Wiley 1967.

Chapter 23

Color Vision Deficiencies

By

LEO M. HURVICH, Philadelphia, Pennsylvania (USA)

With 12 Figures

Contents

I. Description of Color Vision Systems

Color vision deficiencies are inherently intriguing. Perhaps beyond their importance for task performance based on visual discriminations is their significance for color theory. They are, as it were, nature's "test" cases.

Color vision systems are characterized most simply as three-, two-, or one-variable ones. The variables are inferred, alternatively, from the qualitative dimensions of color discrimination (or confusion) or from the number of mixture-stimulus primaries sufficient and necessary to "gauge" or match the visible spectrum. For more precise characterizations, spectral appearance data (including unique hue loci for observers with three-variable systems and spectral neutral points for those with only two variables), luminous efficiency functions, and discrimination functions (wavelength and spectral purity) are determined. Differences in contrast phenomena are also sometimes considered to characterize the different visual systems, although different investigators do not agree on this point

(Tschermak, 1903; Holzlöhner and Stein, 1930/31; Klein and Nordmann, 1948; Engelbrecht, 1948; Chapanis, 1949; Kinney, 1967).

Normal foveal color vision is trivariant and the *normal trichromat* distinguishes colors along the three perceptual dimensions: white-black, red-green, and yellow-blue. The spectral hues, from short to long wavelengths, are ordered in regions that are red-blue (violet), blue-green, green-yellow and yellow-red, with three sharp transition zones, unique blue between violet and blue-green, unique green between blue-green and yellow-green, and unique yellow between green-yellow and orange at average wavelengths about 475, 500 and 580 nm, respectively (see Jameson, chapter 14, this volume, Fig. 7). The normal observer matches the color of any spectral stimulus with appropriate combinations of three selected spectral primaries, and average normal spectral equations have long been established and codified in the form of standard (CIE) color-mixture functions (see Wright, chapter 16, this volume). The normal average photopic luminous efficiency function is shown as Fig. 1 in Le Grand, chapter 15, in this volume. A normal wavelength discrimination curve is given in Fig. 9 (p. 600) and a function representing spectral "saturation" for the normal is shown in Fig. 8 (p. 598).

A group of individuals, roughly, 6% of sampled populations, cannot be characterized by these normal functions, yet has vision that, like the normal's, is trivariant. These anomalous trichromats (König and Dieterici, 1893) also discriminate among whites, blacks, reds, greens, blues, and yellows, but the saturations of spectral lights may differ from normal and the spectral loci of the unique hues vary depending on the type of anomaly (see below, Sec. III). Moreover, the average stimulus-mixture proportions these individuals require for color matching are outside the distribution of normal color equations. Three sub-groupings are conventionally distinguished: protanomalous, deuteranomalous, and tritanomalous (Judd, 1949a; Trendelenburg, 1961; Hsia and Graham, 1965).

Rayleigh Equation. Diagnosis of Protanomaly and Deuteranomaly.

Although a variety of color plates, chips, lanterns and so on are used for color vision testing (see Murray, 1950, 1960; Linksz, 1964; Lakowski, 1969), a single spectral color match, the so-called Rayleigh equation, of the form $a(535\text{ nm}) + b(670\text{ nm}) \equiv c(589\text{ nm})$, serves to differentiate between the normal and each of the two groups of observers labelled protanomalous and deuteranomalous. These spectral stimuli are seen as yellowish-green (535 nm), yellowish-red (670 nm), and reddish-yellow (589 nm) by the average normal observer, but the diagnostic equation is usually loosely characterized as a "red and green mixture" that matches "yellow".

The diagnostic index most widely used to differentiate the different types of color vision is the energy ratio of 670 to 535 nm (or the reciprocal) to match 589 nm. The luminance of the 589 nm test stimulus is sometimes also specified. When the deviant anomalous ratios are expressed relative to ratios obtained by normal observers, the index is called the "anomalous quotient". Pickford (1951) prefers a measure of standard deviations relative to the population distribution, and more recently Lakowski (1969) has proposed expressing the Rayleigh equation data either in dominant wavelength terms or as chromaticities in CIE space. Whatever the units, the 670 nm/535 nm ratios for the deuteranomalous are less than those of the normal group, and the ratios are greater than normal for all protanomalous observers. Frequency distributions of Rayleigh equation mid-point measurements tend to indicate that there is some discontinuity among the normal, protanomalous and deuteranomalous populations, with the possibility that there is a sharper division between normal and deuteranomalous than between normal and protanomalous distributions (TRENDELENBURG and SCHMIDT, 1935; NELSON, 1938; FORSHAW, 1954). However, SCHMIDT's (1955) data throw the differences between groups into greater relief (see Fig. 1).

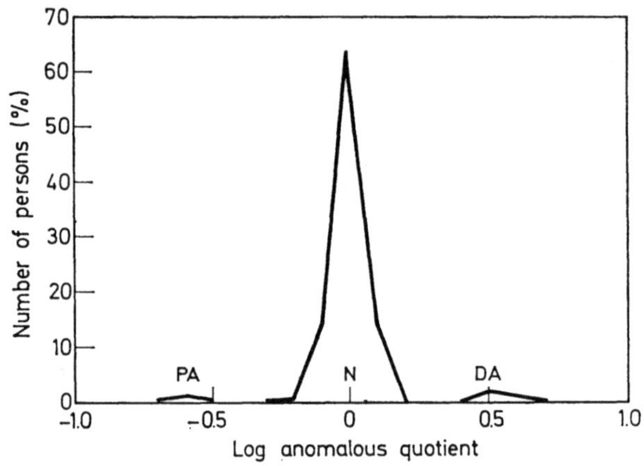

Fig. 1. Distribution of anomalous quotients of 864 males. (SCHMIDT, 1955)

The apparent ease with which these groups are distinguished and pigeonholed in three discrete classes in terms of a simple ratio index masks both an historical fact and an important theoretical issue. The anomalous trichromats have been the most difficult to classify and to understand (v. KRIES, 1924, 1929; JUDD, 1951; ALPERN, 1968). Some researchers interpret them as lying on a continuum between color normals and the dichromats (protanopes and deuteranopes) of their respective classes; others argue that the continuity exists only between the protanomalous and protanope, and deuteranomalous and deuteranope; and still others regard the anomalous as classes distinct from both normals and dichromats.

The root of these difficulties lies in a serious misconception about the meaning of the Rayleigh equation ratio: anomalous color vision tends to be conceptualized by most investigators as "color weakness". If we consider the distribution of Rayleigh equation indices (Fig. 1) we see that deuteranomalous observers require relatively more of the 535 nm stimulus than of 670 nm for a match to 589 nm. They are consequently thought to be "green weak". Protanomalous, on the other hand, who require relatively greater amounts of 670 nm are characterized as "red weak" (WRIGHT, 1947; JUDD, 1949a; MARRIOTT, 1962; BURNHAM *et al.*, 1963).

The misconception has a long history and among the distinguished researchers who held to the view that all anomalous observers were color weak are DONDERS and NAGEL. Others were convinced that color discrimination could be excellent despite deviant or aberrant color equations (see JAMESON and HURVICH, 1956 for details and references). In the first paper reporting the discovery of anomalous observers, RAYLEIGH (1881) noted that one of his deviant observers had difficulty making good observations, whereas in most of his cases the appreciation of small color differences was as distinct as usual. It now seems clear that anomalous observers may be poor ('weak") or good color discriminators. The difficulty stems from interpreting the Rayleigh ratios as a measure of "color weakness", which it is not (HESS, 1922; MÜLLER, 1924; JAMESON and HURVICH, 1956). This measure of "deviance" says nothing about sharpness of discrimination. What is required to determine an index of the observers' relative keenness or weakness of color discrimination is not the midpoint match, but rather the *range* of acceptable 670 nm/535 nm ratios for a match on 589 nm. In principle, such range measures involve the controlled exploration of the match range. The experimenter presents a series of different 670 nm/535 nm mixture ratios, and the observer adjusts the luminance of the 589 nm test field to match the mixture field, if possible. The mixture ratio is varied until the two limits at which matches are no longer possible are reached. The match mid-point is taken to be the ratio value that bisects the experimentally measured range.

The mid-point and range measures may vary independently, hence both are necessary for a proper characterization of the anomaly. Although recent papers have appeared that neglect to measure or report ranges, many investigators have presented both mid-point and range data for large groups of observers for both spectral and filter anomaloscopes. (For example, ROSMANIT, 1914; KÖLLNER, 1914; FRANCESCHETTI, 1928; KÖLLNER and ENGELKING, 1929; TRENDELENBURG and SCHMIDT, 1935; PICKFORD, 1951; WILLIS and FARNSWORTH, 1952; SCHMIDT, 1955; PICKFORD and LAKOWSKI, 1960; see also JAMESON and HURVICH, 1956 where a list of still other investigators who have used both measures can be found.) Fig. 2 summarizes mid-point and range data for 140 observers obtained by WILLIS and FARNSWORTH with the Nagel anomaloscope in an evaluative study of various anomaloscopes and a battery of conventional color vision tests. In the figure, each point and horizontal line represents an individual case as ordered by WILLIS and FARNSWORTH.

The letters P, N, and D represent the protan, normal and deutan classes, respectively, and the letter U was used by WILLIS and FARNSWORTH where classification on the basis of the whole battery of color vision tests was "uncertain" or doubtful. The abscissa values are ratios of 670 nm/535 nm mixtures that match a 589 nm test field and are expressed in comparative scale units where 50 = normal.

To illustrate the extent to which the match mid-point and range indices vary independently, we can regroup the data by visually selecting four range groups and ordering the individual results in accordance with increasing mid-point deviations from the normal ratio of 50% in both directions, i.e., toward 0% and 100%. Replotted in this way the data are shown in thin lines in Fig. 3.

Spectral Luminosity. There is considerable spread, as there is for normals, within a given anomalous class in the peak locus of the spectral luminosity function, but it is generally agreed that the peaks are centered near 540 nm with relative deficit in long-wave luminosity for protanomalous and the maxima are near 560 nm for deuteranomalous individuals. These peaks compare to the normal average at 555 nm (see WYSZECKI and STILES, 1967, p. 504). SCHOBER (1958, p. 180) gives the normal maximum at 550 nm, protanomalous maxima between 520 and 550 nm, and deuteranomalous between 550 and 580 nm.

Spectral Discrimination. The wavelength discrimination functions of deuteranomalous and protanomalous observers may differ considerably both within the anomalous groups and in comparison with those of the normal, and the property of the visual system that reflects itself in the Rayleigh equation range data is also expressed in these discrimination functions (see Fig. 9). Such functions have been measured by ENGELKING (1926); PITT (1935); CORBETT (1937); NELSON (1938); McKEON and WRIGHT (1940); WRIGHT (1947); and McLELLAN (1966, see LAKOWSKI, 1968). Saturation (least colorimetric purity) discrimination functions for anomalous observers are reported by WRIGHT (1947) and his students and CHAPANIS (1944).

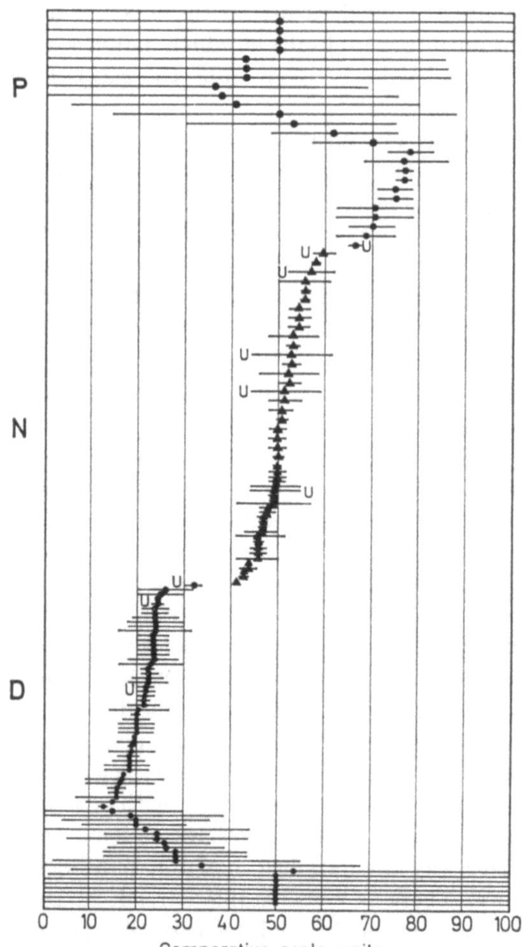

Fig. 2. Replot of Rayleigh-equation data measured with Nagel anomaloscope by WILLIS and FARNSWORTH (1952)

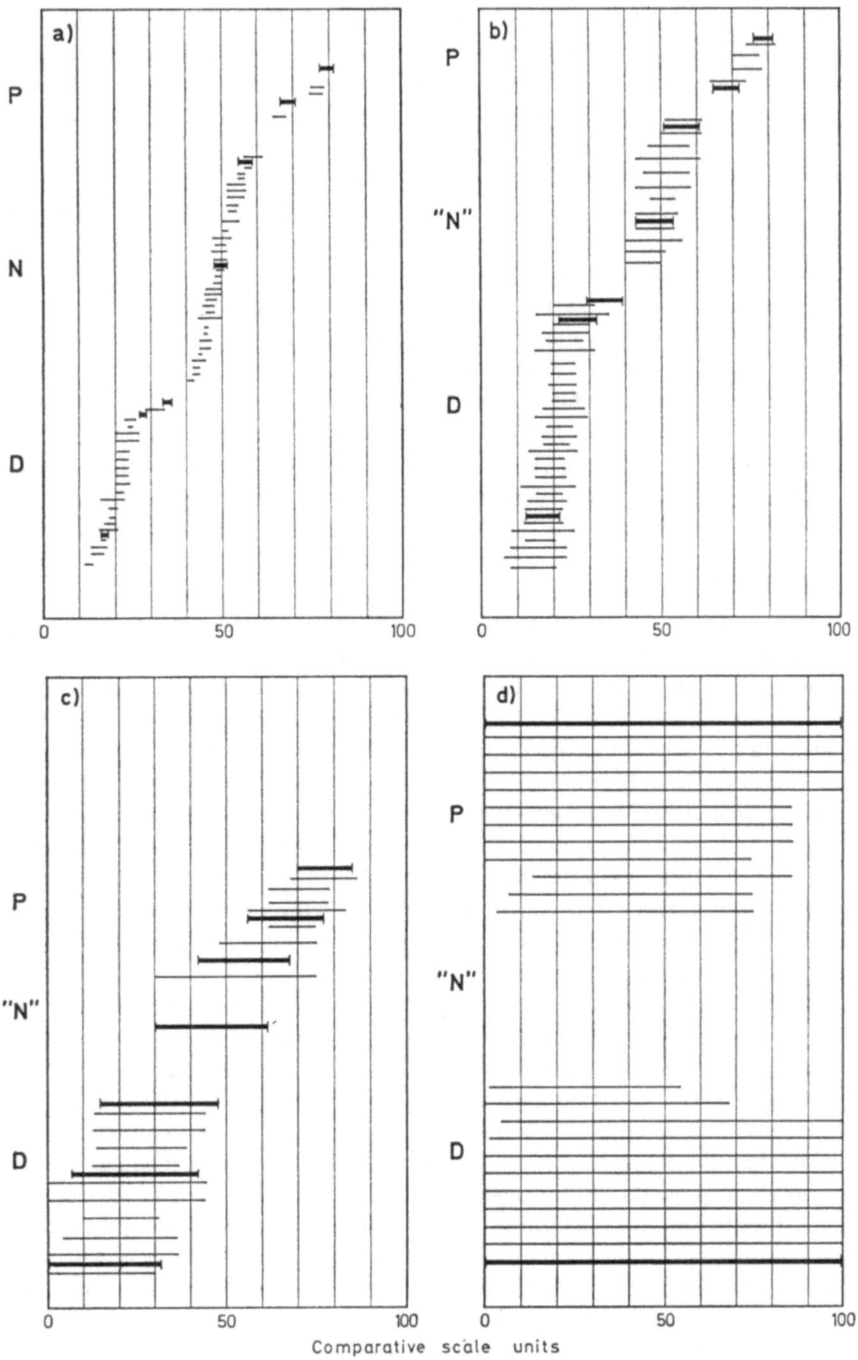

Fig. 3. Normal and abnormal Rayleigh ratios for observers (a) with normal strength red-green response systems, (b) with red-green response systems 0.1 normal strength, (c) 0.03 normal strength and (d) with complete lack of red-green response systems. Heavy lines — predicted by theory. Thin lines — measured by WILLIS and FARNSWORTH (1952)

Contrast and Adaptation. Some investigators believe that anomalous are also differentiated from normals in that they show heightened susceptibility to contrast. (References on p. 583, see also ROSMANIT, 1914; PARSONS, 1924; SCHOBER, 1958; TRENDELENBURG, 1961). But CHAPANIS (1949) questioned this interpretation and found no convincing evidence for differences in contrast-susceptibility in his own study of anomalous observers.

It has also been claimed that anomalous show greater "fatiguability" than normals on continued exposure to a given stimulus (ROSMANIT, 1914). We have noted in our laboratory that individual observers, normal and defective, differ markedly in their degree of desensitization or adaptation („Umstimmung") to continued stimulation. We have even observed cases where almost total color "wash-out" occurs in a matter of seconds. ENGELKING (1933) investigated such individuals and used the term "asthenopes" for them. (See also HARTUNG, 1935; TRENDELENBURG and SCHMIDT, 1935; SCHMIDT, 1935; WAARDENBURG, 1963). Despite its importance, with some notable exceptions (ROGGE, 1946; CIBIS and HUCK, 1949; PICKFORD, 1951; MCCREE, 1960; CLARKE, 1960; CIBIS, 1965) relatively little attention has been given to this temporal "washout" issue, whether in normal or abnormal color vision.

Diagnosis of Tritanomaly

A third, and rarer form of anomalous trichromatic vision that involves primarily the yellow-blue dimension of color perception was first reported by ENGELKING (1925). (See also HARTUNG, 1926; ENGELKING, 1927; ENGELKING and HARTUNG, 1927, and GÖTHLIN, 1937). Although there are diagnostic difficulties in these instances, particularly in disentangling the effects of short-wave absorption by the macular pigment (see RUDDOCK, chapter 17, this volume), other related cases have been reported by MEITNER (1941), OLOFF (1935) and SCHMIDT (1943, 1970). (For a full bibliography up to 1955 on "tritan" defects, both congenital and acquired, see JAEGER, 1955.) Both CRONE (1956) and SPERANSKAYA (1961) have more recently described two congenital cases ("tritanomals"), and COLE *et al.* (1965) have uncovered a family with a pedigree that contains at least 10 "tritans", of whom at least three are thought to be "tritanomalous".

For these individuals, color vision is still three variable and three primaries are necessary to gauge the spectrum, but again the stimulus matching proportions differ from the normals and may exhibit high variability in given spectral regions. A typical colorimetric equation used to detect such anomalies is: 517 nm + 470 nm ≡ 490 nm, and the anomalous observer requires more of the 470 nm stimulus for the match than do normals. As already noted, the presence of macular pigment, which absorbs appreciably in this spectral region and which differs in density from one individual to the next, complicates any diagnosis by such an equation.

Hue naming, spectral unique-hue loci, luminosity functions, wavelength discrimination and saturation discrimination curves are available for various observers among the papers cited above, but the picture of yellow-blue anomaly still remains unclear and will be discussed at greater length below.

Dichromats

In contrast to the normal and anomalous trichromats, a small percentage of the population (estimated as between 2 % and 3 %) is dichromatic. There are two major groups: one fails to make red-green discriminations, the other yellow-blue ones. The former are the protanopes and deuteranopes and the inferences of intelligent, scientifically trained, color defectives (DALTON, 1798; POLE, 1859, 1893; AHLENSTIEL, 1951) that their remaining hue sensations are yellow and blue are confirmed by the reports of rarely occurring unilateral protanopes and deuteranopes who have normal color vision in one of their two eyes (JUDD, 1948; SLOAN and WOLLACH, 1948; GRAHAM *et al.*, 1961; COX, 1961). The yellow and blue spectral regions are demarked by a neutral "gray" or "white" appearing locus, which is on the average at a slightly shorter wavelength for protanopes than deuteranopes. This locus corresponds approximately to the unique green of neutrally-adapted normals, and both types of defective can be shown to have an extra-spectral neutral experience that corresponds to the normal's unique red. Spectral gauging is achieved with only two stimuli, and the luminous efficiency functions of these observers tend to peak at different spectral loci; the protanopic function is displaced toward shorter wavelengths, is depressed relative to the normal at the long-wave end, and peaks at about 540 nm. Since long-wave stimuli of equivalent energies appear darker than they do to normals, these observers have come to be called "red-blind" (TRENDELENBURG, 1961; MARRIOTT, 1962; HSIA and GRAHAM, 1965). This is an inept characterization since it implies absence of red hue experience but fails to make clear that these individuals also lack green hue perception, and that reds, greens and grays of the normal observer can all be perfectly matched to each other by these individuals.

Deuteranopes also fail to perceive red and green hues, but the deuteranopic luminosity function does not fall off in the long-wave region in the way the protanopic one does. However, the precise form and locus of the deuteranopic luminosity function in relation to the normal is a very much unresolved issue at the moment (WILLMER, 1950; GRAHAM and HSIA, 1960; HEATH, 1958, 1960; COLLINS, 1961; GRÜTZNER, 1962; ALPERN *et al.*, 1968). Since the mid-spectral region does not appear dark to these observers in the way that long wavelengths do to their protanopic counterparts, there is still less justification to describe them as "green-blind". They are, however, sometimes so characterized (WALD, 1966) on the assumption that their defect derives from the loss of a mid-spectral visual pigment (see below, Sec. IV). This characterization is similarly inept since it obscures the fact that this type of observer has also lost red sensory experiences, has both a spectral and extra-spectral neutral locus, and that the normal's reds, greens and grays also all match for him.

The second major group of dichromats, the "yellow-blue" defective type, is usually termed tritanopic, but is also sometimes thought to be divisible into two subcategories: tetartanopes and tritanopes. Both types fail to discriminate blues and yellows and see only reds and greens in the spectrum. The tetartanope presumably has two neutral spectral loci (the normal's unique blue and yellow regions) (see below, Sec. IV) and the tritanope a single one in the "yellow" region of the spectrum. The other neutral locus is presumably extra-spectral. In any event, both classes confuse yellows, grays, and blues. Spectral color matching requires only two stimuli, and the measured luminosity functions tend to lie in the normal range with similar peak loci. Among the earliest congenital cases of tritanopia (commonly called "blue blindness" also with singular inappropriateness) are those reported by Vintschgau (1891, 1894); Piper (1905); Levy (1906) and Köllner (Köllner and Engelking, 1929). That the perceptions are restricted to reds and greens is verifiable from the reports by Holmgren and Dieter of unilateral tritanopes (see Judd, 1948 for references).

These types of dichromasy occur much less frequently than protanopia and deuteranopia, but recently many more cases of yellow-blue defects have come to light. Some have been studied intensively, and we now have on hand much additional quantitative data including spectral matching data, luminosity functions, wavelength discrimination, saturation discrimination, increment thresholds, visual fields, and dark adaptation (Judd *et al.*, 1950; Wright, 1952; Fischer *et al.*, 1951; Sperling, 1960; Walls, 1964; Henry *et al.*, 1964; Cole *et al.*, 1965; Cole and Watkins, 1967; Ohta, 1969).

Monochromats

The *typical* monochromat sees the world essentially as the normal does in very dim illumination; no hues are seen but only various shades of black and white. Designations for this color defect include rod monochromasy, achromatopsia, and total color blindness. The spectrum is seen as gray or neutral throughout its entire extent and any wavelength can be matched by any other when adjusted for brightness equality. These individuals have luminosity functions that peak at about 510 nm (approximating the normal scotopic function), they sometimes show evidence of a central scotoma and/or low visual acuity, pupillomotor symptoms, photophobia and nystagmus. There are, however, numerous exceptions, and an individual may, for example, exhibit most of the assorted symptoms but still have good acuity. Francois *et al.* (1955) list some 215 such cases up to the time of their publication, and each passing year sees an occasional additional entry. Podesta (1936) has suggested that these typical monochromats be classified preferably as "complicated", in contrast to the "simple" or "true" totally color-blind most often called *atypical*. The latter type occurs less frequently and up to 1954 only some 25 cases were noted (Baumgardt and Magis, 1954). These observers appear to have foveal vision; they too see only blacks, whites and grays and require a single stimulus, variable in luminance only, to match any spectral light. Their spectral luminosity functions are definitely not scotopic but tend rather to be photopic although not necessarily normal. (See, for example, Sloan and Newhall, 1942; Pitt, 1944; Weale, 1953 and other cases cited in Sec. VI.) Such cases appear to involve cone functions and raise basic theoretical questions.

Tables showing the incidence of various types of defects in various populations can be found in Francois *et al.* (1957); Kherumian and Pickford (1959); Cox (1961); Burnham *et al.* (1963) and Hsia and Graham (1965).

Explanatory Factors

It is generally agreed in principle that normal color vision can be modified by 1) pre-retinal absorption differences that produce selective alterations in stimulus energies incident at the receptors, 2) alterations in the postulated normal receptor mechanisms, 3) losses or reductions of normal receptor and/or neural response, or 4) fusions of two or more receptor and/or response systems. The various possibilities are not mutually exclusive.

A system may be thought of as comprised of various labile photopigments (or receptors) which act as the critical determinants of "visual" events or as comprised of such photopigments linked in specified ways to the neural-retinal-cortical pathways. In either case, the relevant physiological systems and their interactions, whether known or postulated, are expected to provide a coherent account of the perceptions, color-mixture data, luminosity functions, discrimination data, etc., of both normals and individuals with color defective vision.

II. Pre-retinal Absorption Differences

The way in which selective absorption by various pre-retinal elements in the eye, cornea, lens, aqueous and vitreous humors, and macular pigmentation modify the light stimulus prior to incidence at the sensitive surface of the retina are fully discussed in RUDDOCK's chapter 17 in this volume. That color deficiencies of various kinds have been attributed to such selective absorptions is not surprising. In fact, the idea is as old as DALTON's (1798) description of his own dichromacy. DALTON believed his long-wave spectral deficiency (protanopia) was caused by a blue coloration of his vitreous humor, but postmortem examination of his eyes established that the vitreous humor was colorless. WARTMANN (1846), who cites this finding, rejected the absorption argument on the further grounds that the habitual use of blue glasses fails to produce "Daltonism", and that although the lenses in the eyes of older persons may become "amber" tinted, they continue to see objects in their "proper" colors.

Color deficient observers of all types have macular pigmentation and report so-called "Maxwell spots" of various forms when the macula is made visible entoptically. A report by WALLS and MATHEWS (1952) that the entoptic pattern is not visible to deutans (deuteranopes and deuteranomalous) has been acknowledged to be in error (WALLS and HEATH, 1956). As MURRAY (1954) made clear, the visibility of the entoptic pattern with the experimental technique used depends on the color-temperature of the light that illuminates the projection surface.

Since macular pigment absorbs preferentially in the relatively short-wave spectral region, differences in density of this pigment cannot account for the differences in spectral luminosity functions between protanopes and deuteranopes which occur largely in the long-wave spectral region. On the other hand, differential absorption over the short-wave spectral region by all the ocular media, especially by the macular pigment, has long made the rapid diagnosis of tritanopia difficult, and efforts to devise simple instruments using a single color equation such as 517 nm + 470 nm $\equiv$ 490 nm, employed by ENGELKING, have borne little fruit (TRENDELENBURG, 1941a; HAY and ROAF, 1940; CRONE, 1955). No commercial anomaloscope to detect tritoforms with a "blue" equation has yet appeared (RICHTER, 1957).

The role of excessive ocular pigmentation in distorting typical tritanopia is discussed in detail by JUDD *et al.* (1950). To account both for their observer's short-wave luminosity cut-off, and for his somewhat atypical chromaticity confusions, they found it necessary to postulate dense ocular pigmentation.

Differential ocular pigmentation and macular absorption enter importantly in most determinations that have been made of the so-called spectral "neutral points" of protanopes and deuteranopes. Both of these types of red-green defectives, as already mentioned, will match to gray or white a stimulus wavelength in the region of the normal's unique green, and also a stimulus mixture (long-wave + short-wave) that approximates the normal's unique red. All these matched stimuli appear neutral or colorless to the dichromats. Ordinarily, the "neutral point" is limited to seeking out the single spectral stimulus (near 500 nm) that matches a "gray" or "white" broad-band incandescent light source (PARSONS, 1924; HECHT and SHLAER, 1936; JUDD, 1945). The color-temperature of the broad-band light obviously affects the neutral point locus for a given observer, and different amounts of ocular absorption which selectively modify the broad-band distribution also confound interpretation of inter-observer differences. WALLS and HEATH (1956) minimized the effects that pigmentation exerts on matches to broad-band "whites" or "neutrals" by using more broadly selective stimulus mixtures on a color wheel to generate their chromatic stimuli, and then extrapolated to specify the spectral "equivalents". This procedure has the advantage that both broad-band distributions in the match are similarly (although not identically) distorted by the ocular pigments. However, the use of the CIE colorimetric chart to determine spectral loci intercepts in this procedure raises further questions (see below Sec. V). The pigmentation problem could be circumvented by measuring dichromatic neutral points using only spectral stimuli to determine the transition locus between perceived blue and yellow. To the best of our knowledge, no thorough study of this sort with rigorous control of adaptive state to guarantee "neutral tuning" (JAMESON and HURVICH, 1951) has been carried out.

HERING (1885) initially thought that his deuteranomalous and protanomalous observers could be explained in terms of pigmentation differences, particularly macular pigmentation. It is clear on a number of different grounds, however, that this idea is incorrect.

1) The spectral locus of unique yellow differs reliably among normal, protanomalous and deuteranomalous groups. (For example, RUBIN, 1961; HURVICH and JAMESON, 1964). (See Sec. III below.) Since a selective filter cannot affect the composition of a single homogeneous spectral line, factors other than filter selectivity must enter. 2) Differences between anomalous and normal color vision are maintained even in parafoveal comparisons where macular pigmentation is minimal (PARSONS, 1924). 3) The scotopic luminous efficiency function is the same for normal and anomalous observers, hence lenticular absorption differences are not operative (PARSONS, 1924). 4) In "extended Rayleigh equation" matches (where stimulus ratios of the mixture stimuli 670 nm and 535 nm are determined for matches not only to the standard 589 nm test stimulus but also to a series of spectral stimuli intermediate between 670 nm and 535 nm) the normal and anomalous mixture ratios of 670/535 (essentially the "extended anomalous quotient") do not bear a constant relation to each other for all test stimuli in the series. If normals and anomalous differed only because of a selective filter difference, this quotient would be expected to be constant. The variable relation found indicates that an alteration system is responsible (see Sec. III) (v. KRIES, 1919; ENGELKING, 1925, 1927; JAMESON and HURVICH, 1956). 5) The color-mixture data of anomalous

and normals are maximally different in the long-wave spectral regions where the effects of macular pigmentation would be anticipated to be minimal (PITT, 1935). 6) Trans-scleral anomaloscope experiments involving simultaneous viewing of the stimuli by a normal and anomalous observer demonstrate that prereceptoral filters are not responsible for the different Rayleigh equation matches (ALPERN and TORII, 1968a).

III. Alteration Systems (Photochemical; Photochemical plus Neural Decrements)

On the simple assumption that anomalous color vision is intermediate between normal and dichromatic vision, and that the latter comes about through the simple loss of one component of the normal's three-variable system (see Sec. IV. below) it has been proposed on occasion (e.g., PARSONS, 1924, p. 229) that anomalous color vision results from a partial loss or uniform reduction in sensitivity of one of the three-variable systems. But a uniform reduction in sensitivity of any receptor system is equivalent to subtracting the same quality and quantity of excitation from both sides of a color equation, hence such a postulated reduction in receptor activity could not upset a color match. Since anomalous and normal color matches would, except for precision, be essentially the same, the logic of simple reduction is in fundamental contradiction to the fact it sets out to explain, namely that, in general, the normal and anomalous color equations do differ (see Fig. 1). Some sort of qualitative alteration in the anomalous color system is required.

This alteration is usually assumed to occur in the photosensitive absorbing material of the receptors, but the theoretical proposals have varied both in type and in degree of specificity. For example, the peak of one of the distribution functions is assumed to be displaced, the form of one of the functions altered with no shift in peak, form modifications have been assumed to occur together with some degree of sensitivity reduction, and, in some instances, increased relative responsiveness has even been thought to occur. The list of investigators who have proposed receptor sensitivity alterations, in one form or another, is a long one. Among them are: KÖNIG and DIETERICI (1893), GUTTMANN (1908, 1909); ABNEY and WATSON (1913); ROSMANIT (1914); KOHLRAUSCH (1931); KATZIN and MURRAY (1934); TRENDELENBURG and SCHMIDT (1935); NELSON (1938); WRIGHT (1947); DEVRIES (1948); PITT (1949); WALLS and MATHEWS (1952); JAMESON and HURVICH (1956); WALD (1966).

Alteration models based exclusively on receptor photopigment changes cannot cope with all of the measured characteristics of protanomaly and deuteranomaly. For example, PITT (1949), has proposed that the long-wave receptor distribution function undergoes progressive logarithmic reduction to produce protanomaly in varying degrees. This accounts for color equations that deviate progressively from normal, but each reduction in this function must be associated perforce with a loss in long-wave sensitivity. Hence it implies a direct correlation between the Rayleigh equation mid-points and their ranges, a prediction contradicted by the measures presented in Fig. 2. A further difficulty is that progressive reductions in the long-wave receptor distribution function displace perforce the intercept between this curve and the mid-spectral distribution function toward progressively longer wavelengths. The spectral locus of this intercept presumably correlates in Pitt's model with the spectral locus of perceived yellow. Put to direct experimental test, however (Hurvich and Jameson, 1964), as some older data had already indicated (Jameson and Hurvich, 1956), protanomalous yellow loci are found at shorter, *not* longer wavelengths than those of the normal. This is seen in Fig. 4 where the spectral locus of unique yellow is plotted against the Rayleigh mid-point ratio for 40 normals, 6 deuteranomalous and 3 protanomalous observers.

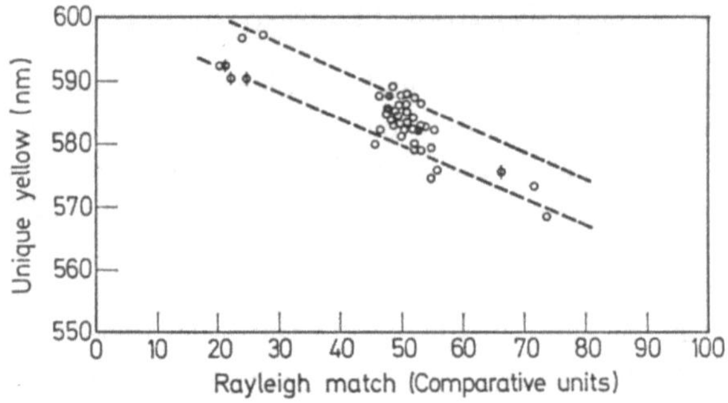

Fig. 4. Rayleigh equation mid-point scores and spectral loci of unique yellow for 49 observers: 40 normals, 6 deuteranomalous and 3 protanomalous (Hurvich and Jameson, 1964)

In a recent study, Alpern and Torii (1968b, c) have also concluded that photopigment alterations are required to account for anomalous color vision. Although protanopes and protanomalous, or deuteranopes and deuteranomalous are "virtually indistinguishable" (Alpern, 1968) in two-color increment threshold measurements (Wald, 1966), by retinal densitometry (Rushton, 1965c), and by luminosity measures using absolute threshold techniques (Alpern and Torii, 1968c), Alpern and Torii were able to show differences between the dichromats and their anomalous counterparts by spectral luminosity functions based on equality-of-brightness. Unfortunately, they did not use a bi-partite foveal test field in these experiments, but rather, a 30′ central test field which was matched in brightness to a surrounding annulus. Measures always began at the short-wave end of the spectrum, the spectrum was traversed in 10 nm steps, and a new annulus color was substituted and matched to the test field six times during the spectral traverse, after which the cascade procedure was repeated in the reverse direction from long to short wavelengths. Although the single standard annulus setting common to all subjects was the short-wave one, the measured functions are locked in mid-spectrum for analysis. The cascade procedure is subject to cumulative error, but more importantly, the center-annulus configuration is ideally suited to reveal inter-observer differences in the gradient of macular pigment density from center to periphery of the foveal pit. Since the same authors conclude in another study that macular pigment is responsible for luminosity differences between what are sometimes described as "class 1" and "class 2" deuteranopes, it is especially unfortunate that their equality-of-brightness data were collected in such a way as to be susceptible of confounding by the same sort of selective filter action. The authors analyze their data, however, in the context of RUSHTON'S conclusions about protanopic and deuteranopic photopigments (see Sec. IV below) and infer the theoretical absorption spectra of the anomalous pigments by examining alternative postulates (Schroedinger and Stiles line-element assumptions) of the way cone mechanisms pool their effects to produce a brightness response. Specifically, they propose that the long-wave photopigment absorption of the protanomalous is approximately like the normal's "green" one but somewhat displaced from it toward longer wavelengths, (that it is a dilute solution of normal "red" pigment seems to them less likely), whereas the absorption spectrum of the deuteranomalous mid-spectral photopigment is very similar to the normal "red" pigment but shifted very slightly toward shorter wavelengths. The consequences of these particular alteration systems for discrimination are not considered.

MÜLLER (1924) and JAMESON and HURVICH (1956), (HURVICH and JAMESON, 1962) have presented theoretical analyses of anomalous color vision that assume alterations in receptor photopigments, but, in addition, consider the effects of neural changes at the post-receptoral, opponent-process level. MÜLLER'S discussion is qualitative only, and JUDD'S (1949b, 1970) quantification of some of MÜLLER'S postulates for normal and dichromatic vision is not extended to include the mechanisms of anomalous trichromasy.

HURVICH and JAMESON'S account of deficient color vision rests on two assumptions, (1) a displacement rule that specifies degrees of spectral photopigment alterations from the normal ones and (2) a reduction postulate that applies to the post-receptoral neural response level and provides for varying degrees of "neural efficiency". The characteristics of the anomalous systems are thus expressed with sufficient precision for evaluation against color-mixture data, luminosity data, perceptual data and discrimination data for various kinds and degrees of defective color vision. The displacement rule in this account differs from other alteration proposals in that it assumes a uniform translation, in units of frequency rather than wavelength, of all three of the normal selective receptor distributions to yield the anomalous receptor system. The normal photopigment absorptions which are taken to be linearly related to the normal color-mixture curves, are also assumed to approximate the DARTNALL (1953) nomogram form, and the translation rule preserves this form. The linear relation to the color-mixture data is not, of course, preserved in this alteration, hence the altered systems yield anomalous color equations. Moreover, since different degrees of alteration, thus different amounts of frequency translation are assumed, anomalous color equations that differ by different amounts from normal proportions are a consequence of this analysis.

The receptor activities are linked to and control the neural activities at the post-receptoral level, and for normal color vision, the responsiveness of the three-variable, paired-opponent neural system (see JAMESON, chapter 14, this volume) is shown in the center block of Fig. 5. The upper and lower blocks of Fig. 5 show the paired chromatic and achromatic response functions for visual systems in which the receptor pigments are altered by frequency shifts that amount to about 15 nm away from 550 nm toward shorter wavelengths (upper block) to yield a protanomalous system, or toward longer wavelengths (lower block) to yield a deuteranomalous system. A comparison of Fig. 5 with Fig. 6 shows the result of the second postulate, reduction, on these curves, and in Fig. 6 the amplitudes of the red-green functions are represented as 0.1 the normal strength.

The functions at the top of Fig. 5 describe a keen protanomalous observer, and those in the bottom block represent a deuteranomalous individual with good discrimination. On the other hand, the anomalous types represented in Fig. 6 would be expected to show significant discrimination losses and red-green weakness.

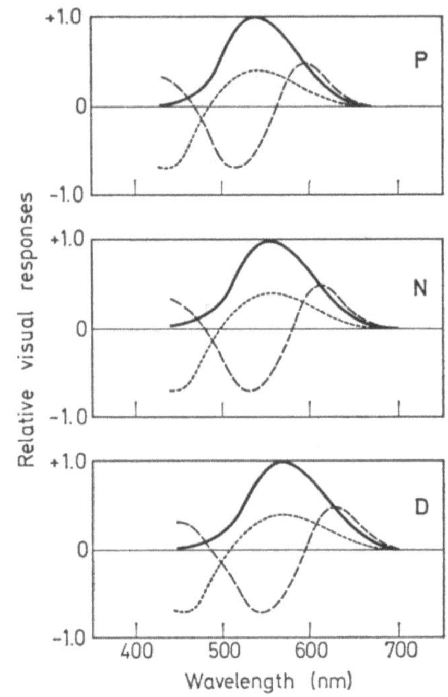

Fig. 5

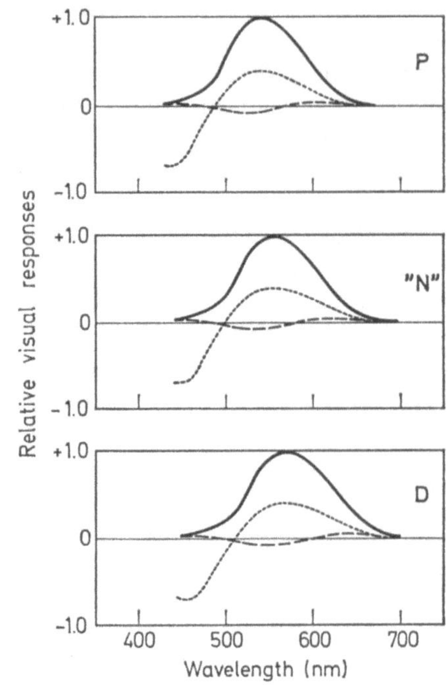

Fig. 6

Fig. 5. Spectral distributions of opponent response processes for observers with protanomalous (upper block), normal (center block) and deuteranomalous photopigments. Normal efficiency of neural response systems in all cases (JAMESON and HURVICH, 1956)

Fig. 6. Spectral distributions of opponent response processes with normal, protanomalous and deuteranomalous photopigments with weak red-green response systems (JAMESON and HURVICH, 1956)

Rayleigh equation mid-points and ranges computed for an average normal observer, for systems with three degrees of photopigment alteration (frequency shifts amounting to 5 nm, 9 nm, and 15 nm from 550 nm) in both the long- and short-wave directions, and for four degrees of red-green responsiveness (normal, 0.1 normal, 0.03 normal, and complete loss of red-green neural response), are shown in the four separate graphs in Fig. 3. The experimental measures for WILLIS and FARNSWORTH's observers are drawn in thin lines, as noted earlier, and the theoretically calculated instances are shown in heavy lines. Crucial to the analysis of data of this sort is the assumption of separate changes in the anomalous visual systems: (1) receptor photopigment alterations that account for the midpoint deviations, and (2) post-receptoral neural efficiency losses that account for the increases in matching range.

Note that in the central block of Fig. 6 the observer has been labelled "N" rather than N. This represents an individual with a normal Rayleigh mid-point but an abnormally large range, and appropriately characterized as color weak. ROSMANIT (1914, p. 107ff.) and MÜLLER (1924, p. 187) have both reported individuals with normal Rayleigh equation mid-points but who exhibited color weakness. Fig. 2 includes at least four such observers about whom WILLIS and FARNSWORTH were uncertain and their data are labelled "U" in the figure. CRONE (1959) also mentions six cases of poor color discrimination with normal Rayleigh ratios. As MÜLLER pointed out, this situation essentially mimics the situation in the periphery of the normal retina (see MORELAND, chapter 20, this volume). To distinguish such individuals from normals we may call them "neuteranomalous" ("Color amblyopes", ENGELKING, 1933).

Alteration systems that postulate shifts in maxima of receptor photopigment distributions anticipate spectral luminosity functions with peaks shifted towards shorter wavelengths for protanomalous, and longer ones for deuteranomalous observers. As noted in Sec. I, protanomalous mean relative luminosity is depressed in the long-wave spectral region and the maximum is displaced toward shorter wavelengths from the average normal peak, whereas the mean deuteranomalous curve peaks at a slightly longer wavelength than normal (WRIGHT, 1947; HARTRIDGE, 1950; JUDD, 1951; SCHOBER, 1958; GRÜTZNER, 1962; WALD, 1966; WYSZECKI and STILES, 1967), Ratio estimates of relative luminosity that use pairs of wavelengths (e.g., 530 nm/650 nm) rather than complete spectral functions can be obtained for large samples of individuals, and such estimates confirm, in general, the displacements of the functions for the three groups (CRONE, 1959). There is, of course, some degree of overlap among the measured functions, and the overlap is more extensive for the deuteranomalous with the normal group. The overlap is not surprising since spectral luminosity measurements show considerable variation within any group (JUDD, 1951; LEE, 1966). These measures vary with psychophysical technique (see above) but more importantly, the form of the function is also affected by both pre-receptoral light absorption and the relative population distributions of the various cone types. Thus, heavy macular pigmentation will decrease the short-wave sensitivity, whereas a selectively reduced population of cones of (say) the long-wave sensitive type would manifest itself in protan-like luminosity curves.

There is, nonetheless, some evidence that the luminosity maximum for protanomalous observers is correlated with the degree of measured color deviance (KOHLRAUSCH, 1931). Furthermore, some recent measures that compare luminosity ratios with the Rayleigh equation values for the same observers tend to support the view that even in normals – there were 197 observers in the study — slight differences in the color systems are associated with slight displacements in spectral luminosity (RUSHTON and BAKER, 1964). In this study, the Pearson product-moment correlation coefficient (r) between Rayleigh mid-point measures and luminosity quotients was $+ 0.40$. A correlation of this magnitude would, in a sample of this size, be expected to occur by chance less than once in a thousand times. (Durup and Piéron, 1943, had failed to find such a correlation in a sample of only 13 normal observers.) A comparable study that included anomalous observers in the measured population would be expected to significantly increase the correlation found by Rushton and Baker.

The chromatic and achromatic response functions for the altered visual systems of Fig. 5 and Fig. 6 have definite implications for the way anomalous observers perceive spectral colors. They indicate, for example, that the spectral unique-hue loci of protanomalous and deuteranomalous observers will be displaced systematically from those of normals. Such comparative measures require that adaptation be rigorously controlled and that the sampled anomalous have fairly good color discrimination (otherwise unique hue transition points are difficult to measure). Group data for all the unique points are rare, and Rubin's (1961) data which do, on the whole, support the theoretically expected hue shifts for the different types, were possibly subject to "anchoring"-type adaptation effects

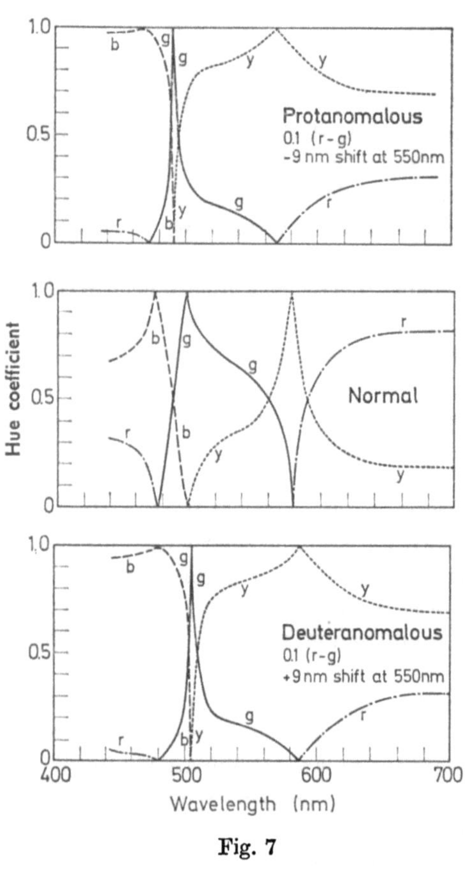

Fig. 7

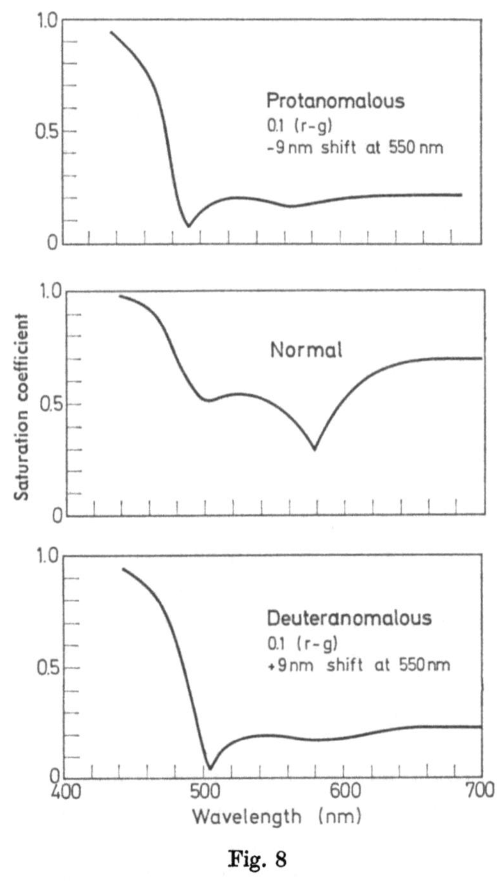

Fig. 8

Fig. 7. Theoretical spectral hue coefficients for normal and abnormal systems as specified in individual graphs (Jameson and Hurvich, 1956)

Fig. 8. Theoretical spectral saturation coefficients for normal and abnormal systems as specified in individual graphs (Jameson and Hurvich, 1956)

(HURVICH *et al.*, 1968). There are, on the other hand, many reports on the locus of unique yellow and these data show a shift in this locus toward shorter wavelengths for protanomalous and toward longer ones for deuteranomalous individuals. See Fig. 4 and data reported by WESTPHAL (1910), ABNEY and WATSON (1913), KÖLLNER (1919), GÖTHLIN (1923), MÜLLER (1924), GOLDMANN (1925), SCHUBERT (1928), HAILWOOD and ROAF (1937), NELSON (1938). (See JAMESON and HURVICH, 1956, for discussion of earlier references.)

The altered systems of the anomalous would be expected to show less clear-cut differences when tested with relatively broad-band stimuli but the spectrally integrated responses would still tend to differ systematically between the normal and each anomalous group. Such a result is reported by WATSON (1914) in a little known paper in which his observers were required to match with a spectral line the "white" of an electric arc filtered through a saturated solution of chromate of potash. Compared to the normal match centered on 578–580 nm, his anomalous observers made equations that moved in the short- and long-wave directions for different groups, and the direction of the displacement correlated directly with their Rayleigh match data.

On the basis of the chromatic and achromatic responsiveness curves (Figs. 5 and 6) coefficient functions can be calculated in order to represent both perceived hue and perceived saturation of spectral lights (HURVICH and JAMESON, 1955; JAMESON and HURVICH, 1959). Such theoretically calculated functions for a protanomalous, normal, and a deuteranomalous system are shown in Figs. 7 and 8.

For the anomalous, receptor photopigment shifts of ± 9 nm from the 550 nm peak have been assumed to occur, and the systems described in Figs. 7 and 8 are assumed to have only 10 per cent of normal *r-g* responsiveness at the neural level.

Table 1. *Reported and predicted sensations of normal and deuteranomalous eyes. Reported appearances for unilateral deuteranomalous from* v. KRIES (1919)

Wave-length nm	Normal eye			Deuteranomalous eye		
	Appearance	Predicted appearance		Appearance	Predicted appearance	
		h. c.	s. c.		h. c.	s. c.
627	red	0.23*y*, 0.77*r*	0.64	considerably yellower	0.77*y*, 0.27*r*	0.20
608	bright red	0.30*y*, 0.70*r*	0.57	yellow (trace of red)	0.87*y*, 0.13*r*	0.19
591	reddish inter-mixture	0.51*y*, 0.49*r*	0.43	pure yellow	0.98*y*, 0.02*r*	0.16
573	slight green yellow	0.75*y*, 0.25*g*	0.33	pure yellow (no difference)	0.93*y*, 0.07*r*	0.18
559	grass green	0.48*y*, 0.52*g*	0.45	almost pure yellow	0.88*y*, 0.12*g*	0.19
535	green	0.34*y*, 0.66*g*	0.53	yellow with slight shimmer of green	0.82*y*, 0.18*g*	0.19
515	green	0.25*y*, 0.75*g*	0.54	greenish yellow (diff. very large)	0.71*y*, 0.29*g*	0.14
505	green	0.15*y*, 0.85*g*	0.52	weak yellow green	1.00*g*	0.04
496	green	0.05*b*, 0.95*g*	0.53	almost colorless (diff. maximal)	0.86*b*, 0.14*g*	0.23
488	blue green	0.43*b*, 0.57*g*	0.60	white (colorless)	0.95*b*, 0.05*g*	0.46
480	green blue	0.88*b*, 0.12*g*	0.69	gray blue	1.00*b*	0.63
464	blue	0.76*b*, 0.24*r*	0.90	perhaps somewhat less blue than left eye	0.97*b*, 0.03*r*	0.86
460	violet	0.74*b*, 0.26*r*	0.93	blue	0.96*b*, 0.04*r*	0.88

For the perceptual qualities reported by observers with anomalous color vision the direct evidence comes from cases where the anomaly occurs in only one eye and the other is normal. Reports of unilateral anomalous individuals are given for example by KOLBE (1887), HAYES (1911), HEGNER (1915), and GOLDSCHMIDT (1919). The only systematically useful reports, however, are those of v. KRIES's (1919) observer REICHERT. (TRENDELENBURG, 1941b, did a follow-up study of REICHERT and his children.) In Table 1 we have reproduced a comparison of this observer's verbal reports for his normal and deuteranomalous eyes with the theoretically derived hue and saturation coefficients of Figs. 7 and 8.

Wavelength discrimination data for anomalous observers have been reported by ENGELKING (1926), SACHS (1928), LADEKARL (1934), CORBETT (1937), NELSON (1938), MCKEON and WRIGHT (1940) and MCLELLAN (see LAKOWSKI, 1968). Illustrative protanomalous and deuteranomalous functions from among ENGELKING's observers (1926) are summarized in Fig. 9. One normal function is also included in the figure. Both the protanomalous and deuteranomalous observers with narrow Rayleigh match ranges have wavelength discrimination functions that resemble the normal one, and the increasing deterioration in discrimination for both types of observer was shown by ENGELKING to be directly correlated with an

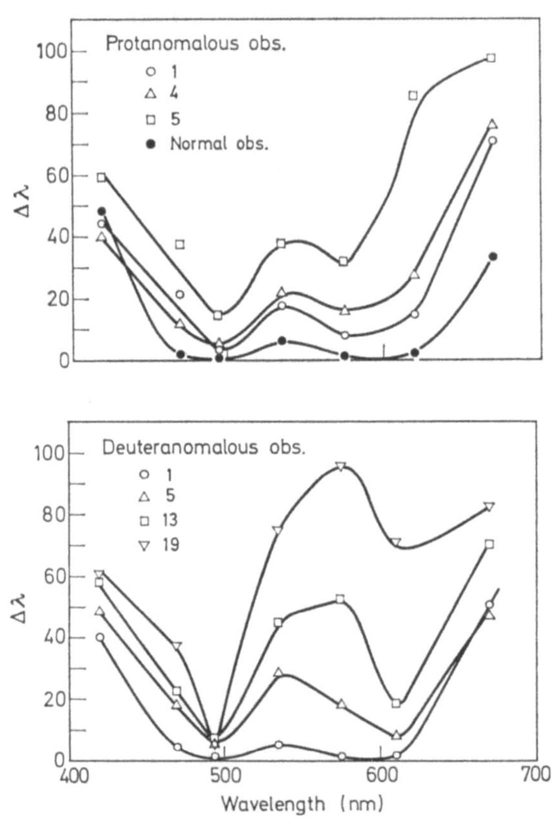

Fig. 9. Illustrative wavelength discrimination functions measured on 1 normal, 3 protanomalous and 4 deuteranomalous observers. (After ENGELKING, 1926)

increase in the Rayleigh equation matching range. Similar comparisons are also available in McLellan's data (Lakowski, 1968). The displacement of the protan and deutan functions from each other in the regions of minimal and maximal sensitivity in the mid- and long-wave regions are in accord with the theoretical responsiveness functions of Figs. 5 and 6 and the hue and saturation coefficient functions (Figs. 7 and 8) on which the individual's discriminative capacities can be shown to rest (Hurvich and Jameson, 1955). Theoretical wavelength discrimination functions for two such observers based on these coefficient functions are shown in Fig. 10. Wavelength discrimination curves measured in the normal periphery where there is also a relative reduction in red and green responsiveness show some general similarities to anomalous curves (Weale, 1953b). (See Fig. 11.)

Saturation or colorimetric purity discrimination for anomalous observers (protans and deutans) have been reported less frequently (Chapanis, 1944; Wright, 1947). Chapanis' data for two anomalous observers are reproduced in

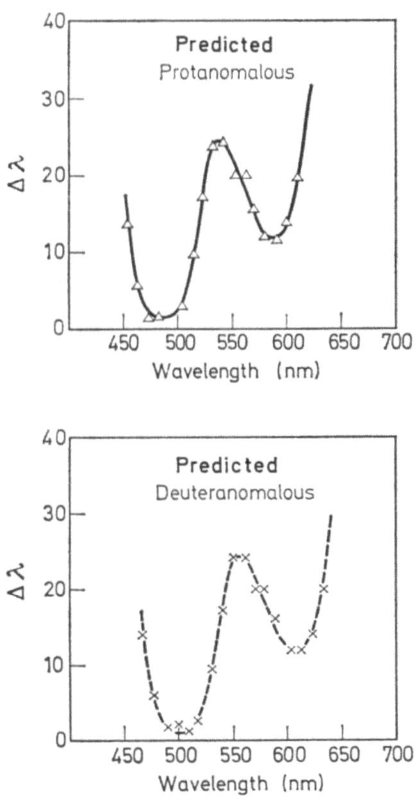

Fig. 10

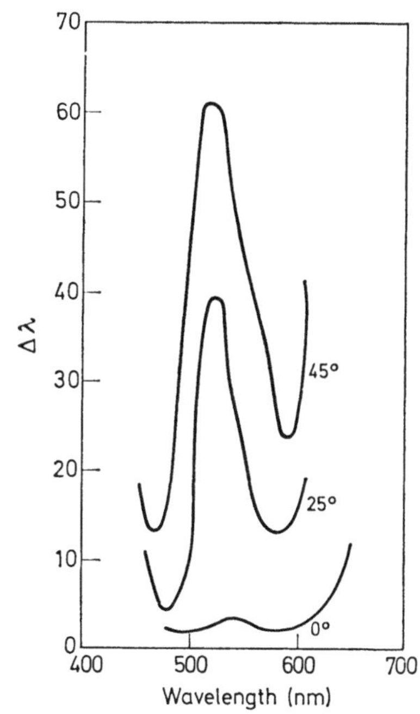

Fig. 11

Fig. 10. Predicted wavelength discrimination functions for 1 protanomalous and 1 deuteranomalous observer based on opponent-process model (Hurvich and Jameson, 1955 and 1962)

Fig. 11. Measured wavelength discrimination functions in fovea and at 2 peripheral retinal loci, 25° and 45° (after Weale, 1953)

Fig. 12a, and theoretical functions calculated for the anomalous systems are shown in Fig. 12b (JAMESON and HURVICH, 1956; HURVICH and JAMESON, 1962).

It should be noted that the comparisons between calculated and measured features of the color anomalies given above are based on assumed alteration and/or reduction systems in which receptor alterations are postulated for all three cone photopigments. Shifted absorption spectra for all three visual pigments was, in fact, the only reasonable hypothesis to explore at the time this model was first developed and when it also seemed reasonable to assume that the normal cone

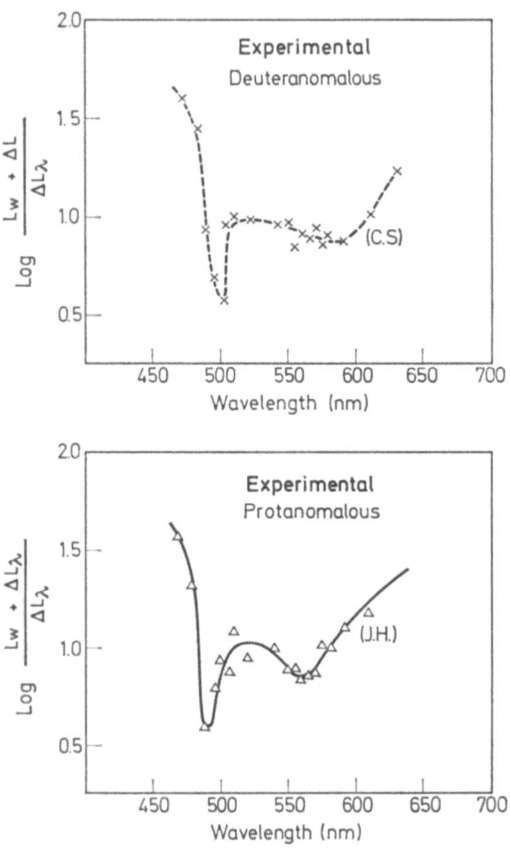

Fig. 12a

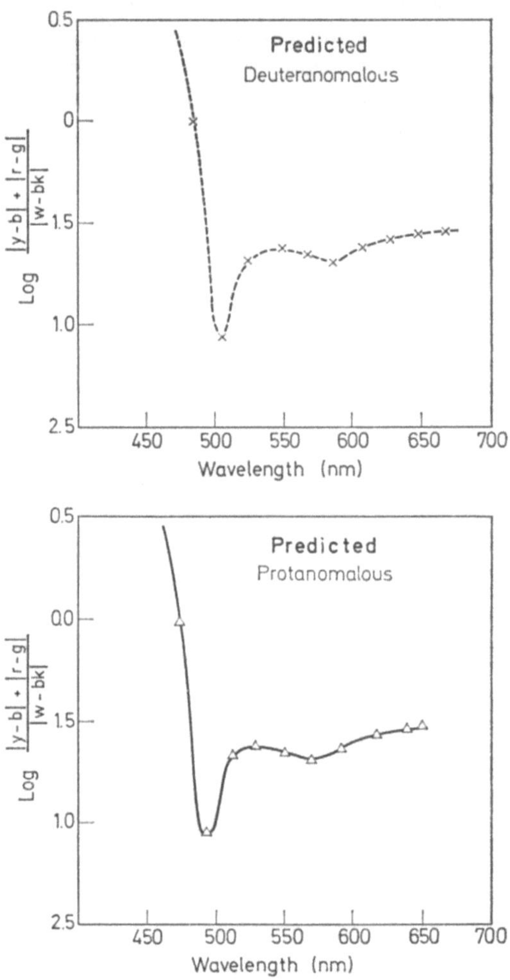

Fig. 12b

Fig. 12a. Measured saturation discrimination thresholds (least colorimetric purity) for 1 deuteranomalous (C.S.) and 1 protanomalous (J.H.) observer (after CHAPANIS, 1944)

Fig. 12b. Predicted saturation discrimination thresholds (least colorimetric purity) for 1 deuteranomalous and 1 protanomalous observer. Based on opponent-process theory (HURVICH and JAMESON, 1955 and 1962)

pigments closely overlapped with one another. (See JAMESON, chapter 14, this volume). Information on cone photopigment absorptions collected over the last ten years, however, makes such close overlap for normals unlikely (JAMESON and HURVICH, 1968), and therefore reopens the possibility that a shifted absorption spectrum for only one, rather than all three, of the cone pigments may be responsible for the receptor alterations of anomalous color systems, as envisaged, for example, by ALPERN and TORII (see above). Since analyses that assume alterations in a single pigment have not yet considered the consequences of such presumed systems for altered discrimination capacities in the anomalous individuals, it is not yet clear that they could yield the necessary degree of independence to account for the separate manifestation of color deviance and red-green weakness by different individuals within the protanomalous and deuteranomalous groups.

The third type of anomalous trichromasy, tritanomaly, is both more rare and less well understood than protanomaly or deuteranomaly. It was ENGELKING (1925) who first uncovered this form of defect and, working in the theoretical context of protanopia, deuteranopia, and tritanopia as "loss" of systems underlying red, green or blue sensations, respectively (see Sec. IV.), he tended to emphasize the "blue" deficiency of this type of observer. He called the deficiency "tritanomaly" and regarded it as expressing an alteration in the form of the short-wave photopigment absorption function. However, the anomalous individual studied by ENGELKING was, as he states, both *yellow* and blue defective.

The case reported by MEITNER (1941) does not, however, show the paired discrimination deficiencies described by ENGELKING. The impairment seems, rather, to consist largely of abnormal responses to short-wave stimuli, and hence MEITNER's case would seem to fall properly in a category of anomalous trichromasy that results from alterations in the receptor pigment with maximal absorption in the 440–450 nm region.

Although MEITNER suggested that his observer be called "atypical tritanomalous" to differentiate him from ENGELKING's case, if tritanomaly is taken to describe anomalous short-wave responses, the "atypical" designation seems inappropriate. Moreover, if the rarely used fourth designation, *tetartanomaly* is interpreted to mean functional losses or reduced efficiency at the paired neural response level, then a careful reading of ENGELKING's report leads us to concur with LINKSZ's (1964) suggestion that "the first case ever labelled a tritanomal actually was tetartanomalous." Not only is there "blue" loss, there is clearly "yellow" loss. For example, bluish-reds and yellowish-reds are difficult to distinguish. Furthermore, short-wave spectral stimuli are reported as "reddish". Thus it would seem that this case involved a relative reduction in responsiveness in the "yellow-blue" coded neural system as well as possible alterations in the short-wave receptor photopigment.

What appears to be a clear-cut unilateral tetartanomalous case was first described by HERMANN (1882), but surprisingly, this report has received little attention. The detailed color naming of this observer on two different spectral apparatuses makes it clear that his right eye was completely normal and trichromatic. With the defective left eye he saw the entire hue gamut, but at about 583–588 nm the yellow was dull ("matt tone of sepia") and at about 465 nm he saw a dull blue. This case also implies deficits at the neural level of "yellow-blue" coding, and poses serious difficulties for interpretations that rely exclusively on short-wave photopigment losses of varying degrees.

A final note. In the above discussion of anomalous color vision which treats the red-green and yellow-blue chromatic systems as independently variable, response decrements in the red-green coded neural system are assumed to occur in the face of a fully active, fully efficient yellow-blue system and vice versa, i.e., yellow-blue decrements to occur in the face of a 100 % efficient red-green system. It is, however, also possible that reduced responsiveness may occur concurrently in the two paired chromatic systems. Anomalous individuals of this sort include one of STILLING's (1910) yellow-blue defectives and the cases that JAEGER (1955) describes as showing depression of the yellow-blue sense along with red-green disturbances. HESS (1922) argues the general case that the two dichromatic systems probably vary independently.

IV. Loss and Fusion Systems (Photochemical; Receptoral)

"Loss" and "fusion" concepts have a long history and have played an important role in color theorizing particularly about the relation between normal and deficient color vision. From a stimulus-mixture point of view, dichromasy is obviously a "loss" system in the sense that such visual systems operate in terms of one less stimulus variable than the normal complement of three. But from the point of view of the mechanisms there is a rather wide variety of assumptions about what specifically is lost (fundamentals? primaries? color processes? sensations? receptors? photopigments?) or what specifically remains in different classes of two-variable "reduction" forms of color vision, as they are commonly called.

The earliest "loss" notions of congenital dichromasy were expressed in terms of the so-called "fundamental sensations", which were taken to be red, green and blue (or violet). One dichromatic system was assumed to retain the normal green and blue sensations but to lack the "red fundamental" ("red blind"), another was postulated to have normal red and blue sensations but to lack the "green fundamental" ("green blind"), and a third was thought to retain the normal red and green sensations but to lack the "blue fundamental" ("blue blind"). The notion was a simple one and for a time during the last century was rather widely held by authorities such as HELMHOLTZ, DONDERS, KÖNIG, v. KRIES and ABNEY. The difficulties and inconsistencies encountered were so serious, however, that even HELMHOLTZ abandoned the idea (1896) to adopt a modified proposal of the sort labelled as "fusion" or "collapse" hypotheses (FICK, 1874, 1879, 1896; LEBER, 1873).

The loss notion and its geometric interpretation in terms of the color-mixture triangle were clearly spelled out by MAXWELL as early as 1855. If there are three and only three elementary sensations and if all the actual sensations of color are produced by combinations of the three elementary ones, color-mixture results are expressible by assigning each one of the elementary sensations to one apex of a triangle and by applying a weighted center of gravity analysis to determine the resultant. In this view, each plotted point on the limiting sides of the triangle and within the triangle itself represents a different color experience that depends on the proportions of the assumed three fundamental sensations. In such a representation the proportions of all three elements may vary or two of them may be fixed relative to each other with variations occurring in the third only. In the latter instance the represented colors fall on straight lines.

Now for "color-blinds" all colors that look alike are usually said to fall on straight lines in such a color triangle and a whole series of such lines can be found for different series of colors that appear alike. "All the lines either pass through one point or are parallel," wrote MAXWELL, which indicates the "absence of a determinate sensation." The missing color experience is inferred to be one of the normal fundamentals, as are also the two remaining ones in the dichromatic system.

HELMHOLTZ (1866) presented a similar analytical and geometric treatment of "color blindness" as sensation loss systems and his analysis led him to state explicitly and precisely what colors "colorblinds" should see. Thus, "The *red* of the spectrum ... would have to appear to red-blind persons as a *saturated green of low luminosity* ... The yellow of the spectrum will appear as *brilliant saturated green* ... *Green* ... a pale shade of green ..." etc. Experimental determinations of confusion colors for one individual led him to conclude that in this instance "red, and not green, ... is the missing colour" and "On YOUNG's hypothesis, therefore," he went on to say, "red blindness would be explained as a paralysis of the red-sensitive nerves" (1924 V. II, p. 151.).

But such simplistic loss schemas were soon recognized to fly in the face of numerous facts which contradicted some basic postulates of the theoretical position that had been adopted, namely, that perceived yellow arises from a mixture of red and green sensations, and white from a combination of all three basic sensations. For example, normals are able to see yellows in retinal regions where neither red nor green are reported ("peripheral color-blindness"); all color defectives who lack specific hue sensations it is agreed still see "whites"; and finally the perceptual reports of *unilateral* protanopic and deuteranopic color defectives indicate clearly that they see yellows and blues and whites and blacks with the abnormal eye but that they do not see reds or greens (JUDD, 1948).

There are, moreover, difficulties that relate to the measured spectral luminosity data of color deficient observers. GRAHAM (1965), for example, points out that the simplest Young-Helmholtz models (JUDD, 1949a) lead to the expectation in the case of the deuteranope who loses the mid-spectral "fundamental" that the luminosity function will be bimodal — which it is not. And that with later modifications of this basic model in which luminosity is assigned exclusively to the long-wave primary (KÖNIG, 1897), we are led to the even more disconcerting notion that the protanope would be completely blind were he to lose the long-wave "fundamental".

But long before such luminosity problems were encountered, the loss view of color-blindness was seen to require revisions if the contradictions between fact and theory were to be resolved. The Fick-Leber fusion or collapse notions were proposed for precisely this reason. Generally speaking, the terms fusion or collapse are applied to views that assume that the abnormal individual has the same complement of, say, processes or photopigments that the normal has, but that the spectral excitabilities or absorption properties are different functions of wavelength in the color defective than they are in the normal (or to account for the color zones, that they are different functions of wavelength in different regions of the normal retina).

In his initial concern with the peripheral "color blindness" of the normal observer, Fick (1874) proposed that in contrast to the set of the normal functions with different short-, mid- and long-wave peaks, the "R" and "G" curves for these peripheral retinal regions had peaks that coincided in the mid-spectral region. This assumption would account for the yellow and blue (and white and black) colors seen in the mid-zone of the normal periphery. For the extreme periphery, he suggested that all three functions had peaks that were superimposed with respect to spectral locus. Later, for color deficiencies themselves (1896) he considered three cases: for one type he proposed that the excitability of the "red" fibers corresponds to that of the "green" ones, for a second that the "green" shifts to be identical to the "blue", and for the third that the "red" is shifted to the spectral locus of the "blue". Helmholtz (1896) adopted a variant of this mechanism but rather than speaking of fiber types as Fick did he handled the problem in photochemical terms. The differences between the different photopigments, say, the "red" and "green" sensitive ones, were assumed to have vanished, but both were either like the normal's "red" sensitive one or like the normal's "green" sensitive one. This interpretation postulates loss, at the most peripheral level, of the selectivity required for the separate sensations of redness or greenness, but the central connections remain the same as for normals; the photopigments are "R" and "G" regardless of spectral absorption, and each continues to feed into the "red" or "green" centers. Consequently, the hue experiences of these dichromats are the required yellows and blues.

Modern adoptions of "fusion" views (usually to account for deuteranopic vision) are those of Pitt (1935), Willmer (1950), Walls and Mathews (1952), and Graham and Hsia (1958). The latter investigators proposed both a short- and long-wave shift, respectively, of the two relevant photopigment distribution functions in the "red" and "green" receptors to account both for their unilateral observer's luminosity curve as well as yellow and blue perceptions reported by this observer. These overlapping functions of wavelength were generated on a purely *ad hoc* basis, however, as was the proposal that the luminosity function be represented by the average of the two basic overlapping curves.

Recent advances in reflection densitometry (Weale, 1968) and the microspectrodensitometry of individual cones (Wald and Brown, 1965; Marks, Dobelle and MacNichol, 1964) have now made available the first direct measures of the photopigment absorptions in the human eye. What do they tell us about the photopigment situation in color defectives? First, what do the *in situ* reflection density measures on the eyes of color defectives tell us?

Rushton's analysis of his most recent data argues for specific photopigment losses (1963a, b, c, 1965a, b). The measures are interpreted to show a single pigment in the protanope that peaks at 540 nm ("chlorolabe") and a single pigment in the deuteranope that peaks at about 570 nm ("erythrolabe"). Since both types of defective are assumed to have a short-wave pigment (not determinable by reflection densitometry), it is concluded that only a single photopigment is lacking in each instance, the long-wave one for the protanope, the mid-spectral one for the deuteranope. Additional evidence for the loss of a single photopigment comes from the fact that the action spectrum of bleaching agrees with the foveal luminosity curve of the given type of color defective and that in each instance the pigment regenerates in accord with the recovery of sensitivity in the retina.

Two points need to be emphasized. No hue-coding interpretation has been given to these findings. In view of the difficulties faced by early theorists who conceived the color-deficiencies as simple red, green and blue losses, RUSHTON's apparent reluctance to proffer specific proposals is easy to understand. Despite the hard data now in hand, the interpretive issues remain the same and equally contradictory outcomes face the modern investigator who adopts the simplistic coding view that labels photopigments "red", "green", "blue" and ties them with red, green and blue sensations, respectively. The reflection densitometry data *per se* do not reveal any information about presence or absence of specific receptor-neural pathways or functional organizations present in the normal retina. The recorded loss of photopigment absorption at one spectral locus and the recorded presence of photopigment absorption at another says nothing about the receptor-neural organization.

There is in this work, moreover, a major unresolved issue at the experimental level. The "proof" for loss of one of the photopigments is seriously flawed by the fact that the absorption measurements obtained for the dichromats are identical to those for the corresponding types of anomalous trichromats (RUSHTON, 1965c). Trichromacy, whether normal or anomalous, is agreed to require the presence of three differently selective pigments in the retina and yet the anomalous observers can be shown to have only the single pigment of the dichromat by reflection densitometry. Serious limitations are still inherent in the method.

WALD (WALD and BROWN, 1965), like RUSHTON, has now concluded that only a "loss" mechanism produces dichromatic vision. Having established the existence of three photopigments via microspectrodensitometry of single cones in the extracted retina, WALD turned (ironically) to the use of psychophysical techniques to isolate and specify the individual receptor types in normal and color defective humans. Like ALPERN, WALD used the increment threshold technique under conditions of selective adaptation (see ENOCH chapter 21, this volume) and measured foveal spectral thresholds in normals, five protanopes, thirteen deuteranopes and three tritanopes. The adapted sensitivity curves are interpreted as photopigment absorptions following selective bleaching, and, in contrast to the normals who show evidence of the expected three absorbing pigments, the dichromats reveal only two. Deuteranopes show only short- and long-wave ("blue"- and "red"-sensitive pigments, protanopes only "blue"- and "green"-sensitive pigments, and tritanopes only mid- and long-wave ("green"- and "red"-) sensitive pigments.

WALD (1964, 1966) does concern himself with the hue coding problem and his present view of dichromacy is that all three sensory channels are retained and that both protanopes and deuteranopes have the capacity to experience all three primary sensations but that in each case two sensations are excited by a single visual pigment: "... one might assume that in protanopes the green-sensitive pigment, and in the deuteranopes ... the red-sensitive pigment excites indiscriminately the red and green sensations thus yielding a sensation of yellow." This analysis, which assumes that all three "hue-coded" central mechanisms are retained and triggered by only two photopigments is directly comparable to the fusion systems envisaged by FICK, LEBER, and HELMHOLTZ.

WALD himself believes his present evidence argues against fusion hypotheses. However, by "fusion" he means something other than the original usage. For him "fusion" refers to systems that possess all three visual pigments in normal proportions and also all three sensory channels but where the disability "involves only a confusion of the red and green pathways, such that both the red- and green-sensitive pigments, whether in separate cones or mixed in the same cones, excite both pathways indiscriminately and evoke the yellow sensation."

WALD'S evidence for the loss of individual photopigments would seem to resolve the doubts left by the reflection densitometry measures were it not also true that in WALD'S experiments, as in RUSHTON'S, the same psychophysical measures and conditions that reveal only two functions in the dichromat reveal only the same two functions in the corresponding anomalous observers who are known to be trichromatic. We must conclude with ALPERN (1968) that both the fundus reflectometry methods and the increment threshold methods are insufficiently sensitive to decide conclusively about the number of selective photopigments present in any given retina.

We might anticipate that the measured spectral luminosity functions of the color defectives would be of primary importance in helping to clarify the issue of whether or not photopigments are lost, and if they are which ones, simply because their presence or absence would be reflected in such luminosity measures. But as we have already noted in connection with KÖNIG'S view, such analyses depend on how we conceptualize the white (and black) coding mechanisms to be linked to the particular photopigment absorption functions and the conceptualizations are indeed varied. But worse still, even the basic psychophysical facts are in dispute. There is considerable disagreement both about the forms and spectral locations of the dichromatic luminosity functions, particularly those of deuteranopic observers.

WILLMER (1950), for example, reported two types of deuteranope, one with luminosity maximal at 550 nm and indistinguishable from normals (Type I), the other with maximal sensitivity at 570 nm and somewhat depressed sensitivity in the short and extreme long-wave spectral regions (Type II). (Intermediates were also reported.) To accord with these findings, WILLMER postulated both a fusion (Type I) system and a loss (Type II) system. GRAHAM and HSIA'S (1960) threshold data, with one exception, support the "blue-green" losses in luminosity and as already noted above they resorted to an *ad hoc* manipulation of the assumed basic functions in accordance with a fusion hypothesis. ALPERN *et al.* (1968) report that one of their deuteranopes (among eleven tested) exhibits a normal luminosity curve, but their analysis attributes this to the absence of normal amounts of macular pigmentation in a system otherwise identical to the other deuteranopes. The deuteranopic luminosity curves with "blue" and "green" depressions relative to normal are, on the other hand, presumed to arise from loss of the pigment "chlorolabe". One of the major difficulties in seeking to arrive at a clear-cut interpretation of these curves is, of course, the large variability of so-called normal luminosity functions. ALPERN (ALPERN and TORII, 1968) has himself called attention to the fact that 25% of the "normal color vision population ... have a deuteranopic curve" as measured with his brightness matching procedure (LEE,

1966). Thus we are left with deuteranopic curves in the absence of chlorolabe (deuteranopes), deuteranopic curves in the presence of chlorolabe (25 % of normals), and normal curves in the absence of chlorolabe (deuteranope with reduced macular pigment).

The complications increase if we examine measures of spectral luminosity made with flicker techniques (HEATH, 1958, 1960). Using CFF measures, HEATH finds a relative gain in sensitivity in mid-spectral and long-wave regions for deuteranopes, and COLLINS (1961), who has comparative data that emphasize that technique (threshold vs. flicker), flicker rate, and field size generate different data for the same color deficient observer, tends to support the HEATH findings. GRÜTZNER'S (1962) flicker photometry data also support the view that deutans are relatively more sensitive than normals in the long wave regions of the spectrum.

A brief discussion of electroretinography as related to luminosity measures and color defective vision is given in Chapter 27 by RIGGS and WOOTEN, this volume.

There is no fundus reflectometry research on the cone pigments of the tritanope, but a common assumption is that the short-wave photopigment is absent in this condition. Treatments of the color-match data of the tritanope in terms of chromaticity-confusion intersection loci (JUDD *et al.*, 1950; WRIGHT, 1952; THOMSON and WRIGHT, 1953; FARNSWORTH, 1955; SPERLING, 1960) are interpreted as revealing a missing "receptor" or "pigment" in the expected short-wave region of the chromaticity chart and now WALD'S (1964) psychophysical data offer additional support for the "loss" view.

The use of colorimetric charts for the representation of chromaticity-confusion lines and the interpretation of the intersection locus of such lines as defining the null-point of the system or missing element dates back, of course, to MAXWELL'S "absence of a determinate sensation". But in recent treatments such co-punctal points are taken to represent missing receptors, missing photopigments, or "fundamentals", with little explicit recognition of the complex relations between stimuli, physiological mechanisms, and sensations.

Chromaticity-confusion intersection loci were measured for both protanopes and deuteranopes long before data were available for analyzing the tritanopic situation. Among investigators who have reported such data are KÖNIG and DIETERICI (1893), PITT (1935) and NUBERG and YUSTOVA (1955, see JUDD, 1964) (see also WRIGHT, 1947; GRAHAM, 1965).

The use of colorimetric charts in color-deficiency work still needs close scrutiny. HALSEY and CHAPANIS' (1952) experimental research on the isochromaticity lines with precisely specified surface colors showed major differences in some instances from PITT'S data transformed in CIE terms. Some extrapolations of the confusion lines by HALSEY and CHAPANIS even led, in the context in which such data are commonly viewed, to meaningless results. BOYNTON and SCHEIBNER (1967) present individual data of three protanopes on three-color matches to locate the intersection loci and report serious deviations from a single co-punctal point. Even the average intersection loci of their protanopic and deuteranopic observers failed to coincide (SCHEIBNER and BOYNTON, 1968). But to anticipate that any single abnormal observer's data are validly plotted on an average chromaticity chart is to anticipate that any single normal observer's data will traverse a single "white point" in the diagram in a plot, say, of complementary wavelengths. (Pre-retinal absorption differences alone would preclude such a uniform result.) A similar source of error is found in the extrapolated determinations of the "spectral" neutral points of protanopes and deuteranopes made by Walls and Heath (1956). (See above.) The neutral loci were obtained by extending the line connecting the chromaticity matches of an individual observer to the spectrum locus of the CIE chromaticity chart and treating the intercept as the "spectral" neutral locus of the individual observer.

A symposium exchange among Farnsworth (1961), Pitt (1961), and Wright (1961) about the validity of the use of chromaticity data based on averaged color matches to generate isochromatic lines and the meaning of the intersection locus, serves to clarify two points: (1) the dichromatic matching data can validly be plotted on the normal trichromatic chromaticity charts only if the two systems are linearly related and (2) the ocular pigmentation of the two averaged groups is the same. Farnsworth concluded that what is needed is a color-mixture diagram at the receptor level, and this is a reasonable suggestion that has not been followed up for dichromatic analyses. It has been shown, however, that data for small-field chromaticity confusions in the normal eye can be handled in precisely this way (Hurvich and Jameson, 1958).

As already noted, there have been relatively few yellow-blue deficient dichromats reported in the visual literature, but much of the available data conflicts with an interpretation as simple loss of either short-wave pigment or receptor system. If the reported cases are examined carefully, we find that, like Engelking's tritanomalous case which lends itself more reasonably to a "tetartanomalous" diagnosis, the data for diagnosed tritanopes, in many instances, show redness responses in the short-wave spectral region. Thus we find that there are two neutral or gray spectral loci that divide the mid-spectral green from both short-wave and long-wave red regions. Such cases are reported by Stilling (1878; see Müller, 1924, p. 76–77); Hering (1894); Hermann (1882); Kirschmann (1893); Vintschgau (1891–1894); Köllner (1929); Richardson-Robinson (1923); Alrutz (1915; see Müller, 1924; Göthlin, 1943); Sloan and Newhall (1942); Fischer *et al.* (1951). (See also Pickford, 1951, p. 123ff. and François and Verriest's unusual case, 1959).

Precise locations of spectral neutral loci vary slightly from one case to the next but measures on Hermann's yellow-blue deficient dichromatic observer, for example, with one of two spectral apparatuses he used, are definite in showing one neutral locus at 585-588 nm and the other neutral locus at 495–500 nm. Results for the observer's other eye are trivially different, and the results with a second spectrometer were quite similar. Richardson-Robinson's case, studied over a span of more than a decade with various instruments in different laboratories, showed neutral loci both in the 577–589 nm and 478–489 regions. (Jaeger believes this individual had an inherited optic nerve atrophy – Jaeger, 1955.) The Vintschgau-Hering observer (who was also weak in red-green discriminations) had neutral regions at about 571 nm and between 452–460. The case reported by Fisher *et al.* had a neutral locus between 570–580 nm (dependent on the "white" used in the match), and an unsaturated region between 450–480 nm with red seen below 430 nm.

Given the relative infrequency of occurrence of any sort of yellow-blue deficiency, these cases cannot continue to be neglected in theoretical treatments. Their characteristics do not seem consistent with simple loss of the short-wave photopigment, which would be expected to reduce the spectral hues to long-wave red, and green both throughout the mid-spectrum and on to the short-wave extreme. As for the yellow-blue anomalies, the phenomena of tritanopia seem to require for their explanation the consideration of abnormalities both at the photopigment and receptoral level, and at the neural level where the response activities reflect an opponent physiological organization (MÜLLER, 1924; JUDD, 1951; HURVICH and JAMESON, 1955).

V. Loss Systems (Neural)

If interpretations of dichromasy take into account the missing sensory qualities associated with the color discrimination failures, then it seems obvious that in both protanopia and deuteranopia the opponent neural cells that respond in antagonistic fashion to lights that are red or green in normal color vision must lose this function in the red-green deficient dichromats. In the preceding section we have considered the views that the dichromatic loss occurs at the photochemical, receptoral level. Loss of spectrally selective input to opponent cells would, of course, nullify their selective opponent- response characteristics. Alternatively, retention of spectral selectivity in receptor absorption would be nullified if the neural opponent cells were themselves lost. In the latter case, the dichromasies could be conceptualized as extremes of the comparable anomalies where there is evidence of specific neural weakness in addition to photochemical alteration (see above, Section III).

The qualitative and quantitative implications of such a neural loss view to account for red-green deficient dichromats have been spelled out in the HURVICH-JAMESON (1955) model of the opponent-colors theory. The remaining yellow-blue and white-black neural responsiveness functions are assumed to be the same as those two functions illustrated for the comparable types of red-green anomalies in Fig. 6 (Section III). The curves in the upper block would characterize a protanopic system and they specify a protanopic luminosity function with peak displaced from the normal toward shorter wavelengths and a relative loss in luminosity in the long-wave region. An individual classified as deuteranopic might be characterized by y-b and w functions of the sort shown either in the center or lower block of Fig. 6. Those in the center block are generated when no photopigment alteration is assumed, and they are consistent with the characteristics of the Type I deuteranope whose luminosity function approximates the normal one. The curves in the lower block are derived from altered photopigment functions, and, consistent with the characteristics of Type II deuteranopic observers, they specify luminosity functions which, like the deuteranomalous functions, peak at longer wavelengths than normal and show a relative reduction in sensitivity at the shorter wavelengths. Viewed in this way, a more appropriate characterization of the three types might be protanope, neuteranope (Type I deuteranope) and deuteranope (Type II deuteranope).

With respect to the yellow-blue deficient dichromasies, the neural loss view again emphasizes the failure of neural cells whose opponent responses to different wavelength regions suggest a yellow-blue hue coding. If such cells are inoperative in a system that retains the normal photopigments with neither alteration nor loss at the receptor level, the individual would be expected to see red and green hues, with two spectral neutral loci, one near the normal's unique yellow and another near the normal's unique blue, and the short-wave spectral extreme would appear reddish. Reported cases of this sort have been described in Section IV above, where it was suggested that they might appropriately be characterized as tetartanopes. Typical tritanopes, on the other hand, do seem to have suffered a loss of the short-wave receptor pigment in association with the loss of the related opponent-cell function. This assumption generates alterations in the form of the red-green responsiveness function that predict only a single neutral locus in the normally yellow spectral region and luminosity characteristics that correspond to the reported factual situation in tritanopia (HURVICH and JAMESON, 1955).

Theoretical predictions concerning color mixture, perceived hues, luminosity, wavelength and saturation discrimination of various types of dichromats have been presented in quantitative terms (HURVICH and JAMESON, 1955) and compared to the available data from varieties of color defectives. To the experimental measures then available COLE *et al.* (1965) have now added the saturation discrimination data of tritanopes and tritanomalous for comparison with these earlier theoretical derivations.

The Müller model of the opponent-process theory (1924) also assumes loss of the red-green processes beyond the photopigment level to account for protanopia and deuteranopia and loss of the yellow-blue process to account for tetartanopia and tritanopia. In this more complex model the difference between protanopic and deuteranopic systems is established theoretically by assuming that (1) there are two stages of chromatic and achromatic responses which are somewhat different transforms of the photopigment absorption functions and (2) that the response losses occur at different levels for the two types of observers (so-called "outer color-blindness" for protanopes and "inner color-blindness" for deuteranopes). This multi-stage theory also incorporates the concepts of the "brightening" and "darkening" action of spectral lights from different spectral regions and the protanopic luminosity shift toward shorter wavelengths is accounted for in these terms. Protanopia is related to the loss of the intermediate red-green response system in this conceptualization and this is the level at which the "brightening" "darkening" interplay occurs. JUDD has quantified the Müller model and in his most recent publication (JUDD and YONEMURA, 1970) derives protanopic, tritanopic and normal wavelength discrimination functions that agree closely with experimental data in the literature.

Almost all the wavelength discrimination data in the literature for protanopes and deuteranopes are *U*-shaped in form (see BOUMAN-WALRAVEN, chapter 19, this volume) with a minimum at the spectral neutral point of the respective type. Many theoretical accounts, whether conventional Young-Helmholtz or opponent-process, appear adequately to explain them. Recently BALARAMAN *et al.* (1962) reported measures on seven deuteranopes and four protanopes that show deviations from the classical *U* curve for two of the deuteranopes and three of the four protanopes. The usual *U* function is seen but there is also evidence of increased sensitivity in the longwave region: the curves are saw-toothed in appearance but the thresholds tend on the whole to decrease as longer wavelengths are approached. These measures do not resemble those of anomalous observers seen in Fig. 9. Either they reflect saturation differences that are not eliminated by adjusting for luminance equality between the test and comparison fields or the observers could conceivably be sensitive to "reds" in the long-wave extreme. The former possibility might easily have been checked with the simple addition of a variable amount of broad-band "white" to one side of the bipartite field but it was not.

The opponent-process views predicate the retention of three cone photopigment functions in accounting for the red-green deficient dichromacies; what losses occur are at retinal levels beyond where the light is absorbed. But, as already noted, the photopigments are assumed to occupy different positions along the spectral locus in different kinds of deficiencies. Is this "photopigment shift" notion still a viable hypothesis, particularly in the light of the RUSHTON and WALD experiments? The answer depends in large part on how much confidence we are to place in techniques that "prove" that dichromats have only a single pigment in the "red-green" region of the spectrum but which are conceded to be inadequate when they demonstrate the same result for the anomalous trichromats who admittedly have two photopigments in this spectral region. It would seem that new techniques, or perhaps further refinements of the reflection densitometry techniques, will be required before a fully satisfactory and definitive answer is forthcoming on the cone photopigment issue in both dichromats and anomalous trichromats.

It should be said, incidentally, that alteration of the protanopic photopigments from the normal spectral distributions does not conflict with the fact that protanopes may accept normal color matches. Postulation of reduction systems at the neural level can be demonstrated not to conflict with the expectation that dichromats will, on the average, accept Rayleigh equation matches that fall within the normal match range. There is considerable variation in color-matching, whether in a population of normals or in a population of protanopes, for example, but the distribution of matches of the one group overlaps with the distribution of matches of the other, and this is true also for theoretically derived matches based on the neural-loss altered-photopigment model. This issue has been discussed elsewhere (HURVICH and JAMESON, 1962).

It should also be added that the fact that chromaticity confusion intersection loci are commonly used to represent the reduction systems of dichromats as photopigment or receptor losses of specified types does not argue for or against alternative postulates of how the reductions come about.

The red-green and yellow-blue chromatic response systems are independent ones. They not only exhibit varying degrees of responsiveness for unit stimulation in different individuals, they also show specific dependencies upon luminance and area within the summation area (HARTRIDGE, 1950; FARNSWORTH, 1955; HURVICH and JAMESON, 1955, 1957, 1958), and these dependencies can be shown to account for well-known perceptual effects. In normals, for example, the differential rates of response of the paired chromatic systems as functions of luminance have been shown to underlie the Bezold-Brücke hue shift phenomenon (HURVICH and JAMESON, 1955). Taken in conjunction with the even more rapid rate with which the achromatic white-black responses increase compared to the color systems as a function of luminance, the desaturation of high luminance stimuli is also explainable. Not surprisingly, where single paired systems are operative, they seem to behave similarly and related luminance dependencies are seen in dichromats (RAEHLMANN, 1899; STILLING, 1909–1910). Luminance level is obviously critical for diagnostic purposes and since, as we have seen, different anomalous observers manifest varying degrees of responsiveness per unit stimulation, it is not surprising that some dichromats who are diagnosed as red-green deficient on conventional color vision "tests" appear to show residual red-green responsiveness when examined under higher luminance conditions in a spectral color-naming situation (SCHEIBNER and BOYNTON, 1968), even though color naming is notoriously unreliable for studying color deficiencies.

That some dichromats become trichromatic with an increase in stimulus size was first reported by NAGEL (1905, 1907). NAGEL and LENZ (TRENDELENBURG, 1961), one a deuteranope and the other a protanope, both become trichromatic with relatively large increases in stimulus field size (10° or so in NAGEL'S case). NAGEL (1907) collected similar data on 30 other dichromats (both protanopes and deuteranopes) and even had a large field (20°) anomaloscope constructed to investigate the effect of stimulus size (1910). JAEGER and KROKER (1952) have also reported similar instances of what they have labelled "incomplete dichromats". This terminology would, of course, be equally applicable to the various anomalous observers who manifest only *traces* of one paired color system response along with the obvious color signal of the second paired color system.

VI. Loss Systems in Monochromats

FRANÇOIS *et al.* (1955) in their review of "L'achromatopsie congénitale" estimate that up to the year 1955 about 430 cases of this type of color deficiency had been reported in the literature. Individuals with this defect presumably see only whites, grays, and blacks and no hues, and a variety of different names have been used to characterize this condition, for example, achromatopsia, achromacy, total color blindness, monochromatism, cone blindness, cone monochromatism, rod-cone monochromatism, rod monochromacy, etc. The multiplicity of names reflects the fact that this class of color deficiencies expresses itself in a variety of forms — forms that depend on different patterns of related visual responses thought to be connected with the color defect *per se*. The relevant visual properties include acuity, relative luminosity, nystagmus, photophobia, visual fields, adaptation, hue remnants evokable, etc. Since the abnormal manifestations appear to vary somewhat independently of one another, many different combinations produce a variety of syndromes. In an effort to reduce the complexity of the problem, a number of different dichotomous classifications have been proposed by the arbitrary grouping of "symptoms". Thus we have achromatopes who are labelled typical or atypical, incomplete or complete, and simple (true) or complicated. These dichotomous classifications are not necessarily mutually exclusive, and FRANÇOIS *et al.* (1955) prefer three major categories that stress the "completeness" and amblyopic aspects of the defect. Thus they propose: (1) complete congenital achromatopsia with amblyopia, (2) incomplete congenital achromatopsia with amblyopia, and (3) congenital achromatopsia without amblyopia.

Monochromats of the simple, uncomplicated type (PODESTA, 1936; FRANÇOIS *et al's* group 3) can readily be related to anomalous and dichromatic color vision and assumed neural loss of both types of chromatic opponent cells provides a straightforward explanation of this defect. Individuals of this sort gauge the spectrum with any single stimulus and any two compared stimuli can be completely equated simply by adjusting their relative luminances since the individual has no hue discrimination whatsoever. These observers have good foveal vision (no central scotoma), normal acuity, no nystagmus or photophobia.

What is of particular interest is that these cases all show photopic luminosity functions. But that is not all. It appears that the measured luminosity functions have different peak spectral loci that in different cases are comparable to those of the protanope, normal and deuteranope, respectively. The cone monochromats reported by HEINSIUS (1938), PITT (1944), SLOAN (1946) and WEALE (1953a) appear to have protanopic luminosity functions; RAEHLMANN'S (1899) admittedly unusual case (see MÜLLER, 1924 for a full discussion), PIPER'S unilateral case (1905), ABNEY'S (1913), VIERLING'S (1928) and BEST'S (1929, 1948) cases appear to have normal luminosity functions; and one of CRONE'S monochromats (1956) showed a luminosity function with its maximum shifted toward longer wavelengths as compared with the normal curve.

WEALE'S (1953a) detailed analysis of the data of three of his cases led him to conclude that the vision of these observers is not due to the action of only a single pigment and that the locus of the defect is post-receptoral. This was essentially HEINSIUS' conclusion. In a later study WEALE (1959), using fundus reflectometry techniques, concluded that the cone-monochromat has the same photosensitive pigments demonstrable with this technique in the normal, thus supporting the post-receptoral notion. The results on the accommodative reflex (FINCHAM, 1953), selective adaptation (GIBSON, 1962), and electroretinogram (IKEDA and RIPPS, 1966) are interpreted in the same way. These interpretations are in accord with the analysis that assigns color coding and hue losses to the neural mechanisms, but whereas dichromacy involves the retention of one or the other of the two chromatic systems (plus white and black), in the monochromatic cases both chromatic systems are non-functional. The fact that the luminosity functions peak at different loci for different individuals suggests that the photopigments may be altered in the manner assumed to account for the different spectral luminosity curves of the anomalous trichromats and dichromats.

It should be noted, however, that ALPERN (1968) has rejected WEALE'S analysis in favor of a receptor-loss hypothesis both for WEALE'S cases and others described as "blue-cone monochromats" (BLACKWELL and BLACKWELL, 1961; ALPERN *et al.*, 1965). "Blue-cone monochromats" are observers whose measured spectral sensitivity presumably reflects the activity of "blue cones" defined by STILES' "π_1" mechanism (see ENOCH, chapter 21, this volume). ALPERN does not regard WEALE'S cone-monochromats' deficiency as post-receptoral but interprets these cases as reflecting "green-cone" activity only. ALPERN in fact anticipates that in addition to "blue cone-monochromats", and "green cone-monochromats", there will also be found "red cone-monochromats".

It turns out upon closer examination that many cases conventionally categorized as "achromatopsia" show evidence of trace amounts of color response (JAEGER, 1950, 1951; FRANÇOIS and VERRIEST, 1959). The existence of visual systems with only trace hue responses is consistent with interpretations of anomalous color vision where the efficiency of hue-coded neural responses is assumed to express itself in varying degrees of color-weakness. Different cases of so-called "pseudo-monochromacies" where minimal color responses exist are also reported to have luminosity functions that peak at different spectral loci. Thus the König (1894) and Silex (1899) cases (see Jaeger, 1950 for references to these and other cited instances), showed traces of yellow and blue responsiveness and "protanopic" luminosity functions. Becker's (1879) observer, described as "totally" color-deficient and of the simple uncomplicated type had a "normal" luminosity function but also manifested what appears to be a trace amount of yellow-blue response. The pseudomonochromatic cases studied by Guttmann (1907) and Kondo (1931; see Jaeger, 1950) had "deuteranopic" luminosity functions. Other instances of a related sort are reported by Wehrli (1902; see Köllner and Engelking, 1929), Krahnert (1941), Sloan and Newhall (1942), Crone (1956, 1965), Grützner (1965) and Siegel *et al.* (1966).

The luminance and area effects exhibited in the normal and the dichromatic eye also find their counterparts in monochromacy. With an increase in luminance level, some monochromatic observers can be shown to move towards dichromacy, and both Jaeger and Baumgardt report monochromatic cases that show dichromatic vision with an increase in stimulus area. Baumgardt's observer in fact showed integrative effects up to 30° in size. (For summation effects over large areas in normals, see Burnham, 1952).

These effects become truly puzzling, however, when they occur in cases diagnosed as "rod-monochromats", or *typical* achromats. These are individuals characterized mainly (in addition to their lack of color responses) by the fact that instead of the photopic luminosity associated with cone activity, they have scotopic luminosity functions. (See Jaeger, 1950, 1953; and François *et al.*, 1955 for references to various cases.)

The typical achromats constitute the single largest group of totally color deficient observers. Many hundreds of cases have been reported, and in general the condition is characterized, in addition to the scotopic luminosity function, by low visual acuity, photophobia, nystagmus, pupillomotor symptoms and in some cases by a central scotoma. There are apparently no necessary connections among the individual symptoms and specific cases differ in the particular combination of symptoms present (Goodman *et al.*, 1963). There have even been reports of "typical" cases with good visual acuity (e.g., Shindo, 1932; see Jaeger, 1950).

No single satisfactory theoretical account that resolves the many puzzling aspects of this condition has yet been given. The variety of symptoms associated with the defect lend themselves to a ready explanation, namely that there is an absence of cone function. This view was long held and in fact this accounts for the designation "rod-monochromacy" for this type of defect. However, sufficient evidence has built up over the years to cast doubt on this simple interpretation. There is histological evidence of cones, although not necessarily normal in number or appearance (Larsen, 1921; Harrison *et al.*, 1960; Falls *et al.*, 1965); dark-adaptation functions show evidence of the conventional duplex rod-cone break (Sloan, 1954); there is a Stiles-Crawford effect characteristic of cone retina (Alpern *et al.*, 1960); and photopic responses are seen in the electroretinogram (Pabst and Echte, 1962; Dodt *et al.*, 1967).

The favored explanation at the moment appears to be one that emphasizes the presence of two receptor systems that correspond to the normal rod and cone systems but where the cone system exhibits rod properties, e.g., it is characterized by a scotopic spectral sensitivity function. This is essentially equivalent to saying that the cones contain rhodopsin (HECHT *et al.*, 1948; SLOAN, 1954; FALLS *et al.*, 1965; DODT *et al.*, 1967). WALLS and HEATH'S (1954) alternative to this analysis was to argue that the typical achromat's data are accountable for by assuming the presence of "blue-cones" in addition to rods. The problem continues to generate considerable interest.

Acknowledgements. This chapter is based largely on reviews and research carried out jointly with DOROTHEA JAMESON.

I should like to thank ELEANOR DIXON for her assistance with the references.

Preparation of this chapter was supported in part by NIH Grant EY-00249.

References

ABNEY, W. DE W.: Researches in Colour Vision and the Trichromatic Theory. London: Longmans, Green 1913.

— WATSON, W.: A case of trichromatic colour vision due to a shift in the spectrum of the green-sensation curve. Proc. roy. Soc. (Lond.) A **89**, 232—245 (1913).

AHLENSTIEL, A.: Rotgrünblindheit als Erlebnis. Göttingen: Musterschmidt 1951.

ALPERN, M.: Distal mechanisms of vertebrate color vision. Ann. Rev. Physiol. **30**, 279—318 (1968).

— FALLS, H. G., LEE, G. B.: The enigma of typical total monochromacy. Amer. J. Ophthal. **56**, 996—1011 (1960).

— LEE, G. B., SPIVEY, B. E.: π_1 cone monochromatism. Arch. Ophthal. **74**, 334—337 (1965).

— MINDEL, J., TORII, S.: Are there two types of deuteranopes? J. Physiol. (Lond.) **199**, 443—456 (1968).

— TORII, S.: Prereceptor colour vision distortions in protanomalous trichromacy. J. Physiol. (Lond.) **198**, 542—560 (1968a).

— — The luminosity curve of the protanomalous fovea. J. gen. Physiol. **52**, 717—737 (1968b).

— — The luminosity curve of the deuteranomalous fovea. J. gen. Physiol. **52**, 738—749 (1968c).

ALRUTZ, S.: Ett fall at violett-eller gulblablindhet (tritanopi). Psyke (Upsala). 1—101 (1915).

BALARAMAN, S., GRAHAM, C. H., HSIA, Y.: The wavelength discrimination of some color-blind persons. J. gen. Psychol. **66**, 185—201 (1962).

BAUMGARDT, E., MAGIS, C.: Sur un cas exceptionel d'achromatopsie. J. Physiol. (Paris) **46**, 237—240 (1954).

BECKER, O.: Ein Fall von angeborener einseitiger totaler Farbenblindheit. Graefes Arch. Ophthal. **25** (2), 205—212 (1879).

BEST, F.: Ungewöhnliche Form totaler Farbenblindheit. Klin. Mbl. Augenheilk. **82**, 521 (1929).

— Discussion. Ber. dtsch. ophthal. Ges. **54**, 85—86 (1948).

BLACKWELL, H. R., BLACKWELL, O. M.: Rod and cone receptor mechanisms in typical and atypical congenital achromatopsia. Vision Res. **1**, 62—107 (1961).

BOYNTON, R. M., SCHEIBNER, H. M. O.: On the perception of red by "red-blind" observers. Acta chromatica. **1**, 205—220 (1967).

BURNHAM, R. W.: Comparative effects of area and luminance on color. Amer. J. Psychol. **65**, 27—38 (1952).

— HANES, R. M., BARTLESON, C. J.: Color: A Guide to Basic Facts and Concepts. New York: Wiley 1963.

CHAPANIS, A.: Spectral saturation and its relation to color-vision defects. J. exp. Psychol. **34**, 24—44 (1944).

— Simultaneous chromatic contrast in normal and abnormal color vision. Amer. J. Psychol. **62**, 526—539 (1949).

CIBIS, P. A.: Lokaladaptation. Ber. dtsch. ophthal. Ges. **66**, 193—202 (1965).
— HUCK, H.: Raum- und zeitmessende Untersuchungen des Farbensinnes an der Stelle des schärfsten Sehens bei Normalen und angeborenen Farbsinngestörten. Graefes Arch. Ophthal. **149**, 179—198 (1949).
CLARKE, F. J. J.: A study of Troxler's effect. Optica Acta **7**, 219—236 (1960).
COLE, B. L., WATKINS, R. D.: Increment thresholds in tritanopia. Vision Res. **7**, 939—947 (1967).
— HENRY, G. H., NATHAN, J.: Phenotypical variations of tritanopia. Vision Res. **6**, 301—313 (1965).
COLLINS, W. E.: The effects of deuteranomaly and deuteranopia upon the foveal luminosity curve. J. Psychol. **48**, 285—297 (1959).
— Luminosity functions of normal, deuteranomalous and deuteranopic subjects as determined by absolute threshold and C.F.F. measurements. J. opt. Soc. Amer. **51**, 202—206 (1961).
COX, J.: Unilateral color deficiency, congenital and acquired. J. opt. Soc. Amer. **51**, 992—949 (1961).
CRONE, R. A.: Clinical study of colour vision. Brit. J. Ophthal. **39**, 170—173 (1955).
— Combined forms of congenital colour defects. A pedigree with atypical colour blindness. Brit. J. Ophthal. **40**, 462—472 (1956).
— Spectral sensitivity in color-defective subjects and heterozygous carriers. Amer. J. Ophthal. **48**, 231—238 (1959).
— Inkomplette Achromatopsie mit rohrförmigen Gesichtsfeldern. Ber. dtsch. ophthal. Ges. **66**, 176—181 (1965).
DALTON, J.: Extraordinary facts relating to the vision of colors. Mem. Lit. Phil. Soc. (Manchester) **5**, 28—45 (1798).
DARTNALL, H. J. A.: The interpretation of spectral sensitivity curves. Brit. med. Bull. **9**, 24—30 (1953).
DEVRIES, HL.: The fundamental response curves of normal and abnormal dichromatic and trichromatic eyes. Physica **14**, 367—380 (1948).
DODT, E., VAN LIGHT, G. H. M., SCHMIDT, B.: Electroretinographic evaluation of the photopic malfunction in a totally colour blind. Vision Res. **7**, 231—241 (1967).
DURUP, G., PIÉRON, H.: L'équation de Rayleigh et la dissociation des valences chromatique et lumineuse. Rev. Opt. (Paris) **22**, 224—231 (1943).
ENGELBRECHT, K.: Die Kontraststeigerung der anomalen Trichromaten. Ber. dtsch. ophthal. Ges. **54**, 211—219 (1948).
ENGELKING, E.: Die Tritanomalie, ein bisher unbekannter Typ der anomalen Trichromasie. Graefes Arch. Ophthal. **116**, 196—244 (1925).
— Über die spektrale Verteilung der Unterschiedsempfindlichkeit für Farbentöne bei den verschiedenen Formen der anomalen Trichromasie. Klin. Mbl. Augenheilk. **77**, (Suppl.) v. **61** (1926).
— Über den Verlauf der Eichwertkurven bei den anomalen Trichromaten. Klin. Mbl. Augenheilk. **78** (Suppl.), 209—219 (1927).
— Farbenschwäche und künstliche zeitweilige Farbenblindheit. Klin. Mbl. Augenheilk. **90**, 9—21 (1933).
— HARTUNG, H.: Spektraluntersuchungen über die Minimalfeldhelligkeiten des Tritanomalen und seine Unterschiedsempfindlichkeit für Änderungen der Helligkeit. Graefes Arch. Ophthal. **118**, 211—220 (1927).
FALLS, H. F., WOLTER, J. R., ALPERN, M.: Typical total monochromacy. Arch. Ophthal. **74**, 610—616 (1965).
FARNSWORTH, D.: Tritanomalous vision as a threshold function. Farbe **4**, 185—197 (1955).
— Let's look at those isochromatic lines again. Vision Res. **1**, 105 (1961).
FICK, A. E.: Zur Theorie der Farbenblindheit. Verh. phys.-med. Gesell. (Würzb.) **5**, 158—162 (1874).
— Die Lehre von der Lichtempfindung. In: Handbuch der Physiologie. HERMANN, L. (Ed.), Vol. 3, S. 139—234. Leipzig: Vogel 1879.
— Zur Theorie der Farbenblindheit. Pflügers Arch. ges. Physiol. **64**, 313—320 (1896).
FINCHAM, E. F.: Defects of the colour sense mechanisms as indicated by the accommodation reflex. J. Physiol. (Lond.) **121**, 570—580 (1953).

Fischer, F. P., Bouman, M. A., ten Doesschate, J.: A case of tritanopy. Documenta ophthal. **5/6**, 73—87 (1951).

Forshaw, C. R.: A new form of anomaloscope. J. sci. Instrum. **31**, 16—17 (1954).

Franceschetti, A.: Die Bedeutung der Einstellungsbreite am Anomaloskop für die Diagnose der einzelnen Typen der Farbensinnstörungen, nebst Bemerkungen über ihren Vererbungsmodus. Schweiz. med. Wschr. **58**, 1273—1279 (1928).

François, J., Verriest, G.: Contribution à l'étude des dyschromatopsies congénitales à symptomes intermédiaires entre ceux des systèmes dichromatiques classiques et ceux de l'achromatopsie typique: observation personelle et revue de la littérature. Ann. Oculist (Paris) **192**, 81—120 (1959).

— — DeRouck, A.: L'achromatopsie congénitale. Documenta ophthal. **9**, 338—424 (1955).

— — Mortier, V., Vanderdonck, R.: De la fréquence des dyschromatopsies congénitales de l'homme. Ann. Oculist. (Paris) **189**, 5—16 (1957).

Gibson, I. M.: Visual mechanisms in a cone-monochromat. J. Physiol. (Lond.) **161**, 10—11 (1962).

Göthlin, G. F.: Die diagnostische Untersuchung des Farbensinnes mit dem Polarisationsanomaloskop. Hand. Biol. Arbeitsmeth. (Abderhalden), Abt. 5; Teil 6; Hälfte **2**, 903—948 Berlin: Urban and Schwarzenberg 1937.

— An analysis of the perception defect in published and spectroscopically investigated cases of congenital tritanopia. Acta ophthal. (Kbh.) **21**, 88—96 (1943).

Goldmann, H.: Über Dauerwirkungen farbiger Lichter auf das Auge. (Farbige Verstimmung und allgemeine chromatische Lichtwirkung). Pflügers Arch. ges. Physiol. **210**, 70—115 (1925).

Goldschmidt, R. H.: Übungstherapeutische Versuche zur Steigerung der Farbentüchtigkeit eines anomalen Trichromaten. Z. Sinnesphysiol. **50**, 192—216 (1919).

Goodman, G., Ripps, H., Siegel, I. M.: Cone dysfunction syndromes. Arch. Ophthal. **70**, 214—231 (1963).

Graham, C. H.: Color: Data and theories. In: Vision and Visual Perception, Graham, C. H. (Ed.): pp. 414—451. New York: Wiley 1965.

— Hsia, Y.: Color defect and color theory. Science **127**, 675—682 (1958).

— — Luminosity losses in deuteranopes. Science **131**, 414 (1960).

— Sperling, H. G., Hsia, Y., Coulson, A. H.: The determination of some visual functions of a unilateral colorblind subject: method and results. J. Psychol. **51**, 3—32 (1961).

Grützner, P.: Beitrag zur Frage der spektralen Hellempfindlichkeit bei angeborenen Farbensinnstörungen. Graefes Arch. Ophthal. **164**, 411—420 (1962).

— Der normale Farbensinn und seine Abweichungen. Ber. dtsch. ophthal. Ges. **66**, 161—172 (1965).

Guttmann, A.: Ein Fall von Grünblindheit (Deuteranopie) mit ungewöhnlichen Komplikationen. Z. Sinnesphysiol. **41**, 45—56 (1907).

— Untersuchungen über Farbenschwäche. Z. Sinnesphysiol. **42**, 24—64; 250—270 (1908).

— Untersuchungen über Farbenschwäche. Z. Sinnesphysiol. **43**, 146—162; 199—223; 255—298 (1909).

Hailwood, J. G., Roaf, H. E.: The sensation of yellow and anomalous trichromatism. J. Physiol. (Lond.) **91**, 37—47 (1937).

Halsey, R. M., Chapanis, A.: An experimental determination of some isochromaticity hues in color-deficient vision. J. opt. Soc. Amer. **42**, 722—739 (1952).

Harrison, R., Hoefnagel, D., Hayward, J. N.: Congenital total color blindness, a clinicopathological report. Arch. Ophthal. **64**, 685—692 (1960).

Hartridge, H.: Recent Advances in the Physiology of Vision. London: Churchill 1950.

Hartung, H.: Untersuchungen über Farbenasthenopie. Klin. Mbl. Augenheilk. **94**, 21—32 (1935).

— Über drei familiäre Fälle von Tritanomalie. Klin. Mbl. Augenheilk. **76**, 229—240 (1926).

Hayes, S. P.: The color sensations of the partially colorblind. A criticism of current teaching. Amer. J. Psychol. **22**, 269—407 (1911).

Heath, G. G.: Luminosity curves of normal and dichromatic observers. Science **128**, 775—776 (1958).

— Luminosity losses in deuteranopes. Science **131**, 417—418 (1960).

Hecht, S., Shlaer, S.: The color vision of dichromats. I. Wavelength discrimination, brightness distribution, and color mixture. J. gen. Physiol. **20**, 57—82 (1936).
— — Smith, E. L., Haig, C., Peskin, J. C.: The visual functions of the complete colorblind. J. gen. Physiol. **31**, 459—472 (1948).
Hegner, C. A.: Über angeborene einseitige Störungen des Farbensinns. Klin. Mbl. Augenheilk. **54**, 81—89 (1915).
Heinsius, E.: Die einfache unkomplizierte Form der angeborenen totalen Farbenblindheit. Klin. Mbl. Augenheilk. **101**, 489—494 (1938).
Helmholtz, H. L. F. von: Handbuch der physiologischen Optik (1st ed.). Hamburg: Voss 1866.
— Treatise on Physiological Optics. Southall, J. P. C. (Trans.) Rochester: Optical Society of America 1924—1925. 3 vols.
— Handbuch der physiologischen Optik (2nd Ed.). Hamburg: Voss 1896.
Henry, G. H., Cole, B. L., Nathan, J.: The inheritance of congenital tritanopia with the report of an extensive pedigree. Ann. hum. Genet. **27**, 219—231 (1964).
Hering, E.: Über individuelle Verschiedenheiten des Farbensinnes. Lotos, Jb. Naturwiss. N. F. **6**, 142—198 (1885).
— Über einen Fall von Gelb-Blaublindheit. Pflügers Arch. ges. Physiol. **57**, 308—332 (1894).
Hermann, G.: Ein Beitrag zur Casuistik der Farbenblindheit. Thesis. Dorpat: Kaiser University 1882.
Hess, C.: Das Farbensehen der Anomalen. Arch. Augenheilk. **91**, 133—146 (1922).
Holzlöhner, E., Stein, W. H.: Über den gesteigerten farbigen Simultankontrast der anomalen Trichromaten. Z. Sinnesphysiol. **61**, 209—224 (1930/1931).
Hsia, Y., Graham, C. H.: Color blindness. In: Vision and Visual Perception. Graham, C. H. (Ed.), pp. 395—413. New York: Wiley 1965.
Hurvich, L. M., Jameson, D.: Some quantitative aspects of an opponent-colors theory. II. Brightness, saturation, and hue in normal and dichromatic vision. J. opt. Soc. Amer. **45**, 602—616 (1955).
— — An opponent-process theory of color vision. Psychol. Rev. **64**, 384—404 (1957).
— — Further development of a quantified opponent-colours theory. In: Visual Problems of Colour Vol. II, pp. 691—793. London: H. M. Stationery Office 1958.
— — Color theory and abnormal red-green vision. Documenta ophthal. **16**, 409—442 (1962).
— — Does anomalous color vision imply color weakness? Psychon. Sci. **1**, 11—12 (1964).
— — Cohen, J. D.: The experimental determination of unique green in the spectrum. Perc. Psychophys. **4** (2), 65—68 (1968).
Ikeda, H., Ripps, H.: The electroretinogram of a cone-monochromat. Arch. Ophthal. **75**, 513—517 (1966).
Jaeger, W.: Systematische Untersuchungen über inkomplette angeborene totale Farbenblindheit. (Eine Zwischenform zwischen angeborener totaler Farbenblindheit und Protanopie). Graefes Arch. Ophthal. **150**, 509—528 (1950).
— Angeborene totale Farbenblindheit mit Resten von Farbenempfindung. Klin. Mbl. Augenheilk. **118**, 282—288 (1951).
— Typen der inkompletten Achromatopsie. Ber. dtsch. ophthal. Ges. **58**, 44—47 (1953).
— Tritoformen angeborener Störungen. Farbe **4**, 197—216 (1955).
— Kroker, K.: Über das Verhalten der Protanopen und Deuteranopen bei großen Reizflächen. Klin. Mbl. Augenheilk. **121**, 445—449 (1952).
Jameson, D., Hurvich, L. M.: Use of spectral hue-invariant loci for the specification of white stimuli. J. exp. Psychol. **41**, 455—463 (1951).
— — Theoretical analysis of anomalous trichromatic color vision. J. opt. Soc. Amer. **46**, 1075—1089 (1956).
— — Perceived color and its dependence on focal, surrounding, and preceding stimulus variables. J. opt. Soc. Amer. **49**, 890—898 (1959).
— — Opponent-response functions related to measured cone photopigments. J. opt. Soc. Amer. **58**, 429—430 (1968).
Judd, D. B.: Standard response functions for protanopic and deuteranopic vision. J. opt. Soc. Amer. **35**, 199—221 (1945).
— Color perceptions of deuteranopic and protanopic observers. J. Res. nat. Bur. Standards (Wash.) **41**, 247—271 (1948).

Judd, D. B.: Current views on colour blindness. Documenta ophthal. 3, 251—288 (1949a).
— Response functions for types of vision according to the Müller theory. J. Res. nat. Bur. Standards (Wash.) **42**, 1—16 (1949b).
— Basic correlates of the visual stimulus. In: Handbook of Experimental Psychology. Stevens, S. S. (Ed.), pp. 811—867. New York: Wiley 1951.
— Relation between normal trichromatic vision and dichromatic vision representing a reduced form of normal vision. Acta chromatica. **1**, 89—90 (1964).
— Plaza, L., Farnsworth, D.: Tritanopia with abnormally heavy ocular pigmentation. J. opt. Soc. Amer. **40**, 833—841 (1950).
— Yonemura, G. T.: CIE 1960 UCS diagram and the Müller theory of color vision. J. Res. nat. Bur. Standards (Wash.) A **74**, 23—30 (1970).
Katzin, D., Murray, E.: Instability in color-naming in normal and anomalous observers. Amer. J. Psychol. **46**, 611—620 (1934).
Kherumian, R., Pickford, R. W.: Héredité et fréquence des dyschromatopsies. Paris: Vigot Frères 1959.
Kinney, J. A. S.: Induced colors seen by a deuteranope. J. opt. Soc. Amer. **57**, 1149—1154 (1967).
Kirschmann, A.: Beiträge zur Kenntnis der Farbenblindheit. Phil. Stud. 8, 173—230 (1893).
Klein, R., Nordmann, J.: L'exageration du contraste des couleurs chez les dyschromatopes. Bull. Soc. Ophthal. (Paris) **1**, 453—455 (1948).
Köllner, H.: Die Störungen des Farbensinnes. Berlin: Karger 1912.
— Über die Grundlagen, die zu der neuen Anleitung zur Prüfung des Farbenunterscheidungsvermögens mittels des Anomaloskops geführt haben. Z. Bahn. Bahnkassenärzte **9**, 93—100 (1914).
— Engelking, E.: Die Abweichungen des Farbensinnes. In: Handbuch der normalen und pathologischen Physiologie. Bethe, A. *et al.* (Eds.). Vol. 12, Pt. 1, 502—535. Berlin: Springer 1929.
König, A.: Über „Blaublindheit" S.-B. Akad. Wiss. (Berlin) 718—731 (1897).
— Dieterici, C.: Die Grundempfindungen in normalen und anomalen Farbensystemen und ihre Intensitäts-Verteilung im Spectrum. Z. Psychol. Physiol. Sinnesorg. **4**, 241—347 (1893).
Kohlrausch, A.: Tagessehen, Dämmersehen, Adaptation. In: Handbuch der normalen und pathologischen Physiologie. Bethe, A. *et al.* (Eds.) Vol. 12. Pt. 2. 1499—1594. Berlin: Springer 1931.
Kolbe, B.: Ein Fall von angeborener einseitiger Rothgrünschwäche. Zbl. prakt. Augenheilk. **6**, 291—296 (1882).
Krahnert: Totale Farbenblindheit und Hemeralopie. Klin. Mbl. Augenheilk. **107**, 211—212 (1941).
Kries, J. von: Über einen Fall von einseitiger angeborener Deuteranomalie (Grünschwäche). Z. Sinnesphysiol. **50**, 137—152 (1919).
— Normal and anomalous color systems. In: Helmholtz, H. L. F.: Treatise on Physiological Optics (3rd ed.) Vol. II, pp. 395—425. Southall. J. P. C. (Trans.) Rochester: Optical Society of America 1924.
— Zur Lehre von den dichromatischen Farbensystemen. In: Handbuch der normalen und pathologischen Physiologie. Bethe, A. *et al.* (Eds.): Vol. 12. Pt. 1. 585—593. Berlin: Springer 1929.
Ladekarl, P. M.: Über Farbendistinktion bei Normalen und Farbenblinden. Acta ophthal. (Kbh.), Suppl. III. **12**, 9—128 (1934).
Lakowski, R.: The Pickford-Nicholson anomaloscope. Report No. 421. Psychology Laboratory University of Edinburgh 1968.
— Theory and practice of colour vision testing: A review. Brit. J. industr. Med. **26**, Part I, 173—189; Part II, 265—288 (1969).
Larsen, H.: Demonstration mikroskopischer Präparate von einem monochromatischen Auge. Klin. Mbl. Augenheilk. **67**, 301—302 (1921).
Leber, T.: Über die Theorie der Farbenblindheit und über die Art und Weise, wie gewisse, der Untersuchung von Farbenblinden entnommenen Einwände gegen die Young-Helmholtz'sche Theorie sich mit derselben vereinigen lassen. Klin. Mbl. Augenheilk. **11**, 467—473 (1873).

Lee, G. B.: Luminosity curve differences among subjects with normal color vision. J. opt. Soc. Amer. **56**, 1451 (1966).

Levy, M.: Über einen Fall von angeborener beiderseitiger Tritanopie (Blaublindheit). Graefes Arch. Ophthal. **62**, 464—480 (1906).

Linksz, A.: An Essay on Color Vision and Clinical Color-Vision Tests. New York: Grune and Stratton 1964.

Marks, W. B., Dobelle, W. H., MacNichol, E. F., Jr.: Visual pigments of single primate cones. Science **143**, 1181—1183 (1964).

Marriott, F. H. C.: Colour vision: Other phenomena. In: The Eye, Davson, H. (Ed.), Vol. 2. pp. 273—297. New York: Academic Press 1962.

Maxwell, J. C.: On the theory of colours in relation to colour-blindness. In: Suppl. to Researches on Colour-Blindness. Wilson, G. Edinburgh: Sutherland-Knox 1855.

McCree, K. J.: Colour confusion produced by voluntary fixation. Optica Acta **7**, 281—290 (1960).

McKeon, W. M., Wright, W. D.: The characteristics of protanomalous vision. Proc. phys. Soc. (Lond.) **52** (4), 464—479 (1940).

Meitner, H. J.: Über einen eigenartigen Fall von Anomalie des „Blausinns". Klin. Mbl. Augenheilk. **107**, 293—301 (1941).

Müller, G. E.: Darstellung und Erklärung der verschiedenen Typen der Farbenblindheit. Göttingen: Vandenhoeck und Ruprecht 1924.

Murray, E.: Vision: color; tests. In: Medical Physics, Glasser, O. (Ed.), Vol. II. pp. 1161 to 1171. Chicago: Year Book Publishers, 1950.

— Review of Walls, G. L., Mathews, R. N.: New Means of Studying Color Blindness and Normal Foveal Color Vision. Amer. J. Psychol. **67**, 182—188 (1954).

— Vision; color; tests. In: Medical Physics, Glasser, O. (Ed.), Vol. III. pp. 687—692. Chicago: Year Book Publishers, 1960.

Nagel, W. A.: Dichromatische Fovea, trichomatische Peripherie. Z. Psychol. Physiol. Sinnesorg. **39**, 93—101 (1905).

— Neue Erfahrungen über das Farbensehen der Dichromaten auf großem Felde. Z. Sinnesphysiol. **41**, 319—337 (1907).

— Farbenumstimmung beim Dichromaten. Z. Sinnesphysiol. **44**, 5—17 (1910).

Nelson, J. H.: Anomalous trichromatism and its relation to normal trichromatism. Proc. phys. Soc. (Lond.) **50**, 661—697 (1938).

Ohta, Y.: One case of slight hemeralopia with tritanopia. Acta chromatica **2**, 42—47 (1969).

Oloff, H.: Über angeborene blauanomale Trichromasie (Tritanomalie). Klin. Mbl. Augenheilk. **94**, 11—20 (1935).

Pabst, W., Echte, K.: Die Unterschiedsempfindlichkeitsschwelle bei Achromaten, bestimmt mit Hilfe des Elektroretinogramms. Acta ophthal. (Kbh.) Suppl. **70**, 168—175 (1962).

Parsons, J. H.: An Introduction to the Study of Colour Vision. Cambridge: Cambridge University Press 1924.

Pickford, R. W.: Individual Differences in Colour Vision. London: Routledge and Kegan Paul, 1951.

— Lakowski, R.: The Pickford-Nicholson anomaloscope. Brit. J. physiol. Opt. **17**, 131—150 (1960).

Piper, H.: Beobachtungen an einem Fall von totaler Farbenblindheit des Netzhautzentrums im einen und von Violettblindheit des anderen Auges. Z. Sinnesphysiol. **38**, 155—188 (1905).

Pitt, F. H. G.: Characteristics of dichromatic vision. Spec. Rep. Ser. No. 200. Med. Res. Council London: H. M. Stationery Office 1935.

— Monochromatism. Nature (Lond.) **154**, 466—468 (1944).

— Some aspects of anomalous vision. Documenta ophthal. **3**, 307—317 (1949).

— Comments on Dean Farnsworth's paper: Let's look at those isochromatic lines again. Vision Res. **1**, 6—7 (1961).

Podesta, H.: Beitrag zur Frage der Abgrenzung der angeborenen Farbensinnsstörungen, insbesondere der totalen Farbenblindheit. Klin. Mbl. Augenheilk. **96**, 786—796 (1936).

Pole, W.: On colour-blindness. Phil. Trans. B **149**, 323—339 (1859).

POLE, W.: On the present state of knowledge and opinion in regard to colour-blindness. Trans. roy. Soc. (Edinb.) **37**, 441—479 (1893).
RAEHLMANN, E.: Über relativen und absoluten Mangel des Farbensinns. Z. Augenheilk. **2**, 315—340, 403—427 (1899).
RAYLEIGH, LORD (J. W. Strutt). Experiments on colour. Nature (Lond.) **25**, 64—66 (1881).
RICHARDSON-ROBINSON, F.: A case of color-blindness to yellow and to blue. Amer. J. Psychol. **34**, 157—184 (1923).
RICHTER, M.: Die Ausgestaltung des Nagelschen Anomalskops zu einem „Tritoskop". Farbe **6**, 5—6 (1957).
ROGGE, A. J.: On colour asthenopy. Acta ophthal. (Kbh.) **24**, 147—158 (1946).
ROSMANIT, J.: Anleitung zur Feststellung der Farbentüchtigkeit. Leipzig: Deuticke 1914.
RUBIN, M. L.: Spectral hue loci of normal and anomalous trichromats. Amer. J. Ophthal. **52**, 166—172 (1961).
RUSHTON, W. A. H.: A cone pigment in the protanope. J. Physiol. (Lond.) **168**, 345—359 (1963a).
— The density of chlorolabe in the foveal cones of the protanope. J. Physiol. (Lond.) **168**, 360—373 (1963b).
— Cone pigment kinetics in the protanope. J. Physiol. (Lond.) **168**, 374—388 (1963c).
— A foveal pigment in the deuteranope. J. Physiol. (Lond.) **176**, 24—47 (1965a).
— Cone pigment kinetics in the deuteranope. J. Physiol. (Lond.) **176**, 38—45 (1965b).
— Discussion on human colour vision. In: Ciba Foundation Symposium on Colour Vision. DEREUCK, A. V. S., KNIGHT, J. (Eds.) pp. 246—247. Boston: Little-Brown 1965c.
— BAKER, H. D.: Red/green sensitivity in normal vision. Vision Res. **4**, 75—85 (1964).
SACHS, E.: Die Unterschiedsempfindlichkeit für Farbentöne bei verschiedenen Farben-Systemen. Z. Sinnesphysiol. **59**, 243—256 (1928).
SAMOJLOFF, A.: Untersuchung über die spektrale Helligkeitsverteilung beim Protanopen. Klin. Mbl. Augenheilk. **76**, 214 (1926).
SCHEIBNER, H. M. O., BOYNTON, R. M.: Residual red-green discrimination in dichromats. J. opt. Soc. Amer. **58**, 1151—1158 (1968).
SCHMIDT, I.: Über „Ermüdbarkeit" bei normalen Trichromaten. Klin. Mbl. Augenheilk. **94**, 433—442 (1935).
— Über zwei Fälle von angeborener Blau-Gelb-Sehstörung. Klin. Mbl. Augenheilk. **109**, 635—652 (1943).
— Some problems related to testing color vision with the Nagel anomaloscope. J. opt. Soc. Amer. **45**, 514—522 (1955).
— On congenital tritanomaly. Vision Res. **10**, 717—743 (1970).
SCHOBER, H.: Das Sehen. Vol. 2. Leipzig: Fachbuchverlag 1958.
SCHUBERT, G.: Sind urfarbige Lichterpaare komplementär? Pflügers Arch. ges. Physiol. **220**, 82—100 (1928).
SIEGEL, I. M., GRAHAM, C. H., RIPPS, H., HSIA, Y.: Analysis of photopic and scotopic functions in an incomplete achromat. J. opt. Soc. Amer. **56**, 699—704 (1966).
SLOAN, L. L.: A case of atypical achromatopsia. Amer. J. Ophthal. **29**, 290—294 (1946).
— Congenital achromatopsia: A report of 19 cases. J. opt. Soc. Amer. **44**, 117—128 (1954).
— NEWHALL, S. M.: Comparison of cases of atypical and typical achromatopsia. Amer. J. Ophthal. **25**, 945—961 (1942).
— WOLLACH, L.: A case of unilateral deuteronopia. J. opt. Soc. Amer. **38**, 502—509 (1948).
SPERANSKAYA, N. J.: Dokl. Akad. Nauk SSSR **130**, 1362 (1960). (Reported by GRÜTZNER, 1965).
SPERLING, H. G.: Case of congenital tritanopia with implications for a trichromatic model of color reception. J. opt. Soc. Amer. **50**, 156—163 (1960).
STILLING, J.: Über Entstehung und Wesen der Anomalien des Farbensinnes. Z. Sinnesphysiol. **44**, 371—427 (1910).
THOMSON, L. C., WRIGHT, W. D.: The convergence of the tritanopic confusion loci and the derivation of the fundamental response functions. J. opt. Soc. Amer. **43**, 890—894 (1953).
TRENDELENBURG, W.: Ein Anomaloskop zur Untersuchung von Tritoformen der Farbenfehlsichtigkeit mit spectraler Blaugleichung. Klin. Mbl. Augenheilk. **106**, 537—546 (1941a).

Trendelenburg, W.: Über Vererbung bei einem Fall von anomalem Farbensinn des einen und normalen Farbensinn des anderen Auges beim Mann. Klin. Mbl. Augenheilk. **107**, 280—293 (1941b).
— Der Gesichtssinn. 2nd Ed. Monjé, M., Schmidt, I., Schütz, E. (Eds.). Berlin-Göttingen-Heidelberg: Springer 1951.
— Schmidt, I.: Untersuchungen über Vererbung von angeborener Farbenfehlsichtigkeit. Zugleich ein Beitrag zur Theorie der Farbensysteme. S.-B. Akad. Wiss. Berlin phys. math. Kl. 13—81 (1935).
Tschermak, A.: Über Kontrast und Irradiation. Ergebn. Physiol. **2** (1), 726—798 (1903).
Vierling, O.: Über spektrale Wertbestimmung der Farben durch Schwellenmessung mit dem modifizierten Anomaloscop. Z. Bahnärzte **23**, 261—276 (1928).
Vintschgau, M. von: Physiologische Analyse eines ungewöhnlichen Falles partieller Farbenblindheit. (Trichromasie des Spectrums). I. Pflügers Arch. ges. Physiol. **48**, 431—528 (1891); II. **57**, 191—307 (1894).
Waardenburg, P. J.: Genetics and Ophthalmology. Springfield, Ill.: Thomas 1963.
Wald, G.: The receptors of human color vision. Science **145**, 1007—1017 (1964).
— Defective color vision and its inheritance. Proc. nat. Acad. Sci. (Wash.) **55**, 1347—1363 (1966).
— Brown, P. K.: Color vision and color blindness. Cold Spr. Harbor Symp. quant. Biol. **30**, 345—361 (1965).
Walls, G. L.: Notes on four tritanopes. Vision. Res. **4**, 3—16 (1964).
— Heath, G. G.: Typical total color blindness reinterpreted. Acta ophthal. (Kbh.) **32**, 253—297 (1954).
— — Neutral points in 138 protanopes and deuteranopes. J. opt. Soc. Amer. **46**, 640—649 (1956).
— Mathews, R. W.: New Means of Studying Color Blindness and Normal Foveal Color Vision. Berkeley: University of California Press 1952.
Wartmann, M. E.: Memoir on daltonism [or color blindness]. In: Scientific memoirs. Vol. 4. Taylor, R. (Ed.), pp. 166—187. London: Taylor 1846.
Watson, W.: On anomalous trichromatic colour vision. Proc. roy. Soc. (Lond.) A **90**, 443—448 (1914).
Weale, R. A.: Cone-monochromatism. J. Physiol. (Lond.) **121**, 548—569 (1953a).
— Colour vision in the peripheral retina. Brit. med. Bull. **9**, 55—60 (1953b).
— Photosensitive reactions in fovea of normal and cone-monochromatic observers. Optica Acta **6**, 158—174 (1959).
— Photochemistry and vision. Ch. 9. In: Photophysiology, Vol. 4. Giese, E. C. (Ed.). New York: Academic Press 1968.
Westphal, H.: Unmittelbare Bestimmungen der Urfarben. Z. Sinnesphysiol. **44**, 182—230 (1910).
Willis, M. P., Farnsworth, D.: Comparative evaluation of anomaloscopes. Med. Res. Lab. Rep. No. 190, 1—89 Bur. Med. Surg., U.S. Navy Dept.: Washington 1952.
Willmer, E. N.: Further observations on the properties of the central fovea in colour-blind and normal subjects. J. Physiol. (Lond.) **110**, 422—446 (1950).
Wright, W. D.: Researches in Normal and Defective Colour Vision. St. Louis: Mosby 1947.
— The characteristics of tritanopia. J. opt. Soc. Amer. **42**, 509—521 (1952).
— Comments as written to Dean Farnworth in 1958. Vision Res. **1**, 8 (1961).
Wyszecki, G., Stiles, W. S.: Color Science. New York: Wiley 1967.
Young, T.: On the theory of light and colours. In: Lectures in Natural Philosophy. Vol. 2, pp. 613—632. London: Printed for Joseph Johnson, St. Paul's Church Yard, by William Savage 1807.

Chapter 24

Genetics of Congenital Colour Deficiencies

By

W. JAEGER, Heidelberg (Germany)

With 5 Figures

Contents

Genetically there is a fundamental difference between the types of red-green blindness (protanomaly, protanopia, deuteranomaly and deuteranopia) and congenital achromatopsia. The types of red-green blindness are transmitted by a recessive X-linked mode of inheritance, whereas congenital achromatopsia behaves autosomal-recessively. The sensory mechanisms are also fundamentally different: Persons with different types of red-green blindness as well as those with tritan defects have a cone receptor system and have, therefore, normal visual acuity and fixation. Persons affected with congenital achromatopsia, however, use the rod receptor system even in daylight and show, therefore, low visual acuity, nystagmus and photophobia. (For further discussion of psychophysical data, see HURVICH, chapter 23, this volume.)

Tritan defects cannot yet be analysed very reliably as to their mode of genetic transmission. Cone monochromatism seems to follow the same mode of inheritance as the types of red-green blindness. This is true at least of the red-green defect which is included in this deficiency.

Finally, the genetic nature of colour amblyopia and colour asthenopia have not yet been sufficiently explored. This is mainly due to the great difficulties of any precise investigation.

I. Red-Green Deficiencies (Protan and Deutan Defects)

A. Historical Data

In 1777, HUDDART described a family with four affected brothers who could distinguish only between yellow and blue. Two other brothers, one sister and both parents were normal. In 1798, JOHN DALTON, who had one colour-blind brother and one normal brother and sister, published observations on himself. In the same year, GOETHE examined two affected siblings. He had worked out and painted a colour test. Erroneously he thought the deficiency was localized in the perception mechanism for blue (akyanoblepsia) (JAEGER, 1969). In fact, the members of the family described by HUDDART, DALTON and his brother, and the subjects of GOETHE's experiments were protanopes!

The next step was the differentiation of two different types of red-green blindness by SEEBECK (1837). Finally, in 1881, Lord RAYLEIGH was the first to distinguish between dichromasy and anomalous trichromasy when he introduced his spectral colour test (Rayleigh equation).

The manner of hereditary transmission was described by HORNER in 1876: Colour-blindness is inherited by grandchildren from grandfathers via normal daughters. It is the same rule that NASSE had pointed out for hemophilia in 1820. Scientific explanation of this mode of inheritance became possible when in 1910 MORGAN described X-chromosomal transmission in Drosophila melanogaster. In 1911, WILSON suspected that red-green deficiencies might follow the X-chromosomal mode of inheritance. Red-green deficiencies and hemophilia have since become the most popular examples of X-chromosomal transmission (WAARDENBURG, 1963a).

B. X-linked Inheritance

1. General Rules

Since HORNER, protanomaly (PA), protanopia (P), deuteranomaly (DA) and deuteranopia (D) have been classical examples of X-linked inheritance. There are only very few exceptions to, and deviations from, the rules of this mode of inheritance: The gene for red-green deficiency is localized in the X-chromosome. It behaves recessively, the normal allele is dominant. Since males, with the XY-constellation, carry only one X-chromosome, they are colour-blind if the X-chromosome is affected (hemizygous). Females, with the XX-constellation, are colour-blind only if both X-chromosomes carry the gene for red-green deficiency, i.e., if the woman is homozygous for that gene. If only one X-chromosome is affected, the female is phenotypically normal, but a conductor for colour-blindness (heterozygous carrier of the gene).

These rules, however, can be applied only if the same type of red-green deficiency is involved. On this assumption the following combinations exist (TRENDELENBURG, 1941) (Fig. 1): Since it has become possible to distinguish exactly between different types of red-green defects by means of spectral colour matches with the anomaloscope (Rayleigh equation), we know that the offspring of combinations 1 and 2 are always affected with the same type of colour deficiency (intrafamilial stability; FRANCESCHETTI, 1930). Of course, the different X-chromosomes in combinations 3, 4 and 5 may carry the allele for the same type as well as for different types of colour deficiency. If it is of the same type we will also find intrafamilial stability. If, however, different types of colour deficiency occur in one family, one must assume two different X-chromosomes of the parents, each carrying the genes for two different types. This would be possible in combinations 3, 4 and 5.

2. Dominance Relationship of the Different Series of Multiple Alleles: Normal > Anomalous > Anope

Just as the gene for normal colour sense predominates over the gene for colour deficiency, minor disturbances are more prevalent than more serious defects. If,

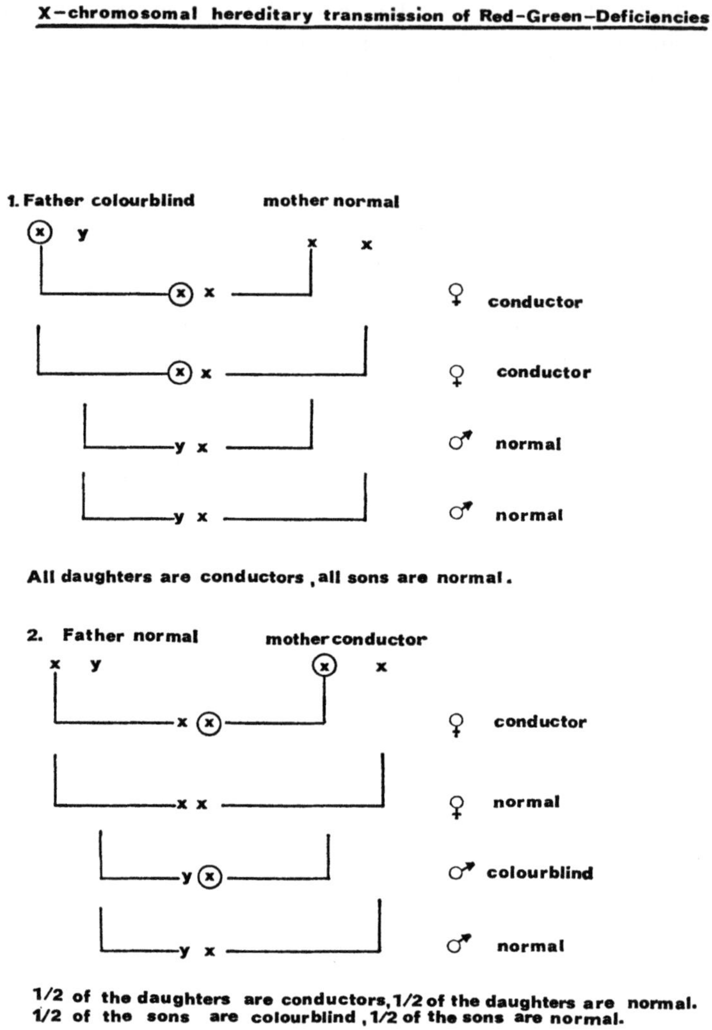

Fig. 1. X-linked recessive transmission of red-green deficiencies

for instance, a female carries the abnormal gene for DA in one X-chromosome and the gene for D in the other, DA will manifest itself. Sons of this female will be half DA and half D. The same rule applies to PA and P. According to this, dominance relationship can be expressed in the following way (protan and deutan types taken separately):

$$\text{normal} > \text{anomalous} > \text{anope}$$

We therefore assume that two series of multiple alleles are localized in two different loci of the X-chromosome (JUST, 1925; WAALER, 1927; FRANCESCHETTI, 1957). There are three members in each series. The genes producing the less marked defect are always dominant over those resulting in more serious deficiencies.

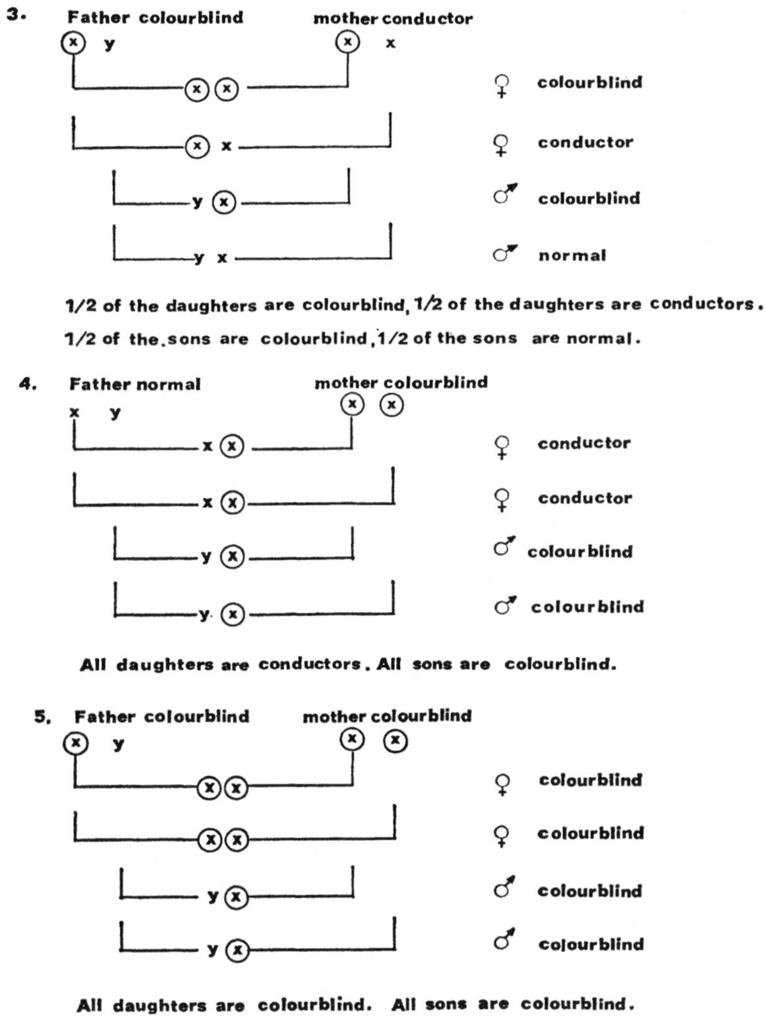

Fig. 1

3. Extreme Anomaly

Klein and Franceschetti (1964) discuss whether there is a further step between anomaly and anopia, the so-called extreme anomaly. In the anomaloscope test, subjects were found who accept one of the two extreme equations – not both of them, because in this case they would have been protanopes or deuteranopes. Protanomalous subjects who accept the equation "red" = "yellow" are called extreme protanomalous; deuteranomalous subjects who accept the equation "green" = "yellow" are called extreme deuteranomalous.

Hereditary transmission of the extreme anomaly seems, however, to be unstable. As a rule, extreme deuteranomaly shows irregular alternation with deuteranomaly, and extreme protanomaly alternates with protanomaly. Besides the gene for the colour defect, a modificator gene (extreme-factor) is possibly transmitted. Data, however, on the rules of hereditary transmission of the "extreme-factor" are still insufficient (Waardenburg, 1963a).

C. Frequency in Males

1. Total Frequency in European and Non-European Countries

The publications of Kherumian and Pickford (1959), Waardenburg (1963a), Klein and Franceschetti (1964) review population studies in European and non-European countries. There exist considerable geographical and racial differences. In males of European races red-green defects occur in about 8 %. With the anomaloscope, rather constant values are obtained. In the Jewish population, too, in Russia as well as in New York, about 8 % were found to be affected.

People of coloured races, however, present a considerably lower incidence of red-green defects than those of the white race: American Negroes about 3.5 %, African Negroes about 2.5 %, Japanese and Chinese between about 4 and 6 %, and Malayan people about 4 %. The lowest percentage was found in American Indian tribes with a maximum of 2.5 %.

It is difficult to compare the different statistics, because European statistics were based on anomaloscope measures, non-European, however, usually on pseudo-isochromatic plate tests only. If, however, comparisons were based on identical tests, the differences between white and coloured races would possibly be even greater. There is no doubt that the white race shows by far the highest incidence of red-green defects.

2. Frequency of the Different Biotypes

Deuteranomaly is the most frequent group among the different biotypes. In all statistics more than 50 % of patients with red-green disturbances are deuteranomalous. In European races the 8 % of red-green defects are distributed in the following way: P 1 %, PA 1 %, D 1 %, DA 5 % (Waaler, 1927).

It is strange that the ratio of anomalous to anope differs in protan and deutan types. This ratio might possibly shift if a larger test field than the one in Nagel's anomaloscope were used. Jaeger and Kroker (1952) were able to demonstrate that 2/3 of protanopic persons would then turn out to be protanomalous, whereas only 2/7 of deuteranopic persons would be found to be deuteranomalous. Thus the ratio PA : P approaches that of DA : D.

D. Frequency in Females

1. Total Frequency

The frequency of affected females is only about 0.4 %. The most reliable statistics carried out with the anomaloscope are those of Waaler (0.44 % $\pm$ 0.07) and von Planta (0.43 % $\pm$ 0.12). Data on the incidence of affected females in coloured races vary considerably and are still insufficient.

2. Frequency of Protan and Deutan Types

Since genes producing less marked defects are dominant over those producing more serious disturbances, the ratios P : PA and D : DA in females will be shifted.

P and D are extremely rare. A compilation of the most reliable European statistics is given by KLEIN and FRANCESCHETTI: P 3.6 %, PA 12.6 %, D 2.7 %, DA 81.1 % (!). Thus the preponderance of deuteranomalous subjects in colour-defective females is even more pronounced than in males.

E. Non-Allelic "Compounds"

1. Discrepancy between the Theoretically Expected Number of Affected Females and the Number Actually Observed

There is no difficulty in calculating the theoretically expected frequency in females on the basis of the frequency in males: 8 % is the frequency in males as well as the frequency of the abnormal gene in the total population. The expected incidence in females would be 0.64 %. This is considerably higher than the actually observed number 0.4 %. By means of WAALER'S and v. PLANTA'S statistics, FRANCESCHETTI (1928), moreover, calculated the theoretically expected frequency of the 10 different genotypical combinations in females:

a) allelic compounds: PAPA, PAP, PP, DADA, DAD, DD
b) non-allelic "compounds": PADA, PAD, PDA, PD.

All non-allelic "compounds" together reach a percentage of 0.2340 %, which is exactly the difference between the theoretically expected and actually observed numbers of affected females. The simplified calculations of STERN (1958) (1 % PA, 1 % P, 1 % D, and 5 % DA) come to the same result: 0.64 % total, 0.4 % allelic compounds, and 0.24 % non-allelic "compounds". Simply by calculation one could expect non-allelic "compounds" to be phenotypically normal.

2. Normal Colour Sense of Non-Allelic "Compounds"

In fact, in 1924 GÖTHLIN found a woman with normal colour vision who had protanopic as well as deuteranopic sons. She must have carried the gene for protanopia in one X-chromosome and the gene for deuteranopia in the other. According to this it can be assumed that a female conductor of a protan and a deutan defect will be normal. This proves that these genes belong to different series of multiple alleles. In this case it does not matter whether it is P or PA, or D or DA.

In earlier publications by WAALER, BRUNNER, KONDO and others, all non-allelic "compounds" were detected when sons with protan as well as deutan defects were found. Finally, FRANCESCHETTI and KLEIN (1957) were able to follow up the histories of protanopic and deuteranopic patients. Occasionally it happened that a protanopic man was married to a deuteranopic woman and a deuteranopic man married to a protanopic woman. He found that the daughters of these families had normal colour sense, although they must have been genotypically "compounds" for P and D.

On the basis of this experience, WAALER developed a model that permitted very precise conclusions. He assumed the normal disposition for colour sense to be an intact square model. A defect on the deutan side could either be minor, leading to DA, or major, resulting in D, whereas a defect on the protan side could lead either to PA or P. Since males have only one X-chromosome, the genotypical

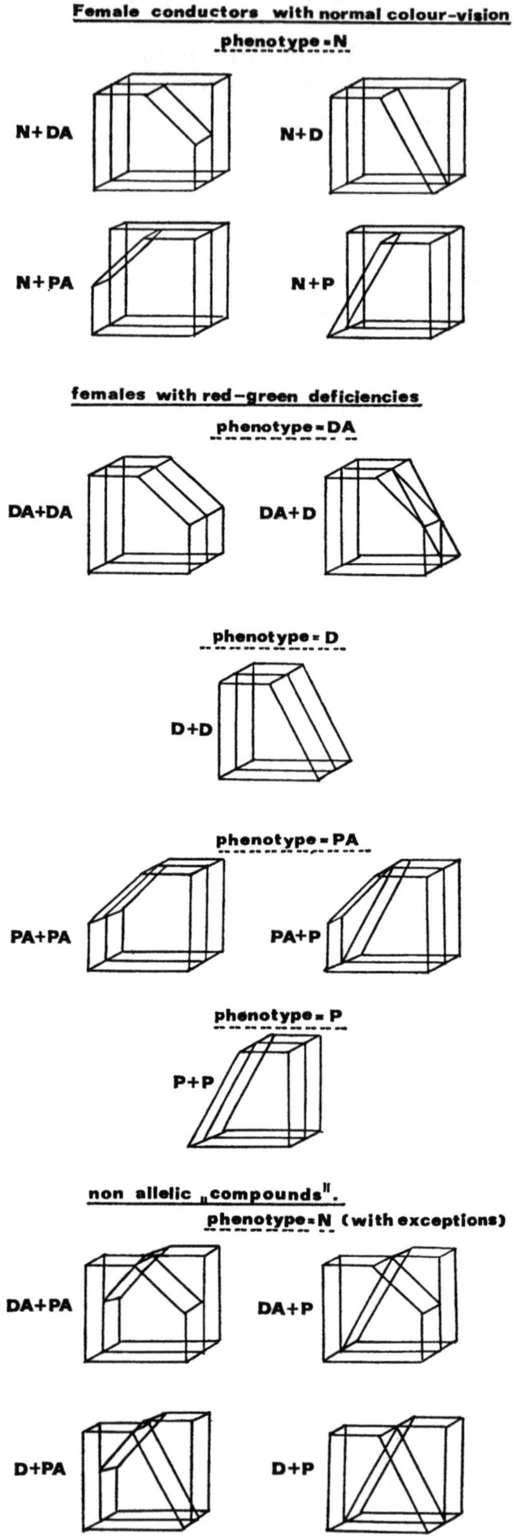

Female conductors with normal colour-vision
phenotype = N
N+DA
N+D
N+PA
N+P
females with red-green deficiencies
phenotype = DA
DA+DA
DA+D
phenotype = D
D+D
phenotype = PA
PA+PA
PA+P
phenotype = P
P+P
non allelic „compounds".
phenotype = N (with exceptions)
DA+PA
DA+P
D+PA
D+P

Fig. 2

situation could be deduced from the phenotype. WAALER's model proved to be reliable for the investigation of colour deficiencies in females as well: If the alleles for D and DA occur together, the less marked defect dominates over the more serious deficiency, in both the protan and deutan series. In the same way, of course, the normal gene is dominant over the affected one. This model allows us to explain the behaviour of non-allelic "compounds", too: If two X-chromosomes, one with a protan, the other with a deutan defect, occur together, they complete each other in the most desirable way. The result is phenotypically normal colour sense (Fig. 2).

This model is diagrammatic, but it can be extrapolated without difficulty to the field of gene localization on the chromosome. The model is an important argument for the assumption that protan and deutan defects are localized in different loci of the X-chromosome.

This two-loci theory has again been confirmed by VANDERDONK and VERRIEST (1960) who found a sibship with D and PA-affected and at the same time two normal sons! (Fig. 3). There is no doubt that the mother was non-allelic "compound". We can only assume that by means of crossing-over some of her X-chromosomes changed into a normal chromosome and one affected with D and PA which would explain the occurrence of normal sons. It is impossible to say what would have happened if the doubly affected X-chromosome had been transmitted to one of the sons. Monochromatism would probably have been the result. In the family investigated by VANDERDONK and VERRIEST, in both cases only the X-chromosome which had become normal by crossing-over had been transmitted to the sons.

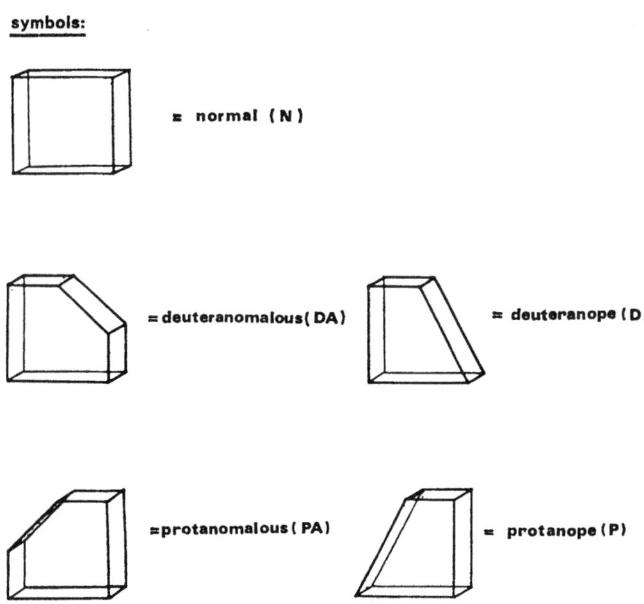

Fig. 2. Waaler's model symbolizing the dominance relationship of the different series of alleles of protan and deutan deficiencies

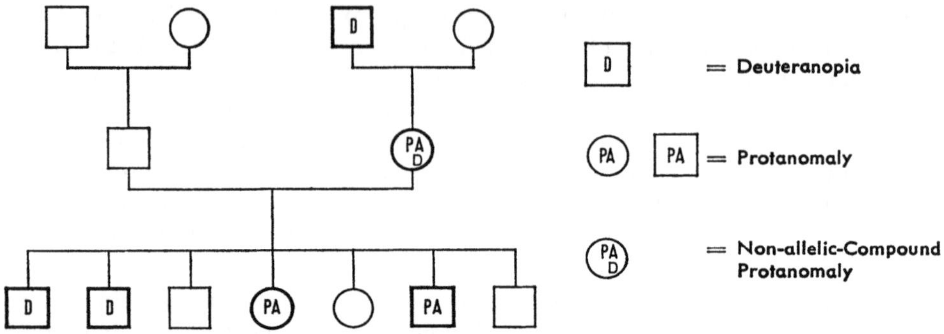

Fig. 3. Non allelic compound with colour-blind and normal sons (VANDERDONK and VERRIEST, 1960)

3. Non-Allelic "Compounds" with Defects of Colour Sense

VANDERDONK'S and VERRIEST'S pedigree is quite extraordinary in an other respect as well: The non-allelic "compound" DPA is not normal as might be supposed, but is herself also PA. This confirms an observation made by JAEGER (1951) (Fig. 4). The phenotypes of non-allelic "compounds" obviously can not be predicted so exactly as in the transmission of colour defects. Two genotypically identical sisters with a combination of P and DA were completely different in their phenotypes: one compound was P, the other compound atypically DA (although to such a small degree that she could have been taken for almost normal after superficial examination). An additional tritanomaly probably led to the manifestation of colour deficiency in both non-allelic "compounds".

Another pedigree was published by WEALE (1953) (Fig. 5), who also found colour deficiency in a non-allelic "compound" for extreme PA and DA. This

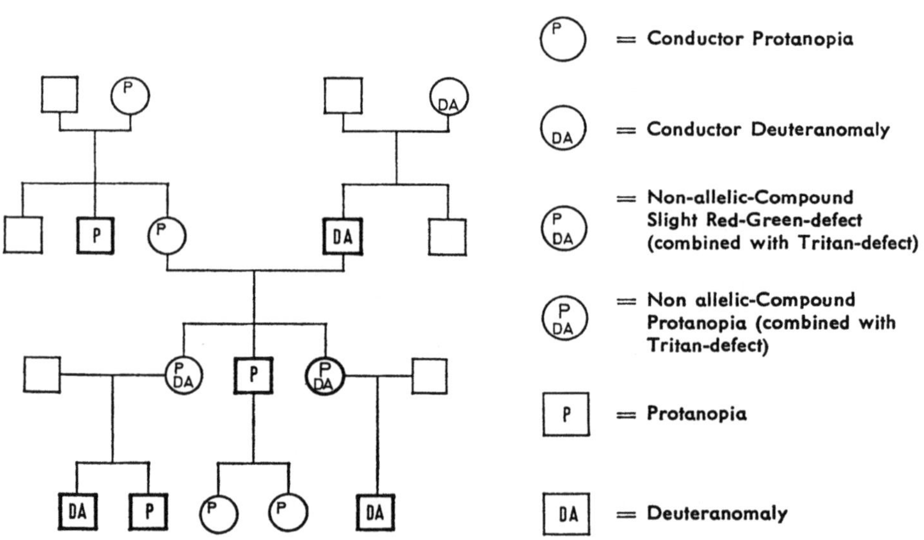

Fig. 4. Non allelic compounds with manifest colour-deficiencies (JAEGER, 1951)

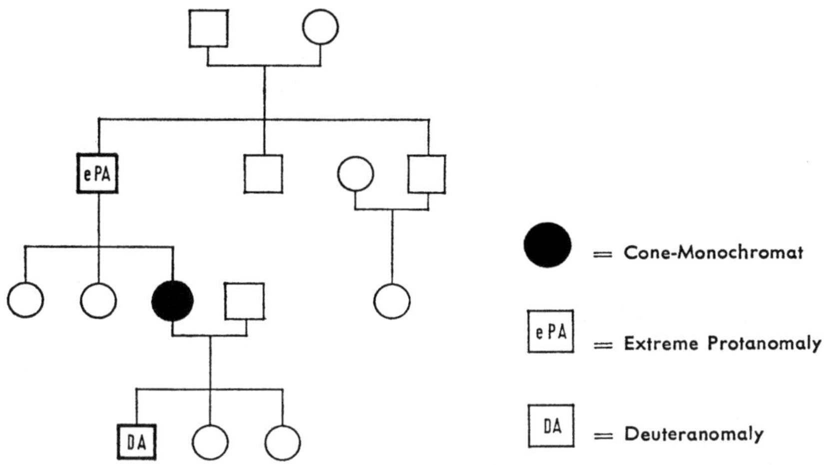

Fig. 5. Cone monochromatism in a case of non allelic compound (WEALE, 1953)

patient had a cone monochromatism with a luminosity curve typical of protan defects.

All these examples show that the dominance relationship in non-allelic "compounds" is less stable than in heterozygotes and allelic compounds. Besides examples with normal colour vision there are a few exceptions, in which non-allelic "compounds" have colour defects of quite different severity. Undoubtedly, these cases of non-allelic "compounds" with defects of colour sense are extremely rare. A further semi-dominant allele or a shifting of dominance induced by exogenic factors is then possibly involved.

F. Deficiencies in Female Conductors

1. Affected Heterozygous Females

Heterozygous females who, contrary to the general rule, are red-green blind, are certainly extremely rare. WAARDENBURG (1963a) has compiled a list of all cases so far published. Of course, the majority have not been examined thoroughly enough. Apart from that, only the fact that a colour-blind woman has normal and colour-blind sons can give clear evidence (Pater semper incertus). Sometimes, however, the early stages of an acquired colour defect may look like a congenital red-green deficiency. In the pedigree described by JAEGER (1952a) a woman had a normal and a DA-son. She herself accepted a wide range of anomaloscope equations. Despite degeneration of the macula of both eyes and vision of 5/25 on either side, DA and not an acquired colour defect was assumed. The mean values of the anomalous quotients obtained with the Helmholtz colorimeter supported this interpretation. Obviously, however, at that time it must have been a very early stage of an acquired defect. In the following years the colour deficiency grew worse, and in the meantime a typical red-green deficiency caused by degeneration of the macula has developed.

This example may show that, despite thorough examination with spectral colours, an early stage of an acquired colour deficiency can simulate DA or PA. All reports on heterozygously affected females with simultaneous involvement of the macula (e.g., FRANCESCHETTI, 1929) must, therefore, be regarded with scepticism. Considering this fact, there is no published case of manifest red-green-defect in heterozygous women which could be accepted without any doubt.

2. Slight Intermediate Deficiencies

Quite another question is the occurrence of minor errors in reading Ishihara plates and a slight shift in the luminosity maximum of protan conductors towards shorter wavelengths (SCHMIDT, 1955). But this "Schmidt's sign" is not always present! Using the flicker-photometric method, CRONE (1959) worked out a luminosity quotient (i.e., the ratio of the luminosity of green of 530 nm and red of 650 nm). The luminosity quotient in deutan heterozygotes was lower than in normals. The quotient in protan heterozygotes was found to be much higher than normal.

G. Genetic Aspects of Unilateral Colour Defects

Unilateral cases are of special interest to the physiologist, because they make it possible to find out how the various hues are seen by subjects with red-green disturbances. But one ought to be very cautious not to overlook remnants of a disease of the optic nerve or retina. Only cases examined with the anomaloscope are of value. Moreover, in the majority of reports in the literature the families were not examined with all methods. WAARDENBURG brings together all the published cases, but he is of the opinion that most of them offer hardly anything of importance to the geneticist.

In cases of unilateral colour defects an acquired colour deficiency should be suspected at the outset. These acquired disturbances can look very much like congenital hereditary defects. Deutan and protan defects with different impairment of the two eyes may possibly also be explained by an additional acquired disturbance. Thus, retinitis centralis serosa can impair hue discrimination to such a degree that DA seems to have turned into D (JAEGER and NOVER, 1951). There remains only one published case of an undoubted genetically conditioned unilateral defect (TRENDELENBURG, 1941). A man with unilateral DA married to a carrier for D had a DA-daughter an a D-son. Unilaterality was not transmitted to the offspring.

Data on female carriers of unilateral atypical D are of special theoretical interest. In these cases, however, test results differ so much from the typical behaviour of D that the disturbance could just as well have been acquired (KLEIN and FRANCESCHETTI, 1964).

H. Crossing-Over

Cases of crossing-over are more frequent than originally expected. This becomes evident in examinations of kindred with hemophilia. In 1937, RIDDELL was the first to find crossing-over in such a patient. A pedigree investigated by RATH (1938) and VERSCHUER (1938) shows all possible combinations of colour deficiency and hemophilia. A female carrier of a protan defect and hemophilia had four sons: 1. hemophilia + P, 2. hemophilia + normal colour sense, 3. normal blood coagulation + PA, 4. normal blood coagulation + normal colour sense (JAEGER, 1952 b). For at least two sons we must assume that crossing-over had taken place during meiosis of the mother.

In cases of protan defects combined with hemophilia, crossing-over is much more frequent than in deutan disturbances. From this we conclude that the locus of the protan defect is farther away from the gene for hemophilia than that of the deutan defect. KLEIN and FRANCESCHETTI (1964) have also compiled literature data on other combinations of colour defects and X-linked hereditary diseases. It is regrettable that in many cases the type of colour defect was not investigated. Now that is certain that protan and deutan defects are localized in two different loci, a differential diagnosis between protan and deutan defects is indispensable in all these cases.

J. Red-Green Defects and Chromosomal Abnormalities

1. Ullrich-Turner Syndrome

We know that patients with gonadal dysgenesis lack one gonosome. In case of an X0-genotype it must a priori be presumed that protan and deutan defects are found with the same frequency as in males. According to FRASER (1963) 76% of the X-chromosomes of X0-patients come from the mothers, 24 % come from the fathers. In fact, since the publication of POLANI *et al.* (1954) a conspicuously high percentage of colour deficiencies in such patients has been reported (KLEIN and FRANCESCHETTI, 1964; SCHAEFER-GEIERSBACH, 1970). In each case of Ullrich-Turner syndrome, the colour sense of the patient and his family should be investigated in order to find out whether the X-chromosome came from the father's or the mother's side.

2. Klinefelter Syndrome

This tubular dysplasia of testes is due to non-disjunction of gonosomes of the X-chromosomes, resulting in the XXY-genotype. Since in 2/3 of XXY-patients the two X-chromosomes derive from the mother, we should assume that red-green defects occur nearly as frequently as in females with the XX-genotype (= 0.4 %). In practice, however, 2.8 % of Klinefelter patients are found to be affected with a red-green defect. The additional Y-chromosome possibly intensifies the effect of the recessive gene. Such chromosome anomalies may possibly help to explain deviations from the regular mode of inheritance of red-green defects (FREY, 1961), although this could not be proven in any of the cases so far published.

II. Tritan Deficiencies

Just as in protan and deutan defects, in tritan disturbances we distinguish between tritanomaly (TA) as the minor and tritanopia (T) as the more serious defect. Compared to protan and deutan types, the genetics of tritan deficiencies are much less explored. The tests are much less reliable and diagnosis much more complicated. Selective absorption in refracting media as well as retinopathies can simulate tritan deficiency. The hereditary transmission of tritan deficiencies is not yet sufficiently explored.

A. Tritanomaly

At first, it looked as if tritanomaly was X-linked similarly to PA and DA (ENGELKING, 1925; HARTUNG, 1926). The frequency of affected women, however, in all families found so far is disproportionately high (JAEGER, 1955). Investigations of offspring of previously diagnosed tritanomalous patients could not confirm X-chromosomal transmission (SCHMIDT, 1970). Although KALMUS (1955) presumes X-chromosomal inheritance, considering the data of WRIGHT'S mass examination, it is just possible that acquired tritan defects have also been included. Thus the mode of inheritance of tritanomaly must still remain unclear.

B. Tritanopia

By analogy with protan and deutan defects, the modes of inheritance of tritanomaly and tritanopia should be assumed not to differ too much from each other. According to the investigations of KALMUS (1955/56), however, tritanopia must be considered to be incompletely autosomal-dominant, although this has occasionally been questioned. Autosomal-dominant infantile optic atrophy causes a tritan defect which very much resembles a congenital tritan deficiency. It is possible that members of the pedigree investigated by KALMUS were affected with such acquired tritan defects.

III. Cone Monochromatism

Undoubtedly, cone monochromates are absolutely colour-blind in the sense that, for them, all hues are perceived as black-and-white gradations. They have normal visual acuity, no nystagmus and no nyctalopia. Spectral sensitivity corresponding to either protan or deutan defects allows us to assume a close relationship to red-green deficiencies. We might suggest a combination of protanopia and tritanopia on the one hand, or of deuteranopia and tritanopia on the other. Neither genetic considerations nor the type of colour deficiency suggest any relationship to congenital achromatopsia.

A. Different Biotypes of Monochromatism

1. Protan Type

The luminosity curve is shifted in the short-wave direction. The long-wave end of the spectrum is shortened. Cases reported by WEALE (1953b) and a patient of PITT (1944) have been examined with special care.

2. Deutan Type

The maximum of the luminosity curve is either normal or shifted in the long-wave direction. One of VIERLING'S (1928) patients seems to manifest this syndrome. The pedigree published by CRONE (1955) was based on careful examinations.

3. Incomplete Types

Following KÖNIG's (1903) example, the name "pseudo-monochromasy" was used in the earlier literature (JAEGER, 1950). The expression "incomplete monochromatism" is, of course, better. We should also distinguish between a protan and a deutan type (WAARDENBURG, 1963b).

B. Genetic Data

Genetic data also support the assumption that in monochromates either protan or deutan defects are combined with tritan deficiencies. CRONE (1955) has reported the most exact genetic family study. It is observed that this accidental combination can be split both in ancestors as well as in offspring. In such cases the X-chromosomal character of protan or deutan defects becomes evident, whereas tritan defects are found to behave autosomally.

IV. Congenital Achromatopsia

A. Historical Data

The clinical picture of congenital achromatopsia has been known since the 17th century. Even in the first descriptions, in addition to total colour-blindness, day-blindness, impaired visual acuity, relatively good vision in dim light and nystagmus are mentioned. Even in daylight such patients see with the rods.

This explains a number of other symptoms: amblyopia, photophobia, maximum of the luminosity curve corresponding to scotopic vision, shortening of the spectrum at the long-wave end, and absence of Kohlrausch's kink (rod-cone break) in the dark-adaptation curve. Histologic investigations (LARSEN, 1921; HARRISON *et al.*, 1960) show that the cones are either reduced in number or that their outer segments are very short or absent.

B. Complete Typical Achromatopsia

In 1955, FRANÇOIS, VERRIEST, and DE ROUCK compiled all the data from the older literature. They were able to show that 70 % of all cases were familial. They found consanguinity of the parents in about 30 %, and females were affected as often as males. This suggests a priori that congenital achromatopsia must follow another mode of inheritance than red-green defects. Congenital achromatopsia is transmitted autosomal-recessively. The largest pedigrees are, therefore, found in inbreeding areas (e.g., the island of Fur/Danmark; FRANCESCHETTI *et al.*, 1958).

C. Incomplete Congenital Achromatopsia

Unlike the complete type, the incomplete type first discovered by FRANCESCHETTI in 1928 is able to distinguish between blue and red hues. Sometimes, however, this works only when large test-fields are used. The luminosity curve is less regular than in the complete type. In cases precisely investigated with spectral lights two maxima could sometimes be observed in the luminosity curve.

The incomplete type is also transmitted autosomal-recessively. As in monochromatism, one can probably differentiate between various forms of the incomplete type (JAEGER, 1953; BLACKWELL and BLACKWELL, 1957). The complete and incomplete types of congenital achromatopsia do not differ genetically. It is just a matter of penetrance of the same gene. Thus FRANCESCHETTI *et al.* (1958) found, in a family with consanguineous parents, two brothers, one affected with complete, the other with incomplete achromatopsia.

V. Concluding Remarks

Our knowledge of the genetics of congenital colour-defects is incomplete, because we have still no information on the mode of inheritance of colour amblyopia and colour asthenopia. Both symptoms are not yet sufficiently explored with respect to their genetics. This is mainly because of the great difficulties encountered in testing by local adaptation of the retina. It is very difficult to maintain fixation exactly for long times. Even with maximal co-operation on the part of the patient it is hard to say whether he is able to see any colour or not. In cases of bad observation, limited co-operation, low intelligence and high suggestibility the situation is quite hopeless. New methods, however, will possibly help to overcome these difficulties and provide exact information on the modes of inheritance of these disturbances.

For all other types of congenital colour-blindness there exist good and reliable test-methods. Since there are such different types of colour deficiency, a diagnosis of the type is always indispensable. Problems of sensory physiology as well as genetic questions cannot be answered until the diagnosis of the type of colour deficiency is absolutely certain.

References

BLACKWELL, H. R., BLACKWELL, O. M.: "Blue mono-cone monochromasy": a new color vision defect. J. opt. Soc. Amer. **47**, 338 (1957).

BRUNNER, W.: Über den Vererbungsmodus der verschiedenen Typen der angeborenen Rot-Grünblindheit. Graefes Arch. Ophthal. **124**, 1—52 (1930).

CRONE, R. A.: Clinical study of colour vision. Brit. J. Ophthal. **39**, 170—173 (1955).

— Combined forms of congenital colour defects. A pedigree with atypical total colour blindness. Brit. J. Ophthal. **40**, 462—472 (1956).

— Spectral sensitivity in colour-defective subjects and heterozygous carriers. Amer. J. Ophthal. **48**, 231—238 (1959).

DALTON, J.: Extraordinary facts relating to the vision of colours. Mem. Lit. Phil. Soc. (Manchester) 5, 28—45 (1798).

ENGELKING, E.: Die Tritanomalie, ein bisher unbekannter Typus anomaler Trichromasie. Graefes Arch. Ophthal. **116**, 196—244 (1926).

FRANCESCHETTI, A.: Die Bedeutung der Einstellungsbreite am Anomaloskop für die Diagnose der einzelnen Typen der Farbensinnstörungen, nebst Bemerkungen über ihren Vererbungsmodus. Schweiz. med. Wschr. **58**, 1273—1279 (1928).

— Über Dominanzverhältnisse bei der Vererbung angeborener Farbensinnstörungen. Ber. ges. Physiol. **50**, 312—313 (1929).

— Die Vererbung von Augenleiden. In: Kurzes Handbuch der Ophthalmologie. SCHIECK and BRÜCKNER, (Eds.) Bd. 1, 663—855. Berlin: Springer 1930.

Franceschetti, A., Jaeger, W., Klein, D., Ohrt, V., Rickli, H.: Etude patho-physiologique de la grande famille d'achromates de l'île de Fur (Danemark). Description d'une nouvelle famille avec achromatopsie totale chez le fils aîné et achromatopsie incomplète chez le frère cadet. XVIII Concilium ophthalmologicum 1958. Belgica, Vol. II, pp. 1582—1588.

— Klein, D.: Two families with parents of different types of red-green blindness. Acta genet. (Basel) **7**, 255—259 (1957).

François, J.: L'hérédité en Ophthalmologie. Paris: Masson 1958.

— Verriest, G., Rouck, A. de: L'achromatopsie congénitale. Documenta ophthal. **9**, 338—424 (1955).

Fraser, G. R. 1963, cited by W. Lenz: Medizinische Genetik. Stuttgart: Thieme 1970.

Frey, R.G.: Chromosomale Anomalien und die Vererbung angeborener Farbensinnstörungen. Graefes Arch. Ophthal. **163**, 117—129 (1961).

Göthlin, G. F.: Congenital red-green abnormalety in colour-vision, and congenital total colour-blindness, from the point of view of heredity. Acta ophthal. (Kbh.) **21**, 15—34 (1924).

Harrison, R., Hoefnagel, D., Hayward, J. N.: Congenital total color blindness. Arch. Ophthal. **64**, 65—72 (1960).

Hartung, H.: Über drei familiäre Fälle von Tritanomalie. Klin. Mbl. Augenheilk. **76**, 229—240 (1926).

Horner, J. F.: Die Erblichkeit des Daltonismus. Ein Beitrag zum Vererbungsgesetz. Amtl. Ber. Verwaltung d. Medizinalwesens d. Kantons Zürich, 208 (1876).

Huddart, J.: An account of persons who could not distinguish colours. Phil. Trans. (Lond.) **67**, I, 260—265 (1777).

Jaeger, W.: Systematische Untersuchungen über inkomplette angeborene totale Farbenblindheit. Eine Zwischenform zwischen angeborener totaler Farbenblindheit und Protanopie. Graefes Arch. Ophthal. **150**, 509—528 (1950).

— Gibt es Kombinationsformen der verschiedenen Typen angeborener Farbensinnstörung? Graefes Arch. Ophthal. **151**, 229—248 (1951).

— Werden die angeborenen Störungen des Rot-Grünsinns ausnahmslos rezessiv-geschlechtsgebunden vererbt? Graefes Arch. Ophthal. **152**, 397—384 (1952a).

— Beitrag zur Frage der Genlokalisation der Farbensinnstörungen. Graefes Arch. Ophthal. **152**, 385—388 (1952b).

— Typen der inkompletten Achromatopsie. Ber. dtsch. Ophthal. Ges. **58**, 44—47 (1953).

— Tritoformen angeborener und erworbener Farbensinnstörungen. Farbe **4**, 197—215 (1955).

— Studien Goethes an Personen, die gewisse Farben nicht unterscheiden können. Documenta Ophthal. **26**, 264—272 (1969).

— Kroker, K.: Über das Verhalten der Protanopen und Deuteranopen bei großen Reizflächen. Klin. Mbl. Augenheilk. **121**, 445—449 (1952).

— Nover, A.: Störungen des Lichtsinns und Farbensinns bei Chorioretinitis centralis serosa. Graefes Arch. Ophthal. **152**, 111—120 (1951.)

Just, G.: Zur Vererbung der Farbensinnstufen beim Menschen. Arch. Augenheilk. **96**, 406—418 (1925).

Kalmus, H.: The familial distribution of congenital tritanopia. With some remarks on some similar conditions. Ann. hum. Genet. **20**, 39—56 (1955—1956).

Kherumian, R., Pickford, R. W.: Hérédité et fréquence des dyschromatopsies. Paris: Vigot 1959.

Klein, D., Franceschetti, A.: Mißbildungen und Krankheiten des Auges. In: Humangenetik, Vol. 4, pp. 1—247. Becker, P. E. (Ed.) Stuttgart: Thieme 1964.

König, A.: Gesammelte Abhandlungen, p. 322. Leipzig: Barth 1903.

Kondo, T.: Untersuchungen bei angeborenen Farbensinn-Anomalien. Acta Soc. Ophthal. Jap. **36**, 1337—1346 (1932) and German summary, pp. 101—102.

Larsen, H.: Demonstration mikroskopischer Präparate von einem monochromatischen Auge. Klin. Mbl. Augenheilk. **67**, 301—302 (1921).

Nasse, C. F.: Von einer erblichen Neigung zu tödlichen Blutungen. Arch. med. Erfahr. (Berlin) Nr. 1, 385—434 (1820).

Pitt, F. H. G.: Monochromatism. Nature (Lond.) **154**, 466 (1944).

PLANTA, P. VON: Die Häufigkeit der angeborenen Farbsinnstörungen bei Knaben und Mädchen und ihre Feststellung durch die üblichen klinischen Proben. Graefes Arch. Ophthal. **120**, 253—281 (1928).
POLANI, P. E., HUNTER, N. E., LENNOX, B.: Chromosomal sex in Turner's syndrome with coarctation of the aorta. Lancet **1954 II**, 120—121.
RATH, B.: Rot-Grünblindheit in der Kalmbacher Blutersippe. Arch. Rass.-Gesellschaftsbiol. **32**, 397—407 (1938).
RAYLEIGH, LORD (STRUTT, J. W.). Experiments on colour. Nature (Lond.) **25**, 64—66 (1881).
RIDDEL, W. J. B.: Haemophilia and colour-blindness occurring in the same family. Brit. J. Ophthal. **21**, 113—116 (1937).
SCHAEFER-GEIERSBACH, U.: Das Erscheinungsbild der Gonadendysgenesie. Eine klinische und zytogenetische Untersuchung. Dissertation, Heidelberg 1970.
SCHMIDT, I.: Über zwei Fälle von angeborener Blaugelbsehstörung. Klin. Mbl. Augenheilk. **109**, 635—652 (1943).
— A sign of manifest heterozygosity in carriers of color deficiency. Amer. J. Optom. **32**, 404—408 (1955).
— On congenital tritanomaly. Vision Res. **10**, 717—743 (1970).
SEEBECK, A.: Über den bei manchen Personen vorkommenden Mangel an Farbensinn. Ann. Phys. Chem. **42**, 177—233 (1837).
STERN, C.: Colourblindness in Klinefelter's syndrome. Nature (Lond.) **183**, 1452—1453 (1959).
— Le daltonisme lié au chromosome X a-t-il une localisation unique ou double? J. Génét. hum. **7**, 302—307 (1958).
— The chromosomes of man. Amer. J. hum. Genet. **11**, 301—314 (1959).
TRENDELENBURG, W.: Über Vererbung bei einem Fall von anomalem Farbensinn des einen und normalem Farbensinn des anderen Auges beim Mann. Klin. Mbl. Augenheilk. **107**, 280—293 (1941).
VANDERDONCK, R., VERRIEST, G.: Femme protanomale et hétérozygote mixte (gènes de la protanomalie et de la deuteranopie en position de répulsion) ayant deux fils deutéranopes, un fils protanomale et deux fils normeaux. Biotypologie **21**, 110—120 (1960).
VERSCHUER, O. VON: Der erste Nachweis von Faktorenaustausch (crossing-over) beim Menschen. Erbarzt **5**, 3—4 (1938).
VIERLING, O.: Über spektrale Wertbestimmung der Farben durch Schwellenmessung mit dem modifizierten Anomaloskop. Z. Bahnärzte **23**, 261—276 (1928).
WAALER, G. H. M.: Über die Erblichkeitsverhältnisse der verschiedenen Arten von angeborener Rot-Grünblindheit. Acta ophthal. (Kbh.) **5**, 309—345 (1927).
WAARDENBURG, P. J.: Colour Sense and Dyschromatopsia. In: Genetics and Ophthalmology, Vol. 2, pp. 1425—1566. Assen: van Gorcum **1963** a.
— Achromatopsia congenita. In: Genetics and Ophthalmology, Vol. 2, pp. 1695—1718. Assen: van Gorcum **1963** b.
WALLS, G., MATTHEWS, R. W.: New Means of Studying Color-Blindness and Normal Foveal Color Vision. Berkeley: Univ. Calif. Press 1952.
WEALE, R. A.: Some aspects of total colour-blindness. Trans. ophthal. Soc. U.K. **73**, 241—249 (1953).
— Cone-monochromatism. J. Physiol. (Lond.) **121**, 548—569 (1953).
WILSON, E. B.: The sex chromosomes. Arch. mikr. Anat. **77**, II, 249—271 (1911).
WRIGHT, W. D.: The characteristics of tritanopia. J. opt. Soc. Amer. **42**, 509—521 (1952).

Chapter 25

Acquired Color Vision Defects

By

PETER GRÜTZNER, Freiburg (Germany)

With 8 Figures

Contents

A. Introduction

Acquired defects of color vision are common. Their frequency, however, is not generally appreciated. Like all functions of the eye, color vision is influenced by many diseases, congenital abnormalities and even physiological processes such as aging.

Functional disturbances are based on alterations of the anatomical structure. The more we learn about the normal anatomy and physiology of the eye, the easier it will be to understand the abnormal. Conversely, abnormalities such as acquired color vision defects may contribute to a better understanding of the normal. In addition to its scientific value, the evaluation of a color vision defect provides an important addition to the differential diagnostic and prognostic abilities of the ophthalmologist.

B. General Characteristics of Acquired Color Vision Defects

Only rarely are acquired color vision defects as clear-cut as inherited ones. Therefore, some authors see such deficiencies as very insignificant and fail to identify them as a specific type of color vision defect. In fact, patients with the same disease will sometimes have differing kinds of color vision defects, depending on the stage of the disease and on the method of investigation. Even psychological variables have to be taken into consideration (LAKOWSKI, 1970). The severity or degree of the deficiency will change if the process is active. It may be unilateral or localized to only parts of the visual field. These findings, which are not characteristic of inherited defects, are helpful in our diagnostic and prognostic efforts.

In general, patients with an acquired color vision defect are not as sensitive to differences in brightness as are individuals with inherited defects. Moreover, they do not perceive color contrasts as do individuals with congenital protanomaly or deuteranomaly who are supersensitive in this respect. These facts may be considered as specific signs of such an acquired deficiency. Usually a patient with an acquired color vision defect has other functional disturbances. He will name a color as he perceives it. A person with a similar but congenital abnormality names colors as learned through education from "normal" people (KÖLLNER, 1912).

However, there are exceptions. Some diseases of the eye lead to acquired defects of color vision before other functions are markedly disturbed. Intoxications or degenerative processes usually involve both eyes. In degenerative diseases color vision may be altered so early in childhood that these persons either cannot remember or never develop normal perception. It is in these cases that we have great difficulty in distinguishing the acquired from the inherited defects (JAEGER and GRÜTZNER, 1963).

C. Methods of Examination

In both congenital and acquired defects the methods of investigation are the same. An ophthalmological consulting room should contain pseudo-isochromatic plates such as Ishihara, AO H-R-R, Stilling-Hertel, Boström-Kugelberg, etc. They help to screen color defectives, regardless of etiology, from those non-affected. However, one is seldom able to make an accurate diagnosis or even to get reproducible responses with these plates. The Nagel anomaloscope is often very useful to get comparable results. However, among the acquired color vision defectives, there are many who have difficulties in the short-wave, blue end of the spectrum and this region is not covered by the instrument. To detect such deficiencies, Farnsworth-Munsell tests should be used.

Until some 20 years ago colored stimuli were often used to detect functionally disturbed areas of the visual field (ENGELKING, 1921). Today we are unfamiliar with this type of investigation because we are able to change the size and brightness of the "white" stimulus light. However, for special purposes (FRANÇOIS *et al.*, 1966), or on some instruments such as Haitz's device (GÄRTNER, 1957), colored targets are still useful to detect small functional disturbances.

For more extensive evaluation of color vision defects and for research purposes, more sophisticated equipment such as a photometer and/or a color-mixture apparatus may be used.

D. Types of Acquired Color Vision Defects

Often, in any one disease, several or all components responsible for the perception of colors are involved. Nonetheless, some order or classification in the acquired deficiencies of color vision, may be made. They may be classified as protan-, deutan- or tritan-like defects, depending on the similarity of the responses to those of the inherited forms. I will discuss the different deficiencies in the anatomical sequence of the visual pathway, because we can often determine through objective findings the tissue which is involved.

1. Acquired Color Vision Defects in Diseases of the Optic Media

The optic media may act as optic filters. Corneal diseases have no specific influence on color vision. Of greater interest is the slow and gradual change with age in the color of the lens. It becomes more and more yellow, thereby hindering short-wave light from stimulating the retina (LAKOWSKI, 1962; RUDDOCK, 1965; see also RUDDOCK, chapter 17, this volume). Because this progresses slowly, most older people are not aware of any change in color perception. If a patient has diminished visual acuity and the sensation of looking through a red filter, blood in the vitreous might be expected. To establish this diagnosis it is not necessary to check the color vision.

2. Acquired Color Vision Defects in Diseases of the Retina

It is more difficult to explain color vision deficiencies caused by involvement of the nervous tissue itself. If the retina is affected, often a tritan-defect will result (Table 1). This tendency is sometimes called the rule of KÖLLNER, who was the first to make this association. Various diseases of the retina can cause such tritan-defects, including inflammatory and degenerative processes, intoxication and detachment. The functional defect is usually called "uncharacteristic", meaning that it is not specific for a particular disease. Yet, color vision examination may, for example, support the diagnosis of an early Chloroquine retinopathy

Table 1. *Acquired color vision defects in diseases of the retina*

Diagnosis	Type of color vision defect	Preferred methods of investigation
diffuse degenerative processes; intoxication; inflammation; detachment	tritan-like	Farnsworth-Munsell tests; determination of hue discrimination; determination of saturation discrimination
	Exceptions	
central serous retinopathy	protan-like and tritan-like	Nagel anomaloscope; Farnsworth-Munsell tests
juvenile macular degeneration	protan-like	Nagel anomaloscope; determination of the luminosity curve

or a diffuse retinal degeneration *sine pigmento* (GRÜTZNER, 1969). These patients may have difficulty in reading pseudo-isochromatic plates, even though they are constructed for the detection of congenital red-green color deficiencies. However, their errors are uncharacteristic of such inherited abnormalities. On the Ishihara-plates patients with acquired defects may read neither the numbers visible to the normal, nor the picture-puzzle visible to congenital color defectives. Such responses should prevent us from classifying these cases in the wrong group.

Some pseudo-isochromatic plates show greenish or bluish figures against a grayish background as on Stilling- or H-R-R plates. Patients with tritan defects may have more trouble detecting such figures than people with a congenital red-green color defect. Some plates are specifically constructed for the detection of tritan-defects, both congenital and acquired. They may be helpful. But the diagnosis of a tritan-defect using only pseudo-isochromatic plates is always less certain than the corresponding result for red-green color defectives.

For the purpose of demonstrating a tritan defect it is much more helpful to use one of the Farnsworth tests (Panel D-15 or 100-hue test). Patients with an acquired tritan defect arrange the caps of the Panel D-15 test so that when the response is charted there are confusion lines in the horizontal axis (Fig. 8).

We obtain more accurate data if we determine hue discrimination over the whole spectrum (Fig. 1). With this method, such patients will demonstrate a

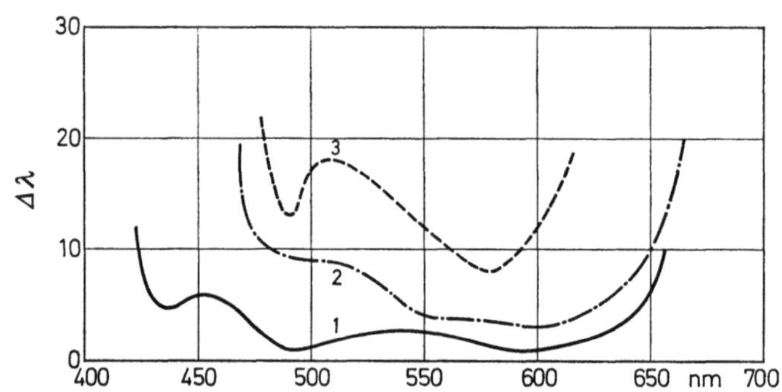

Fig. 1. Hue discrimination curves in patients with retinal diseases (3 = chloroquine retinopathy, 2 = choroideremia) compared with the responses of a normal person (No. 1)

diminished ability to distinguish different wavelengths, especially in the "blue" end of the spectrum. The maximum discriminability in the "orange" area, though not normal, is satisfactory. The reduction in sensitivity over the whole spectrum explains the difficulties in reading pseudo-isochromatic plates. The characteristic deficiency at shorter wavelengths may also be demonstrated by measuring the discrimination efficiency for saturation (Fig. 2).

Sometimes the color vision is disturbed to such a degree that the results of testing correspond to those from individuals with inherited dichromatopsia. Such individuals are able to match each wavelength with a mixture of only two selected colors or stimuli (KÖLLNER, 1912). The reason for this is quite different in inherited and acquired defects. Therefore, the same data call for different conclusions.

In inherited forms of dichromatopsia such measurements are usually interpreted to mean that only two different pigments are active. In advanced cases of acquired color vision defects all colors are perceived as unsaturated, and this enables the individual to perform such matches.

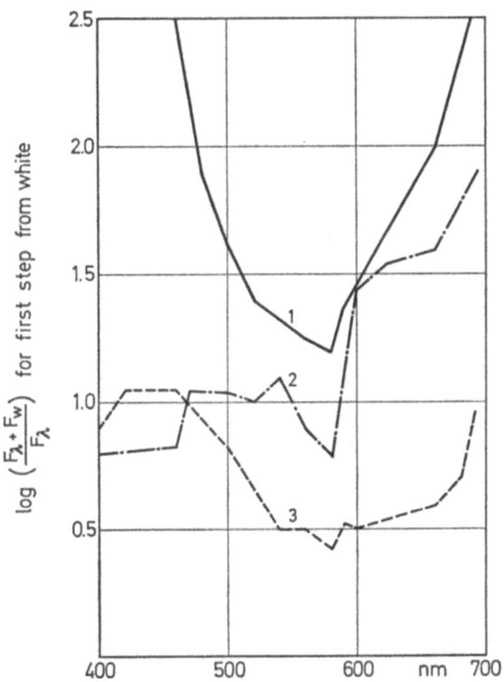

Fig. 2. Saturation discrimination curves in patients with retinal diseases (2 = hypertensive retinopathy, 3 = pigmentary retinopathy) compared with the curve of a person with normal color vision (No. 1) (from MARRÉ, 1969)

One of the best verifications that all kinds of cones or selective visual pigments are involved in acquired color vision deficiencies was demonstrated by MARRÉ (1969; Fig. 3, Table 2). She used WALD's (1966) technique and bleached two of the visual pigments with appropriate color stimuli. Then the increment treshold for different wavelengths across the entire spectrum was determined. It is assumed that the resulting curve shows the relative sensitivity of the remaining, non-bleached pigment. There was a remarkable difference in sensitivity between normal persons and those with retinal diseases. The sensitivity of the "blue" receptor was particularly diminished.

In diseases of the retina, why is the sensitivity for shorter wavelengths predominantly diminished? It may be argued that the rods are responsible for sensitivity in this range of the spectrum. Deterioration of the rods in diseases of the retina can often be proven by a diminished dark adaptation. This argument seems to be supported by evidence derived from degenerative processes such as choroideremia. The more advanced the concentric contraction, the more pronounced is the tritan defect (see WAARDENBURG, 1963). However, if we use a

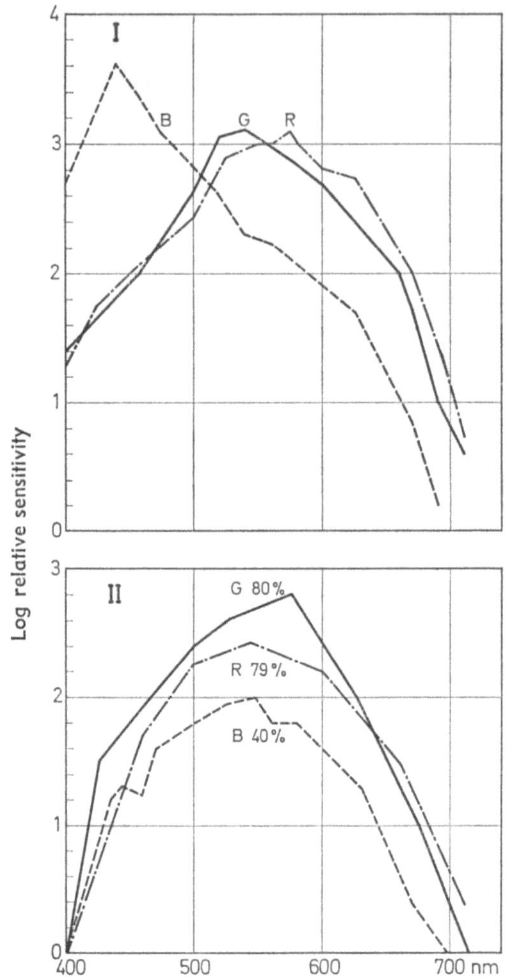

Fig. 3. Spectral sensitivities of the "blue"-, "green"-, and "red"-receptor mechanisms (B, G, R). Two mechanisms have been depressed respectively. I = mean curves from 11 persons with normal color vision, II = responses from a patient with pigmentary retinopathy. The percentage indicates the sensitivity in comparison with the measurements in normal persons (from Marré, 1969)

central target with a diameter of only 1.5 or 2 degrees and if the stimulus is bright enough, rod activity is essentially inhibited. Furthermore, acquired tritan defects have been described in patients with affections of the retina whose dark adaptation is not diminished and who have a normal ERG (König, 1897; Köllner, 1912; Engelking and Schreck, 1938; François et Verriest, 1957; Cox, 1961). This may be explained when we learn more about the anatomical and functional connections between the different tissue layers.

For example, when discussing the threshold effect of colored targets, Brindley (1960) implied that the receptors for short wavelengths are more interconnected than the other cones. If one of these cells is damaged, the whole group may de-

Table 2. *Spectral sensitivities of the "blue"-, "green"-, and "red"-receptor mechanisms (B, G, R). Measurements on patients with retinal diseases. The percentage indicates the aera under the curve, as compared with that of normal persons (from* Marré, 1969*)*

Diagnosis	Visual acuity	B%	G%	R%
postoperative retinal detachment	0.4	87	100	99
	0.7	82	102	97
	0.6	72	96	100
	0.6	97	106	95
chloroquine retinopathy	0.7	60	97	94
	1.0	57	93	95
diabetic retinopathy	1.0	88	99	96
	1.0	33	88	91
	0.3	40	82	92
hypertensive retinopathy	0.3	10	30	22
	1.0	30	81	87

teriorate via retrograde degeneration. From another point of view Wald (1966) in studies of inherited color vision defects, assumes that "any functional attack on cone vision is likely to result in the loss of the blue-receptor, while leaving representation of red- and green-receptors".

An exclusive tritan defect should not alter color perception for longer wavelengths. However, Köllner (1912) long ago documented that many patients with an acquired tritan defect do not accept the normal Rayleigh match on the Nagel anomaloscope. They use more long-wave light than normals to match the "yellow" comparison light (Fig. 4). These results may indicate that the "red-sensitive" system is affected. Responses on the Nagel anomaloscope should depend only upon the "red"- and on the "green-sensitive" cones, of which we find a high density in the center of the macular area (Wald, 1967). As yet, we do not know why the "red-sensitive" mechanism seems to be more vulnerable than the "green-sensitive" system.

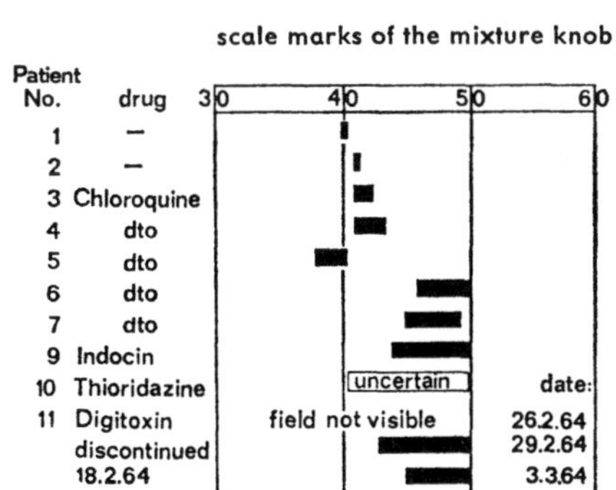

Fig. 4. Matches on the Nagel anomaloscope. Nos. 1 and 2 were healthy individuals with normal color vision. No. 3 to 11 had different degrees of drug retinopathy and acquired tritan defects (Grützner, 1969)

If the macular area is specifically affected we often find a more pronounced protan-like color vision defect. In central serous retinopathy the responses on the Nagel anomaloscope are quite characteristic. The amount of shift toward the long-wave component and the range of the matches provide a very sensitive measure for determining improvement or deterioration (JAEGER and NOVER, 1951). However, in such cases the Farnsworth test will show a tritan defect as in other retinal diseases (ZANEN and MEUNIER, 1965; KÖHLER, 1968).

Most striking and diagnostic are the findings in patients with juvenile macular degeneration. Their responses on the Nagel anomaloscope often cannot be distinguished from those of persons with an inherited protan defect. In advanced cases the results look like those of individuals with achromatopsia (Fig. 5). As might be expected, with this latter finding, there is often a shift of the luminosity curve toward shorter wavelenghts. The explanation proposed is that the cones sensitive to long-wave light may also be responsible for the sensation of brightness. If they are damaged, the visible spectrum is shortened at the long-wave end and the maximum of the luminosity curve (V_λ) is shifted, as in protanopia or even as in achromatopsia. Only in the periphery of the fundus does the spectral sensitivity remain in the normal range (GRÜTZNER, 1961). When these same patients are tested on the Goldmann Perimeter there is a broad central scotoma for the brigh-

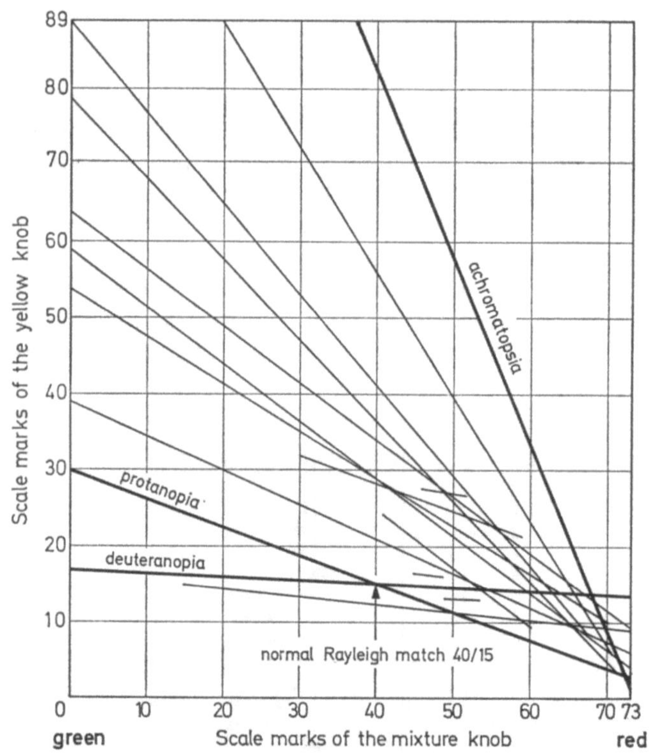

Fig. 5. Matches on the Nagel anomaloscope in patients with juvenile macular degeneration (thin lines, the lengths indicate the range of the accepted matches) in comparison with matches of persons with congenital dichromatopsia and achromatopsia (wider lines)

test and largest red stimulus. A person with inherited achromatopsia however, is unable to see this light even in the periphery of the visual field.

Contrary to these statements, MARRÉ (1969), utilizing a different technique, found a predominantly tritan defect in patients with juvenile macular degeneration (Table 3). Her measurements were made only in early stages when central fixation was still possible. The protan-like responses of such patients on the anomaloscope are not as pronounced as those for advanced stages of macular degeneration. These individuals cannot fixate with their fovea. But this fact is no explanation for the described shift of the luminosity curve. The perception of brightness should be the same in the center as well as in the periphery of the retina as long as photopic conditions are maintained.

Of special interest are the findings in patients with a macular form of diffuse tapeto-retinal degeneration (GRÜTZNER, 1962). The tritan defect, usually found in patients with diffuse degeneration of the retina, combines with the protan-like defect characteristic of alterations in the macular area. The residual function looks like that of a patient with an inherited achromatopsia. In both abnormalities the ERG findings are similar and evoked only with single flashes.

Table 3. *Spectral sensitivities of the "blue"-, "green"-, and "red"-receptor mechanisms (B, G, R). Measurements on patients with juvenile macular degeneration. The percentage indicates the area under the curve, as compared with that of normal persons (from* MARRÉ, *1969)*

Visual acuity	B%	G%	R%
0.7	69	104	105
0.4	87	103	100
0.9	48	100	104
1.5	81	105	108

3. Acquired Color Vision Defects in Diseases of the Optic Nerve

According to the rules of KÖLLNER, diseases of the optic nerve lead to an acquired red-green type of color vision defect (Table 4). More specifically, there is an acquired deutan-like deficiency. This implies that the spectral luminosity curve (V_λ), has the same relative distribution as in normals, even if all colors are perceived as being darker by these patients. In determining such responses, and particularly in patients with a central scotoma, it is important that photopic conditions are maintained. Otherwise a shift of the luminosity curve occurs due to the influence of dark adaptation.

The results of the pseudo-isochromatic plates, or the Farnsworth tests, may be similar to those of persons with inherited red-green color defects. On the anomaloscope, the normal match will be accepted. However, the range of the match is markedly enlarged, particularly if the target is fixated for longer than two seconds. This enlargement is usually more toward the "green" component than toward the "red". In advanced cases either of the two mixture lights alone can be matched with the "yellow" comparison light. The luminance of the "yellow" light is always in the same range as in congenital deuteranopia. This is simply an indication that the luminosity curve has not shifted.

Table 4. *Acquired color vision defects in diseases of the optic nerve*

Diagnosis	Type of color vision defect	Preferred methods of investigation
retrobulbar neuritis tobacco-alcohol amblyopia Leber's optic atrophy neoplasm trauma	deutan-like	pseudo-isochromatic plates Nagel anomaloscope determination of hue discrimination determination of the neutral zone
	Exceptions	
glaucoma	tritan-like	Farnsworth-Munsell tests determination of hue discrimination
infantile optic atrophy with dominant inheritance	tritan-like	Panel D-15 test determination of hue discrimination determination of the neutral zone
rare type of the above degenerative disease	protan-like	Nagel anomaloscope

The hue discrimination of patients with diseases of the optic nerve usually shows a markedly decreased minimum in the middle of the spectrum (around 530 nm) (Fig. 6). In far advanced cases even the maximum of discrimination in the "orange" region at 590 nm will be lost, but not the maximum in the "blue-green" range (at 490 nm).

Even with such time-consuming procedures, we may have difficulty in differentiating between an inherited deuteranopia and an acquired one. However, we are able to make a decision through a determination of the neutral zone. For such a purpose we present "white" light (e. g. 3200° K) in one half of a visual field and a spectral light in the other half. By ranging over the entire spectrum, we will find the area where the patient is unable to distinguish the spectral light from "white", as long as the brightness is the same. Patients with optic atrophy are often able to match "white" with lights from the middle of the spectrum, where their *minimum* of hue-discrimination is located (Fig. 7). Colors are perceived as being so desaturated that they cannot be distinguished from pure white light. The extent of the neutral band correlates with the diminution of visual acuity, and this depends upon the size of the central scotoma. In advanced cases the neutral band extends to the long-wave end of the spectrum. But such patients will always recognize blue as being a color and name it as such.

A person with congenital dichromatopsia (protanopia or deuteranopia) also has a neutral area, but it is very small. This neutral point is situated in the "blue-green" region of the spectrum, at his *maximum* of hue discrimination. Presumably both residual pigments, or cone populations, are stimulated to the same degree by this wavelength.

Patients with optic atrophy of varying origins exhibit acquired color vision defects which are quite similar. They do not depend upon the etiology which may

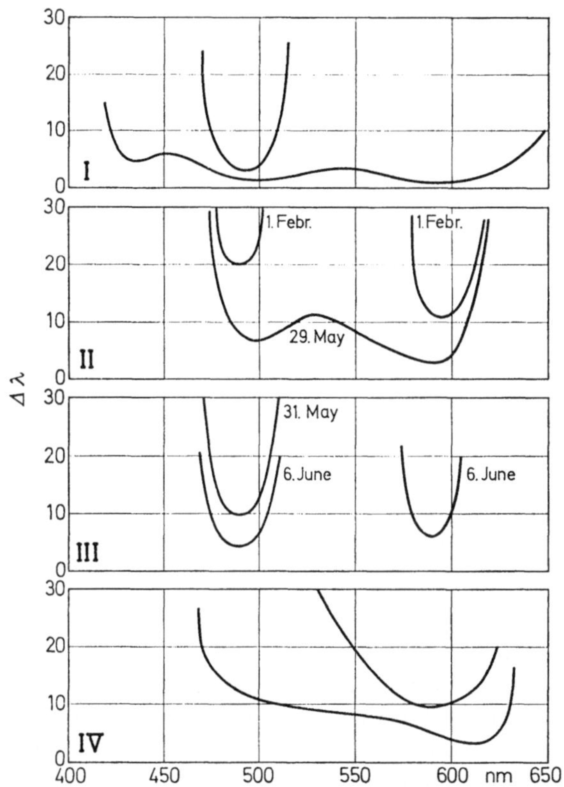

Fig. 6. Hue discrimination curves in patients with diseases of the optic nerve. I: in comparison with the responses of a person with normal color vision, and of an individual with congenital deuteranopia. II: responses of a patient with diminishing retrobulbar neuritis (visual acuity on Febr. 1st = 5/7.5, on May 29th = 5/4). III: responses of a patient with tobacco-alcohol amblyopia (visual acuity on May 31st = 5/35, on June 6th = 5/15). IV: results of two patients with infantile optic atrophy with dominant mode of inheritance

be trauma, intoxication, inflammation, or neoplasm. The location of the defect has no influence on the functional disturbance. The nerve fibers may be interrupted at the optic disc, in the chiasm, or just before the geniculate body with no discernible differences in the resultant abnormalities. Even an interruption of the visual pathway at a higher level may cause such an acquired color vision defect (Ohta and Kurata, 1967).

The resultant color vision deficiency seems to depend greatly on visual field defects. The deficiency is most pronounced in an eye where the papillomacular bundle is disturbed (e. g., by retrobulbar neuritis, tobacco-alcohol amblyopia, Leber's optic atrophy). Rählmann (1875) and Nagel (1905) long ago noted a similarity between the acquired color vision defect in patients with retrobulbar neuritis and the diminished color perceptions in the periphery of the normal retina. The low visual acuity of the periphery of the normal fundus is associated with a decrease of hue discrimination especially in the middle of the spectrum. (See Moreland, chapter 20, this volume).

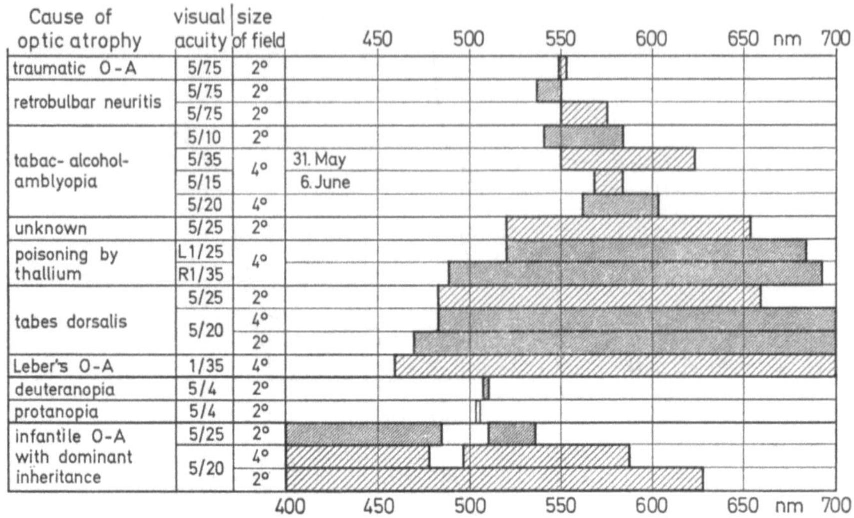

Fig. 7. Neutral bands in patients with diseases of the optic nerve, in comparison with the results in persons with congenital dichromatopsia (color temperature for the white light 3200° K)

Apparently many receptors must be stimulated for the perception of colors. Even a normal person cannot perceive a centrally located color if the stimulus is very small (SIEBECK, 1907), or if the time of exposure is very short (ZAHN, 1912). In patients with diseases of the optic nerve many fibers are interrupted. Only a few of them can forward the response received from the receptors to a higher level. If the stimulated area is large enough (i. e. if the responses of enough cones are integrated), colors are perceived. In the macular area of an eye with a relative scotoma resulting from optic atrophy, we note conditions similar to those found in the normal periphery of the fundus. The functioning cones are less dense than in the normal macular area. If there is a central scotoma, by definition we always do the measurements in a paracentral area.

However eccentric fixation by itself cannot be the cause for the pronounced color vision defect in patients with optic atrophy. Support for this statement is found in patients with strabismus and eccentric fixation where we see no remarkable deviation of color perception (OPPEL, 1963; FRANÇOIS and VERRIEST, 1967). Furthermore, in patients with inherited juvenile macular degeneration and central scotoma, there is a quite different type of acquired color vision defect.

Individuals with diseases of the optic nerve often perceive the ends of the visible spectrum as being colored even if the middle of the spectrum cannot be distinguished from white light (NAGEL, 1909). This is due to the fact that short or long wavelengths stimulate primarily only one of the three types of photoreceptors that are active under daylight conditions. The "green" mid-spectral lights stimulate all kinds of these receptors. Therefore these colors are most desaturated. A normal individual perceives white if all his receptors are stimulated to the same degree. This occurs for a light source characterized by a continuous spectrum, such as sunlight. Other broad-band distributions, such as the light from a fluorescent tube, may or may not have the same effect.

It is remarkable that in very advanced cases of such an acquired color vision deficiency "red" cannot be distinguished from "white", but "blue" is always perceived as a color. One explanation for this fact may be that the receptors sensitive to short-wave light (see p. 648) are more interconnected than those which are sensitive to the longer wavelengths. This "blue-system", therefore, has more avenues to advance the stimuli than do receptors which are more sensitive to the longer wavelengths.

Some patients with advanced diseases of the optic nerve are able to distinguish only two colors. Like persons with congenital dichromatopsia, they can match all colors of the spectrum with a mixture of two colors, taken from different portions of the spectrum – one on either side of the neutral zone (KÖLLNER, 1909, 1912). This is particularly true if the stimuli are complementary colors. The reasons for such measurements differ according to the color vision defect. For patients with optic atrophy, such measurements can be obtained because they perceive colors in the middle of the spectrum as highly desaturated. The results are proof of only a strongly diminished discrimination for hue and saturation. Therefore, the resulting curves do not really indicate the coefficient curves as they do in individuals with congenital dichromatopsia, where only two photosensitive pigments are presumably active.

It is rare that a traumatic optic atrophy is followed by a concentric contraction of the visual field. If there is such a field defect, it may be associated with a tritan defect (MARRÉ, 1969; GRÜTZNER, 1966). In our considerations of functional disturbances, the large group of patients with glaucoma belong to this category of optic atrophy. In glaucomatous eyes "the most characteristic finding in the retina is degeneration of the nerve fiber and ganglion cell layer" (HOGAN and ZIMMERMAN, 1962). The first functional disturbances in this disease are paracentral scotomas, and in advanced cases we also find a concentric contraction of the visual field. When color vision has been evaluated, the abnormality noted is most often a tritan defect (FRANÇOIS et VERRIEST, 1959; DUBOIS-POULSEN et MAGIS, 1961; VAN REY-KOKOTT, 1964; KURATA, 1967). Only ZIMMERMANN (1966), using the colored dots of TRENDELENBURG, described acquired red-green defects in such patients.

From a functional point of view, in glaucoma we have a situation similar to that seen in purely retinal diseases. Here, as there, we find paracentral scotomas and tritan defects. Such a combination of functional disturbances cannot be accidental. The different receptor systems seem to differ in their vulnerability. This may be responsible for the functional responses.

MARRÉ (1969) using WALD's bleaching method, found a general diminution of short-wave sensitivity to be prominent in diseases of the optic nerve, as is usually the case in diseases of the retina (Table 5). This was particularly true of patients with papilledema. It may be that the retina itself was affected by the edema. However, MARRÉ is convinced that this high vulnerability of the "*blue*" receptor can also be demonstrated in different forms of optic atrophy. MARRÉ's findings seem to be in direct opposition to the rest of the published findings. Although this supports the statement that acquired color vision defects never are as clear-cut as the inherited variety, some explanation is necessary.

Table 5. *Spectral sensitivities of the "blue"-, "green"-, and "red"-receptor mechanisms (B, G, R). Measurements on patients with diseases of the optic nerve. The percentage indicates the area under the curve, as compared with that of normal persons (from* Marré, *1969)*

Diagnosis	Visual acuity	B%	G%	R%
papilledema by intracranial pressure	0.9	83	99	95
	0.9	78	100	96
	1.0	78	92	99
	0.9	75	91	102
	1.0	66	94	105
	1.0	37	90	98
	0.7	74	77	95
optic atrophy	0.7	53	84	93
	0.2	37	35	34
	0.4	6	42	43
optic neuritis	0.6	57	61	71

Each disease process will damage all the structures where it is located and this is certainly the case if the fibers of the optic nerve are interrupted. It is unlikely, for example, that an inflammation would damage only special fibers. Since different fibers may be related to different kinds of stimuli, it seems reasonable to expect that the whole function of color vision will be diminished, and all colors will look desaturated. However, this will be more pronounced in the middle of the spectrum, where the absorption curves of the three pigments overlap and where the "normal" person's minimum of saturation is located. It is our present concept, that only one pigment is active at each end of the spectrum. Therefore, these wavelengths will be perceived as the "proper" color for a long time, even if the bleaching method shows that the elements responsible for blue perception are more affected than the others.

From a practical point of view, ophthalmologists test color vision to make a more accurate diagnosis or to make an estimate of progression or improvement in an affected eye. For this reason we use methods which are applicable in an ophthalmological office, such as pseudo-isochromatic plates, the Farnsworth-Munsell tests, and the Nagel anomaloscope. We always have to keep in mind, that acquired color vision defects have origins which are different from those of the inherited types.

Many patients with optic nerve diseases have functional responses similar to those of deutan defects. However, there is an exception in patients with an infantile optic atrophy with dominant mode of inheritance. These patients have very pronounced tritan defects. Their arrangement of the colors in the Farnsworth D-15 test is quite characteristic (Fig. 8), and their hue discrimination is remarkable diminished in the region of shorter wavelengths (Fig. 6). If a neutral band is found, it always begins at the short-wave end of the spectrum (Fig. 7). In contrast to the results obtained in patients with other types of optic atrophy, this along with other functional destruction may be an indication that this inherited disease is primarily

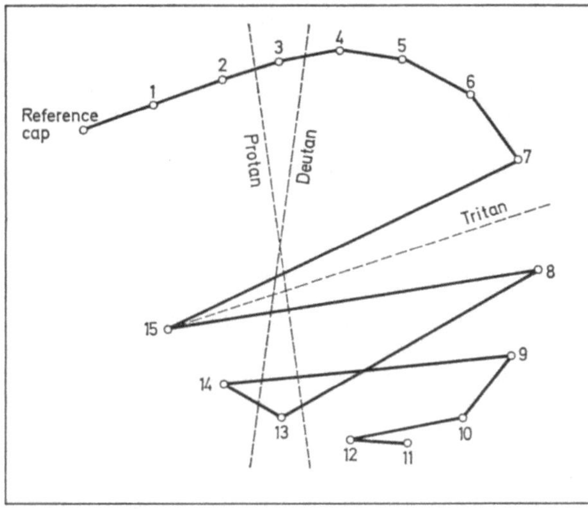

Fig. 8. Panel D-15 test from a patient with infantile optic atrophy with dominant mode of inheritance

one of retinal degeneration (JAEGER, 1954; GRÜTZNER, 1963). Yet, the only objective change is the pallor of the optic disk.

In one family with infantile optic atrophy and a dominant mode of inheritance, the affected members had an acquired protan-like defect. This finding was previously thought to be characteristic of and found only in juvenile macular degeneration (AULHORN and GRÜTZNER, 1969). These results seem to indicate that there are different genes causing the various types of infantile optic atrophy. The genotypes can be distinguished only by the different functional disturbances.

E. Differential Diagnostic Problems between Congenital and Acquired Color Vision Defects

Acquired color vision deficiencies are very common, and may imitate a congenital defect. If an "unusual" color vision defect is encountered, it is important to consider this possibility. Several papers dealing with monocular color vision deficiencies exemplify cases in which the possibility of an acquired defect was not considered. Without an ophthalmological examination and without the determination of other functional studies, it is definitely not justifiable to conclude a monocular and congenital color vision defect. In fact, a critical study demonstrated that the majority of such cases may have been acquired color vision defects (WEIL, 1964).

Tritan defects are quite common but are almost always acquired. Only a few of the so-called inherited tritanopes have been seen by an ophthalmologist and a definite diagnosis established (OHTA, 1969).

To evaluate the incidence of inherited color vision defects in the population one must use more than pseudo-isochromatic plates. One cannot distinguish between the inherited and the acquired defects by utilizing only these plates.

References

Aulhorn, E., Grützner, P.: Infantile optic atrophy with dominant mode of inheritance, accompanied by an acquired protanopia. (Proc. 2nd Congr. Neuro-Ophthal. and Neuro-Genetics, Montreal 1967). Internat. Congr. Ser. No. 176, Vol. II, 128—132. Amsterdam: Excerpta Medica Foundation 1969.

Brindley, G. S.: Physiology of the Retina and the Visual Pathway, pp. 248—249. London: Arnold 1960.

Cox, J.: Colour vision defects acquired in diseases of the eye. Brit. J. physiol. Opt., N. S. **17**, 195—216 (1960); **18**, 3—32, 67—79 (1961).

Dubois-Poulsen, A., Magis, C.: La dyschromatopsie du glaucome. Bull. Mém. Soc. franç. Ophthal. **74**, 25—31 (1961).

Engelking, E.: Über den methodischen Wert physiologischer Perimeterobjekte. Erfahrungen mit peripheriegleichen, invariablen Farben bei den angeborenen und erworbenen Störungen des Farben- und Lichtsinnes. Graefes Arch. Ophthal. **104**, 75—132 (1921).

— Schreck, E.: Über Farbensinnstörungen bei Netzhautoperierten. 52. Ber. dtsch. ophthal. Ges. 271—279 (1938).

François, J., Verriest, G.: Les dyschromatopsies acquises. Ann. Oculist. (Paris) **190**, 713—746, 812—859, 893—943 (1957).

— — Les dyschromatopsies acquises dans le glaucome primaire. Ann. Oculist. (Paris) **192**, 191—199 (1959).

— — La discrimination chromatique dans l'amblyopie strabique. Documenta Ophthal. **23**, 318—328 (1967).

— — Israel, A.: Périmétrie statique colorée effectuée à l'aide de l'appareil de Goldmann. Résultats obtenus en pathologie oculaire. Ann. Oculist. (Paris) **199**, 113—154 (1966).

Gärtner, J.: Technische Verbesserungen am Stereokampimeter nach Haitz. Klin. Mbl. Augenheilk. **131**, 676—678 (1957).

Grützner, P.: Typische erworbene Farbensinnstörungen bei heredodegenerativen Macula-leiden. Graefes Arch. Ophthal. **163**, 99—116 (1961).

— Maculäre Form der diffusen tapeto-retinalen Degeneration. Graefes Arch. Ophthal. **165**, 227—245 (1962).

— Über Diagnose und Funktionsstörungen bei der infantilen, dominant vererbten Opticus-Atrophie. 65. Ber. dtsch. ophthal. Ges. 268—273 (1963).

— Über erworbene Farbensinnstörungen bei Sehnervenerkrankungen. Graefes Arch. Ophthal. **169**, 366—384 (1966).

— Acquired color vision defects secondary to retinal drug toxicity. Ophthalmologica (Basel) Suppl. **158**, 592—604 (1969).

Hogan, M. J., Zimmerman, L. E.: Ophthalmic Pathology, 2nd Edition, pp. 714—716. Philadelphia: Saunders 1962.

Jaeger, W.: Dominant vererbte Opticusatrophie. Unter besonderer Berücksichtigung der dabei vorhandenen Farbensinnstörung. Graefes Arch. Ophthal. **155**, 457—484 (1954).

— Grützner, P.: Erworbene Farbensinnstörungen. In: Entwicklung und Fortschritt in der Augenheilkunde, Fortbildungskurs für Augenärzte, Hamburg, 1962, pp. 591—614. Stuttgart: Enke 1963.

— Nover, A.: Störungen des Lichtsinns und Farbensinns bei Chorioretinitis centralis serosa. Graefes Arch. Ophthal. **152**, 111—120 (1951).

Köhler, U.: Erworbene Farbsinnstörungen bei Erkrankungen des Sehnerven und der Macula mit dem Farbfleckverfahren nach Trendelenburg. Klin. Mbl. Augenheilk. **152**, 578—584 (1968).

Köllner, H.: Beiträge zur Pathologie des Farbensinnes. Erworbene totale Farbenblindheit mit Bericht über einen weiteren Fall. Z. Augenheilk. **21**, 193—204, 309—326 (1909).

— Die Störungen des Farbensinnes, ihre klinische Bedeutung und ihre Diagnose. Berlin: Karger 1912.

König, A.: Über „Blaublindheit". S.-B. Akad. Wiss., (Berlin) 718—731 (1897).

Kurata, K.: Study of color discrimination of subjects with acquired anomalous color vision. II. Color confusion in glaucomatous eyes due to fluctuation of brightness. Acta Soc. Ophthal. Jap. **71**, 223—229 (1967).

LAKOWSKI, R.: Is the deterioration of colour discrimination with age due to lens or retinal changes? Farbe **11**, 69—86 (1962).
— Psychological variables in colour vision testing. In: International Colour Meeting Stockholm 1969, pp. 79—86. Göttingen: Musterschmidt 1970.
MARRÉ, M.: Versuch einer quantitativen Analyse erworbener Farbensehstörungen. Wiener Ophthal. Ges., Wien 14. April 1969.
— Die Darstellung von drei Farbseh-Mechanismen bei erworbenen Farbenssehstörungen. In: International Colour Meeting Stockholm 1969, pp. 97—104. Göttingen: Musterschmidt 1970.
NAGEL, W.: Einige Beobachtungen über die Farbensinnstörung im Netzhautzentrum bei retrobulbärer Neuritis. Klin. Mbl. Augenheilk. **43 I**, 742—751 (1905).
— Über typische und atypische Farbensinnstörungen. Z. Sinnesphysiol. **43**, 299—309 (1909).
OHTA, Y.: One case of slight hemeralopia with tritanopia. Acta Chromatica **2**, 42—47 (1969).
— KURATA, K.: Studies on acquired anomalous color vision. Color sense anomalies in patients with lesions of the optic nerve, optic chiasme and post-occipital center. Acta Soc. Ophthal. Jap. **71**, 771—778 (1967).
OPPEL, O.: Vergleichende Farbsinnuntersuchungen zwischen normalen und schielamblyopen Augen. Graefes Arch. Ophthal. **165**, 387—391 (1963).
RÄHLMANN, E.: Über den Farbensinn bei Sehnervenerkankungen. Graefes Arch. Ophthal. **21**, II, 27—66 (1875).
REY-KOKOTT, U. VAN: Über erworbene Farbensinnstörungen bei Glaukom. Inaug. Diss. Med. Fak. Heidelberg 1964.
RUDDOCK, K. H.: The effect of age upon colour vision. II. Changes with age in light transmission of the ocular media. Vision Res. **5**, 47—58 (1965).
SIEBECK, R.: Über Minimalfeldhelligkeiten. Z. Sinnesphysiol. **41**, 89—101 (1907).
WAARDENBURG, P. J.: Genetics and Ophthalmology. Vol. II, p. 1583. Assen, Netherlands: Royal Van Gorkum 1963.
WALD, G.: Defective color vision and its inheritance. Proc. nat. Acad. Sci. (Wash.) **55**, 1347 to 1363 (1966).
— Blue-blindness in the normal fovea. J. opt. Soc. Amer. **57**, 1289—1301 (1967).
WEIL, K.: Gibt es eine angeborene, einseitige Farbensinnstörung? Inaug. Diss. Med. Fak. Heidelberg 1964.
ZAHN, A.: Über die Helligkeitswerte reiner Lichter bei kurzen Wirkungszeiten. Z. Sinnesphysiol. **46**, 287—300 (1912).
ZANEN, J., MEUNIER, A.: La perception colorée et les seuils absolus et chromatiques dans la rétinopathie séreuse centrale. Bull. Soc. Belge Ophthal. **140**, 359—369 (1965).
ZIMMERMAN, U.: Farbsinnstörungen bei Glaukom. Klin. Mbl. Augenheilk. **148**, 845—850 (1966).

Added in proof. For further information see: Proceedings of the International Symposium on Acquired Colour Vision Deficiencies, Ghent 1971. Modern Problems of Opthalmology, Vol. 11. Basel: Karger 1972.

Chapter 26

Visual Scaling

By

David H. Krantz, Ann Arbor, Michigan (USA)

Contents

"Scaling" refers to a family of procedures that attempt to give quantitative descriptions of perceptual attributes. The first part of this chapter discusses the three main families of scaling procedures: confusability scaling, direct estimation, and multidimensional scaling. Several applications of these procedures are described in the second part: scaling of brightness, hue and saturation, and color differences are discussed in some detail, and brief mention is made of work on space and form perception.

Scaling Methods

Confusability Scaling I: Parallel Psychometric Functions

The simplest way to obtain a scale based on stimulus confusions is by defining the just-noticeable difference (JND) as a unit of "sensation" difference. One then counts numbers of JND's to establish the scale. For example, take an arbitrary luminance x as the zero-point of an interval scale of brightness. If y is a light that is just-noticeably brighter than x, then y has brightness 1; if z is just-noticeably brighter than y (two JND's above x), z is assigned brightness 2; etc.

A more precise formulation of the above procedure requires specification of two things:

(i) the method by which discrimination is tested;

(ii) the numerical value of confusion probability, or of some other discriminability index, which is taken to define just-noticeable differences.

The scale constructed by counting JND's will be quite useless unless it remains invariant, or at least transforms in a simple way, when these two specifications are changed. These invariance requirements will now be considered in more detail.

First, suppose that there is a fixed method of testing discrimination, which leads to a numerical index $r(y, x)$ of the discriminability of y from x. For example, in one method of testing luminance discrimination, $r(y, x)$ might be the probability that y is judged brighter than x; in another method, $r(y, x)$ might be the value of d' obtained by signal detectability methods. (See NACHMIAS, chapter 3, this volume); or still another method would take $r(y, x)$ to be the speed of reaction when x is replaced by y. The arguments x, y are considered to be values on an ordered continuum, such as luminance; the index r is an increasing function of the first variable, and a decreasing function of the second one; and $r(x, x)$ is a constant, independent of x. For a fixed x, the function plotting $r(y, x)$ against y is called the *psychometric function* (an indefensible, but seemingly well-established term).

For a fixed method, any value of r except $r(x, x)$ can be taken to define a JND (of course, values near $r(x, x)$, or values in the range of near-perfect discrimination, are impractical). For a fixed value of r (say, $r(y, x) = s$), the increment in x needed to produce that fixed value of discriminability is denoted $\Delta_s(x)$, and is called the Weber function. That is, for all x,

$$r[x + \Delta_s(x), x] = s. \tag{1}$$

Weber's Law is the generalization that Weber functions have the following form:

$$\Delta_s(x) = k(s)\,(x + x_0), \tag{2}$$

where x_0 is a constant (usually interpreted as internal noise) independent of s. The proportionality constant $k(s)$ is called the Weber fraction. A more familiar form of the same law is $\Delta x/(x + x_0) = k$. The insertion of x_0 accounts for the rise in $\Delta x/x$ for small values of x, and yields a good approximation to a wide range of discrimination data from different modalities.

Using the psychometric function, $r(y, x)$, and the Weber function, $\Delta_s(x)$, we can now return to the question of how the JND scale changes when varying numerical values of r are used to define a JND. The desired result, of course, is that changes in the numerical definition of JND cause all JND-scale differences to be multiplied by a constant factor, representing the value of the old unit difference (old JND) in terms of the new units. LUCE and EDWARDS (1958) showed that a necessary and sufficient condition for JND scales to transform in this way, with changes in the defining numerical value of r, is that there exists a transformation,

$$x \to u(x),$$

of the physical continuum that renders all psychometric functions parallel. Mathematically, there must be a solution (u, g) to the following equation:

$$r(y, x) = g^{-1}[u(y) - u(x)]. \tag{3}$$

Intuitively, Eq. (3) says that equal u-scale differences are discriminated equally well; the function g^{-1} is the psychometric function relating u-scale difference to discriminability. Using Eq. (1), we can rewrite Eq. (3) as

$$g(s) = u[x + \Delta_s(x)] - u(x), \tag{3'}$$

i. e., $g(s)$ is the u-scale difference (sensation difference?) corresponding to discriminability level s. The conditions under which the u-transformation exists have been investigated by FALMAGNE (1971) and LEVINE (1970). In general, the u-transformation, if it exists at all, is unique up to changes of origin and unit.

If Eq. (3) has a solution, then any JND-scale is linear with the u-scale. Thus, one way to proceed is to use one or more JND-scales to estimate the u-scale, and then to test whether the u-scale, so estimated, renders all the psychometric functions parallel. If so, then the JND-scales for different numerical criteria are mutually consistent.

If the Weber function, $\Delta_s(x)$, is given as a definite function of s and x, then one can apply FALMAGNE's criteria to determine whether a solution to Eq. 3 exists, and one can calculate the solution (the u-scale) from $\Delta_s(x)$ by various means. One method is to approximate $u(x)$ by

$$\int \frac{dx}{\Delta_s(x)};$$

if the approximations are normalized to have fixed zero and unit, then they converge to the u-scale as $g(s) \to 0$ (KRANTZ, 1971). This seems to have been FECHNER's idea, when he passed from Weber's Law to his famous logarithmic law. In fact, if one substitues Eq. (2) in the integrand, one obtains

$$\int \frac{dx}{k(s)\,(x + x_0)} = [1/k(s)] \log (x + x_0)\,.$$

Normalizing removes the factor $[1/k(s)]$; in this case no passage to the limit is needed. By substituting in Eq. (3), using Eq. (2), one can easily verify that

$$\begin{aligned} u(x) &= a + b \log (x + x_0), \\ g(s) &= b \log [1 + k(s)] \end{aligned} \tag{4}$$

is a solution to Eq. (3). The logarithmic relation between u and x is known as FECHNER's Law.

Other methods for obtaining u from $\Delta_s(x)$ are discussed by LUCE and EDWARDS (1958), FALMAGNE (1971), and LEVINE (1970). It should be emphasized, however, that in general, no u-scale can be had; even for Weber functions as simple as

$$\Delta_s(x) = k(s)[x + x_0(s)], \quad \text{or} \quad \Delta_s(x) = k(s)\,(x + x_0)^n,$$

no solution to Eq. (3) exists (unless $x_0(s)$ is constant or unless $n = 1$, respectively).

This concludes our discussion of invariance of JND-scales under changes in the numerical definition of the JND.

Next, consider two different methods of evaluating discriminability, leading to different indices, r and r', and correspondingly, to different Weber functions, $\Delta_s(x)$ and $\Delta'_{s'}(x)$. Invariance demands that the same scale u render both sets of psychometric functions parallel, i. e., that (u, g) and (u, g') be respectively solutions to Eq. (3) with the unprimed and primed Weber functions. Conditions leading to such u-scale invariance were studied by FALMAGNE (1971). In particular, he investigated the case where the ratio $\Delta_s(x)/\Delta'_{s'}(x)$ is independent of x. This finding was reported by PIÉRON (1936), for luminance discrimination, with response speed and probability as the two indices. The equation expressing this finding,

$$\frac{\Delta_s(x)}{\Delta'_{s'}(x)} = h(s, s'), \tag{5}$$

is called Piéron's Law, by FALMAGNE. FALMAGNE proved that, under rather general conditions, Piéron's Law implies that Weber's Law [Eq. (2)] holds for both Δ and Δ', with the same value of x_0, and hence, that the logarithmic transformation renders both sets of psychometric functions parallel.

Clearly, if the transformation $x \to u(x)$ renders parallel the psychometric functions obtained by a particular method, and remains invariant with changes in method, then it is a valuable device for organizing and simplifying discrimination data. Whether such a u-scale should be called "sensation" is another matter. In my view, "sensation" should only be defined in the context of a *theory* relating stimulus intensity to discrimination or to other kinds of psychophysical judgments. The next subsection, therefore, presents Thurstone's theory of discrimination. In the context of this theory, a "sensation" function is defined that under some conditions (Thurstone Case V) coincides with the u-scale, but otherwise may differ from it.

Confusability Scaling II: Discriminal Processes

This section has two purposes. First, it illustrates the importance of a theory of discrimination for the interpretation of confusability scaling. Second, it introduces the principal methods of Thurstonian scaling, which are still among the mainstays of psychometrics. For a more general survey of discrimination theory, consult LUCE and GALANTER (1963a).

THURSTONE (1927a, b) postulated that each stimulus produces a variable effect on an hypothetical scale of internal effects, or "sensation". The variability is described by a normally distributed random variable, called a *discriminal process*. If a subject is asked whether x or y is more intense, he samples randomly from the bivariate normal distribution defined by the two discriminal processes, and chooses whichever value is higher. Suppose that the means and standard deviations of the two discriminal processes are respectively $S(x)$, $\sigma(x)$ and $S(y)$, $\sigma(y)$ and that the correlation is $\varrho(y, x)$. The probability that y is judged more intense than x, denoted $P(y, x)$, is simply the probability that the difference between the sampled y sensation and the sampled x sensation is positive. This sample difference has a normal distribution, with mean $S(y) - S(x)$ and with standard deviation $\sigma(y, x)$, where

$$\sigma(y, x) = [\sigma(y)^2 - 2\varrho(y, x)\,\sigma(y)\,\sigma(x) + \sigma(x)^2]^{1/2}. \tag{6}$$

Therefore

$$P(y,x) = f^{-1}\left[\frac{S(y) - S(x)}{\sigma(y,x)}\right], \tag{7}$$

where f^{-1} denotes the cumulative normal distribution function, i. e.,

$$f^{-1}(t) = \int_{-\infty}^{t} (2\pi)^{-1/2}\, e^{-w^2/2}\, dw.$$

The analogy between Eq. (7) (Thurstone's Law of Comparative Judgment) and Eq. (3) is obvious. In particular, if both $\sigma(x)$ and $\varrho(y, x)$ are constant, then $\sigma(y, x)$, defined by Eq. (6), is constant, and Eq. (7) reduces to Eq. (3). This is called Thurstone's Case V. In this case, $u(x)$ can be identified with $S(x)$, the mean of the discriminal process (and the u-scale psychometric function, g^{-1}, becomes the normal ogive, f^{-1}). If the discriminal process were considered to represent random variation in sensation, then $u(x) = S(x)$ would be the mean sensation evoked by x. Thus, Fechner's Law of sensation would be justified.

On the other hand, if Thurstone's Law of Comparative Judgment [Eq. (7)] holds, but Case V is inapplicable, i. e., $\sigma(y, x)$ is nonconstant, then we have a basis for distinguishing between the u-scale and sensation; in fact, the S-scale (mean of discriminal process) may better represent sensation, in this theoretical context. A case of particular interest is the assumption that the correlation, $\sigma(y, x)$, is a function of the discriminability, $P(y, x)$, i. e., for some function h,

$$\varrho(y, x) = h[P(y, x)].$$

In this case, it can be shown that Eqs. (3) and (7) (with $P = r$) are satisfied simultaneously [with a suitable g in Eq. (3)] for

$$\begin{aligned} u(x) &= a' + b' \log (x + x_0), \\ S(x) &= a + b(x + x_0)^B, \\ \sigma(x) &= c(x + x_0)^B. \end{aligned} \tag{8}$$

Eq. (8) mean that Weber's Law holds, that Fechner's Law (the logarithmic transform) renders the psychometric functions parallel, but that the *standard deviation* σ *of the discriminal process is a linear function of its mean,* $\sigma = (c/b)\ (S - a)$, and that sensation, S, follows a *power law.* (Stevens, 1959, referred to this as "Case VI" of Thurstone's Law of comparative judgment.) The power function, in a slightly different form, is called Stevens' Law, though it is usually based on direct estimation rather than on confusability scaling.

The usual methods of obtaining scale values from the Law of Comparative Judgment [Eq. (7)] do not involve measurement of psychometric functions; rather, they make direct use of special cases of Eq. (7). For example, for Thurstone's Case V we have

$$S(y) - S(x) = \sigma \cdot f[P(y, x)], \tag{9}$$

where σ is a constant, which can be normalized at 1. Thus, the difference between the scale values of two stimuli is given directly as the inverse normal transform, f, of the pairwise choice probability. In the *method of paired comparisons*, one observes $P(x_i, x_j)$ for all $n(n - 1)/2$ pairs of n stimuli, $x_1, \ldots, x_n$. Equation 9 is applied to get $n(n - 1)/2$ estimates $S(x_i) - S(x_j)$. There are really only $n - 1$

independent parameters — the differences $S(x_{i+1}) - S(x_i)$ — so the parameters are overdetermined, and one can test the applicability of Eq. 9. Even if $\sigma(x)$ is not assumed constant, so that $\sigma(x_i)$ is estimated, $i = 1, ..., n$, there are still many fewer parameters than estimation equations, if n is at all large. (This latter situation is called Case III.) Methods for estimation and statistical testing in these cases are given by TORGERSON (1958) and by BOCK and JONES (1968).

The method of paired comparisons is very economical compared with laborious determination of many psychometric functions, and moreover, is applicable to cases where there is no natural physical continuum ordering the stimuli (e. g., to judgments of emotionality of faces). Because of this last feature, Thurstone's methods produced a great wave of psychometric research beginning in the 1930's. Their economy and extended applicability are bought, however, at the price of strong assumptions. While minor violations of the normality assumption are probably unimportant, constancy of correlations, $\varrho(y, x)$, is often violated very systematically (see next subsection, on criticisms of confusability scaling).

A popular alternative to the method of paired comparisons is the *method of category rating*. Subjects are presented one stimulus at a time and respond with one of m categories, $1, ..., m$, under instructions to put more intense stimuli in higher categories. The Thurstonian model for this task postulates that the underlying sensation continuum is partitioned by the subject into m regions, by $m - 1$ category boundaries, and that the subject samples randomly from a discriminal process and responds according to the position of the sampled sensation relative to the category boundaries. The data are nm frequencies — $n(m - 1)$ of them independent — i. e., the frequencies that the ith stimulus evokes response category j. In addition to the stimulus parameters, $S(x_i)$ and possibly $\sigma(x_i)$, one must estimate positions (and sometimes variances also) of the category boundaries. The virtue of this method is economy; if m is sufficiently smaller than n, estimation of mn frequencies is very economical compared with performing $n(n - 1)/2$ pair comparisons; and if some of the frequencies are zero, little harm is done [whereas, if $P(y, x)$ is estimated to be 0, or nearly zero, then the pair comparison observations on the pair y, x are rather uninformative]. The disadvantage of the category method is that the postulated model is an unlikely one (see next subsection) for replicated data from individual subjects.

An alternative to the normal-distribution assumptions was introduced by BRADLEY and TERRY (1952), LUCE (1959), and RASCH (1960). In its simplest form, it merely substitutes the logistic for the normal distribution, but there are many rich offshoots, especially well-developed by LUCE. For recent work on this model, see BRADLEY (1966), RASCH (1966), and THOMPSON and SINGH (1967).

Criticisms of Confusability Scaling

The main criticism of confusability scaling is that discriminability of stimuli is related only in an indirect and complex way (if at all) to the sensations evoked by them (STEVENS, 1961). Some of the possible complexities of this relation are incorporated into the Thurstone theory [e. g., nonconstancy of $\sigma(y, x)$ in Eq. (7) above]; within the framework of this theory, it became clear that one ought not identify JND-scale values, or Case V scale values, as sensation measures, without critically examining the Case V assumption. Still, even the general Thurstone model in Eq. (7) cannot cope with the possible issues that may arise.

First, in many paradigms of discrimination testing, discrimination is based on detection of the "transients" produced by a shift in stimulus level. The size of such "transients" may bear a very complex relation to the steadystate "sensations" evoked by each stimulus level in isolation.

A second factor that decouples discriminability from sensations is the presence of irrelevant dimensions. For example, suppose that we tried to use the paired comparison method to establish a brightness scale for monochromatic lights of varying wavelength. Consider four lights: $x = (560\text{ nm}, 100\text{ mL})$, $y = (560\text{ nm}, 101\text{ mL})$, $z = (600\text{ nm}, 110\text{ mL})$, $w = (600\text{ nm}, 111.1\text{ mL})$. Because the difference in hue between x and z makes the brightness judgment more difficult, we might well have $P(y, x) = P(z, x) = P(w, z)$, even when the brightness difference between z and x is considerably larger than those between y and x or between w and z. It is impossible to account for this type of effect by any conceivable values of $\sigma(x)$, $\sigma(y)$, etc. One could postulate that ϱ decreases as the hue difference increases, but the quantitative manner in which this occurs remains to be elucidated before Thurstonian methods can be applied. This type of problem is especially prevalent in just those situations — having complex, multidimensional stimuli — where Thurstonian methods were once hailed as revolutionary. Demonstrations of this point, in situations where confusability scaling has been seriously proposed, are discussed by COOMBS (1964, Chap. 23), KRANTZ (1964, pp. 25–27 and 1967a) and TVERSKY and RUSSO (1969). These results suggest that confusability scaling must either (i) be restricted to cases where there are no "irrelevant" dimensions or where "irrelevant" dimensions produce only small effects, or (ii) be preceded by a careful study of the ways in which ϱ and σ vary. The worthwhileness of the latter type of study must be judged on its own merits in each case.

Apart from the role of irrelevant dimensions, there are other complicating factors that may influence stimulus confusions, e. g., memory, adaptation level, and response biases. It is not possible to enter here into a detailed analysis of these factors (for references, see discussion of direct estimation below). However, it is obvious that if the subject remembers one or more previous "sensations," and his responses to them, and judges a given stimulus relative to these, then the Thurstone model for category rating (involving only comparison of sensations with boundaries) can be a gross oversimplification of the actual process of assigning categories. This sort of difficulty is probably minimized in signal-detection paradigms (see NACHMIAS, chapter 3, this volume), where normal distribution assumptions are tested and shown to fit quite nicely, and is maximized in uncritical application of the method of category rating.

Two conclusions concerning confusability scaling seem justified:

1. If a u-scale exists, which renders psychometric functions parallel, and which is invariant over several methods, then its usefulness as a rescaling device is undeniable.

2. The interpretation of u-scale values, or scale values derived from variants of Thurstone's theory, as measures of an internal process labelled "sensation,"

depends, in each case, on careful, detailed examination of the empirical validity of the theory used to account for the subjects' judgments. The presence of factors such as "transients", irrelevant dimensions, memory, bias, etc. means that a simple Thurstonian theory is likely to be applicable only for very carefully designed experiments, if at all.

Direct Estimation I: Methods und Results

TORGERSON (1958) discusses details of a variety of direct estimation methods. A summary of results and theories may be found in LUCE and GALANTER (1963b). Here, discussion is confined to three methods: magnitude estimation, cross-modality matching, and category rating.

In *magnitude estimation* of brightness (for example), lights of different luminance are presented singly, and the subjects are instructed to assign numbers to them "in proportion to the apparent brightness" (J. C. STEVENS and S. S. STEVENS, 1963). In the second method, *cross-modality matching* (J. C. STEVENS *et al.*, 1960; S. S. STEVENS, 1966), subjects are instructed to produce a stimulus on one continuum that matches a given stimulus on another continuum (e. g., to match the brightness of a light by adjusting the loudness of a tone or the force on a handgrip). Finally, the method of *category rating* was discussed above as a method of confusability scaling – subjects attempt to divide the intensive continuum into categories. It becomes a method of direct estimation if observers are instructed, or instruct, themselves, to use category ratings that are "equally spaced" with respect to "sensation."

It has not generally been recognized that all direct estimation methods implicitly force the observer to make *comparative judgments of two or more pairs of stimuli*. For example, the instruction to assign numbers "in proportion" clearly means that the observer must not respond only to the present stimulus in isolation, rather, he must remember the brightness of one or more previous stimuli, and the corresponding number(s) previously assigned, and must match the ratios of present to previous numbers to the "ratios" of present to previous brightnesses. The observer, in trying to match a pair of numbers (one of them remembered) to a pair of brightnesses (one of them remembered), must make a comparative judgment (of equality) of two pairs. The above argument is even more obvious when it comes to cross-modality matching, where, for example, a pair of brightnesses is matched to a pair of loudnesses. In category rating, observers try to match the difference, rather than the ratio, of category numbers to the "difference" in sensation.

From the above standpoint, the critical question for interpretation of direct estimation results is the following: *What properties of stimulus pairs form the basis for ordering and matching them, and how are such properties of pairs related to "sensation?"* Before dealing with this question, we should briefly consider the various empirical results that bear on it.

Since Weber's Law [Eq. (2)] holds, to a rough approximation, for luminance discrimination (LE GRAND, 1968, Chap. 11; see also BLACKWELL, chapter 4, this volume), the Fechnerian function $u(x) = \log(x + x_0)$ renders psychometric functions approximately parallel. However, superficial examination of a series of gray papers, spaced equally on a log scale of reflectance, or a series of lights spaced by equal logarithmic steps, suffices to indicate that the logarithmic scale is somehow "wrong" as a description of sensation. The logarithmic scale for lightness was rejected very early by PLATEAU (1873) and later by MUNSELL (1915). The basis for rejecting it consists of the judgment that the pairs of stimuli, separated by equal logarithmic steps, are nonetheless unequal in respect to some perceptual property or properties pertaining to pairs. The direct estimation methods require observers to deal with precisely such perceptual properties of pairs ("sensation ratios" or "sensation differences"). We turn therefore to a brief summary of the results using direct estimation.

STEVENS (1957) summarized evidence that for a great many (so called Class I, or *prothetic*) one-dimensional stimulus continua, the mean (or median) magnitude estimate $\psi(x)$ increases approximately as a power function of stimulus intensity x:

$$\psi(x) \approx bx^B. \tag{10}$$

The exponent, B, he considers to characterize the continuum (though it may vary somewhat with individuals or with stimulating conditions, e. g., state of adaptation). This exponent is generally estimated from the slope of the function in log-log coordinates, i. e., from

$$\log \psi(x) \approx \log b + B \log x. \tag{10'}$$

Variants of Eq. (10), that produce better fits for low values of x, are

$$\psi(x) \approx b(x - x_0)^B, \tag{11}$$

$$\psi(x) \approx bx^B - \psi_0, \tag{12}$$

$$\psi(x) \approx b[(x + x_0)^B - x_0^B]. \tag{13}$$

Eq. (11) is used regularly by STEVENS. JAMESON and HURVICH (1964) favor Eq. (12), because the subtractive constant ψ_0 gives a good account of simultaneous contrast effects; they present a theory by which its value can be predicted. Eq. (13) is a special case of the form given above in Eq. (8), which arises from the combination of Weber's Law and Thurstone's Law of Comparative Judgment. In situations where simultaneous or successive contrast is involved, the virtues of Eqs. (12) and (13) may need to be combined, by use of the general form given in Eq. (8). All the variants in Eqs. (10—13) have asymptotic slope B when log ψ is plotted against $\log x$; for $0<B<1$, the slopes for small values of x are steeper than B, which is what is needed to fit most data.

Studies of cross-modality matching (J. C. STEVENS *et al.*, 1960; S. S. STEVENS, 1966) show that the matching-stimulus intensity grows approximately as a power function of test-stimulus intensity, with exponent roughly equal to the ratio of the exponents obtained from magnitude estimation for the two continua. For example, let x denote luminance, y force of handgrip, and let ψ_L denote the magnitude-estimation scale for brightness and ψ_F the same scale for perceived force. We have

$$\psi_L(x) \approx b_L x^{0.33},$$

$$\psi_F(y) \approx b_F y^{1.7}.$$

Setting $\psi_L = \psi_F$ (cross-modality matching), we have

$$y \approx bx^{0.33/1.7} \approx bx^{0.20}$$

(where $b = [b_L/b_F]^{1/1.7}$). The obtained slope (J. C. STEVENS *et al.*, 1960) when log matching handgrip force is plotted against log luminance is precisely 0.20. As illustrated, then, the results of magnitude estimation and cross-modality matching yield a very consistent picture.

Although the results of magnitude estimation and of cross-modality matching yield a pretty picture of consistency, the relation of these results to category rating remains an outstanding puzzle. It is possible to analyze category data in two ways: by estimating the means of the (assumed) underlying normal distributions (and their variances, and the category boundaries) or more simply, by calculating the mean category response to each stimulus. The former (Thurstonian) analysis assumes that the subjects can judge the *order* between a momentary sampled sensation and the remembered sensation corresponding to a category boundary; while the second analysis makes the assumption that subjects' category responses are based on *equating (hence, ordering) sensation differences*. The second method of analysis, based on assumptions closely related to those of magnitude estimation, yields scale values for stimuli that are nonlinearly related to the corresponding magnitude estimation values. The scales constructed by these two types of analyses are sometimes referred to as processed category scales and (equi) partition scales, respectively.

Direct Estimation II: Ideal Theory

This subsection sketches a theory of "ideal" direct estimation behavior. The sense in which the "ideal" differs from actual direct estimation behavior will be brought out in the succeeding subsection. The theory sketched here is based on unpublished work by R. N. SHEPARD (see KRISTOF, 1967, and KRANTZ, 1972). Its ground is the observation noted earlier, that all direct estimation methods implicitly force the observer to order or equate *pairs* of stimuli.

Suppose that the subject judges stimuli that may be drawn from any one of n continua, $X_1, X_2, \ldots, X_n$. Physical measures of stimuli on continuum X_i are denoted x_i, y_i, etc. The continuum X_1 is the one that controls the subject's use of numbers in magnitude estimation; most likely, X_1 is line length. Any pair (w_i, x_i) of stimuli in X_i can be ordered relative to any pair (y_j, z_j) in X_j (where possibly $i = j$). This ordering is based on some unknown property of stimulus pairs, which we shall call a "sensation ratio." Thus, $(w_i, x_i) \geqq (y_j, z_j)$ means that the "sensation ratio" of w_i to x_i is at least as large as the "sensation ratio" of y_j to z_j.

In a cross-modality matching experiment involving continua X_i and X_j, the subject, having matched x_i with z_j, and being presented w_i to match, searches for y_j such that $(w_i, x_i) = (y_j, z_j)$ (with respect to this underlying ordering of pairs). In magnitude estimation, the subject performs cross-modality matching between X_i and X_1, basing his numbers on learned numerical relations in X_1. Thus, luminance w_i is judged to be "twice as bright" as luminance x_i provided that, with respect to the underlying "sensation ratio" property of pairs, (w_i, x_i) is matched by a pair of lines whose physical ratio is two to one.

The basic law of this theory is the following:

$$\textit{If } (x_i, x_i') \geqq (y_j, y_j') \textit{ and } (x_i', x_i'') \geqq (y_j', y_j''), \quad \textit{then } (x_i, x_i'') \geqq (y_j, y_j''). \tag{14}$$

A closely related law was tested by FAGOT and STEWART (1969). If (14) is valid, and if certain other technical axioms are valid, then it can be shown (see KRANTZ, 1972) that there exist scales ψ_i on X_i such that

$$(x_i, x_i') \geqq (y_j, y_j') \textit{ if and only if } \psi_i(x_i)/\psi_i(x_i') \geqq \psi_j(y_j)/\psi_j(y_j'). \tag{15}$$

Moreover, these scales are unique up to transformations of the form $\psi_i \to a_i \psi_i^B$. If the scale ψ_1 on X_1 can be taken to be the identity function (e. g., judgments of line-length ratios are veridical), then the ψ_i are ratio scales and are given directly by magnitude estimation.

The additional property that Stevens' Law holds can be characterized easily as follows:

$$\textit{For any positive } t, (x_i, y_i) = (tx_i, ty_i). \tag{16}$$

This is equivalent to Eq. 10; it can easily be adapted for other forms of Stevens' Law [Eqs. (8), (11), (12), or (13)].

This ideal theory, then, asserts that magnitude estimation and cross-modality matching are based on an *ordering of the pairs of stimuli* within each modality, with numbers assigned according to their learned use in a special modality such as line length (perhaps numerousness could be used instead). The ordering satisfies property (14), and perhaps, to a good approximation, (16) or some variant of it.

The theory accounts for STEVENS' main results from cross-modality matching and magnitude estimation experiments. If it is accepted, it raises a further puzzle: what is the sensory basis of the underlying ordering of stimulus pairs? Resolution of this latter question may be quite important in determining whether the scale values obtained by direct estimation should be called "sensation," since we do not know how the ordering of stimulus pairs relates to other sensory processes, like discrimination. Some of the results to be discussed in the sections on brightness and hue scaling suggest, however, that the relation to other sensory processes is a quite natural one.

Among the things that require clarification is the relation of the above ordering of pairs to the results of category rating experiments. Three views have been proposed.

STEVENS (1957) believes that subjects really can judge "sensation differences," i. e., can establish an ordering of pairs distinct from the ordering of "sensation ratios." Implicitly, he must assume that the two orderings of pairs interlock in the right way so that a single sensation scale can predict the "ratio" judgments by ratios of scale values and the "difference" judgments by differences of scale values. In this view, one should expect the partition scale (average category ratings) to be consistent with the magnitude estimation scale. STEVENS explains the observed nonlinear relation between these scales by arguing that subjects are "misled" by discriminability to stretch the lower end of the scale, where discriminability is better, thus distorting the true scale.

The other two views assume that the true relation between magnitude and category scales is not linear but rather is approximately logarithmic (deviations from this logarithmic relation being the distortions). TORGERSON (1961) derives this by assuming that subjects really order pairs in the same way when they are asked to judge "differences" as when they are given "ratio" instructions. Since the theorist varies the representation according to the instructions given, representing the pair (x_i, y_i) by either $\psi_i(x_i)/\psi_i(y_i)$ or by $\psi_i'(x_i) - \psi_i'(y_i)$, one obtains the relation $\psi_i' = \log \psi_i$.

The other derivation of the logarithmic relation is based on the idea that the Thurstonian model of category rating describes behavior. That is, subjects are not judging "differences" at all; discrimination, STEVENS' "distorting factor," now becomes the sole explanatory factor for the observations. The logarithmic relation is based on subjects' tendency to make the same average error at all points on the scale ("equiprecision" scale). If the true scale of mean sensation is a power function, and standard deviations grow linearly with the means, then [see Eq. (8) above] the logarithmic transformation renders psychometric functions identical at all points of the scale. Under these circumstances, the JND scale will be logarithmic, as pointed out earlier; but furthermore, it is assumed that subjects reproduce the JND scale in their category ratings, i. e., they impose the logarithmic transformation on their sensations in order to obtain an "equiprecision" scale. (The same result can be derived without assuming that sensation is a power function.) This is essentially the view espoused by EISLER (1962a, 1963a, 1965) and by HELM *et al.* (1961). Empirical support for this view has been obtained from careful studies of category rating by GALANTER and MESSICK (1961) and by EISLER (1962b, 1963b). EISLER has taken particular pains to account for the fact that partition scales are not precisely the same as JND scales; GALANTER and MESSICK obtained processed category scales that are logarithmically related to magnitude estimation scales from the same subjects.

Although this third view seems to have won the field, there are still some puzzles. For one thing, if it is really true that subjects judge sensation pairs, then the relation of the sensation scale, constructed from these pair judgments, to discrimination needs to be rethought. Perhaps the discrimination index $r(y, x)$ simply orders pairs in much the same way as do the supraliminal judgments of "sensation ratios." No logarithmic transformation for equipartition need be assumed. Secondly, it may still be that subjects can order pairs in another way, when instructed to judge "sensation differences;" more empirical work on this is needed. If two different empirical orderings of pairs, $\geqq$ and $\geqq'$, are to be describable by means of the same scale ψ, the first ordering using ψ-ratios and the second one using ψ-differences, then a critical interlocking property must be satisfied:

If $(x, x^\star) = (y, y^\star) = (z, z^\star)$ (equal "sensation ratios"), then $(x, y) \geqq' (y, z)$ ("sensation differences") if and only if $(x^\star, y^\star) \geqq' (y^\star, z^\star)$. Even if this property holds, and both $\geqq$ and $\geqq'$ satisfy Eq. (14), the scales constructed from "sensation ratios" and from "sensation differences" may need to be modified before they coincide: the "ratio" scale can be changed by an arbitrary power transformation (same exponent on all continua that have been interlocked by cross-modality matching) and the "difference" scale can be changed by an arbitrary translation (choice of zero).

Further work is needed to elucidate the various bases on which stimulus pairs can be ordered and the relation of such orderings to "sensation."

Factors Affecting Direct Estimation Judgments

It is well established that the basis for direct estimation judgments is more complex than mere matching of stimulus pairs. For example, magnitude estimates are affected by the size of the first stimulus pair (x, x') that is judged (i. e., by the first stimulus, x', and the second stimulus, x), and by the total range of stimuli presented. A very interesting theory of range effects has been developed by R. TEGHTSOONIAN (1972). Also noteworthy are POULTON'S (1968) review and earlier studies of adaptation level by HELSON (1964).

Subjects in direct estimation experiments show, of course, considerable variability in response when the same stimulus is repeated; one may attempt to analyze this variability more closely to separate the roles of sensory and nonsensory factors. See LUCE and GALANTER (1963b) and LUCE and MO (1965).

Finally, consideration of the two conceptually distinct theories of category rating – the Thurstone theory of comparison with category boundaries, and the theory sketched above, of comparison of pairs – suggests that some subjects may mix the two processes. Even in magnitude estimation or cross-modality matching, a subject may sometimes try directly to match a given "sensation ratio" with a numerical ratio or a "sensation ratio" on another modality, but he may at other times merely judge the position of the present stimulus relative to remembered category boundaries. J. E. KEITH SMITH has coined a felicitous phrase for this latter strategy: "making the category error."

As POULTON has said, "...a magnitude estimate is a mixture between 'how it seems' and 'how I judge it.' S. S. STEVENS' simple transducer theory is only part of the truth... Central processes involving judgment cannot be understood entirely in terms of the behavior of the sense organs" (1968, p. 17).

Nevertheless, it must be noted that the mere demonstration that judgmental factors can seriously influence subjects' responses does not entail that these factors play any major role in affecting the outcomes of STEVENS' experiments. Indeed, STEVENS regards these effects as "second order," to be avoided by suitably randomizing and averaging. Whatever one may think of randomization as a device to overcome systematic errors, the fact remains that none of the "judgment theorists" has even attempted to account for the remarkable regularities of STEVENS' results in terms of nonsensory factors. The mere demonstration of possible influences of extraneous factors, without attempting to account for the main, "first-order" findings, seems to be a very fruitless strategy. The only attempts to combine sensory and nonsensory factors in a single framework are those of LUCE and his coworkers, and of R. TEGHTSOONIAN, cited above. The latter theory involves the distortion of (numerical-valued) sensation ratios by multiplicative factors that vary as a function of the stimulus range.

The working assumption for the present, then, is that magnitude estimation and cross-modality matching are heavily based on matching of stimulus pairs, in terms of some, as yet poorly understood, sensory property of such pairs, and that the ordering based on this property satisfies the condition (14). Thus, magnitude estimates yield an index ψ of sensory function, satisfying (15), and related to physical energy approximately by Eqs. (8), (10), (11), (12), or (13). However, the details of the index ψ may be influenced by nonsensory factors.

Multiplicity of Perceptual Attributes: Multidimensional Scaling

Direct estimation and confusability scaling are both concerned with the description of quantitative changes in sensation as stimuli are varied along a single attribute. Suppose that an observer is asked to judge or to match the brightness of a monochromatic light, the luminance of which is varied. Variations in luminance produce variations in brightness, but they also produce variations in hue (the Bezold-Brücke effect, see JAMESON, chapter 14, this volume) and in saturation. Thus, there is considerable difference between varying a light along a single physical dimension (radiance, say) and varying a light along a single perceptual attribute (say, brightness). In either case, the subject can be required to judge a single perceptual attribute, ignoring concomitant variations (if any) along other attributes. How well he can do this is a matter for experimental test; as will be shown below, for brightness, it works quite well.

Another question concerns the identification of all the various perceptual attributes evoked by a given stimulus. In the case of color, trichromacy of color matching (see WRIGHT, chapter 16, this volume) entails that there be exactly three *independent* perceptual attributes; but the three can be chosen in various ways: hue, saturation, and brightness; redness/greenness, yellowness/blueness, and whiteness/blackness; etc. (see chapter 14). Indeed, if we know the quantities of any three color attributes, the others can be predicted (at least in principle). For example, if we know the saturation, redness, and whiteness of an orange color, then its yellowness is determined: since we know the relation of total redness plus yellowness to whiteness (saturation) and we know two of the three quantities that enter this relation (redness, whiteness), we can solve for the third, the yellowness. Then, having the redness and yellowness, the hue is determined.

In other domains, however, there are cases where we do not know what perceptual attributes, or even how many, are involved in perception of a given stimulus. It is hard even to give a good general criterion for what constitutes a perceptual attribute.

Multidimensional scaling is an indirect technique for determining the number, and possibly the nature, of perceptual attributes evoked by stimuli of a given class. The most common method now used in practice (due to SHEPARD, 1962a) is as follows. For each pair of stimuli, some measure of "proximity" is obtained (various ones have been used). One then searches for a configuration of points in Euclidean space, one point corresponding to each stimulus, such that the ordering of proximities between stimuli is reproduced as faithfully as possible by the ordering of inverse distances between the corresponding points. One tries to obtain such a faithful reproduction of the proximity ordering in as small a number of dimensions (of the Euclidean space) as possible. If a good fit is obtained for dimensionality $\geqq n$, but the fit falls apart suddenly for dimensionality $n-1$, then one concludes that the proximities are based on variations in n independent perceptual attributes. Frequently, a further inference is drawn, as to the nature of the attributes, by a kind of informal "principal axes" analysis.

A large number of computational schemes have been devised for finding appropriate configurations of points, starting with proximities; one of the ones in most frequent use is that of KRUSKAL (1964). A good deal of work has been done on the development of analogous schemes that substitute other kinds of assumptions for the Euclidean distance model, but these have not as yet found widespread application. Prior to SHEPARD's work, multidimensional scaling had been based on finding Euclidean configurations with inverse distances linear with (rather than monotonic with) observed proximities (see TORGERSON, 1958). Such methods are still used quite frequently, although the assumption that any particular proximity measure is actually linear with Euclidean distance is rather hard to justify (see KRANTZ, 1967a).

The basic idea of inferring perceptual attributes from proximity, or similarity data has much to recommend it. If two stimuli x and y are each just as similar to u as to v, but x and y are dissimilar from one another, then u and v must differ from one another in a way that is quite different from the way that x and y differ. (For if only one attribute were involved, then x and y would have to be midway between u and v on that attribute, hence, identical to one another.) Hence, the difference between proximities that can be represented by distances on a line, and proximities that require more than one dimension, is very simple. However, the justification for using formal geometric n-dimensional models is much less evident. This problem has been considered in some detail by BEALS *et al.* (1968) and TVERSKY and KRANTZ (1970). They recommend increased effort toward identifying perceptual attributes in terms of qualitative properties of similarity data, rather than fitting specific models, such as the Euclidean model. Another foundational study, in which the geometry of the space is related to distributions of attention over perceptual attributes, was recently published by MICKO and FISCHER (1970).

Applications in Vision

Brightness I: The Munsell System

One of the most ambitious attempts to generate a comprehensive scale of brightness is embodied in the MUNSELL Book of Color (1929). In the Munsell system, the interval between 0% and 100% reflectance is divided into ten perceptually equal steps. The nine intervening levels are called Munsell Value /1, /2, ..., /9. At each Value level, achromatic and colored samples are prepared, for all attainable colors. (For a detailed description, see NEWHALL *et al.*, 1943, and JUDD and WYSZECKI, 1963.) A Munsell Value level is specified by a value of luminous reflectance[1], Y, between 0 and 1.0. This works because samples

[1] Of course, luminous reflectance is specified for a standard light source, in this case, a type of artificial daylight; use of the colored samples in any other illuminant may destroy the brightness matches.

of equal luminous reflectance, differing in color, are generally judged to be about equal in "lightness" or Value.

To a first approximation, at least, the equal-spacing property of the Munsell Values is independent of the overall *level* of illumination. Independence of this kind can occur only if the relation between brightness and luminance is given by a logarithmic or a power function. For if $\psi(x)$ denotes the brightness corresponding to x, then the fact that the spacing between x and z equals that between z and y is given by the equation

$$\psi(x) - \psi(z) = \psi(z) - \psi(y),$$

which reduces to

$$z = \psi^{-1}\left[\frac{\psi(x) + \psi(y)}{2}\right]. \qquad (17)$$

If this equality of spacing is preserved when x, y, and z are multiplied by a common factor t, we have

$$\psi(tx) - \psi(tz) = \psi(tz) - \psi(ty),$$

which reduces to

$$tz = \psi^{-1}\left[\frac{\psi(tx) + \psi(ty)}{2}\right]. \qquad (18)$$

Eliminating z between Eqs.(17) and (18) yields, for any x, y, and t,

$$\psi^{-1}\left[\frac{\psi(tx) + \psi(ty)}{2}\right] = t \cdot \psi^{-1}\left[\frac{\psi(x) + \psi(y)}{2}\right]. \qquad (19)$$

It is known (Aczel, 1966, p. 152) that the only continuous functions ψ satisfying Eq. (19) are given by

$$\psi(x) = a + b \log x,$$

$$\psi(x) = a + bx^B.$$

In point of fact, the relation between Munsell Values and the corresponding value of luminous reflectance is well approximated by the power function, with $B = 0.5$. (For a summary of attempts to obtain a more precise lightness scale, see Judd and Wyszecki, 1963.)

Brightness II: Context Effects

A systematic study of the brightness of (more or less achromatic) selfluminous sources, in varying viewing contexts, has been carried out by S. S. Stevens and his collaborators, using magnitude estimation methods. (J. C. Stevens and S. S. Stevens, 1963; Aiba and S. S. Stevens, 1964; S. S. Stevens and Diamond, 1965). They invariably fit power functions of the form of Eq. (11), i. e.,

$$\psi(x) = b(x - x_0)^B. \qquad (11)$$

For a moderate-sized target (5.7°), presented for 2 seconds in an otherwise dark field to a dark-adapted or slightly light-adapted eye, the exponent B is around 0.33. For smaller or briefer targets, or higher adaptation level, or with a glare source in the field, they find increases in the exponent, and sometimes changes in b and x_0 as well. These increases are documented thoroughly in the above references. However, Jameson and Hurvich (1964) question whether the exponent does really change, contending that at least in the case of contrast effects, it can be kept constant by use of Eq. (12) instead of Eq. (11), i. e.,

$$\psi(x) = bx^B - \psi_0. \tag{12}$$

In view of the fact that the constant x_0 in Eq. (11) does not have any convenient interpretation (the interpretation as a luminance "threshold" is nonsense, since the "threshold" is a statistical fiction, and since anyway the values of x_0 rarely correspond to directly measured "thresholds"), while ψ_0 is incorporated into a theory of simultaneous contrast, and in view of the invariance of the exponent, JAMESON and HURVICH have a bit the better of the argument. However, systematic attempts to explore different forms of equation in a wide variety of settings are still needed. A form that I think is particularly promising is given by Eq. (8), recast in the form

$$\psi(x) = b[(x + x_0)^B - x_0^B] - \psi_0. \tag{8'}$$

Here, b (sensitivity) and x_0 (luminance equivalent of internal noise) may vary with adaptation, while ψ_0 (inhibition) may vary with simultaneous and successive contrast; B should be fixed under variations in these factors.

Without worrying too much about the exact parametric form for the brightness function, and the way in which the parameters transform, we can still note one very positive aspect of all these results. Brightness estimates, obtained by magnitude estimation, successfully predict cross-context brightness matches (e. g., haploscopic matches with different conditions in the two eyes). This has been found repeatedly by STEVENS and his collaborators and independently confirmed by ONLEY (1961) and JAMESON (1969). This is a striking result, since cross-context matches are a highly reliable, standard procedure for evaluating the effects of viewing context on brightness.

Brightness III: Chromatic Stimuli

Brightness is a quality of colored stimuli as well as of achromatic stimuli. Lights that differ widely in color may be matched in brightness. However, there has been considerable debate about the uniqueness and stability of the criterion adopted for such heterochromatic matches, and about the generalizations that are appropriate from such matches. One of the main issues revolves around the question of the validity of Abney's Law of additivity of heterochromatic brightness matches (see LE GRAND, chapter 15, this volume). If lights u and v match in brightness, and u' and v' match in brightness, then do the additive mixtures $u + u'$ and $v + v'$ also match in brightness?

In the Munsell system, as noted above, Value is identified with luminous reflectance; hence, the system provides evidence that equiluminous stimuli are approximately equally bright. This could happen if the CIE luminosity function, which is used to calculate the luminous reflectance of the Munsell samples, did in fact correspond to the inverse radiances for equal brightness of spectral stimuli, and if in addition, additivity held for mixtures of spectral stimuli. Both assumptions, however, are quite implausible, because of evidence cited below. Another possible explanation is that the deviations from these two assumptions, large as they are, are insufficient to produce really marked discrepancies in the Munsell samples; to some extent, averaging over large numbers of wavelengths in the rather nonselective stimuli produced by Munsell samples may eliminate some of the discrepancies. Still a third explanation will be offered below.

The most clearcut evidence of brightness nonadditivity is due to GUTH *et al.* (1969). If equally bright lights u_1, u_2, of wavelengths λ_1, λ_2 are added to a light u_3 of wavelength λ_2, the heterochromatic sum $u_1 + u_3$ is generally less bright than the monochromatic sum $u_2 + u_3$; if λ_1 is sufficiently far from λ_2, $u_1 + u_3$ *may even be less bright than* u_3 *itself*. In other words, monochromatic lights of a given luminance seem to be brighter than mixed lights of the same total luminance. It has sometimes been argued that this kind of effect is due to a "confusion" of brightness with saturation, i. e., to ambiguity as to what "brightness" is. However, GUTH *et al.* and BOYNTON *et al.* (1964), showed exactly the same effects for threshold luminous efficiency measurements; i.e., in the above example, with overall intensities greatly reduced, $u_1 + u_3$ is less detectable than $u_2 + u_3$ and may even be less detectable than u_3 itself. WILSON (1964), whose work is discussed below in more detail, showed that threshold and equal-brightness luminous efficiency functions, obtained under identical viewing conditions, are nearly identical, and so it is very hard to argue that the "brightness criterion" is faulty. If luminous efficiency is defined by relative energies for threshold, then highly saturated monochromatic lights are no brighter than less saturated (yellow) monochromatic lights of the same (threshold) luminous efficiency. But threshold luminous efficiency matches, hence also suprathreshold brightness matches, are nevertheless nonadditive.

It has long been known that additivity can be improved if the standard heterochromatic matching task is abandoned; flicker photometry was considered to be the best alternative (the criterion of equality is no longer "equal brightness" but minimization of flicker between two alternating lights). Recently, BOYNTON and KAISER (1968) showed that additivity can be produced by a much simpler criterion: minimization of the distinctness of the border in a bipartite field.

It is my guess that two somewhat different properties of lights are involved in these studies. One of them, which might be called "whiteness," is additive with respect to color mixture (like the other opponent-process attributes, redness/greenness and yellowness/blueness). This "whiteness" property is chiefly involved in minimization of flicker, in minimization of the distinctness of borders, and in the equating of Munsell samples at constant Value; it is moderately well represented by the CIE luminance function. "Perceived whiteness" grows approximately as the 0.50 power of the luminance, as indicated by the Munsell system. The other property, brightness, is a weighted combination of the *absolute values* of the opponent processes, whiteness/blackness, redness/greenness, and yellowness/blueness[2]. It is the property involved in threshold detection and in suprathreshold matching: It accounts for the wide deviations of luminosity functions based on these methods from the CIE form based on flicker photo-

[2] GUTH takes the implicit position that these absolute values need to be squared, then added, then the square root extracted, since he uses an Euclidean model. I am not prepared to argue this point; further work will be needed to find the exact combination rule yielding brightness.

metry. It is nonadditive because the absolute-value function is nonadditive: a red and a green light have high absolute values of redness/greenness, but their additive mixture has a lower absolute value than one or both of the two components. Perceived brightness grows (in a dark surround) approximately as the 0.33 power of radiance (for monochromatic lights or for any other fixed spectral energy distribution, with total radiance varied).

One of the most beautiful studies of heterochromatic brightness was performed by WILSON in her doctoral dissertation (1964)[3]. She measured spectral luminous efficiency functions by three methods: thresholds, heterochromatic matching, and magnitude estimation. For heterochromatic matching, she employed a bipartite field, matching the brightness of a variable wavelength in the left half of the field to that of a fixed wavelength (at fixed radiance) (550 nm) on the right. To keep the same viewing conditions in the other two methods, the same fixed 550 nm stimulus filled the right half of the field, even though, as far as the observers were concerned, the right field was irrelevant to the detection of the stimulus on the left. For magnitude estimation, the right field served as the standard. The results may be summarized briefly: the luminous efficiency functions measured by the three methods were virtually identical. In particular, this means that heterochromatic matching can predict the magnitude estimation function for one wavelength from the magnitude estimation function for another. When different wavelengths are equated for luminous efficiency (either threshold or equal-brightness), and viewing conditions are kept the same as in the luminous efficiency measurements, magnitude estimates of brightness are independent of wavelength.

Earlier, EKMAN, EISLER, and KÜNNAPAS (1960) found brightness functions for monochromatic lights with approximately the same exponent (0.33) for all wavelengths.

WILSON's results leave little doubt that the attribute brightness can be abstracted from color in a highly consistent manner and measured in a meaningful way by magnitude estimation. The consistencies found by WILSON with heterochromatic matching reinforce the ones found by cross-context matching (as cited above) and by cross-modality matching.

Hue and Saturation

Hue is widely considered to be a metathetic continuum, i. e., one on which the quality, rather than the quantity of sensation is changing. The proper representation of hue is generally considered to be the color circle. Starting with any hue, one can go through a long series of hues, separated by very small steps, and return ultimately to the starting point, without ever retracing. For example, starting with red, one goes through reddish-orange, orange, yellowish-orange, ..., and finally returns via reddish-purple back to red. From this standpoint, the scaling of hue involves two steps. First, a nominal scale of hue is developed: we identify colors that match in hue (for example we obtain suitable matches between red and pink, between purple and lavender, etc.). Second, the different

[3] See also JAMESON (1970) for a brief summary of WILSON's work and a discussion of Eq. (12).

hue names are arranged in a circle, such that equal spacing along the circle (distances measured by shorter arc, of course) represents equal perceptual steps.

The MUNSELL Book of Color (1929) contains one of the best known and most carefully constructed scales of this sort. The colored samples for any constant Munsell Value (see discussion above, under Brightness) are arranged in constant-hue radii. There are forty such radii, chosen for equal perceptual spacing. They are labelled by five cardinal hue names (red, yellow, green, blue, purple, or R, Y, G, B, and P) and five intermediate names (YR, GY, BG, PB, RP). Each of these ten names corresponds to 10% of the circle and includes five numerically labelled radii (e. g., 0 YR, 2.5 YR, 5 YR, 7.5 YR, and 10 YR; where 0 YR coincides with 10 R and 10 YR coincides with 0 Y). The nominal scale (equality of hue along each radius) and the perceptual-difference scale have been subjected to intensive study by NEWHALL (1939, 1940). He had subjects make quantitative judgments (by drawing arrows of appropriate lengths and directions) of the deviations from constancy of hue and from equal hue spacing. The results of these studies were summarized in the Optical Society of America Subcommittee Report (NEWHALL *et al.*, 1943) and were adopted by the Optical Society of America as the Munsell Renotation. These results have been reproduced in many standard reference works by means of chromaticity charts showing loci of Munsell Renotation Hue contours.

The Munsell hue scale can be extremely useful in any application, practical or scientific, where it is desired to determine whether and by how much two colors differ in hue. It can be used in two ways. In the first, colorimetric measurements are converted to Munsell Renotation. The second method requires the subjects to scale the colors directly, using Munsell names. In the first method, one must be quite careful about viewing conditions. Tristimulus values (Chap. 16) can be obtained and converted to Munsell Renotation, but the results may not be useful unless the color in question is viewed under the conditions in which the Munsell Renotation scale is valid (daylight adaptation, neutral surround). (Note that the color stimulus can be measured by visual colorimetry under any viewing conditions, but the Renotation coordinates still apply to that same stimulus viewed under the aforementioned standard conditions; this point is obvious in the case of photoelectric colorimetry.) If colors are viewed in other conditions, then one must use cross-context colorimetry. The simplest method is to use the Munsell samples themselves as the colorimeter: a given color, under arbitrary viewing conditions, is matched to a Munsell sample viewed under daylight or artificial daylight illumination, with daylight adaptation and neutral surround. (Note that this does not give the Munsell scale directly; one must still check the Renotation.) Another caution is that results obtained by this method are subject to errors due to individual differences in perceived hues.

The second method, direct scaling, is easier to implement, and avoids problems of viewing conditions. However, it relies on the subjects' ability to remember the assignment of responses to percepts in the Munsell system. In practice, the great precision of the Munsell scale would be illusory, and therefore it is just as well to use a simpler system of color names. A good example is found in the study of the Bezold-Brücke hue shift by BOYNTON and GORDON (1965). They allowed the subjects a choice among only twelve responses: four cardinal names, R, G, B, and Y, and eight pairwise combinations, RB, RY, GB, GY, BR, BG, YR, and YG; where RB means red-blue, predominantly red, while BR means red-blue, predominantly blue. The fine discriminations between two similar hues were based on differences in the distributions of names. For example, two different blue-greens might each elicit responses B, BG, GB, and G, from a single subject, but the distribution of responses over these four categories would be somewhat different.

In the framework of opponent-colors theory, hue is no longer considered to be a metathetic continuum, rather, it is analyzed as the relation between two prothetic, or quantitative continua: redness/greenness and yellowness/blueness. From this standpoint, a blue-green has its hue defined, not by a distribution of responses over color names, but by the relative amounts of perceived blueness and greenness (JAMESON and HURVICH, 1959). Alternatively, each component of the perceived hue can be scaled separately, for example, by direct estimation methods.

YAGER and TAYLOR (1970) obtained magnitude estimates of yellowness and greenness, as functions of radiance, at unique[4] yellow and unique green wavelengths, respectively. They obtained good fits with Eq. (12), rewritten in the form

$$\begin{aligned} \psi_Y(x) &= \psi_{0,Y}[(x/x_{0,Y})^B - 1], \\ \psi_G(x) &= \psi_{0,G}[(x/x_{0,G})^B - 1]. \end{aligned} \tag{20}$$

(If $\psi = bx^B - \psi_0$, then $\psi = \psi_0[(x/x_0)^B - 1]$ where x_0 is defined by $\psi_0 = bx_0^B$, i. e., as the value where $\psi = 0$.) They used the magnitude estimation data only to estimate B and to confirm that Eq. 20 gives a good fit, with the same B for yellowness as for greenness ($B = 0.28$). They then assumed that Eq. 20 would continue to be valid, with the same value of B, for yellowness and greenness of a yellow-green wavelength (550 nm) as its energy, x, was varied. For this wavelength, $x_{0,Y}$ and $x_{0,G}$ were measured by determining the energies at which the stimulus appeared "just noticeably yellow" and "just noticeably green" (assuming $\psi = 0$ at such thresholds). They had subjects judge *relative proportions* of yellow and green, for the 550 nm stimulus, as a function of energy. The ratio $\psi_{0,Y}/\psi_{0,G}$ was estimated by writing

$$\psi_Y(x_{0.50}) = \psi_G(x_{0.50}),$$

where $x_{0.50}$ denotes the energy at which the hue was judged to be 50% yellow and 50% green. With these determinations of the constants in Eq. (20), they could predict percentage hue reports for all energies x above the yellow threshold at 550 nm, by the formula

$$H = \frac{\psi_Y(x)}{\psi_Y(x) + \psi_G(x)} \,. \tag{21}$$

Empirically, 550 nm yields a large Bezold-Brücke hue shift. The "yellow threshold," $x_{0,Y}$, is larger than the "green threshold," $x_{0,G}$, by a factor of more than 30 (1.5 $\log_{10}$ units), so for low energies, the stimulus is nearly pure green. The proportion of yellow rises to about 30% at 0.3 $\log_{10}$ units above the yellow

[4] A unique yellow/blue is defined as a color which appears neither reddish nor greenish; a unique red/green appears neither yellowish nor bluish.

threshold, and is still rising steadily, but less rapidly, at around 75% yellow, 2.1 $\log_{10}$ units above the yellow threshold.

Eqs. (20) and (21) predict a shift of this kind, since at the yellow threshold, $H = 0$, and H increases to an asymptote for large x. Quantitatively, however, the prediction is imperfect, since the predicted H rises slightly too fast and then levels off to an asymptote, while the observed H rises more steadily.

YAGER and TAYLOR interpret this discrepancy in terms of an assumed interaction between yellowness and greenness in which the hue component with the larger magnitude "masks" the other component. Although this hypothesis is somewhat ad hoc, it could be tested in a number of ways, e. g., by directly scaling yellowness and greenness in yellow-green lights, rather than at unique hue loci. Moreover, there is other evidence for such an interactive or "masking" effect. For example, HURVICH and JAMESON (1951) showed that broad-band lights (2842–10,000 °K) may appear non-achromatic at low luminance levels but appear white at high luminance. Thus, perceived redness and yellowness (for a tungsten source, say) are actually decreased for sufficient increases in energy, indicating a kind of "masking" by white.

From the opponent-colors standpoint, saturation is also a relation between prothetic continua. The saturation of a green depends on the relative quantities of perceived greenness and perceived whiteness. Thus, in the YAGER-TAYLOR study, subjects had to judge greenness, not saturation; as the energy of their green light increased, both greenness and whiteness increased; judgments of saturation would not have increased as sharply under those circumstances.

In some other scaling experiments (PANEK and STEVENS, 1966; INDOW and STEVENS, 1966) the instructions to the subjects were to judge amount of hue, and "to assign numbers proportional to your impression of the saturation," and the stimuli varied in colorimetric purity, rather than luminance. That is, if the stimulus is considered as a mixture of a monochromatic and a neutral light (to which it is metameric), then as the luminance of the monochromatic component was increased, the luminance of the neutral component decreased, in such a way as to keep the sum of the luminances constant. If the judgment of greenness (for example) depends only on the luminance of the monochromatic component, then the results should be identical with the results of YAGER and TAYLOR, for a corresponding variation of the luminance of a monochromatic light. On the other hand, if the subjects in the colorimetric purity experiments judged the relation between greenness and whiteness, then one might expect a much steeper slope for judged "greenness" as a function of the luminance of the green component, because whiteness would be decreasing at the same time as greenness increased.

In fact, the slopes found by STEVENS and his coworkers are approximately six times as large as those found by YAGER and TAYLOR. Besides the possible explanation just indicated, i. e., that subjects in the purity experiment judged a relation between hue components and white rather than judging the hue components themselves, there are various other factors that may contribute to this enormous discrepancy. One, which is closely related to the "masking" explanation offered by YAGER and TAYLOR to account for their underprediction of the Bezold-Brücke effect, is "masking" of weak hue components by strong white components. This possibility was noted above in discussing the studies of whiteness by HURVICH and JAMESON. Another possible factor is the overall luminance range, which was much larger in the YAGER and TAYLOR study. Minor factors are the difference in level of luminance and the possible nonneutralness of the desaturating light in the purity experiments.

It should be emphasized that the internal consistency of INDOW and STEVENS' data is extraordinarily impressive; particularly, their use of many different colors and their elaborate checks by heterochromatic and heteroluminous matching. The validity of their data is not in doubt; but their interpretation, in terms of the various qualities being judged, and interactive dynamics, may be quite complicated.

It is clear that direct estimation of hue components and their relations (hue, saturation) may be a powerful tool for investigating color perception, but that the effects of different instructions and the interactions among chromatic and achromatic components need further investigation.

Finally, it should be noted that the Munsell system also includes a saturation scale. Samples on any constant-hue radius are designed to be equally spaced in Munsell Chroma, giving rise to equally spaced concentric constant-Chroma circles. The Chroma spacing was also studied by NEWHALL, in the papers cited above. There are also valuable hue and saturation scales in other color-order systems (see WYSZECKI and STILES, 1967, Sec. 6.5).

Color Differences

Two kinds of scaling can be attempted for color differences. In one hand, one can try to develop a scale for *magnitude of color difference*, analogous to a scale for brightness or for redness. This can be attempted either by confusability scaling or by direct estimation. In confusability scaling, for example, one may ask subjects to make pair comparisons of color differences, or category ratings of color differences, and apply Thurstonian or other appropriate models. For example, the Thurstone Case V procedure would be to estimate color-difference-scale values $u(x, y)$ and $u(x', y')$ such that

$$P[(x, y,) \, (x', y')] = \int_{-\infty}^{u(x,y)-u(x',y')} (2\pi)^{-\frac{1}{2}} e^{-\frac{1}{2}w^2} \, dw,$$

where $P[(x, y), (x', y')]$ is the probability that the color difference between x and y is judged greater than that between x' and y', and $u(x, y)$, $u(x', y')$ are color-difference-scale values. In direct estimation, one can have subjects make magnitude estimates or cross-modality matches to color differences.

Secondly, one can try *multidimensional scaling of color differences* to develop a (vector) scale for the colors themselves, such that distances between vectors correspond to color differences. If one starts with only an ordering of color differences, then the distance between vectors constitutes a ratio scale for color differences; hence, in ordinal multidimensional scaling, one of the byproducts of the scale for colors is a scale of the former type, i. e., a scale for magnitude of color differences. Earlier methods of multidimensional scaling, which are still used somewhat, require that the scale for magnitude of color differences be obtained as a prior step, since they attempt to find a linear, rather than merely a monotonic relation between vector distances and the color-difference measure.

Most attempts to scale magnitude of color difference have been motivated primarily by an interest in multidimensional scaling rather than in the color-difference scale itself. An exception to this was my doctoral dissertation (KRANTZ, 1964, 1967a, 1967b), which tested whether a reasonable scale could be constructed encompassing both small differences [ones which are confusable with a "zero-difference" (x, x)] and large ones. Although this proved to be possible (1967b), it was found that models of the Thurstone type fit very poorly (1967a), mainly because of "difficulty of choice" factors of the kind cited above among the criticisms of confusability scaling.

Another study of color-difference scales was performed by HELM (1964), who compared Thurstonian analysis of category ratings with direct estimation, and found a linear relation after an exponential transformation was applied to the Thurstonian scale. The same exponential transformation reduced the dimensionality of the Euclidean multidimensional scale from 12 to 2 (HELM, 1960).

Turning to multidimensional scaling of color differences, we may note first that there is no real doubt, in the case of colors, as to the number of *independent* perceptual attributes. The number is three, as dictated by the trichromacy of color matching and the invariance of topological dimension. Furthermore, there is no question of identifying "the three" attributes, since there are many possible choices of three (hue, brightness, saturation; redness/greenness, yellowness/blueness, whiteness/blackness; etc.) Thus, multidimensional scaling of color differences can have three purposes: validation of the multidimensional scaling method, in a situation where the proper results are more or less known; development of practical scales for specifying color tolerances; and investigating the underlying basis of color similarity.

The very fact that so much is already known about color attributes is particularly useful in validation of new scaling methods. Quite a number of studies of color differences have been performed with this in mind, including those of RICHARDSON (1938), TORGERSON (1951, 1958), EKMAN (1954), and MESSICK (1956). Where a method gives the "wrong" answer (EKMAN obtained a five-dimensional solution by factor analysis) and reanalysis of the same data by another scaling method gives the "right" answer (SHEPARD, 1962b), the latter method (in this case, SHEPARD's method of ordinal multidimensional scaling) is supported.

Practical scales for color differences have focused on the construction of a three-dimensional coordinate system, related in a simple manner to coordinate systems already in use, which can give a reasonable approximation to color differences. The most common proposals involve transformations of either the CIE coordinate systems or of the Munsell Hue, Chroma, Value coordinates. A good summary may be found in JUDD and WYSZECKI (1963, pp. 271–300).

Finally, we come to multidimensional scaling that is directed toward elucidation of the underlying basis of color similarity. One set of studies tests the appropriateness of distance geometries, especially Euclidean ones, as models of color similarity. HELM (1960), INDOW and KANAZAWA (1960), INDOW and UCHIZONO (1960), SHEPARD (1962b), and WRIGHT (1965) all obtained support for a Euclidean model. Previously, MACADAM (1943) and BROWN and MACADAM (1949) had rejected the Euclidean model for small differences. Recently, theoretical advances in multidimensional scaling (described in the section on scaling methods) have permitted a more refined analysis of distance geometries as models. I recently was able to show that lightness differences and chromaticness differences do not act orthogonally in determining overall color differences. For example, many chromaticness differences make smaller contributions to color difference when the pair of colors is of high lightness than when the same chromaticness pair is judged at lower lightness.

Space and Form

Colors are characterized very naturally in terms of multiple subjective attributes. When we move to the areas of space and pattern vision, the relevance of scaling paradigms is less salient. Indeed, it may be more useful to consider patterns as bundles of discrete features or gestalten, rather than as points in some low-dimensional vector space.

I think that this issue is far from settled, and shall not try to force a settlement here. Rather, this section merely illustrates a few of the results obtained from scaling experiments with other visual qualities.

Scaling of length seems to show that perceived length grows very nearly proportionally to physical length (KÜNNAPAS, 1958; EKMAN and JUNGE, 1961; STEVENS and GUIRAO, 1963; TEGHTSOONIAN, 1965; TEGHTSOONIAN and TEGHTSOONIAN, 1965). This holds for horizontal or vertical lines, felt lines or seen lines, and appears to be independent of factors, such as stimulus range, which seem to affect other modalities more seriously. These results form part of the rationale of the "ideal" theory for magnitude estimation that I sketched in the methods section. According to this view, subjects use numbers, in magnitude estimation, by matching a given "sensation ratio" (of brightnesses, say) to the "sensation ratio" of a pair of lines. Line length "sensation ratios" are translated veridically into numbers because there is an "algorithm" for doing so – by visually laying off the smaller length several times along the larger one, etc.

The scale for perceived area is less well agreed-on; a major factor is its dependence on the shape of the objects being judged. EKMAN and JUNGE (1958) found exponents of about 1.0, but TEGHTSOONIAN (1965) argues convincingly that such results depend on the presence of a common linear dimension and the instruction to judge physical area. In effect, subjects can be induced to judge squared length. Judgments of apparent size, on the other hand, seem to be better described by the exponent 0.8 (see also STEVENS and GUIRAO, 1963).

EKMAN and JUNGE also obtained scales of apparent volume for three-dimensional cubes (exponent about 1.0) and for drawings of cubes and spheres (exponents around 0.75). In view of the findings of TEGHTSOONIAN for area, these exponents may turn out to be different when subject are instructed differently or are deprived of common linear extents.

Apparent distance has been scaled by GILINSKY (1951) and by KÜNNAPAS (1960), but they obtained widely different results, using very different methods, and it does not seem feasible at this time to make any general statement. STERN-

BERG (1966) analyzed size and distance estimates obtained by R. and M. TEGHTSOONIAN, in which perceived area increased as the 0.82 power of physical area (at fixed distance), perceived distance increased as the 1.16 power of physical distance, and perceived size increased as the 0.11 power of distance when actual size was fixed. The most likely interpretation of these results is that *retinal* size is corrected for *perceived* distance *before* the perceived size power transformation is performed.

Perceived velocity was found to vary as the 1.77 power of physical velocity, by EKMAN and DAHLBÄCK (cited by STEVENS, 1957).

If we turn from perception of static and dynamic qualities of visual space, to that other vast area of perception, visual form, we may well ask, to begin with, whether there is anything at all to be gained by scaling. It is possible to think of shapes as being analyzed into discrete features, each of which is either present or absent, not scalable on any continuum. We recognize a chair, for example, by means of the presence of one of several alternative conjunctions of features; the "chairness" of a stool might be rated higher than that of a table, but the ratings probably reflect the presence or absence of distinctive features (backrest) or the quantity of certain other features (length of legs, size of horizontal surface).

KÜNNAPAS (1966) had subjects judge nine alphabetic characters, demanding both similarity judgments and "ness" judgments of the kind just discussed, e. g., the "*I*-ness" of a *J*, etc. Factor analysis yielded three factors, "rectangularity (E-ness)," "roundness (*O*-ness)," and "vertical linearity (*I*-ness)." Of course, these results, in which three factors are used to describe nine stimuli, are not very convincing; they are cited here to illustrate a point of view, rather than for their inherent value. The point of view is that the "code" for visual form consists, at least in large part, of a set of relatively independent, quantitatively variable "codes" for subjective dimensions. Thus, just as the "code" for orange consists of certain quantitative values on three independent "codes" (redness, yellowness, and whiteness), so the "code" for an ice-cream cone shape consists of quantitative values of elongation, circularity, triangularity, etc. These subjective values may be related to others, e.g., circularity to variance in perceived curvature, elongation to perceived height and perceived width, etc.

A recent study by BROWN and ANDREWS (1968) illustrates the systematic program being conducted by BROWN to elaborate an approach to form perception along the lines just described. They used reaction time in a matching task as an index of "proximity" of randomly generated polygons, and analyzed the proximities by ordinal multidimensional scaling. They found that "attributes" such as compactness, jaggedness, and elongation contributed importantly to the ordering of proximities. However, the attempt to establish these qualities as quantitatively variable attributes, and to relate them to physical dimensions, is not very convincing, as BROWN and ANDREWS recognize in their discussion.

The theoretical work on multidimensional scaling by TVERSKY and KRANTZ (1970) suggests certain formal characteristics that perceptual attributes should satisfy. TVERSKY and I tried to apply this analysis to form perception by testing whether similarity judgments of rectangles satisfy these formal characteristics better when analyzed in terms of perceived height and width or in terms of perceived area and height/width ratio. For some subjects, a clearcut decision seemed possible. Generally, however, these were subjects who paid attention to area at the expense of height/width ratio or vice-versa. These results also do not lend very strong support to the idea of analyzing form in terms of quantitative perceptual attributes. The ultimate value of that approach remains to be determined.

Acknowledgement. Preparation of this chapter was supported in part by NSF grant GB 4947 to the University of Michigan.

References

Aczél, J.: Lectures on Functional Equations and Their Applications. New York: Academic Press 1966.

Aiba, T. S., Stevens, S. S.: Relation of brightness to duration and luminance under light- and dark-adaptation. Vision Res. **4**, 391—401 (1964).

Beals, R., Krantz, D. H., Tversky, A.: Foundations of multidimensional scaling. Psychol. Rev. **75**, 127—142 (1968).

Bock, R. D., Jones, L. V.: The Measurement and Prediction of Judgment and Choice. San Francisco: Holden-Day 1968.

Boynton, R. M., Gordon, J.: Bezold-Brücke hue shift measured by color-naming technique. J. opt. Soc. Amer. **55**, 78—86 (1965).

— Ikeda, M., Stiles, W. S.: Interactions among chromatic mechanisms as inferred from positive and negative increment thresholds. Vision Res. **4**, 87—117 (1964).

— Kaiser, P. K.: Vision: the additivity law made to work for heterochromatic photometry with bipartite fields. Science **161**, 366—368 (1968).

Bradley, R. A.: Another interpretation of a model for paired comparisons. Psychometrika **30**, 315—318 (1966).

— Terry, M. E.: Rank analysis of incomplete block designs. I. The method of paired comparisons. Biometrika **39**, 324—345 (1952).

Brown, D. R., Andrews, M. H.: Visual form discrimination: Multidimensional psychophysics. Perc. Psychophys. **3**, 401—406 (1968).

Brown, W. R. J., MacAdam, D. L.: Visual sensitivities to combined chromaticity and luminance differences. J. opt. Soc. Amer. **39**, 808—834 (1949).

Coombs, C. H.: A Theory of Data. New York: Wiley 1964.

Eisler, H.: On the problem of category scales in psychophysics. Scand. J. Psychol. **3**, 81—87 (1962a).

— Empirical test of a model relating magnitude and category scales. Scand. J. Psychol. **3**, 88—96 (1962b).

— Magnitude scales, category scales, and Fechnerian integration. Psychol. Rev. **70**, 243—253 (1963a).

— A general differential equation in psychophysics: Derivation and empirical test. Scand. J. Psychol. **4**, 265—272 (1963b).

— The connection between magnitude and discrimination scales and direct and indirect scaling methods. Psychometrika **30**, 271—289 (1965).

Ekman, G.: Dimensions of color vision. J. Psychol. **38**, 467—474 (1954).

— Eisler, H., Künnapas, T.: Brightness scales for monochromatic light. Scand. J. Psychol. **1**, 41—48 (1960).

— Junge, K.: Psychophysical relations in visual perception of length, area, and volume. Scand. J. Psychol. **2**, 1—10 (1961).

Fagot, R. F., Stewart, M.: Tests of product and additive scaling axioms. Perc. Psychophys. **5**, 117—123 (1969).

Falmagne, J.-C.: The generalized Fechner problem and discrimination. J. math. Psychol. **8**, 22—43 (1971).

Galanter, E., Messick, S.: The relation between category and magnitude scales of loudness. Psychol. Rev. **68**, 363—372 (1961).

GILINSKY, S.: Perceived size and distance in visual space. Psychol. Rev. **58**, 460—482 (1951).
GUTH, S. L., DONLEY, N. J., MARROCCO, R. T.: On luminance additivity and related topics. Vision Res. **9**, 537—575 (1969).
HELM, C. E.: A successive intervals analysis of color differences. Office of Naval Research Technical Report (Contract Nonr 1858-15), Princeton University 1960.
— Multidimensional ratio scaling of perceived color relations. J. opt. Soc. Amer. **54**, 256—262 (1964).
— MESSICK, S., TUCKER, L. R.: Psychological models for relating discrimination and magnitude estimation scales. Psychol. Rev. **68**, 167—177 (1961).
HELSON, H.: Adaptation-Level Theory. New York: Harper & Row 1964.
HURVICH, L. M., JAMESON, D.: A psychophysical study of white. I. Neutral adaptation. J. opt. Soc. Amer. **41**, 521—527 (1951).
INDOW, T., KANAZAWA, K.: Multidimensional mapping of Munsell colors varying in hue, chroma, and value. J. exp. Psychol. **59**, 330—336 (1960).
— STEVENS, S. S.: Scaling of saturation and hue. Perc. Psychophys. **1**, 253—271 (1966).
— UCHIZONO, T.: Multidimensional mapping of Munsell colors varying in hue and chroma. J. exp. Psychol. **59**, 321—329 (1960).
JAMESON, D.: Brightness scales and their interpretation. In: International Colour Meeting Stockholm 1969, pp. 377—385. Göttingen: Musterschmidt 1970.
— HURVICH, L. M.: Perceived color and its dependence on focal, surrounding, and preceding stimulus variables. J. opt. Soc. Amer. **49**, 890—898 (1959).
— — Theory of brightness and color contrast in human vision. Vision Res. **4**, 135—154 (1964).
JUDD, D. B., WYSZECKI, G.: Color in Business, Science, and Industry. New York: Wiley 1963.
KRANTZ, D. H.: The scaling of small and large color differences. Ph. D. thesis, University of Pennsylvania. Ann Arbor: University Microfilms 1964.
— Rational distance functions for multidimensional scaling. J. math. Psychol. **4**, 226—245 (1967a).
— Small-step and large-step color differences for monochromatic stimuli of constant brightness. J. opt. Soc. Amer. **57**, 1304—1316 (1967b).
— Integration of just-noticeable differences. J. math. Psychol. 8, 591—599 (1971).
— A theory of magnitude estimation and cross-modality matching. J. math. Psychol. **9**, in press (1972).
KRISTOF, W.: A foundation of interval scale measurement. Educational Testing Service Research Bulletin RB 67-22, Princeton, 1967.
KRUSKAL, J. B.: Nonmetric multidimensional scaling: A numerical method. Psychometrika **29**, 115—129 (1964).
KÜNNAPAS, T.: Measurements of subjective length in the vertical-horizontal illusion. Acta Psychologica **14**, 371—374 (1958).
— Scales for subjective distance. Scand. J. Psychol. **1**, 187—192 (1960).
— Visual perception of capital letters: Multidimensional ratio scaling and multidimensional similarity. Scand. J. Psychol. **7**, 189—196 (1966).
LE GRAND, Y.: Light, Colour, and Vision. (2nd. Ed.) London: Chapman and Hall 1968.
LEVINE, M. V.: Transformations that render curves parallel. J. math. Psychol. **7**, 410—443 (1970).
LUCE, R. D.: Individual Choice Behavior. New York: Wiley 1959.
— EDWARDS, W.: The derivation of subjective scales from just noticeable differences. Psychol. Rev. **65**, 222—237 (1958).
— GALANTER, E.: Discrimination. In: Handbook of Mathematical Psychology, Vol. 1. LUCE, R. D., BUSH, R. R., GALANTER, E. (Eds.): New York: Wiley 1963a.
— — Psychophysical scaling. In: Handbook of Mathematical Psychology, Vol. 1. LUCE, R.D., BUSH, R. R., GALANTER, E. (Eds.) New York: Wiley 1963b.
— Mo, S. S.: Magnitude estimation of heaviness and loudness by individual subjects: A test of a probabilistic response theory. Brit. J. math. stat. Psychol. **18**, 159—174 (1965).
MACADAM, D. L.: Specification of small chromaticity differences. J. opt. Soc. Amer. **33**, 18—26 (1943).
MESSICK, S. J.: An empirical evaluation of multidimensional successive intervals. Psychometrika **21**, 367—376 (1956).

MICKO, H. C., FISCHER, W.: The metric of multidimensional psychological space as a function of differential attention to subjective attributes. J. math. Psychol. **7**, 118—143 (1970).

Munsell Book of Color. Baltimore: Munsell Color Co. 1929.

MUNSELL, A. H.: Atlas of the Munsell Color System. Boston: 1915.

NEWHALL, S. M.: The ratio method in the review of the Munsell colors. Amer. J. Psychol. **52**, 394—405 (1939).

— Preliminary report of the O. S. A. subcommittee on the spacing of the Munsell colors. J. opt. Soc. Amer. **30**, 617—645 (1940).

— NICKERSON, D., JUDD, D. B.: Final report of the O. S. A. subcommittee on the spacing of the Munsell colors. J. opt. Soc. Amer. **33**, 385—418 (1943).

ONLEY, J. W.: Light adaptation and the brightness of brief foveal stimuli. J. opt. Soc. Amer. **51**, 667—673 (1961).

PANEK, D. W., STEVENS, S. S.: Saturation of red: a prothetic continuum. Perc. Psychophys. **1**, 59—66 (1966).

PIÉRON, H.: Récherches sur la latence de perception des accroissements de luminosité. Ann. Psychol. (Paris) **37**, 1—16 (1936).

PLATEAU, J.: Über die Messung physischer Empfindungen und das Gesetz, welches die Stärke der Empfindung mit der Stärke der erregenden Ursache verknüpft. Ann. Physik **150**, 465—475 (1873).

POULTON, E. C.: The new psychophysics: six models for magnitude estimation. Psychol. Bull. **69**, 1—19 (1968).

RASCH, G.: Probabilistic Models for Some Intelligence and Attainment Tests. Copenhagen: Nielsen and Lydiche 1960.

RASCH, G.: An item analysis which takes individual differences into account. Brit. J. math. stat. Psychol. **19**, 49—57 (1966).

RICHARDSON, M. W.: Multidimensional psychophysics. Psychol. Bull. **35**, 659—660 (1938).

SHEPARD, R. N.: The analysis of proximities: Multidimensional scaling with an unknown distance function. I. Psychometrika **27**, 125—140 (1962a).

— The analysis of proximities: Multidimensional scaling with an unknown distance function. II. Psychometrika **27**, 219—246 (1962b).

STERNBERG, S.: Four theories of the effect of distance on apparent size. Psychonomic Society Meetings, 1966.

STEVENS, J. C., MACK, J. D., STEVENS, S. S.: Growth of sensation on seven continua as measured by force of handgrip. J. exp. Psychol. **59**, 60—67 (1960).

— STEVENS, S. S.: Brightness function: Effects of adaptation. J. opt. Soc. Amer. **53**, 375—385 (1963).

STEVENS, S. S.: On the psychophysical law. Psychol. Rev. **64**, 153—181 (1957).

— Sic transit gloria varietatis? (Review of L. L. THURSTONE, The measurement of values.) Contemp. Psychol. **4**, 388—389 (1959).

— To honor Fechner and repeal his law. Science **133**, 80—86 (1961).

— Matching functions between loudness and ten other continua. Perc. Psychophys. **1**, 5—8 (1966).

— DIAMOND, A. L.: Effect of the glare angle on the brightness function for a small target. Vision Res. **5**, 649—659 (1965).

— GUIRAO, M.: Subjective scaling of length and area and the matching of length to loudness and brightness. J. exp. Psychol. **66**, 177—186 (1963).

TEGHTSOONIAN, M.: The judgment of size. Amer. J. Psychol. **78**, 392—402 (1965).

— TEGHTSOONIAN, R.: Seen and felt length. Psychon. Sci. **3**, 465—466 (1965).

TEGHTSOONIAN, R.: Range effects in psychophysical scaling and a revision of Stevens' law. Amer. J. Psychol. **85**, in press (1972).

THOMPSON, W. A., SINGH, J.: The use of limit theorems in paired comparison model building. Psychometrika **32**, 255—264 (1967).

THURSTONE, L. L.: A law of comparative judgment. Psychol. Rev. **34**, 273—286 (1927a).

— Psychophysical analysis. Amer. J. Psychol. **38**, 368—389 (1927b).

TORGERSON, W. S.: A Theoretical and Empirical Investigation of Multidimensional Scaling. Ph. D. thesis, Princeton University 1951.

Torgerson, W. S.: Theory and Method of Scaling. New York: Wiley 1958.
— Distances and ratios in psychophysical scaling. Acta Psychologica **19**, 201—205 (1961).
Tversky, A., Krantz, D. H.: The dimensional representation and the metric structure of similarity data. J. math. Psychol. **7**, 572—596 (1970).
— Russo, J. E.: Substitutability and similarity in binary choices. J. math. Psychol. **6**, 1—12 (1969).
Wilson, B. C.: An experimental examination of the spectral luminosity construct. Ph. D. thesis, New York University. Ann Arbor: University Microfilms 1964.
Wright, H.: Precision of color differences derived from a multidimensional scaling experiment. J. opt. Soc. Amer. **55**, 1650—1655 (1965).
Wyszecki, G., Stiles, W. S.: Color Science. New York: Wiley 1967.
Yager, D., Taylor, E.: Experimental measures and theoretical account of hue scaling as a function of luminance. Perc. Psychophys. **7**, 360—364 (1970).

Chapter 27

Electrical Measures and Psychophysical Data on Human Vision

By

LORRIN A. RIGGS and BILLY R. WOOTEN, Providence, Rhode Island (USA)

With 14 Figures

Contents

Introduction

This chapter compares psychophysical methods of studying human vision with more objective methods, especially that of recording electrical responses from the visual system. Two sites are available for obtaining these responses without

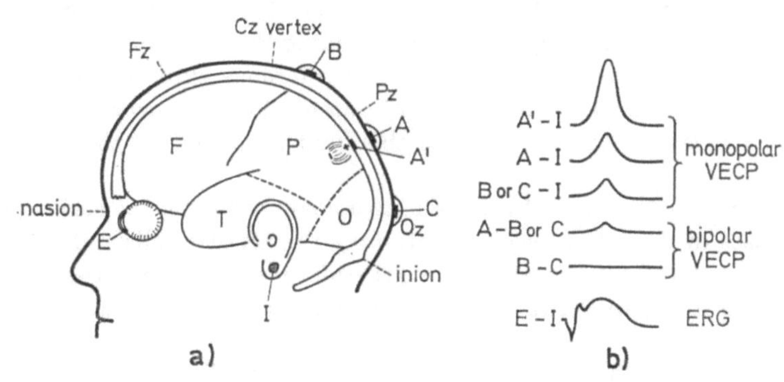

Fig. 1. a) Placement of gross electrodes for recording light-elicited electrical responses from the eye and brain of human subjects. The ERG is recorded with the active electrode, *E*, embedded in a scleral contact lens and the indifferent electrode, *I*, in contact with the cheek, forehead, or (as shown here) the earlobe. The VECP may be recorded with any of several active-electrode configurations as discussed in the text. Some typical placements are represented by *A*, *B*, and *C*; as with the ERG, the earlobe is frequently used as the indifferent site. *A'* represents a hypothetical electrode placed directly on the cortical surface. b) Hypothetical responses resulting from the use of the designated pairs of electrodes, in conjunction with differential amplification, assuming, for simplicity, that a simple source-sink is located as shown, directly beneath electrodes *A* and *A'*. The actual VECP wave is complex, and may include potentials generated in the various lobes of the brain (*F*, frontal; *P*, parietal; *T*, temporal; *O*, occipital). These are shown in (a), together with the major. midline designations according to standard EEG terminology (Jasper, 1958). Position *Oz* is located at 10% of the distance from the inion (the most prominent part of the external occipital protuberance) to the nasion (middle point of nasofrontal suture) *Pz* at 30%, *Cz* at 50%, and *Fz* at 70%. The ERG is generated by various types of neurone within the retina of the eye (region shown by hatching) The electrical properties of volume conduction are such, however, that it can be recorded as a response potential wave appearing between the gross electrodes at *E* and *I*

undue discomfort or injury to the subject. These are (*1*) the cornea of the eye and (*2*) the scalp over the occipital cortex, as shown in Fig. 1. Accordingly, we give separate consideration to each of these sites, covering the topics of (a) the nature of the response recorded there, (b) techniques of eliciting and recording the response, and (c) resulting data, in comparison with psychophysical results under similar conditions.

Other chapters in this volume give more extensive coverage of the psychophysical data on visual problems; and chapters in other volumes are concerned with visual neurophysiology, including the electrophysiology of human vision. Thus the present coverage is confined mainly to the relation between the two, namely the extent to which psychophysical and electrophysiological methods can be combined for a better understanding of the visual process. Ideally, this means the simultaneous use of the two methods on the same subjects, but we have extended our coverage to include data that are obtained under comparable, though not identical conditions.

The Nature of the Responses

The Electroretinogram (ERG)

Experiments on animals (see chapters in the volume of visual neurophysiology) have shown that the cornea of the vertebrate eye is in relatively good electrical contact with the anterior (vitreal) surface of the retina. The posterior (choroidal) retinal surface, on the other hand, is in good electrical contact with the bloodstream and hence with the body tissues surrounding the eye. Thus an active corneal electrode can be used, in conjunction with a reference skin electrode, to obtain reasonably faithful records of differences of potential that appear across the retina itself. The ERG is a composite wave of this kind produced by the action of light on the eye.

Experiments on the eyes of animals have also shown that a major portion of the ERG arises in the retinal layers containing the bipolar cells and their connections with the rod and cone receptors. We therefore conclude that the human ERG can be used to measure events occurring at an early retinal stage in the visual pathways.

The waveform of the ERG is typically complex. Fig. 2 shows human ERG waves elicited by flashes of light. By convention, downward deflections (*a*-waves) indicate negativity, while upward ones (*b*-waves) show positivity of the cornea electrode with respect to the reference electrode on the skin. There is evidence that, at least in the eyes of mammals, the early negative portions of the response originate in the receptors, while the later positive portions arise in the bipolar layer (Granit, 1947; Auerbach and Burian, 1955; Brown and Wiesel, 1961). Conditions that favor photopic (cone receptor) stimulation lead to small, diphasic responses of short latency. Stimulation of the scotopic (rod-receptor) system produces relatively large response components of longer latency (Adrian, 1945, 1946).

A light flash of very high luminance is capable of producing an "early receptor potential" (ERP) having no measurable latency (Brown and Murakami, 1964; Cone, 1964) in the eyes of experimental animals. The ERP does not usually appear on human ERG records such as those in Fig. 2 but has been elicited in the normal human eye (Galloway, 1967; Yonemura and Kawasaki, 1967) with sufficiently intense flashes. Data are not yet available, however, on the relation of the ERP to visual sensitivity.

Summaries by Kohlrausch (1931), Granit (1947, 1955, 1962) and Riggs (1965) may be consulted for surveys of the ERG literature, and Brown (1968) has recently discussed the origins of components of the ERG.

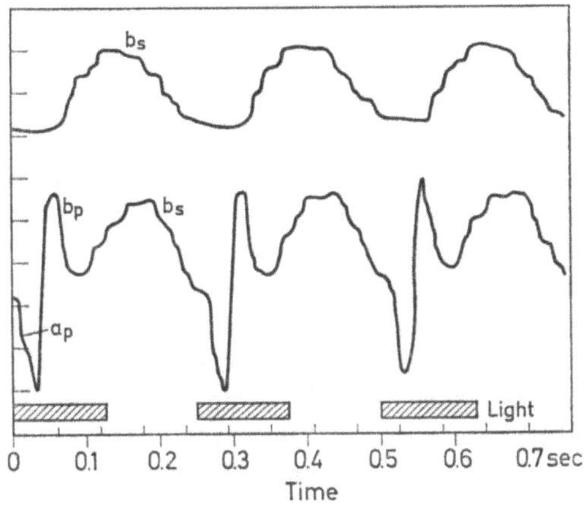

Fig. 2. Records of the human ERG. Upper tracing: Slow, scotopic b-waves (b_s) obtained with violet light flashes (410 nm) that stimulate mainly the rod receptors. Lower tracing: Complex waveform resulting from flashes of orange light (610 nm) that stimulates both rods and cones. Waves a_p and b_p are the relatively quick photopic components resulting from cone stimulation, while b_s is mainly a slower scotopic component similar to that in the upper trace. (After Riggs, 1965)

The Visually Evoked Cortical Potential (VECP)

A transient electrical change can be recorded with gross electrodes from the exposed occipital cortex of an animal as a result of stimulating the retina with light. Although such evoked potentials are superimposed on the spontaneous electrical activity of the brain (the electroencephalogram or EEG) they are distinguished from it by having a definite temporal relation to the eliciting stimulus. It is known that the evoked potential is cortical in origin (Bergamini and Bergamasco, 1967), but the actual cellular electrogenesis is poorly understood. Most workers do agree that evoked potentials represent the summated pre- and postsynaptic graded potentials of many cortical neurons rather than summated action potentials (Bremer, 1961; Creutzfeldt and Kuhnt, 1967). Fox and O'Brien (1965) have shown a close correspondence between the waveform of the visually evoked potential and the frequency distribution of the firing of a single cell recorded with the same microelectrode. Thus, whatever potential sources contribute to the evoked potential wave, they are intimately related to single cell firing patterns. (See Creutzfeldt's chapter in Vol. VII/3 of this series for a fuller discussion of this problem.)

The amplitude of the evoked potential recorded directly from cortex may reach several hundred microvolts. Recorded with scalp electrodes, however, it is so severely attenuated due to the intervening tissue and bone that its amplitude is considerably lower than the background electrical noise from EEG and muscle activity. It is therefore necessary to resort to signal averaging techniques (see p. 696) to obtain reliable records. Thus the averaged evoked potential is really a statistical abstraction. Nevertheless, studies comparing scalp recording with direct cortical recording in patients undergoing brain surgery have shown that the former is essentially an attenuated version of the latter (e. g., Rayport *et al.*, 1964; Cooper *et al.*, 1965).

The light-elicited potential recorded with scalp electrodes over the occipital cortex has been variously called the visual evoked response, cortical evoked potential, cortical response, occipital response, occipitogram or simply the evoked potential. We propose "visually evoked cortical potential" (VECP) as a term that most accurately describes the recorded electrical change as both visual and cortical in origin and elicited rather than spontaneous.

The waveform of the VECP is complex and variable. It is dependent on electrode placement, bipolar or monopolar mode of recording and stimulus conditions. Since no standard recording procedure has evolved, the literature is replete with a variety of waveforms and it is difficult to specify "the" VECP. Nevertheless certain consistent features are evident. Fig. 3, a record from Gastaut and Régis (1964), serves to illustrate a typical waveform when slow, repetitive flash stimulation is used. The early waves labeled *1*, *2*, and *3* represent what Cigánek (1961) and others have called the "primary response" and the later waves, *4* and *5*, the "secondary response". The rhythmic waves beginning with *6* have been called the "after-discharge".

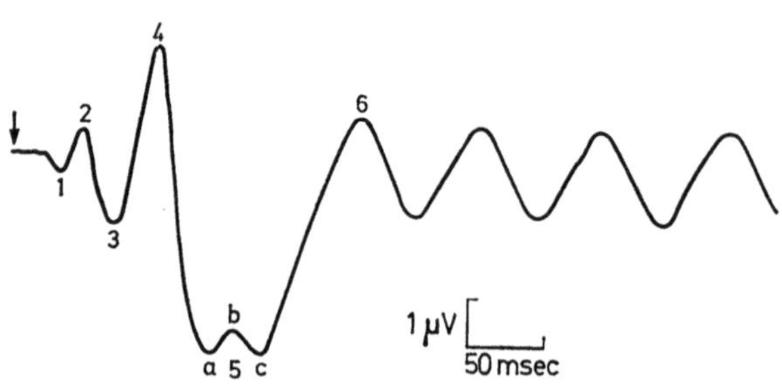

Fig. 3. VECP recorded with a monopolar electrode (inion-ear). Cumulation of 50 sweeps of the computer. (From Bergamini and Bergamasco, 1967; after Gastaut and Régis, 1964)

The question of which cortical structures generate the various waves of the VECP is still in controversy. Cigánek (1961) concluded that the primary response represents specific activity of the visual cortical area while the secondary response represents non-specific activity of diffuse pathways. More recently Cigánek (1965) has even included the primary response in the non-specific category since he could record temporally comparable auditory evoked potentials with the same electrodes. Rémond (1964) has made extensive mapping studies and has shown that visually evoked potentials can be recorded from virtually any area of the scalp, although the waveform varies from area to area.

Important considerations with regard to the origin of VECP waves are the number and positions of the electrodes in relation to underlying structures. These two factors are critical because two different kinds of potential are most certainly present: (a) specific, occipital responses via the classical pathways of retina to lateral geniculate nucleus to occipital cortex, and (b) non-specific, non-occipital responses via the retina to reticular nucleus to diffuse thalamic projection system. With gross electrodes located anywhere but directly over occipital cortex, including bipolar electrodes with one lead over non-occipital regions, these non-specific potentials would clearly contribute partially or wholly to the waveform of the VECP. In fact, due to volume conduction effects, even a monopolar, occipital recording could be compounded of both types of response. Gastaut and Régis (1964) have, however, presented evidence that such monopolar recordings are strongly localized over the occipital region, retaining large amplitude and invariant waveform only within a 3 cm semicircle with the inion[1] as center. These findings are also consistent with the results of a case of "cortical blindness" reported by Kooi and Sharbrough (1966). They recorded VECP's from a subject who was temporarily blinded as a result of a head injury. During the period of total blindness there was no detectable VECP with a monopolar electrode at the inion. However, with a similar electrode at the vertex (over parietal cortex) a sizable response could be elicited with either visual or auditory stimuli. As vision gradually returned a detectable VECP from the occipital region appeared. This clinical case is of particular interest since it indicates that the occipital VECP can be recorded without confounding with the non-occipital response.

A tentative, but reasonable, conclusion is that both the primary and secondary responses are specific occipital responses when recorded with monopolar electrodes with the active lead near the inion. Bipolar recordings, such as Cigánek's, where one lead is near the inion and the other near the vertex are probably compounded of the specific, occipital response and the non-specific parietal response. This is consistent with the well-documented rich projection of the diffuse thalamic system to the parietal region.

Experimental Methods

Standard reference books may be consulted on the general procedures for electrophysiological amplification, electrical shielding and recording (Donaldson, 1958; Cornsweet, 1963; Sidowsky, 1966; Venables and Martin, 1967).

ERG Electrodes

A corneal electrode for the human eye is conveniently provided by embedding a metallic electrode in a scleral contact lens. Properly fitted, such an attachment to the eye (see Fig. 1) is sufficiently comfortable to permit recording sessions of two or three hours' duration (Riggs, 1941). An isotonic contact lens solution is used to fill the space between the cornea and the surface of the electrode, thus providing stable electrical contact with the cornea. More complex contact lens electrodes have been designed for clinical use (Karpe, 1945; Henkes, 1951; Burian, 1953; Burian and Allen, 1954). In clinical practice, short test sessions are the rule. The patient's cornea is anesthetized and no attempt is made to achieve an individual fit. Instead, some form of suction is often applied to the lens, and the lids may also be retracted in an attempt to hold the lens in place.

Standard skin electrodes, of the form used in EEG recording, may be used for reference leads in ERG experiments. One such electrode may be placed on the earlobe, or on the forehead near the eye; the ERG is recorded as a momentary change in the difference of potential between it and the electrode on the contact

[1] See Fig. 1 for a diagram showing the location of the inion and vertex.

lens. To minimize the effects of unwanted electrical noise or interference, a balanced (differential) amplifier input circuit may be used. This requires a third (ground) electrode which may be a skin electrode clipped to the other earlobe or taped elsewhere on the head.

VECP Electrodes

The usual EEG scalp electrodes (metallic disks a few mm in diameter) are used in VECP recording. A slightly abrasive and highly conductive paste is applied to the scalp and the electrodes, coated with the same paste, are placed usually over the occipital region and held there with collodion or a headpiece. The configuration of electrodes markedly affects the shape of the response and is a factor responsible for the wide variety of waveforms reported in the literature. Fig. 1a is a greatly oversimplified diagram which illustrates some basic principles of volume conduction. The source and sink[2] are assumed to be localized within the cerebral cortex. The size and shape of the recorded potential clearly depend upon the placement of electrodes relative to the source-sink. Monopolar recording ($A - I$, $B - I$, or $C - I$) reflects most accurately the amplitude of the potential. Bipolar recording ($A - B$, $A - C$, or $B - C$) gives much more exact information on the location of the potential. This figure also shows that the more distant the electrode from the potential field ($A - I$ compared to $A' - I$) the smaller the recorded amplitude, although the shape is preserved. With the addition of many sources and sinks located at various depths due to the complicated convolutions of the cerebral cortex, the recording situation becomes extremely complex. Hence it is not surprising that the VECP has a complex waveform which is highly dependent on recording conditions.

Signal-Averaging Techinques

Whereas ERG waves may approach 1 mv in amplitude for a fully dark-adapted eye, some of the most interesting responses from the photopic system are in the range from 0 to 10 μv. Moreover, VECP amplitudes seldom exceed this range under any conditions. Thus both ERG and VECP are typically below the level of random electrical fluctuation ("noise") due to involuntary muscle potentials and to inherent instability of electrodes and amplifiers. As a result it is virtually impossible to measure such responses without resorting to some form of signal-averaging procedure.

A convenient arrangement for recording average response potential waves from the eye is shown in Fig. 4. Repetitive flashes of light are delivered to the eye by a shutter mechanism that also operates a trigger circuit for the activation of a response-averaging computer.

Several models of computer are now available for this task; but all of them operate on the same basic principle. The time axis is digitized or broken up into some finite number (e. g. 400) of discrete intervals for each of which there is a "bin" or electronic storage compartment. The voltage level of the electrical signal during each interval is sampled and stored in the corresponding bin. Since each bin maintains a constant time relation to the onset of the stimulus, any time-locked stable signal, such as the ERG or VECP, will tend to fill or not-fill specific bins as the stimulus is repeated again and again. On the other hand any electrical

[2] The "source" is the origin of current flow and the "sink" is the place to which it flows.

activity which occurs randomly with respect to the eliciting stimulus, such as the EEG, muscle activity or amplifier drift, will tend to fill each bin equally in the long run. Thus, as the cumulation process proceeds, the "signal" will emerge as the dominant waveform and the "noise", even though much larger, will tend to average out to zero. The result is therefore a summed digital conversion of a series of continuously varying (analog) signals. This digital representation is finally converted back to an analog signal and recorded, with an $X - Y$ plotting device, to produce permanent records such as those appearing in Figs. 2 and 3.

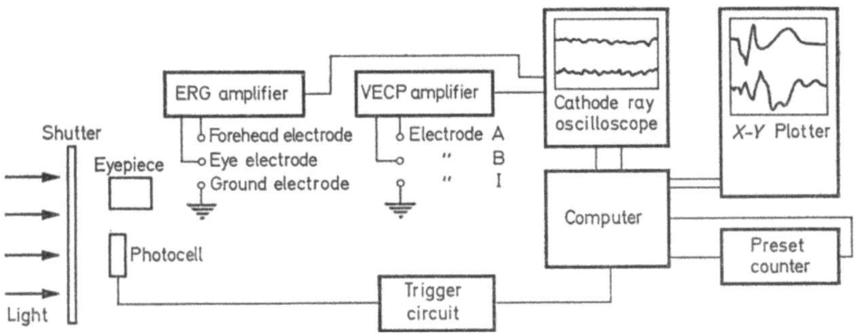

Fig. 4. Diagram of arrangements for plotting ERG and VECP potential waves. See text for details. (Adapted from RIGGS, 1965)

The signal-averaging procedures just outlined contribute immensely to the usefulness of ERG and VECP recording from the human visual system. Responses to stimuli at moderate luminance levels are now easily measurable, while without the averaging procedures they are completely obscured by random noise. The averaging procedures represent a technical advance, in the last few years, that is comparable in significance to the much earlier appearance of amplifiers and oscillographs for recording gross electrical responses. We must not forget, however, that new artifacts may readily creep into our new recording devices. Any event that is synchronized with the stimulus must now be suspect. Vibration or electromagnetic signals from the shutter, photoelectric potentials from the electrodes, reflex muscular responses to the light: all these and many other unwanted effects must be checked by running appropriate control experiments.

ERG Findings in Relation to Psychophysics

Stimulus Variables under Scotopic Conditions

Vision requires that the rod and cone receptors be acted upon by light in such a way as to initiate neural activity within the afferent visual system. The ERG is an early sign of such activity, and it is of interest to observe the dependency of the ERG on characteristics of the stimulus such as energy level or luminance (L), duration (t), wavelength (λ), area (A) and frequency (ν) of flashes of light. These aspects of the stimulus have different effects under scotopic and photopic conditions of stimulation.

Energy Level or Luminance. In the dark-adapted eye, moderate flashes of light produce ERG waves in which the scotopic b-wave (b_s) predominates. The amplitude of b_s grows linearly with log energy of stimulation over a range of about two log units (see Fig. 5). Above that range b_s rises no further and may indeed decline at high flash energies, where the negative *a*-wave has become very large (RIGGS and JOHNSON, 1949; BOYNTON and RIGGS, 1951; CRAMPTON and ARMINGTON, 1955).

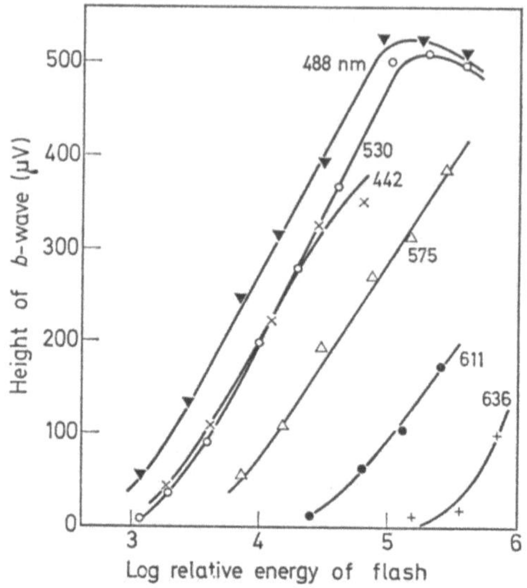

Fig. 5. Magnitude of the scotopic *b*-wave of the ERG as a function of log energy of stimulus flash. Each curve is for the designated wavelength of light. (From RIGGS and JOHNSON, 1949)

Duration. For flash durations of 0.1 sec or less, the effectiveness of the flash for eliciting a b_s wave increases with stimulus duration (MÜLLER-LIMMROTH, 1953). Over a considerable range the height of b_s is proportional to log total energy, i. e. $b_s = k \log (It)$ (JOHNSON and BARTLETT, 1956; ALPERN and FARIS, 1956).

Area. Area and energy have also been shown to be interchangeable stimulus parameters for eliciting b_s waves (BOYNTON and RIGGS, 1951; WIRTH and ZETTERSTRÖM, 1954; CRAMPTON and ARMINGTON, 1955; JOHNSON, 1958). To a first approximation, then, it is the total quantity of light $(I \cdot t \cdot A)$ that determines its effectiveness for eliciting the scotopic ERG; and over a dynamic range of about two log units it is approximately true that $b_s = k \log(I \cdot t \cdot A)$.

Stray Light. Under conditions of full dark adaptation, the retinal rods become so sensitive that they respond not only to patches of light focused on them, but also to non-focal light scattered from the main beam as it traverses the lens and other optic media of the eye and is partially reflected from that part of the retina on which it is focused. A bright flash of light that is deliberately focused on the blind spot of the eye can be shown, indeed, to arouse a b_s wave as large as those produced when the same patch is moved onto normally sensitive regions of the retina (ASHER, 1951; BOYNTON and RIGGS, 1951). This result emphasizes the fact that more than 100 million rod receptors are available for stimulation by light that scatters throughout the retina; it is therefore of trivial significance whether light is focused on the blind spot where there are no rods at all, or on a peripheral region of equivalent size that contains fewer than 1% of the whole number of rods in the retina.

Wavelength. Standard spectral sensitivity curves show that a wavelength of about 505 nm is maximally effective for stimulating human vision at scotopic levels (WALD, 1945) and this is true with respect to the b_s wave as well (ADRIAN, 1944, 1945; RIGGS and JOHNSON, 1949). A more detailed comparison of spectral sensitivity functions has revealed, moreover, a good agreement throughout most of the spectrum between standard psychophysical curves and curves based on the absorption spectrum of rhodopsin on the one hand (DARTNALL, 1962) and the scotopic ERG results on the other (RIGGS *et al.* 1949). In the case of the ERG results, however, there is a discrepancy in the direction of excess sensitivity for wavelengths below 500 nm. This discrepancy results in part from the fact that short-wave light is scattered more effectively than lights of higher wavelengths (BOYNTON and RIGGS, 1951). Fluorescence may also play a part (DODT and WALTHER, 1958). Through the use of large stimulus fields, BOYNTON (1953) was able to minimize the effects of scatter. The final results showed good agreement between psychophysical and ERG determinations of human scotopic spectral sensitivity, and this finding is amply substantiated by later experiments (ARMINGTON, 1959; GRANDA and BIERSDORF, 1966; VAN LITH, 1966).

Stimulus Variables under Photopic Conditions

We have seen that ERG waves of scotopic origin are readily obtained by the use of relatively large stimuli delivered to a fully dark-adapted eye. It is not easy, however, to isolate for measurement the purely photopic components of the ERG. Early investigators (MOTOKAWA and MITA, 1942; ADRIAN, 1945) noted the appearance of such components in the response potential waves of their human subjects. Unfortunately, however, the scotopic components of the human ERG are so large that they obscure and distort the photopic ones (see Fig. 2) even under high levels of illumination. Perhaps this is because there are relatively few cone receptors in the human eye. In any case, rather special conditions of stimulation are required to evoke purely photopic human ERG's.

Intermittent Flashes. One method by which scotopic responding can be minimized is to use high rates of intermittent flashes (ADRIAN, 1945, 1946; DODT, 1951; BORNSCHEIN and SCHUBERT, 1953). This procedure has been used to yield ERG potentials on which to base spectral sensitivity curves (JOHNSON and CORNSWEET, 1954; ARMINGTON, 1955; ARMINGTON and BIERSDORF, 1956; HECK, 1957; DODT *et al.*, 1958). Done before averaging techniques were available, these experiments required the use of large areas and high energies of stimulus flash. Nevertheless the results are in close agreement with the assumption that rates of 20 to 25 flashes per second are sufficiently high to yield ERG waves that are produced entirely by the photopic system. The explanation seems to be that the scotopic system is a slow-acting one in which there is insufficient time for a response to occur to one flash before another flash comes along (JOHNSON, 1958). Photopic responses occur more quickly; hence the photopic system can respond separately to each flash even at relatively high flicker rates.

Background Illumination. A second method for producing purely photopic responses is the use of single test flashes surrounded by steady, intense illumination of the peripheral retina. Early attempts by RIGGS *et al.* (1949) and ARMINGTON *et al.* (1961) were not very successful, since scotopic responses were found to persist until the background illumination became so high as to reduce all responses to a level too low to be measured.

Later experiments have been based on the cumulation of large numbers of response potential waves (BRINDLEY and WESTHEIMER, 1965). With this technique, stray light effects were nearly eliminated by the use of intense backgrounds of steady illumination. Small test spots elicited ERG's of an amplitude that was easily measured, by the technique of signal-averaging, when the light was directed within the fovea. Very little response was obtained with stimuli centered on the blind spot, but other peripheral locations yielded responses of an amplitude dependent on the nearness of the stimulus to the fovea. Thus it became possible to use ERG recording as a clinical technique for the objective mapping of retinal scotomata. (See also COPENHAVER and BEINHOCKER, 1963; and GOURAS *et al.*, 1964).

Experiments by AIBA *et al.* (1967) also made use of steady background illumination to facilitate the recording of responses to small test patches of light. Using blue light as a background they were able to demonstrate an approximate agreement between psychophysical and ERG determinations of photopic spectral sensitivity functions. They concluded that their blue background was sufficiently intense to suppress the activity of the scotopic visual system without unduly depressing photopic receptors, which are much less sensitive to blue light.

Alternating Stripe Pattern. A third solution to the problem of confining the ERG responses to the photopic system is to make use of a stimulus field in which the stimulus fluctuates within small areas while the total energy remains constant. This has the effect that the large numbers of rod receptors in the peripheral retina are electrically silent, since the stray light reaching them from the test patch is of

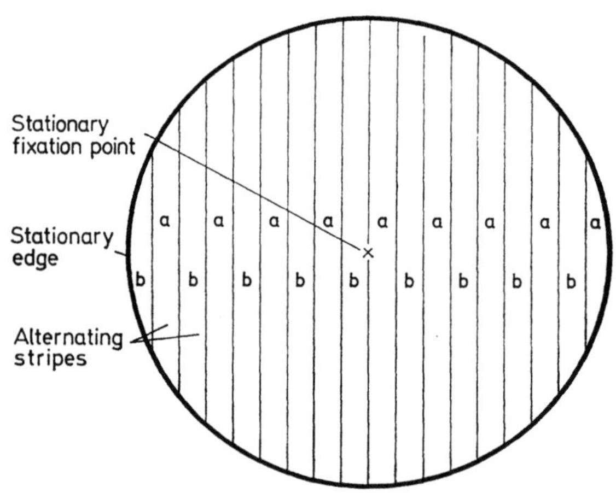

Fig. 6. Alternating stripe pattern used to isolate photopic ERG responses. At one instant the *a* stripes are of one color and the *b* stripes of a second color. At the next instant there is a reversal so that the *a* stripes have the second color and the *b* stripes the first. Continued alternation of this kind, as the eye fixates on a stationary point X, exposes each point on the retina to an alternation between the two colors at a rate of about 10 alternations per sec. The field size is approximately 19° and stripe width 1°7′. (From RIGGS, JOHNSON, and SCHICK, 1966)

constant energy. In one series of experiments (Riggs *et al.*, 1964, 1966; Johnson *et al.*, 1966) the test field was made up of a series of narrow, parallel stripes as shown in Fig. 6. Within each stripe the light was made to fluctuate, in energy or wavelength, at a rate of about 10 fluctuations per second. The fluctuations of odd- and even-numbered stripes were made to be 180° out of phase, so that as half the stripes shifted from one color to a second color, the other half shifted from the second to the first. Thus each receptor within the field was alternately exposed to the two colors, while the total amount of light within the whole field remained constant.

Two lines of evidence lead to the conclusion that the alternating stripe pattern elicits only photopic ERG responses. First, spectral sensitivity data obtained in this way are in good agreement with psychophysical (brightness-matching) data obtained on the same subjects with the same stimulus field (Johnson *et al.*, 1966). Second, the directional sensitivity of the receptors, as determined by the use of the stripe pattern for ERG recording, agrees closely with psychophysical data on the same subjects, using standard photopic procedures (Stiles and Crawford, 1933; see also Crawford, chapter 18, this volume) for observing the directional properties of the retinal cones (Armington, 1967; Sternheim and Riggs, 1968). Evidently the spatial resolution of the scotopic system is unable to cope with the relatively fine dimensions of the stripe pattern, just as the scotopic temporal resolution is insufficient to mediate fast flicker.

As a method for isolating photopic responses, alternating stripe stimulation has the advantages that it does not require the use of a white or blue background, and is not restricted to high frequencies of flash. The method is not, however, very useful with foveal stimulus patches; even with the aid of an average response computer relatively large stimulus fields are needed to generate sizable responses. With a typical rate of about ten alternations per second the ERG responses are nearly sinusoidal in waveform with peak-to-trough amplitudes that seldom exceed six or eight microvolts. The latencies and amplitudes of response waves vary systematically with luminance, but no major variations of waveform are found due to wavelength, even with stimulus fields as large as 20° in diameter (Johnson, *et al.*, 1966). The foveal cones make little contribution to the response, since ERGs from a 2° foveal field are barely discernible (Armington, 1968). Hence we conclude that the responses to alternating-stripe stimuli are primarily those resulting from the arousal of large numbers of parafoveal cone receptors.

Energy Effects. Numerous studies attest to the fact that a curve of increasing slope is obtained when photopic ERG potentials are plotted against log energy. This is true of the older single-flash data on *a*-wave and photopic *b*-wave portions of the ERG (Armington and Thiede, 1954; Crampton and Armington, 1955). It is also true for small responses to sinusoidal flicker (Aiba *et al.*, 1966) where log ERG amplitude is found to be linearly related to log energy for all wavelengths over a range of about two log energy units. These photopic results are all in marked contrast with the corresponding semi-logarithmic relations that we have already noted above for the scotopic responses in full dark adaptation (see Fig. 5).

Area Effects. Under photopic conditions, the fovea yields maximum ERG potentials, with a rapid drop-off as the test spot is moved out into the periphery (Brindley and Westheimer, 1965). This result, too, is in marked contrast to old single-flash scotopic data showing reciprocity of area and energy (see above). Armington (1968) using an alternating stripe procedure, has shown that photopic

ERG amplitudes are linearly related to the number of cone receptors lying within the area of stimulation.

Variables Related to the Human Subject, under Scotopic Conditions

We have enumerated some of the aspects of the ERG that we can easily relate to stimulus variables. We now turn to effects in which the main interest lies in processes within the subject, such as light and dark adaptation, color discrimination, and certain visual defects.

Dark Adaptation. As we have noted, the b_s wave of the ERG is usually its most prominent feature, particularly in a fully dark-adapted eye. This wave is therefore easy to use as a measure of scotopic activity in the eye. The magnitude of b_s grows progressively during the course of dark adaptation (Adrian, 1945; Karpe and Tansley, 1947; Schubert and Bornschein, 1952; Bornschein, 1953). Experiments can therefore be designed to yield a quantitative comparison of dark adaptation curves based on determinations of test light energies necessary to (a) elicit a b_s of specified amplitude and (b) reach an absolute threshold for the same subject to report that he sees the test flash.

Dark adaptation curves based on b_s waves for normal human subjects run roughly parallel with psychophysical threshold curves on the same subjects (Johnson, 1949; Johnson and Riggs, 1951; Best, 1953; Alpern and Faris, 1954). Exact parallels are not found, however; some of the discrepancies are no doubt due to the fact that relatively bright test flashes were required to elicit ERG's as compared to those used to establish psychophysical thresholds (Johnson and Riggs, 1951; Shipley, 1966). Very limited dark adaptation is shown by certain congenitally night-blind subjects; for them, ERG and psychophysical results yield similarly curtailed recovery curves (Riggs, 1954; Armington and Schwab, 1954; Goodman and Bornschein, 1957; Carr and Siegel, 1964; Carr *et al.*, 1966). One rod monochromat has been found, however, who shows an unusually early *b*-wave recovery during her dark adaptation. This may signify that in the absence of cone vision the rods can function more effectively (Elenius and Heck, 1957).

Clinical Conditions. The correlation between psychophysical threshold data and ERG data on visual sensitivity breaks down under certain unusual conditions. A brief period of retinal anoxia, for example, may produce a temporary loss of sight even though the ERG remains normal (Noell and Chinn, 1950). Similarly, permanent blindness due to glaucoma may not entail loss of the ERG (Karpe, 1945; Burian, 1953). In both these cases the explanation would appear to lie in the fact that vision fails when ganglion cells show an early failure to function under conditions of oxygen deficiency. As long as receptor and bipolar function are still maintained, the ERG may remain normal even after vision has been lost. There is also evidence that photopic ERG components may be more easily affected than is the scotopic *b*-wave by anoxia (Brown *et al.*, 1957).

Retinitis pigmentosa is a familial degenerative disease in which the scotopic *b*-wave may appear to be lost even when vision is still relatively normal (Karpe, 1954; Riggs, 1954). Response-averaging techniques may reveal, however, that the loss is not complete and that a small residual wave may still be measured. As the disease invades more and more of the retina there is a fairly close correlation between the magnitude of the ERG on the one hand and the extent of the remaining visual field on the other (Gouras *et al.*, 1964).

We may summarize by saying that the studies cited, and many others as well, point to the scotopic *b*-wave as representing the mass activity of cells activated by the retinal rods. Related animal work also attests to the validity of the *b*-wave as an index of sensitivity and of the bleaching and regeneration of photopigments (Granit *et al.*, 1939; Dowling, 1967). We have noted, however, that exact parallels are not found between ERG and psychophysical threshold findings with regard to scotopic sensitivity. Among the factors accounting for the discrepancy are the relatively great effectiveness of stray light in arousing the ERG, the fact that the ERG is greatly depressed by certain retinal diseases such as retinitis pigmentosa, and the relatively slight effect on the ERG of equally serious conditions such as glaucoma.

Variables Related to the Human Subject under Photopic Conditions

We have seen that early portions of the ERG wave are mainly due to photopic activity, and we have noted that techniques are now available for isolating the photopic ERG by the use of stimulus fields that fail to arouse the scotopic system. We have also noted that spectral sensitivity curves based on the use of these stimulus fields are closely similar to psychophysical spectral sensitivity curves. We are therefore in a position to apply the new techniques to such photopic visual problems as normal and defective color discrimination and the critical frequency of flicker fusion.

Cavonius (1962) and Aiba *et al.* (1967) have obtained photopic ERG responses to intermittent stimulation of the eye. They have found that the various wavelengths of light, when adjusted for equal photopic luminance, produce ERG waves that are nearly identical in their latency and waveform. It thus appears that the specific wavelength differences noted by earlier investigators (e.g. Motokawa and Mita, 1943; Adrian, 1945) were mainly due to the fact that various proportions of scotopic and photopic activity were evoked by the various wavelengths.

Purely photopic waves are now shown to have rather similar shapes for all wavelengths. With respect to differences in phase and latency, small but reliable differences have been measured (Aiba *et al.*, 1967) but differences due to wavelength appear in various amounts and directions from one subject to another. Since all these subjects have normal color vision and spectral sensitivity curves, the weight of the evidence of this study, consistent with earlier ones (Armington, 1955; Cavonius, 1964; Gouras and Gunkel, 1964) is that specific wavelength effects are not significantly coded by the temporal pattern of responding at the level of the ERG.

Color-Differentiating Responses. We have noted above that photopic ERG waves do not show systematic dependency of waveform, phase or latency on wavelength of the stimulating light. There is ample evidence, of course, that color responses are coded spatially rather than temporally at the retinal level, i.e. that there are separate classes of cone receptor which respond selectively to lights from particular regions of the spectrum. If that is the case, the various classes should respond differentially, and ERG waves should be produced at any time when wavelength changes are made in a stimulus field. Furthermore, the responses may be designated as color-discriminating, rather than luminance-discriminating, if the stimulus change is between two wavelengths that have been adjusted for equality of luminance.

The alternating-stripe pattern previously described can readily be used for wavelength-difference experiments. In one set of experiments (RIGGS *et al.*, 1966) monochromatic light from one region of the spectrum was used to illuminate one set of stripes, while the other set was illuminated with another wavelength of light. The whole spectrum was explored in this way, each wavelength being paired with each other wavelength at 15 nm intervals. Within each stripe of the pattern there was an alternation between the two wavelengths of each pair at the rate of about 10 alternations per second. Lights of all wavelengths were adjusted for equality of luminance.

Wavelength-alternation produced ERG responses the magnitude of which depended on the wavelength separation. Responses of maximum amplitude were obtained only with separations of 150 nm or more. Responses of minimum measurable amplitude were obtained with wavelength separations of about 15 nm in the most favorable region of the spectrum (about 590 nm). In less favorable regions larger separations were required, as shown by the ERG curve of Fig. 7, to elicit a measurable ERG response. The results are understandable in terms of the assumption that each of the two wavelengths in the pattern must arouse different classes of cone receptors if it is to produce responses of maximum amplitude. Thus the

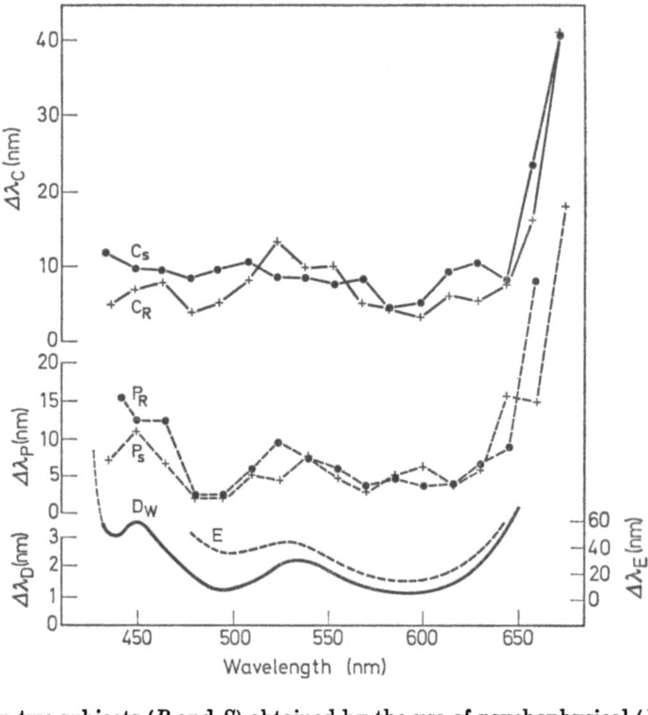

Fig. 7. Data on two subjects (*R* and *S*) obtained by the use of psychophysical (*P*) and evoked cortical (*C*) potential methods for measuring the effects of differences in wavelength ($\Delta\lambda$) that are needed to achieve a criterion response at various wavelengths (nm) throughout the spectrum. Note also the relatively finer $\Delta\lambda$ steps in standard wavelength discrimination studies such as those of WRIGHT and PITT (curve *Dw*). Also note very much coarser wavelength difference steps needed to produce measurable responses at the level of the ERG (curve *E*, scale at right). (From RIGGS and STERNHEIM, 1969)

shift from one wavelength to the other is equivalent to turning the light on for one class of cones while turning it off for another. Fairly good fits to the experimental data are obtained, in fact, by the use of a simple trichromatic model describing the relative contributions of three different color mechanisms that are differentially activated by various wavelengths of light.

Comparisons with VECP and Psychophysical Data. Wavelength-difference experiments have also been carried out with VECP recording. Here it is found that measurable responses can be obtained with alternating stripe patterns even when they are composed of two wavelengths that are relatively close together. Fig. 7 shows, for example, that differences as small as 4 nm may result in measurable responses in favorable regions of the spectrum. It therefore seems that a considerable sharpening or refinement of the wavelength-discriminating signal takes place between the stages in the processing of the visual signals for color from which the ERG and VECP arise.

Fig. 7 shows psychophysical data for comparison with the ERG and VECP results. The curves labelled P_R and P_S were obtained by a matching procedure in which the subject judged the amount of the color difference present in the stripe pattern by comparison with a standard color difference appearing at the same time in another part of the field. Note that the resulting curves are in qualitative agreement with the electrical results and with the wavelength-discrimination results of Wright and Pitt as shown by curve D_w in Fig. 7. That is, each curve shows very poor wavelength discrimination above 630 nm, good discrimination in the regions of 495 and 595 nm, and fairly poor discrimination near 540 nm and below 480 nm.

Dichromasy. Now that purely photopic ERG measurements can be made it should be possible to obtain detailed information on retinal function in dichromats, along the lines of the experiments just described on normal trichromats. Sachs (1929), Armington (1952) and Schubert and Bornschein (1952) have all noted deficiencies in the photopic portion of the *b*-wave when flashes of long-wave light were delivered to protanopic eyes. Dodt *et al.* (1958) moreover, have used 32 Hz intermittent flashes to obtain truly photopic ERG's from normal, protanomalous and protanopic eyes. They found a close agreement between ERG and psychophysical measurements of sensitivity loss, with protanopes showing progressively greater deficiency as the wavelength increases over the range from 520 nm to beyond 650 nm. Deuteranopia and deuteranomaly appear to involve a definite sensitivity loss near 540 nm in individual cases (Copenhaver and Gunkel, 1959), but show less marked deviations from normal responding (Heck and Rendahl, 1957; Rendahl, 1958). Thus ERG results to date are generally in harmony with earlier psychophysical data with respect to spectral sensitivity functions on color deficient subjects. Discrepancies between ERG and psychophysical functions have been reported by Jaeger *et al.* (1961) for color-deficient subjects but they attribute these discrepancies to the fact that their ERG measurements were made with 40° stimulus fields rather than the 2° fields used for the psychophysical determinations.

Selective Adaptation. Stiles (1959) and many other investigators have successfully used selective adaptation to explore the fundamental color response mechanisms by the use of differential threshold procedures. (See Enoch, chapter 21, this volume.) A given wavelength is used as a background against which to measure the increment threshold energies of test patches of the same and other wavelengths. It is found, in general, that test patch thresholds are raised by the presence of a background, and that a maximum effect is exerted by a background of the same wavelength as that of the test. In other words, the background has a wavelength-selective effect such that it light-adapts those particular receptor mechanisms that are most strongly affected by it and has less of a masking effect upon other receptor mechanisms.

Electrophysiological experiments to date have not been so successful. At the level of the ERG it is found that threshold energies of test flash are indeed raised by steady background illumination (Johnson and Riggs, 1951; Boynton and Triedman, 1953; Biersdorf and Armington, 1960; van Lith, 1966). But numerous experiments have shown very slight wavelength-selectivity in the effects of background on ERG responses to a test flash (Armington and Biersdorf, 1956; Cavonius, 1964). Recent additional experiments in our laboratory confirm this conclusion. Background illumination raises the test flash threshold roughly in proportion to the background luminance, irrespective of the specific wavelengths used for background and test. Slight selective effects are found, however, in individual subjects. With intermittent monochromatic test flashes and computer averaging, many of the ERG responses are found to be more strongly depressed by a background of the same wavelength than by one of a different wavelength, when the luminances of the backgrounds are carefully matched for their overall effectiveness in depressing responses to the various wavelengths of test flash.

Critical Frequency of Fusion (CFF). Psychophysical data on flicker (e. g. Hecht and Shlaer, 1936) typically reveal a limit of about 60 flashes per second as the maximum rate for which flicker is perceived, even at high levels of stimulation. The CFF declines to about 20 flashes per sec at low photopic levels, and to still lower frequencies in the scotopic range. (See Kelly, chapter 11, this volume for fuller discussion.) Karpe (1958) has reported ERG data in good agreement with these psychophysical results. He used 100 subjects and plotted the highest frequency of flashes, at each luminance level, that produced measurable ERG response waves. The flashes were diffused over the entire surface of the retina by the use of a milky plastic type of contact lens. Previous investigators (e.g., Dodt and Wadenstein, 1954) had obtained lower CFF values using more restricted stimulus areas.

Future work on the relation of ERG to spatial and temporal resolution will undoubtedly take the form of determining modulation transfer functions to compare with those obtained with psychophysical methods (e.g., De Lange, 1958). A beginning of this sort has already been made (van der Tweel, 1964).

VECP Findings in Relation to Psychophysics

Stimulus Variables

Just as the ERG reflects gross neural activity at an early level in the visual system, the VECP represents the response of many neural elements at a relatively late level. Since the physiology of the VECP is poorly understood, as mentioned above, it is limited as a tool for investigating visual mechanisms. Nevertheless it is unique as an electrical visual response from the cerebral cortex of normal, sentient man. For this reason, if for no other, it is of interest to observe the dependency of the VECP on such stimulus aspects as energy level, duration, area, frequency and wavelength.

In examining the relation between the VECP and the various stimulus parameters most investigators have confined their attention to the secondary response

(Fig. 3). This is strictly an utilitarian choice in that the smaller primary response is totally obscured by noise in many subjects. The secondary response, on the other hand, is always present.

Utility has also dictated the features of the waveform most often measured. While many attributes of the VECP should or could potentially be examined, such as area under the waves or Fourier components, typically only amplitude and/or implicit time[3] have actually been used. Thus most of the following discussion will be based upon these two characteristics.

Energy Level or Luminance. A small but reliable VECP can be recorded when the flash energy is only about 0.3 log unit above psychophysical threshold. Above this level the effect of flash energy on amplitude is highly variable both between and within subjects. ARMINGTON (1964), for example, reported that individual subjects differed markedly with respect to the shape of the curve relating VECP amplitude to stimulus energy. WICKE *et al.* (1964) found a non-monotonic amplitude-intensity function for the major deflection but a monotonic one for an earlier, smaller deflection. Many studies (e. g. CHAPMAN and BRAGDON, 1964) have shown that amplitude is also affected by such subjective factors as attention and fatigue (see pp. 718, 719); other relevant factors are those of electrode placement and size of the stimulus field.

The implicit time of the various waves, on the other hand, bears a much more orderly relation to flash energy: as the flashes are made more and more intense, the implicit times of all the waves monotonically decrease until a seemingly irreducible minimum value is reached. Fig. 8 is from VAUGHAN *et al.* (1966) and shows VECP's recorded from two subjects over a luminance range of 5 log units. Notice that although the waveforms exhibited by the subjects are somewhat different, the implicit time of the first positive deflection, marked by arrows, shows an orderly relation to luminance. VAUGHAN *et al.* found that when the log of the reducible portion of the implicit time[4] was plotted against log luminance a linear function with a slope of about $-1/3$ resulted, i.e., the relation is a power function in which response times vary with the cube root of the stimulus luminance except at low luminance levels where an inflection is found. Fig. 9 illustrates this relation with a compilation of the results of several investigators.

The discontinuity of the implicit-time curves is interpreted by VAUGHAN *et al.* as due to a change from a predominantly photopic response to a predominantly scotopic one. This notion is consistent with the results of RIETVELD and TORDOIR (1965) shown as filled squares on Fig. 9, since they used a considerably larger field (about 25°) than did other investigators (about 6°). This large field would presumably stimulate many more rods, thus prolonging the lower segment of the curve and moving the point of inflection to a higher luminance level. It is also consistent with the finding by VAUGHAN *et al.* that no discontinuity occurs when the stimulus is reduced to a 1.5° foveal field so as to stimulate almost entirely cones. In addition, WOOTEN (1968) has subsequently shown that the low-energy limb obtained with a 5° foveally fixated field has a spectral sensitivity that closely matches the C.I.E. scotopic luminosity function.

---

[3] Most authors have used "latency" to designate the time between stimulus onset and the peak of a given positive or negative wave. But, strictly speaking this term applies to the time that something is present but simply hidden or dormant. Since the peak of a wave cannot be described in this fashion we prefer the term "implicit time" to refer to this interval.

[4] The reducible implicit time is found by subtracting the asymptotic implicit time from each value. In practice the asymptotic value, estimated graphically, is defined as the final minimum level shown by an implicit time-log luminance plot.

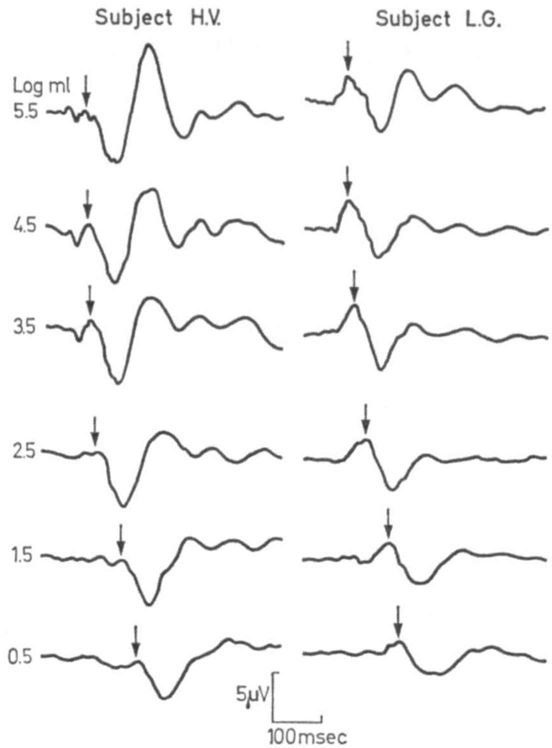

Fig. 8. Examples of VECP's recorded over a 5 log unit luminance range. The arrows indicate the peak of the wave for which implicit times were measured. (After Vaughan *et al.*, 1966)

The exponent of the power function is of particular interest since similar values have been obtained in animal physiological and human psychophysical experiments dealing with response speed. As Vaughan *et al.* pointed out, the latency data on the *Limulus* optic nerve fibers (Hartline, 1934) and both conger eel (Adrian and Matthews, 1927) and frog (Bernhard, 1940) whole optic nerve discharges exhibit power functions with slopes of about $-1/3$. In the same experiment Vaughan *et al.* also showed that data relating reaction times of their human subjects to flash luminance are well described by the same power function. Finally, the curve relating sensation time to stimulus luminance that can be derived from Lit's (1949) work on the Pulfrich stereophenomenon[5] is also a power function with a slope of close to $-1/3$. Thus the rule that response speed in the visual system is related to the cube root of luminance seems to be true whether response speed is defined psychophysically or neurophysiologically.

[5] When the bob of a pendulum which is oscillating in a plane perpendicular to an observer's line of sight is viewed binocularly with a filter over one eye, the bob seems to describe an elliptical path. This effect has been explained on the basis of increased sensation time associated with the filtered eye. If the pendulum's speed is known and the apparent excursion of the bob is determined psychophysically for a range of filter values the relation between sensation time and luminance can be determined. See Lit (1949).

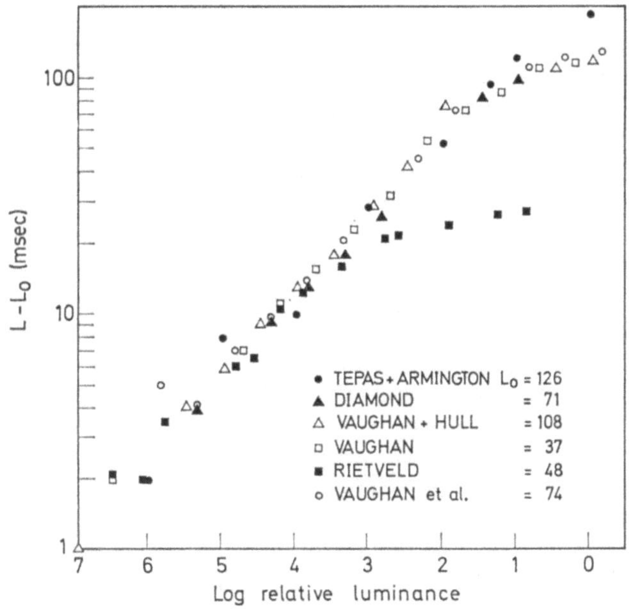

Fig. 9. Reducible implicit time of the VECP as a function of relative luminance. The plot is a compilation of the results of several investigators. In the terminology used here L and L_0 refer to implicit time and irreducible implicit time, respectively. $L - L_0$, then, is the reducible implicit time. The sets of data from the different studies were arbitrarily shifted on the abscissa so as to overlap. The differing values of L_0 reflect the different waves of the VECP chosen for measurement as well as differences in stimulus and recording conditions. (From VAUGHAN *et al.*, 1966)

Wavelength — Spectral Sensitivity. As we have seen, with simple flash stimulation the ERG (b_s) reflects very strongly the activity of the rods, and only with more elaborate stimulating arrangements, such as the alternating-stripe pattern, can purely cone ERG responses be elicited.

The situation with the VECP is quite opposite to that found with the ERG; under most stimulus conditions the response is primarily photopic. This was first indicated by ARMINGTON (1964) who simultaneously recorded ERG's and VECP's elicited with a 3.5° field centered on the fovea. Using a constant amplitude criterion for both responses he found that the ERG's spectral sensitivity curve, as expected, closely matched the C.I.E. scotopic luminosity function. The VECP curve, however, was much closer to the C.I.E. photopic luminosity function, departing from it only in the 425-nm to 475-nm region by exhibiting about .5 log unit greater sensitivity. This slightly high short-wave sensitivity may or may not reflect some scotopic contribution; it is also observed in most psychophysical determinations done with parafoveal stimulation under photopic conditions. In a later study ARMINGTON (1966) extended these findings by moving the 3.5° stimulus field 15° into the temporal retina in one experiment and on to the optic disc in another. The ERG results were essentially the same as when the stimulus was centered on the fovea. The VECP curve was considerably higher (about 1.5 log units) than the C.I.E.

photopic function in the short-wave region. But considering the numerical advantage of the rods as compared to the cones in this region of the retina it is perhaps surprising that the sensitivity of the VECP to the short-wave end of the spectrum was not still higher. Even with conditions so favoring the scotopic system the VECP predominantly reflects photopic activity.

SIEGFRIED (1967) has confirmed the close correspondence between the spectral sensitivity of the VECP and the photopic system in a study comparing the electrical response with a psychophysical response from the same subjects. In this study a 1.5° circular, foveally-fixated, "white" field of constant luminance was alternated (at 1 Hz) with a chromatic field of the same size and falling on the same retinal region. The chromatic field was varied both in wavelength and luminance. VECP's could be detected as a result of switching from the "white" standard field to the chromatic test field and vice versa. The VECP spectral sensitivity function was determined by finding the energy value for each test wavelength which when switched from "standard" to "test" produced the same amplitude of response as when switched from "test" to "standard". The psychophysical function was determined during the same sessions by simply having the subjects indicate when the two alternating fields appeared equally bright. The two methods gave results which were virtually identical. Considering the relatively small field employed and the alternating nature of the stimuli it is safe to assume that the psychophysical response was entirely photopic. In view of the exact correspondence of the VECP with the psychophysical response we conclude that it too was entirely photopic.

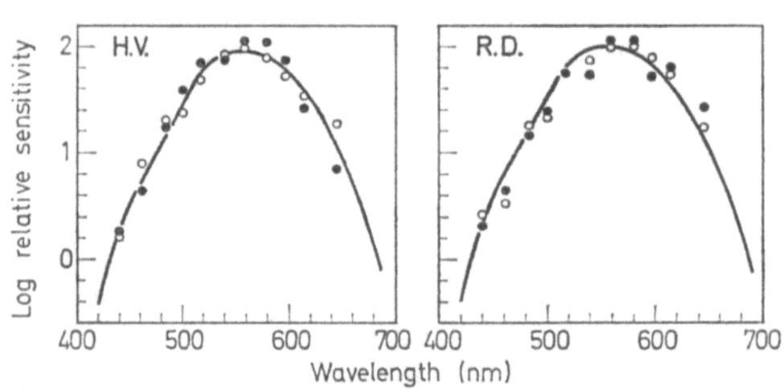

Fig. 10. Photopic spectral sensitivity data based on psychophysical thresholds (open circles) and VECP implicit times of 130 msec (filled circles). Ordinate scales are log reciprocal of relative energy necessary to meet the threshold and implicit time criteria. A centrally-fixated, 45′ circular field was used. The curve drawn through the data points represents the C.I.E. photopic luminosity function. (From DEVOE *et al.*, 1968)

Similar findings have been reported by DE VOE *et al.* (1968) using the implicit time of the first positive wave as the measure of luminous efficiency. Fig. 10 shows their results based on a criterion implicit time of 130 msec and with a 45′ foveally-fixated field. The psychophysically determined (threshold) data points and the electrophysiologically determined ones match quite well. Both sets of data also agree closely with the C.I.E. photopic luminosity function which is also shown in the figure.

In this same study DEVOE *et al.* also underscored the photopic nature of the VECP by taking advantage of the well-documented fact that the Stiles-Crawford effect is a property only of the photopic system. They compared the magnitude of the Stiles-Crawford effect on luminous efficiency as defined by a psychophysical threshold response and a VECP implicit-time criterion. As with the spectral sensitivity results the two sets of data were in excellent agreement.

The results of DEVOE *et al.* strongly imply not just that the VECP reflects photopic activity but that it is primarily elicited by stimulation of the *foveal* cones. Admittedly, stray light from entoptic scatter would certainly stimulate neighboring parafoveal regions, even though the light is focused on a 45′ spot at the center of the fovea. But if this indirect stimulation were important, the spectral sensitivity function of the VECP would have shown an excess short-wave sensitivity that characterizes the parafoveal region (WALD, 1945). Since the spectral sensitivity function agrees instead with that of the fovea, we may conclude that parafoveal cones do not make a major contribution to the response. Studies using stimuli of different sizes and on various retinal loci confirm the foveal domination of the VECP.

All of these studies, then, confirm the photopic nature of the VECP. But all of them were done under conditions which favor the photopic system, i.e. light adaptation, foveal stimulation and/or relatively intense stimuli. WOOTEN (1968) has shown, on the other hand, that if conditions are chosen which strongly favor the scotopic system a purely scotopic VECP results. In this study the subjects were dark adapted for 1 hour and low energy stimuli were used, thus preventing excessive light adaptation during the averaging period. In addition a 5° foveally-centered field was used which, according to calculations from ØSTERBERG'S (1935) data, is an area containing equal numbers of rods and cones. Fig. 11 shows that the resulting spectral sensitivity data (filled circles) based on a constant-criterion implicit time of 250 msec, corresponds well to the C.I.E. scotopic luminosity function except for higher sensitivity at the long-wave end of the spectrum. This high long-wave sensitivity was believed to represent a photopic contribution since it is well known that in this spectral region the cone and rod systems are about equally sensitive. This hypothesis was confirmed by moving the Maxwellian entry beam to the edge of the dilated pupil. This maneuver reduces the cone response (Stiles-Crawford effect) without affecting the rod response. The result is shown in Fig. 11 by the open circles: the sensitivity of the VECP is reduced in the long-wave region and the data are then well described by the C.I.E. scotopic curve. The sensitivity of the VECP in other spectral regions is unaffected, giving additional evidence that purely scotopic mechanisms are reflected.

The data just described show that an entirely scotopic VECP can be elicited under special conditions. But other results from the same study confirm the essentially photopic nature of the response under more usual conditions. When the stimulus intensity was raised to a level about 3 log units above cone threshold and an implicit-time criterion of 150 msec was employed, the resulting spectral sensitivity curve appeared to be purely photopic. The sensitivity curve was somewhat higher in the short-wave region than was the DEVOE et al. curve; but it was no higher than expected on the basis that the larger field used would stimulate parafoveal as well as foveal cones. Thus it appears that once cone threshold is reached the VECP reflects just photopic mechanisms even though the stimulus excites both cones and rods. This may be due to a simple overpowering of the small scotopic response by the much larger photopic response or to inhibition in the retina of the rod-initiated neural events by cone-initiated activity. GOURAS and LINK (1966) have presented some retinal microelectrode evidence that supports the latter hypothesis.

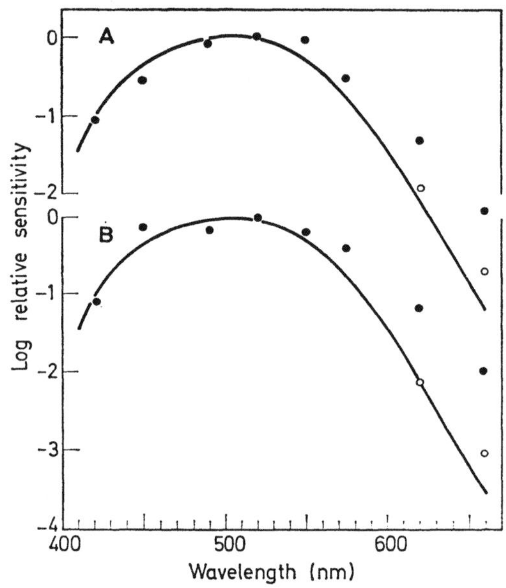

Fig. 11. Spectral sensitivity of two dark-adapted human subjects, *A* and *B*, based on log reciprocal of relative energy necessary to meet an implicit time criterion of 200 msec for the principal wave of the VECP. A concentrated (Maxwellian) stimulus beam entered the dilated pupil either through its center (filled circles) or through a point 3.5 mm off-center (open circles). The curve drawn through the data points represents the C.I.E. scotopic luminosity function. (From WOOTEN, 1968)

Wavelength — Effects on VECP Waveform. As discussed above the energy level of the eliciting flash affects the waveform of the VECP: the implicit time of each component wave is inversely related to luminance and the amplitude may be inversely or directly related to luminance depending on the specific wave examined. The question naturally arises as to whether wavelength *per se* affects the morphology of the response. That is, is there some aspect of the VECP which correlates with the different chromatic sensations experienced as a result of using various monochromatic flashes of equal brightness?

SHIPLEY *et al.* (1965, 1966, 1968) have diligently pursued the waveform problem and have concluded that the VECP "is complexly dependent upon the wavelength of the stimulus light." In their most recent study VECP's were elicited with various narrow waveband lights ranging over the visible spectrum. The 11° stimulus fields were centrally fixated and were equated for brightness by a direct match to a xenon "white" standard. The wavelength dependency of the VECP morphology was clearly apparent in the records from most of the color-normal observers: as the wavelength was changed from long to short the prominent positive peak with an implicit time of about 175 msec fell in amplitude and a second positive peak with a longer implicit time (about 225 msec) emerged and eventually dominated the waveform. This effect was absent in some of the color-normal subjects and in all of the color deficients (dichromats). It was most apparent with short duration (10 msec) flashes and seemed to be independent of electrode position. The authors term this wavelength dependence "color coding" and imply that the various peaks reflect the contribution of different color-vision subsystems, e.g., the first positive peak which is most prominent with long-wave light represents the red-sensitive mechanism.

SHIPLEY *et al.* have clearly established wavelength-specific effects on the VECP, at least under their stimulus conditions. It seems unnecessary to assume, however, that these effects reflect neural color coding. A simpler interpretation is based on the fact that the relatively large (11°) stimulus field that they used may have stimulated markedly heterogeneous regions of the retina in terms of the spectral sensitivities of the constituent receptors. The spectral sensitivity of foveal cones is considerably lower in the short-wave spectral region than is that of the parafoveal cones (WALD, 1945) and of course the rods, to the extent that they may contribute to the VECP (WOOTEN, 1968) have a very different spectral sensitivity function. Furthermore, the foveal cones contribute a disproportionately large share of the amplitude of VECP waves (see Fig. 12 and discussion below). Hence the situation is entirely different from the large-area conditions for ERG experiments with a striped pattern (see p. 700) in which the foveal cones and the rod receptors play no significant role. Thus even though a psychophysical match was made in order to equate for brightness, this does not serve to balance the contributions of those

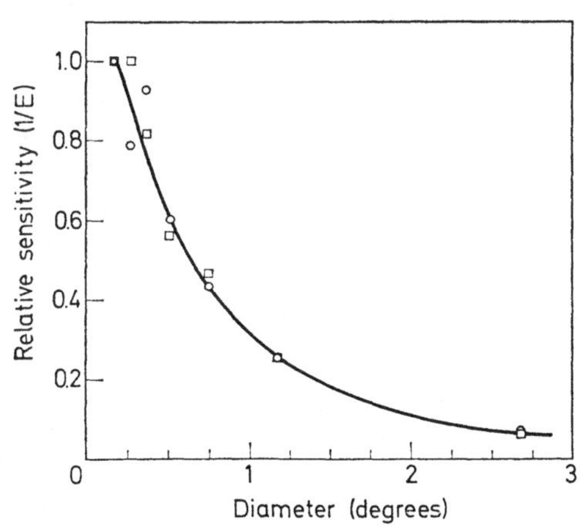

Fig. 12. VECP and psychophysical sensitivity for centrally-fixated, circular stimuli. The ordinate is relative sensitivity based on the reciprocal of the total luminous flux ($1/E$) necessary to elicit a VECP implicit time of 130 msec (circles) or to reach psychophysical threshold (squares). The two types of data have been set equal to a relative sensitivity value of 1.0 for the smallest (10′) stimulus condition. In absolute values the VECP points are about 1 log unit above the corresponding psychophysical ones. (The data are from DEVOE *et al.*, 1968, and were originally plotted as log luminance versus log retinal area)

different regions to the VECP. The wavelength dependency of the response, then, is at least partially explained in terms of inequalities in the degrees of arousal of these regions of differing spectral sensitivity.

The above interpretation is given strong support by an experiment in which Siegfried (1967) compared the results of a large (9°) and a small (2°) field. The 13 monochromatic stimuli were equated for luminous efficiency on the basis of a spectral sensitivity function previously determined (discussed above). Short (20 msec) flashes were used which are optimal for obtaining the wavelength effect. Siegfried's results were similar to those of Shipley *et al.* where the large field was employed, i.e., in the long-wave spectral region the response was dominated by a large positive peak which was gradually replaced by one of longer implicit time as the wavelengths of the stimuli were shortened. With the 2° field, however, no such trends were apparent. Siegfried's data clearly imply that the VECP does not reflect neural color coding since it is in the fovea that chromatic sensations are most highly developed. From this point of view, the waveform dependency of the VECP on wavelength appears to result from the complexities of recording from regions large enough to involve mixed populations of rods and cones.

Selective Adaptation. In contrast to the results with the ERG, discussed above, relatively strong selective adaptation effects are shown by VECP recording. Burkhardt and Riggs (1967) elicited responses with 10°, monochromatic, flickering stimuli (17.5 Hz) superimposed on 16°, monochromatic, steady backgrounds of equal luminance. They found that the largest VECP's occurred when the wavelengths of the stimulus and the background differed by a large amount (usually > 100 nm), and that these responses were often larger than those elicited by the same test stimulus with no background. In addition wavelength-dependent temporal effects were found: shifts as large as 0.5 cycle in the phase relation of the response wave to the stimulus flash occurred when the background wavelength differed appreciably from the stimulus wavelength. Regan (1968b) has shown that the effects of selective adaptation on the VECP amplitude are strongly dependent on modulation frequency. He compared the responses elicited by a red, sinusoidally flickering, 60° field when superimposed on a steady background of the same color or one of a different color (blue). Regan found that the heterochromatic stimulation produced larger responses than the homochromatic when the stimulus was modulated at about 10 Hz, but considerably smaller ones when modulated at 16 Hz.

These two experiments, then, have clearly shown that under certain conditions the amplitude and phase of the VECP is dependent on the wavelength of the background. This is a particularly interesting finding in view of the largely negative results at the ERG level and may indicate that some aspects of selective adaptation or color contrast arise at a level beyond that of the second-order neurons in the processing of color information. But since in both of these studies large stimulus fields were employed, the same consideration of mixed receptor populations discussed above, for simple wavelength effects, apply. It is of great interest to know, therefore, whether or not these selective effects would still occur if the stimulus fields were restricted entirely to the fovea.

Duration. The primary and secondary responses of the VECP are essentially responses to transient increases in the level of illumination and, therefore, identical waveforms result from long (e.g., 1 sec) and relatively short (e.g., 200 msec) flashes. WICKE *et al.* (1964) and VAUGHAN (1966) found, however, that a given amplitude of the secondary response is dependent on the product of energy and duration for flashes briefer than about 100 msec. To a first approximation, then, the amplitude of the VECP parallels the psychophysical relation known as Bloch's Law: The brightness of a short (< about 100 msec) flash can be maintained by any reciprocal manipulation of duration and energy. As mentioned above, this result also holds for the scotopic *b*-wave of the ERG. The data of WICKE *et al.* and VAUGHAN are seemingly contradictory regarding VECP implicit time. The former find that implicit time is determined solely by the flash energy level but the latter reports that it follows the reciprocity relation just as amplitude does. The reason for this discrepancy is not clear.

Flicker. Most of the VECP data discussed in this review concern responses elicited with slowly repetitive flashes, e.g., 1 flash/sec. It is also possible to elicit stable and measurable VECP's at high rates of flicker. VAN DER TWEEL and LUNEL (1965) have emphasized the use of sinusoidally modulated light, pointing out that this kind of stimulus is simpler than the more usual square-wave flicker in that it contains only one frequency (in terms of a Fourier analysis). (See also KELLY, chapter 11.) These investigators varied modulation rate and amplitude, and mean luminance level, and found that responses could be recorded at many frequencies above the critical fusion frequency (CFF). For example, with their conditions (25% modulation, 6000 trolands) CFF was about 40 Hz but VECP's could be elicited up to about 70 Hz. These findings have been confirmed and extended by SPEKREIJSE (1966) and REGAN (1968a, 1968b) for a wide range of stimulus conditions. The fact that VECP's can be elicited above CFF may indicate that even though fast-flicker information is carried to a high level in the brain, it is not effectively available to the mechanisms of perception. Alternatively, the averaging technique may reveal higher frequency responding than single-cell or psychophysical determinations because it may involve larger numbers of neural units, each of which may respond to an occasional flash.

Field Size. The studies on spectral sensitivity, discussed above, clearly showed the dominance of the photopic system in generating the VECP. The work of DEVOE *et al.* with a 1°, centrally-fixated field further indicated that the fovea itself is the most sensitive area of the retina for eliciting a VECP in that neighboring retinal regions stimulated by stray light did not appear to contribute to the spectral sensitivity function. This conclusion is further supported by a number of studies with larger fields which directly stimulated the parafovea as well as the fovea. RIETVELD *et al.* (1965) employed foveally-centered circular stimuli ranging from 28′ to 7° 38′ in diameter. They found that the contribution that a given retinal region makes to response amplitude diminishes rapidly with distance from the center of the fovea, e.g., a unit retinal area 25′ from the foveal center contributes only 1/10 as much as the center itself. This is not to say, however, that the parafoveal contribution as a whole is unimportant. From the function of RIETVELD *et al.* relating VECP amplitude to field size, it can be calculated that the center 2° of a 5° field contributes about 65% of the amplitude. The results of ARMINGTON (1968) are substantially the same: the response amplitude increased by only about 30% when the field was increased in size from 2° to 12°.

DEVOE *et al.* (1968) have shown this same foveal dependency and in addition the close correspondence between the VECP and the psychophysical area-luminance relation in the fovea. Fig. 12 is a replot, on linear coordinates, of their data relating sensitivity to stimulus area. The psychophysical (squares) and the electrophysiological responses (circles) are well described by the same curve and are highly foveally dependent. Increases in field size beyond about 1° contribute relatively little to either lowering the psychophysical threshold or reducing the implicit time of the VECP. In this respect implicit time appears to be more clearly determined by foveal elicitation than is amplitude.

Contour Effects. In most of the studies discussed so far the eliciting stimuli have consisted of simple, homogeneous fields of various sizes. To the extent that the VECP is related to cortical single-unit activity (FOX and O'BRIEN, 1965) and in view of the well-known work of HUBEL and WIESEL (1968) on visual cortex cells, it would be expected that such fields should be relatively poor VECP stimuli. In fact, most cells examined by HUBEL and WIESEL in both cat and monkey were totally unresponsive to diffuse retinal illumination, and were activated only by lines or edges flashed or moved on to the receptive fields. Recent studies have confirmed this expectation with respect to the human VECP by demonstrating that moving or highly patterned fields are particularly effective in eliciting the response.

SPEHLMAN (1965) originally demonstrated the effectiveness of contour content by comparing the VECP's recorded with progressively finer checkerboard patterns. Such a stimulus is convenient since the amount of contour can easily be varied while holding constant both luminance and total luminous flux. He found that response amplitude increased as check size decreased. Furthermore, SPEHLMAN noted that a large response could be markedly reduced in amplitude by degrading the retinal image of the pattern by the addition of a + 10 diopter lens in the optical path. Later studies have confirmed and quantified these results. SPEKREIJSE (1966), RIETVELD *et al.* (1967) and HARTER and WHITE (1969) have all found that the relation between VECP amplitude and check size is described by a curve that rises to a maximum for checks of about 20′ subtense and falls again for still larger checks. HARTER and WHITE (1968), using a graded series of ophthalmic lenses, have shown that the VECP amplitude is exquisitely sensitive to the degree of focus. Fig. 13 illustrates these findings and shows the interaction between degree of focus and check size. With the coarser patterns (60′–120′ check size and the diffuse field) the response amplitude is almost unaffected by image degradation. But with the most effective pattern (10′–20′ check size) a degradation of only 1 diopter causes an amplitude reduction of approximately 25 per cent. This interaction of check-size and degree of focus on the VECP was consistent with subjective reports that indicated the check size for peak amplitude to be the smallest for which pattern was still perceived in each condition. Both of these effects, as well as their interaction, underscore the importance of the presence and sharpness of contours in VECP elicitation. HARTER and WHITE interpret these findings in terms of receptive field properties, pointing out that the check size (10′–20′) that gives the largest VECP amplitude is approximately the same as the receptive field diameter estimated by psychophysical methods (BRYNGDAHL, 1966; ANDREWS, 1967).

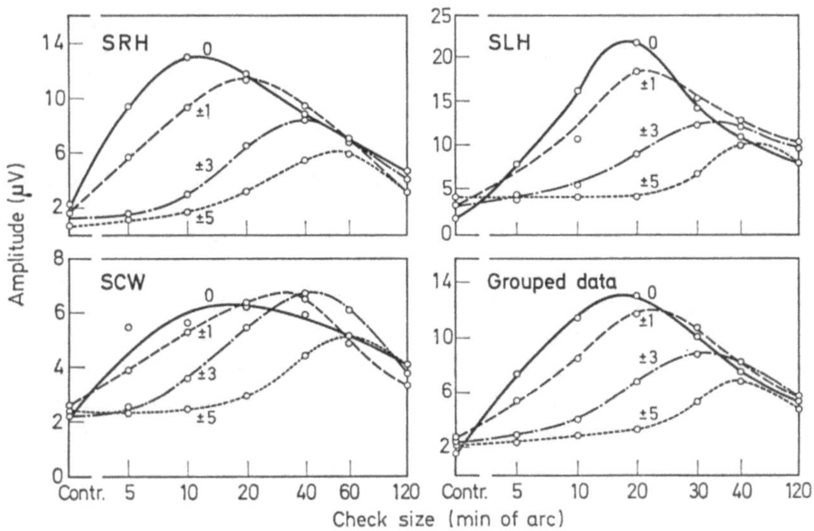

Fig. 13. Amplitude of VECP (at an implicit time of about 180 msec) as a function of induced refractive error (diopters) and check-size (min of arc) of a checkerboard stimulus. Each point in individual figures is the mean of 4 averaged responses, except 0 diopter conditions which are based on 2 responses. Diopter values disregard sign, e. g., the data for +3 and —3 are pooled. (From Harter and White, 1969)

A number of studies (e.g., MacKay and Rietveld, 1968; Dawson *et al.*, 1968) have shown that a small (several minutes of arc) moving spot or line generally results in a larger VECP than a simple flash which is many times larger and more intense. The extraordinary sensitivity of the VECP to stimuli moving across the retinal mosaic has been demonstrated by Gaarder *et al.* (1964). Rather than using stimulus movements to elicit a response these investigators used eye movements. A computer was triggered by saccades which were monitored by light reflected from a mirror embedded in a tightly-fitting contact lens and the stimulus was simply a continuously-fixated 5° field which had an internal grid structure consisting of 20′, circular spots. The results clearly showed that a "normal" and reliable VECP is produced by the extremely fine retinal image displacements caused by saccadic eye movements. These results are particularly interesting since they indicate as the authors point out, "that the nervous-system discharge accompanying vision may not be solely continuous, but instead may be characterized by more or less discontinuous bursts related in time to saccades."

Subjective Variables

Thus far we have considered primarily the dependency of the VECP on a number of physical variables related to the stimulus. The waveform of the response is also affected by a number of other factors related not to the stimulus, but to the subject. We include in this latter category dark- and light-adaptation, complex psychological variables (such as "attention"), and the subjective fading of stimuli (as in binocular rivalry). The waveform of the VECP, a response apparently originating in the cerebral cortex, is dependent on such "central factors" as attention and binocular rivalry. Although the functional significance of this dependency is unknown, the VECP does, to some extent, seem to reflect aspects of the neural state related to these "subjective" variables.

Light- and Dark-Adaptation. Systematic studies relating the VECP to the process of dark adaptation seem to be lacking. This may partially be due to the difficulty of studying such a dynamic process with the response-cumulation procedure which tends to interfere with the very phenomenon being examined, i.e., the considerable number of repetitive flashes needed for computer-averaging tend to retard the progress of dark-adaptation. The VECP studies have therefore been unable to adopt a meaningful "minimum response" criterion and cannot be quantitatively compared with classical psychophysical threshold data. PERRY *et al.* (1968) elicited the VECP with a flash of constant luminance and found that its amplitude doubled after 40 min of dark adaptation, with most (about 80%) of the increase occurring during the first 10 min of adaptation. The stimulus was a 2° 15′, foveally-centered field of 1.4 log foot-lamberts.

WOOTEN and GARTHWAITE (1969) observed similar amplitude changes in responses elicited with a 5° central field at 10 trolands immediately after viewing a 10°, 5 log troland, adapting field for 7 min and after 50 min of dark adaptation. Although the responses obtained after dark adaptation were larger than those obtained after light adaptation, the average implicit time of the first major peak was about 8 msec longer (153 vs. 145 msec). This increase in implicit time is in qualitative agreement with psychophysical studies indicating an increase in latency with dark adaptation. For example, ROCK and FOX (1949) reported that a Pulfrich effect can be observed when one eye is dark-adapted relative to the other and that the direction of apparent rotation is as if a filter were placed before the dark-adapted eye. In addition, STANDING *et al.* (1968) have recently shown that the magnitude of the depth effect increases as the eye becomes more and more dark adapted. Thus, even though the dark-adapted eye is more sensitive to light, it responds more slowly to any given stimulus luminance. ARMINGTON (1964) has reported some effects on the VECP amplitude as a result of what might be called short-term light adaptation. He recorded the responses to trains of 5 flashes and found that the response to the first flash in the train was always larger than the others. Simultaneously recorded ERG's showed the same effect.

Complex Psychological Variables. We use this term to designate such factors as habituation, attention, vigilance, meaningfulness, and expectancy. In more operational terms, we mean those factors that clearly have an effect on the waveform of the VECP in addition to the effects, already discussed, due to either the physical aspects of the stimulus or simple physiological mechanisms, such as adaptation. There are many studies in the literature dealing with this topic and we shall now consider some illustrative examples.

HAIDER *et al.* (1964) have shown that the VECP amplitude is correlated with the degree of vigilance manifested in tedious light detection experiments and that changes in VECP waveform may provide a "measure of fluctuations in focal attentiveness." SPONG *et al.* (1965) and DONCHIN and COHEN (1967), using intermixed auditory and visual stimuli and intermixed visual stimuli of different kinds in experiments where the observer was under instruction to attend to one of the alternating stimuli and to ignore the other, found that the "respond" condition resulted in larger VECP's than the "ignore" condition. Other experiments indicate that the amplitude of the VECP is modulated by the "meaningfulness" or "relevance" of stimuli to a specific problem-solving task (CHAPMAN and BRAGDON, 1964; CHAPMAN, 1965; CHAPMAN, 1966).

From the experiments cited above it is apparent that the waveform of the VECP is dependent on many factors in addition to the physical aspects of the stimulus. These "complex psychological variables" may be of little interest to the sensory physiologist or psychologist, but any visual experiment involving the VECP can be confounded by these "non-sensory" factors. It is necessary, then, when relating the VECP to such basic stimulus variables as the wavelength or the luminance of the light to control for these other influences by such procedures as the counterbalancing of conditions or the use of a "standard stimulus" presented periodically during the experimental sessions.

Subjectively Faded Stimuli — Binocular Rivalry. We now consider certain procedures in which a stimulus of constant physical characteristics fades or disappears from view. The question of interest is: How does the VECP correlate with the altered sensation? We shall consider the effects of binocular rivalry, image stabilization and saccadic eye movements.

When widely disparate patterns are presented to the two eyes the subjective result is binocular rivalry in which one pattern or the other is seen to dominate the field at any given moment. The dominance of one pattern may entail a complete disappearance of the other. VAN BALEN (1964) produced a similar effect by presenting one page of reading matter under steady illumination to the left eye and another in flickering light, to the right eye. The subject was instructed to attend to one or the other passage of reading matter at different times. The VECP's elicited by the flicker stimulation to the right eye were 20 to 40 per cent smaller when the subject attended to the steadily illuminated reading matter presented to the left eye. Simultaneously recorded ERG's did not show the effect. COBB *et al.* (1967a) replicated VAN BALEN'S experiment on six subjects but failed to confirm his conclusion: only two of the subjects showed any tendency to exhibit larger responses while reading with the "flickered" eye. These investigators also pointed out that this situation cannot be regarded as true binocular rivalry in that dominance was not allowed to occur spontaneously but was forced. Thus, any positive results could be attributed to selective attention, which has been shown to affect VECP amplitude.

In order to produce true binocular rivalry, COBB *et al.* (1967a) presented vertical bars to one eye and horizontal ones to the other. The stimuli were small (1° 42′ to 4°) and were transilluminated at the rate of 10 per sec with brief flashes which were 180° out of phase. Under these conditions complete suppression usually occurred. The subject controlled a switch allowing him to sort the responses to one channel of the computer when the left eye was dominant and to another channel when the right was dominant. The resulting records are shown in Fig. 14a along with responses recorded when each eye was stimulated alone. Notice that the two monocular records exhibit roughly sinusoidal waves that are 180° out of phase. If, then, the subjects were perfect at sorting, and if suppression involved complete loss of response to stimulation, the sorted VECP's recorded during rivalry would have exactly the same amplitude and phase as their monocular counterparts. In fact, though, as can be seen in Fig. 14a, the responses recorded under rivalry conditions showed no such trend, tending instead to cancel. Similar experiments with larger fields have been reported by KAUFMAN *et al.* (1965) and by RIGGS and WHITTLE (1967). In these studies subjects were presented with steady illumination to one eye and flicker of various rates to the other. The fields contained lines that were oriented one way for one eye and at right angles for the other eye,

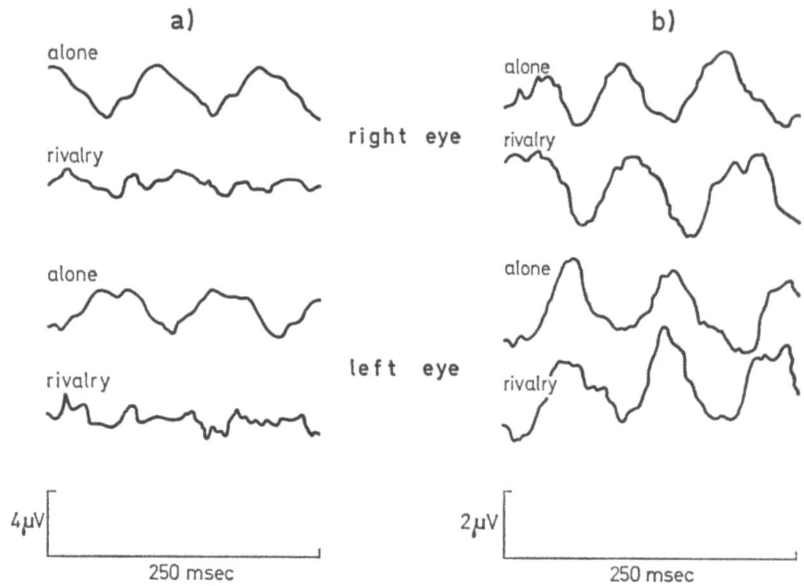

Fig. 14. a) The effect of binocular rivalry on the VECP elicited with 10 Hz flicker. The stimuli were presented to each eye alone or to both eyes simultaneously and were 180° out of phase. The simultaneous condition produced binocular rivalry and responses were averaged for a given eye only when that eye was dominant. See text for details. Each trace is the average of 100 sweeps of the computer. (After COBB *et al.*, 1967a.) b) The effect of binocular rivalry on the VECP elicited with 12 Hz pattern reversal. Stimulus presentation conditions same as above. See text for details. Each trace is the average of 128 sweeps of the computer .(After COBB *et al.*, 1967b)

so that rivalry occurred. For part of the session, the subjects pressed a key during the time the eye receiving the flicker was dominant, and responses were cumulated. For other parts of the session, the subjects pressed the key during the time that eye was suppressed. No reliable differences were apparent, in either amplitude or waveform between the records obtained during dominance and those obtained during suppression. It is therefore clear from these studies that the VECP, elicited by flicker, is not diminished when binocular rivalry causes a substantial amount of subjective disappearance of the flicker-illuminated pattern.

On the other hand COBB *et al.* (1967b) have shown that the VECP elicited by an alternating-stripe stimulus similar to that of RIGGS *et al.* (1964) is strongly affected by binocular rivalry. The particular targets used by COBB *et al.* consisted of small (56′) circular fields made up of dark and light stripes (4′ subtense). Horizontal stripes were presented to the right eye and vertical stripes to the left. Responses were elicited by rapidly moving the target one stripe width, so that a given retinal region was alternately stimulated by the dark and light stripes. One type of experiment was similar to the RIGGS and WHITTLE (1967) design mentioned above: only one of the targets flickered and the subjects sorted the responses by indicating which eye was dominant, so that records were obtained for the stimulated eye in the dominant and suppressed states. For all five subjects there was a clear reduction in amplitude for the responses recorded when the stimulated eye was suppressed. In another type of experiment targets were moved at 12 Hz but were 180° out of phase. VECP's were recorded for each eye alone and for each eye in rivalry, using the sorting procedure mentioned above (COBB *et al.*, 1967a). Fig. 14b shows both kinds of response. Notice that the amplitude and the phase of the responses are the same for a given eye, whether stimulated alone or during its dominant phase of rivalry. This result clearly implies that suppression of the VECP was complete, since anything less than complete suppression would result in partial cancellation due to the phase differences. This finding is in marked contrast to the results, shown in Fig. 14a, of the experiment discussed above, in which simple flicker was used. The authors conclude that dominance and suppression can be successfully revealed by the VECP under conditions of pattern reversal but not under conditions of simple luminance modulation (flicker). This finding implies that pattern information and luminance change are processed differently in the visual system. This same conclusion was reached by MACKAY (1968) using a quite different procedure.

The studies discussed above clearly show that the VECP elicited by flashes in one eye while viewing a steady field with the other is independent of any binocular rivalry that may be induced. KAUFMAN *et al.* (1965) and RIGGS and WHITTLE (1967) have shown, however, that the amplitude of the VECP response to flashes delivered to one eye is larger in the monocular condition than when the other eye is presented with a steady field of light. LEHMANN *et al.* (1967b); LEHMANN and FENDER (1968) extended this finding by varying the complexity of the steady field; to a field that was initially a blank they added first a small black dot, then a cross, and finally a grid. A large VECP was elicited by the flashes in one eye when the other eye was given the steady blank field, somewhat smaller responses with the dot, smaller yet with the cross, and smallest with the grid. The authors attribute the progressive decrease in VECP amplitude to an increased load of visual information on central neural elements which have binocular input. Hence the number of neural elements available for responding in synchrony with the flashes is reduced in proportion to the complexity of the steady, contralateral field.

Subjectively Faded Stimuli — Optically Stabilized Images. Subjective disappearance may also be achieved by stabilizing the retinal image. Here, eye movements are prevented from having their normal effect of shifting the retinal image from one set of receptors to another (DITCHBURN and GINSBORG, 1952; RIGGS *et al.*, 1953). In the absence of image motion, there is a gradual fading and often a complete disappearance of a pattern that had first appeared sharp and clear to the observer. Although the physiological basis for this effect is not known, a common interpretation has been that retinal adaptation takes place. In addition, several experiments (KRAUSKOPF and RIGGS, 1959; LEHMANN *et al.*, 1967a; KEESEY and NICHOLS, 1967) have demonstrated that at least a small portion of the disappearance can be attributed to central, rather than retinal events. We might expect, then, that the VECP would reflect, perhaps by a reduction in amplitude, the adaptation process underlying image disappearance.

RIGGS and WHITTLE (1967) have recorded the ERG and the VECP elicited by stabilized and by unstabilized retinal stimuli. Since both responses are transients resulting from some sort of stimulus change, it was necessary to use temporally modulated stimuli. They employed a flickering pattern of fine black lines and an alternating pattern of light and dark stripes. In order to achieve disappearance of the stabilized image relatively high rates of flicker (> 10 flashes/sec) and stripe-alternation (about 50 square-wave shifts/sec) were needed. Image stabilization was achieved by a contact lens carrying a plane mirror in conjunction with the usual compensating optical system. "The results may be summarized with the statement that no diminution was found to occur in the . . . [ERG or the VECP]. This generalization holds despite the fact that the subjects reported a marked difference in the subjective appearance of the stripes under the two conditions. The stabilized condition produced fading of the image that sometimes amounted to virtually complete disappearance. The persistence of the electrical activity was also found under a variety of conditions of stimulation with respect to frequency, intensity and wavelength."

The results with image stabilization are difficult to integrate with some of the data, discussed above, on binocular rivalry. In the binocular rivalry experiments (e. g. COBB *et al.*, 1967b) the VECP elicited with pattern-alternation was correlated with the disappearance of the stimuli but the response elicited with ordinary flicker was not. On this basis, some workers have suggested that luminance and pattern information are represented by different neural systems. The results of RIGGS and WHITTLE on image stabilization, however, do not fit neatly into such a hypothesis because the VECP's elicited by pattern alternation were no more affected than those elicited by flicker under conditions leading to the subjective disappearance of the stimuli. This may mean that the pattern-disappearance resulting from binocular rivalry occurs earlier in the neural channel than the disappearance caused by image stabilization and that the latter occurs, neurally, after the generation of the VECP. The discrepancy may also be related to the differences in modulation rate since COBB *et al.* (1967b) used 1–20 alternations/sec and RIGGS and WHITTLE used about 50/sec.

The Riggs and Whittle experiment was done with monocular stimulation. LEHMANN *et al.* (1967a) have demonstrated an effect on the VECP resulting from stabilizing a steady, contralateral field. They found no correlation with the disappearance phases of the field, i.e., responses averaged when the steady pattern was perceived were not any smaller than those averaged when the pattern had faded. However, they did find, as mentioned earlier, that the VECP was reduced in amplitude when the steady, structured field was presented to the "non-flickered" eye. Furthermore, if this field was stabilized the response amplitude increased. The authors interpret these results to mean that the disappearance of the stabilized field had the effect of reducing the informational load on the central, data-handling mechanisms, thereby allowing the flashes to excite more neurons.

Subjectively Faded Stimuli — Eye Movements. It has long been known that visual perception is suppressed during rapid eye movements (saccades), thus accounting for continuously "clear" vision even though the stimulus image is undoubtedly blurred as it streaks across the retinal mosaic. DODGE (1900, 1905) and WOODWORTH (1906) argued that the blurring *per se* accounts for the suppression whereas HOLT (1903) believed that there is, in addition, a central inhibitory mechanism. Later investigators (e.g. VOLKMANN, 1962; LATOUR, 1962; and VOLKMANN *et al.*, 1968) used flashes which were too brief to allow any significant amount of blur and found that there remained a significant amount of suppression for stimulus fields presented shortly before, during, and immediately after voluntary saccades. ZUBER *et al.* (1966) also showed that saccadic suppression is accompanied by a reduction in the amplitude of the pupillary reflex.

Several recent experiments have shown that the waveform of the VECP is altered during saccadic suppression. MICHAEL and STARK (1967) presented brief flashes 50–60 msec before and at the onset of voluntary saccades, and found complex gross alterations in the waveform of the response. DUFFY and LOMBROSO (1968) performed a similar experiment but quantified the results by calculating the total power (i.e., the integral of voltage with respect to time) which was attributable to the effects of the light flashes. Their results roughly parallelled the psychophysical data of LATOUR (1962) and VOLKMANN *et al.* (1968) in that the magnitude of the VECP decreased significantly 20–60 msec before the onset of eye movement and did not return to the control level until 160–200 msec after the onset of eye movement. GROSS *et al.* (1967) elicited VECP's by quickly interchanging (from 15 to 215 msec after the onset of a voluntary saccade) the dark and light portions of a continuously viewed, horizontal grating pattern. They reported that the amplitude of the responses correlated well with the detection of the pattern reversal, both being minimal immediately after the onset of the saccades and maximal about 200 msec after the onset.

Current interpretations of suppression are mainly along the lines of the central inhibitory mechanisms suggested by HOLT (1903), though a retinal explanation has been attempted (RICHARDS, 1968). Control experiments by LEDERBERG (1970) showed that the suppression effect is a specific effect of eye movements and not merely an attentional failure.

Conclusions

In comparing ERG and VECP data with psychophysical data we conclude that several close parallels have been established. However, a full appreciation of the unique characteristics of each form of investigation is needed in order to avoid misunderstandings that have plagued this field in the past. Some workers have been led to the conclusion that the ERG is a sort of epiphenomenon, bearing no understandable relation to actual visual experiences. Others have rejected the VECP as too variable and quixotic a response to be used in any serious scientific investigation.

At the outset it is clear that the VECP is far more foveally dependent than the ERG. This accounts for the fact that the early spectral sensitivity studies based on single flashes of monochromatic light yielded VECP curves in good agreement with the photopic C.I.E. luminosity function while the ERG curves even under the same high levels of adaptation tended to approximate the scotopic C.I.E. function. These results are interpretable on the basis of the relation between the recording electrodes and the anatomy of the visual system. The electrode used to record the

ERG is probably equally affected by action potentials from all areas of the retina. This means that with simple flash stimulation, in which light is scattered across the retina, far more rods than cones are stimulated since there are approximately 20 times more rods than cones (Østerberg, 1939). Furthermore, the all-cone foveal region comprises less than 1/30,000th of the whole area of the retina. It is not surprising, then, that only with special and elaborate conditions can the response to stray light be abolished and purely photopic ERG waves attained.

The situation for the VECP, on the other hand, is almost reversed since the ratio of foveal to extra-foveal area representation is increased by a factor of about 1000 at the area striata (calculated by DeVoe *et al.*, 1968, based on Talbot and Marshall, 1941; Whitteridge and Daniel, 1961; and Cowey, 1964). In addition to the "cortical magnification" factor, the fovea is favored because its projection to the area striata is located superficially at the occipital pole whereas the projection area of the more peripheral retinal regions lies deeper in the occipital lobe (on the lips of and buried in the calcarine fissure). Hence, the cortical elements representing the fovea are relatively close to the scalp electrode(s) which is usually placed directly over the occipital pole. Only by setting up very special conditions of stimulation and recording has it been possible to attain purely scotopic signals in the VECP.

In addition to the anatomical factors favoring the fovea in VECP recording, Gouras and Link (1966) have demonstrated rod-cone interactions at the level of the retina which give a functional interpretation of the fact that the VECP is dominated by the photopic system. They simultaneously recorded ganglion cell spikes and ERG's in the rhesus monkey retina. Their main finding was that with stimuli above cone threshold the ERG showed both photopic and scotopic components but the ganglion cell records displayed only photopic activity. The faster, cone signal appears to render the ganglion cell refractory for a short time thereby preventing the slower, rod signal from exciting it. The "inhibition" of the rod signal by the cone signal at the ganglion cell level thus accounts for the finding that bright flashes of light evoke large scotopic responses in the ERG (a pre-ganglion-cell response) while the VECP (a post-ganglion-cell response) is responding primarily to photopic activity.

Finally, it is clear that other visual functions appear quite differently at the levels of the ERG and VECP. Already there is evidence that the VECP signals manifest comparatively greater sensitivity to small differences in wavelength, contour and motion of the stimulus pattern. Furthermore, they are more subject to such neural interaction effects as binocular rivalry, attentional factors and habituation. Looking simultaneously at those signs of retinal and occipital activity that we can measure objectively in human subjects, we gain insight into the processing of information that underlies our subjective visual experiences.

The ERG and the VECP are the only two physiological measures of visual system activity which can be used routinely in human beings. Therefore, it is fortunate that these two types of responses show so many parallels to psychophysical aspects of vision. To the extent that the ERG and VECP differ from one another, scientists can gain even more information about the functioning of the visual system. The purpose of this chapter has been to show the similarities and the differences between the ERG and the VECP, and also the correlations of these physiological measures with psychophysical ones. It is clear not only that the work which has been done with these physiological tools has added greatly to our knowledge and understanding of the visual system, but also that a lot of work remains to be done.

Acknowledgements. This chapter was prepared in the Hunter Laboratory of Psychology at Brown University in Providence, Rhode Island, U.S.A. Preparation of this chapter was aided by the U.S. Public Health Service through grant NB 01453 and by the Office of Naval Research through a contract with Brown University.

References

ADRIAN, E. D.: Rod and cone responses in the human eye. Nature (Lond.) **154**, 361—362 (1944).
— Electric responses of the human eye. J. Physiol. (Lond.) **104**, 84—104 (1945).
— Rod and cone components in the electric response of the eye. J. Physiol. (Lond.) **105**, 24—37 (1946).
— MATTHEWS, R.: The action of light on the eye. Part 1. The discharge of impulses in the optic nerve and its relation to the electric changes in the retina. J. Physiol. (Lond.) **63**, 378—414 (1927).
AIBA, T. S., ALPERN, M., MAASEIDVAAG, F.: The electroretinogram evoked by the excitation of human foveal cones. J. Physiol. (Lond.) **189**, 43—62 (1967).
ALPERN, M., FARIS, J.: Note on the electrical response of the human eye during dark adaptation. J. opt. Soc. Amer. **44**, 74—79 (1954).
— — Luminance-duration relationship in the electrical response of the human eye during dark adaptation. J. opt. Soc. Amer. **46**, 845—850 (1956).
ANDREWS, D. P.: Perception of contour orientation in the central fovea. Part II. Spatial integration. Vision Res. **7**, 999—1013 (1967).
ARMINGTON, J. C.: A component of the human electroretinogram associated with red color vision. J. opt. Soc. Amer. **42**, 393—401 (1952).
— Amplitude of response and relative spectral sensitivity of the human electroretinogram. J. opt. Soc. Amer. **45**, 1058—1064 (1955).
— Chromatic and short term dark adaptation of the human electroretinogram. J. opt. Soc. Amer. **49**, 1168—1175 (1959).
— Adaptational changes in the human electroretinogram and occipital response. Vision Res. **4**, 179—192 (1964).
— Spectral sensitivity of simultaneous electroretinograms and occipital responses. Clinical Electroretinography (Suppl. to Vision Res.) 225—233 (1966).
— Pupil entry and the human electroretinogram. J. opt. Soc. Amer. **57**, 838—839 (1967).
— The electroretinogram, the visual evoked potential, and the area-luminance relation. Vision Res. **8**, 263—276 (1968).
— BIERSDORF, W. R.: Flicker color adaptation in the human electroretinogram. J. opt. Soc. Amer. **46**, 393—400 (1956).
— SCHWAB, G.: Electroretinogram in nyctalopia. Arch. Ophthal. **52**, 725—733 (1954).
— TEPAS, D. I., KROPFL, W. J., HENGST, W. H.: Summation of retinal potentials. J. opt. Soc. Amer. **51**, 877—886 (1961).
— THIEDE, F.: Selective adaptation of components of the human ERG. J. opt. Soc. Amer. **44**, 779—786 (1954).
ASHER, H.: The electroretinogram of the blind spot. J. Physiol. (Lond.) **112**, 40P (1951).
AUERBACH, E., BURIAN, H. M.: Studies on the photopic-scotopic relationships in the human electroretinogram. Amer. J. Ophthal. **40**, 42—60 (1955).
VAN BALEN, A. T. M.: The influence of suppression on the flicker ERG. Documenta Ophthal. **18**, 440—446 (1964).
BERGAMINI, L., BERGAMASCO, B.: Cortical Evoked Potentials in Man. Springfield: Thomas 1967.
BERNHARD, C. G.: Contributions to the neurophysiology of the optic pathway. Acta physiol. scand. **1**, Suppl. **1** (1940).

Best, W.: Das menschliche Elektroretinogramm während der Dunkeladaptation. Acta Ophthal. **31**, 95—116 (1953).

Biersdorf, W. R., Armington, J. C.: Level of light adaptation and the human electroretinogram. J. opt. Soc. Amer. **50**, 78—82 (1960).

Bornschein, H.: Der Einfluß von Adaptationszustand und Reizintensität auf die Komponenten des menschlichen Elektroretinogramms. Z. Biol. **105**, 454—463 (1953).

— Schubert, G.: Das photopische Flimmer-Elektroretinogramm des Menschen. Z. Biol.**106**, 229—238 (1953).

Boynton, R.: Stray light and the human electroretinogram. J. opt. Soc. Amer. **43**, 442—449 (1953).

— Riggs, L. A.: The effect of stimulus area and intensity upon the human retinal response. J. exp. Psychol. **42**, 217—226 (1951).

— Triedman, M. H.: A psychophysical and electrophysiological study of light adaptation. J. exp. Psychol. **46**, 125—134 (1953).

Bremer, F.: Neurogenic factors influencing the evoked potentials of the cerebral cortex. In: Sensory Communications, Rosenblith, W. A. (Ed.). New York: Wiley 1961.

Brindley, G. S., Westheimer, G.: The spatial properties of the human electroretinogram. J. Physiol. (Lond.) **179**, 518—537 (1965).

Brown, J. L., Hill, J. H., Burke, R. E.: The effect of hypoxia on the human electroretinogram. Amer. J. Ophthal. **44**, 57—67 (1957).

Brown, K. T.: The electroretinogram: Its components and their origins. Vision Res. **8**, 633—677 (1968).

— Murakami, M.: A new receptor potential of the monkey retina with no detectable latency. Nature (Lond.) **201**, 626—628 (1964).

— Wiesel, T. N.: Analysis of the intraretinal electroretinogram in the intact cat eye. J. Physiol. (Lond.) **158**, 229—256 (1961).

Bryngdahl, O.: Perceived contrast variation with eccentricity of spatial sine-wave stimuli. Vision Res. **6**, 553—565 (1966).

Burian, H. M.: Electroretinography and its clinical application. Arch. Ophthal. **49**, 241—256 (1953).

— Allen, L.: A speculum contact lens electrode for electroretinography. EEG clin. Neurophysiol. **6**, 509—511 (1954).

Burkhardt, D. A., Riggs, L. A.: Modification of the human visual evoked potential by monochromatic backgrounds. Vision Res. **7**, 453—459 (1967).

Carr, R. E., Ripps, H., Siegel, I. M., Weale, R. A.: Rhodopsin and the electrical activity of the retina in congenital night blindness. Invest. Ophthal. **5**, 497—507 (1966).

— Siegel, I. M.: Electrophysiologic aspects of several retinal diseases. Amer. J. Ophthal. **58**, 95—107 (1964).

Cavonius, C. R.: The effects of chromatic adaptation upon the human electroretinogram. Unpublished Ph. D. thesis, Brown University (1962).

— Color sensitive responses in the flicker ERG. Documenta Ophthal., Separ. **18**, 101—113 (1964).

Chapman, R. M.: Evoked responses to relevant and irrelevant visual stimuli while problem solving. Proceedings of the 73rd Annual Convention of the American Psychological Association, 177—178 (1965).

— Human evoked responses to meaningful stimuli. XVIII International Congress of Psychology, Moscow. **6**, 53—59 (1966).

— Bragdon, H. R.: Evoked responses to numerical and non-numerical visual stimuli while problem solving. Nature (Lond.) **203**, 1155—1157 (1964).

Ciganek, L.: The EEG response (evoked potential) to light stimulus in man. EEG clin. Neurophysiol. **13**, 165—172 (1961).

— A comparative study of visual and auditory EEG responses in man. EEG clin. Neurophysiol. **18**, 625—629 (1965).

Cobb, W. A., Ettlinger, G., Morton, H. B.: Visual evoked potentials in binocular rivalry. EEG clin. Neurophysiol. Suppl. **26**, 100—107 (1967a).

— Morton, H. B., Ettlinger, G.: Cerebral potentials evoked by pattern reversal and their suppression in visual rivalry. Nature (Lond.) **216**, 1123—1125 (1967b).

CONE, R. A.: The early receptor potential of the vertebrate retina. Nature (Lond.) **204**, 736—739 (1964).

COOPER, R., WINTER, A. L., WALTER, W. G.: Comparison of subcortical and scalp activity using chronically indwelling electrodes in man. EEG clin. Neurophysiol. **18**, 217—228 (1965).

COPENHAVER, R. M., BEINHOCKER, G. D.: Evoked occipital potentials recorded from scalp electrodes in response to focal visual illumination. Invest. Ophthal. **2**, 393—406 (1963).

— GUNKEL, R. D.: The spectral sensitivity of color-defective subjects determined by electroretinography. Arch. Ophthal. **62**, 55—68 (1959).

CORNSWEET, T. N.: The Design of Electric Circuits in the Behavioral Sciences. New York: Wiley 1963.

COWEY, A.: Projection of the retina onto striate and prestriate cortex in the squirrel monkey *Saimiri sciureus*. J. Neurophysiol. **27**, 366—393 (1964).

CRAMPTON, G., ARMINGTON, J.: Area-intensity relation and retinal location in the human electroretinogram. Amer. J. Physiol. **181**, 47—53 (1955).

CREUTZFELDT, O. D., KUHNT, U.: The visual evoked potential: Physiological, developmental and clinical aspects. EEG clin. Neurophysiol. Suppl. **26**, 29—41 (1967).

DARTNALL, H. J. A.: The properties of visual pigments in photoreceptors. In: The Eye, DAVSON, H. (Ed.). Vol. 2, pp. 473—522. New York: Academic Press 1962.

DAWSON, W. W., PERRY JR., N. W., CHILDERS, D. G.: Flash and scan stimulation of retinal fields and evoked response repoduction. EEG clin. Neurophysiol. **24**, 467—473 (1968).

DELANGE, H.: Research into the dynamic nature of the human fovea-cortex systems with intermittent and modulated light. J. opt. Soc. Amer. **48**, I. 777—784, II. 784—789 (1958).

DEVOE, R. G., RIPPS, H., VAUGHAN JR., H. G.: Cortical responses to stimulation of the human fovea. Vision Res. **8**, 135—147 (1968).

DITCHBURN, R. W., GINSBORG, B. L.: Vision with a stabilized retinal image. Nature (Lond.) **170**, 36—37 (1952).

DODGE, R.: Visual perception during eye movement. Psychol. Rev. **7**, 454—465 (1900).

— The illusion of clear vision during eye movement. Psychol. Bull. **II**, 193—199 (1905).

DODT, E.: Cone electroretinography by flicker. Nature (Lond.) **168**, 738—739 (1951).

— COPENHAVER, R. M., GUNKEL, R. D.: Photopischer Dominator und Farbkomponenten im menschlichen Elektroretinogramm. Pflügers Arch. ges. Physiol. **267**, 497—507 (1958).

— WADENSTEN, L.: The use of flicker electroretinography in the human eye. Acta Ophthal. **32**, 165—180 (1954).

— WALTHER, J. B.: Fluorescence of the crystalline lens and electroretinographic sensitivity determinations. Nature (Lond.) **181**, 286—287 (1958).

DONALDSON, P. E. K.: Electronic Apparatus for Biological Research. London: Butterworths 1958.

DONCHIN, E., COHEN, L.: Averaged evoked potentials and intramodality selective attention. EEG clin. Neurophysiol. **22**, 537—546 (1967).

DOWLING, J. E.: The site of visual adaptation. Science **155**, 273—279 (1967).

DUFFY, F. H., LOMBROSO, C. T.: Electrophysiological evidence for visual suppression prior to the onset of a voluntary saccadic eye movement. Nature (Lond.) **218**, 1074—1075 (1968).

ELENIUS, V., HECK, J.: Relation of size of ERG to rhodopsin concentration in normal human beings and one totally colour blind. Nature (Lond.) **180**, 819 (1957); also Vergleich zwischen der b-Wellenamplitude und dem Verlauf der Sehpurpurregeneration bei Achromaten und Gesunden. Ophthalmologica (Basel) **136**, 145—150 (1958).

FOX, S. S., O'BRIEN, J. H.: Duplication of evoked potential waveform by curve of probability of firing of a single cell. Science **147**, 888—890 (1965).

GAARDER, K., KRAUSKOPF, J., GRAF, V., KROPFL, W., ARMINGTON, J. C.: Averaged brain activity following saccadic eye movement. Science **146**, 1481—1483 (1964).

GALLOWAY, N. R.: Early receptor potential in the human eye. Brit. J. Ophthal. **51**, 261—264 (1967).

GASTAUT, H., RÉGIS, H.: Visually-evoked potentials recorded transcranially in man. In: Symposium on the analysis of central nervous system and cardiovascular data using computer methods. Washington: NASA, SP72 (1964).

GOODMAN, G., BORNSCHEIN, H.: Comparative ERG studies in congenital night blindness and total color blindness. Arch. Ophthal. 58, 174—182 (1957).

GOURAS, P., ARMINGTON, J. C., KROPFL, W. J., GUNKEL, R. D.: Electronic computation of human retinal and brain responses to light stimulation. Ann. N. Y. Acad. Sci. 115, 763—775 (1964).

— GUNKEL, R. D.: The frequency response of normal, rod achromat and nyctalope ERGs to sinusoidal monochromatic light stimulation. Documenta Ophthal., Separ. 18, 137—150 (1964).

— LINK, K.: Rod and cone interaction in dark-adapted monkey ganglion cells. J. Physiol. (Lond.) 184, 499—510 (1966).

GRANDA, A. M., BIERSFORF, W. R.: The spectral sensitivity of the human electroretinogram during the temporal course of dark adaptation. Vision Res. 6, 507—516 (1966).

GRANIT, R.: Sensory Mechanisms of the Retina. New York: Oxford University Press 1947.

— Receptors and Sensory Perception. New Haven: Yale University Press 1955.

— The visual pathway. In: The Eye, DAVSON, H. (Ed.), Vol. 2, pp. 537—763. New York: Academic Press 1962.

— MUNSTERHJELM, A., ZEWI, M.: The relation between concentration of visual purple and retinal sensitivity to light during dark adaptation. J. Physiol. (Lond.) 96, 31—44 (1939).

GROSS, E. G., VAUGHAN, H. G., Jr., VALENSTEIN, E.: Inhibition of visual evoked responses to patterned stimuli during voluntary eye movements. EEG clin. Neurophysiol. 22, 204—209 (1967).

HAIDER, M., SPONG, P., LINDSLEY, D. B.: Attention, vigilance, and cortical evoked-potentials in humans. Science 145, 180—182 (1964).

HARTER, R. M., WHITE, C. T.: Effects of contour sharpness and check-size on visually evoked cortical potentials. Vision Res. 8, 701—711 (1968).

— — Research communication 1969.

HARTLINE, H. K.: Intensity and duration in the excitation of single photoreceptor units. J. cell. comp. Physiol. 5, 229—246 (1934).

HECHT, S., SHLAER, S.: Intermittent stimulation by light. V. The relation between intensity and critical frequency for different parts of the spectrum. J. gen. Physiol. 19, 965—979 (1936).

HECK, J.: The flicker electroretinogram of the human eye. Acta physiol. scand. 39, 158—166 (1957).

— RENDAHL, I.: Components of the human ERG. Acta physiol. scand. 39, 167—175 (1957).

HENKES, H. E.: Use of electroretinography in measuring the effect of vasodilation. Angiology 2, 125—131 (1951).

HOLT, E. B.: Eye-movement and central anaesthesia. Harvard Psychol. Stud. 1, 3—45 (1903).

HUBEL, D. H., WIESEL, T. N.: Receptive fields and functional architecture of monkey striate cortex. J. Physiol. (Lond.) 195, 215—253 (1968).

JAEGER, W., LUX, P., GRÜTZNER, P., JESSEN, K.-H.: Subjektive und objektive spektrale Helligkeitsverteilung bei angeborenen und erworbenen Farbensinnstörungen. In: The Visual System: Neurophysiology and Psychophysics, JUNG R., KORNHUBER, H. (Eds.). Berlin: Springer 1961.

JASPER, H. H.: Report of the committee on methods of clinical examination in electroencephalography. EEG clin. Neurophysiol. 10, 370—375 (1958).

JOHNSON, E. P.: The electrical response of the human retina during dark adaptation. J. exp. Psychol. 39, 597—609 (1949).

— The character of the *B*-wave in the human electroretinogram. Arch. Ophthal. 60, 565—591 (1958).

— BARTLETT, N.: Effect of stimulus duration on electrical responses of the human retina. J. opt. Soc. Amer. 46, 167—170 (1956).

— CORNSWEET, T. N.: Electroretinal photopic sensitivity curves. Nature (Lond.) 174, 614—616 (1954).

— RIGGS, L. A.: Electroretinal and psychophysical dark adaptation curves. J. exp. Psychol. 41, 139—147 (1951).

JOHNSON, E. P., RIGGS, L. A., SCHICK, A. M. L.: Photopic retinal potentials evoked by phase alternation of a barred pattern. Clinical Electroretinography. Proc. Third Intl. Symp., BURIAN, H. M., JACOBSON, J. H. (Eds.) (Suppl. to Vision Res.) pp. 75—91 (1966).

KARPE, G.: The basis of clinical electroretinography. Acta ophthal. (Kbh.) Suppl. **24**, 1—118 (1945).

— Indications for clinical electroretinography. Arch. Ophthal. **60**, 889—896 (1958).

— TANSLEY, K.: The relationship between the change in the electroretinogram and the subjective dark-adaptation curve. J. Physiol. (Lond.) **107**, 272—279 (1947).

KAUFMAN, L., PITBLADO, C., MILLER, J. F., Jr.: Perceptual phenomena and evoked cortical potentials resulting from binocular stimulation with flickering light. Report SRRC-RR 65—101, Sperry Rand Research Center, Sudbury, Mass. (1965).

KEESEY, U. T., NICHOLS, D. J.: Fluctuations in target visibility as related to the occurrence of the alpha component of the electroencephalogram. Vision Res. **7**, 859—877 (1967).

KOHLRAUSCH, A.: Elektrische Erscheinungen am Auge. In: BETHE, A. *et al.* (Eds.), Handbuch der normalen und pathologischen Physiologie. Vol. 12, Section 2, pp. 1394—1496. Berlin: Springer 1931.

KOOI, K. A., SHARBROUGH, F. W.: Electrophysiological findings in cortical blindness: report of a case. EEG clin. Neurophysiol. **20**, 260—263 (1966).

KRAUSKOPF, J., RIGGS, L. A.: Interocular transfer in the disappearance of stabilized images. Amer. J. Psychol. **72**, 248—252 (1959).

LATOUR, P. L.: Visual threshold during eye movements. Vision Res. **2**, 261—262 (1962).

LEDERBERG, V. S.: Color recognition during voluntary saccades. J. opt. Soc. Amer. **60**, 835—842 (1970).

LEHMANN, D., BEELER, G. W., Jr., FENDER, D. H.: EEG responses to light flashes during the observation of stabilized and normal retinal images. EEG clin. Neurophysiol. **22**, 136—142 (1967a).

— — — Monocularly evoked electroencephalogram potentials: Influence of target structure presented to the other eye. Nature (Lond.) **215**, 204—205 (1967b).

— FENDER, D. H.: Component analysis of human averaged evoked potentials: dichoptic stimuli using different target structure. EEG clin. Neurophysiol. **24**, 542—553 (1968).

LIT, A.: The magnitude of the Pulfrich stereophenomenon as a function of binocular differences of intensity at various levels of illumination. Amer. J. Psychol. **62**, 159—181 (1949).

VAN LITH, G. H. M.: Simultane Bestimmung der elektroretinographischen und sensorischen Reizschwelle. Vision Res. **6**, 185—197 (1966).

MACKAY, D. M.: Evoked potentials reflecting interocular and monocular suppression. Nature (Lond.) **217**, 81—83 (1968).

— RIETVELD, W. J.: Electroencephalogram potentials evoked by accelerated visual motion. Nature (Lond.) **217**, 677—678 (1968).

MICHAEL, J. A., STARK, L.: Electrophysiological correlates of saccadic suppression. Exp. Neurol. **17**, 233—246 (1967).

MOTOKAWA, K., MITA, T.: Über eine einfachere Untersuchungsmethode und Eigenschaften der Aktionsströme der Netzhaut des Menschen. Tohoku J. exp. Med. **42**, 114—133 (1942).

MÜLLER-LIMMROTH, W.: Der Einfluß der Dauer des Reizlichtes auf das Elektroretinogramm. Pflügers Arch. ges. Physiol. **257**, 35—47 (1953).

NOELL, W., CHINN, H. I.: Failure of the visual pathway during anoxia. Amer. J. Physiol. **161**, 573—590 (1950).

ØSTERBERG, F.: Topography of the layer of rods and cones in the human retina. Acta Ophthal. Suppl. **6** (1935).

PERRY, N. W., Jr., CHILDERS, D. G., DAWSON, W. H., STEWART, H. L.: Dark-adapted visual evoked response. Proceedings, 76th Annual Convention of the American Psychological Association, 315—316 (1968).

RAYPORT, M., VAUGHAN, G. ROSENGART, C. L.: Simultaneous recording of visual averaged responses to flashes from scalp and calcarine cortex in man. EEG clin. Neurophysiol. **17**, 806—611 (1964).

REGAN, D.: A high frequency mechanism which underlies visual evoked potentials. EEG clin. Neurophysiol. **25**, 231—237 (1968a).

— Chromatic adaptation and steady-state evoked potentials. Vision Res. 8, 149—158 (1968b).

Rémond, A.: Level of organisation of evoked responses in man. Ann. N. Y. Acad. Sci. **112**, 143—159 (1964).

Rendahl, I.: Components of the human ERG. Acta physiol. scand. **44**, 189—202 (1958).

Richards, W.: Visual suppression during passive eye movement. J. opt. Soc. Amer. **58**, 1159—1160 (1968).

Rietveld, W. J., Tordoir, W. E. M.: The influence of flash intensity upon the visual evoked response in the human cortex. Acta Physiol. Pharmac. Neerl. **13**, 160—170 (1965).

— — Duyff, J. W.: Contribution of fovea and parafovea to the visual evoked response. Acta Physiol. Pharmacol. Neerl. **13**, 330—339 (1965).

— — Hagenouw, J. R. B., Lubbers, J. A., Spoor, A. C.: Visual evoked responses to blank and to checkboard pattern flashes. Acta Physiol. Pharmacol. Neerl. **14**, 259—270 (1967).

Riggs, L. A.: Continuous and reproducible records of the electrical activity of the human retina. Proc. Soc. exp. Biol. Med. (N. Y.) **48**, 204—207 (1941).

— Electroretinography in cases of night blindness. Amer. J. Ophthal. **38**, 70—78 (1954).

— Electrophysiology of vision. In: Vision and Visual Perception, Graham, C. H. (Ed.). New York: Wiley 1965.

— Berry, R. N., Wayner, M.: A comparison of electrical and psychophysical determinations of the spectral sensitivity of the human eye. J. opt. Soc. Amer. **39**, 427—436 (1949).

— Johnson, E. P.: Electrical responses of the human retina. J. exp. Psychol. **39**, 415—424 (1949).

— — Schick, M. L.: Electrical responses of the human eye to moving stimulus patterns. Science **144**, 567 (1964).

— — — Electrical responses of the human eye to changes in wavelength of the stimulating light. J. opt. Soc. Amer. **56**, 1621—1627 (1966).

— Ratliff, F., Cornsweet, J. C., Cornsweet, T. N.: The disappearance of steadily fixated visual test objects. J. opt. Soc. Amer. **43**, 495—501 (1953).

— Sternheim, C. E.: Human retinal and occipital potentials evoked by changes of the wavelength of the stimulating light. J. opt. Soc. Amer. **59**, 635—640 (1969).

— Whittle, P.: Human occipital and retinal potentials evoked by subjectively faded visual stimuli. Vision Res. **7**, 441—551 (1967).

Rock, M. L., Fox, B. H.: Two aspects of the Pulfrich phenomenon. Amer. J. Psychol. **62**, 279—284 (1949).

Sachs, E.: Die Aktionsströme des menschlichen Auges, ihre Beziehung zu Reiz und Empfindung. Klin. Wschr. **8**, 136—137 (1929). (Cited in Kohlrausch, 1931.)

Schubert, G., Bornschein, H.: Beitrag zur Analyse des menschlichen Elektroretinogramms. Ophthalmologica (Basel) **123**, 396—413 (1952).

Shipley, T.: Dark-adaptation and summed visual potentials. In: Clinical Electroretinography (Suppl. to Vision Res.) 263—273 (1966).

— Jones, R. W., Fry, A.: Evoked visual potentials and human color vision. Science **150**, 1162—1164 (1965).

— — — Intensity and the evoked occipitogram in man. Vision Res. **6**, 657—667 (1966).

— — — Spectral analysis of the visually evoked occipitogram in man. Vision Res. **8**, 409—431 (1968).

Sidowsky, J. B. (Ed.): Experimental Methods and Instrumentation in Psychology. New York: McGraw-Hill 1966.

Siegfried, J. B.: Spectral sensitivity of the human visual system as measured from both evoked cortical potentials and psychophysical responses. Unpublished Ph. D. thesis Brown University (1967.)

Spehlmann, R.: The averaged electrical responses to diffuse and to patterned light in the human. EEG clin. Neurophysiol. **19**, 560—569 (1965).

Spekreijse, H.: Analysis of EEG responses in man. Thesis, University of Amsterdam (1966).

Spong, P., Haider, M., Lindsley, D. B.: Selective attentiveness and cortical evoked responses to visual and auditory stimuli. Science **148**, 395—397 (1965).

Standing, L. G., Dodwell, P. C., Lang, D.: Dark adaptation and the Pulfrich effect. Perc. Psychophys. **4**, 118—120 (1968).

Sternheim, C. E., Riggs, L. A.: Utilization of the Stiles-Crawford effect in the investigation of the origin of electrical responses of the human eye. Vision Res. **8**, 25—33 (1968).

STILES, W. S.: Color vision: The approach through increment-threshold sensitivity. Proc. nat. Acad. Sci. (Wash.) **45**, 100—114 (1959).
— CRAWFORD, B. H.: The luminous efficiency of rays entering the eye pupil at different points. Proc. roy. Soc. (Lond.) B **112**, 428—450 (1933).
TALBOT, S. A., MARSHALL, W. H.: Physiological studies on neural mechanisms of visual localization and discrimination. Amer. J. Ophthal. **24**, 1255—1264 (1941).
VAN DER TWEEL, L. H.: Relation between psychophysics and electrophysiology of flicker. Documenta Ophthal. **18**, 287—304 (1964).
— VERDUYN LUNEL, H. F. E.: Human visual responses to sinusoidally modulated light. EEG clin. Neurophysiol. **18**, 587—598 (1965).
VAUGHAN, H. G., Jr.: The perceptual and physiological significance of visual evoked responses recorded from the scalp in man. Clinical Electroretinography (Suppl. to Vision Res.) 203—223 (1966).
— COSTA, L. D., GILDEN, L.: The functional relation of visual evoked response and reaction time to stimulus intensity. Vision Res. **6**, 645—656 (1966).
VENABLES, P. H., MARTIN, I.: Manual of Psycho-Physiological Methods. Amsterdam: North Holland; New York: Wiley 1967.
VOLKMANN, F. C.: Vision during voluntary saccadic eye movements. J. opt. Soc. Amer. **52**, 571—578 (1962).
— SCHICK, A. M. L., RIGGS, L. A.: Time course of visual inhibition during voluntary saccades. J. opt. Soc. Amer. **58**, 562—569 (1968).
WALD, G.: Human vision and the spectrum. Science, N. Y. **101**, 653—658 (1945).
WHITTERIDGE, D., DANIEL, P. M.: The representation of the visual field on the calcarine cortex. In: The Visual System: Neurophysiology and Psychophysics. JUNG, R., KORNHUBER, H. (Eds.), pp. 222—228. Berlin: Springer 1961.
WICKE, J. D., DONCHIN, E., LINDSLEY, D. B.: Visual evoked potentials as a function of flash luminance and duration. Science **146**, 82—85 (1964).
WIRTH, A., ZETTERSTRÖM, B.: Effect of area and intensity on the size and shape of the ERG. Brit. J. Ophthal. **38**, 257—265 (1954).
WOODWORTH, R. S.: Vision and localization during eye movements. Psychol. Bull. **3**, 68—70 (1906).
WOOTEN, B. R.: Photopic and scotopic contributions to the human visual evoked cortical potential. Unpublished M. Sc. thesis, Brown University (1968).
— GARTHWAITE, C. R.: Unpublished observations, 1969.
YONEMURA, D., KAWASAKI, K.: The early receptor potential in the human electroretinogram. Jap. J. Physiol. **17**, 235—244 (1967).
ZUBER, B. L., STARK, L., LORBER, M.: Saccadic suppression of the pupillary light reflex. Exp. Neurol. **14**, 351—370 (1966).

Chapter 28

Visual Psychophysics in Animals

By

Donald S. Blough and Dean Yager, Providence, Rhode Island (USA)

With 11 Figures

Contents

Animal psychophysics is essentially the same as human psychophysics; both reduce to the study of relations between stimulus variables (usually of a highly restricted sort) and simple responses (even more restricted). Although one may say he is determining what the human or animal "sees," the inference is indirect in both cases. The inference may seem more direct in the human instance because the response is often verbal, and because relations between stimulus and response behavior are, as a rule, easier to set up with human subjects. Much of this chapter will discuss ways to establish stimulus-response relations in animals that might be established with humans simply by saying "look there and say yes if you see the light," or some such simple instruction.

In this sense, work with human subjects is much easier than work with animals. The advantages of animal work, however, are well known. It makes possible the comparison of anatomical, physiological, and behavioral information in the same species, and comparison across species; the selection of subjects uniquely suited to a given problem; the undertaking of experiments too damaging, dangerous or arduous for human subjects.

This chapter will first outline several broad categories of methods that have been used effectively by investigators of visual function. These methods will be illustrated by a few from among the very many experiments in this rapidly growing literature. Next will come comment upon some of the general problems that one is apt to encounter when he sets out to communicate with his animal subjects. The chapter concludes with a selective review of literature that illustrates the fruitful interaction of behavioral with physiological data, one of the main justifications of the whole enterprise.[1]

Basic Methods of Animal Psychophysics

Animal methods fall naturally into two groups characterized by the means by which stimulus-response relations are developed: (a) "reflex" methods, in which the animal enters the experiment equipped to respond appropriately to the stimuli; and (b) training methods, in which the necessary relations are established either through Pavlovian (also called "classical" or "respondent") conditioning, or through Thorndikian reward ("operant" or "instrumental") conditioning.

Reflex Methods

These methods depend upon reflex or stereotyped reactions to changes in the visual field. They attract the investigator because training is not required to prepare the subject, and no reinforcement is needed to maintain the behavior. Their use is limited, however, for the investigator will only rarely find an easily-measured response elicited by just that stimulus aspect of interest to him.

A group of reflexes that have long been used to study acuity, motion perception, contrast thresholds, and color discrimination are the "optomotor responses," — movements of the eyes, head or body in response to moving visual patterns. A common experimental arrangement is illustrated by recent research on bats (SUTHERS, 1966). The bat was placed in a transparent chamber at the center of a large vertical cylinder. Vertical black and white stripes of equal width alternated

[1] The proceedings of a recent symposium on animal psychophysics have been published in book form (STEBBINS, 1970), and provide a detailed description of a wide variety of methods and results in animal experimentation.

around the inner walls of the cylinder, illuminated by an overhead light. The experimenter waited until the bat was motionless and then rotated the cylinder at about six revolutions per minute. The bats usually responded by turning their heads, and often their whole bodies, in the direction of rotation of the cylinder. Suthers used stripes of various widths, and the narrowest stripe that yielded a clear response provided an estimate of minimum separable visual angle. The estimate was between 0.7 and 6.0 degrees, depending upon species, although 0.7 represents the narrowest stripe used.

The threshold is defined in terms of the response that is recorded, and different responses may yield different results. This point is illustrated in optokinetic work of Schlieper (1927) on the color vision of insects, fish, and a lizard. Even though at least some of his species are known to discriminate colors under other circumstances, Schlieper reported that when the stripes on the drum in which the animal was placed were alternately colored and gray, there was always some shade of gray that abolished the subject's movements. Thus, the optokinetic response in this case might define a brightness match but not a color match. Similarly, in the acuity work, it might turn out that training methods would yield responses to stripes too narrow to elicit an optomotor response. Special care must also be taken to exclude variability due to irrelevant factors affecting the emission of the response. In the case of the bats, Suthers reports that the response was sometimes absent "because of a low degree of interest on the part of the animal." If a certain stripe width produced no response, it was recorded as below the acuity threshold only if its presentation was immediately preceded and followed by trials that elicited clear responses to moving stripes.

The unconditioned reflex method was used by Hecht (1934) in his classical study of adaptation in mollusks, and a recent example is Cronly-Dillon's study (1966) of spectral sensitivity in the scallop. The scallop, *Pecten maximus*, has an image-forming eye and closes its shell in response to a specific visual stimulus; namely, a sudden diminution in light intensity. Again, of course, the threshold depended upon the response, and, as in other reflex cases, the experimenter was somewhat at the mercy of the response mechanism. For example, a refractory period of at least five minutes followed each shell closure, so relatively long periods had to elapse between trials.

A final experiment illustrates another difficulty that may be particularly onerous in the reflex-based methods. Muntz (1962) reports data on the positive phototactic behavior of frogs. His subjects (*Rana temporaria*) tended to jump through appropriately placed illuminated windows, a response that might seem suitable for measuring spectral sensitivity or other threshold functions. However, although the response was elicited more easily by blue light than by other colors, this finding did not demonstrate a higher sensitivity to short wavelengths, since a given "blue" was also chosen in preference to a mixture of the same amount of "blue" plus additional "green" light energy.

Training Methods

Classical and operant training methods are characterized by stimulus-response relations specifically tailored to the problem at hand. Verbal instructions usually establish such relations with human subjects, and these may include rewards of a non-specific nature ("you are doing well") or information about correctness of response. In animal experiments, the contingency between stimulus and reinforcement defines the instructions and also maintains the animal's behavior. For example, a rat might receive food for a right turn to an intense stimulus, and for a left turn to a less intense one; such "instructions" are equivalent to those given verbally to a human subject. In most psychophysical experiments, the information of interest is the stimulus value at which the animal ceases to follow instructions. This would be the stimulus intensity at which the rat ran left as often as right.

Training methods may be classified conveniently into those based on unconditioned reflexes, which involve Pavlovian conditioning methods, and those using an operant response maintained by reinforcement such as food reward or avoidance of shock.

Pavlovian Conditioning Methods

The Pavlovian conditioned reflex is established by correlating the occurrence of a neutral stimulus – in the present case, a visual stimulus – with an unconditioned stimulus that predictably elicits some conveniently measurable response. After conditioning, the neutral stimulus also elicits the response, and the response then indicates detection of the stimulus. Although Pavlov is famous for his work with the salivary response, it is a good deal more convenient to use a motor response.

Operant methods are more commonly used, but under certain circumstances the Pavlovian technique is the method of choice. For example, certain species are quiescent or sluggish; they emit little behavior that one can strengthen through reward. Reward may prove difficult, as in species that do not feed readily in captivity, satiate quickly, or require troublesome reinforcers such as moving insects. Granda and his coworkers (1965) recently chose a classical method for their studies of visual processes in turtles, because these animals are sluggish, eat irregularly, and satiate quickly. (However, we shall see that operant methods have also proved effective with turtles.)

Granda *et al.* used as their unconditioned reflex the withdrawal of the turtle's head to a shock through the jaw. Two small screws set in the turtle's jaw held a line to a response recorder; the screws also served as electrodes through which the shock could be delivered. The scheme is diagrammed in Fig. 1. Elastic bands held the turtle down, and a spring on the line drew the turtle's head into position such that the left eye was in front of a circular stimulus patch. As shown in Fig. 1, the conditioned stimulus (CS), a light, was followed after 5 sec by a shock (US). Head withdrawal during the light exposure stopped the shock from occurring. Zwick and Granda (1968) measured light thresholds for the turtle by establishing conditioned head withdrawal to a succession of lights of decreasing intensity. They then traced dark adaptation following periods of light adaptation. Thresholds were obtained by an up-down tracking method, with stimulus intensity decreasing 0.2 log unit after each head withdrawal, and increasing by 0.2 log unit following failure to withdraw.

In most animals shock produces autonomic effects such as changes in respiration and heart rate; when conditioned, these changes may serve as indicator responses in psychophysical studies. MCCLEARY and BERNSTEIN (1959) used this method with goldfish. Shock delivered across the fish's body produced heart-rate deceleration; implanted electrodes registered the change on an electrocardiograph. In these experiments, the fish was fixed in place, and colored lights that appeared from behind a screen provided the conditioned stimuli. Other experiments have used general activity as the response, and either food or shock as the unconditioned stimulus (BITTERMAN, 1966).

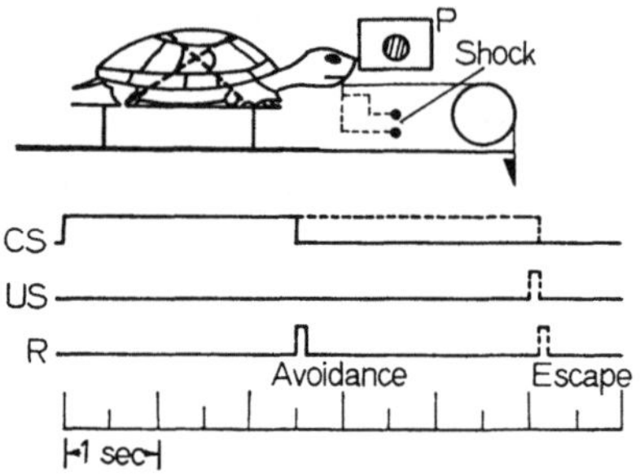

Fig. 1. Above, method by which a turtle's head withdrawal is used to indicate detection of a visual stimulus presented to the left eye, at P. As shown below, withdrawals to this stimulus could precede, and thus avoid the unconditioned shock stimulus. (After GRANDA *et al.*, 1965)

A very promising method measures classical conditioning through its effect on ongoing operant behavior. This method is based on the "conditioned suppression" phenomenon, in which an operant response, such as bar pressing or key pecking, is suppressed by a conditioned stimulus (CS) that precedes a shock. The amount of this suppression (decrease in rate of response to the CS) serves as a measure of the conditioned response to the CS. Extensive studies of conditioned suppression (e.g., KAMIN, 1963) have shown that suppression to the conditioned stimulus follows the classic laws of Pavlovian conditioning.

A paper by HENDRICKS (1966) describes the suppression method as applied to determination of critical flicker thresholds in pigeons. The first step in the procedure establishes the behavior to be suppressed. In most studies the baseline behavior is the rate of a free operant response, such as a lever press or a key peck, maintained by intermittent food reinforcement. In HENDRICKS' study, for example, pigeons were trained to peck an illuminated key for 25 or more one-hour sessions. Over this time they developed a regular rate of response, maintained by a variable interval (VI) schedule of reinforcement (FERSTER and SKINNER, 1957) that provided one reinforcement every 2 min on the average (VI 2 min). For suppression training, the steady illumination of the key was interrupted at random intervals by a 20 sec presentation of a stimulus flickering at 10 cps, followed by a 45 msec shock delivered through electrodes implanted in the bird's tail region on 60% of the trials. An average of 30 such trials was given over each hourly session for 12 sessions.

Pigeons trained in the manner just described peck at a moderate, rather steady, rate at the steadily illuminated key, but when the key light begins to flicker, they emit few or no responses until after shock that terminates the trial. Suppression is measured by comparing the response rate during the 20 sec flickering CS with the

20 sec period immediately preceding the CS. The ratio

$$\frac{\text{(pre-flicker responses)} - \text{(flicker responses)}}{\text{(pre-flicker responses)}}$$

provides a quantitative measure of suppression.

Training proceeded with gradually increasing flicker rates until the suppression ratios fell below 0.5 consistently within a range of 6 cps. Thresholds were then determined, with threshold defined as the lowest flicker frequency that yielded a suppression ratio of 0.5 or below on at least three of a block of five trials. To minimize disruption of the birds' behavior, shocks were omitted on test trials during which no suppression occurred. To control for artifacts, sham trials of 220 cps flicker, far above the CFF, were periodically given. HENDRICKS tested at a number of luminance levels with very regular and stable results. Her records show abrupt failure of suppression as the flicker threshold is exceeded by only one or two cps. The range of thresholds within subjects averaged less than 4 cps, and inter-subject variability did not exceed 5 cps at any luminance level.

Several aspects of this method deserve comment. First, suppression was enhanced by omitting food reinforcement during the flicker stimulus, so that flicker signalled the absence of food as well as oncoming shock. Second, as compared with other training methods, relatively short training may be adequate. However, flicker vs. no-flicker on a pecking key is a very "easy" discrimination for the pigeon. With these stimuli brief training might also suffice with other methods. HENDRICKS also remarks that the subjects never lost their differential response to the flicker, and periodic retraining was unnecessary. Such retraining is often necessary with difficult discriminations or aversive training procedures.

Two-Choice Operant Methods

The two-response, forced-choice procedure is among the commonest methods for studying visual problems with animal subjects. It is also one of the oldest. YERKES used an early version in his animal discrimination studies in which the animal chose one of two paths that led to food past appropriate visual displays (LASHLEY, 1912). However, animals learned much faster in the later Lashley jumping stand (LASHLEY, 1938). The differences between the Yerkes box and the Lashley stand are instructive. In the Lashley stand, the animal jumps directly at the stimulus, rather than running past it; thus, the animal is reinforced immediately for correct responses, not later in another location as in the Yerkes box. Wrong responses may be punished, as the animal bumps its nose on a locked door and falls into a net. The gap over which the animal jumps serves to keep the subject at a constant viewing distance prior to choice. This gap also favors the development of appropriate observing behavior; other two-choice methods are often plagued by the tendency for the subject to respond too quickly, "without looking."

The Lashley stand illustrates many of the features that favor good animal discrimination, and in one variant or another it is still used. However, it is clearly unsuitable for some species and problems, it is relatively slow, and it requires the constant attention of an experimenter (who may unwittingly introduce variability and response biases in his handling of the animals.) To minimize the latter difficulties, automatic two-choice equipment is now used in many studies. Such equipment is exemplified by an apparatus for turtles devised by BITTERMAN (1964). GRAF (1967) used flicker photometry in this apparatus to determine spectral sensitivity in the turtle *Chrysemys picta picta*. Turtles were trained to take pieces of hamburger from the edge of a disk that projected into a slot between two Plexiglas response keys. The turtle held its head between the keys, upon which the choice stimuli were projected. On one key a standard white light alternated with darkness at 45 cps, on the other the flicker rate was 13 cps. The turtles were given a bit of hamburger if they pressed the panel illuminated with the more rapidly alternating light. If they made an error, the stimuli were presented again after a 35 sec interval of darkness. This interval of darkness provided a mild "punishment" for errors, and the correction procedure — repetition of the same stimuli following an error — forced the turtle to respond to each side, an important feature to which we shall return.

Sensitivity was determined (as in standard flicker-photometry) by substituting monochromatic light of variable energy for the dark interval in each stimulus beam, (see LE GRAND, chapter 15, this volume). Changing the density in the monochromatic light beam produced a psychometric function, with percent correct plotted against density, as in Fig. 2. From the point of minimal flicker, as shown in the figure, the energy for each stimulus wavelength was determined and a spectral sensitivity function was plotted for 11 wavelengths from 575 to 715 nm.

GRAF's turtles failed to make reliable discriminations at wavelengths below 585 nm. One of the possible reasons suggested for this finding calls attention once again to the fact that unlearned preferences or reflexes may intrude upon the data gathered by a training technique. In the present case, GRAF suggests that high-intensity, short wavelength lights are aversive to turtles.

Many psychophysical tasks require more complex responses than simply detecting a stimulus, but an operant two-choice method can often be adapted to meet the required conditions. For example, SCOTT and POWELL (1963) undertook to measure

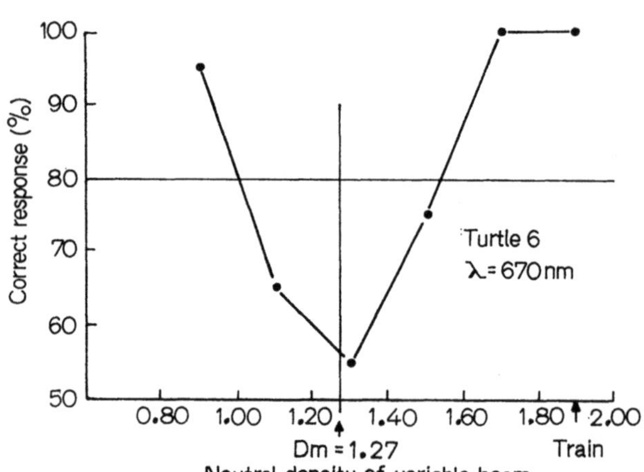

Fig. 2. Sample psychometric function resulting from GRAF's flicker experiment with the turtle. Monochromatic light alternated rapidly with white light. Flicker was hardest to discriminate at a certain intensity of the monochromatic light; this intensity was used in the construction of a spectral sensitivity function. (After GRAF, 1967)

the spiral after-effect in monkeys. The procedure required the monkey first to fixate a rotating adaptation stimulus for a time, and then to respond differentially to a target stimulus that was either expanding or contracting. If an after-effect is present, the perceived expansion or contraction is modified by the direction of rotation of the adaptation spiral. This task took several months for the monkeys to learn. A three-field mirror tachistoscope presented a rotating spiral adaptation stimulus, a circular test stimulus that expanded or contracted at different rates, and a fixation spot, at an optical distance of five feet. The monkey, seated in a restraining chair, fixated a spot of light at the center of the rotating spiral for 10 seconds. Then the spiral vanished and a bright circle appeared. If this circle (traced on an oscilloscope face) was expanding, a press on a right-hand lever was correct; if the circle was contracting, a left-lever press was correct. Equal numbers of left and right responses imply a stationary target. Every second correct press produced a food pellet, while presses of the wrong lever or in the presence of the spiral yielded a mild shock. A lever response turned off the circle and the spiral reappeared for the next trial.

This experiment required explicit training of an observing response. At first, only the fixation point was presented, without the spiral, and when the animal fixated it, the circle was turned on. Later in training the spiral was introduced. One of the advantages of an operant technique such as this is the possibility of conditioning explicit observing behavior, and the use of "conditioned reinforcers" (here, the appearance of the circle) in such a way that rather complex chains of behavior may be maintained if necessary.

In the test series, the rate of expansion or contraction of the circle was varied over a range of values, and there resulted a psychophysical function relating the proportion of left lever presses to the rate of change of the circle. Figure 3 shows

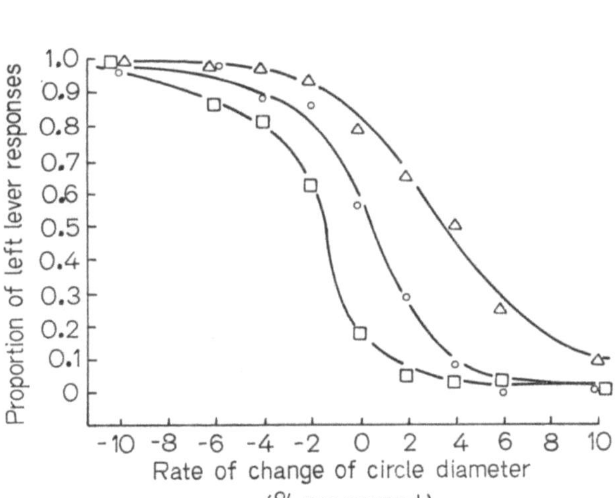

Fig. 3. For a monkey viewing a circle changing in the manner shown on the abscissa, the curves show the proportion of left lever ("contracting") responses following exposure to a spiral that was "contracting" (squares); stationary (circles); "expanding" (triangles). Relative displacement of the curves indicates the extent of the motion aftereffect. (After SCOTT and POWELL, 1963)

the results for three different pre-exposure conditions. It is evident that pre-exposure to the "expanding" or "contracting" spiral shifted, in the expected direction, the point at which the monkey judged the circle "stationary", and the data are regular enough to yield a quantitative statement of the motion after-effect.

Multiple-choice Methods

Increasingly in modern research, multiple stimulus and response alternatives are presented to the animal subject, rather than a simple choice of two. This complicates apparatus construction, but the benefits of multiple response methods may outweigh the cost. First the probability of being correct by chance is reduced from 1/2 to 1/N, where N is the number of response alternatives. Thus, in a four-choice task, the probability of reinforcing a chance response is reduced from 1/2 to 1/4, and this decreases the likelihood that spurious factors such as position will continue to control the animal's behavior. It also yields a wider working range over which to follow the subject's performance, which may vary between 25 % (chance) and 100 % correct.

Another interesting advantage of the multiple choice procedure is that, at least in some subject species, it may enhance transfer from one problem to another. This might be desirable if several visual functions are of interest. For example, in work of DeValois and his associates on primate color vision, a four-choice task was

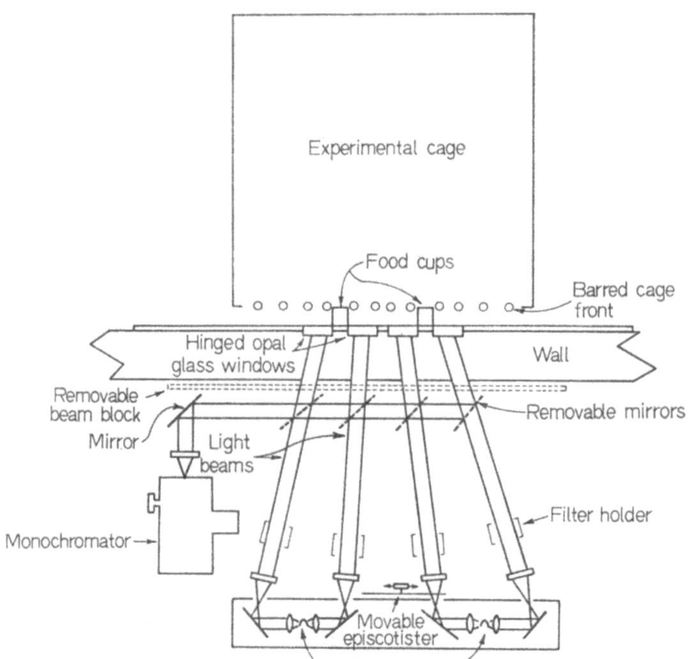

Fig. 4. Four-choice apparatus used to determine visual functions of monkeys. One of the four windows differed from the others in some characteristic of its illumination such as flicker or spectral composition. (After DeValois, 1965)

employed (1968). The monkey, in a darkened cage, faced four hinged windows of opal glass. These were illuminated simultaneously, and the monkey pressed one. If the pressed stimulus was correct, a pellet dropped into an adjacent food cup (Fig. 4). Although several visual functions were studied, all could be defined in the same way, namely, "choose that stimulus of the four which differs from the other three." Thus, in one task, monkeys chose the flickering stimulus from among steady lights; in another, they chose the spectral stimulus from white lights; in another, an analogue of the anomaloscope used with human subjects, three windows were illuminated with monochromatic yellow light and a fourth with a variable mixture of yellow-red and yellow-green lights. A considerable amount of research has shown that primates, given enough such problems, can learn the "oddity concept," and in such an array will pick the stimulus that differs from all the rest without regard to the specific characteristic in which the difference lies. This ability is useless in the two-choice test, where each problem must be redefined in specific terms.

Although the oddity task appears to be useful as a psychophysical technique with monkeys, most animals have great difficulty learning such abstract "concepts." Oddity learning, in the sense of forming a concept that transfers readily to new tasks, has been convincingly demonstrated only in primates. Pigeons, for example, when taught oddity problems, tend to learn each as a separate task, and their discrimination breaks down when they are transferred to a new problem (Cumming and Berryman, 1961). This difficulty in the use of abstract stimulus characteristics constitutes one of the few real differences between animal and human psychophysics; we shall examine it in more detail below.

In the great majority of applications, the two-choice or multiple choice methods require the animal to respond "to" a correct stimulus – jump at a door illuminated by the stimulus, press a panel upon which it appears, push a lever under it, and so on. It is also possible for the animal to make different responses in association with different aspects of a single stimulus array, while not responding directly to the stimulus. For example, Yarczower *et al.* (1966) required a monkey to press a lever located below a peephole in order to illuminate a Landolt C. The gap in the C faced either left or right, and when it appeared, the monkey chose a lever indicating the direction of the opening in the C. Graham *et al.* (1968) used four C orientations and four levers. Such tasks, in which the response manipulanda are spatially distant from the stimulus, are much harder to learn than those in which the animal responds directly to the stimulus.

Discrete-Trial Single-Response Methods

The procedures just described involve a symmetrical choice among alternatives. Single response procedures analogous to the "yes-no" methods of human psychophysics may also be used. In such cases, "percent correct" is the usual response measure. In addition, latency or reaction time can yield important information. An example is provided in a study by Moody (1969), which is especially informative because it illustrates the flexibility which the operant method can bring to the whole experimental situation.

Moody's method derives from work of Stebbins and his associates that was concerned with equal loudness contours (1966). In Moody's application, equal brightness functions for the rat are derived from latencies of bar release. The basic assumption here is that equal latency of bar release to stimuli indicates equal brightness of the stimuli.

MOODY trained his rats to enter a viewing tunnel inserted in the wall of an experimental chamber. At the far end of the tunnel was a frosted glass screen for the visual stimuli. About halfway down the tunnel, a response lever projected up through the floor; above the lever was a loudspeaker, and a water delivery mechanism was located in the chamber near the tunnel opening. The rats were reinforced for a chain of behavior: in the presence of a white noise from the speaker, they pressed the lever, and then released it when a light appeared on the glass screen. Water reinforcement followed lever releases in the presence of the light. Since visual stimuli were not presented unless the lever was held down (for a variable interval of 0.2 to 3.0 sec), this procedure kept the rat in about the same position from trial to trial. The intertrial interval without noise lasted 20 sec; the light went out after 1 sec if the rat did not release the lever within that time.

By varying the energy of light at each of several wavelengths, MOODY obtained a family of latency curves. Latency decreased over an effective range of about 0.7 sec to 0.4 sec with increase in stimulus energy. Equal latency cuts through this family of curves at several points yielded a family of "equal brightness functions" similar to those in the literature for the human periphery and for rat electroretinograms.

In his discussion of the method applied by MOODY, STEBBINS (1966) points out that the human reaction-time experiment is also a chain of events, for the subject is ordinarily given a "ready" signal and at this time prepares himself to respond "quickly" after a second stimulus is given. In animal work, the stimulus is presented only when the animal has pressed the lever and is "ready" to react, a procedure that reduces the variability of the data. Variability may be further reduced by differentially reinforcing short latencies (MILLER *et al.*, 1966).

It is possible, of course, to use negative as well as positive reinforcement in the single response procedure. We have already seen that conditioned suppression (classical conditioning) methods make effective use of aversive stimuli. Some experimenters, however, report difficulties during attempts to use aversive stimuli in operant experiments. For example, SIDLEY *et al.* (1965) gave restrained monkeys a shock 2 sec after each of a series of test flashes, unless the monkey pressed a lever in the interim and had not pressed the lever for 2 sec before the flash. A descending sequence of energies was used to determine thresholds at 20 stimulus wavelengths, and threshold was defined as that level of energy at which the monkey received three shocks in a row. Although the data obtained in this way were satisfactory, the investigators report that the animals became harder and harder to handle, and the method was switched to one that used positive reinforcement. The new method was much like that developed by STEBBINS and used by MOODY, with a "ready" lever press, followed by lever release to a light flash. The latter response was reinforced with orange juice. A spectral sensitivity function was derived, again by a descending method of limits.

Single-Response Methods Using Rate

In many studies that make only a single response lever available, stimuli are presented for extended periods and the rate of the response becomes an important variable. Responses are permitted at any time and reinforcements are delivered on an intermittent schedule. Often, but not always, explicit discrimination training is also introduced; one or more negative stimuli replace the positive stimulus, and no reinforcement follows responses to the negative stimuli. After such training, the animal responds in the presence of the positive training stimulus, and responds to a lesser extent to stimuli different from the positive stimulus. This stimulus-response relation may be clearly defined by the "generalization gradient" that results from varying the stimulus along one or more dimensions of interest.

Experimenters have used this method under circumstances in which, were their subjects human, they might ask for "similarity judgments." When training has produced a stable rate of response in the presence of the positive stimulus, and a generalization test is run, reinforcement ceases, and the stimulus is varied over a range of values (MOSTOFSKY, 1965). The rate at which responses occur to a stimulus may be taken as a measure of the similarity of that stimulus to the positive, training stimulus. For example, MELLO (1966) studied transfer between eyes in the pigeon, as follows: Pigeons were fitted with goggles that restricted vision to the anterior visual field of one eye. They were then reinforced for pecking at a line tilted at 45° (the positive stimulus, or "S+"), with food delivered on an average of once per minute. Five minute presentations of this 45° S+ were alternated with presentations of a line tilted the opposite way (135°) during which no reinforcements were delivered; in fact, pecks during the S− presentation delayed the return of the S+ for 1 minute. Such a delay following an incorrect response is often used in psychophysical studies, and speeds the acquisition of the desired discrimination. (See GRAF's turtle study, above.)

Generalization tests are usually carried out during extinction. Reinforcement is discontinued because the experimenter cannot specify which stimulus is "correct" during the test – this would be like informing the human subject which stimuli he should judge similar to the standard. Since no food is forthcoming the response eventually extinguishes, but if intermittent schedules of reinforcement are used in training, there are enough responses during extinction to provide informative data. However, if the test situation differs substantially from the training situation, additional steps may be taken to assure adequate responding. In MELLO's experiment, for example, birds tend to respond rather little following monocular training, when the untrained eye is exposed and the trained eye occluded. Hence, MELLO provided a day of key-peck experience for the untrained eye, and reinforced responses to a plain white key on a VI 1 min schedule. Each test session was then also preceded by a 10 min warmup on the white key.

MELLO followed the usual generalization test procedure, presenting in randomized sequence six angles of tilt that ranged between 15° and 165° in 30° steps. Each stimulus appeared for 30 sec. Each bird was tested first with its untrained eye alone open, then with its trained eye open, on each of three successive days. MELLO found that with the trained eye open the birds responded most to the 45° line on which they had been trained, but with the untrained eye open, they responded most to the 135° line, the mirror image of the training pattern. This striking finding suggests the power of the generalization procedure, through it is open to conflicting interpretations (p. 749). Among other problems to which the method has been recently applied is the perception of the visual vertical (THOMAS and

Lyons, 1968). A two-key adaptation of the method was applied by Boakes (1969) to the bisection of brightness intervals. Many studies of wavelength generalization have been conducted, but unfortunately few of these have been done in a way that generated clear information relevant to color vision. For example, luminance is usually uncontrolled when wavelength is varied in the test situation.

Generalization is but one way of using free-operant single-response procedures. For example, Mello and Peterson (1964) used a single-response method with a different measure to shed light on the paradoxical case of color vision in the cat. Cones have been found in the cat retina, and certain electrophysiological responses suggest wavelength discrimination, but cats have failed to discriminate color in most behavioral tests. Mello and Peterson trained cats to press a panel next to a stimulus display on which lights of variable wavelength and energy could be projected. The cats were allowed to press the panel freely, and received food on the average of once per minute (VI 1 min schedule). In testing sessions, responses to red stimuli continued to be reinforced, while 3 min presentations of green, blue or yellow were never accompanied by reinforcement. Human observers provided matched brightnesses of these colors, but because these could not be assumed to be correct for the cat, the energies of the stimuli presented to the cats were varied over a wide range around the human brightness matches, so that discrimination could not be based on brightness alone. Records of response rate to each stimulus were made during training with food reinforcement. These results were checked in subsequent extinction tests, which eliminated the possibility of differential responding on the basis of reinforcement itself. The rate of response was found in both cases to vary systematically with wavelength, being high for "red" and lower for other colors. Rate did not vary systematically with luminance. Mello and Peterson comment that previous behavioral studies may have failed to show color discrimination because they used discrete-trial, forced-choice procedures, relatively brief training, and inadequate food deprivation. They, on the contrary, used the free-operant method described, their cats had some $1^1/_2$ years of experience on color problems, and were run 22 hours hungry and at 80 % of their free-feeding weight. We see no particular reason why the operant method they used should be more effective than a good two-choice method (cf. Brown and Sechzer, 1964), but we agree with Mello and Peterson that food deprivation is probably the major factor that made possible their results. Many investigators fail to deprive their subjects enough to produce high levels of discrimination behavior for food reinforcement. Mello and Peterson report that cats less deprived than their test animals perform capriciously even on easy discrimination tasks.

Operant Tracking

Little has been said thus far about the sequence and control of stimuli. Variants of the classical methods of limits or constant stimuli are often used; we shall touch on this matter below. Where it is necessary to get an estimate of a threshold rapidly or continuously over a period of time, the subject may be trained to adjust the stimulus to values near the critical level. Békésy's (1947) method for tracking the human auditory threshold is such a procedure, and Blough (1957, 1958) adapted this technique for animal work. The essential idea is that of a feedback loop: the stimulus controls the animal's behavior as a result of discrimination training, and the animal's behavior adjusts the value of the stimulus via automatic apparatus.

Blough (1958) tracked the absolute visual threshold of the pigeon as follows. The bird was reinforced on an intermittent schedule for pecking one response key (key A) when the stimulus patch was visible and another (key B) when the patch was dark. The peck on key A reduced the luminance of the stimulus, while the pecks on key B increased it. These contingencies caused the stimulus luminance to vary up and down across the pigeon's threshold. Figure 5 shows a schematic picture of the apparatus.

The response sequence used in tracking was maintained by a chain of events similar to those used to maintain observing responses. The animal is reinforced for "observing" (e.g., holding down a lever, as in Stebbins' method) by the eventual appearance of the stimulus; this leads to a detection response reinforced with food. In threshold tracking, response to key A, which reduces stimulus luminance, is reinforced intermittently by darkness – a shutter turns out the light – and a response indicating detection of "light out" (key B) brings food. This reinforcement sequence is imposed intermittently on the basic tracking task in order to keep the animal responding properly. The key to the method lies in the fact that the animal cannot discriminate shutter closure (the condition under which food follows key B responses) from the dimming of the light to subthreshold levels.

The tracking method has been used successfully in a number of studies with various animal species and stimulus parameters (e.g., Gourevitch *et al.*, 1960; Elliott *et al.*, 1962). Some investigators have found it difficult to train animals in tracking, and the method should probably be chosen only where rapid estimates of threshold or continuous threshold tracking are important. The time course of drug effects and the course of dark adaptation are two such situations (Blough, 1956, 1958).

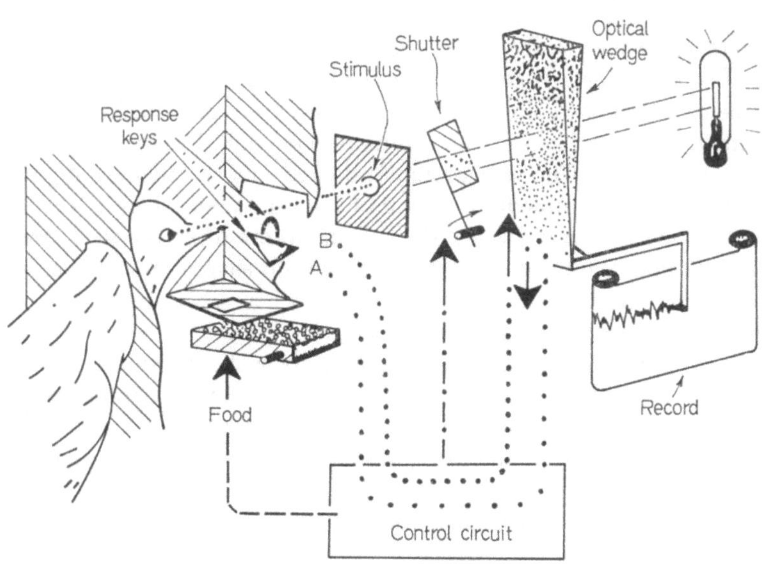

Fig. 5. A schematic picture of the apparatus used to track visual thresholds in the pigeon. (After Blough, 1958)

Methodological Review

The Choice of a Method

The types of problems that can be studied by reflex methods are limited. These methods are used either when they happen to be so appropriate that conditioning is unnecessary, or when it is not clear that the animal can be conditioned. If a training method seems called for, one must decide between classical and operant methods. Again, the species may limit the choice. Frogs seem difficult if not impossible to train in the operant manner; no one seems to have been able to teach them to do anything to produce food, water, shock termination, etc. However, it seems possible that classical conditioning of heart rate or respiration might be accomplished with a visual conditioned stimulus, and this would give the investigator a potential response indicator. Even if operant behavior is available and conditionable, it may be ill-advised. If the animal is sluggish or skittish, hard to deprive without risk to life or health, satiates quickly with known reinforcers, or requires very long deprivations, ordinary positive reinforcement may be difficult. If, in addition, the subject is highly stressed by known aversive stimuli, or does not readily avoid them, negative reinforcement of operant behaviors may be out of the question, and the investigator may adopt the classical paradigm.

Usually, however, operant training procedures make it possible for the investigator to fit his method most appropriately to his problem. An arbitrary indicator response suited to the species and the problem may be selected. Also, ancillary behavior that positions the animal properly and indicates his readiness to respond may be conditioned, or more complex tasks such as tracking may be used. We consider next some of the general issues that arise in operant work.

Motivation and Reinforcement Variables

All operant methods assume an active and attentive subject. In studies using positive reinforcers such as food, it is urgent that the subjects be highly deprived and that they work for a highly preferred incentive. As we saw above, there is reason to believe that the color vision of cats may have remained obscure because the subjects in early studies were not motivated enough. Preliminary work with a new species is essential. The indicators of adequate motivation are high activity, swift response, and the immediate taking of the reinforcer when it is offered. For hunger motivation in many species, the rule of thumb often is "80 % free-feeding weight, and 24 hours hungry," but this will be too severe in some cases, and in others longer periods without any food may be necessary. (Graf used a week without food in his turtle work discussed above.)

When a correct response is made, the reinforcer should appear immediately. Usually, this is best done by using one or more conditioned reinforcers — signals that are followed by food. Thus, when an animal pushes the correct lever, a tone might sound, indicating that food is available in a nearby cup. The tone can be sounded within a fraction of a second after the response; if the animal does not move immediately to the cup when the tone sounds, further training or more deprivation is necessary.

Sometimes operant behavior is maintained by the avoidance of shock rather than by positive reinforcement. In other cases investigators couple reinforcement for correct responses with punishment for incorrect ones. Mild punishment seems often to improve performance, perhaps by encouraging the animal to "look before it leaps." This is literally true in the Lashley stand, where punishment is a bump on the nose and a fall into the net below. Care is necessary, especially in the use of punishment alone. Discriminations may become erratic or the animals intractable, as SIDLEY *et al.* reported (1965).

A "punishment" that seems effective is the imposition of a delay following incorrect responses. This prevents the spurious reinforcement of incorrect responses which comes about through conditioned reinforcement: "getting on to the next trial when the current discrimination is difficult." Such delay is particularly necessary for free-response methods as in MELLO and PETERSON's work on cats (see above).

Observing Behavior

Experimenters commonly report difficulty in teaching tasks that force the subject to respond to a stimulus spatially separated from the response manipulandum. This probably happens because animals tend to look in the place where they respond. An effective method encourages the subject to look at the stimuli; it also reduces variability by creating constant conditions (such as body position) at the time of stimulus presentation.

Operant methods permit explicit conditioning of appropriate observing behavior. A number of the studies mentioned above exemplify this procedure: SCOTT and POWELL trained their monkeys to look at a fixation point; rats positioned themselves and pressed a "ready" lever in MOODY's brightness studies; pigeons inserted their heads through a positioning hole in BLOUGH's tracking experiments. After pretraining, no additional reinforcement is ordinarily needed to maintain such observing behavior. It is maintained as an early link in a response chain, and it is reinforced by the subsequent appearance of the visual display to which the animal makes discriminative responses (WYCKOFF, 1952).

Stimulus Preferences and Response Bias

A number of variables control an animal's response. The probability of discriminative responses established through conditioning will depend upon reinforcement contingencies set up by the experimenter, but this probability may also be a function of prior learning, genetic factors, or other variables. For example, operant conditioning may establish lever release to stimulus onset, and built-in mechanisms presumably account for the fact that with increasing intensity, response latency diminishes. This regular relation yields psychophysical functions. However, unlearned control can be a confounding factor; HERTER (1953: pp. 155 to 195) gives a thorough review of experiments on vision in fish which depend on spontaneous responses to many different kinds of visual stimuli. MUNTZ and CRONLY-DILLON (1966) found that goldfish learn a color discrimination faster if blue is the positive stimulus than if blue is negative. Similarly, several investigators (MUNTZ, 1962; CHAPMAN, 1966) report that frogs prefer to jump to certain wavelengths rather than others, which (if the frog could be trained) would interfere with choice procedures. The generalization procedures may be particularly susceptible to preference effects, for training often does not involve procedures that strictly define the controlling stimulus.

Response biases – usually position preference – often plague experimenters attempting to develop difficult discriminations in animal subjects. In a simple two-choice task, repetition of a single choice may bring reinforcement on half of the total trials. Such intermittent reinforcement is often enough to keep the subject repeating that choice indefinitely unless counter-measures are taken. The most common of these is the "trial rerun" correction procedure. When the animal makes a mistake, the same stimulus pattern is repeatedly presented until at length the subject makes the correct response and is reinforced. This method forces the animal to choose the non-preferred as well as the preferred position, and it assures equal reinforcement on each. Of course, responses on the rerun trials cannot be included in the data analysis, since the correction response may simply follow the rule "switch sides if no reinforcement." A more sophisticated sequencing of trials to avoid response bias is described by Jenkins (1965).

Response bias in the single-response ("yes-no" or "go-no/go") situation is familiar to students of human psychophysics, who may use signal detectability analysis to separate sensory effects from bias (Green and Swets, 1966). (See Nachmias, chapter 3, this volume.) Some signal detection analyses of single-response animal data have been suggested (Hack, 1963; Blough, 1967) but for practical applications it seems more effective to minimize bias by forcing choices between two or more response alternatives.

Stimulus Ordering

Discussions of standard methods of human psychophysics concentrate on stimulus variables. Much of what is said in this context can be applied rather directly to animal experiments and does not warrant repetition here (Woodworth and Schlosberg, 1954). We should note, however, that in discrete trial procedures many investigators prefer the "descending method of limits" to other, more symmetrical procedures. We saw this in several of the studies cited earlier. Typically, a session starts with highly discriminable stimuli which are made progressively more difficult until some error criterion is reached; often, at this point, the stimulus difference is again made highly discriminable. At least since Pavlov it has been recognized that an animal, when forced to its discriminative limits, may cease to discriminate effectively and require retraining even on stimuli that it formerly discriminated with ease. This effect may be largely due to the extinction of observing behavior. The extinction commences when stimuli cease to be discriminable (Ziegler and Wyckoff, 1961). Observing behavior is presumably maintained by warmup trials with highly discriminable stimuli and by frequent retreat to such stimuli during testing.

Stimulus Definition

This chapter began with the remark that the essence of a psychophysical experiment is the same, whether human or animal serves as subject. Once a "language" is established, through which the experimenter can give instructions and the subject can report what he sees, the experiment proceeds to determine systematic stimulus-response relations. However, an important limitation seems to be imposed by the manner in which species categorize stimuli. Roughly speaking, humans readily "abstract" characteristics of stimulus arrays. Other primates are considerably less efficient at this, and the ability to abstract seems rapidly to diminish in simpler forms. For example, it is easy for a human subject to choose the "odd" stimulus from an array, and a monkey may learn this after extensive practice, but the task may be beyond the reach of pigeons. This is not to say that a line can be drawn between those species that respond to relations and those that do not. Stimuli are always relationally defined – "brightness" for example is determined partially by conditions of surround and prior stimulation – and the process of "abstracting" characteristics of interest appears to begin at the retina. But with progressively higher-order relations the abilities of simple species become strained, and they may fail to respond according to the stimulus as defined by the human investigator.

A consequence of this awkward situation is the current status of "psychophysical scaling" with animals. (Compare KRANTZ, chapter 26, this volume.) Although some experimenters have tried (cf. HERRNSTEIN and VAN SOMMERS, 1962), no one has satisfactorily demonstrated scaling in animals apart from confusability. The most promising recent attempts have been experiments on the bisection of brightness intervals (BOAKES, 1969).

Threshold studies ordinarily do not raise such problems of stimulus categorization. Typically, the subject reports any difference it may detect between two stimulus situations. Information of a somewhat different sort may be provided by the suprathreshold methods. In the examples cited above, this method is represented by the latency technique used by MOODY and the generalization tests of MELLO. In such work, the stimulus varies over a wider range than in the case where it only "crosses the threshold," and responses also vary more widely, so that we end up not simply with information about the "resolving power" of the organism, but also with information about what the stimulus "looks like."

Suprathreshold data must be interpreted with care, because the subject's definition of the stimulus may differ from that of the experimenter. The interpretation of MELLO's "mirror-image" work mentioned above (p. 743) is a case in point. MELLO's pigeons, when trained on a 45° line with one eye, responded most to the mirror image – a line tilted at 135° – with the other eye. The human observer is intrigued by this apparent "mirror-image" transfer. However, BEALE and CORBALLIS (1968) suggested that the bird actually learns an invariant discrimination between up and down. If a bird trained with the right eye attended only to the right half of the stimulus key, a 45° line would be "stimulus in the upper part of the field" and a 135° line would be "stimulus in the lower part of the field." If the bird then attended to the left half of the key when its left was eye exposed, the 135° line would be "stimulus in the upper part of the field" and the obtained transfer would follow. At the present writing, the nature of the effective stimulus has not been determined with certainty in this case, but it is clear that careful tests varying stimulus aspects independently are necessary to define the stimulus in such an instance.

Physiological Bases of Psychophysical Discriminations

The study of the retina and higher visual centers by the microelectrode technique has reached a high degree of sophistication (see volume VII/3, on neurophysiology of vision), but the value of this work in understanding the phenomena of vision depends on the validity of the linking hypotheses by which the data are interpreted in terms of visual function. Animal psychophysical techniques such as those described in the first part of this chapter make it possible to compare electrophysiological data with parallel psychophysical data obtained from the same species. If precise psychophysical and electrophysiological data are obtained from the same species, it is possible to look for isomorphisms between electrophysiological results and behaviorally determined functions. It is also possible to test theoretical models by attempting to predict psychophysical functions from physiological data.

This section of the chapter will therefore consider several different types of visual functions which have been investigated from both the behavioral and physiological points of view in the same species. The number of studies eligible for consideration is so large that no comprehensive review can be attempted here, but illustrative studies of spectral sensitivity, color discriminations, and flicker discrimination will be described.

Spectral Sensitivity

Cat

In the cat retina, Granit (1945) found cells which responded to light throughout the whole length of the spectrum. In the dark-adapted eye cells were maximally sensitive to light of a wavelength of about 500 nm, and their sensitivity fell off monotonically on both sides of the maximum; these cells he called scotopic "dominators." In 1952, Gunter obtained psychophysical spectral sensitivity functions from the cat. He used a two-response, forced-choice procedure in a Y-maze, and determined the energies of various wavelengths of light which were of equal brightness to the cat. Gunter's behavioral data for the cat in the dark-adapted state are shown in Fig. 6 along with Granit's data for the spectral sensitivity of the scotopic dominator, and the absorption spectrum of extracted rhodopsin, the rod visual pigment. It is clear that the behavioral luminosity measures are closely related to the spectral sensitivity of the scotopic dominator cells in the retina, and that both these measures are in turn closely related to the absorption spectrum of rhodopsin.

Pigeon

A similar comparison can be made for the scotopic spectral sensitivity of the pigeon. These results are also presented in Fig. 6. Again it can be seen that the spectral sensitivity of the dark-adapted eye measured behaviorally by Blough (1956, see p. 745 for method) agrees closely with the spectral sensitivity of ganglion cells in the retina recorded by Donner (1953). These two measures of spectral sensitivity are again in good agreement with the spectral absorption characteristics of the rod photopigment in this species as determined by Bridges (1962).

The results from these two species are typical of what is found in a wide variety of experiments on scotopic spectral sensitivity. There is strict isomorphism between receptor light absorption and neural activity in the retina, and the isomorphism is maintained between the most peripheral elements of the visual system and the visual discriminations of the intact animal.

Photopic spectral sensitivity is less simply determined. BLOUGH'S (1957) measures of spectral sensitivity in the light-adapted pigeon are also shown in Fig. 6. The wavelength of maximal sensitivity for the pigeon is shifted toward longer wavelengths compared to the dark-adapted state, just as with human spectral sensitivity functions. This change in relative spectral sensitivity with light adaptation is closely paralleled by the responses of light-adapted retinal neurons, as shown by GRANIT'S (1942) measures in Fig. 6. The Purkinje shift is related to a

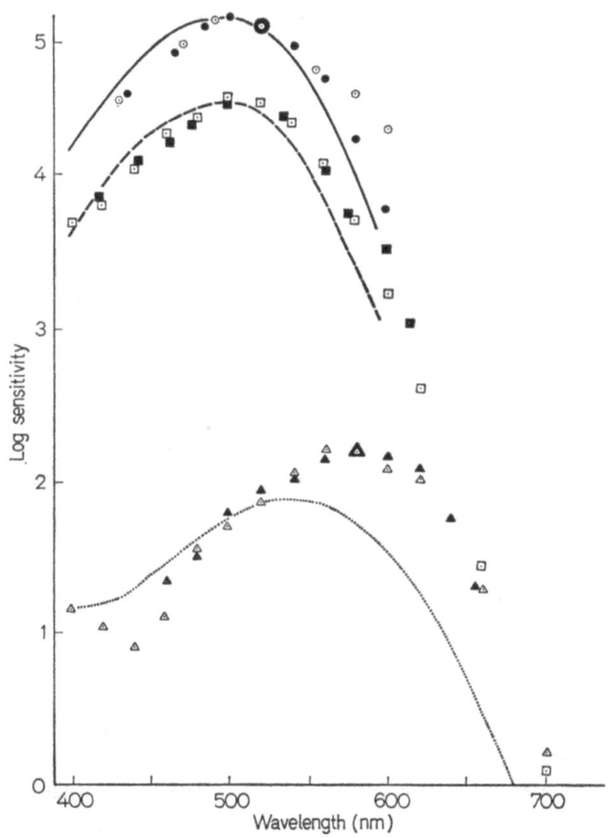

Fig. 6. *a* Behavioral equal-brightness function for dark-adapted cats: ⊙ (GUNTER, 1952). *b* Spectral sensitivity of ganglion cells in dark-adapted cat retina: ● (GRANIT, 1945). *c* Absorption spectrum of rhodopsin: solid curve. *d* Behavioral scotopic spectral sensitivity function for pigeons: ⊡ (BLOUGH, 1957). *e* Spectral sensitivity of ganglion cells in dark-adapted pigeon retina: ■ (DONNER, 1953). *f* Absorption spectrum of pigeon rod pigment: dashed curve (BRIDGES, 1962). *g* Behavioral photopic spectral sensitivity function for pigeons: △ (BLOUGH, 1957). *h* Spectral sensitivity of ganglion cells in the light-adapted pigeon retina: ▲ (GRANIT, 1942). *i* Absorption spectrum of pigeon cone pigment: dotted curve (BRIDGES, 1962)

change from rod vision while dark-adapted, to photopic cone vision. The photopic measures do not, however, agree with the single cone pigment found in the pigeon eye by Bridges (1962).

The cone receptor characteristics in pigeons and other birds are altered by the presence of colored oil droplets in these eyes. Moreover, in animals that have color vision there is usually more than one spectrally selective cone photopigment. Hence, the analysis of photopic spectral sensitivity may be appropriately considered in the more general context of mechanisms of color discrimination.

Color Discrimination

In the last decade a great deal of physiological information had been obtained from the visual systems of several species which suggests mechanisms for discriminating between lights on the basis of their spectral compositions. In two species, namely, goldfish and monkeys, the absorption characteristics of single cones have been measured, and a variety of response characteristics have been recorded from single cells by the use of microelectrodes. We shall therefore limit our review of behavioral measures of color discrimination to results obtained in these two species.

Goldfish

There have been many behavioral studies of visual discriminations in a variety of fish in which a variety of reflex and training methods have been used. The most extensive review of the earlier work is given by Herter (1953), and other reviews can be found in Warner (1931), Walls (1942), Brett (1957), Autrum (1960), and Viaud (1960).

A number of studies have been concerned specifically with color vision in the goldfish. As an example, McCleary and Bernstein (1959) used a conditioned autonomic response to measure goldfish discrimination. Fish were trained to discriminate between a red and a green stimulus. These animals were then tested with bright and dim red, and bright and dim green stimuli, and they were found to generalize perfectly according to hue. Using an operant discrimination procedure, Muntz and Cronly-Dillon (1966) showed that goldfish could discriminate between pairs of panels painted with different colors when brightness cues were eliminated. Their data are consistent with trichromatic color vision, although, taken alone, they do not rigorously establish this (Yager and Jameson, 1968). The same investigators (Cronly-Dillon and Muntz, 1965) had previously obtained a spectral sensitivity function for the goldfish. Yarczower and Bitterman (1965) measured a wavelength discrimination function for the goldfish which suggests that this species can discriminate among wavelengths throughout the spectral region they investigated (450 to 630 nm). They did not control for brightness cues, so their function may reflect brightness discriminations as well as color differences.

Yager (1967) used a two-choice operant method to measure both photopic spectral sensitivity and saturation discrimination in the goldfish. In the former experiment, light-adapted fish were trained to choose between an illuminated, reinforced target, and a non-illiminated, non-reinforced one. A modified method of constant stimuli was used to determine the stimulus energy at each wavelength required for 75 % choice of the illuminated target. In the saturation (least-colorimetric-purity) experiment, the choice was between two illuminated targets, one of which was illuminated by "white" light (2850° K) alone, and the other by a mixture of "white" light with varying amounts of monochromatic light. The targets were maintained at a constant luminance for the fish on the basis of their spectral sensitivity data. An observing response was used in both experiments, which served both to initiate a trial and to extinguish the adapting light during the presentation of the test stimuli.

The form of the spectral sensitivity function was accounted for by a trichromatic model of the visual system that postulates a summation of responses from the three different types of cones whose spectral absorptions were measured by LIEBMAN and ENTINE (1964) and MARKS (1965). Recordings from single ganglion cells in the goldfish retina by MACNICHOL *et al.* (1961) have also shown that some cells respond with either "on" or "off" responses to all spectral wavelengths, and these cells are usually interpreted as reflecting combined inputs from the different cone receptors. From other cells, they have recorded wavelength-dependent opponent responses, with on-discharges to short wavelengths and off-discharges to long wavelengths, or vice versa. These cells must also be related to more than one type of cone, and they are presumably concerned with the process of hue coding.

YAGER'S model for photopic spectral sensitivity assumes that

$$S_\lambda = K_1 \alpha_\lambda + K_2 \beta_\lambda + K_3 \gamma_\lambda \qquad (1)$$

where S_λ is psychophysical sensitivity with an equal quantum intensity spectrum at the retina, α, β, and γ are percentage absorption functions for the three selective cone photopigments with maxima at 455, 530 and 620 nm, and K_1, K_2, K_3 are factors which express the spectral absorptions of the three photopigments relative to each other. Estimates of K_1, K_2, and K_3 were obtained by a least-squares fit to the spectral sensitivity data.

For spectral saturation discrimination, YAGER'S model includes both the non-opponent, luminosity responses and the opponent, chromatic responses. The assumptions of the model are similar to those made by HURVICH and JAMESON in their theoretical analyses of human color vision (1955, 1957, 1968, see also JAMESON, chapter 14, this volume). If a, b, c, and d are names for chromatic responses for the fish and w is the achromatic response, then

$$a_\lambda - b_\lambda = K_2\beta_\lambda - K_1\alpha_\lambda, \qquad (2)$$

$$c_\lambda - d_\lambda = K_2\beta_\lambda - K_3\gamma_\lambda, \qquad (3)$$

$$w_\lambda = K_1\alpha_\lambda + K_2\beta_\lambda + K_3\gamma_\lambda, \qquad (4)$$

where $K_1 \alpha$, $K_2 \beta$, and $K_3 \gamma$ are the best fitting photochemical absorptions for the spectral sensitivity function. JAMESON and HURVICH (1955) have shown that, for the human, saturation discrimination is predicted by the ratio of total chromatic sensitivity to achromatic sensitivity at each wavelength. Written on the basis of Eq. (2), (3) and (4) for the goldfish, we have

$$\frac{|K_2\beta_\lambda - K_1\alpha_\lambda| + |K_2\beta_\lambda - K_3\gamma_\lambda|}{K_1\alpha_\lambda + K_2\beta_\lambda + K_3\gamma_\lambda}\,. \qquad (5)$$

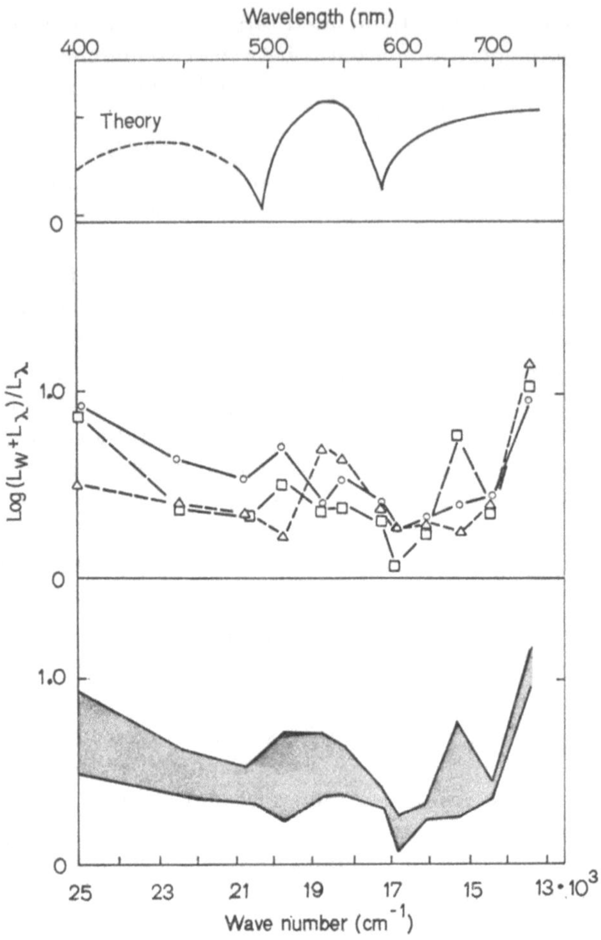

Fig. 7. Top: Theoretical saturation discrimination function for goldfish, from the opponent-colors theory. Bottom: spectral saturation discrimination functions for three fish. (After YAGER, 1967)

This function is shown in a logarithmic plot in the upper part of Fig. 7, and the behavioral discrimination data are shown in the lower part of the same figure.

The functions show two minima with a mid-spectral maximum, and rise toward the two ends of the spectrum. The theoretical visual response functions Eqs. (2), (3) and (4) are plotted in Fig. 8. Electrophysiological data from SVAETICHIN (1956), MACNICHOL *et al.* (1961), and JACOBSON (1964), show retinal and tectal single-cell responses with gross, qualitative similarities to those specified in the model, although differences in the stimulating and adapting conditions make quantitative comparisons difficult.

Monkey

The research reported by DEVALOIS and his co-workers (DEVALOIS, 1965; DEVALOIS and JACOBS, 1968; DEVALOIS *et al.*, 1966) is an example of the most

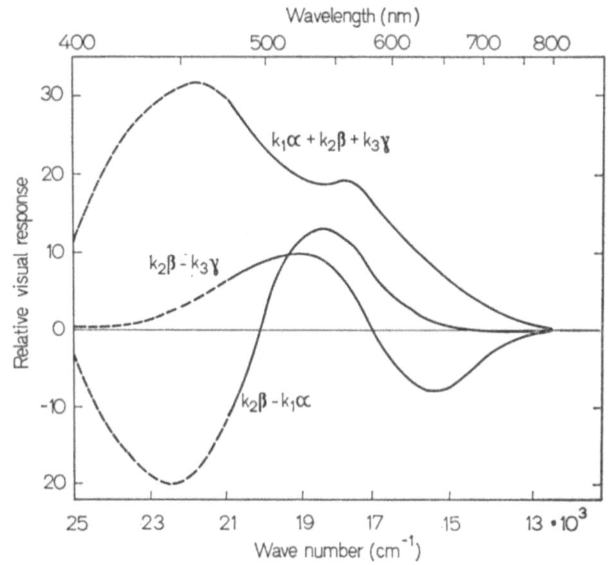

Fig. 8. Visual response functions for goldfish from the opponent-colors theory (YAGER, 1967)

logical way to approach the study of physiology of a sensory system. They obtained both psychophysical discrimination data and electrophysiological recordings from the visual systems of tje same species, in the same laboratory, and they have also related their data to the monkey cone photopigments measured by MARKS *et al.* (1964). This sort of research program provides the best chance of discovering the interrelations between the physiology and psychophysics of vision.

DEVALOIS and his associates have made a detailed analysis of the response characteristics of single cells in the lateral geniculate nucleus of the macaque monkey. On the basis of their responses the cells were divided into two general classes: a) spectrally non-opponent cells which respond to all wavelengths with either an increase or decrease from the spontaneous firing rate; b) spectrally opponent cells which respond with an increase in firing rate to some parts of the spectrum and with a decrease to others. Four types of opponent cells were found: "red" excitatory and "green" inhibitory; "green" excitatory and "red" inhibitory; "yellow" excitatory and "blue" inhibitory; "blue" excitatory and "yellow" inhibitory. If the spectral sensitivities of the opponent cells are plotted as a function of wavelength as shown in Fig. 9, except for a missing short-wave "red" limb, they exhibit a striking resemblance to human psychophysical chromatic response functions as reported by JAMESON and HURVICH (1955). (See JAMESON, chapter 14).

The psychophysical functions investigated by these experimenters on this same species include: 1) spectral sensitivity; 2) wavelength discrimination; 3) saturation discrimination. The same type of apparatus was used in all behavioral experiments (see Fig. 4). The method, which was described in the first part of this chapter, was an operant-conditioning technique in which the monkey was required to solve an oddity problem.

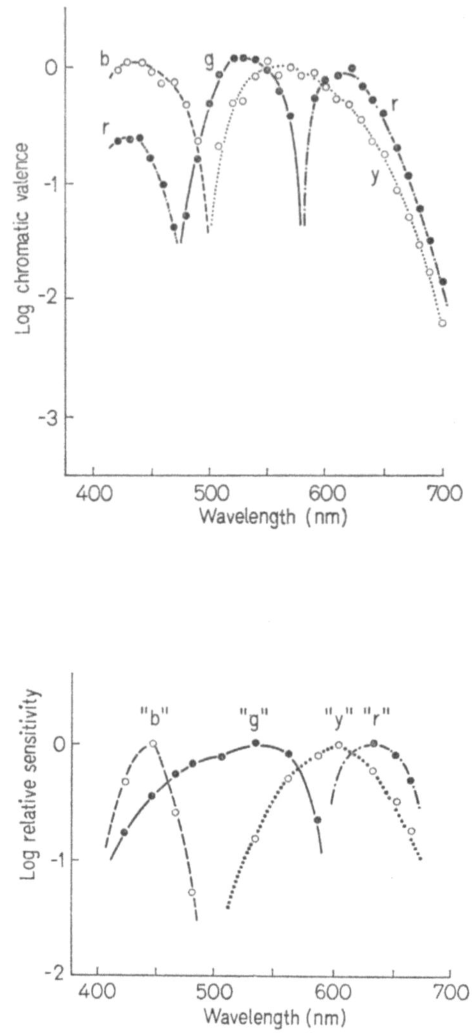

Fig. 9. Top: Log chromatic response functions. Observer. J (Jameson and Hurvich, 1955). Bottom: Equal response spectral sensitivity curves for the excitatory components of each of the four types of opponent cells; criterion = 15 spikes/sec increase. (DeValois, Abramov, and Jacobs, 1966)

In the spectral sensitivity experiment the animals were presented with one flickering light and three steady lights, all of the same wavelength. They had to choose the flickering light to receive reward. On successive blocks of trials, all four lights were dimmed until an energy level was reached at which the animal could no longer discriminate the flickering light. To determine the photopic spectral sensitivity curve high flicker rates were used: high light energies are required to detect fast flicker. Macaques were found to have approximately the same photopic spectral sensitivity function as human beings with normal vision, and this function was

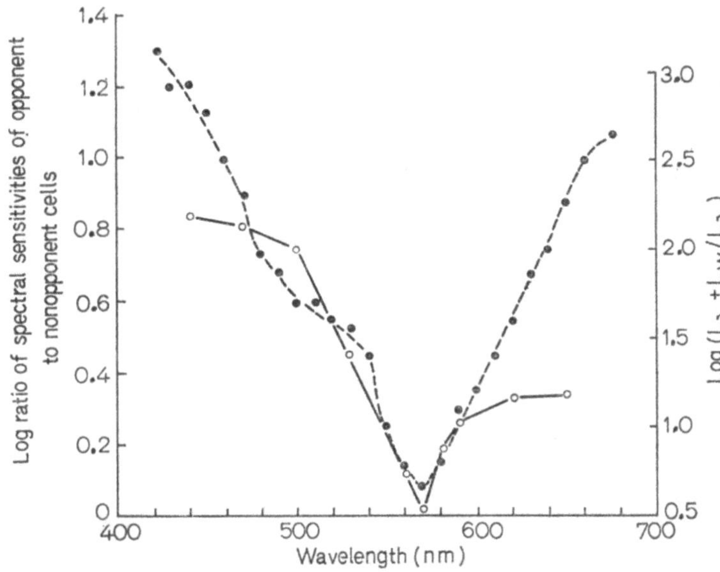

Fig. 10. Comparison of the relative saturation of various spectral lights, as determined in psychophysical tests of the macaque, with the relative sensitivities of macaque opponent and nonopponent cells at various wavelengths. Macaque cells: ●; Macaque behavioral data: ⊙. The ordinate at right, for the behavioral data, and the ordinate at left, for cell responses, have been adjusted for best fit. (After DeValois and Jacobs, 1968)

closely related to the spectral sensitivity of the non-opponent cells. This indicates that the non-opponent cells are carrying an achromatic, or brightness, signal.

The spectral wavelength discrimination function was examined in this species (DeValois and Jacobs, 1968) by illuminating three of the stimulus patches with a given wavelength and the fourth stimulus patch with light of a different wavelength. In successive blocks of trials the wavelength of the test light was shifted in small steps closer and closer to that on the other patches until the animal could no longer discriminate the odd stimulus. The results indicate that macaque monkeys have wavelength discrimination ($\Delta\lambda$) functions similar to those of normal human trichromats, with two minima, at about 490 nm and 580 nm, maxima at the spectral extremes, and a secondary maximum in the mid-spectral region. DeValois, *et al.* (1967) synthesized a wavelength discrimination function for the macaque by determining wavelength shifts necessary to produce criterion responses in wavelength-opponent geniculate cells. They assume that wavelength discrimination is mediated only by the most sensitive mechanism at a given wavelength. This assumption differs from theoretical accounts of human wavelength discrimination based on opponent color mechanisms (Hurvich and Jameson, 1955).

The saturation discrimination function of the macaque was found by training the animal to select a chromatic light presented with three white lights. Once the subject could do this, white light was added to the chromatic light in succeeding trials, and the amount of monochromatic light correspondingly decreased. This procedure was continued until the animal could no longer discriminate the colored light, now highly desaturated, from the three white lights. It was found for the macaque, as for the normal human, that all spectral wavelengths except a small region around 570 nm were quite highly saturated, with saturation increasing monotonically toward the two ends of the spectrum (Fig. 10).

If the opponent cells signal hue and the non-opponent cells signal achromatic brightness, then one might suppose that the saturation of the stimulus would be coded by the ratio between opponent and non-opponent cell activities. The function given by this ratio at different wavelengths satisfactorily describes the behavioral saturation discrimination curve (Fig. 10). This analysis is similar to the account of human saturation discrimination by Jameson and Hurvich (1955).

Flicker Discrimination

Pigeon

Hendricks (1966) used a conditioned suppression paradigm to determine critical flicker frequency (CFF) at several different stimulus luminances for three white Carneaux pigeons. This elegant technique is described in detail on p. 736. The bird pecked a steadily illuminated key for food reinforcement. Occasionally the steady light was replaced by a square-wave flickering stimulus of the same average luminance, and an electric shock followed on 60 % of these trials. After the training, presentation of the flickering light without shock led to a suppression of responding on the key for food. The CFF was taken as that flicker frequency which would produce a suppression ratio (see p. 737) of 0.5, for a particular level of stimulus luminance.

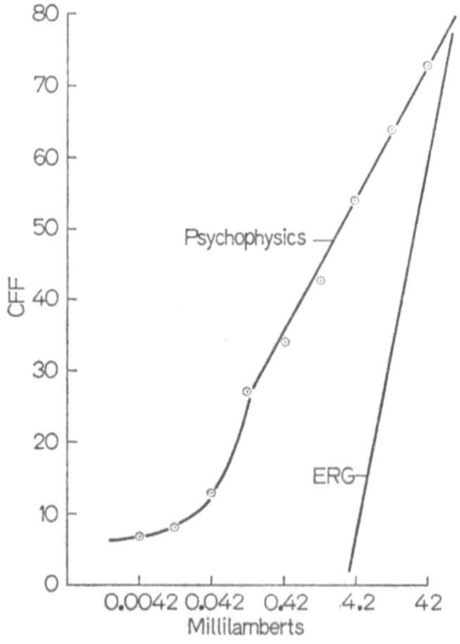

Fig. 11. Median psychophysical CFF for three pigeons as a function of log luminance (Hendricks, 1966). The heavy line describes the CFF function for the pigeon ERG (Dodt and Wirth, 1953)

Median CFF's determined in this way for three subjects are plotted as a function of log stimulus luminance in Fig. 11. The CFF function conformed to the Ferry-Porter law above about 0.4 ml, that is, it increased linearly with log luminance. There is a suggestion of a discontinuity or inflection between 0.04 and 0.4 ml; the function may consist of two limbs, as it often does in human studies (see KELLY, chapter 11, this volume).

There are few electrophysiological studies of responses of the pigeon visual system to flickering light. GRANIT (1935) and DODT and WIRTH (1953) report studies of CFF in the electroretinogram (ERG) of the pigeon. Although ERG studies are often difficult to interpret in psychophysical terms, (see RIGGS and WOOTEN, chapter 27, this volume), the results of DODT and WIRTH (Fig. 11) also conform to the Ferry-Porter law, although with a greater slope and over-all lower CFF, than HENDRICKS' behavioral data. This could be due partially to differing conditions of adaptation and stimulus size as well as the nature of the response.

It is assumed, of course, that modulations of the ERG are correlated with modulations in the firing rate of neurons of the optic nerve and higher visual center, and that these modulations of nervous activity lead to the behavioral discrimination of flicker. This correspondence between ERG and single-cell modulations does exist in some vertebrates, although it has yet to be demonstrated in the pigeon.

Monkey

A conditioned suppression technique has also been used by SHUMAKE *et al.* (1968) to determine CFF for three rhesus monkeys over a 10 log unit range of stimulus luminance. Again, at high luminances the data conformed to the Ferry-Porter law, with a much more obvious break in the function at about 0.1–0.4 ml, and 30 cps. The rod system is probably operating at the low luminances and frequencies, whereas only the cone system is able to follow the high frequencies (see KELLY, chapter 11). This confirms earlier, but less complete, results on monkeys obtained by BRECHER (1935) and SYMMES (1962), who used different methods.

WALKER *et al.* (1943) investigated the extent to which various visual pathway structures could follow a flickering light, in this same species. Responses were recorded simultaneously from large numbers of neurons, and it was found that, with a stimulus luminance of about 10 ml, the optic nerve and lateral geniculate could be driven at maximum rates of 62 cps and 59 cps, respectively, rates that are near the psychophysical CFF for the monkey at this luminance as determined by SHUMAKE *et al.* The striate cortex, however, could be driven at a maximum rate of only 34 cps, which is lower than the behaviorally determined CFF. This type of comparison between psychophysical and neural responses to flicker stimulation can help to indicate where in the visual system fusion of flicker occurs; this cannot be revealed by electrical recording alone.

Cat

In the cat, a great deal is known about the physiological mechanisms of flicker discrimination. Most of the important studies have been reviewed by BROWN (1965). (See also volume VII/3.) Various electrophysiological experiments (GRÜSSER, 1957, 1960; LINDSLEY, 1953) lead to predictions about psychophysical flicker functions, which differ depending on the postulated locus of fusion in the visual system. Such psychophysical functions have not yet been extensively determined, but one early experiment (Kappauf, 1936) does provide data on CFF for three different stimulus luminances.

Kappauf used a two-choice procedure, in which the cat was trained to discriminate between a frosted glass panel that was illuminated by flickering light and one illuminated by steady light. When the cat pressed the lever in front of the flickering panel, it received food reinforcement, and when it chose the panel illuminated with steady light, it received foot shock. The CFF was taken as the frequency at which choice responding approached chance level. For three stimulus luminances, CFF was a monotonic increasing function of luminance and was comparable to the pigeon and monkey functions reported above. The stimulus values were, however, too widely spaced to show the presence or absence of a break in the function.

Dodt and Enroth (1953) reported that the CFF for the ERG of the cat was also a monotonically increasing function of stimulus luminance, with a frequency of about 70 cps at a luminance of about 500 ml. There was a definite discontinuity in the function at about 20 ml and 30 cps. (This relatively high luminance for the break in the function probably reflects the dominance of rod photoreceptors in the cat eye, as compared to the pigeon and monkey.) Retinal ganglion cells exhibited similar response patterns: the extent to which the ERG followed luminance changes was closely related to the ability of retinal ganglion cells to emit at least one action potential per cycle. Grüsser and Creutzfeldt (1957) further reported that single cortical neurons in the cat could follow flicker frequencies up to about 50 cps at 50 ml, and that at lower luminances the CFF declined.

Because of the incompleteness of the cat behavioral data, it is not yet possible to determine which level of the nervous system mediates the fusion of a flickering light. Psychophysical functions are also needed to compare with extensive data available on other temporal characteristics of single cell responses in the cat. These include results that suggest a mechanism for the Brücke-Bartley brightness enhancement effect (Grüsser and Creutzfeldt, 1957), and modulation transfer functions for responses to sinusoidally flickering light (Cleland and Enroth-Cugell, 1966).

Acknowledgement. The preparation of this chapter was supported in part by grants MH-02456 and EY-00400 from the United States Public Health Service.

References

Autrum, H.: Vergleichende Physiologie des Farbensehens. Fortschr. Zool. **12**, 176—205 (1960).

Beale, I. L., Corballis, M. C.: Beak shift: an explanation for interocular mirror-image reversal in pigeons. Nature (Lond.) **220**, 82—83 (1968).

Bitterman, M. E.: An instrumental technique for the turtle. J. exp. Anal. Behav. **7**, 189—190 (1964).

— Animal learning. In: Experimental Methods and Instrumentation in Psychology. Sidowski, J. B. (Ed.): New York: McGraw-Hill 1966.

Blough, D. S.: Dark adaptation in the pigeon. J. comp. physiol. Psychol. **49**, 425—430 (1956).

— Spectral sensitivity in the pigeon. J. opt. Soc. Amer. **47**, 827—833 (1957).

— A method for obtaining psychophysical thresholds from the pigeon. J. exp. Anal. Behav. **1**, 31—43 (1958).

— Stimulus generalization as signal detection in pigeons. Science **158**, 940—941 (1967).

BOAKES, R. A.: The bisection of a brightness interval by pigeons. J. exp. Anal. Behav. **12**, 201—209 (1969).
BRECHER, G. A.: Die Verschmelzungsgrenze von Lichtreizen beim Affen. Z. vergl. Physiol. **22**, 539—547 (1935).
BRETT, J.: The eye. In: Physiology of Fishes, Vol. 2. New York: Academic Press 1957.
BRIDGES, C. D. B.: Visual pigments of the pigeon (*Columba livia*). Vision Res. **2**, 125—137 (1962).
BROWN, J. L.: Flicker and intermittent stimulation. In: Vision and Visual Perception. (GRAHAM, C. H. Ed.) New York: Wiley 1965.
— SECHZER, J.: Color discrimination in the cat. Science **144**, 427—429 (1964).
CHAPMAN, R. M.: Light wavelength and energy preferences of the bullfrog: Evidence for color vision. J. comp. physiol. Psychol. **61**, 429—435 (1966).
CLELAND, B., ENROTH-CUGELL, C.: Cat retinal ganglion cell responses to changing light intensities: sinusoidal modulation in the time domain. Acta physiol. scand. **68**, 365—381 (1966).
CRONLY-DILLON, J. R.: Spectral sensitivity of the scallop *Pecten maximus*. Science **151**, 345—346 (1966).
— MUNTZ, W.: The spectral sensitivity of the goldfish and clawed toad tadpole under photopic conditions. J. exp. Biol. **42**, 481—493 (1965).
CUMMING, W. W., BERRYMAN, R.: Some data on matching behavior in the pigeon. J. exp. Anal. Behav. **4**, 281—284 (1961).
DEVALOIS, R. L.: Behavioral and electrophysiological studies of primate vision. In: Contributions to Sensory Physiology, Vol. 1. NEFF, W. D. (Ed.): New York: Academic Press 1965.
— ABRAMOV, I., JACOBS, G.: Analysis of response patterns of LGN cells. J. opt. Soc. Amer. **56**, 966—977 (1966).
— — MEAD, W.: Single cell analysis of wavelength discrimination at the lateral geniculate nucleus in the macaque. J. Neurophysiol. **30**, 415—433 (1967).
— JACOBS, G. H.: Primate color vision. Science **162**, 533—540 (1968).
DODT, E., ENROTH, C.: Retinal flicker response in cat. Acta physiol. scand. **30**, 375—390 (1953).
— WIRTH, A.: Differentiation between rods and cones by flicker electroretinography in pigeon and guinea pig. Acta physiol. scand. **30**, 80—89 (1953).
DONNER, K.: The spectral sensitivity of the pigeon's retinal elements. J. Physiol. (Lond.) **122**, 524—537 (1953).
ELLIOTT, D. N., FRAZIER, L., RIACH, W.: A tracking procedure for determining the cat's frequency discrimination. J. exp. Anal. Behav. **5**, 323—328 (1962).
FERSTER, C. B., SKINNER, B. F.: Schedules of Reinforcement. New York: Appleton-Century-Crofts 1957.
GOUREVITCH, G., HOCK, M. H., HAWKINS, J. E., JR.: Auditory thresholds in the rat measured by an operant technique. Science **131**, 1046—1047 (1960).
GRAF, V.: A spectral sensitivity curve and wavelength discrimination for the turtle. *Chrysemys picta picta*. Vision Res. **7**, 915—928 (1967).
GRAHAM, E. S., MCVEAN, G. W., FORRER, D. N.: Near and far visual acuity in rhesus monkeys *(Macaca mulatta)*. Perc. Motor Skills **26**, 1067—1072 (1968).
GRANDA, A. M., MATSUMIYA, Y., STIRLING, C. E.: A method for producing avoidance behavior in the turtle. Psychon. Sci. **2**, 187—188 (1965).
GRANIT, R.: Two types of retinae and their electrical responses to intermittent stimuli in light and dark adaptation. J. Physiol. (Lond.) **85**, 421—438 (1935).
— The photopic spectrum of the pigeon. Acta physiol. scand. **4**, 118—124 (1942).
— Color vision mechanisms of the mammalian retina. J. Neurophysiol. **8**, 195—210 (1945).
GREEN, D. M., SWETS, J. A.: Signal Detection Theory and Psychophysics. New York: Wiley 1966.
GRÜSSER, O. J.: Rezeptorpotentiale einzelner Zapfen der Katze. Naturwissenschaften **44**, 522 (1957).

GRÜSSER, O. J., CREUTZFELDT, O.: Eine neurophysiologische Grundlage des Brücke-Bartley-Effektes: Maxima der Impulsfrequenz retinaler und corticaler Neurone bei Flimmer-Licht mittlerer Frequenzen. Pflügers Arch. ges. Physiol. **263**, 668—681 (1957).
— Rezeptorabhängige Potentiale der Katzenretina und ihre Reaktionen auf Flimmerlicht. Pflügers Arch. ges. Physiol. **271**, 511—525 (1960).
GUNTER, R.: The spectral sensitivity of dark-adapted cats. J. Physiol. (Lond.). **118**, 395—404 (1952).
HACK, M. H.: Signal detection in the rat. Science **139**, 758 (1963).
HECHT, S.: The nature of the photoreceptor process. In: Handbook of General Experimental Psychology. MURCHISON, C. (Ed.): Worcester, Mass.: Clark University Press 1934.
HENDRICKS, J.: Flicker thresholds as determined by a modified conditioned suppression procedure. J. exp. Anal. Behav. **9**, 501—506 (1966).
HERRNSTEIN, R. J., VAN SOMMERS, P.: Method for sensory scaling with animals. Science **135**, 40—41 (1962).
HERTER, K.: Die Fischdressuren und ihre sinnesphysiologischen Grundlagen. Berlin: Akademie-Verlag 1953.
HURVICH, L., JAMESON, D.: Some quantitative aspects of an opponent-colors theory. II. Brightness, saturation, and hue in normal and dichromatic vision. J. opt. Soc. Amer. **45**, 602—616 (1955).
— — An opponent-process theory of color vision. Psychol. Rev. **64**, 384—404 (1957).
JACOBSON, M.: Spectral sensitivity of single units in the optic tectum of the goldfish. Quart. J. exp. Physiol. **49**, 384—393 (1964).
JAMESON, D., HURVICH, L.: Some quantitative aspects of an opponent-colors theory. I. Chromatic responses and spectral saturation. J. opt. Soc. Amer. **45**, 546—552 (1955).
— — Opponent-response functions related to measured cone photopigments. J. opt. Soc. Amer. **58**, 429—430 (1968).
JENKINS, H. M.: Measurement of stimulus control during discriminative operant conditioning. Psychol. Bull. **64**, 365—376 (1965).
KAMIN, L. J.: Backward conditioning and the conditioned emotional response. J. comp. physiol. Psychol. **56**, 517—519 (1963).
KAPPAUF, W. E.: Flicker discrimination in the cat. Psychol. Bull. **33**, 597—598 (1936).
LASHLEY, K. S.: Visual discrimination of size and form in the white rat. J. anim. Behav. **2**, 310—331 (1912).
— The mechanism of vision: XV. Preliminary studies of the rat's capacity for detail vision. J. gen. Psychol. **18**, 123—193 (1938).
LIEBMAN, P., ENTINE, G.: Sensitive low-light-level microspectrophotometer: detection of photosensitive pigments of retinal cones. J. opt. Soc. Amer. **54**, 1451—1459 (1964).
LINDSLEY, D. B.: Effect of photic stimulation on visual pathways from retina to cortex. Science **117**, 469 (1953).
MACNICHOL, E., WOLBARSHT, M., WAGNER, H.: Electrophysiological evidence for a mechanism of color vision in the goldfish. In: Light and Life, MCELROY, W. D., GLASS, B. (Eds.). Baltimore: Johns Hopkins Press 1961.
MARKS, W. B.: Visual pigments of single goldfish cones. J. Physiol. (Lond.) **178**, 14—32 (1965).
MCCLEARY, R. A., BERNSTEIN, J. J.: A unique method for control of brightness cues in the study of color vision in fish. Physiol. Zool. **32**, 284—292 (1959).
MELLO, N. K.: Interocular generalization: A study of mirror-image reversal following monocular training in pigeon. J. exp. Anal. Behav. **9**, 11—16 (1966).
— PETERSON, N. J.: Behavioral evidence for color discrimination in the cat. J. Neurophysiol. **27**, 323—333 (1964).
MILLER, J. M., GLICKSTEIN, M., STEBBINS, W. C.: Reduction of response latency in the monkey by a procedure of differential reinforcement. Psychon. Sci. **5**, 177—178 (1966).
MOODY, D. B.: Equal brightness functions for supra-threshold stimuli in the pigmented rat: a behavioral determination. Vision Res. **9**, 1381—1389 (1969).
MOSTOFSKY, D.: Stimulus Generalization. Stanford: Stanford University Press 1965.
MUNTZ, W. R. A.: Effectiveness of different colors of light in releasing the positive phototactic behavior of frogs, and a possible function of the retinal projection to the diencephalon. J. Neurophysiol. **25**, 712—720 (1962).

MUNTZ, W. R. A., CRONLY-DILLON, J.: Color discrimination in goldfish. Anim. Behav. **14**, 351—355 (1966).

SCHLIEPER, C.: Farbensinn der Tiere und optomotorische Reaktionen. Z. vergl. Physiol. **12**, 1—77 (1927).

SCOTT, T. R., POWELL, D. A.: Measurement of visual motion aftereffect in the rhesus monkey. Science **140**, 57—59 (1963).

SHUMAKE, S. A., SMITH, J. C., TAYLOR, H. L.: Critical fusion frequency in rhesus monkeys. Psychol. Rec. **8**, 537—542 (1968).

SIDLEY, N. A., SPERLING, H. G., BEDORF, E. W., HISS, R. H.: Photopic spectral sensitivity in the monkey: Methods for determining and initial results. Science **150**, 1837—1839 (1965).

STEBBINS, W. C.: Auditory reaction time and the derivation of equal loudness contours for the monkey. J. exp. Anal. Behav. **9**, 135—142 (1966).

— Animal Psychophysics. New York: Appleton-Century-Crofts 1970.

SUTHERS, R. A.: Optomotor responses by echolocating bats. Science **152**, 1102—1104 (1966).

SVAETICHIN, G.: Spectral response curves from single cones. Acta physiol. scand. **39**, Suppl. 134, 17—46 (1956).

SYMMES, D.: Self-determination of critical flicker frequencies in monkeys. Science **136**, 714—715 (1962).

TEITELBAUM, P.: Physiological Psychology. Englewood Cliffs, N. J. Prentice-Hall 1967.

THOMAS, D. R., LYONS, J.: Further evidence of a sensory-tonic interaction in pigeons. J. exp. Anal. Behav. **11**, 167—171 (1968).

VIAUD, G.: La vision chromatique chez les animaux (sauf les insectes). In: Mechanisms of Colour Discrimination. GALIFRET, Y. (Ed.). New York: Pergamon Press 1960.

WALKER, A. E., WOOLF, J. I., HALSTEAD, W. C., CASE, T. J.: Mechanism of temporal fusion effect of photic stimulation on electrical activity of visual structures. J. Neurophysiol. **6**, 213—220 (1943).

WALLS, G.: The Vertebrate Eye and its Adaptive Radiations. New York: Hafner 1963.

WARNER, L.: The problem of color vision in fishes. Quart. Rev. Biol. **6**, 329—348 (1931).

WOODWORTH, R. S., SCHLOSBERG, H.: Experimental Psychology. New York: Holt, Rinehart and Winston 1954.

WYCKOFF, L. B.: The role of observing responses in discrimination learning, Part I. Psychol. Rev. **59**, 431—442 (1952).

YAGER, D.: Behavioral measures and theoretical analysis of spectral sensitivity and spectral saturation in the goldfish, *Carassius auratus*. Vision Res. **7**, 707—727 (1967).

— JAMESON, D.: On criteria for assessing type of colour vision in animals. Anim. Behav. **16**, 29—31 (1968).

YARCZOWER, M., BITTERMAN, M.: Stimulus generalization in the goldfish. In: Stimulus Generalization. MOSTOFSKY, D. (Ed.). Stanford: Stanford University Press 1965.

— WOLBARSHT, M. L., GALLOWAY, W. D., FLIGSTEN, K. E., MALCOLM, R.: Visual acuity in a stumptail macaque. Science **152**, 1392—1393 (1966).

ZIEGLER, H., WYCKOFF, L. B.: Observing responses and discrimination learning. Quart. J. exp. Psychol. **13**, 129—140 (1961).

ZWICK, H., GRANDA, A. M.: Behaviorally determined dark adaptation functions in the turtle, *Pseudemys*. Psychon. Sci. **11**, 239—240 (1968).

Author Index

Page numbers in *italics* refer to the bibliography

Subject Index

Compiled by

Katherine Frost Bruner, Cambridge, Massachusetts (USA)

Page numbers in parentheses refer to material in figures

MIX
Papier aus verantwortungsvollen Quellen
Paper from responsible sources
FSC® C105338

If you have any concerns about our products,
you can contact us on
ProductSafety@springernature.com

In case Publisher is established outside the EU,
the EU authorized representative is:
Springer Nature Customer Service Center GmbH
Europaplatz 3, 69115 Heidelberg, Germany

Printed by Libri Plureos GmbH
in Hamburg, Germany